OPHTHALMOLOGY

PRINCIPLES AND CONCEPTS

Eighth Edition

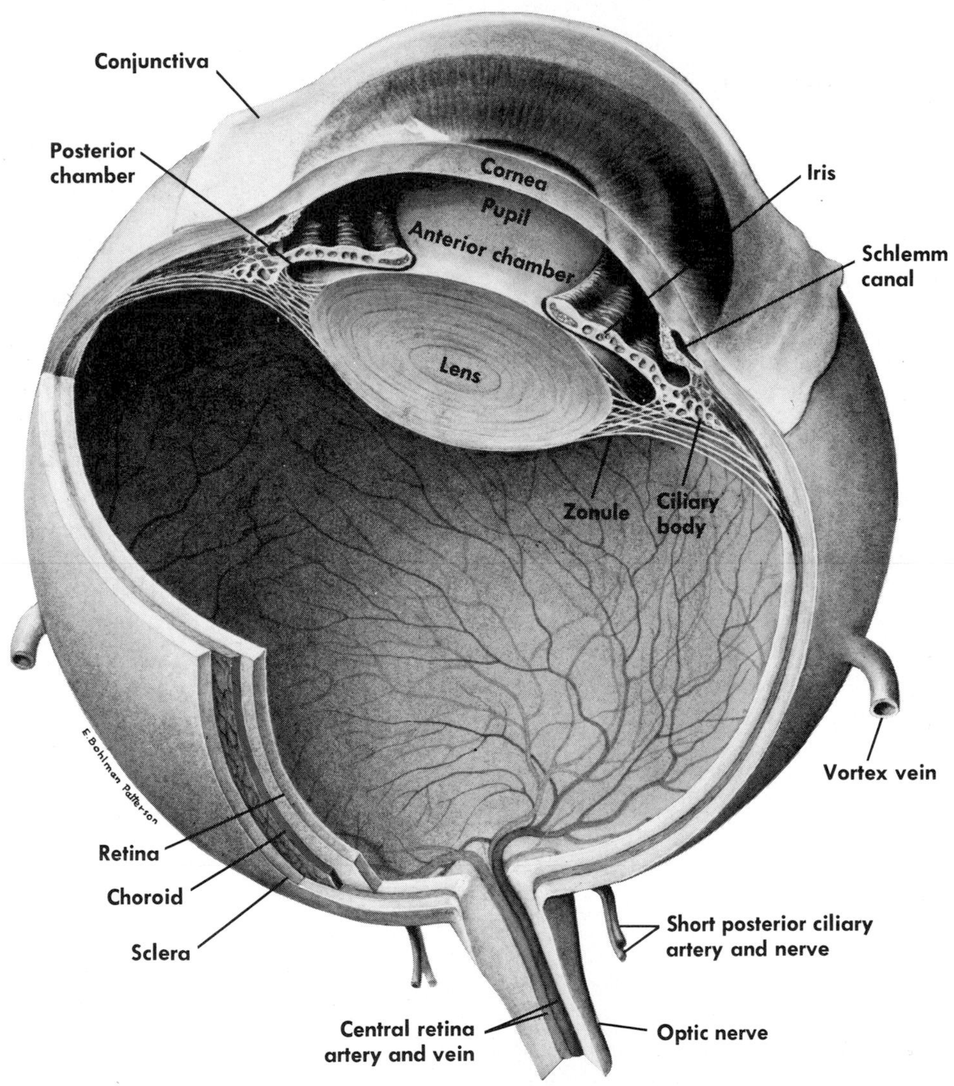

THE HUMAN EYE

OPHTHALMOLOGY
PRINCIPLES AND CONCEPTS

Frank W. Newell, M.D., M.Sc. (Ophth.)

The James N. and Anna Louise Raymond Professor Emeritus

Department of Ophthalmology and Visual Science

The University of Chicago

Chicago, Illinois

EIGHTH EDITION

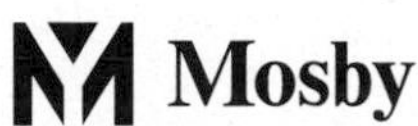

St. Louis Baltimore Boston

Carlsbad Chicago Naples New York Philadelphia Portland

London Madrid Mexico City Singapore Sydney Tokyo Toronto Wiesbaden

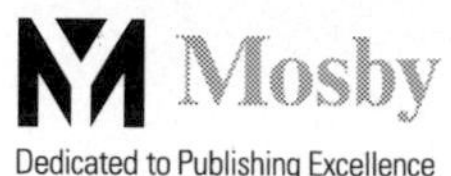

Dedicated to Publishing Excellence

A Times Mirror Company

Publisher: Anne S. Patterson
Senior Editor: Laurel Craven
Developmental Editor: Kimberley Cox
Project Manager: Linda Clarke
Associate Production Editor: Deborah Ann Cicirello
Designer: Carolyn O'Brien
Manufacturing Manager: William A. Winneberger, Jr.

EIGHTH EDITION

Printed in the United States of America
Composition by Graphic World, Inc.
Printing/binding by Maple-Vail Book Manufacturing Group

Mosby–Year Book, Inc.
11830 Westline Industrial Drive
St. Louis, Missouri 63146

Library of Congress Cataloging-in-Publication Data
Newell, Frank W.
Ophthalmology : principles and concepts / Frank W. Newell ; -- 8th ed.
p. cm.
Includes bibliographical references and index.
ISBN 0-8151-7093-9
1. Ophthalmology. I. Title.
[DNLM: 1. Eye Diseases. WW 140 N544o 1996]
RE46.N57 1996
617.7--dc20
DNLM/DLC
for Library of Congress 96-5854
CIP

96 97 98 99 00 / 9 8 7 6 5 4 3 2 1

To Frankie, Arien, Johnny,
Daniel, and Lilly

PREFACE

It is a particular privilege to revise this textbook some 31 years after it first appeared. Since the publication of the first edition in 1965, ophthalmology and medicine have undergone a host of changes. The National Eye Institute was established in 1968, and the increased emphasis on research dealing with ocular disease and function has provided rich rewards. The medical literature is quickly and easily available through Medline, Grateful Med, and other retrieval services, which permit the practitioner a rapid review of current medical and scientific journals. A rich variety of books provides detailed information concerning a host of ophthalmic disorders.

As previously, I have been impressed with the detailed textbooks assigned for medical student study. They range from anatomy, biochemistry, physiology, pharmacology, pathology, medicine, surgery, and pediatrics, to special fields. I have tried to simplify the study of ophthalmology by bringing the lessons of these volumes to this textbook. The current emphasis on managed care requires that every practitioner be more familiar with disorders of the eye and other organs than in past years.

As with earlier editions, students past and present have been attentive in detecting errors and suggesting changes. Daniel Snydacker, M.D., with whom I collaborated over 40 years ago in writing "Refraction," has reviewed many chapters and suggested clarifications and practical approaches to many topics. As with prior editions, Mrs. Mary L. Borysewicz corrected galley proofs and reviewed sections of the typescript. Mrs. Karin Cassel, my secretary for more than 30 years, when I served as chairman of the Department of Ophthalmology of the University of Chicago, reviewed and corrected my computer-generated prose. Ms. Nicole Netter provided skilled redaction. Ms. Crista Wellman, of the audiovisual department of the University of Chicago generously assisted with illustrations. Dr. Samir Patel, head of the retina service of the Department of Ophthalmology and Visual Science of the University of Chicago, assembled the material for the clinical atlas. As with editions one to seven, the editorial and production staff at Mosby–Year Book provided professional and gentle direction.

Frank W. Newell, M.D., M.Sc.(Ophth.)

CONTENTS

PART 1

BASIC MECHANISMS

1

ANATOMY AND EMBRYOLOGY

ANATOMY

Dissection of a fresh rabbit or cattle eye readily discloses the interrelationship of intraocular structures and the organization of the eye as a multichambered, nearly spherical organ. The surface anatomy of the eyelids and the globe is easily studied in a living subject by direct inspection, with a small penlight used for illumination and a +20-diopter lens for magnification.

THE EYE

The eye (see frontispiece) rests on a hammock of fascia, in the anterior one half of the cavity of the bony orbit. The exposed anterior one third of the eye consists of a central transparent portion, the cornea, through which the colored iris that surrounds the black pupil is visible. The cornea is surrounded by the white sclera, which is covered by the bulbar conjunctiva. The bulbar conjunctiva is continuous with the palpebral conjunctiva, which lines the inner surface of the protective tissue curtains, the eyelids. Normally the eyelids conceal the upper and lower margins of the cornea with the sclera.

The posterior one half of each bony orbit contains the optic nerve (N II), the blood vessels, the extraocular muscles, the sensory and motor nerves, and the orbital fat. The bony orbit separates its contents from the intracranial cavity, the nasal accessory sinuses, and the nasal cavity.

The anterior pole of the eye is the center of curvature of the cornea. The posterior pole of the eye is the center of curvature of the sclera. It is located slightly lateral to the optic nerve. The geometric axis of the eye is a line that connects these two poles. The anteroposterior dimension of the normal eye, measured by ultrasonography or radiography, is 22 to 26 mm.

The equator of the eye encircles the globe midway between the two poles (Fig 1-1). In the average eye (24 mm in length), the equator is located on the surface of the sclera 16 mm posterior to the junction of the clear cornea and the white sclera (the limbus corneae). Measured on the surface of the eye, the posterior pole is 32 mm from the corneoscleral limbus. The circumference of the eye at the equator measures 69 to 81 mm (22 × pi [3.1416] or 24 × pi).

Within the eye the termination of the corneal endothelium marks its peripheral margin. The anterior termination of the sensory retina is at the ora serrata. The distance separating these structures is 6.23 mm on the temporal side of the eye and 5.75 mm on the nasal side. The more anterior termination of the retina on the nasal side accounts, in part, for the more extensive temporal visual field.

The globe has three main layers (Table 1-1), each of which is further divided. The outer layer, the supporting coat, consists of the transparent cornea, the opaque sclera, and their junction, the corneoscleral limbus.

The middle layer, the uvea, consists of the iris, the ciliary body, and the choroid. The iris, the highly colored structure located between the cornea and the crystalline lens, encloses the opening, the pupil, which constricts with contraction of the sphincter pupillae muscle (parasympathetics, N III) and dilates in response to the dilatator pupillae muscle (sympathetics). The ciliary body secretes the aqueous humor and, in accommodation to near and far vision, changes the shape and thickness of the crystalline lens, to which it is connected by zonular fibers. The choroid furnishes the blood supply to the adjacent retinal pigment epithelium and to the outer layers of the sensory retina.

The inner layer, the retina, is composed of an outer layer (nearest the choroid), the retinal pigment epithelium, and an inner layer, the sensory retina, which is composed of many layers.

The lens is a transparent tissue located immediately posterior to the iris. It consists of an outermost capsule that surrounds a lens cortex and a central lens nucleus. It is supported in position by a series of fine fibers, the zonule, which insert into the valleys between the ciliary processes and into the lens capsule at its equator.

TABLE 1-1.
Layers of the Eye

I. Outer layer
  A. Cornea
  B. Sclera
  C. Their junction: limbus corneae
II. Middle layer (uvea)
  A. Iris
  B. Ciliary body
  C. Choroid
III. Inner layer
  A. Retinal pigment epithelium
  B. Sensory retina
    1. Anterior margin: ora serrata

The eye encloses three chambers: (1) the vitreous cavity, (2) the posterior chamber, and (3) the anterior chamber (see frontispiece). The *vitreous cavity,* by far the largest, is located behind the lens and zonule and is adjacent to the sensory retina. The *posterior chamber* is minute in size and is bounded by the lens and zonule behind and the iris in front. The *anterior chamber* is located between the iris and the posterior surface of the cornea and communicates with the posterior chamber through the pupil.

The outer coat

The outer coat of the eye consists of relatively rigid fibrous tissues, the cornea and the sclera (Table 1-2). The transparent cornea constitutes the anterior one sixth of the globe, and the white, opaque sclera, the posterior five sixths. The cornea has a radius of curvature of about 7.5 mm and the sclera has a radius of curvature of about 13 mm.

The sclera.—The sclera, a dense connective tissue structure, forms the "white" of the eye. Its anterior surface is covered with the conjunctiva, the fascia bulbi (Tenon capsule), and the richly vascular episclera. The delicate blood vessels of the episclera are visible anteriorly deep to the larger blood vessels of the translucent conjunctiva. Posteriorly, the fascia bulbi attach to the sclera with fine, loose collagen fibers.

The sclera has two large openings, the anterior and posterior scleral foramina. The anterior scleral foramen is bridged by the transparent

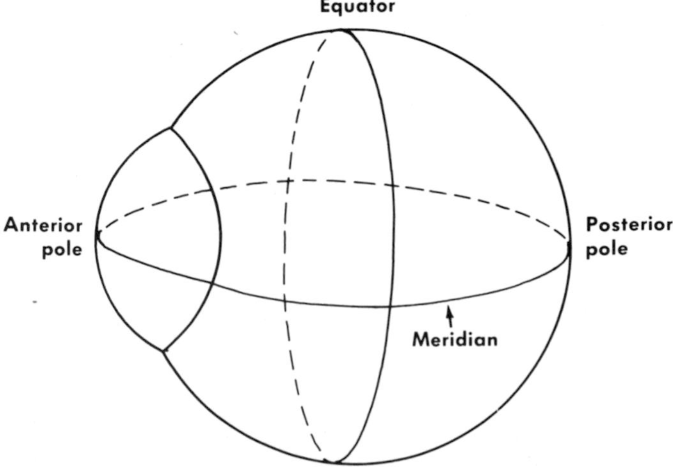

FIG 1-1.
Principal coordinates of the eye. The visual line that connects an object in space with the fovea centralis does not correspond exactly to the geometric axis, which connects the anterior to the posterior pole.

TABLE 1-2.
Layers of Cornea and Sclera

- I. Precorneal tear film
  - A. Oil layer (from meibomian glands)
  - B. Aqueous layer (from lacrimal glands)
  - C. Mucoid layer (from goblet cells)
- II. Cornea
  - A. Epithelium
    1. Surface cell layer
    2. Wing cell layer
    3. Basal cell layer (columnar cells)
    4. Basement membrane
  - B. Stroma
    1. Anterior condensation (Bowman zone)
    2. Lamellar stroma
  - C. Mesothelium (endothelium)
    1. Descemet membrane (basement membrane) between endothelium and stroma
- III. Sclera
  - A. Episclera
  - B. Scleral stroma
  - C. Lamina fusca

cornea. The periphery of the anterior scleral foramen is a transitional area, the corneoscleral limbus. The inner surface of the sclera, immediately posterior to the corneoscleral limbus, is thickened into a ridge, the scleral spur (see Fig 1-11). It borders on the canal of Schlemm and supplies the attachments for the trabecular meshwork and the longitudinal portion of the ciliary muscle.

The sclera is perforated 3 mm medial to the posterior pole by the posterior scleral foramen, the canal through which the optic nerve and central retinal vein leave the eye and through which the central retinal artery enters the eye. The canal is cone-shaped and measures 1.5 to 2.0 mm in diameter on the inner surface of the sclera and 3.0 to 3.5 mm on the outer surface. The posterior scleral foramen is bridged by a sievelike structure, the lamina cribrosa (Fig 1-2), the most posterior portion of which is

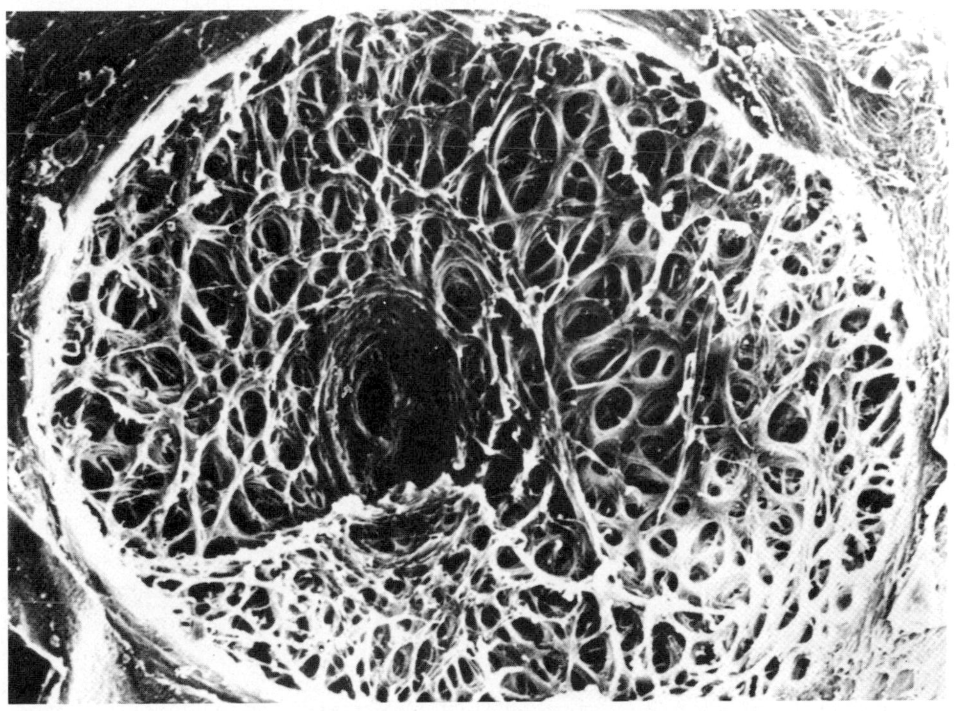

FIG 1-2.
Scanning electron micrograph of the human posterior scleral foramen viewed from the vitreous cavity. The opening is bridged by a sievelike structure, the lamina cribrosa. It is composed of some 10 stacked sheets of connective tissue collagen (types I and III) that contain 200 to 400 pores through which pass optic nerve fiber bundles and central retinal blood vessels. On the inner surface are abundant astrocytes and much elastic tissue derived from Bruch membrane. (*From Miller NR:* Walsh and Hoyt's clinical neuro-ophthalmology, *ed 4, vol 1, Baltimore, 1982, Williams & Wilkins. Used by permission.*)

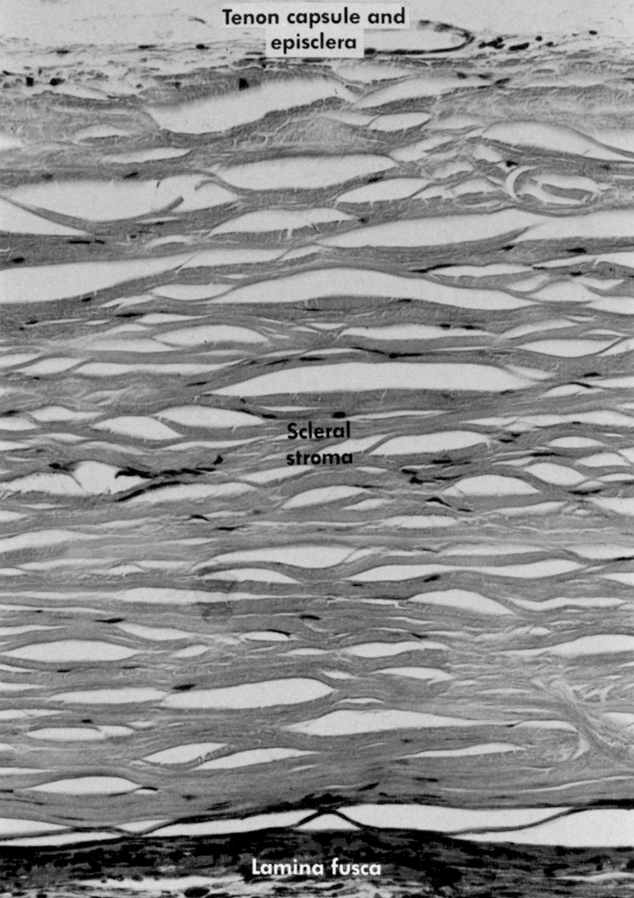

FIG 1-3.
A transverse section through the sclera anterior to the equator of the eye (Masson trichrome, ×160).

formed by scleral fibers. The anterior portion, rich in elastic tissue, is derived from the choroid and Bruch membrane.

About 4 mm posterior to the corneoscleral limbus and just anterior to the insertions of the recti muscles, the anterior ciliary arteries pierce the sclera at sites sometimes marked with a visible dot of pigment 2 to 4 mm from the corneoscleral limbus. About 4 mm posterior to the equator of the eye in the region between the recti muscles are the openings for the vortex veins that are the collecting channels for choroidal veins. In the area surrounding the optic nerve, the sclera is perforated by the long and short ciliary nerves and the long and short posterior ciliary arteries.

The sclera is thickest (1.0 mm) in the region surrounding the optic nerve, where the meningeal coverings (mainly dura mater) of the optic nerve blend into the sclera. It is thinnest (0.3 mm) immediately posterior to the insertions of the recti muscles.

Structure.—The sclera (Fig 1-3) has three layers: (1) the episclera, (2) the scleral stroma, and (3) the lamina fusca.

The *episclera* is the outermost layer. It is a moderately dense, vascularized connective tissue that merges with the scleral stroma and sends connective tissue bundles into the fascia bulbi (Tenon capsule). The anterior portion of the episclera has a rich blood supply that may become markedly congested in inflammation. The episclera and the fascia bulbi are attenuated behind the ocular equator, which accounts for the relative avascularity of the posterior sclera.

The dense *scleral stroma* consists mainly of types I and III collagen fibers (Fig 1-4) that vary in diameter from 10 to 16 μm and in length from 30 to 140 μm. The fibers are oriented parallel to the corneoscleral limbus to form an interlacing basketlike weave in that region. In the region of the insertion of the extraocular muscles, they become more meridional, apparently in response to mechanical stresses induced by trac-

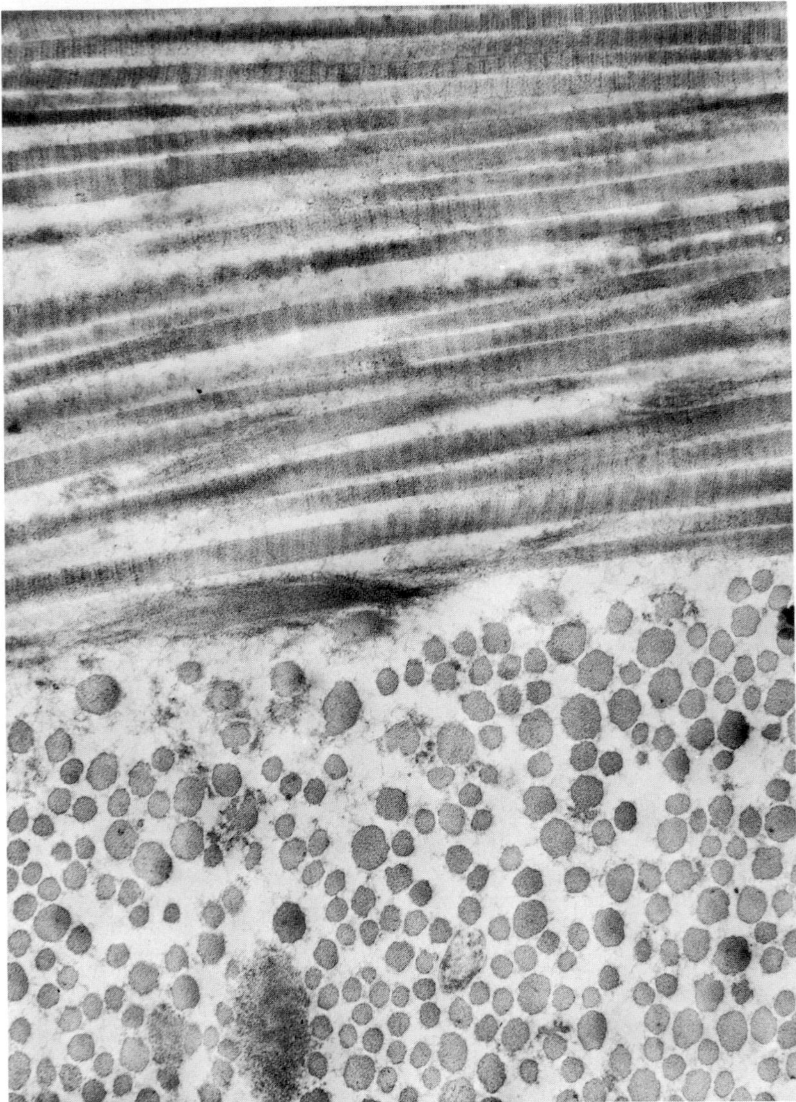

FIG 1-4.
Transmission electron micrograph of scleral stroma showing collagen bundles. Collagen fibrils in the lamellae are of variable diameters and much more irregularly arranged than those of the cornea (×45,000). *(Courtesy of Ramesh C. Tripathi, M.D.)*

tion of the ocular muscles and intraocular pressure. The sclera is white because of the variable diameter and irregular arrangement of the collagen fibers of the stroma. When the water content of the sclera (usually between 65% and 70%) is reduced to less than 40% or increased to more than 80%, the sclera becomes transparent.

The *lamina fusca,* the innermost layer of the sclera, is as much a part of the outer portion of the uvea, to which it is adjacent, as the sclera. It is composed of fine collagen fibers derived from the sclera, and it provides delicate connections between the sclera and the uveal tract. Enmeshed within these fibers are melanocytes and mesodermal tissue derived from the choroid and the ciliary body.

Blood supply.—The blood supply of the scleral stroma is provided by the episcleral and choroidal vascular networks. Anterior to the insertions of the recti muscles, the anterior ciliary arteries form a dense episcleral plexus. These vessels become congested in "ciliary injection." Small branches of the long and short posterior ciliary arteries supply the scleral stroma posterior to the recti muscles.

Sensory nerve supply.—The anterior sclera is mainly innervated by the two long ciliary nerve branches of the nasociliary nerve (N V_1). Inflammations of the anterior sclera may be exceptionally painful. The posterior sclera is mainly innervated by sparse short ciliary nerves.

The cornea.—The cornea forms the anterior, transparent, one sixth of the globe. At its periphery it merges with the sclera to form the corneoscleral junction (the limbus corneae). The superficial margins are not distinct. The intraocular portion of the corneoscleral limbus terminates at the trabecular meshwork, through which most of the aqueous humor leaves the eye. The cornea separates air, which has an index of refraction of 1.00, and the aqueous humor, which has an index of refraction of 1.33. It is the main refracting surface of the eye. The anterior surface of the cornea measures about 10.6 mm vertically and 11.7 mm horizontally; the conjunctival covering makes exact measurement difficult. The intraocular surface is circular and has a diameter of 11.7 mm. The central optical portion is 0.52 mm thick and has nearly parallel external and intraocular surfaces. The peripheral portion thickens to about 1.0 mm, and the surfaces are not parallel.

The radius of curvature of the external surface is 7.8 mm, and the radius of curvature of the concave intraocular surface is 6.2 to 6.8 mm. Variations in the radius of curvature in the different meridians of the cornea change their refractive power and cause astigmatism.

Structure.—The cornea (Fig 1-5) has three layers: (1) an anterior layer, the epithelium and its basement membrane; (2) a middle layer, the substantia propria (stroma) and its anterior condensation, Bowman zone; and (3) a lining layer, the mesothelium (endothelium) and its basement membrane (Descemet membrane), which separates the endothelium from the stroma (see Table 1-2).

The *epithelium* is 50 to 90 μm thick and covers the stroma anteriorly. It is continuous with the epithelium of the conjunctiva. It is composed of stratified squamous epithelium that is five to seven cell layers thick centrally and seven to ten layers thick at its periphery, where it is continuous with the epithelium of the conjunctiva. The corneal epithelium consists of three layers: (1) a superficial layer of flattened cells, two cell layers thick; (2) a midzone layer formed by two or three layers of polyhedral cells (wing cells); and (3) a basal germinal layer, one cell thick, that rests on a thin basement membrane attached to the underlying Bowman zone of the stroma. The epithelial cells originate in the deep basal layer, become progressively flatter as they are displaced anteriorly, and are shed from the superficial layer 7 days later.

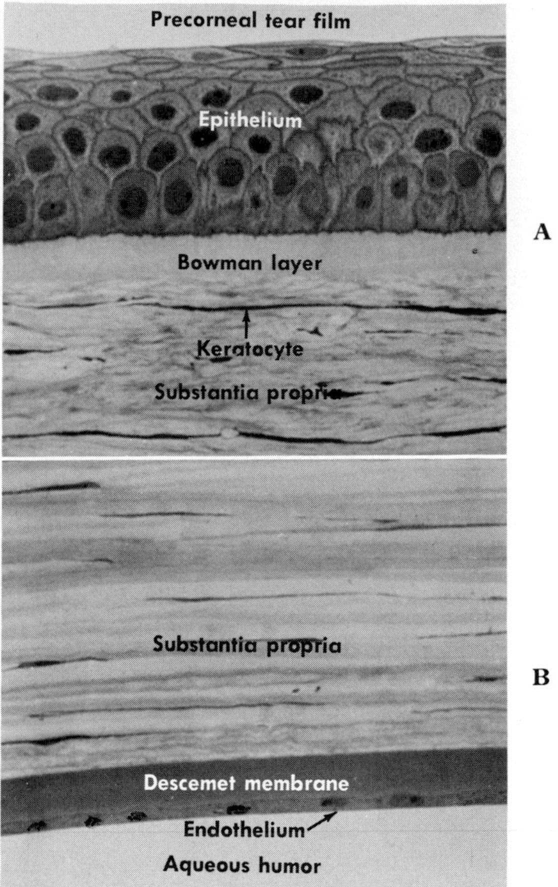

FIG 1-5.
Cross section of the axial area of the cornea. The *substantia propria* constitutes 90% of the thickness. **A,** The basement membrane of the epithelium is firmly adherent to the *Bowman zone,* the anterior condensation of the substantia propria. **B,** The lamellae of the posterior substantia propria are much more regularly arranged than those of the anterior substantia propria (×500). *(Courtesy of Ramesh C. Tripathi, M.D.)*

The squamous cells of the surface layer are flat, and have horizontal nuclei (Fig 1-6). Their superficial surfaces have many microplicae and microvilli, which may be responsible for adher-

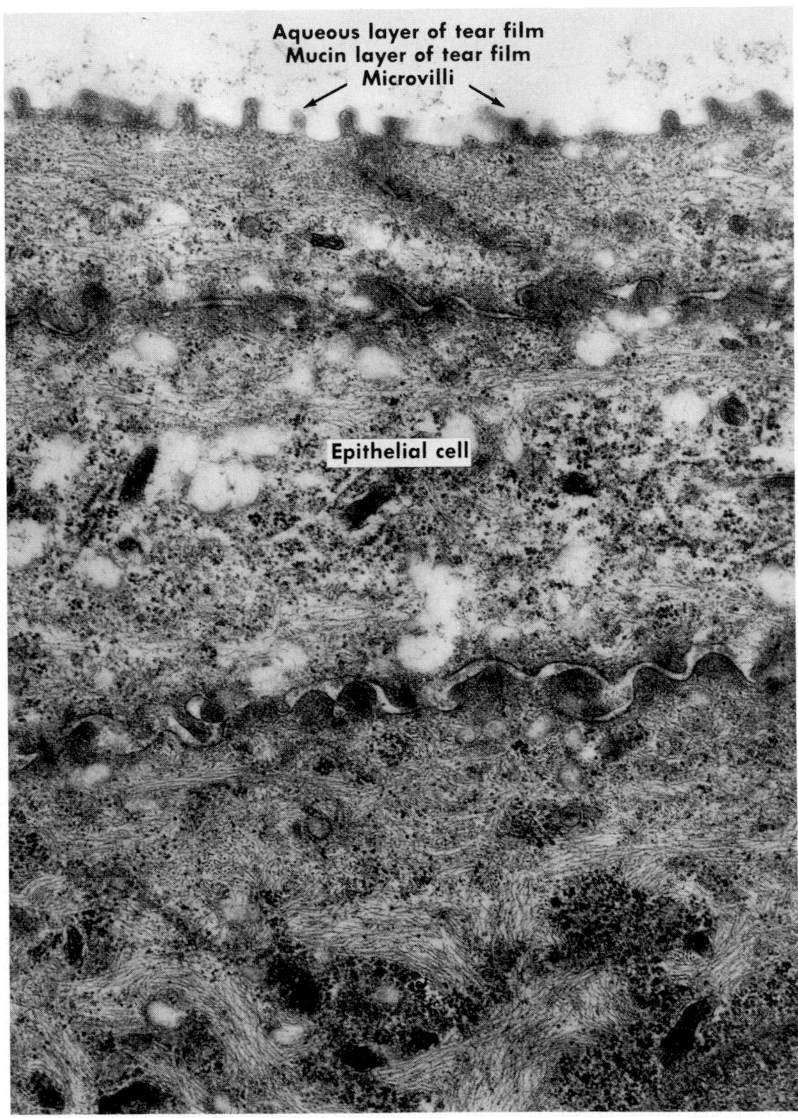

FIG 1-6.
Transmission electron micrograph of corneal epithelium with the surface cells *(top)* showing microvilli. The surface barrier of the epithelium is formed by the integrity of the most anterior squamous cells that are bound together by terminal bars (×37,000). *(Courtesy of Ramesh C. Tripathi, M.D.)*

ence of the precorneal tear film (see Fig 2-2). As surface cells age, they lose their interdigitations and disintegrate or are swept away by the eyelids during blinking.

The wing cells in the midzone are polyhedral with a convex anterior surface, parallel with the surface of the cornea, and a concave posterior surface. Those immediately adjacent to the inner basal cell layer have round nuclei that become successively flatter as the cells approach the surface of the cornea. The cells are joined together from base to apex by desmosomes. Centrally, the wing cell layer is two or three cell layers thick, whereas it may be five or six cell layers thick at the corneal periphery.

The basal cells in the deepest epithelial layer are tall and columnar and often show mitosis. Their interdigitating lateral cell borders are joined by desmosomes. The cells are attached to their basement membrane by hemidesmosomes, anchoring filaments, and the adhesive glycoproteins, laminin and fibronectin.

The basement membrane is positive to periodic acid-Schiff stain (PAS) and is composed of type IV collagen. It is firmly attached to the underlying anterior condensation of the substantia propria (Bowman zone) by anchoring filaments composed of type VII collagen. After injury these attachments may take as long as 6 weeks to be reestablished. The basement membrane is essential in attaching the epithelium to the underlying stroma. It does not regenerate after injury.

The *substantia propria* (Fig 1-7), or stroma, constitutes 90% of the corneal thickness. Its anterior portion, the Bowman zone (Bowman membrane or layer to the light microscopist), is made up of randomly oriented collagen fibers that form an acellular region resistant to deformation, trauma, and the passage of foreign bodies or infecting organisms. Once damaged, its typical architecture is not restored and causes corneal opacification and an irregularity in corneal thickness that results in irregular astigmatism (see Chapter 24).

The stroma is composed of lamellae of collagen fibrils of uniform diameter and regular spacing that extend the entire width of the cornea. They have a periodicity typical of embryonic collagen. In the posterior cornea, the lamellae are of almost equal thickness; they become more irregular in the anterior portion. All fibers within a lamella are parallel—but at a right angle—to fibers in the adjacent lamellae. They are enmeshed in glycosaminoglycans. Scattered throughout are fixed, long, and flat cells known as keratocytes or corneal corpuscles, which function as fibroblasts do in other tissues. There are also a few wandering cells (leukocytes and macrophages).

The corneal stroma in humans is composed of type I collagen (50% to 55%), type VI collagen (30% to 40%), and type V collagen (5% to 10%). Type III collagen may be present in the human fetal cornea and after injury. The lamellae are enmeshed in macromolecules, the proteoglycans, in which high-molecular-weight glycosaminoglycans are linked to a core protein. Acetylglucosaminoglycan, in which keratan sulfate is the amino sugar, and acetylgalactosaminoglycan, in which chondroitin 4 (6) sulfate (dermatan/chondroitin sulfate) is the amino sugar, act as anions and bind cations and water.

The posterior surface of the cornea is lined with a loosely attached, PAS-positive, glassy membrane, the Descemet membrane. It is the basement membrane of the endothelial cells that line the cornea. After injury, the Descemet membrane regenerates readily and may form glass membranes that extend into the anterior chamber. Descemet membrane terminates

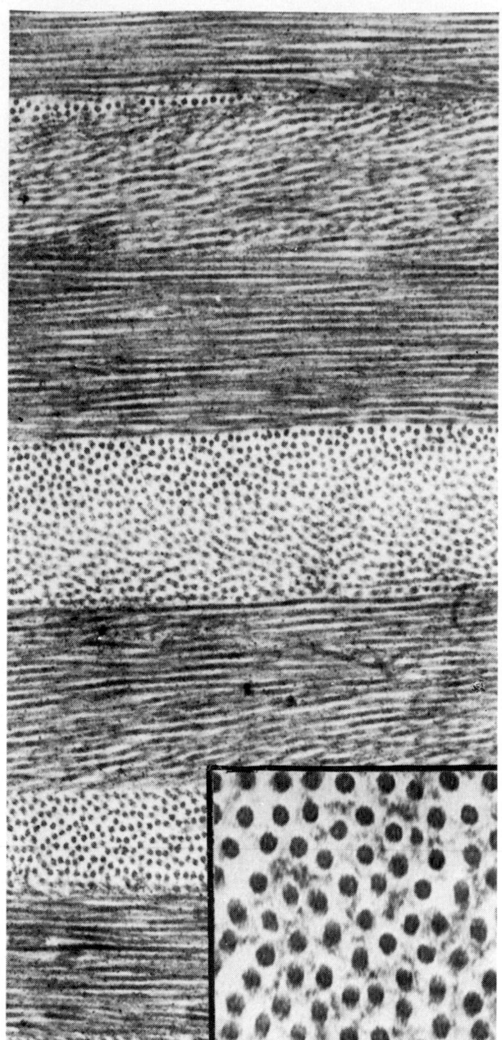

FIG 1-7.
Cross section of the substantia propria of the cornea. The collagen fibers are in bundles of approximately 200 lamellae that are arranged tangentially and at right angles to each other. Collagen fibrils (types I, V, and VI) are embedded in proteoglycans and are separated by a distance of about 200 nm (one half the wavelength of blue light, so that the cornea is transparent). The collagen fibrils (*inset, bottom right,* ×90,000) generally are of uniform size; interspersed among them is a microfibrillar structure that may be a precursor of collagen (×32,500). *(Courtesy of Ramesh C. Tripathi, M.D.)*

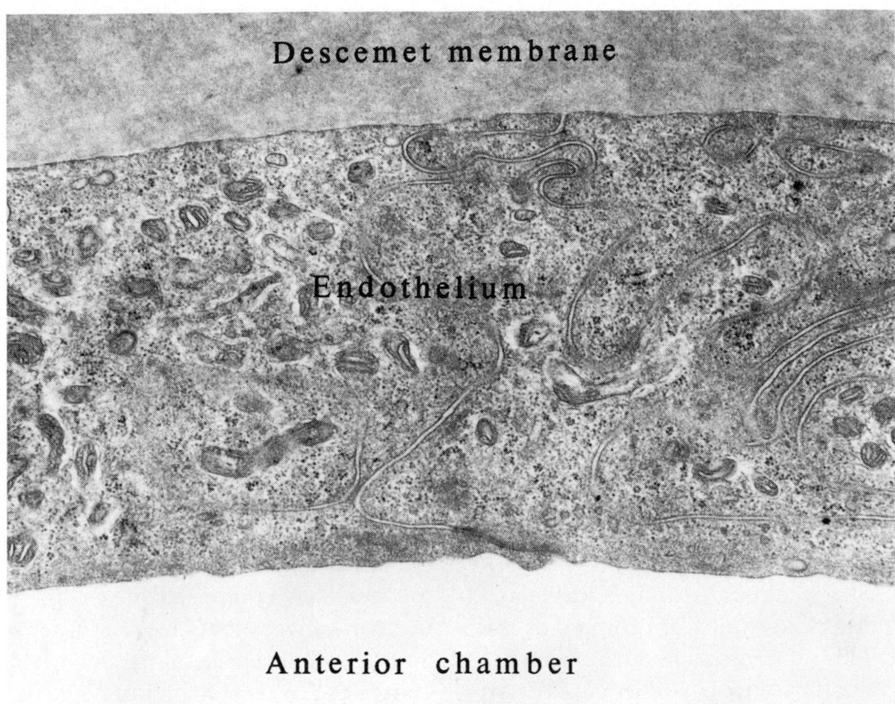

FIG 1-8.
Corneal mesothelium (endothelium). The cells are rich in organelles; adjacent cell borders are markedly convoluted but parallel and are attached by terminal bars near the anterior chamber aspect (×24,000). *(Courtesy of Ramesh C. Tripathi, M.D.)*

abruptly at the periphery of the cornea to form the line of Schwalbe, the anterior border of the trabecular meshwork.

The *endothelium* of the cornea is a single layer of mesothelium (Fig 1-8). The apices of the endothelial cells are in direct contact with the aqueous humor and have occasional microvilli. The cells are tightly bound together with desmosomes (maculae adherentes); near the apical region a terminal bar is constantly present. The cells contain large oval nuclei and are rich in intracellular organelles. The endothelium regulates the exchange of electrolytes and fluid between the cornea and the aqueous humor in the anterior chamber and constitutes the chief mechanism of corneal dehydration (deturgescence; see Chapter 2). Injury to the endothelium results in edema of the corneal stroma. The corneal endothelium does not regenerate in adult humans.

At the corneal periphery, the Bowman zone and the Descemet membrane stop abruptly. A line connecting these terminations constitutes the anterior margin of the corneoscleral limbus.

Blood supply.—The central cornea is avascular, but the corneoscleral limbus is generously supplied by the anterior conjunctival branches of the anterior ciliary arteries. These vessels course circumferentially around the corneoscleral limbus, giving off small radial branches that end in either the deep or the superficial corneal plexus with recurrent branches that anastomose with posterior conjunctival arteries.

Nerve supply.—The cornea is richly innervated by corneal nerves that send afferent impulses through the long ciliary nerves (N V_1). Within the cornea the nerves are not myelinated, but they acquire a myelin sheath at the corneoscleral limbus. Most are concentrated in the anterior stroma immediately beneath the Bowman zone and send branches forward into the epithelium with either beadlike thickening or bare fibers. Descemet membrane and the endothelium are not innervated.

Corneoscleral junction.—The limbus (junction) corneae is the 1- to 2-mm-wide transitional zone between the cornea and the sclera,

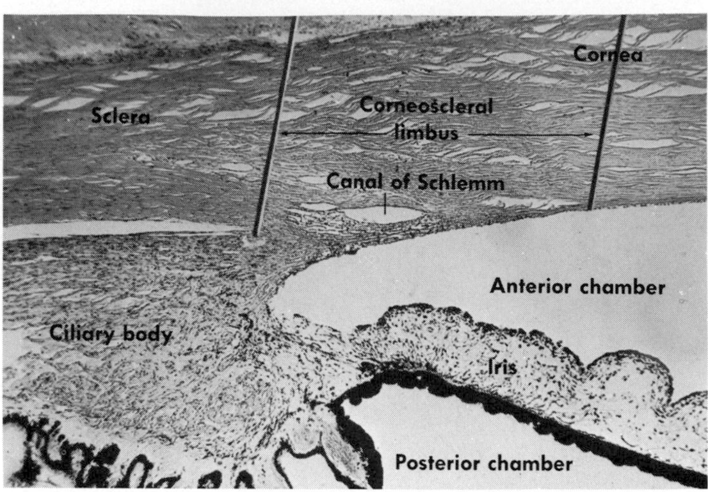

FIG 1-9.
Corneoscleral limbus. The central margin of the corneoscleral limbus is a line drawn between the termination of the Bowman zone and the point where the Descemet membrane becomes discontinuous (line of Schwalbe). The posterior margin is a line drawn parallel to the central margin and passing through the root of the iris (hematoxylin and eosin, ×105).

which contains the trabecular meshwork through which the aqueous humor leaves the anterior chamber. Externally, it is covered by the conjunctiva. Here the corneal epithelium loses its regular structure and becomes continuous with the conjunctival epithelium that contains goblet cells and lymphatic channels.

The corneal stroma ends abruptly in a loose arrangement of collagen fibers, filaments, and amorphous material. The regularity of the corneal lamellae is lost, the collagen bundles vary in diameter, and some resemble those of the central cornea and others those of the sclera. The continuity of the Descemet membrane ceases (the line of Schwalbe) and it splits into narrow bands that supply the anterior chamber surface of the trabecular meshwork. The corneal endothelium loses its continuity and continues as the endothelium that covers each of the bands of the trabecular meshwork.

The anterior border of the corneoscleral limbus is an imaginary line drawn between the terminations of the Bowman zone and the Descemet membrane (Fig 1-9). The posterior margin is a line drawn parallel to the anterior border that passes through the root of the iris. Enmeshed in the corneoscleral limbus are the trabecular meshwork and the canal of Schlemm, the drainage system of the anterior chamber. Clinically, the area is viewed with a goniolens.

Trabecular meshwork.—The trabecular meshwork surrounds the circumference of the anterior chamber (Fig 1-10). The aqueous humor of the anterior chamber filters through the trabecular meshwork to pass to the canal of Schlemm and its collector veins. The trabecular meshwork is composed of two portions: (1) a uveal meshwork that faces the anterior chamber and (2) a corneoscleral meshwork that is adjacent to the canal of Schlemm. The uveal portion of the meshwork extends from the termination of the Descemet membrane (the line of Schwalbe) to the scleral spur, the anterior face of the ciliary body, and the root of the iris. The corneoscleral portion of the meshwork extends from the line of Schwalbe to the base of the scleral spur.

The meshwork consists of a number of superimposed circular, oval, and rhomboidal fibrocellular cords (Latin *trabecula:* diminutive of beam; plural *trabeculae*) (Fig 1-11). Near the scleral spur the meshwork contains approximately 12 layers of cords, whereas there are only two or three near the line of Schwalbe. Each cord is covered by endothelium and contains a collagen core surrounded by a thin matrix of fibrils. Connective tissue elements are adherent to a variety of glycosaminoglycans, with hyaluronic acid being the most abundant in the human. The extracellular matrix contains laminin and type IV collagen, which are not present in the sclera.

The trabecular meshwork is innervated by the two long ciliary nerves (N V_1) in a plexus of delicate axons that terminate without specialized endings.

Canal of Schlemm.—The canal of Schlemm (Fig 1-11) is a channel, oval in cross section, that encircles the entire circumference of the anterior chamber. It is lined with a single layer of endothelial cells that contain

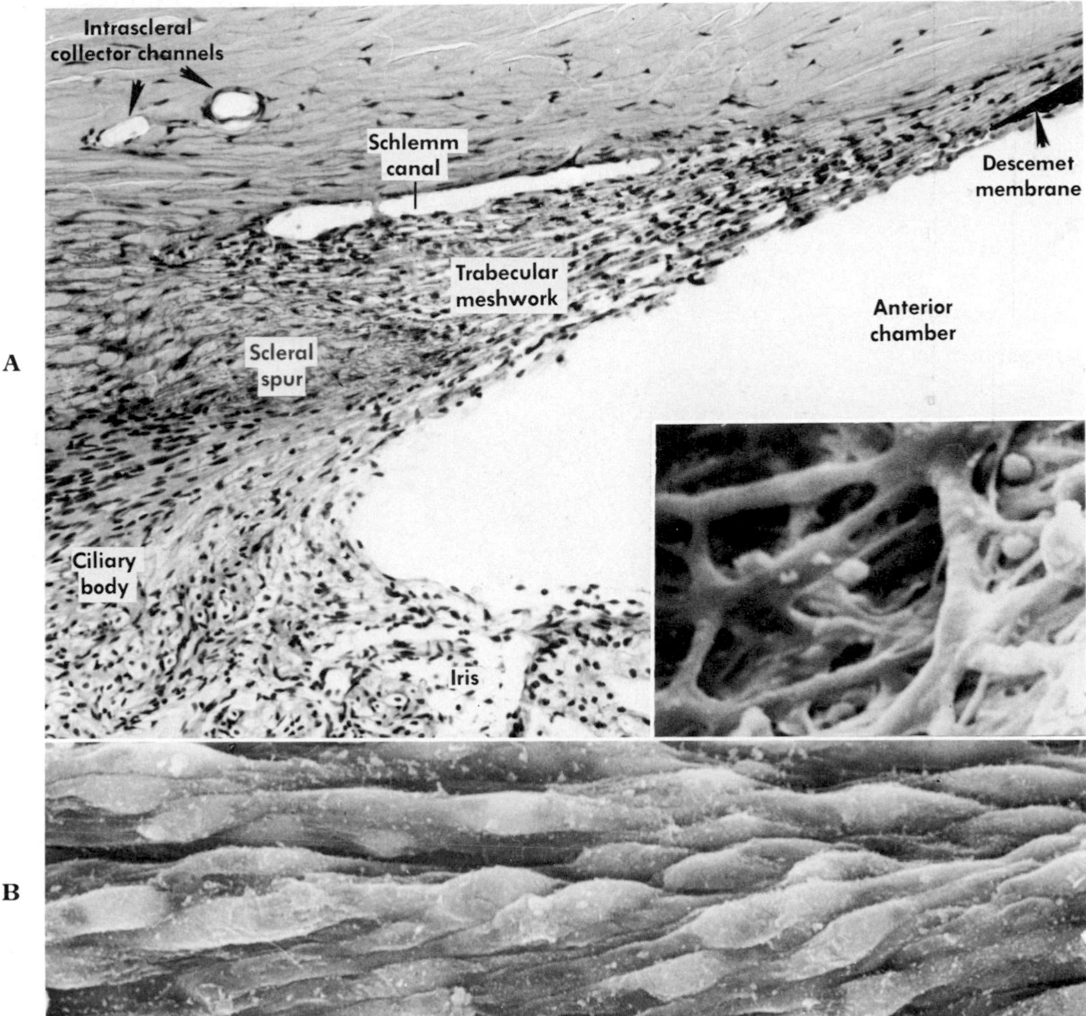

FIG 1-10.

A, Meridional section of human trabecular meshwork. The aqueous drainage pathway consists of the trabecular meshwork, canal of Schlemm, and intrascleral collector channels. The trabecular meshwork, located in the inner corneoscleral limbus, extends from the scleral spur, anterior face of the ciliary body, and iris root to the deeper corneal lamellae and peripheral termination of Descemet membrane (×138). The inset shows the rounded trabeculae from the anterior chamber aspect. **B,** Scanning electron micrograph of the endothelial lining of the trabecular wall (inner) of the canal of Schlemm viewed from inside the canal. Note the crypts between cells, their spindle shape, and the central bulges that correspond to the location of nuclear and macrovacuolar structures. The long axes of the cells usually parallel the canal circumference. (*From Tripathi RC: Pathologic anatomy of the outflow pathway of aqueous humor in chronic simplex glaucoma,* Exp Eye Res Suppl *25:403, 1977. Used by permission.*)

giant vacuoles. On the surface facing the anterior chamber, the canal is adjacent to the trabecular meshwork through which aqueous humor passes. On the scleral surface its wall is buried in the stroma of the corneoscleral limbus. The canal of Schlemm connects with the anterior ciliary veins and episcleral veins through the scleral plexus that is composed of anastomoses of 25 to 30 collector channels.

Several collector channels may bypass this plexus in some eyes and continue to the surface of the sclera. They may be seen beneath the bulbar conjunctiva as minute vessels, the aqueous veins, and contain clear aqueous humor.

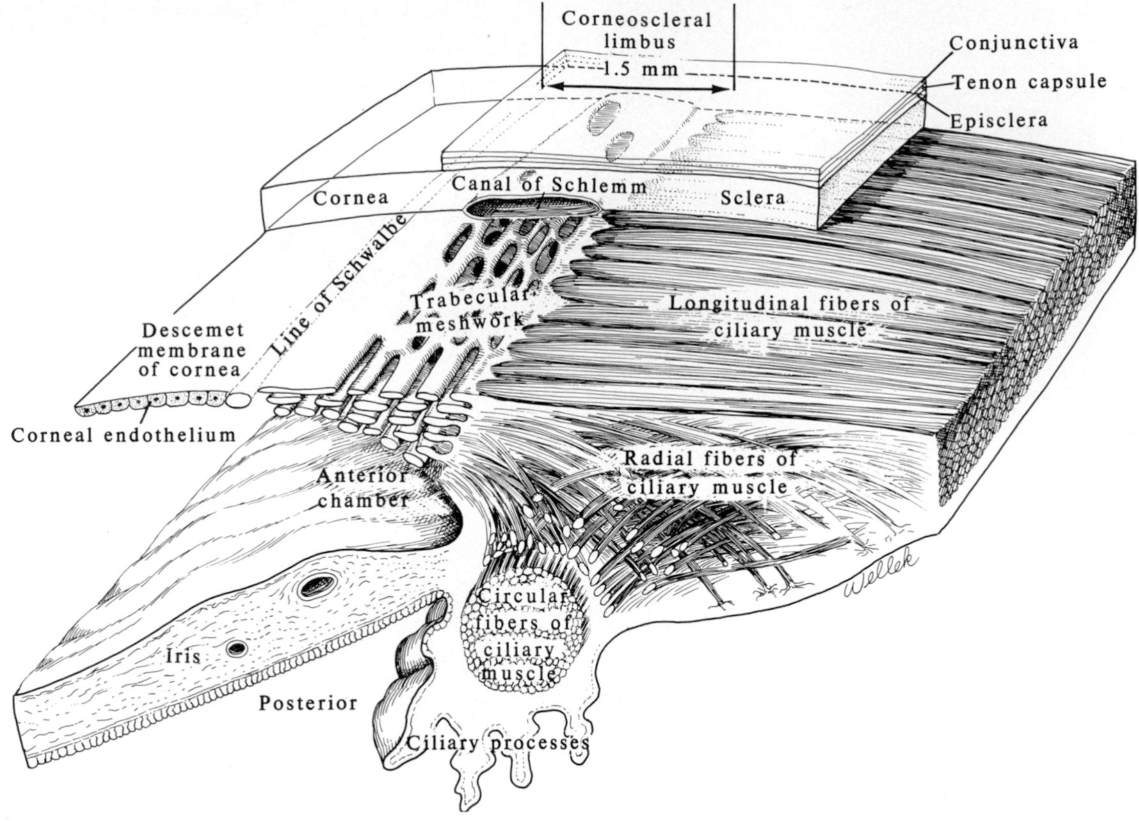

FIG 1-11.

Schematic construction of the ciliary body and angle recess in humans. Anteriorly the area is covered by the cornea and posteriorly by the sclera, which contains the canal of Schlemm. The termination of the corneal endothelium is marked by the line of Schwalbe. The ciliary muscle consists of longitudinal fibers, which are mainly parallel to the sclera; radial fibers, which are intermediate; and a circular muscle, which is most internal. The corneoscleral trabecula provides a filtering area between the anterior chamber angle and the canal of Schlemm. (*Redrawn from Rohen JW:* Das Auge und seine Hilfsorgane. *In Von Mollendorf W, Bargmann W, editors:* Handbuch der mikroskopischen Anatomie des Menschen, *Berlin, 1964, Springer-Verlag. Used by permission.*)

TABLE 1-3.

Layers of Uvea and Bruch Membrane

I. Uvea
  A. Choroid
    1. Lamina fusca
    2. Layer of large veins (of Haller)
    3. Layer of smaller veins (of Sattler)
    4. Choriocapillaris (blood supply of the outer retina)
  B. Ciliary body
    1. Uveal portion
      a. Lamina fusca
      b. Vessel layer
      c. Ciliary muscle
        (1) Longitudinal
        (2) Radial
        (3) Circular
    2. Epithelial portion
      a. Pigmented epithelium
      b. Nonpigmented epithelium
  C. Iris
    1. Anterior border layer (fibroblasts and melanocytes, absent in pupillary zone)
    2. Stroma (connective tissue, blood vessels, sphincter pupillae muscle [N III])
    3. Epithelium
      a. Anterior (myoepithelium: dilatator pupillae muscle [sympathetics])
      b. Posterior pigmented layer
II. Bruch membrane (lamina basalis choroideae)
  A. Basement membrane or choriocapillaris endothelium
  B. Outer collagen layer
  C. Elastic layer
  D. Inner cuticular layer
  E. Basement membrane of pigment epithelium

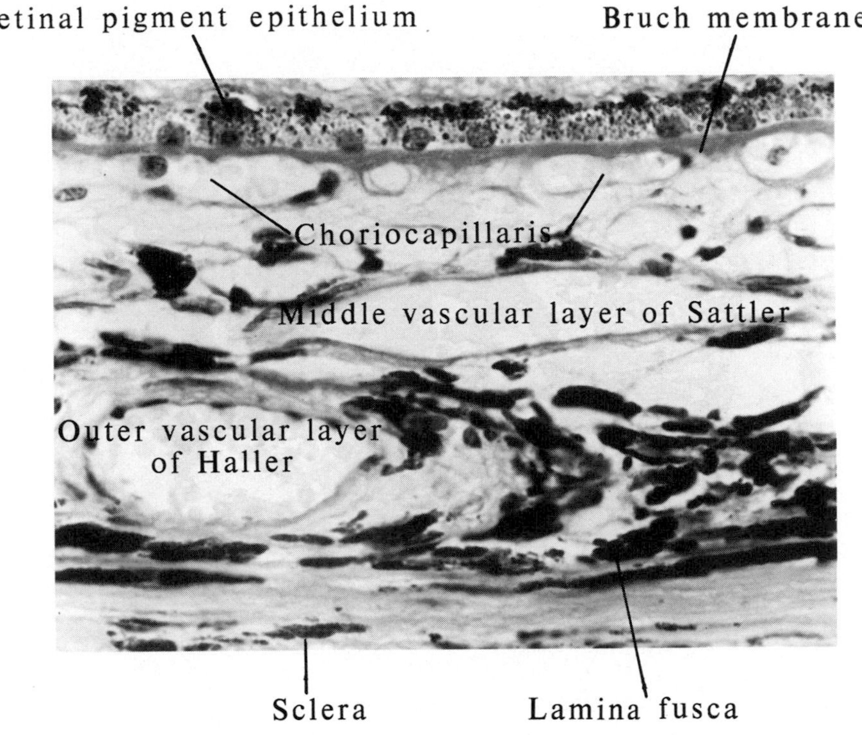

FIG 1-12.
Transverse section of the choroid. The veins in the outer vascular layer (of Haller) lead to vortex veins; the middle vascular layer (of Sattler) drains the choriocapillaris (hematoxylin and eosin, ×625).

They terminate in conjunctival veins within a few millimeters of the corneoscleral limbus.

Fibers of the longitudinal portion of the ciliary muscle insert into the scleral spur adjacent to the canal of Schlemm. Possibly the muscle affects the rate of outflow of aqueous humor from the anterior chamber through the canal of Schlemm.

Middle coat

The middle, or uveal, coat of the eye (Latin *uva:* grape) consists of the choroid, the ciliary body, and the iris (Table 1-3). The choroid is a layer of blood vessels surrounded by pigment that provides the blood supply to the retinal pigment epithelium and the outer half of the sensory retina, which is adjacent to it. The ciliary body secretes aqueous humor into the posterior chamber and contains smooth muscle that changes the shape of the crystalline lens to provide clear vision at different distances (accommodation). The iris surrounds the pupil, a central opening that controls the amount of light entering the eye.

The choroid.—The choroid (Fig 1-12) is located between the sclera on its outer side and the retinal pigment epithelium on its inner side. It extends anteriorly from the periphery of the optic nerve to the ora serrata, the scalloped margin located at the junction of the sensory retina with the ciliary body. The choroid is composed of an innermost layer of large (21 μm) capillaries, and successively larger collecting veins arranged approximately in two layers. It is thickest (0.25 mm) at the posterior pole and gradually thins anteriorly (0.10 mm). It is attached firmly to the sclera in the region surrounding the posterior scleral foramen, where the posterior ciliary arteries enter the eye, and also at the points of exit of the vortex veins.

Structure.—The three layers of blood vessels of the choroid have supporting structures on either side: the suprachoroid (lamina fusca) on the outer (scleral) side and the basal lamina (Bruch membrane) on the inner (retinal) side.

The outermost layer, the *suprachoroid (lamina fusca),* is made up of lamellae composed of elastic and collagenous fibers to form a syncy-

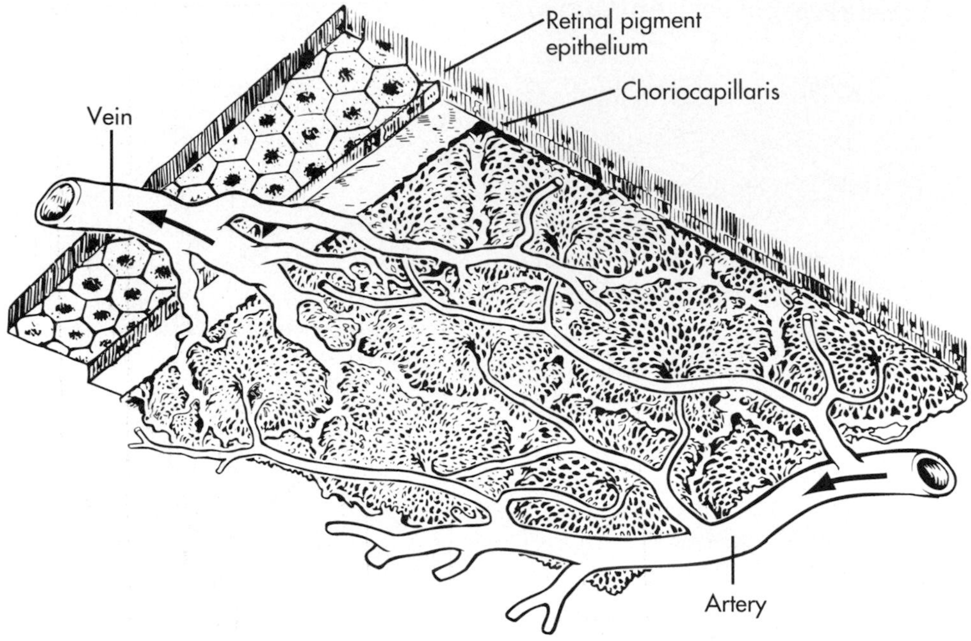

FIG 1-13.
Lobular structure of the choroidal circulation viewed from the scleral side. The short posterior ciliary arteries divide soon after their entry into the eye and send branches to the center of each lobule, which drains into peripheral veins. *(Courtesy of Lee Allen.)*

tium that is dense posteriorly and becomes looser anteriorly. Melanocytes (fibroblasts that contain pigment) are abundant in this layer and decrease in number in the vascular layers. Located in this layer are smooth muscle fibers, fibroblasts, endothelial cells, the long and short posterior ciliary arteries, and nerves. The short posterior ciliary arteries have but a short course in the suprachoroid and extend directly to the choriocapillaris.

The blood vessel layer has three components: (1) the outer (nearest the sclera) vessel layer (of Haller), which consists of large veins that have no valves and lead to the vortex veins; (2) the middle vessel layer (of Sattler), which consists of medium-sized veins and some arterioles and which contains a loose, collagenous stroma with many elastic fibers, fibroblasts, and melanocytes; and (3) the choriocapillaris, which consists of large fenestrated capillaries that form a dense, flat vascular network that extends from the margin of the optic nerve to the ora serrata. The blood vessels are arranged in lobules with a central arteriole and draining venules at the periphery (Fig 1-13).

Bruch membrane.—Bruch membrane (lamina basalis choroideae) (Fig 1-14) separates the choriocapillaris from the retinal pigment epithelium. It is about 2.0 μm thick in early childhood and increases to 4.7 μm thick by the seventh decade. It is composed of five layers to which both the choriocapillaris and the retinal pigment epithelium contribute. The outer layer, nearest the choroid, consists of the basement membrane of the endothelial cells of the choriocapillaris. Next to the outer layer is a delicate layer of collagen fibers. Centrally, a layer of elastic tissue fibers extends outward to form the supporting structure for the capillaries of the choriocapillaris. The inner (cuticular) layer originates from the retinal pigment epithelium and is composed of collagen fibers surrounded by glycosaminoglycans. Resting on this layer is the thin basement membrane of the retinal pigment epithelium.

The elastic layer of the Bruch membrane provides supporting fibers to the lamina cribrosa, but other layers stop at the disk margin. Anteriorly, at the ora serrata, the Bruch membrane loses the layer contributed by the chorio-

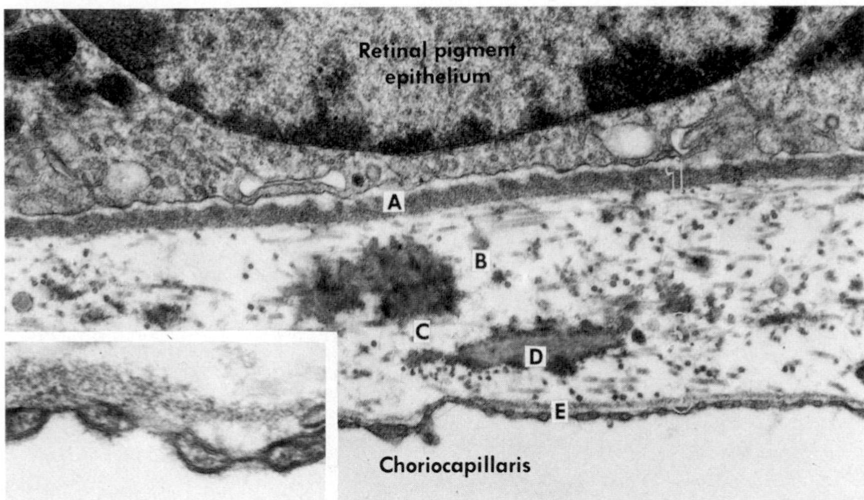

FIG 1-14.
Electron micrograph of the Bruch membrane, which separates the choriocapillaris from the retinal pigment epithelium. *A,* Basement membrane of the retinal pigment epithelium; *B,* inner collagen layer; *C,* elastic layer; *D,* outer collagen layer; *E,* basement membrane of the choriocapillaris (×21,000). *Insert,* The choriocapillaris, showing fenestrations bridged by membranous diaphragms (×77,000). *(Courtesy of Ramesh C. Tripathi, M.D.)*

capillaris and the elastic tissue layer. The cuticular and basement membrane layers derived from the retinal pigment epithelium continue anteriorly as the basement membrane of the pigment epithelium of the ciliary body.

Blood supply.—The blood supply of the choroid is derived from the short posterior ciliary arteries, the two long posterior ciliary arteries, and their seven anterior ciliary arteries (Fig 1-15). The short posterior ciliary arteries originate as two or three branches of the ophthalmic artery. These branches subdivide into 10 to 20 branches that perforate the sclera around the circumference of the optic nerve. The majority pass at once into the choroid and communicate directly with the central portion of the lobules of the choriocapillaris layer.

The medial and lateral long ciliary arteries perforate the sclera just medial and lateral to the optic nerve. They pass forward in the medial and lateral regions of the suprachoroidal space (between the choroid and the sclera) to the ciliary body. There each divides into two branches that extend circumferentially to form the major arterial circle of the iris (Fig 1-22) that is located in the ciliary body. Branches extend anteriorly to the iris. Recurrent choroidal branches extend posteriorly to terminate in the choriocapillaris.

The anterior ciliary arteries are the terminal branches of the two muscular arteries of each rectus muscle (except the lateral rectus muscle, which has but one muscular artery). The anterior ciliary arteries bifurcate into vessels that penetrate the sclera and nonpenetrating vessels that extend toward the cornea. The penetrating vessels provide the blood supply to the ciliary body and send recurrent branches to the anterior extremity of the choriocapillaris and to the major arterial circle of the iris. The nonpenetrating vessels extend forward as anterior conjunctival arteries. They anastomose with posterior conjunctival arteries, and terminate in the superficial (conjunctival) and deep (episcleral) pericorneal plexus (see conjunctival blood supply and Fig 1-22).

Venous blood from the choroid, ciliary body, and iris is collected by a series of veins of increasingly large diameter. These lead to four or more large vortex veins located behind the equator of the globe. The vortex veins empty into the superior and inferior ophthalmic veins, which drain into the cavernous sinus.

Nerve supply.—The choroid is innervated mainly by sympathetic nerves that have synapsed in the superior cervical ganglion and have passed through the ciliary ganglion without

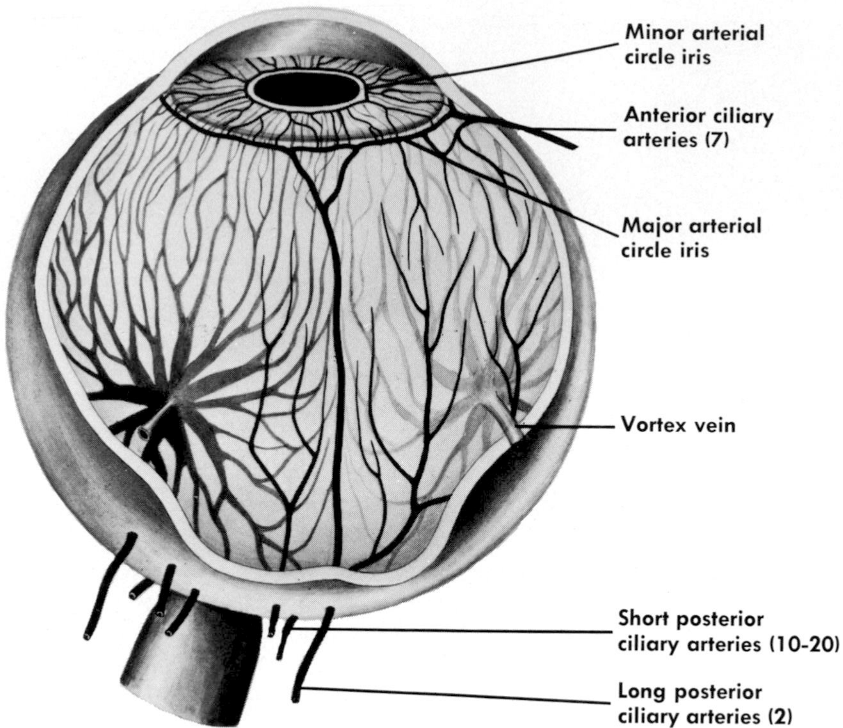

FIG 1-15.
The blood supply of the uveal tract. The two long ciliary arteries mainly supply the iris. The anterior ciliary arteries supply the ciliary body, whereas the short posterior ciliary arteries supply the choroid. Note that there are no corresponding veins. Venous blood is collected into four or more vortex veins that empty into the superior and inferior ophthalmic veins, which drain into the cavernous sinus.

synapse. They are distributed to the choroid by the short ciliary nerves. As they enter the suprachoroid, they lose their myelin sheaths and branch repeatedly to form a plexus. The nerve endings contact both pigment cells and the smooth muscle in the walls of arterioles.

The ciliary body.—The ciliary body (Figs 1-16 and 1-17) extends between the termination of the retina at the ora serrata and the scleral spur. It is divided into the following: (1) an epithelial portion that is adjacent to the vitreous cavity and the equator of the crystalline lens and (2) a uveal portion that is adjacent to the sclera. The epithelial portion is further divided into the following: (1) the pars plana (orbiculus ciliaris) and (2) the pars plicata (corona ciliaris).

Epithelial portion.—The pars plana is about 4 mm wide and extends anteriorly from the ora serrata margin of the retina to the pars plicata portion of the ciliary body. Its posterior margin is scalloped to correspond to the margin of the termination of the sensory retina. In this region the sensory retina abruptly changes into a single layer of elongated cells, the nonpigmented epithelium of the ciliary body. The retinal pigment epithelium continues anteriorly as the pigment epithelium of the ciliary body. The choriocapillaris ends at the sensory retina. Bruch membrane and its inner cuticular layer, which originates from the retinal pigment epithelium, continues forward as the basement membrane of the pigmented epithelium of the ciliary body. Surgical instruments are introduced into the vitreous cavity or into the crystalline lens through the sclera overlying the pars plana.

The pars plicata forms the most anterior portion of the ciliary body. It consists of 60 to 70 folds, the ciliary processes, which secrete the posterior aqueous humor into the posterior chamber. Each ciliary process is composed of a finger of tissue covered with a single layer of

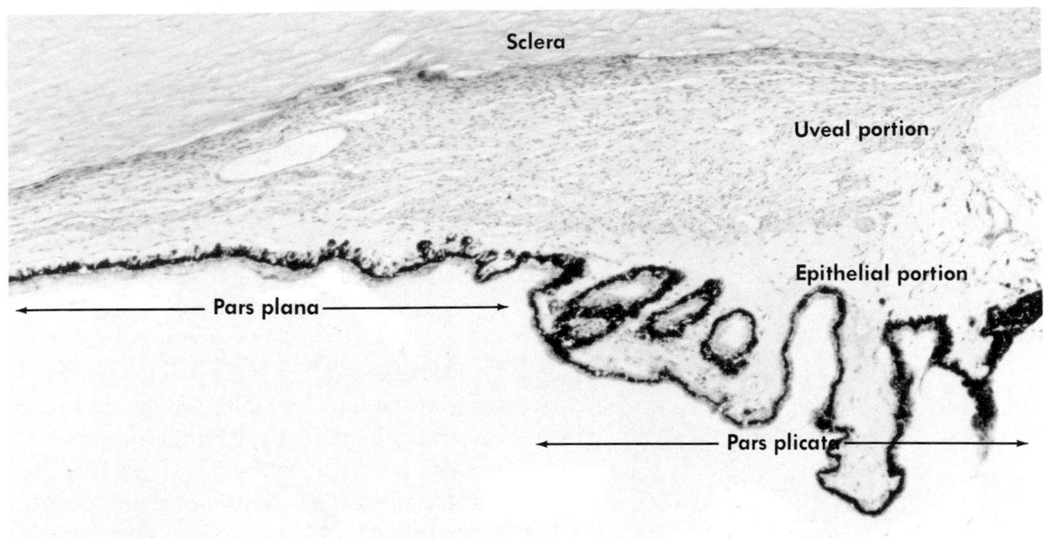

FIG 1-16.
Cross section of the ciliary body that encircles the eye. The pars plicata portion is about 2 mm in width, the pars plana about 4 mm. Intraocular surgeons often use an incision through the sclera and the adjacent pars plana (hematoxylin and eosin, ×60).

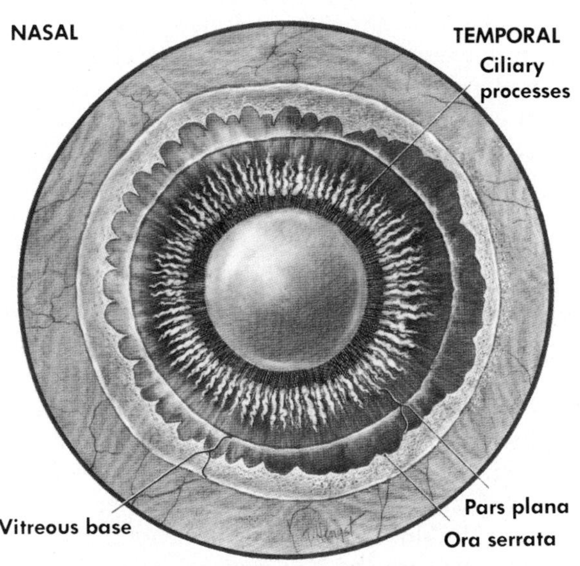

FIG 1-17.
View from behind the epithelial portion of the ciliary body. The indentations of the ora serrata are irregular. The vitreous humor has firm attachments (vitreous base) to the periphery of the sensory retina and the posterior pars plana (orbiculus ciliaris). (*From Michels RG:* Vitreous surgery, *St Louis, 1981, Mosby–Year Book. Used by permission. Artwork © The Johns Hopkins University.*)

nonpigmented epithelium that covers a layer of pigmented epithelium that surrounds a central vascular core (Fig 1-18). Each process measures about 0.8 mm in height and 1 mm in width.

Uveal portion.—The ciliary muscle (Fig 1-11) is the most prominent structure in the uveal portion of the ciliary body. It is composed of three groups of smooth muscle: (1) the longitudinal fibers (Brücke muscle), which are the outermost, parallel the surface of the overlying sclera, and constitute the main bulk of the muscle; (2) the radial fibers, which originate from the anterior portion of the longitudinal fibers and run obliquely to become continuous with circular fibers; and (3) the circular fibers (Müller muscle), which are the innermost portion and parallel the lens equator.

The ciliary zonule supports the crystalline lens in its position immediately posterior to the iris (see lens and zonule this chapter and Chap-

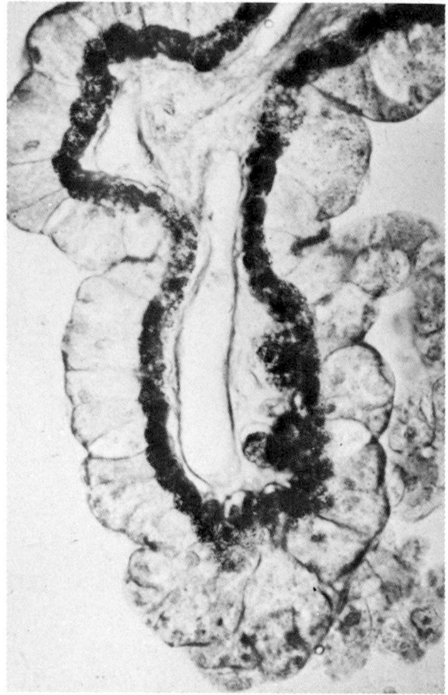

FIG 1-18.
Cross section of ciliary processes. Nonpigmented epithelium is on the surface; its base faces the posterior chamber, and the cell apex faces the pigmented epithelium. The nonpigmented epithelium is a forward extension of the sensory retina, whereas the pigmented epithelium is continuous with the retinal pigment epithelium (periodic acid-Schiff stain, ×63).

ter 21). The zonule is composed of pure fibrillin fibers that extend from the valleys between the ciliary processes to insert into the anterior and posterior lens capsule at the equator of the lens. Contraction of the circular fibers of the ciliary muscle relaxes the lens zonule, which allows the greater curvature of the lens, thereby increasing its refractive power (accommodation, see Fig 24-2).

The scleral surface of the ciliary body is the suprachoroid (lamina fusca). The vessel layer is composed mainly of the major arterial circle of the iris, its tributaries, and veins. There is no choriocapillaris.

Blood supply.—The blood supply of the ciliary body is mainly from the major arterial circle of the iris, formed by the two long ciliary arteries and the penetrating branches of the seven anterior ciliary arteries.

Nerve supply.—The parasympathetic nerve supply to the ciliary muscle originates in the Edinger-Westphal portion of the nucleus of the oculomotor nerve (N III). Within the orbit the sympathetic axons pass in the inferior branch of the oculomotor nerve to the short (motor) root of the ciliary ganglion. The axons synapse in the ciliary ganglion, and postganglionic fibers are distributed to the ciliary muscle and the sphincter pupillae muscle. Reflecting the difference in size of the structures, some 97% of the fibers go to the ciliary muscle and the remainder to the sphincter pupillae muscle.

The iris.—The iris is a diaphragm that lies in front of the lens and ciliary body and separates the anterior chamber from the posterior chamber. Its posterior surface rests on the anterior surface of the lens. Without this support the iris is tremulous (iridodonesis). The iris extends through the anterior chamber face of the ciliary body to insert into the scleral spur. Located slightly to its nasal side is a circular opening, the pupil, which controls the amount of light entering the eye.

The anterior iris surface (Fig 1-19) is divided by the collarette into a central pupillary zone, from which the anterior border layer is absent, and a peripheral ciliary zone. The collarette, a circular ridge, marks the site of the minor vascular circle of the iris, from which the pupillary membrane originated in embryonic life. Atrophy of the pupillary membrane begins in the seventh gestational month and is usually completed by 8 ½ months. Sometimes a few delicate strands persist and extend from the collarette to the anterior lens capsule.

The pupillary zone of the iris is relatively flat, and its width varies with the degree of atrophy of the anterior border layer and of pupillary dilation. The ciliary zone contains many radial interlacing ridges, giving a gossamer appearance. In blue irises, concentric contraction furrows may be seen. The color of the iris depends on the amount of melanin in the anterior border layer: if slight, reflection from the pigment of the pigmented epithelium causes scattering and a blue color. If there is a moderate amount of melanin, the iris is hazel (green); if there is a large amount, the iris is brown.

Structure.—The iris consists of two layers: (1) stroma, located anteriorly and originating from mesoderm; and (2) pigmented epithelium, located posteriorly and originating from neural ectoderm (Fig 1-20).

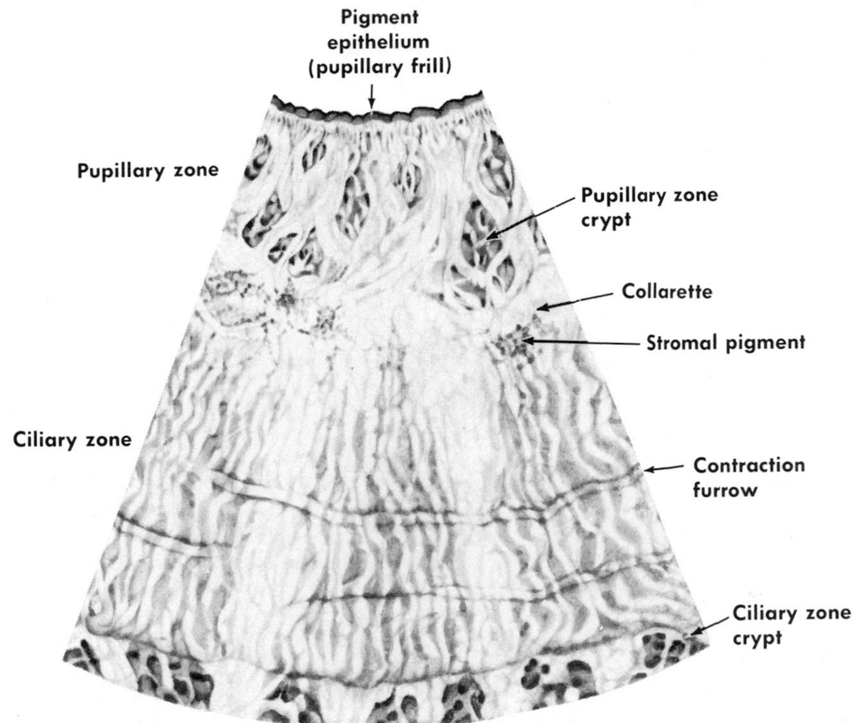

FIG 1-19.
Surface pattern of the iris. The collarette divides the pupillary zone from the ciliary zone and marks the position of the minor vascular circle of the iris, from which the pupillary membrane originated in fetal life.

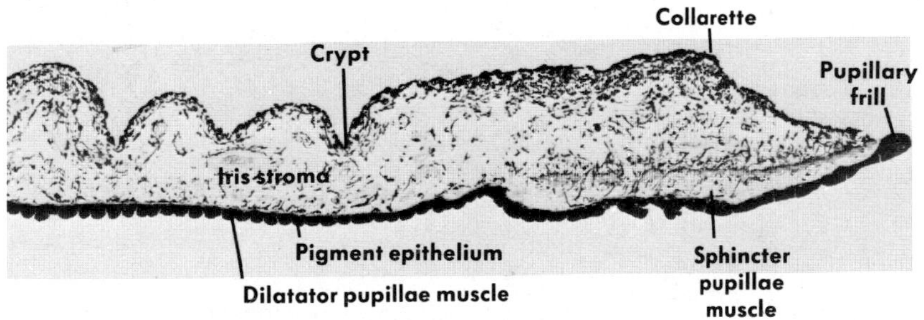

FIG 1-20.
Transverse section of the iris. The stroma is derived from mesoderm, whereas the pigment epithelium constitutes a fusion of the two layers of the primitive optic vesicle. It is a forward extension of both the sensory retina and retinal pigment epithelium. The pupillary zone extends from the pupillary frill to the collarette. The ciliary zone of the iris extends from the collarette to the peripheral termination of the iris (hematoxylin and eosin, ×43).

The stroma may be divided into an anterior border layer and a deeper stroma proper. The anterior border layer of the iris is a loose collagen tissue in which pigmented or nonpigmented cells are densely packed. This layer develops maximally about the seventh month of fetal life. Thereafter, generalized atrophy occurs, forming the pupillary zone that measures about 1.5 mm in width. The remaining, much wider iris is the ciliary zone. Irregular atrophy in the ciliary zones forms iris crypts. In brown irises the surface is smooth and heavily pigmented; in blue or hazel irises it is irregular with crypts. The anterior border layer ends abruptly at the iris root, but spokelike processes may continue as iris processes to the line of Schwalbe.

The stroma proper has a similar appearance irrespective of the color of the iris. It is visible in the pupillary zone and in the depth of iris crypts. It consists of bundles of collagen fibrils arranged in columns around blood vessels, nerves, pigment cells, and nonpigmented cells, all enmeshed in a hyaluronidase-sensitive glycosaminoglycan. The stroma proper contains more elastic tissue and fewer pigment cells than the anterior border layer. Its capillaries are not fenestrated, and have a structure similar to that of other nonfenestrated capillaries.

The *iris pigmented epithelium* consists of two layers of cells that constitute a fusion of the two layers of the primitive optic vesicle. They are densely packed with melanin. The anterior layer of pigment cells intermingles with the dilatator pupillae muscle and is absent in the region of the sphincter pupillae muscle. The posterior layer of epithelium is covered on its lenticular surface with a basement membrane continuous with that of the retina and the ciliary body. Often the pupillary margin has a pigment frill continuous with the ectodermal pigmented epithelium that constitutes the anterior extremity of the optic cup.

The sphincter pupillae muscle (N III) is located in the pupillary zone of the posterior stroma. It is a smooth muscle about 1 mm wide that forms a sphincter surrounding the pupillary margin. The dilatator pupillae muscle (sympathetics) is a thin sheet of smooth muscle (myoepithelium) located between the stroma and the posterior layer of the pigmented epithelium. It extends from the iris root at the ciliary body as far as the sphincter pupillae muscle. Both muscles are derived from neural ectoderm from the outer layer of the optic cup.

Blood supply.—The blood supply of the iris is provided by radial vessels in the stromal layer that extend from the major arterial circle of the iris (circulus arteriosus iridis major), located in the ciliary body (Fig 1-21). The major arterial circle of the iris is formed by the two long

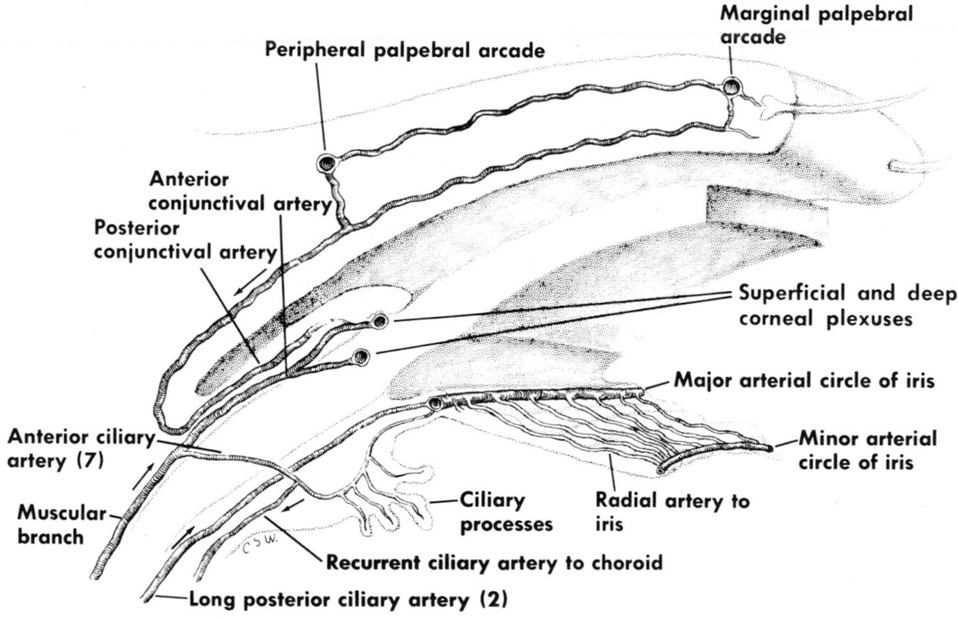

FIG 1-21.
Blood supply of the anterior ocular segment. Two anterior ciliary arteries arise from the muscular branches of each rectus muscle except for the lateral rectus muscle, which contributes only one. Two long posterior ciliary arteries enter the globe on the nasal and temporal sides of the optic nerve and extend forward in the suprachoroidal space to the ciliary body. The vascular arcades of the eyelid are derived from the lateral palpebral branches of the lacrimal artery and the medial palpebral branches of the dorsonasal artery. They have generous anastomoses with branches of the external carotid artery distributed to the face.

posterior ciliary arteries and the seven anterior ciliary arteries. The iris blood vessels pass radially in a corkscrew pattern toward the pupillary margin, creating the meridional striations of the ciliary portion of the iris. At the collarette they anastomose to form the incomplete minor vascular circle of the iris. The vessels have thick collagen adventitia and a thin muscularis layer. The endothelial cells of the veins have a perivascular sheath. They drain into the vortex veins.

The endothelial cells of the capillaris are not fenestrated, with junctional complexes that prevent the passage of large molecules. This vascular endothelium, together with the tight junctions of the pigment epithelium of the ciliary body processes and iris, forms the blood-aqueous barrier. The ciliary body vessels, like those of the choroid, are fenestrated.

Nerve supply.—The iris is richly innervated by the short ciliary (N III) and the two long ciliary (N V_1), and sympathetic nerves. The nerves are partially medullated and have a thick neurilemma. The motor innervation of the dilatator pupillae muscle emerges from sympathetic nerves that accompany the long ciliary arteries. The sphincter pupillae muscle is innervated by cholinergic fibers from the Edinger-Westphal nucleus of the oculomotor nerve that synapse in the ciliary ganglion and are distributed with short ciliary nerves (see Chapter 7). The adrenergic (sympathetic) nerve supply of the arteries of the iris is carried by the short ciliary nerves.

Inner coat: the retina

The retina develops from invagination of the primitive optic vesicle to form two layers: (1) an outer layer, the retinal pigment epithelium, and (2) an inner layer, the sensory retina. The sensory retina is stratified into many layers, but the retinal pigment epithelium is only one layer thick (Table 1-4). The layers of the retina nearest the choroid are designated as the outer layers, and those nearest the vitreous humor are the inner layers. The sensory retina extends from the optic nerve posteriorly to its scalloped margin (the ora serrata) anteriorly.

Retinal pigment epithelium.—The retinal pigment epithelium (Fig 1-22) is a single layer of

TABLE 1-4.
Layers of the Retinal Pigment Epithelium and Sensory Retina

- I. Retinal pigment epithelium (outer layer of optic vesicle)
  - A. Base (plasma membrane, mitochondria)
  - B. Body (nucleus, endoplasmic reticulum, lipofuscin)
  - C. Apex (pigment, ingested outer segment [phagosomes])
    - 1. Microvilli
    - 2. Lateral terminal bars (zonula adherens and zonula occludens)
- II. Sensory retina (inner layer of optic vesicle)
  - A. Photoreceptor cells (nuclei form the outer nuclear layer)
    - 1. Outer segment (rods and cones)
    - 2. Cilium
    - 3. Inner segment
      - a. Ellipsoid
      - b. Myoid
      - c. Outer fiber (surrounded by terminal bars of Müller cells)
      - d. Cell body (nucleus), the outer nuclear layer
      - e. Inner fiber
      - f. Synaptic vesicle
  - B. Modular cells (the nuclei form the inner nuclear layer)
    - 1. Bipolar*†
      - a. Midget
      - b. Flat midget
      - c. Diffuse
      - d. Interplexiform
    - 2. Horizontal*
    - 3. Amacrine†
  - C. Transmitter cells
    - 1. Ganglion†
      - a. Nerve fiber layer (axons of ganglion cells)
  - D. Skeletal support
    - 1. Müller cells (nuclei within inner nuclear layer)
    - 2. Internal limiting membrane (retinal basement membrane)
    - 3. Accessory glia
      - a. Small astrocytes
      - b. Oligodendrocyte-like cells

*The axons of photoreceptor cells and horizontal cells and the dendrites of bipolar cells and horizontal cells form the outer plexiform layer of the retina (the outer molecular layer).

†The axons of bipolar cells and processes of amacrine cells and the dendrites of ganglion cells form the inner plexiform layer (the inner molecular layer).

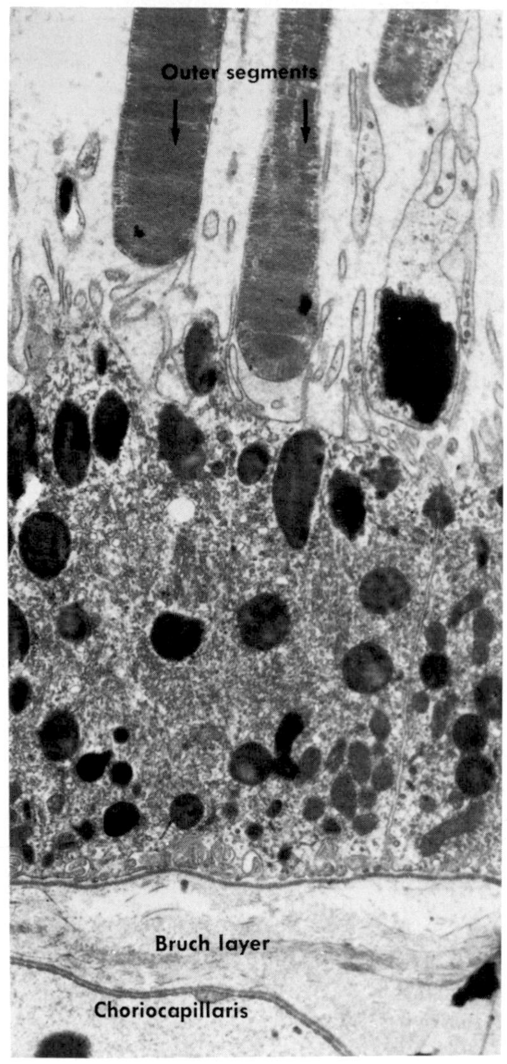

FIG 1-22.
Electron micrograph of the human retinal pigment epithelium. Microvilli at the apex of the pigment epithelial cell surround the outer segments of the photoreceptors. The extracellular fluid is the interphotoreceptor matrix. The Bruch membrane separates the retinal pigment epithelium from the choriocapillaris (×8,250). *(Courtesy of Ramesh C. Tripathi, M.D.)*

cells that extends to the optic nerve margin posteriorly and to the ora serrata anteriorly, where it fuses with the anterior continuation of the sensory retina and continues forward as the pigmented ciliary epithelium.

The apices of the retinal pigment cells enmesh the terminal ends of the outer segments of the rods and cones in an interphotoreceptor retinoid-binding protein that maintains contact between the two layers derived from the primitive optic cup. The retinal pigment epithelium supports the metabolism of the outer portion of the sensory retina and has special binding sites to transport vitamin A from the circulating blood to the rods and cones. The cells of the retinal pigment epithelium contain varying amounts of melanin, which, on ophthalmoscopic examination, give a granular appearance to the fundus. The pigment is of neural ectodermal origin and not of neural crest origin. The cells are generally hexagonal in flat section, but individual cells may have four to eight sides. The cells fit together, like cobblestones, in a regular arrangement. In the central region the cells are slender and tall. In the periphery they are more cuboid in shape. They are divided into a base, a body, and an apex.

The base is adjacent to the cuticular portion of Bruch membrane, to which its basement membrane is firmly attached. The base contains prominent infolding of the basal plasma membrane, many mitochondria, and little or no pigment.

The body contains the cell nucleus, many organelles, and lipofuscin. The lipofuscin become prominent in the retinal pigment epithelium underlying the central retina in individuals older than 30 years. On fluorescein angiography (see Chapter 6), a diagnostic technique for visualizing retinal and choroidal vascular abnormalities, lipofuscin, and melanin in the retinal pigment epithelium obscure the fluorescence from the underlying choroid.

The apices are topped with microvilli in which the outer segments of the rods and cones are imbedded in the interphotoreceptor matrix. There are no specialized attachments between the photoreceptors and the retinal pigment epithelium. The cytoplasm of the apical portion of the cell contains ovoid pigment granules and the partially digested disks of the outer segments of rods and cones.

The lateral surfaces of the apices of adjacent cells (but not the microvilli) are bound together by terminal bars that are composed of a basilar portion and an apical portion. There is no intercellular space at the level of these junctions, and together with the nonfenestrated retinal blood vessels they constitute the blood-retinal barrier.

Sensory retina.—The sensory retina (pars optica retinae) develops from the inner wall of

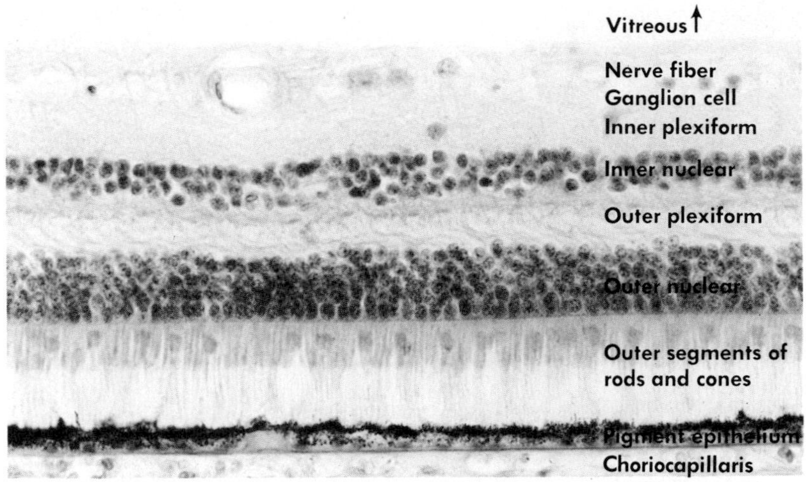

FIG 1-23.
Cross section of the human retina (hematoxylin and eosin, ×625).

the secondary optic vesicle. Its outermost layer adjacent to the retinal pigment epithelium consists of photoreceptor cells, the rods and cones. The innermost retinal layer is the nerve fiber layer, which forms the optic nerve. The sensory retina may be divided into three layers of nuclei and three layers of nerve fibers. Conventionally the layers closest to the retinal pigment epithelium are the outer layers and the layers closest to the vitreous cavity are the inner layers.

The three nuclear layers are (1) the outer nuclear layer, which contains the nuclei of photoreceptors (rods and cones); (2) the inner nuclear layer, which contains the nuclei of bipolar, horizontal, amacrine, and Müller cells; and (3) the ganglion cell layer, which contains the nuclei of ganglion cells. The three nerve layers are (1) the outer plexiform layer, where there is synapsis between rods and cones and the dendrites of bipolar cells and horizontal cells; (2) the inner plexiform layer, where there is synapsis between bipolar cells, amacrine cells, and ganglion cells; and (3) the nerve fiber layer, composed of axons of ganglion cells.

Functionally, the retina is divided into temporal and nasal portions by a line drawn vertically through the center of the fovea. Light impulses originating from photoreceptors temporal to this line pass to the lateral geniculate body on the same side. Light impulses originating from cells nasal to this line cross in the optic chiasm to the opposite side of the brain.

Ophthalmoscopically, the clinician uses the optic nerve as a hub to divide the retina into superior and inferior temporal portions, superior and inferior nasal portions, and a central area. The different quadrants are further divided into the regions posterior and anterior to the equator.

Rods and cones.—The outermost layer of the sensory retina consists of photoreceptor cells, the rods and cones. The axons of these cells synapse with cells that modulate their response (Fig 1-23). The modulator cells in turn synapse with cells that transmit spike discharges to the brain. The rod and cone cells correspond to the sensory nerve endings elsewhere in the nervous system. The glial system of the Müller cells provides mechanical support to the retina.

The rods and cones may be divided into the following parts (Fig 1-24): (1) an outer segment, the distal portions of which are surrounded by the interphotoreceptor matrix and the microvilli of the retinal pigment epithelium cells; (2) a cilium, a tubular structure that connects the outer to an inner segment; (3) an inner segment, which consists of an ellipsoid and a myoid portion; (4) the outer rod (or cone) fiber, which connects the inner segment to the cell body; (5) the cell body, which contains the nucleus; and (6) the inner rod (or cone) fiber, which terminates in a specialized synaptic ending.

The *outer segment* consists of a vertical stack of 700 to 1,000 flattened sacs (disks) that contain the light-sensitive photopigments. They are enmeshed in cytoplasm that contains the sodium,

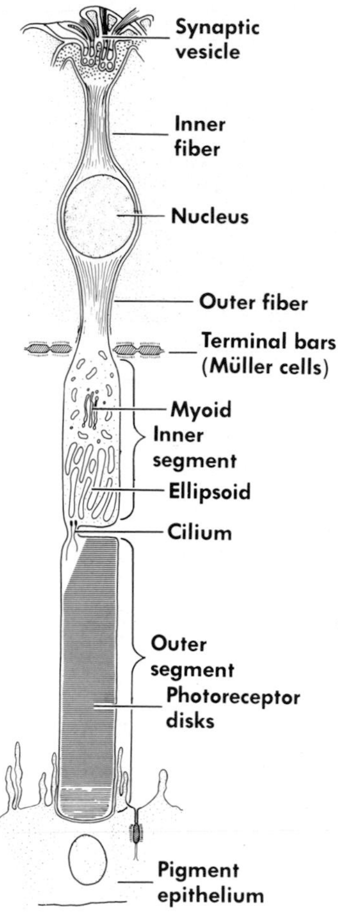

FIG 1-24.
Diagram of a rod photoreceptor cell. Photoreceptor disks of the outer segment form in the inner segment and migrate in the outer segment to the retinal pigment epithelium where they are phagocytized. The visual cell does not undergo mitosis but constantly forms new photoreceptor disks. The terminal bars of the outer process of Müller cells orient the outer segments vertically for maximal visual efficiency.

calcium, and magnesium ions concerned with the gated channels, which control the hyperpolarization of the plasma membrane, which initiates the nervous impulse stimulated by light. The disks and the cytoplasm are surrounded by a plasma membrane that is continuous with the disks of cones but separate from the disks of rods (see Chapter 2). The light-sensitive photopigment in the approximately 110 million rods, in humans, is rhodopsin. The cones contain three different photopigments concerned with color vision. The cone outer segments (6.3 to 6.8 million) have a conical shape with the apex pointing toward the sclera. In the foveal region (see Figs 1-26 and 1-27) the cones are more slender than elsewhere and resemble the cylindrical shape of rods. Outside of the fovea centralis, the tapered portion of the cone is short and the microvilli of the retinal pigment epithelium are longer, to reach the cone outer segment.

The interface between the microvilli of the apices of the retinal pigment epithelium and the distal ends of the outer segments of the photoreceptors reflects the apposition of the outer and inner layers of the primitive optic cup. The extracellular fluid is the interphotoreceptor matrix, which surrounds the microvilli of the apices of the retinal pigment epithelium and the distal portions of the rod and cone outer segments. It is composed of a mixture of proteoglycans, a glycoprotein, the interphotoreceptor retinoid-binding protein, lysosomes, and detached photoreceptor disks. The proteoglycans and lysosomes originate with the retinal pigment epithelium. The interphotoreceptor retinoid-binding protein originates with the rods. It is exceptionally antigenic, and the injection of a minute amount into experimental animals excites a severe bilateral inflammation of the uveal tract (uveitis). As photoreceptor disks detach, they are engulfed by the microvilli and digested by intracellular lysosomes of the retinal pigment epithelium.

The *cilium* connects the outer segment to the inner segment. It contains nine pairs of microtubules but lacks the central pair seen in mobile cilia. This structure transmits cellular components from the inner segment and cell nucleus to the disks and their plasma membrane.

The *inner segment* is divided into a refractile outer ellipsoid portion and a nonrefractile, basophilic inner myoid portion. The ellipsoid contains mitochondria grouped around the base of the cilium. Sodium-calcium channels in this portion of the cell are active in visual transduction. The myoid portion (contractile in some amphibia) contains free and membrane-bound ribosomes, Golgi complexes, and a variety of vesicles and vacuoles. The division into ellipsoid and myoid portions is more distinct in rods than in cones.

The inner segment is connected to the cell body by a rod or cone *outer fiber*. This fiber may be long or short, depending on the distance between the myoid and the cell body. Most outer

A

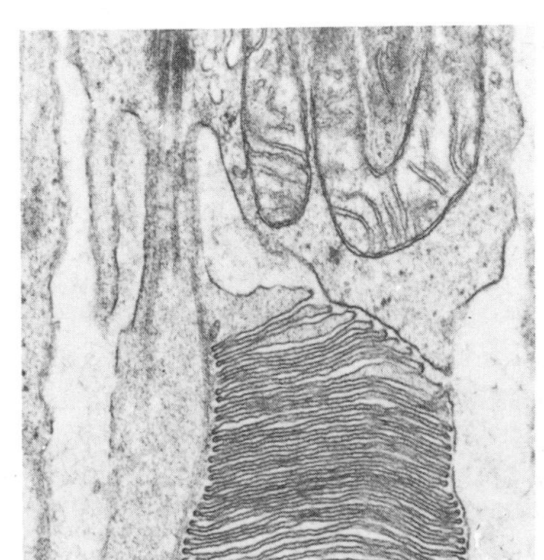

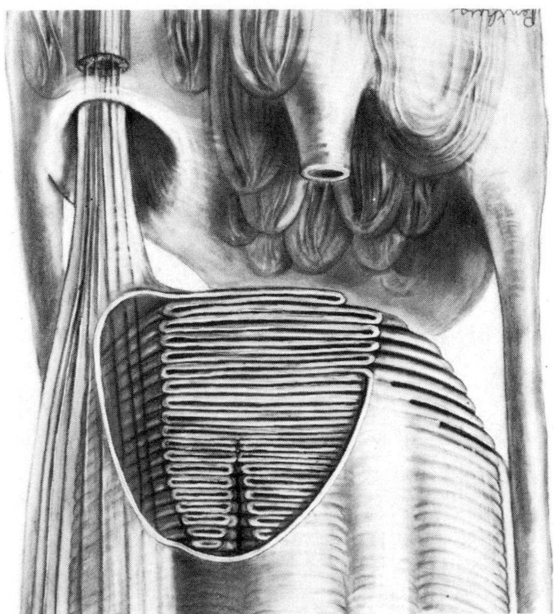

B

FIG 1-25.
A, Electron micrograph showing the junction of the outer and inner segments of retinal rod of the rhesus monkey. The membranous disks form by inward folding of the outer cell membrane adjacent to the inner segment. As the disks mature they are displaced away from the base by newer disks and lose their attachment to the outer membrane and to each other. **B,** Drawing of this region reconstructed from electron micrographs to illustrate the process of disk formation. (*From Young RW: Visual cells and the concept of renewal,* Invest Ophthalmol Vis Sci *15:700, 1976. Used by permission.*)

fibers of cones are shorter than those of rods. The outer fiber is surrounded by the terminal bars of Müller cells. In light microscopy this is the external limiting membrane. These bars provide a vertical orientation for the photoreceptors.

The *cell body* located in the outer nuclear layer, consists almost entirely of nucleus.

An *inner fiber* (rod or cone inner fiber) passes in the outer plexiform layer and terminates in a synaptic expansion, the rod spherule, or in a cone pedicle, the cone-foot. These expansions synapse in the outer plexiform layer with cells having their nuclei in the inner nuclear layer. There are several types of synaptic endings, and it is possible that at this level the nerve impulse is both integrated and inhibited. At this level, also, chemical intermediates are secreted that are involved in the synaptic transmission of nerve impulses.

Mature visual cells do not replicate, and their deoxyribonucleic acid (DNA) is stable. In contrast, ribosomal ribonucleic acid (RNA), transfer RNA, and messenger RNA are constantly renewed by the cell nucleus and passed to the myoid. The organelles of the myoid synthesize the visual pigments, the phospholipids and proteins of the outer segments, and the interphotoreceptor matrix. Proteins reach the outer segment through the connecting cilium (Fig 1-25). The oldest disks of rods and cones, which are surrounded by the microvilli of the retinal pigment epithelium, are detached in small groups from the tip of the cell. They are phagocytized and digested by the pigment epithelium.

Modulator cells.—The nervous signal initiated by stimulation of the outer segment is transmitted by three different cell types: (1) bipolar cells; (2) horizontal cells; and (3) amacrine cells. Their nuclei are located in the inner nuclear layer. A basketlike configuration of the dendrites at the border of the inner and middle thirds of the outer plexiform layer forms a dense structure that divides the sensory retina into inner and outer portions. In humans the outer portion of the retina is nurtured by the choriocapillaris and the inner portion by the capillaries of the central retinal artery.

In primates there are four types of bipolar cells: (1) midget; (2) flat midget; (3) diffuse; and (4) interplexiform bipolar cells. Their dendrites attach to photoreceptor synaptic vesicles with desmosomes. Synapsis with horizontal cells is by desmosomes and gap junctions.

All cones synapse with at least one midget bipolar cell and often with other bipolar cells, but midget bipolar cells generally synapse with a single cone. There are many more ganglion nuclei than there are cones in the human foveal area. There are enough ganglion cells to transmit the information from closely spaced foveal cones to both ON- and OFF-channels (see Chapter 2).

Bipolar axons terminate in synaptic vesicles comparable to those of photoreceptors. In the inner plexiform layer they synapse with the dendrites of ganglion cells and the processes of amacrine cells.

The nuclei of *horizontal cells* are located in the outer portion of the inner nuclear layer. Both their axons and dendrites are located in the outer plexiform layer. Horizontal cell dendrites synapse with several closely adjoining photoreceptors, and their axons synapse with several photoreceptors in a distant part of the retina. Other axons synapse with bipolar cells. Possibly, horizontal cells act as condensers in an electric circuit, collect impulses from a group of photoreceptors, and, with discharge, trigger a visual impulse.

Amacrine cells are oriented in the wrong direction in terms of the transmission of the light impulse. The amacrine cell processes synapse with ganglion cells and bipolar cells. Their cell bodies lie at the inner portion of the inner nuclear layer, and their processes are directed inward toward the ganglion cell layer. Some contain large vesicles in their nuclei and cell processes that may contain dopamine. They may inhibit the integration of the visual impulse.

Transmitter cells.—Ganglion cells are the transmitter cells of the retina. Their nuclei are located in the innermost cellular layer of the retina and their axons form the nerve fiber layer. The nerve fibers form the optic nerve, which transmits spiked discharges that synapse in the lateral geniculate body and other centers in the midbrain.

The inner layers of the retina are absent in the fovea centralis (see below) but, in the region surrounding the fovea centralis, the ganglion cell layer is five to seven cell layers thick. In the retinal periphery the ganglion cell layer is but a single cell thick. Ganglion cells may be classified anatomically on the basis of their dendrites: nonstratified, multistratified, diffuse, small, or large. Ganglion cell dendrites synapse with the axons of bipolar cells and the axons of amacrine cells in the inner plexiform layer. Physiologically, ganglion cell axons may be divided into those that transmit visual impulses and those that transmit afferent impulses that control the constriction of the pupil by light. Axons subserving vision synapse in the lateral geniculate bodies. Those transmitting impulses that control pupillary size synapse in the pretectal nuclei in the midbrain (see Chapter 7).

The axons of ganglion cells form the nerve fiber layer. This layer is sometimes visible in red-free light and may often be seen ophthalmoscopically in black individuals. The nerve fibers originating from ganglion cells of the fovea centralis extend directly medially to the optic nerve. Axons from the temporal retina arch above and below these fibers but do not cross the horizontal raphe of the retina, which extends temporally from the fovea centralis to the ora serrata. The fibers from the nasal side of the optic disk have an approximately straight radial course. The distribution is important in the configuration of visual field defects in glaucoma. The major branches of the central retinal artery and vein are located in the nerve fiber layer.

The supporting astroglia.—The structural support of the sensory retina is supplied mainly by large astrocytes (Müller cells), which are partially aided by smaller glial and fibrous and protoplasmic astrocytes in the inner plexiform, ganglion cell, and nerve fiber layers of the retina. The nuclei of Müller cells are located in the middle portion of the inner nuclear layer of the retina. Terminal bars of the outer processes attach to the outer fibers of the photoreceptors and orient the outer segments for maximum visual efficiency. Inner processes extend toward the nerve fiber layer, where their footplates separate this layer from the internal limiting lamina. Many filaments of the inner processes pass between axons of the nerve fiber layer.

Müller cells furnish the enzymes for glycolysis. They accumulate retinal potassium and pass it to the vitreous (in some species).

Regions of the retina.—The sensory retina is divided histologically and functionally as follows: (1) the central retina, often called the macula, which surrounds the fovea centralis; (2) the peripheral or extracentral retina; and (3) the ora serrata, the scalloped anterior termination of the sensory retina.

Central retina.—The central retina measures about 4.5 mm in diameter. (The optic disk is about 1.5 mm in diameter and is the unit used clinically to describe the size of retinal lesions.) The central retina extends from the fovea centralis, at its center, nasally almost to the optic disk. It extends, between the superior and inferior temporal blood vessels, about the same distance temporally. Except at the fovea centralis, the ganglion cell layer in the central retina has two or more layers of ganglion cell nuclei. The retina in the central region between the outer nuclear layer and the nerve fiber layer contains a yellow carotenoid pigment, xanthophyll, and

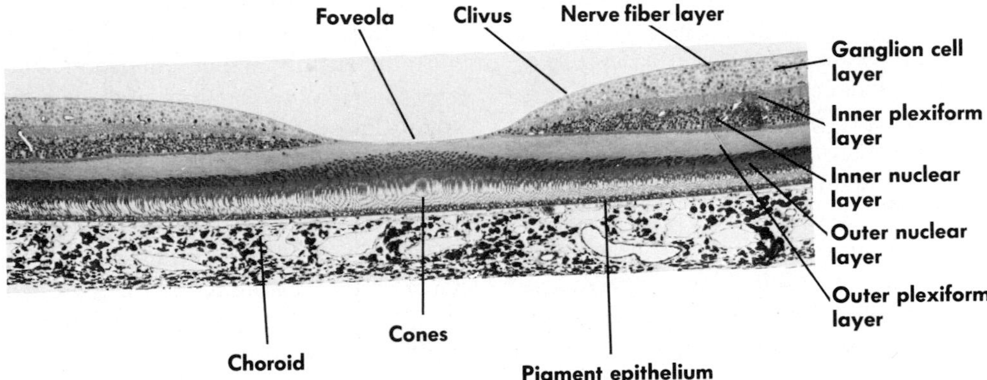

FIG 1-26.
Human fovea centralis. The fovea centralis is a depression with sloping walls, the clivus. The floor of the fovea centralis, the foveola, is flat. The fibers of the outer plexiform layer are tangential to the surface of the retina. The inner layers of the retina are absent, so that light falls directly upon the cones. The floor of the fovea centralis corresponds closely to the capillary-free region of the retina, and this area is nurtured solely by the choriocapillaris (×105). *(Courtesy of Ramesh C. Tripathi, M.D.)*

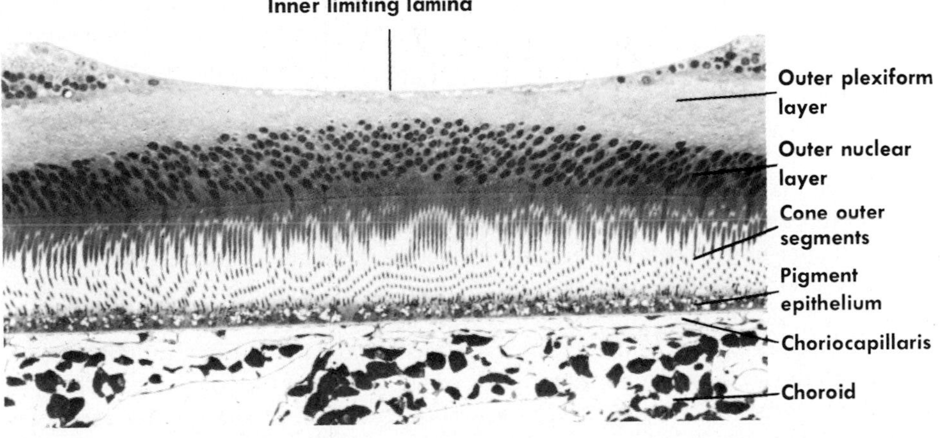

FIG 1-27.
The human foveola. The outer segments of cones of the foveola are densely packed, thin, long, and attenuated. The inner layers of the retina are absent and only the outer nuclear layers and the outer plexiform layer are present (×350). *(Courtesy of Ramesh C. Tripathi, M.D.)*

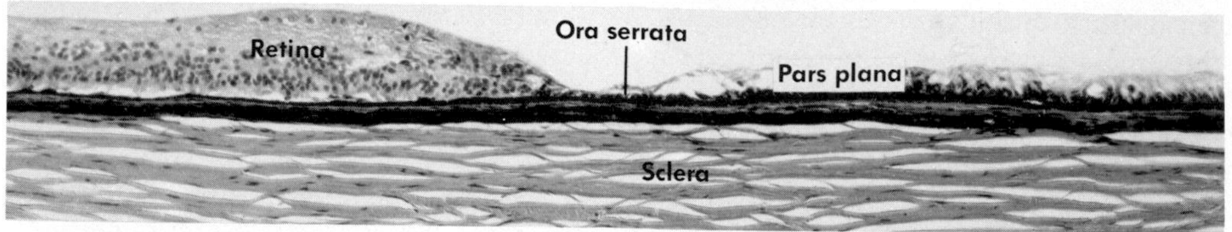

FIG 1-28.
The laminated sensory retina terminates in a serrated border at the ora serrata and continues forward as the epithelium of the pars plana portion of the ciliary body. The retinal pigment epithelium continues as the pigment epithelium of the ciliary body (hematoxylin and eosin, ×43).

this region is called the macula lutea (yellow spot).

The fovea centralis (Fig 1-26) is a depressed area located in the central retina about 3 mm temporal to the optic disk and 0.8 mm below the horizontal meridian. It measures 1.5 mm in diameter. The slope of the depression is called the clivus. Its center is the foveola, which measures about 0.4 mm in diameter. The fovea centralis is composed exclusively of cones, the photoreceptors for colors. The outer segments of the cones in the foveola are long, thin, attenuated, and densely packed together (Fig 1-27).

The foveola is nurtured solely by the choriocapillaris of the choroid and does not contain the capillaries of the sensory retina. The inner cell layers are displaced peripherally, and only the layer of cones, their nuclei in the outer nuclear layer, and their connections in the outer plexiform layer are present. The fibers in the outer plexiform layer extend radially to the inner nuclear layer.

Peripheral retina.—In the peripheral retina the photoreceptors are mainly rods, and the outer segments of the few scattered cones present are thicker than those in the central retina. The outer plexiform layer is vertically arranged, and the inner nuclear layer has a regular orientation. The ganglion cells are larger than those in the central retina, and their cell bodies are arranged in a single layer.

Ora serrata.—The ora serrata is the anterior termination of the sensory retina. It consists of a scalloped (dentate) fringe adjacent to the pars plana of the ciliary body (Fig 1-28; see Fig 1-17) and is located about 6 mm from the corneoscleral limbus.

In this area the sensory retina abruptly loses its laminated structure, and the two layers of the primitive optic vesicle fuse and continue forward as the ciliary epithelium.

Blood supply.—The outer and inner portions of the retina each have a separate blood supply. This is not a double blood supply; each must be intact to maintain retinal function. The outer portion is nurtured by the choriocapillaris layer of the choroid. The inner portion of the retina is nurtured by the branches of the central retinal artery. The border between the two blood supplies is the basketlike configuration of bipolar cell dendrites at the junction of the outer and middle thirds of the outer plexiform layer. These layers are absent at the fovea centralis so that the foveal layers receive their blood supply only from the choriocapillaris.

The central retinal artery is a branch of the ophthalmic artery, which is given off by the internal carotid artery as it emerges from the cavernous sinus. (See the section on blood supply in this chapter.) The ophthalmic artery enters the orbit through the optic foramen, below and lateral to the optic nerve. It crosses to the medial side of the orbit either above or below the optic nerve and gives off the central retinal artery, which enters the optic nerve about 12 mm posterior to the globe. The central retinal artery extends forward to the optic disk, where it bifurcates into superior and inferior papillary branches. As the vessel passes through the lamina cribrosa, its wall is reduced to about half its previous thickness, the internal elastic lamella is lost, and the medial muscle coat becomes incomplete. Thus, its major branches within the eye are arterioles and not arteries.

The superior and inferior papillary branches of the central retinal artery bifurcate within the optic nerve or on the surface of the optic disk to form nasal and temporal branches. The nasal

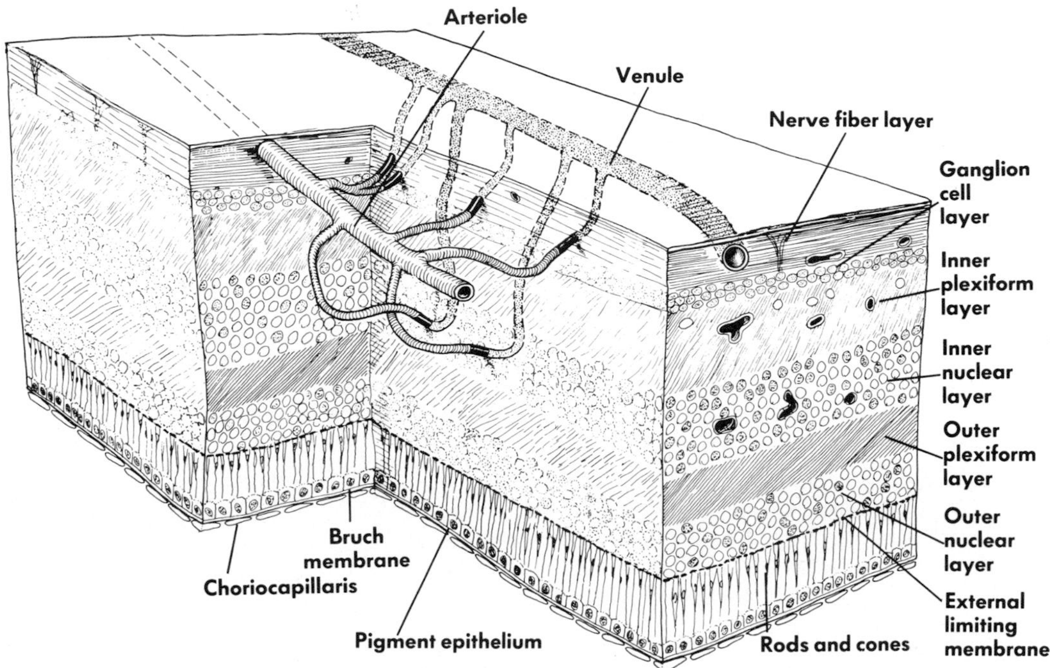

FIG 1-29.
Retinal arterioles provide two major capillary layers in the retina: one in the nerve fiber layer and one in the inner nuclear layer. In general, diseases affecting primarily the arteries, such as vascular hypertension, involve the capillary network in the nerve fiber layer, whereas predominantly venous diseases, such as diabetes mellitus, involve the layer of capillaries in the inner nuclear layer. The photoreceptors together with their cell bodies in the outer nuclear layer and the outer one third of the outer plexiform layer are nurtured by the choriocapillaris of the choroid. Both systems are necessary to the function of the retina.

branches follow a relatively direct course to the periphery. The temporal vessels arch above and below the fovea centralis and pass to the periphery.

Capillaries.—The retinal capillaries are distributed in two layers: (1) a superficial network at the level of the nerve fiber layer and (2) an intraretinal network at the level of the inner nuclear layer (Fig 1-29). The intraretinal capillaries receive blood from the capillaries in the nerve fiber layer. Arterial abnormalities (such as vascular hypertension) tend to involve the capillaries in the nerve fiber plexus, whereas venous abnormalities (such as diabetes mellitus) tend to involve capillaries located in the inner nuclear layer. The arterioles have a capillary-free zone surrounding them.

The endothelial cells that line retinal capillaries are regularly arranged with their nuclei parallel to the direction of the vessel. The vessel wall contains pericytes (mural cells) that are separated from the endothelium by its basement membrane. The endothelial cells are joined by terminal bars and constitute, together with the tight junctions of retinal pigment epithelium, the blood-retinal barrier.

Veins.—The veins in the retina essentially follow the distribution of the arteries. They consist of an endothelial coat supported by a small amount of connective tissue. At points in the retina where arteries cross veins, the vessels are bound together with a common adventitial sheath. The central vein exits from the optic nerve about the same region the central retinal artery enters, some 12 mm behind the globe. The superior and inferior branches often join within the nerve to form two papillary branches, which then join to form the central retinal vein. In its exit from the nerve, the central retinal vein must pass through the meninges sheathing the nerve, where it is vulnerable to increases in intracranial pressure, a factor important in the production of papilledema.

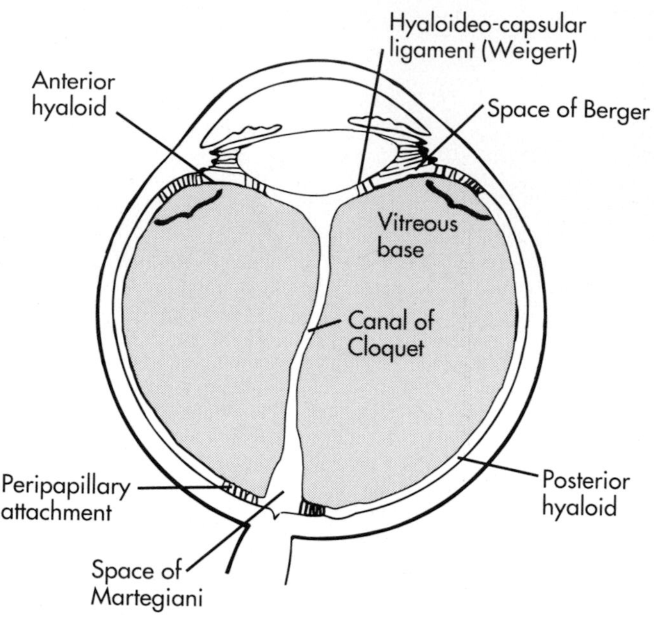

FIG 1-30.

Schematic drawing of vitreous humor. The canal of Cloquet is mainly a theoretical structure, which marks the course of the hyaloid vasculature in the embryonic eye. Fibrils extend between the vitreous humor and (1) the posterior capsule of the lens (hyaloideocapsular ligament of Weigert); (2) the pars plana of the ciliary body and the periphery of the retina (the vitreous base); and (3) the periphery but not the surface of the optic disk. Inflammatory cells may sometimes be seen in the space of Martegiani in optic neuritis. The thin layer of cortical vitreous humor surrounds the entire vitreous body, normally in contact with the retina and posterior lens surface. The central portion of vitreous constitutes its major part.

Chambers of the eye

The eye contains three chambers: the anterior chamber, the posterior chamber, and the vitreous cavity (see frontispiece).

Anterior chamber.—The anterior chamber is bounded anteriorly by the cornea, posteriorly by the front surface of the iris and lens, and peripherally by the anterior chamber angle, which contains the trabecular meshwork. The anterior chamber is deepest in its central portion (3 mm) and shallowest at the peripheral insertion of the iris. In humans, its volume is approximately 0.2 mL.

Posterior chamber.—The posterior chamber is bounded anteriorly by the iris, peripherally by the ciliary processes, and posteriorly by the anterior lens capsule and the zonule. In human adults, its volume is about 0.06 mL. Posterior aqueous humor is secreted by the nonpigmented epithelium of the ciliary processes into the posterior chamber and flows through the pupil into the anterior chamber.

Vitreous cavity.—The vitreous cavity is the largest chamber of the eye. It is bounded anteriorly by the lens, zonule, and ciliary body and posteriorly by the retina and optic nerve. It has a volume of 4.5 mL.

The vitreous cavity contains the vitreous humor, a transparent gel composed of a random network of uniformly thin collagen fibrils suspended in a highly dilute solution of salts, protein, and hyaluronic acid. Its main component is water (98.5% to 99.7%). In young adults about 80% is gel and the remainder liquid vitreous humor that contains hyaluronic acid without collagen fibrils. With aging, the liquid component increases to about 50%.

The vitreous humor is shaped like a sphere with the anterior portion removed to form a saucer-shaped depression for the crystalline lens (anterior hyaloid lenticular fossa). In the region of the depression, the vitreous humor is condensed and described clinically as the anterior hyaloid face (Fig 1-30). The peripheral portion of the anterior hyaloid may be loosely attached to the posterior lens capsule to form the annular hyaloid ligament of Weigert. The vitreous humor adheres firmly to the margin of the optic

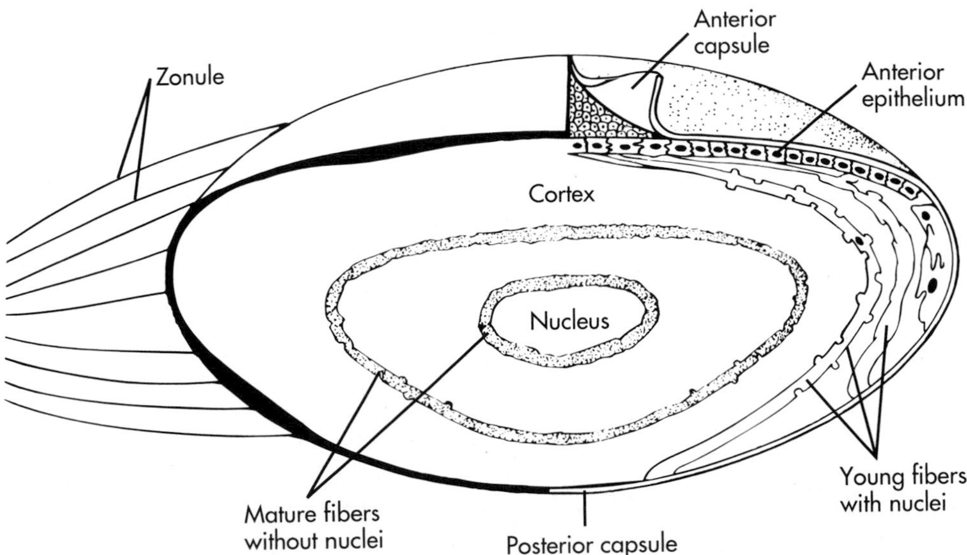

FIG 1-31.
Cross section of the crystalline lens. In humans, new lens cells (fibers) form at the equator throughout life. Older fibers migrate toward the center of the lens (nucleus) where at the center one may see lens fibers that formed in fetal life. The nuclei of the newly formed cells are located at the equator of the lens. The posterior lens process is attached to its basement membrane, the posterior lens capsule. The anterior lens process extends into the cortex. The lens fibers in the cortex and nucleus do not have nuclei and do not attach to the posterior capsule. The anterior epithelial cells do not have lens processes and are in intimate contact with their basement membrane, the anterior lens capsule.

disk, to the peripheral retina near the ora serrata, and to the ciliary epithelium in the region of the pars plana (the vitreous base). Sometimes it is firmly attached to retinal blood vessels.

In the normal eye, the vitreous humor is in contact with the entire retina and is attached to the internal limiting lamina of the retina by scattered collagenous filaments. If the vitreous humor degenerates and shrinks (vitreous detachment), the filamentary attachments may adhere to the sensory retina and cause a retinal hole that may lead to a retinal detachment.

The vitreous humor may be divided into two portions: (1) a cortical portion, which surrounds the entire vitreous body adjacent to the lens and retina; and (2) a central portion. The vitreous base is a 4-mm band of vitreous that straddles both the ora serrata and the pars plana ciliaris, to which it is attached by many fibrils. At the periphery of the optic disk, fibrils extend between the vitreous and the footplates of Müller cells. Embryologically, the vitreous is divided into three parts: (1) primary (mesenchymal, canal of Cloquet); (2) secondary (most of the adult vitreous); and (3) tertiary (the lens zonule).

The structure of the central vitreous is less dense with fewer fibrils than the vitreous of the cortex. The vitreous cortex contains a few cells called "hyalocytes," which are believed to be macrophages.

Lens and zonule

The crystalline lens.—The crystalline lens (Fig 1-31) is a grossly transparent, biconvex structure, located directly behind the iris and pupil and anterior to a shallow depression in the anterior face of the vitreous humor, the anterior hyaloid lenticular fossa. It is held in position by its suspensory ligament, the ciliary zonule. The zonular fibers blend into the anterior and posterior lens capsule near the equator. The zonular fibers extend further over the anterior lens capsule than the posterior lens capsule.

The center of curvature of the anterior surface is the anterior pole; the posterior pole is the corresponding point on the posterior surface.

The anterior surface has a radius of curvature of 10 mm. The posterior pole has a radius of curvature of 6 mm. The equator is separated from the free edge of the processes of the ciliary body by a distance of 0.5 mm.

The lens forms new cells throughout life. In humans old lens processes are compressed centrally to form an increasingly large, inelastic lens nucleus. Although the normal lens appears brilliantly transparent when viewed grossly, biomicroscopy discloses minute opacities and concentric areas with different indices of refraction.

The lens is composed of the following: (1) a lens capsule, which envelops the entire lens and is divided into a thick anterior capsule and a thin posterior capsule; (2) epithelial cells located just beneath the anterior capsule and lens cells with their nuclei near the equator of the lens; (3) lens substance consisting of the cortex, which is composed of lens fibers that have their nuclei near the equator of the lens and their posterior processes attached to the posterior capsule; and (4) a central region called the nucleus, composed of lens fiber membranes that are no longer attached to a cell nucleus or to the posterior capsule.

The lens capsule is a smooth, homogeneous, acellular structure. It is thickest on the anterior and posterior surfaces just central to the insertion of the zonular fibers. The anterior capsule is the basement membrane of the anterior lens epithelium; it is the thickest basement membrane in the body. The posterior capsule is the basement membrane of lens cells that have their nuclei in the nuclear bow near the lens equator. The anterior lens epithelial cells consist of a single row of cuboidal cells of regular shape, having numerous interdigitations and their bases adjacent to their basement membrane, the anterior lens capsule. The cells rarely show mitotic figures and are responsible for the metabolism of the entire lens. In humans, each lens cell (called a lens fiber) consists of a cell nucleus and anterior and posterior membranous processes. The nuclei of the most immature cells are located near the equator.

As new lens cells form, their nuclei displace the older cell nuclei inward to form a "nuclear bow." The posterior lens process of each nucleated cell is in contact with the posterior capsule, which constitutes its basement membrane. The anterior process extends forward in the anterior lens cortex. Each lens process is a curved, hexagonal prism, 8 to 10 µm wide and 2 µm thick. The lens processes have numerous ridges and knobs together with socket invaginations to receive the knobs, particularly at the lateral margins. Their apical ends are flat with lobulated margins. When first formed, the lens processes are short but gradually become 3.5 to 5 mm long. Lens cells multiply throughout life in the entire circumference of the lens, and the junctions of their processes form complex patterns.

The posterior processes gradually extend until they reach the posterior pole of the lens, at which time they lose their nuclei, their contact with the posterior capsule, and are displaced inward. Such mature lens fibers, including both the anterior and posterior lens processes, form most of the substance of the lens. They are packed into an increasingly dense central region, called the lens nucleus.

In fetal life, the apices of lens processes join at the anterior central area and maintain junctions with cells extending from corresponding cells of the opposite side to form the upright, anterior Y-suture of the lens. When cells lose their nuclei, the posterior fibers are detached from the posterior capsule and are pushed deeper into the central zone to form the inverted Y-shaped posterior suture. After the fetal nucleus forms, the fibers that originate from the entire circumference of the lens form more complicated junctions than the Y-sutures.

The zonule.—The lens zonule (zonule of Zinn, or suspensory ligament of the lens; Fig 1-32) supports the lens in position and connects the lens to the ciliary muscle. It is composed of a series of fine fibrils of fibrillin that insert at the equator on the outer surface of the lens capsule. The zonules attach to the lamellar portion of the lens capsule on either side of the equator and to the basement membrane of the ciliary epithelium in the valleys between the ciliary processes. The ciliary attachment is long, and fibers may extend to the pars plana of the ciliary body. Other fibers may attach to the anterior vitreous face. The lens insertion extends about 2 mm in front of and 1 mm behind the lens equator.

THE ORBIT

The eyes rest in the anterior portion of two bony cavities, the orbits (Fig 1-33), located on

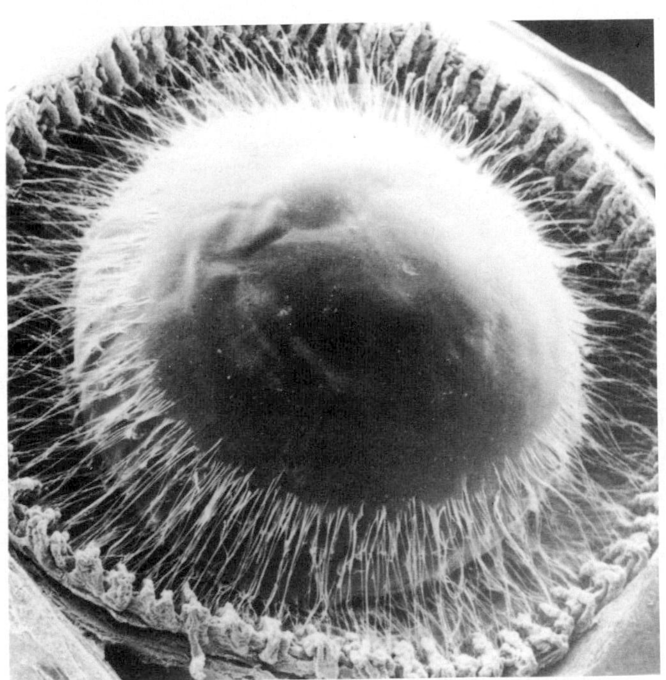

FIG 1-32.
Scanning electron micrograph of the zonular insertion to the anterior lens capsule after removal of the cornea and iris. The anterior heads of the ciliary processes are free of zonules, and the angle between the anterior and the posterior zonules is evident. The lens is 25% smaller than normal owing to processing shrinkage (×25). (*From Streeten BW:* Zonular apparatus. *In Duane TD, Jaeger EA, editors:* Biomedical foundations of ophthalmology, *vol 1, New York, 1983, Harper & Row. Used by permission.*)

either side of the nose. Although each orbit appears to be positioned directly forward, only the medial walls are parallel, and the lateral walls diverge at an angle of about 45°. The posterior openings of each orbit, the optic foramen and the superior orbital fissure, are located medial to the eye. The optic nerve, blood vessels, and ocular muscles are directed laterally, a factor in ocular rotations.

Each wall of the orbit, except the medial, is approximately triangular, with the base forming the anterior margin. The anterior two thirds of each orbital wall are roughly the shape of a truncated quadrilateral pyramid, with each base measuring about 35 to 40 mm. The posterior one third narrows to the shape of a triangular pyramid. The orbit measures 35 to 40 mm in height, width, and depth, and has a volume of about 30 mL.

Structure

The anterior bony margin of each orbit is thickened to protect the eye. The lateral bony margin is formed by the zygomatic bone and the zygomatic process of the frontal bone. The entire superior margin, the heaviest, is formed by the frontal bone. At the junction of the medial one third with the lateral two thirds is the supraorbital notch (or sometimes foramen) that transmits the supraorbital blood vessels and nerve. The medial margin is formed by the angular process of the frontal bone and the frontal process of the maxillary bone. The bony fossa of the lacrimal sac makes the medial margin poorly defined. The inferior margin is formed by the zygomatic bone laterally and the body of the maxillary bone medially.

The anterior one third of the lateral wall is formed by the zygoma, and the posterior two thirds are formed by the greater wing of the sphenoid bone. The zygoma is dense bone that separates the orbit from the fossa of the temporalis muscle, while the greater wing of the sphenoid is extremely thin and separates the orbit from the temporal lobe of the brain. The lateral orbital tubercle is situated on the anterior margin of the zygoma. To it is attached the aponeurosis of the levator palpebrae superioris muscle, the suspensory ligament of the globe (the ligament of Lockwood), the check ligament of the lateral rectus muscle, and the lateral palpebral (canthal) ligament.

The roof of the orbit is mainly formed by the orbital plate of the frontal bone. The lesser wing of the sphenoid bone contributes slightly to the apex. On its lateral side, the orbital roof forms sutures with the zygoma anteriorly and the greater wing of the sphenoid posteriorly. The bony fossa for the lacrimal gland is located in its anterior lateral portion. On its medial side, the

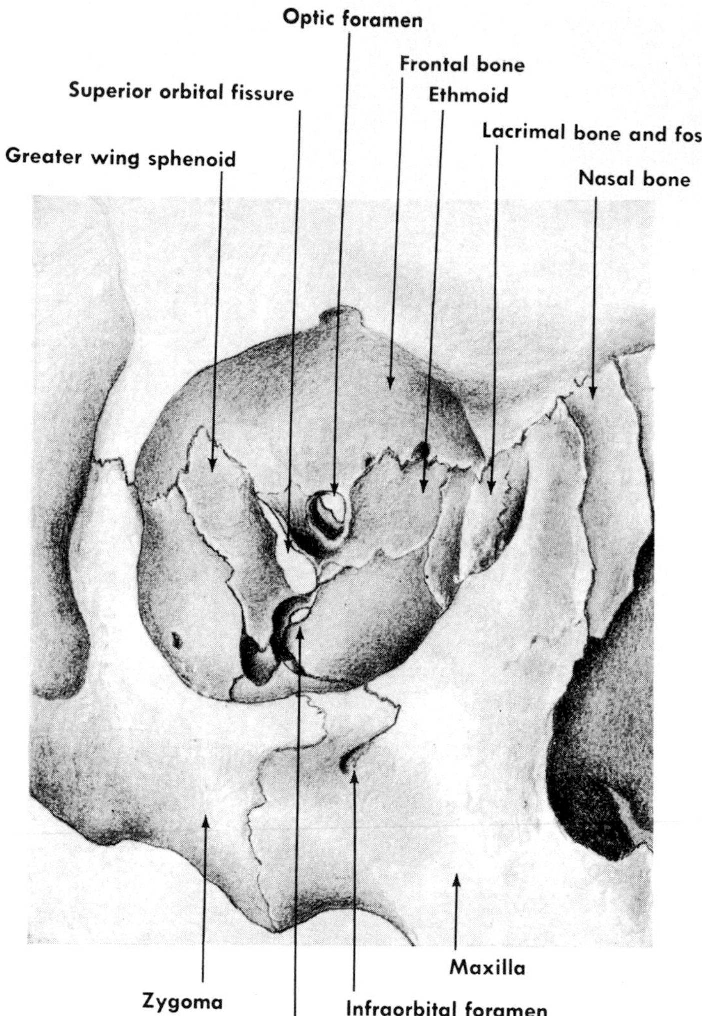

FIG 1-33.
The bony orbit.

frontal bone forms sutures with the lacrimal bone anteriorly and the ethmoid bone posteriorly. The trochlea, a fibrous structure that forms a pulley for the tendon of the superior oblique muscle, is located near the anterior, medial margin of the roof of the orbit. Located immediately above the roof of the orbit is the frontal nasal sinus anteriorly and the front lobe of the brain posteriorly.

The medial wall is quadrilateral. It is formed mainly by the orbital plate of the ethmoid bone, which has sutures anteriorly with the lacrimal bone and posteriorly with the body of the sphenoid bone. The lamina papyracea of the ethmoid bone is extremely thin, and the sinus may rupture into the orbit when inflamed. When the lamina papyracea is fractured, it allows air to enter the orbit (emphysema of the orbit). In the anterior portion of the orbit, the bony fossa of the lacrimal sac is located between the anterior lacrimal crest of the frontal process of the maxilla and the posterior lacrimal crest of the lacrimal bone. The lacrimal sac occupies this fossa and extends downward through the nasal lacrimal duct into the nose. The two leaves of the medial canthal ligament insert into the anterior and posterior lacrimal crests. The posterior portion of the medial wall of the orbit formed by the body of the sphenoid bone contains the optic foramen.

The orbital floor does not extend to the apex. The floor is formed mainly by the orbital plate of the maxilla. The orbital surface of the zygoma extends laterally, and the orbital process of the

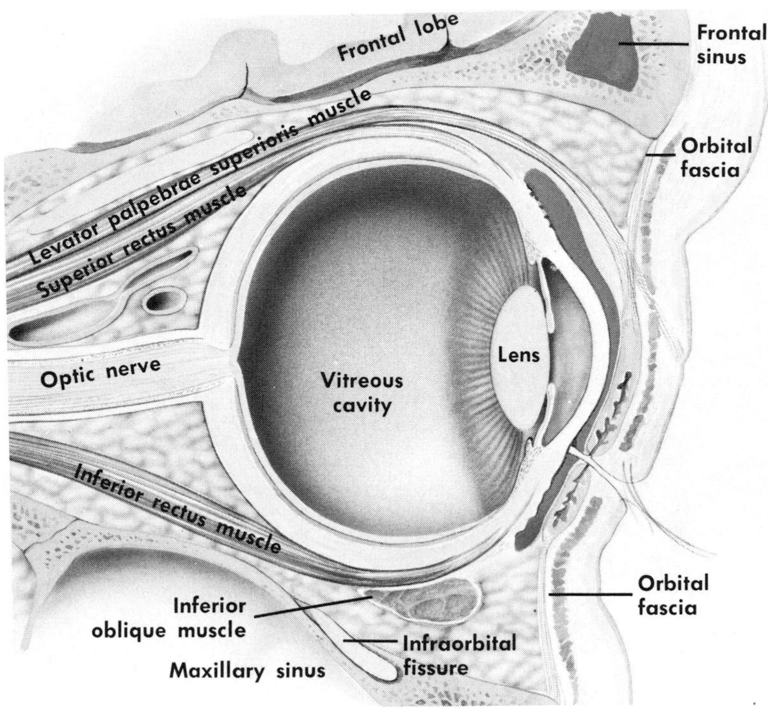

FIG 1-34.
Sagittal section of the orbit. The infraorbital fissure is the weakest area of the orbit and may incarcerate the inferior rectus muscle in fractures (blowout) of the floor of the orbit.

palatine bone extends medially. Posteriorly, the infraorbital sulcus (Fig 1-34) extends across the floor of the orbit from the infraorbital fissure. It transmits the infraorbital artery and maxillary nerve (N V_2). At about the midpoint of the orbit, the sulcus becomes a canal that opens on the face, the infraorbital foramen, and transmits the infraorbital artery and nerve.

OPTIC FORAMEN AND ORBITAL FISSURE

The optic foramen, the opening of the optic canal into the orbit, is located at the posterior medial aspect of the orbit. The optic canal measures 4 to 10 mm in length and is formed between the upper and lower processes of the small wing of the sphenoid bone. Through the canal passes the optic nerve en route to the brain, the ophthalmic artery that nurtures the orbital contents, the central retinal vein, and the sympathetic nerves from the carotid plexus.

Just lateral to the optic foramen is the superior orbital fissure that divides the greater and lesser wings of the sphenoid bone. The fissure is divided into medial and lateral portions by a fibrous band of tissue, the annulus of Zinn (annulus tendineus communis), from which the recti muscles originate. Passing through the medial portion of the superior orbital fissure, within the annulus of Zinn, are the following: (1) the oculomotor nerve (N III); (2) the abducent nerve (N VI); (3) the nasociliary branch of the ophthalmic branch of the trigeminal nerve (N V_1); and (4) the sympathetic root of the ciliary ganglion. Passing superior and lateral to the annulus of Zinn are the following: (1) the lacrimal and frontal branches of the ophthalmic branch of the trigeminal nerve; (2) the trochlear nerve (N IV); and (3) the superior ophthalmic vein (Fig 1-35).

The inferior orbital fissure (sphenomaxillary) is formed at the junction of the orbital plate of the greater wing of the sphenoid bone and the lateral margin of the orbital process of the maxillary bone. It transmits the infraorbital nerve of the second (maxillary) branch of the trigeminal nerve and the infraorbital artery. Anastomoses between the inferior orbital vein and the pterygoid plexus occur through the inferior orbital fissure. The fissure is covered by the smooth muscle of Müller, which has a questionable function in humans. It is the analogue of the retractor bulbi of lower animals.

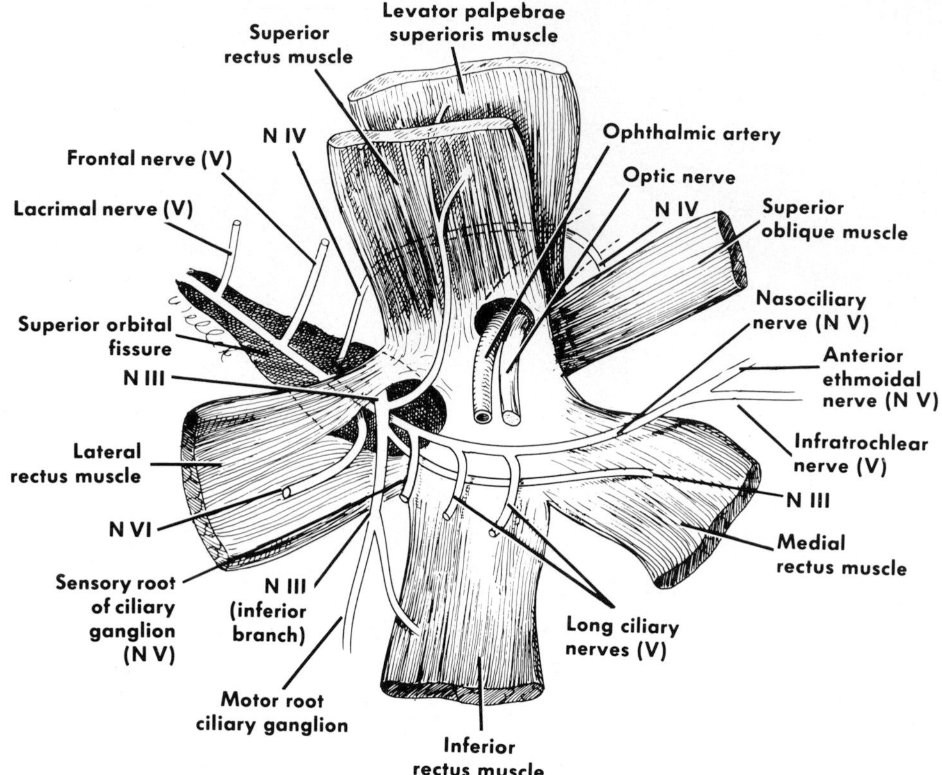

FIG 1-35.
Apex of the right orbit. The optic nerve, ophthalmic artery, and sympathetic nerves are transmitted through the optic foramen. The optic foramen and the medial portion of the superior orbital fissure are encircled by the annulus of Zinn. The lacrimal and frontal branches of the ophthalmic division of the fifth nerve and the trochlear nerve (N IV) enter the orbit in the lateral portion of the superior orbital fissure outside of the annulus. The other branches of the ophthalmic division of the fifth nerve and the oculomotor (N III) and abducent (N VI) nerves enter the orbit more medially within the annulus. The maxillary, or second, division of the trigeminal nerve enters the orbit through the inferior orbital fissure and emerges on the face at the intraorbital foramen. The lateral rectus muscle is divided into upper and lower origin by the annulus of Zinn as it bridges the superior orbital foramen. The superior oblique muscle is exceptional in receiving its motor nerve, the trochlear (N IV), on its orbital surface. All the other muscles are innervated on the side closest to the globe.

The dura mater of the meninges that surrounds the optic nerve in the optic foramen divides into two layers at the orbital apex. One portion lines the orbit as the periosteum; the other continues forward as the dural sheath of the optic nerve. The annulus of Zinn inserts medially into the cleft formed by this splitting; laterally, it is attached at the spina recti lateralis at the tip of the greater wing of the sphenoid. Each rectus muscle originates at the annulus of Zinn. The origin of the lateral rectus muscle is divided into an upper and a lower head by the superior orbital fissure.

ORBITAL FASCIA

The orbital contents are bound together and supported by connective tissues that divide the orbit into spaces of clinical importance in limiting the spread of hemorrhage and inflammation. The main orbital fasciae are (1) the periorbita (periosteum of the orbit); (2) the orbital septum (palpebral fascia); (3) the bulbar fascia (Tenon capsule); and (4) the muscular fascia.

The *periorbita (periosteum of the orbit)* is the periosteal lining of the orbit. It is derived from the dura mater, which splits at the optic foramen into two layers, one constituting the periosteum

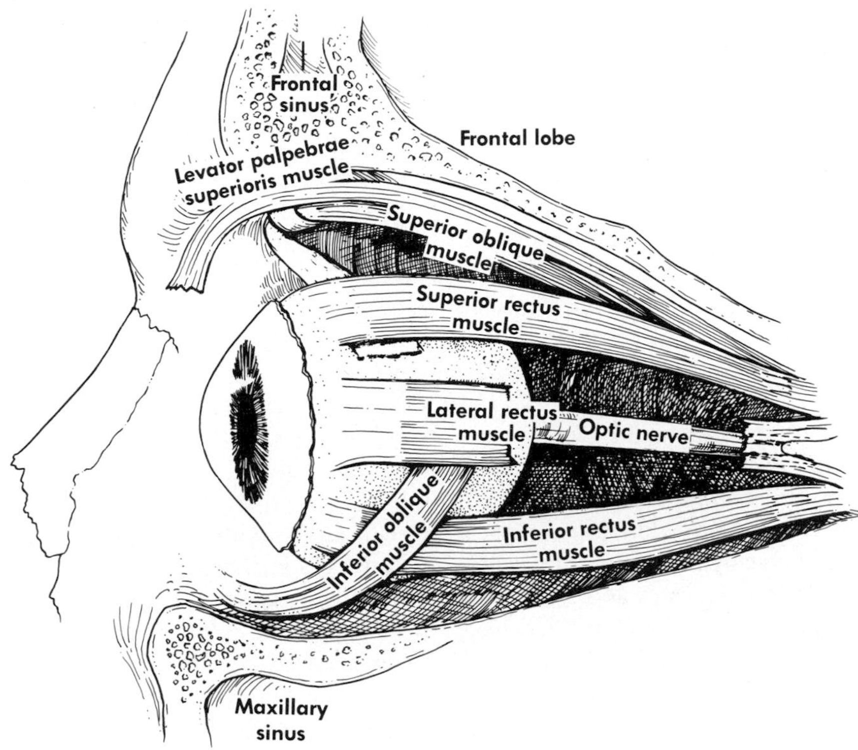

FIG 1-36.
Extrinsic muscles of the eye. Both oblique muscles insert behind the equator of the globe. The inferior oblique muscle passes inferior to the body of the inferior rectus muscle but beneath the lateral rectus muscle. The numbers indicate the distance of the insertion from the corneoscleral limbus and the length of the muscle tendon.

and the other continuing as the dural sheath of the optic nerve.

The *orbital septum (palpebral fascia)* extends from the bony margins of the orbit to the eyelid in close relationship with the posterior surface of the palpebral portion of the orbicularis oculi muscle. It divides the orbit into anterior and posterior portions. The septum prevents orbital fat from entering the eyelids and limits the spread of inflammation from the eyelid into the orbit.

The *bulbar fascia (Tenon capsule)* separates the globe from orbital fat and provides the socket in which the eye rotates. It extends anteriorly to the insertion of the conjunctiva at the corneoscleral limbus. Its lower portion is thickened to form a sling (the ligament of Lockwood), on which the globe rests. Posteriorly, the fascia is thin and perforated by the structures passing to or from the eye.

The *muscular fascia* surrounds the ocular muscles, particularly their anterior portions. The portion that covers the medial and lateral recti muscles sends expansions to the orbital margins as check ligaments. Other fibers extend to the conjunctiva and hold it taut in ocular rotation.

EXTRINSIC MUSCLES

The extrinsic muscles of the eye (Fig 1-36) are the four recti and the two oblique muscles. (The ciliary muscles and the sphincter pupillae and dilatator pupillae muscles are the intrinsic muscles.)

Origin

The four recti muscles originate at the apex of the orbit from the ligament of Zinn (annulus tendineus communis), which encircles the optic foramen and the medial portion of the superior orbital fissure (see Fig 1-35). The superior oblique muscle originates at the apex of the orbit from the periorbita of the lesser wing of the sphenoid bone medial to and above the optic foramen. The inferior oblique muscle originates on the floor of the orbit from the periorbita covering the anteromedial portion of the maxilla. The four recti muscles insert into the sclera anterior to the equator of the globe. The two oblique muscles insert into the sclera posterior to the equator.

The ocular muscles are the most highly differentiated of all striated muscles. On their outer surface are slow fibers that are capable of graded contracture. These fibers correspond to red muscle fibers and contain many mitochondria and a high content of oxidative enzymes. The fibers are innervated by grapelike motor nerve terminals. Centrally the muscles are composed of fast fibers responsible for rapid movements. These fibers correspond to white muscle fibers and contain more glycolytic enzymes and glycogen and less oxidative enzymes and mitochondria than do the slow fibers. The fast fibers have plaquelike motor nerve endings.

Recti muscles

The recti muscles are as follows: (1) the medial rectus muscle; (2) the lateral rectus muscle; (3) the superior rectus muscle; and (4) the inferior rectus muscle. They originate from the ligament of Zinn and pass forward in the orbit, gradually diverging to form the ocular muscle cone. Recti muscles are about 40 mm long and about 10 to 11.5 mm wide at their insertion into the sclera. By means of a tendon, the muscles insert into the sclera between 5.3 and 7.9 mm from the corneoscleral limbus (Fig 1-37).

Their main functions in rotating the eye are as follows: adduction; abduction; elevation; depression; incycloduction (rotation of the superior meridian of the eye medially); and excycloduction (rotation of the superior meridian of the eye laterally [Table 1-5]). The superior and inferior recti and oblique muscles do not form right angles with the superior sagittal diameter of the globe. Thus, their maximal action varies with the rotation of the eye.

The *medial rectus muscle* originates from the medial portion of the ligament of Zinn in close contact with the optic nerve. (Rotation of the eye in retrobulbar neuritis [see Chapter 20] is painful because of the close relationship of the superior and medial recti muscles with the optic nerve.) It is innervated by the inferior division of

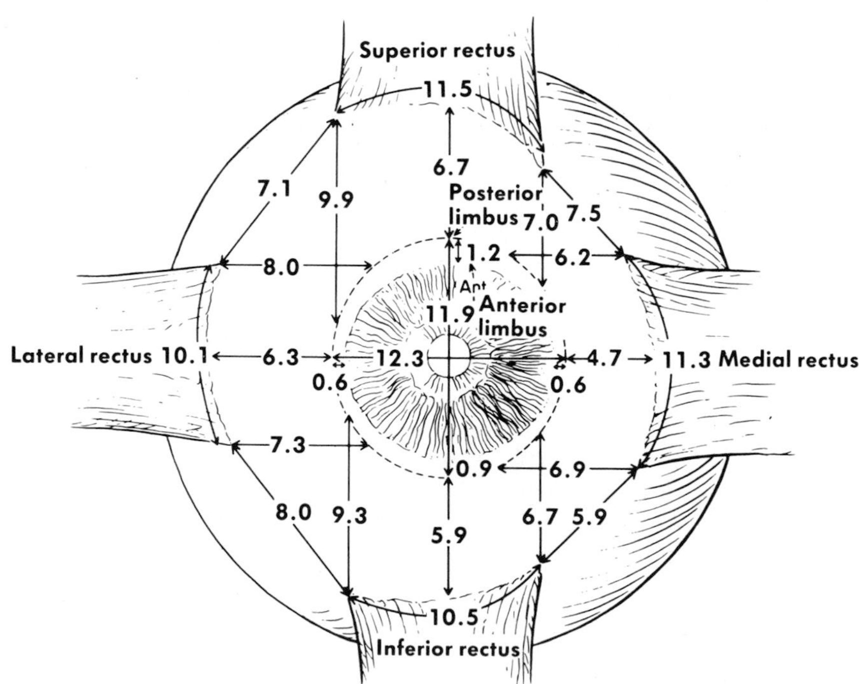

FIG 1-37.
Insertion of rectus muscles into the sclera. (*From Apt L: An anatomic reevaluation of rectus muscle insertions,* Trans Am Ophthalmol Soc *78:365, 1980. Used by permission.*)

the oculomotor nerve (N III), which enters the muscle on its bulbar surface. Medial rotation (adduction) of the globe is its only action.

The *lateral rectus muscle* originates from two heads from the lateral aspect of the upper and lower portions of the ligament of Zinn, where the ligament bridges the superior orbital fissure. It passes forward, over the insertion of the inferior oblique muscle, to insert into the sclera. It is innervated by the abducent nerve (N VI), which enters on its bulbar surface at about the middle. Lateral rotation (abduction) of the globe is its only action.

The *superior rectus muscle* originates from the superior portion of the ligament of Zinn in close contact with the meningeal sheaths surrounding the optic nerve. The muscle passes forward and laterally from the ligament and forms an angle of 23° with the sagittal diameter of the globe. Superiorly, it is beneath the levator palpebrae superioris muscle throughout its course. The superior rectus muscle is innervated by the superior division of the oculomotor nerve, which enters its bulbar surface at the junction of the anterior one third with the posterior two thirds.

The main function of the superior rectus muscle is upward rotation of the eye, an action that becomes maximal in abduction and decreases in adduction. The muscle rotates the superior meridian of the cornea inward (incycloduction). When the eye rotates medially, the superior rectus muscle aids in adduction.

The *inferior rectus muscle* originates from the inferior portion of the ligament of Zinn and passes forward and laterally, forming an angle of 23° (as does the superior rectus muscle) with the sagittal diameter of the globe. It is innervated by the terminal branch of the inferior division of the oculomotor nerve, which enters on its superior (bulbar) side at the junction of its anterior one third with the posterior two thirds.

The main function of the inferior rectus muscle is downward rotation of the eye, an action that becomes maximal in abduction and decreases in adduction. The muscle rotates the superior meridian of the cornea outward (excycloduction). When the eye rotates medially, the inferior rectus muscle aids in adduction. Through fibrous tarsal and subconjunctival attachments, it also acts as a retractor of the lower eyelid.

Oblique muscles

There are two oblique muscles: the superior oblique and the inferior oblique.

The *superior oblique muscle* originates from the periosteal covering of the lesser wing of the sphenoid bone above and medial to the optic foramen. It consists of two parts: (1) a direct muscular portion that extends from its origin to the trochlea; and (2) a reflected portion, composed entirely of tendon, that extends from the trochlea beneath the superior rectus muscle to its insertion at the globe.

The direct muscular portion passes forward in the angle between the roof and the medial wall of the orbit to the trochlea. The trochlea is a synovial-lined fibrous tissue sling attached to the trochlear spine of the medial aspect of the frontal bone a few millimeters behind the superior orbital margin. The tendon of the superior oblique muscle begins about 10 mm behind the trochlea. From the trochlea the tendon passes downward, laterally, and posteriorly beneath the superior rectus muscle to be inserted on the

TABLE 1-5.
Actions of the Extraocular Muscles

Muscle	Primary Function	Secondary Function	Tertiary Function
Medial rectus	Adduction (in)		
Lateral rectus	Abduction (out)		
Superior rectus	Elevation	Incycloduction	Adduction
Inferior rectus	Depression	Excycloduction	Adduction
Superior oblique	Incycloduction	Depression	Abduction
Inferior oblique	Excycloduction	Elevation	Abduction

The vertical recti muscles are adductors.
The oblique muscles are abductors.
The superior muscles are incycloductors.
The inferior muscles are excycloductors.

upper outer quadrant of the eye posterior to the equator. The tendon is a fibrous cord, about 1 by 2 mm in size, that becomes flatter and wider as it approaches the medial margin of the superior rectus muscle.

The superior oblique muscle is innervated by the trochlear nerve (N IV). The nerve enters the orbit through the lateral portion of the superior orbital fissure, outside the annulus of Zinn. It enters the muscle on its orbital surface, the only extraocular muscle that does not receive its innervation on the bulbar surface.

The main function of the superior oblique muscle is rotation of the superior meridian of the cornea inward (incycloduction). When the eye is rotated medially, the superior oblique muscle rotates the eye downward. In the straight-ahead position, the muscle aids in abduction.

The *inferior oblique muscle* originates at the periosteum covering the orbital plate of the maxilla a few millimeters behind the orbital margin and near the orifice of the nasolacrimal duct. It passes laterally and posteriorly between the inferior rectus muscle and the floor of the orbit in a tunnel in the fascia that envelops the inferior rectus muscle. It then curves upward around the globe to insert into the posterior sclera on the inferior lateral surface of the globe. The muscle fibers have a broad insertion into the sclera. The muscle has no tendon. It is innervated by the inferior division of the oculomotor nerve (N III), which enters its bulbar surface just after the muscle has passed to the lateral side of the inferior rectus muscle.

The main function of the inferior oblique muscle is rotation of the superior meridian of the cornea outward (excycloduction). When the eye is rotated medially, the inferior oblique muscle rotates the eye upward. In the straight-ahead position, the muscle aids in abduction.

EYELIDS

The eyelids (Fig 1-38) are thin curtains of skin, muscle, fibrous tissue, and mucous membrane that protect the eye from external irritation, interrupt and limit the amount of light entering the eye, and distribute tears over the surface of the globe. The upper eyelid is limited above by the eyebrow; the lower eyelid merges with the cheek. Each eyelid is divided by a horizontal furrow (sulcus) into an orbital and a tarsal portion. The upper eyelid furrow is formed by the insertions of the levator palpebrae superioris muscle into the skin of the eyelid at the level of the attached border of the tarsus. The lower eyelid furrow is poorly defined and is

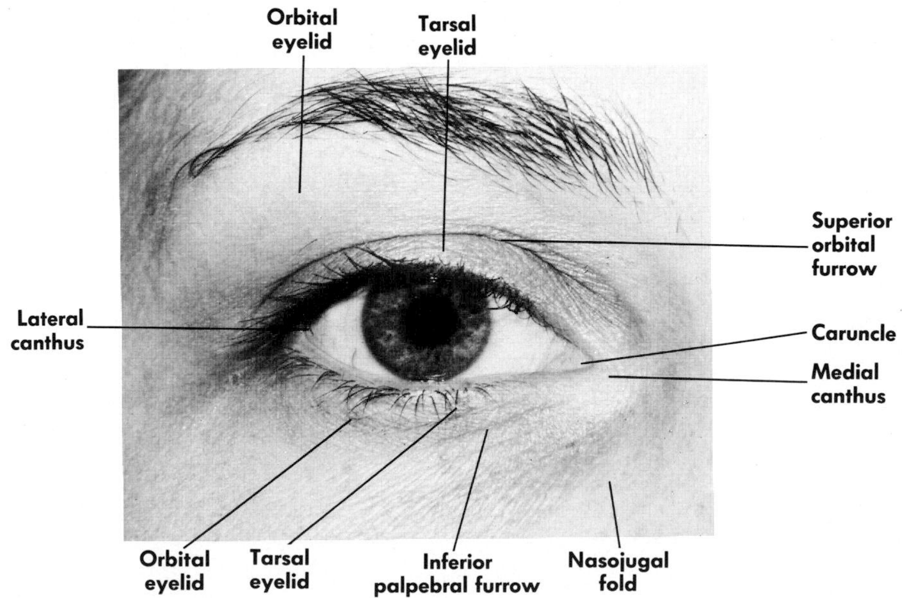

FIG 1-38.
The eyelids and the palpebral sulcus. The superior and inferior palpebral sulci (furrows) divide the eyelids into tarsal and orbital portions.

formed by a few cutaneous connections from the orbicularis oculi muscle. The corneoscleral limbus is covered above and below by the eyelids.

When open, the eyelids form an elliptic opening, the palpebral fissure, which measures about 12 × 30 mm. Laterally the fissure forms a 60° angle; medially it is rounded. The lateral margin (canthus) is about 2 mm higher than the medial margin except in Asians, in whom it may be 5 mm higher. The fissure is widest at the junction of the inner one third with the outer two thirds. In Asians the fissure is highest in its middle, and the medial margin may be obscured by a characteristic vertical fold of skin (epicanthus). When present in infants, an epicanthus may cause the eyes to appear to be deviated inward (pseudostrabismus). The skin fold disappears with the growth of the face.

The margin of each eyelid is 2 mm thick and 30 mm long. Five millimeters from the medial angle of each eyelid is a small eminence, the papilla lacrimalis. In each is the lacrimal punctum, the minute external opening of the superior or inferior lacrimal canaliculus (Fig 1-39). The medial one sixth of the eyelid, or the lacrimal portion, has no cilia or gland openings, and the margins of the eyelid are rounded. The lateral five sixths of the eyelid margin, the ciliary portion, have squared edges.

The intramarginal sulcus, or gray line, of the margin of the eyelid divides the eyelid into an anterior leaf containing muscle and skin and a posterior leaf containing tarsus and conjunctiva. The eyelashes originate anterior to the gray line, and the orifices of the tarsal glands open posterior to it. The junction of the conjunctiva and the stratified epithelium of the skin is at the level of the orifices of the tarsal glands.

The eyelashes (cilia) on the upper eyelid margin curve upward and are more numerous than those on the lower eyelid margin, which curve downward. Opening into the follicle of each cilium are the ducts of the sebaceous glands of Zeis. Large sweat glands (of Moll) open either into these follicles or directly onto the eyelid margin between the cilia.

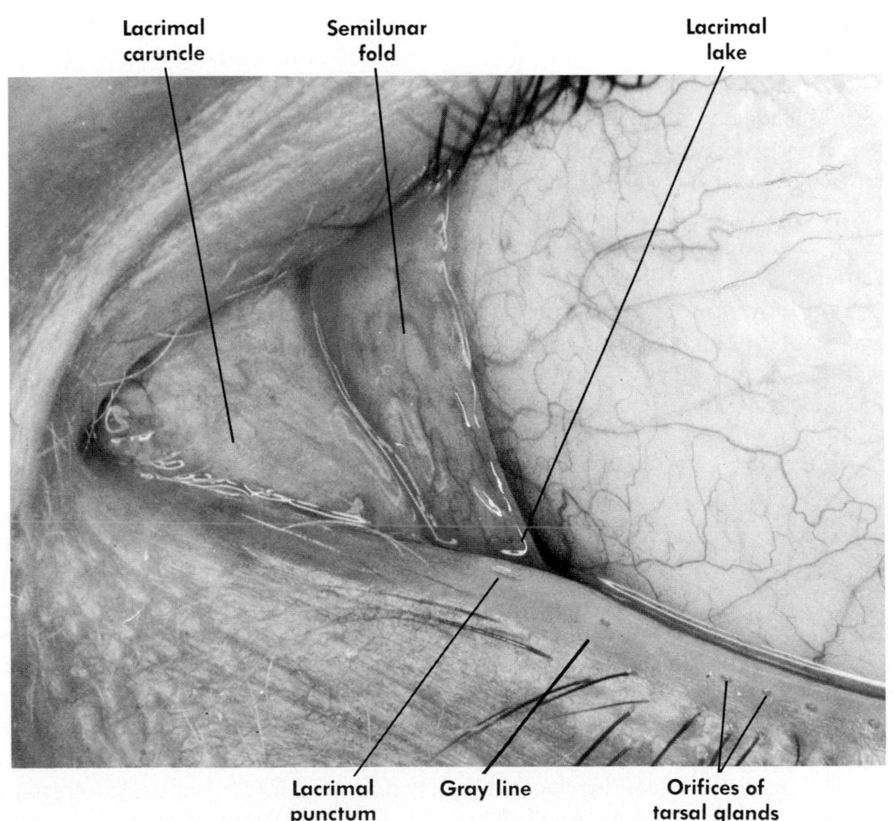

FIG 1-39.
Lacrimal portion of the eyelid margin.

Structure

The eyelids contain the following parts (Fig 1-40):

- Skin
- Muscles
  - Orbicularis oculi (N VII)
  - Eyelid retractors
    - Levator palpebrae superioris muscle (N III)
    - Superior tarsal muscle (sympathetic)
    - Inferior rectus muscle (N III)
    - Inferior tarsal muscle (sympathetic)
- Fibrous tissue
  - Septum orbitale (palpebral fascia)
  - Tarsal plates
- Conjunctiva

The skin of the eyelids is the thinnest in the body. There is no fat in the subcutaneous areolar area, and the skin is thrown into numerous folds. It may be markedly distended by blood or fluid and, because of its thinness, underlying blood vessels may appear as dark blue channels.

The orbicularis oculi muscle (N VII), the sphincter of the eyelids, is a thin oval sheet of striated muscle composed of concentric muscle fibers that surround the palpebral fissure. It is divided into a peripheral orbital portion, which functions in forcible closure of the eyelids and a central palpebral portion that functions in involuntary blinking. The orbital part of the muscle originates from the medial margin of the orbit and the anterior surface of the medial palpebral (canthal) ligament. It inserts into the periorbita of the superior and inferior orbital margin and into the lateral palpebral (canthal) ligament.

The palpebral part of the orbicularis oculi muscle is divided into a preseptal portion overlying the orbital septum and a pretarsal part overlying the upper and lower tarsal plates. The upper and lower preseptal portions have deep heads that originate in the region of the posterior lacrimal crest and superficial origins from the medial palpebral ligament. The preseptal portions of the orbicularis oculi muscle pass laterally anterior to the orbital septum and join to form the lateral palpebral raphe that inserts into the fascia investing the orbital margin of the zygomatic bone. The upper and lower pretarsal muscles originate from the posterior lacrimal crest and from the medial canthal ligament that inserts into the anterior lacrimal crest. They sweep laterally to insert into the lateral canthal ligament that inserts into the lateral orbital tubercle. The fibers at the medial canthus surround the lacrimal puncta and with each blink create suction in the lacrimal sac.

The facial nerve (N VII), the motor innervation of the orbicularis oculi muscle, emerges from the skull through the stylomastoid foramen, turns forward on the base of the styloid process, and enters the parotid gland, where it divides into temporofacial and cervicofacial divisions. The temporofacial division gives off temporal and zygomatic (malar) branches. The temporal branch joins with the zygomaticotemporal (orbital) branch of the maxillary nerve (N V_2) to innervate the orbicularis oculi, frontalis, and supercilii muscles. The zygomatic branch joins the lacrimal branch of the ophthalmic nerve (N V_1) to innervate the orbicularis oculi and zygomaticus muscles.

The orbital septum separates the eyelids from the contents of the orbit. In the upper eyelid it fuses with the aponeurosis of the levator palpebrae superioris muscle slightly above the upper level of the tarsus. It attaches laterally to the lateral canthal ligament and to the periorbita overlying the orbital tubercle. Nasally the orbital septum attaches to the posterior lacrimal crest. In the lower eyelid the orbital septum attaches to the lateral reticulum along the entire width of the lower border of the tarsus and to the posterior lacrimal crest.

The levator palpebrae superioris muscle (N III) is closely related to the superior rectus muscle in its origin and its course. It originates from the periosteal covering of the lesser wing of the sphenoid bone. Its origin blends with that of the superior rectus muscle below and the superior oblique muscle medially. It runs forward beneath the roof of the orbit to a point about 10 mm behind the septum orbitale, where it expands into an aponeurosis, which passes through the orbital septum. The aponeurosis inserts into the skin of the eyelid to form the superior palpebral furrow, into the anterior surface of the tarsal plate, and into the medial and lateral palpebral ligaments. The nerve supply is from the superior division of the oculomotor nerve (N III), which passes through the underlying superior rectus muscle to reach the inferior surface of the levator muscle.

The capsulopalpebral fascia in the lower eye-

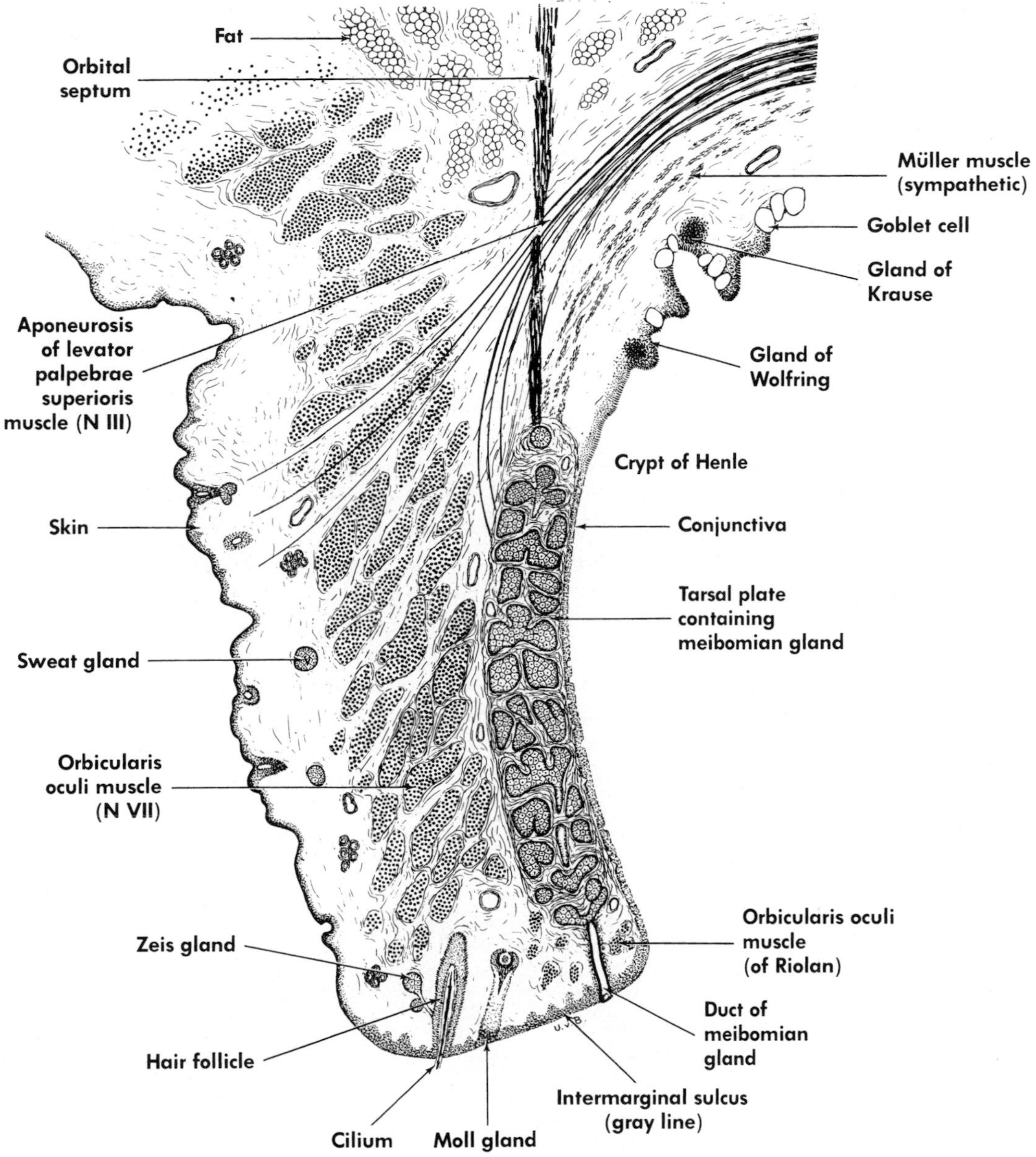

FIG 1-40.
The eyelid in cross section. The orbital septum separates the intraorbital contents from the eyelid. The intermarginal sulcus provides a line of surgical dissection separating the anterior structures of the eyelid from the tarsus and tarsal conjunctiva.

lid corresponds to the aponeurosis of the levator palpebrae superioris muscle in the upper eyelid. It extends between the fascia of the inferior oblique and inferior rectus muscles, Tenon capsule, the inferior transverse ligament (of Lockwood), and the inferior border of the lower tarsus. The connection with the tarsus makes this fascia the principal retractor of the lower eyelid.

The inferior tarsal muscle originates from the inferior rectus muscle sheath, where it surrounds the inferior oblique muscle. It courses upward and forward and inserts into the bulbar conjunctiva and to the expansion of the fascia of the inferior rectus muscle that inserts into the tarsus. Its fibers are continuous over the lateral orbital rim.

The superior and inferior palpebral smooth muscles of Müller (sympathetics) are small sheets of smooth muscle located immediately beneath the orbital portion of the palpebral conjunctiva. The superior palpebral muscle originates from the undersurface of the levator palpebrae superioris muscle. The sympathetic innervation of these smooth muscles is distributed with the branches of the ophthalmic artery to the eyelid.

The fibrous tissue of the eyelids consists of a peripheral layer, the palpebral fascia or septum orbitale, and a thickened central portion, the tarsal plates.

The tarsal plates consist of firm connective tissue (not cartilage) that gives form and density to the free margin of the eyelids. Each tarsal plate is about 1 mm thick and 25 to 30 mm long. The upper tarsal plate is about 11 mm wide and the lower tarsal plate about 5 mm. The plates extend from the lacrimal puncta medially to the lateral canthus.

The free edge of the tarsal plate extends the length of the ciliary portion of the eyelid margin. The posterior surface of the tarsus is firmly attached to the tarsal conjunctiva and conforms to the curvature of the globe. The anterior surface of the tarsus is separated from the orbicularis oculi muscle by loose areolar tissue, so that the muscle moves freely over its surface. The attached margin of the tarsus gradually merges into the orbital septum. Medially and laterally, the tarsal plates attach to palpebral ligaments.

Each tarsus contains sebaceous (meibomian) glands, the ducts of which open onto the eyelid margin. These glands are arranged in a single row in the tarsal plate, and each consists of 10 to 15 acini placed irregularly around a central canal that opens onto the eyelid margin. The sebaceous secretion prevents the overflow of tears, makes possible an airtight closure of the eyelids, and provides the external layer of the precorneal tear film, which prevents the rapid evaporation of tears.

Blood supply.—The blood supply to the eyelids is derived from marginal and peripheral vascular arcades. These are formed by the lateral palpebral branches of the lacrimal artery and the medial palpebral branches of the dorsonasal artery, both of which are derived from the internal carotid artery through the ophthalmic artery. There is a wide anastomotic circulation provided by branches of the external carotid

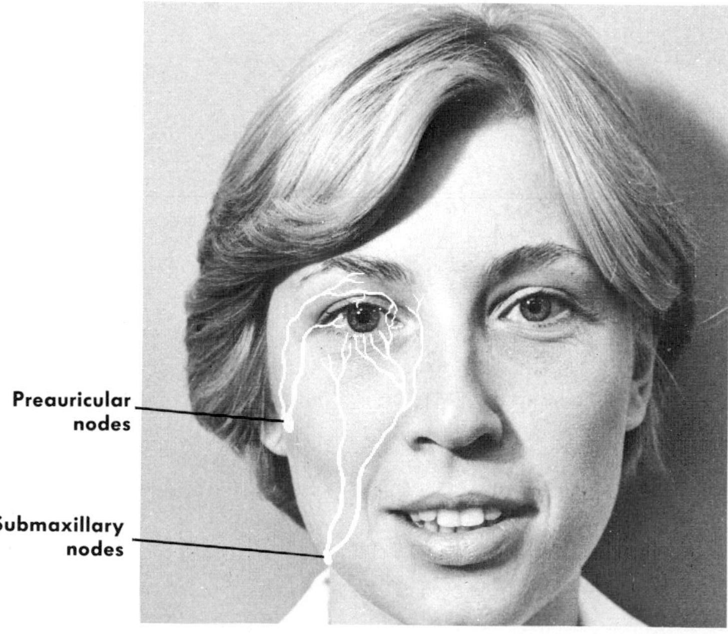

FIG 1-41.
Lymphatic drainage of the eyelids and conjunctiva. The orbit and the globe and its contents have no lymphatics.

artery through the facial, superficial temporal, and infraorbital arteries.

Nerve supply.—The ophthalmic (first) division of the trigeminal nerve (N V_1) provides the sensory innervation to the upper eyelid and to a small lateral portion of the lower eyelid. Innervation of the remaining medial portion of the lower eyelid is by the maxillary (second) division of the trigeminal nerve (N V_2) through branches of the infraorbital nerve. The facial nerve (N VII) innervates the orbicularis oculi muscle, and the oculomotor nerve (N III) supplies the levator palpebrae superioris muscle. Postganglionic sympathetic fibers from the superior cervical ganglion innervate the palpebral muscles of Müller. They enter the orbit with the ophthalmic artery and are distributed with the palpebral branches of the lacrimal artery and the palpebral branches of the dorsonasal artery.

Lymphatic supply.—The eyelids are drained by two groups (Fig 1-41) of lymphatic vessels: (1) a medial group drains the medial two thirds of the lower eyelid and the medial one third of the upper eyelid into the submaxillary lymph nodes; and (2) a lateral group drains the lateral one third of the lower eyelid and lateral two thirds of the upper eyelid into the preauricular lymph nodes.

THE CONJUNCTIVA

The conjunctiva is a thin, translucent mucous membrane (Fig 1-42) that lines the inner surface of the eyelids and covers the anterior portion of the sclera. Its epithelium is continuous with that of the cornea and with the lacrimal drainage system through the puncta. The conjunctiva is divided into three regions: (1) the palpebral conjunctiva; (2) the superior and inferior fornices; and (3) the bulbar conjunctiva.

The *palpebral conjunctiva* is divided into marginal tarsal and orbital portions. The tarsal portion is closely adherent to the tarsal plate, from which it can be removed only with difficulty. The orbital portion is thrown into many folds.

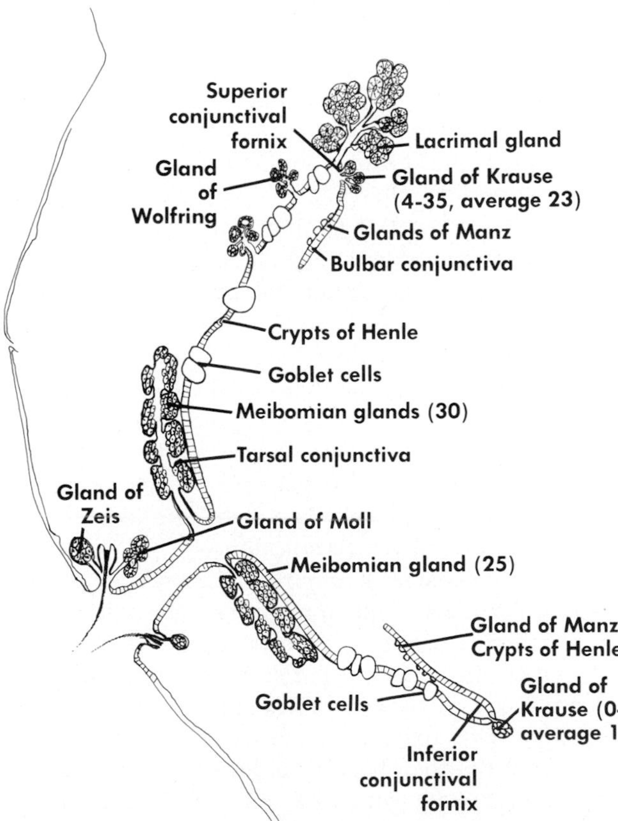

FIG 1-42.
Sagittal section of the eyelids to show the glandular structures of the conjunctiva. Mucin, the wetting agent of the precorneal tear film, is mainly secreted by goblet cells, with minor amounts secreted by the glands of Wolfring and Manz. The lacrimal gland and the glands of Krause secrete the aqueous portion of tears. The meibomian glands secrete the oily exterior layer of the tear film.

The *conjunctiva of the superior and inferior fornices* forms transitional areas between the palpebral and bulbar conjunctivae. It is but loosely attached to the underlying tissue and may become markedly swollen.

The *bulbar conjunctiva* is adjacent to the sclera, which can be seen as the "white" of the eye through the translucent conjunctival tissue.

At the medial angle of each eye are two specialized structures formed in part by the conjunctiva: the semilunar fold and the lacrimal caruncle. The semilunar fold (plica semilunaris) consists of a delicate vertical crescent of conjunctiva, the free edge of which is concave and concentric with the corneal margin. It is separated from the bulbar conjunctiva by a 2-mm-deep cul-de-sac. The lacrimal caruncle is a minute piece of modified skin located medial to the semilunar fold. It is covered by stratified epithelium that is not keratinized. It contains large sebaceous glands similar to meibomian glands and has delicate hairs with sebaceous glands similar to the glands of Zeis. The caruncle is conspicuous when the eye is rotated laterally.

Structure

Similar to other mucous membranes, the conjunctiva is composed of two layers: (1) stratified columnar epithelium and (2) lamina propria composed of an adenoid and a fibrous layer.

The *stratified epithelium* varies in thickness from two cell layers in its upper tarsal portion to five to seven layers at the corneoscleral junction. It is never keratinized in healthy individuals. After 3 months of age, the development of the adenoid tissue makes the conjunctival surface moderately irregular.

The *lamina propria* is composed of connective tissue that contains blood vessels, nerves, glands, mast cells, macrophages, and polymorphonuclear leukocytes. The bulbar conjunctiva and the orbital portion of the palpebral conjunctiva contain adenoid tissue with many lymphocytes enmeshed in a fine reticular network. True lymphatic follicles are not present except in childhood and in response to inflammation (follicular conjunctivitis). The *fibrous layer* of the conjunctiva is continuous with the inner margins of the tarsal plates and contains the smooth palpebral muscles of Müller (sympathetic nervous system).

Glands

The conjunctival epithelium contains many glands (see Fig 1-42) responsible for maintaining moisture and secreting the constituents of the precorneal tear film. Unlike the corneal epithelium, the conjunctival epithelium contains numerous unicellular mucous glands (goblet cells) that secrete mucin, the wetting agent of the precorneal tear film. The glands are most numerous in the conjunctival fornices, occur less frequently in the bulbar conjunctiva, and are absent at the eyelid margins and corneoscleral limbus.

The accessory lacrimal glands of Krause are located deep in the substantia propria, particularly in the fornices. They have the histologic structure and secretion of the lacrimal gland proper. Most are located in the temporal one third of the conjunctiva. The glands of Wolfring and Manz are less common and secrete a mucinous substance similar to that produced by goblet cells. The conjunctiva has a papillary pattern, the crypts of Henle, above and below the tarsal plates.

The blood supply of the palpebral conjunctiva is from the peripheral and marginal arterial arcades of the eyelid. The marginal arcade nurtures the margins of the eyelids and part of the tarsal area of the palpebral conjunctiva. The bulbar and fornix conjunctiva is nourished by the peripheral arcade.

The posterior conjunctival branches of the peripheral arterial arcade provide the blood supply of the peripheral bulbar conjunctiva. These vessels are superficial and nearly invisible, and extend to within 4 mm of the corneoscleral limbus. In the area adjacent to the corneoscleral limbus, the anterior conjunctival branches of the seven anterior ciliary arteries divide to form a superficial (conjunctival) and a deep (episcleral) pericorneal plexus. The anterior and posterior conjunctival vessels anastomose.

The posterior conjunctival vessels are dilated when there is inflammation of the bulbar conjunctiva. Because of their superficial position, they appear bright red and move with the conjunctiva. They are most evident in the fornices and fade toward the corneoscleral limbus. Because of their superficial location, they may be constricted with the topical instillation of 1 : 1,000 epinephrine.

The superficial (conjunctival) pericorneal

plexus, which is derived from the anterior ciliary arteries, is injected in inflammations of the cornea (ciliary injection). The deep (episcleral) pericorneal plexus is injected in inflammations of the iris and the ciliary body and in closed-angle glaucoma. Because of their deep position, these vessels appear dull red to purple and do not move with the conjunctiva. They are not constricted by topical epinephrine. These vessels are most evident near the corneoscleral limbus and fade toward the fornices. Because of the generous anastomoses between the anterior and posterior conjunctival arteries, severe inflammations always cause injection of both ciliary and conjunctival vessels.

Nerve supply

The bulbar conjunctiva is innervated by sympathetic nerves that accompany blood vessels and sensory nerves. Sensory innervation of the superior palpebral conjunctiva is from the frontal nerve medially and lacrimal nerve laterally. Sensory innervation of the inferior palpebral conjunctiva is from the lateral palpebral branch of the lacrimal nerve laterally (ophthalmic division; N V_1) and the infraorbital nerve (maxillary division; N V_2) medially. The sensory innervation of the conjunctiva in the region of the corneoscleral limbus is by branches of the long ciliary nerves.

LACRIMAL APPARATUS

The lacrimal apparatus consists of a secretory and a collecting portion. The secretory portion is composed of the lacrimal gland. The collecting portion consists of the canaliculi with their orifices (the puncta), the lacrimal sac, and the lacrimal duct, which has its opening in the inferior nasal meatus. (Note that, in addition to originating in the lacrimal gland, tears are derived from glands in the margin of the eyelids and accessory lacrimal glands in the conjunctiva.)

Secretory portion

Lacrimal gland.—The lacrimal gland is located in the anterior lateral portion of the roof of the orbit in the lacrimal fossa. It is divided into a large orbital portion and a small palpebral portion by the lateral part of the aponeurosis of the levator palpebrae superioris muscle. The lacrimal gland is of the tubuloalveolar type and has numerous acini composed of a double layer of cells surrounding a central canal. The canals open into the larger ducts that in turn open into excretory ducts. Three to five ducts drain the orbital portion of the gland, and five to seven ducts drain the palpebral portion. The ducts of the orbital portion pass through the palpebral lobe, and each of the ducts opens separately into the superior temporal conjunctival fornix.

The secretory innervation to the lacrimal gland begins in the lacrimal (salivatory) nucleus of the facial nerve (N VII) on the floor of the fourth ventricle and extends with the facial nerve to the geniculate ganglion. The lacrimal fibers do not synapse here but leave the facial pathway by way of the greater superficial petrosal nerve to synapse in the sphenopalatine (Meckel) ganglion. From here, postganglionic fibers are distributed to the lacrimal gland, passing either directly or with the zygomaticotemporal branch of the maxillary branch of the trigeminal nerve (N V). Postganglionic sympathetic fibers from the superior cervical ganglion pass by way of the deep petrosal nerve to the sphenopalatine ganglion, where they are distributed with fibers destined for the lacrimal gland. The sympathetic innervation is mainly to blood vessels of the gland and has no direct effect on secretion.

Collecting portion

The collecting portion of the lacrimal apparatus (Fig 1-43) is composed of the puncta, the canaliculi, the lacrimal sac, and the nasolacrimal duct.

Puncta.—The puncta are slightly elevated, round or slightly oval openings about 2 mm in size, located on the upper and lower eyelid margins about 6 mm from the medial canthus. The openings are surrounded by relatively dense, avascular connective tissue. The puncta openings of the lacrimal canaliculi are inverted into the lacrimal lake with closure of the eyelids. The surrounding orbicularis oculi muscle prevents their collapse.

Canaliculi.—The upper and lower canaliculi each consist of a vertical portion 2 to 3.5 mm in length and a horizontal portion directed medially for about 8 mm where the two join to form the common canaliculus. Each canaliculus is about 0.5 mm in diameter, lined by stratified squamous epithelium, and surrounded by elastic tissue.

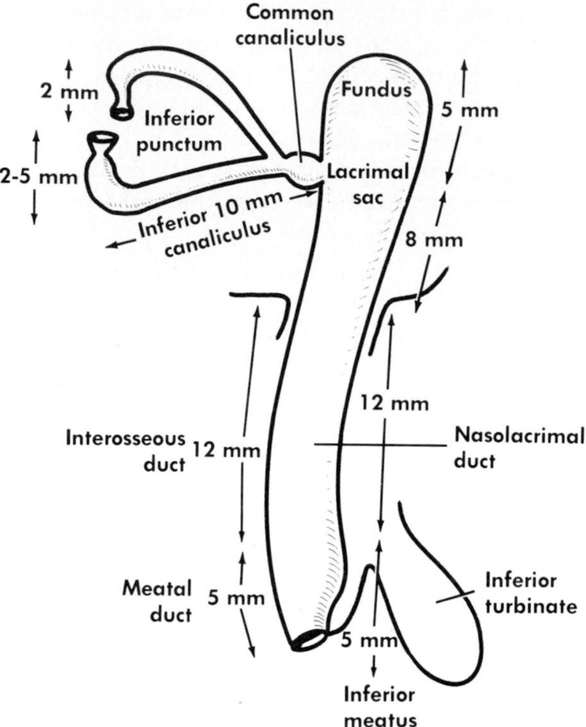

FIG 1-43.
The collecting portion of the lacrimal apparatus. Tears enter the canaliculi through the puncta and then pass through the lacrimal sac and nasolacrimal duct to the inferior nasal meatus.

Lacrimal sac.—The lacrimal sac is located in the medial portion of the orbit in the lacrimal fossa between leaves of medial palpebral ligament. The ligament attaches to the anterior lacrimal crest, and a portion is reflected to the posterior lacrimal crest. The fundus of the sac rises 3 to 5 mm above the palpebral ligament. Immediately posterior to the ligament the sac receives the canaliculi. Inferiorly the sac is continuous with the nasolacrimal duct.

Nasolacrimal duct.—The nasolacrimal duct is a downward extension of the sac and opens into the inferior nasal meatus. The duct is surrounded by the bone of the nasolacrimal canal, and it opens in the inferior nasal meatus at the anterior portion of the lateral wall. The duct may pass for several millimeters in the nasal mucous membrane before the opening. A variety of constrictions and folds in the sac and the nasolacrimal duct are described as "valves."

BLOOD SUPPLY

Arteries

The structures of the orbit usually receive their main blood supply from the ophthalmic artery. There are many variations, the most common being the substitution of the lacrimal artery for the ophthalmic artery. The eyelids and conjunctiva have a generous anastomotic supply from the branches of both the external carotid and the ophthalmic arteries.

Ophthalmic artery.—The ophthalmic artery is the first intracranial branch of the internal carotid artery and originates just as the artery exits from the cavernous sinus. The ophthalmic artery enters the orbit through the optic foramen below and lateral to the optic nerve, turns forward and upward, and passes over the optic nerve to its medial side. It ascends to the medial wall of the orbit, passes forward with the nasociliary nerve between the medial rectus and the superior oblique muscles, and terminates by dividing into dorsonasal and supratrochlear branches (Fig 1-44).

The majority of branches of the ophthalmic artery are given off while the vessel is lateral to the optic nerve. These branches include the following arteries (Table 1-6).

1. The *central retinal artery* sends nutrient vessels to the optic nerve. It divides into superior and inferior branches (papillary), which in turn divide into nasal and tem-

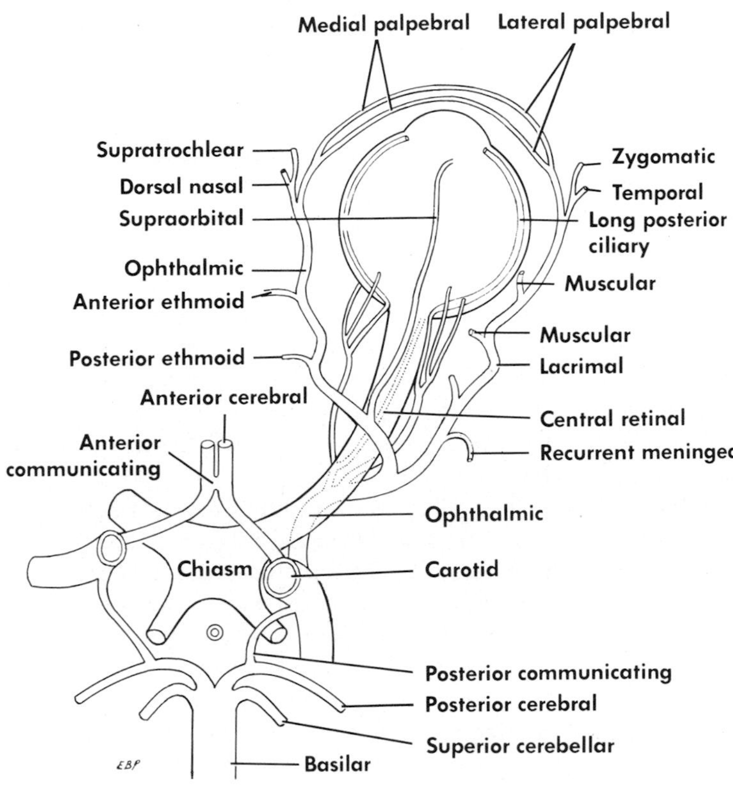

FIG 1-44.
Arteries that supply blood to the orbit and the ocular adnexa. There are many variations.

TABLE 1-6.
The Ophthalmic Artery

- I. Ophthalmic artery
  - A. Central retinal artery (1)
    - 1. Superior and inferior papillary arteries (2)
      - a. Temporal and nasal retinal arteries (4)
  - B. Supraorbital artery (1)
    - 1. Anastomoses with superficial temporal and superficial trochlear arteries
  - C. Medial and lateral ciliary arteries (2)
    - 1. Medial and lateral long ciliary arteries (2)
      - a. Posterior ciliary arteries (6-20)
  - D. Lacrimal artery (1)
    - 1. Recurrent meningeal artery (anastomosis with middle meningeal branch of maxillary artery)
    - 2. Superior and inferior muscular arteries
      - a. Anterior ciliary arteries (7)
        - (1) Circulus arteriosus iridis
    - 3. Tarsal and peripheral palpebral arcades
  - E. Anterior and posterior ethmoidal arteries
  - F. Superior and inferior palpebral arteries
  - G. Dorsonasal artery
    - 1. Anastomosis with angular artery
      - a. Inferior palpebral arcade
  - F. Supratrochlear artery

poral branches that provide blood to the inner layers of the retina.

2. The *medial and lateral ciliary arteries* enter the globe on either side of the optic nerve and pass forward in the suprachoroidal space as the long ciliary arteries to the ciliary body. Here they anastomose with the anterior ciliary arteries to form the circulus arteriosus iridis major. Before penetrating the globe, they give off 6 to 20 posterior ciliary arteries that enter the globe to be distributed to the choroid and optic disk.
3. The *lacrimal artery and its branches* provide much of the blood supply to orbital structures other than the eye itself. Its recurrent meningeal branch passes into the cranial cavity through the superior orbital fissure. It anastomoses with the middle meningeal branch of the maxillary artery, which is the terminal branch of the external carotid artery. There is often a superior and inferior muscular branch together with a branch to the lateral rectus muscle. The superior branch is distributed to the superior rectus, superior

oblique, and levator palpebrae superioris muscles. The inferior branch is distributed to the inferior oblique, the medial rectus, and the inferior rectus muscles.

The arterial branches to the recti muscles provide the anterior ciliary arteries. Each rectus muscle has two muscular arteries, except the lateral muscle, which has one. The anterior ciliary vesicles extend to the corneoscleral limbus as the anterior conjunctival arteries and form the pericorneal arcade. The anterior conjunctival arteries anastomose with the posterior conjunctival arteries derived from the palpebral arcade. About 4 mm from the corneoscleral limbus, branches of the anterior ciliary arteries penetrate the sclera to contribute, together with long posterior ciliary arteries, to the circulus arteriosus iridis major to provide blood vessels to the ciliary processes.

The lacrimal artery terminates in temporal and zygomatic branches that anastomose with the anterior deep temporal and transverse facial arteries. These form lateral palpebral branches that anastomose with medial palpebral arterial arcades of the eyelid. Branches of the peripheral arterial arcade are distributed to the conjunctiva as the posterior conjunctival arteries.

4. The supraorbital artery originates from the ophthalmic artery where it is superior to the optic nerve. It extends anteriorly to anastomose with the superficial temporal and superficial trochlear arteries in the scalp.
5. As the ophthalmic artery courses medial to the optic nerve it gives off the anterior and posterior ethmoidal arteries. Superior and inferior palpebral branches anastomose through the tarsal and peripheral palpebral arcades with the corresponding branches of the lacrimal artery. The ophthalmic artery terminates in two branches: (1) the dorsonasal artery, which is distributed to the skin of the nose and anastomoses with the angular artery, the terminal branch of the facial artery; and (2) the supratrochlear artery, which supplies the forehead and scalp.

External carotid artery.—The blood supply to the eye and eyelids from branches of the external carotid artery originates from (1) the external maxillary (facial) artery; (2) the superficial temporal artery; and (3) the internal maxillary artery.

The *external maxillary (facial) artery* has a number of branches to the face. Its terminal branch is the angular artery, which anastomoses at the medial canthus with the dorsonasal branch of the ophthalmic artery to provide blood for the inferior arterial arcades of the eyelids. It also anastomoses with the infraorbital artery, a branch of the maxillary artery.

The *superficial temporal artery* is a small terminal branch of the external carotid artery. The transverse facial artery, the largest branch of the superficial temporal artery, anastomoses with the infraorbital and angular arteries. The zygomatico-orbital artery anastomoses with the lacrimal artery and its palpebral branches to participate in the arterial arcade of the eyelids. The frontal artery anastomoses with the supraorbital and frontal branches of the ophthalmic artery and with the corresponding artery from the opposite side.

The *internal maxillary artery* is the larger of the terminal branches of the external carotid artery. Its largest branch is the middle meningeal artery, which supplies the bone and dura mater at the base of the skull. The internal maxillary artery sends an orbital branch through the superior orbital fissure that anastomoses with a recurrent branch of the ophthalmic artery. The infraorbital artery originates in the pterygopalatine (sphenomaxillary) fossa, enters the orbit through the infraorbital fissure, runs in the infraorbital sulcus and canal in the orbital plate of the maxilla, and passes forward to emerge on the face from the infraorbital foramen. The infraorbital branch anastomoses with the angular branch of the external maxillary (facial) artery, the transverse facial branch of the superficial temporal artery, and the lacrimal and dorsonasal branches of the ophthalmic artery.

Veins

Venous drainage of the orbit is mainly through the superior and inferior orbital veins. These are markedly tortuous, have no valves,

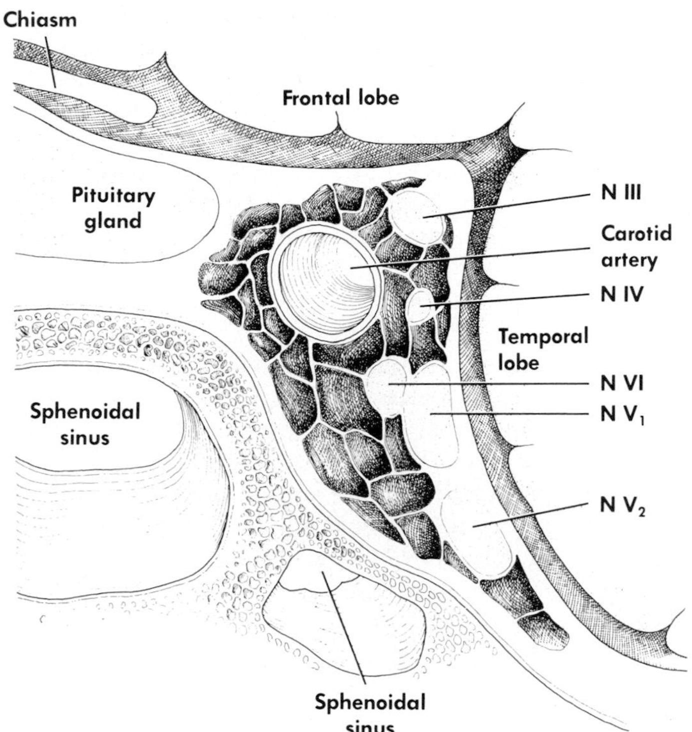

FIG 1-45.
Coronal section of the cavernous sinus posterior to the orbit. It is almost continuous with the superior orbital vein.

and pass through the superior orbital fissure to empty into the cavernous sinus. The superior orbital vein communicates with the angular vein, which is continuous with the facial vein. The two or more superior vortex veins empty into the superior orbital vein, and the two or more inferior vortex veins join the inferior orbital vein. The inferior ophthalmic vein communicates with the pterygoid plexus through the inferior orbital fissure and may either connect directly with the cavernous sinus or empty into the superior ophthalmic vein. The central retinal vein usually exits the optic nerve close to the entrance of the artery. It enters the cavernous sinus separately or empties into the superior ophthalmic vein.

The cavernous sinus (Fig 1-45) is an irregular-shaped, endothelium-lined venous space situated between the meningeal and periosteal layers of the dura mater on either side of the body of the sphenoid bone. It extends from the medial end of the superior orbital fissure to the apex of the petrous bone behind. Anteriorly it receives the superior orbital vein, with which it is almost continuous. Medially it communicates with the opposite sinus, and posteriorly, with the superior and inferior petrosal sinuses. The internal carotid artery passes through the cavernous sinus on its medial wall; the abducent nerve (N VI) is just lateral to the artery. The oculomotor nerve (N III) and trochlear nerve (N IV) are in its lateral wall on its superior aspect, whereas the ophthalmic and maxillary branches of the trigeminal nerve (N V) are located lateral to and below the artery. One or more of these nerves may be affected by inflammation of the cavernous sinus or an internal carotid artery fistula or aneurysm.

NERVES OF THE EYE

The eye and the orbital contents are richly innervated with motor nerves (oculomotor, N III; trochlear, N IV; abducent, N VI); mixed motor and sensory nerves (trigeminal, N V; and facial, N VII); autonomic nerves (parasympathetic, N III, N VII, and sympathetic); and visual nerves (optic, N II).

Motor nerves

The motor nerves innervate the ocular muscles and the levator palpebrae superioris muscle that elevates the eyelid (Table 1-7).

Oculomotor (third cranial) nerve.—The oculomotor nerve supplies the inferior oblique

TABLE 1-7.
Motor Nerves of the Eye

I. Oculomotor nerve (N III)
  A. Nuclei
    1. Superior medial cell group (nucleus Edinger-Westphal)
      a. Neurons in inferior branch N III synapse in ciliary ganglion and distributed with short ciliary nerves to sphincter pupillae and ciliary muscles.
    2. Inferior cell group
      a. Connected to nuclei N IV and N VI through medial longitudinal fasciculus. Sends neurons to extraocular muscles.
    3. Orbital branches
      a. Superior branch
        (1) Superior rectus muscle
        (2) Levator palpebrae muscle
      b. Inferior branch
        (1) Medial rectus muscle
        (2) Inferior oblique muscle branch
          (a) Short root ciliary ganglion: short ciliary nerves to sphincter pupillae and ciliary muscle
          (b) Inferior oblique muscle
        (3) Inferior rectus muscle
II. Trochlear nerve (N IV)
  A. Nucleus (in line with cells of N III)
  B. Nerve
    1. Within brain: totally decussates
    2. Within orbit
      a. To superior oblique muscle
III. Abducent nerve (N VI)
  A. Nucleus (in line with cells N III, N IV, and N XII)
    1. Fibers to nucleus N III in medial longitudinal fasciculus (not to N IV)
  B. Nerve (within orbit)
    1. Lateral rectus muscle

muscle; the superior, medial, and inferior recti muscles; and the levator palpebrae superioris muscle. Its visceral efferent fibers innervate the ciliary muscle and the sphincter pupillae muscle after synapse in the ciliary ganglion.

Nucleus.—The oculomotor nuclear complex (Fig 1-46) is a small (5 to 6 mm) collection of cells arranged medial to the diverging medial lateral fasciculi and beneath the aqueduct of Sylvius at the level of the superior colliculus. The trochlear nerve nucleus is continuous caudally with the nucleus of the oculomotor nerve. An unpaired mass of cells located caudally and centrally sends efferent fibers to the levator palpebrae superioris muscles. The motor cell pool of the superior rectus muscle sends efferent fibers to the contralateral superior rectus muscle. Paired lateral nuclei send efferent fibers to the ipsilateral medial and inferior recti muscles and the inferior oblique muscle. A pair of nuclei (Edinger-Westphal) located rostrally and ventrally sends preganglionic parasympathetic fibers to the ciliary ganglion, where they synapse and are then distributed to the ciliary muscle (accommodation) and the sphincter pupillae muscle (constriction).

The medial (posterior) longitudinal fasciculus connects motor cells of the oculomotor complex to each other, the nuclei of the trochlear and abducent cranial nerves, the supranuclear centers for gaze, the cerebellum, and the sensory nuclei of the trigeminal nerve (see Fig 23-3). This important fiber tract transmits stimuli that coordinate conjugate movements of the eyes

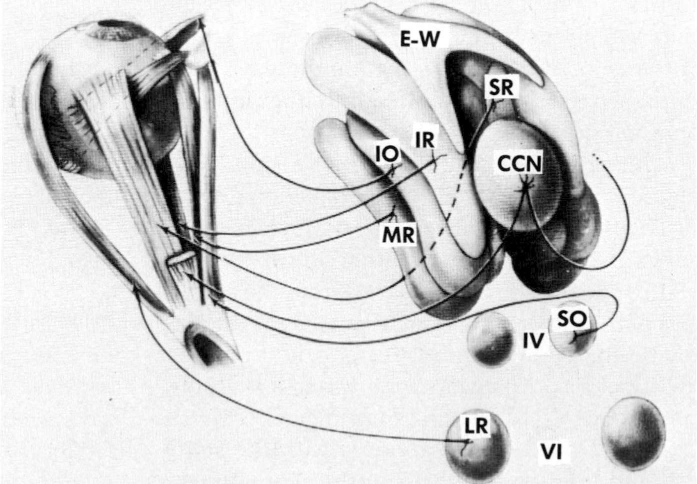

FIG 1-46.
Organization of the oculomotor nucleus viewed from above, left posterior. *E-W,* Edinger-Westphal parasympathetic subnucleus; *IR,* inferior rectus muscle nucleus; *IO,* inferior oblique muscle nucleus; *MR,* medial rectus muscle nucleus. The efferent fibers of superior rectus, *SR,* and superior oblique, *SO* (N IV), motor pools innervate muscles on the opposite side. *CCN,* the caudal nucleus, is distributed to the levator palpebrae superioris on both sides. *LR,* abducent nucleus (N VI) for lateral rectus muscle. (*From Glaser JS:* Neuro-ophthalmology, *ed 2, New York, 1990, Harper & Row. Used by permission.*)

(eyes right, eyes left, eyes up, or eyes down). Axons from the abducent nuclei decussate to the opposite medial fasciculus bundle and are distributed mainly to the medial rectus muscle nucleus. Thus, on the signal "eyes left," the left lateral rectus muscle contracts, as does the right medial rectus muscle. (A lesion in an abducent nucleus thus causes a failure to rotate both eyes to the right or to the left. A lesion in an abducent nerve affects only the lateral rectus muscle of that side.) Anterior lesions of the medial longitudinal fasciculus produce an internuclear ophthalmoplegia in which convergence is normal but, on attempts to turn the eyes laterally, the adducting eye does not pass beyond the midline and there is a coarse nystagmus of the abducting eye.

Intracerebral course.—From the third cranial nerve nuclei, efferent fibers run through the tegmentum, red nucleus, and substantia nigra and leave the midbrain in the interpeduncular fossa between the cerebral peduncles.

Intracranial course.—In their intracranial course, the oculomotor nerves are closely associated with the posterior cerebral arteries above and the superior cerebellar arteries below. From the midbrain, the oculomotor nerves pass forward, outward, and downward to pierce the dura mater and enter the roof and lateral wall of the cavernous sinus about midway between the anterior and posterior clinoid processes. In the cavernous sinus, each nerve is close to the trochlear nerve and ophthalmic division of the trigeminal nerve.

Orbital distribution.—Each oculomotor nerve leaves the cavernous sinus near the lesser wing of the sphenoid bone and enters the orbit through the superior orbital fissure. Here it divides into a small superior and larger inferior division. The superior division is distributed to the superior rectus muscle on its bulbar surface and passes through this muscle to terminate in the levator palpebrae superioris muscle. The inferior division is distributed to the medial and inferior recti muscles. Its terminal branch ends in the posterior border of the inferior oblique muscle. This terminal branch to the inferior oblique muscle sends the short or motor root branch, which carries preganglionic, parasympathetic nerve fibers, to the ciliary ganglion.

Ciliary ganglion.—The ciliary ganglion is located in the posterior orbit, about 6 mm anterior to the superior orbital fissure, to the lateral side of the optic nerve and between the optic nerve and the lateral rectus muscle. It is quadrilateral in shape and measures about 2×2 mm. It has three roots: motor, sensory, and sympathetic.

The *motor root* consists of visceral motor fibers (Edinger-Westphal nucleus) given off by the terminal branch of the inferior division of the oculomotor nerve, which ends in the inferior oblique muscle. After synapse in the ciliary ganglion, emerging fibers are distributed with the short ciliary nerves as postganglionic cholinergic fibers to the ciliary muscle (accommodation) and the sphincter pupillae muscle (pupillary constriction).

The *sympathetic root* consists of fibers derived from the cavernous sinus and internal carotid artery plexuses. The sympathetic nerves are postganglionic fibers that synapse in the superior cervical ganglion and thus pass through the ciliary ganglion without synapse (see Fig 1-47). These fibers mainly provide vasoconstrictor fibers to choroidal blood vessels.

The *sensory root* is derived from the nasociliary branch of the ophthalmic division of the trigeminal nerve; these fibers do not synapse. The sensory root also contains sympathetic fibers that may entirely replace the separate sympathetic root.

The branches of the ciliary ganglion are 6 to 20 short ciliary nerves that branch and pierce the sclera around the optic nerve. They are distributed to the vasculature of the uvea (sympathetic) and to the ciliary muscles (accommodation) and the sphincter pupillae muscle (pupillary constriction).

Trochlear (fourth cranial) nerve.—The trochlear nerve innervates the superior oblique muscle only. Its fibers decussate in the anterior medullary vellum, and it is the only cranial nerve to emerge from the dorsal surface of the brain.

Nucleus.—The nuclei of the trochlear nerve are a small group of cells located at the posterior end of the lateral (paired) portions of the oculomotor nerve. They are located beneath the cerebral aqueduct of Sylvius near its connection with the fourth ventricle, at about the level of the inferior colliculus. The cells are connected by the medial longitudinal fasciculus to the oculomotor nucleus (but not the abducent nucleus), the vestibular nuclei, and the trigeminal sensory nucleus.

Course in the brain stem.—The trochlear is the sole cranial nerve to decussate dorsally. The axons pass laterally and then curve around the aqueduct of Sylvius, progressing caudally and passing over the aqueduct, at which point they leave the brain stem.

Intracranial course.—After emerging from the brain stem on its dorsal surface, the trochlear nerve passes as a slender filament around the cerebral peduncle to reach the ventral surface of the brain just posterior to the oculomotor nerve. It enters the dura mater posterior to the entrance of the oculomotor nerve at about the level of the posterior clinoid process. It is located in the lateral wall of the cavernous sinus somewhat below the oculomotor nerve. The trochlear nerve emerges from the cavernous sinus and enters the lateral portion of the superior orbital fissure outside the ligament of Zinn. In the orbit it passes anteriorly and medially, crossing above the oculomotor nerve, the levator palpebrae superioris muscle, and the superior rectus muscle. It enters the superior oblique muscle on its orbital surface. This is the only extraocular muscle that does not receive its innervation on its bulbar aspect.

Abducent (sixth cranial) nerve.—The abducent nerve has the longest intracranial course of any of the motor nerves of the eye. It makes a sharp turn over the petrous ridge, which makes it vulnerable to trauma and increased intracranial pressure.

Nuclei.—The nuclei of the abducent nerves (N VI) are located in the gray matter of the floor of the fourth ventricle lateral to the medial longitudinal fasciculus. The genu of the facial nerve curves over the dorsal and lateral surfaces of each abducent nucleus. These structures produce an eminence on the floor of the fourth ventricle described as the facial colliculus.

The abducent nerve is unique, because destroying a nucleus impairs not only abduction of the lateral rectus muscle on the same side but also adduction of the medial rectus muscle on the opposite side. Destruction of an abducent nerve root impairs only the lateral rectus muscle on the same side. This occurs because axons from each abducent nerve nucleus cross the midline to ascend in the medial longitudinal fasciculus to the medial rectus motor cells in the oculomotor nuclear complex. The signal to the lateral rectus muscle to abduct the eye is thus sent equally to the medial rectus muscle of the fellow eye causing it to adduct.

Course in the brain stem.—The axons of the abducent nucleus pass forward and downward through the pons on the medial side of the superior olivary nucleus and on the lateral side of the pyramidal tract. They emerge on the ventral surface of the brain stem in a deep groove between the pons anteriorly and the medulla posteriorly.

Intracranial course.—The axons of the sixth cranial nerve pass anteriorly on the surface of the pons, to which they are bound by the anterior inferior cerebellar artery, the first branch of the basilar artery. Each nerve then pierces the dura mater and passes vertically over the posterior part of the petrous portion of the temporal bone to enter the cavernous sinus. Just before entering this sinus, each nerve passes under the petrosphenoid ligament. In the cavernous sinus the abducent nerve is located just below the carotid artery and is the most inferiorly located of the motor nerves to the eye. Each nerve enters the orbit through the superior orbital fissure between the two heads of the lateral rectus muscle. It passes forward and laterally in the orbit to innervate the lateral rectus muscle from its bulbar surface.

Mixed nerves

The facial nerve and the trigeminal nerve are both motor and sensory.

Facial (seventh cranial) nerve.—The facial nerve supplies derivatives of the second branchial arch. It is mainly motor to the muscles of the face and scalp, but it has a small sensory component that transmits sensations of taste from the anterior two thirds of the tongue. Additionally, it carries fibers that stimulate the maxillary and sublingual salivary glands and the lacrimal gland.

Nuclei.—The motor nuclei of the facial nerve are located in the pons medial to the spinal trigeminal tract and lateral to the fibers of the abducent nerve. The gustatory (taste) nuclei receive fibers from cranial nerves VII, IX, and X. The cell bodies are located in the geniculate ganglia, and the axons extend centrally to the gustatory nuclei in the medulla. Fibers that stimulate salivary and lacrimal secretions originate in the salivary nuclei.

Course in the brain stem.—The motor axons pass medially and posteriorly to the floor of the fourth ventricle to form a compact genu around each abducent nucleus. The axons pass laterally to emerge from the ventral surface of the brain stem at the inferior border of the pons, considerably lateral to the abducent nerve.

Intracranial course.—On emerging from the brain stem, the motor fibers of each facial nerve pass in the posterior cranial fossa anterior and lateral to the internal auditory meatus, which they enter in company with the acoustic and vestibular nerves and the intermediate nerve of Wrisberg. The facial nerve makes a sharp backward bend in the temporal bone to enter the dorsal aspect of the middle ear. It emerges from the temporal bone at its lower portion through the stylomastoid foramen.

The nerve then immediately turns anteriorly around the base of the styloid process to enter the parotid gland, where it divides into its terminal divisions, the upper temporofacial and the lower cervicofacial divisions. The temporofacial division gives off temporal and zygomatic branches supplying the orbicularis oculi, the frontalis, the corrugator supercilii, and the anterior and superior auricularis muscles. The cervicofacial division supplies the lower face. These upper and lower divisions have separate areas of origin in each facial nucleus. The upper division has cortical connections with both hemispheres, but the lower division has connections only with the opposite motor cortex. Thus, in a unilateral supranuclear lesion, the muscles innervated by the upper division (orbicularis oculi, frontalis, and corrugator supercilii) are not affected. Those muscles innervated by the lower division are affected.

Motor fibers to the salivary and lacrimal glands are contained in the intermediate nerve of Wrisberg, which passes with the facial nerve into the internal auditory meatus. As the facial nerve turns to enter the facial canal, most of the visceral efferent fibers leave at the apex of the angle as the greater superficial petrosal nerve, which runs forward through the petrous bone to reach the intracranial cavity. The greater superficial petrosal nerve then runs under the semilunar ganglion and emerges from the cranial cavity through the foramen lacerum. It then passes through the pterygoid canal to join the sphenopalatine ganglion. Motor fibers to the lacrimal gland join the maxillary branch of the trigeminal nerve, and its zygomaticotemporal branch to the acrimal nerve (N V_1) contains postganglionic parasympathetic fibers from the sphenopalatine ganglion to the lacrimal gland.

Trigeminal (fifth cranial) nerve.—The trigeminal nerve has a complicated structure (Table 1-8). It is the only sensory nerve of the face and head, but it also sends motor fibers to the muscles of mastication. It has extensive central connections with reflex arcs associated with cranial nerves III to XII.

Motor nucleus and root.—The masticator nerve is the motor portion of the trigeminal nerve. Its nucleus is located cephalad to the facial nerve nucleus near the floor of the cerebral aqueduct of Sylvius. The fibers are distributed with the mandibular nerve and innervate the muscles that move the mandible and the muscles of mastication: the masseter, the temporalis, the internal pterygoid, the mylohyoid, the anterior belly of the digastric, and the external pterygoid. Additionally, motor fibers supply the tensor tympani muscle, which tenses the eardrum, and the tensor veli palatine muscle, which stretches the soft palate.

The mesencephalic root of each trigeminal nerve is situated between the main sensory and the motor nuclei. Fibers of this root are distributed with each of the main divisions of the trigeminal nerve. In the act of biting, impulses pass to the mesencephalic root.

Sensory nuclei.—The principal sensory nucleus of each trigeminal nerve is located near the point of entry of the sensory root into the pons; it lies near the lateral surface of the pons close to the margin of the inferior cerebral peduncle. Functionally, it appears related to tactile impulses.

The nucleus of each spinal trigeminal tract extends down to the second cervical segment of the spinal cord and becomes continuous with the substantia gelatinosa of the dorsal horn. It is functionally associated with the sensation of pain and temperature.

The sensory root is composed of fibers that originate in the semilunar (gasserian) ganglion,

TABLE 1-8.
Trigeminal Nerve (N V)

I. Motor
  A. Muscles of mastication
  B. Tensor tympani muscle
  C. Tensor veli palatine muscle
II. Mesencephalic root
  A. Proprioceptive and deep from tendons and muscles of mastication
III. Gasserian ganglion: cell bodies of neurons mediating touch, pain, and temperature sensation
  A. Ophthalmic branch (N V_1)
    1. Frontal nerve
      a. Supraorbital nerves
        (1) Medial and lateral frontal nerves: skin and conjunctiva of medial upper eyelid, forehead, scalp, frontal sinus
      b. Supratrochlear nerve
        (1) Conjunctiva of medial upper eyelid, forehead, side of nose
    2. Lacrimal nerve
      a. Superior branch
        (1) Lateral palpebral nerves: skin, conjunctiva of lateral eyelid
      b. Inferior branch
        (1) Zygomaticotemporal twig from N V_2
          (a) Postganglionic efferent nerves to reflex lacrimation (N V_2)
    3. Nasociliary nerve
      a. Nasal nerves
        (1) Anterior and posterior ethmoidal nerves: nasal septum mucosa, middle and inferior turbinates, lateral wall of nose
      b. Internal nasal nerves
        (1) Nasal mucosa
      c. External nasal nerve
        (1) Tip of nose
    4. Infratrochelar nerve
      a. Superior and inferior palpebral nerves: canaliculi, caruncle, lacrimal sac, skin and conjunctiva of medial canthus
    5. Sensory (short) root from ciliary ganglion
      Sensation from short ciliary nerves of ciliary ganglion
    6. Long ciliary nerves (2)
      Ciliary body, iris, and cornea; sympathetic impulses to dilatator pupillae muscle
  B. Maxillary branch (N V_2)
    1. Zygomaticotemporal twig to inferior branch of lacrimal nerve
      a. Parasympathetic fibers to lacrimal gland
    2. Infraorbital nerve
      a. Inferior palpebral nerve: lower eyelid
      b. Nasal: side of nose
      c. Superior labial: upper eyelid

together with a few fibers from the ciliary ganglion and possibly from other ganglia. The sensory root extends from the posterior border of the semilunar ganglion to the pons. As it leaves the semilunar ganglion, it pierces the dura mater under the attached border of the tentorium, which contains the superior petrosal sinus. The sensory root lies on the trochlear nerve and then crosses over the facial and auditory foramina. It is then related to a groove in the medial aspect of the petrous portion of the temporal bone lateral to the abducent nerve.

The sensory root of the trigeminal nerve enters the brain on the lateral surface of the pons about midway between its anterior and posterior margins. Inside the pons it divides into ascending and descending tracts. The thick ascending fibers terminate almost immediately in the principal sensory nucleus. The thin descending fibers are adjacent to the nucleus of the spinal trigeminal tract.

Semilunar ganglion.—The semilunar ganglion is a crescent-shaped mass of cells lying in the Meckel cave, which is a cleft located between layers of dura mater in the middle fossa of the skull on a depression on the anterosuperior surface of the petrous bone. At its anterior concave aspect, the semilunar ganglion receives three branches: the ophthalmic division (N V_1), the maxillary division (N V_2), and the mandibular division (N V_3).

The ophthalmic division, the smallest branch of the semilunar ganglion, is located in the lateral wall of the cavernous sinus (see Fig 1-45). Just posterior to the superior orbital (sphenoidal) fissure, the semilunar ganglion receives the frontal, lacrimal, and nasociliary nerves. The frontal and lacrimal nerves leave the orbit above the ligament of Zinn, whereas the nasociliary branch leaves through the annulus of the ligament.

The *frontal nerve* is located in the roof of the orbit between the levator palpebrae superioris muscle and the periosteum. The supraorbital and supratrochlear are its major branches. The supraorbital nerve enters the orbit through the supraorbital notch. Its major branches, the medial and lateral frontal nerves, receive sensory impulses from the forehead, scalp, and upper eyelid. The supratrochlear nerve contains sensory nerves from the medial scalp, eyelid, and conjunctiva that enter the orbit near the trochlea.

The *lacrimal nerve* follows the upper border of the lateral rectus muscle accompanied by the lacrimal artery. Its superior branch originates as the lateral palpebral nerve, receiving sensory impulses from the skin and conjunctiva of the upper and lower eyelids. The inferior branch receives a twig from the zygomatico-temporal branch of the maxillary division (N V_2) of the trigeminal nerve, which contains secretory innervation to the lacrimal gland.

The *nasociliary nerve* has a course similar to that of the ophthalmic artery. Its long ciliary nerves provide the sensory innervation of the globe. It receives the long (sensory) root of the ciliary ganglion at the superior orbital fissure. Its nasal branch has anterior and posterior ethmoidal branches and internal and external nasal branches.

The two long ciliary nerves form the nasociliary nerve as it crosses above the optic nerve. They emerge from the sclera with the short ciliary nerves and accompany the long posterior ciliary arteries. The fibers are mainly sensory, but they also carry the sympathetic fibers to the dilatator pupillae muscle. The short ciliary nerves carry the motor fibers to the sphincter pupillae and ciliary muscle.

Autonomic nervous system

The autonomic nervous system is a subdivision of the motor portion of the nervous system that carries impulses to smooth muscles, cardiac muscle, and glands. In contrast to skeletal muscle, in which a single neuron extends from the central nervous system to the muscle fiber, the autonomic nervous system is composed of a two-neuron chain. The first, or preganglionic, neuron has its cell body in the central nervous system and synapses with postganglionic neurons in an autonomic ganglion. The neuron has its cell body in the autonomic ganglion and terminates in smooth muscle, cardiac muscle, or glands.

The autonomic nervous system is composed of two parts: (1) visceral efferent fibers in cranial nerves III, VII, IX, X, and XI and sacral nerves II, III, and IV, which comprise the parasympathetic portion (craniosacral division); and (2) visceral efferent fibers of the thoracic and lumbar nerves, which comprise the sympathetic system (thoracolumbar division).

Parasympathetic nervous system.—The visceral efferent branch of the oculomotor nerve originates from cell bodies located in the Edinger-Westphal nuclei. Its axons pass, together with the inferior division of the oculomotor nerve, to the inferior oblique muscle and form the preganglionic motor root (short) of the ciliary ganglion. The fibers synapse in the ciliary ganglion with the cells of postganglionic fibers, which pass with the short ciliary nerves to innervate the ciliary and sphincter pupillae muscles.

Sympathetic nervous system.—The sympathetic nervous system (Fig 1-47) has centers located in the hypothalamus and the medulla: (1) the superior ciliospinal center and (2) the inferior ciliospinal center (of Budge). The *superior ciliospinal center* is located near the nucleus of the hypoglossal nerve. The *inferior ciliospinal center* is located in the upper portion of the spinal cord. Sympathetic efferent fibers originate in the anterior lateral columns and leave the spinal cord in the ventral roots of thoracic I to lumbar II spinal nerves. These fibers pass with the anterior rami lateral to the vertebral column until they leave the anterior rami in the white ramus communicans. The white rami turn at right angles at the vertebral column to form the sympathetic nerve trunk, which extends from the base of the skull to the tip of the coccyx. Within the trunk are ganglia in which synapse is made with peripheral postganglionic sympathetic nerves.

The ganglia at the level of cervical I, II, and III spinal nerves fuse to form the superior cervical ganglion. Most of the preganglionic fibers that synapse in the superior cervical ganglion have left the spinal cord at the level of the first two thoracic nerves and have coursed upward in the sympathetic nerve trunk.

The superior cervical ganglion is 2.5 to 3.7 cm long and is located ventral to the transverse processes of the second (axis) and third cervical vertebrae and dorsal to the sheath of the great vessels of the neck. It is in close proximity to the subclavian artery (see Fig 7-4).

Postganglionic fibers from the superior cervical ganglion are widely distributed. The internal carotid branch extends intracranially with fibers distributed to the internal carotid artery and the cavernous plexus. These fibers provide almost all of the sympathetic nerve branches to the eye and the orbit. Fibers for sweating of the face, however, are distributed with the external carotid artery.

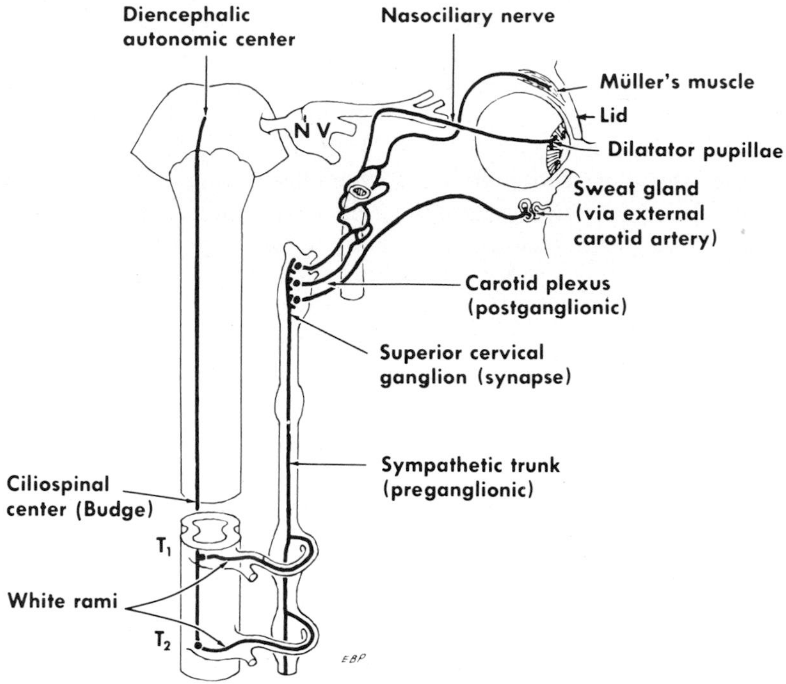

FIG 1-47.
Sympathetic nervous system of the eye. Efferent fibers synapse in the superior cervical ganglion. Postganglionic fibers then pass to the sweat glands of the face and eyelids along the external carotid artery. Other branches extend intracranially with the internal carotid artery and pass with the ophthalmic artery into the orbit. Vasomotor fibers are distributed by the short ciliary nerves to blood vessels in the choroid. Fibers to the dilatator pupillae muscle do not pass through the ciliary ganglion and are carried to the globe by the long ciliary branches of the nasociliary nerve (N V). The smooth muscles of the eyelids are innervated by sympathetic fibers that accompany branches of the ophthalmic artery to the eyelid.

Sympathetic nerve fibers pass through the ciliary ganglion without synapse. They are mainly vasomotor and are distributed by the short ciliary nerves to the uveal blood vessels.

Fibers to the dilatator pupillae muscle pass to the eye in the two long ciliary nerve branches of the nasociliary nerve (N V) and do not pass through the ciliary ganglion.

VISUAL PATHWAYS

Visual stimuli, which originate in each retina, are transmitted to the brain by the axons of retinal ganglion cells, in the optic nerves. The optic nerves originate at the optic disks, located at the same level as the nerve fiber layer of the retina, slightly nasal to the posterior pole of the eye. Retinal axons that originate from ganglion cells located nasal to a vertical line that passes through the center of the fovea centralis decussate in the optic chiasm. They join uncrossed axons from the temporal one half of the retina of the fellow eye to form the optic tract. The axons terminate in the lateral geniculate body (form and motion) and the pretectal nuclei (pupil). Axons from the lateral geniculate body pass in the optic radiation to the visual cortex located in the occipital cortex (Fig 1-48). The pupillary fibers pass in the brachium of the superior colliculi to their synapse in the pretectal nuclei.

Optic nerve

The optic nerve is a portion of a white fiber tract of the central nervous system composed of axons of retinal ganglion cells.

The optic nerve is divided into four parts. The intraocular portion, which measures about 1.0 mm in length and 1.0 to 1.7 mm in diameter, has been intensively studied as the major landmark of the ocular fundus in ophthalmoscopy

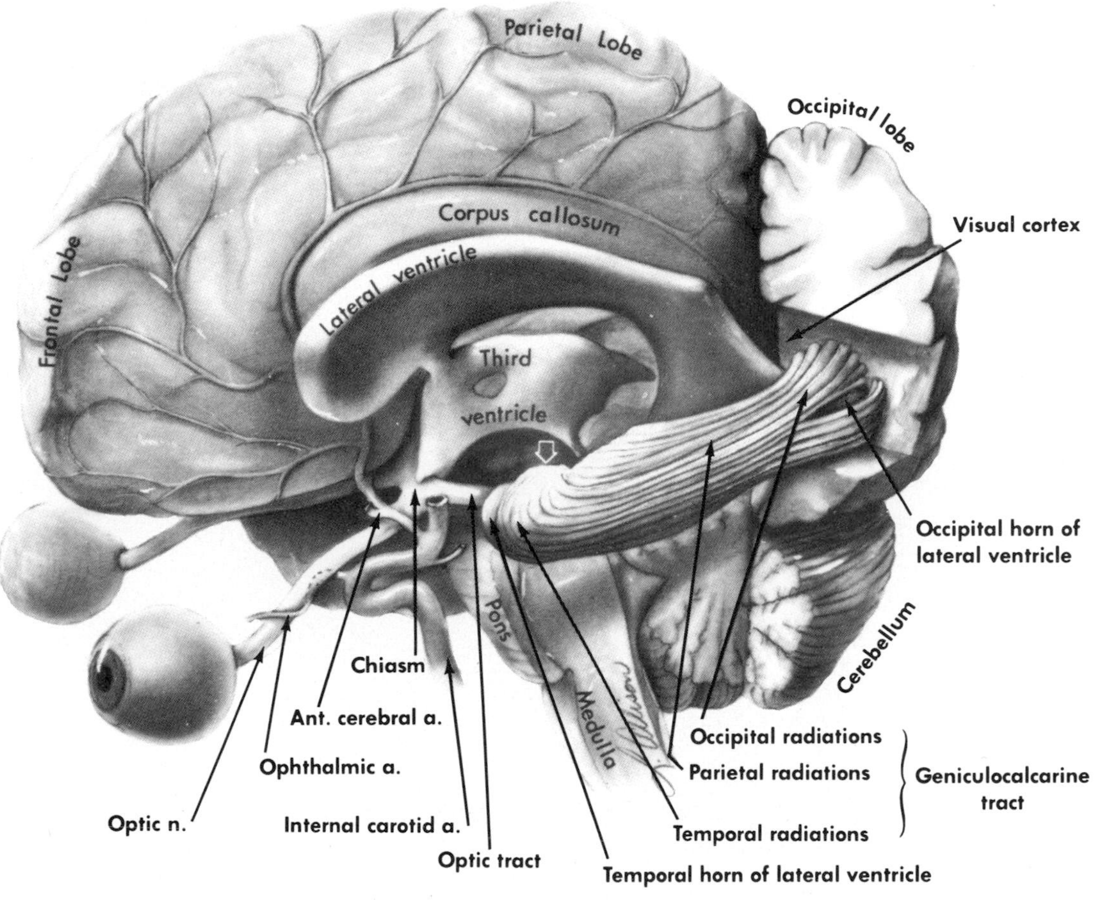

FIG 1-48.
The visual-sensory system viewed from the left side. The left cerebral hemisphere has been removed except for a portion of the occipital lobe and the ventricular system. The arrow beneath the third ventricle points to the lateral geniculate body. The cerebral falx and the cerebellar tentorium are not shown. (*From Glaser JS:* Neuro-ophthalmology, *ed 2, New York, 1990, Harper & Row. Used by permission.*)

and because of its vulnerability to damage in optic atrophy, particularly that secondary to glaucoma (see Chapter 22). The intraocular portion is divided into (1) the optic disk; (2) prelaminar, the portion between the optic disk and the lamina cribrosa; (3) laminar, the portion within the lamina cribrosa; and (4) postlaminar, the intraocular portion located posterior to the lamina cribrosa that is still within the scleral canal.

The intraorbital portion measures about 40 mm in length and increases in diameter to 3.0 to 4.0 mm as the result of myelination of its axons and the meningeal sheaths that contain the subarachnoid space continuous with that of the brain. The intracanicular portion is the 5.0-mm segment within the optic canal. The intracranial portion extends between the cranial opening of the optic canal and the optic chiasm. It is about 10 mm long and 3.0 mm in diameter, the nerve having lost its meningeal sheaths.

The optic disk, the surface of the optic nerve within the eye (see Fig 6-7), is the major ophthalmoscopic landmark of the ocular fundus. Here the ganglion cells' axons in the nerve fiber layer of the retina and the central retinal vein make a right-angle turn to enter the posterior scleral canal. The central retinal vein is just temporal to the central retinal artery within a central depression of the optic disk, the physiologic cup. The edges of the physiologic cup parallel the margins of the posterior scleral canal and mirror its size and the angle the optic nerve

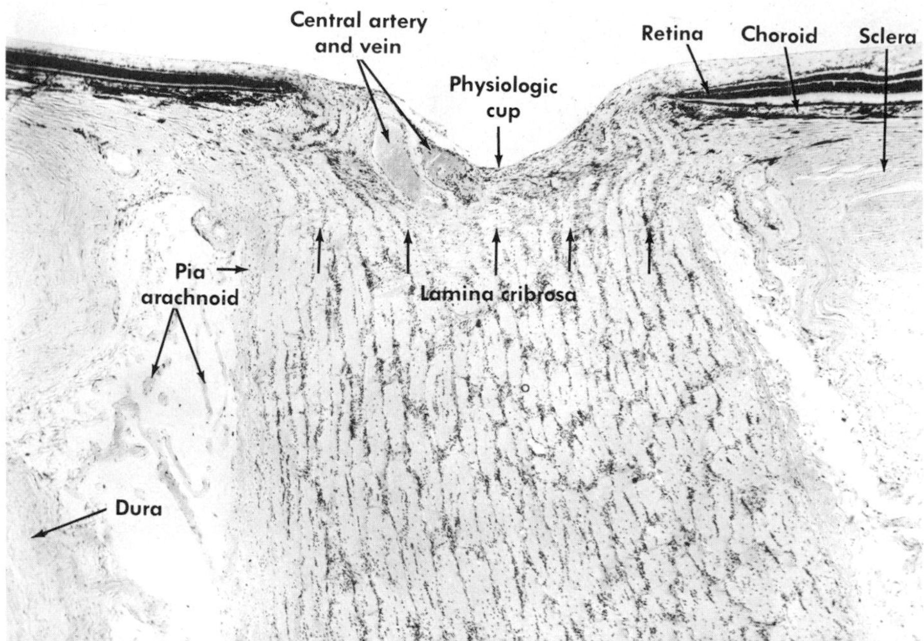

FIG 1-49.
Optic disk and optic nerve (hematoxylin and eosin, ×43).

makes with the globe. The physiologic cup is lined with astrocytes. When numerous they obliterate the cup. When scanty they permit ophthalmoscopic visualization of the perforations of the lamina cribrosa.

The optic disk is not elevated above the surrounding nerve fiber layer of the retina, and the term "optic papilla" is a misnomer. Nonetheless, the central artery and vein divide into papillary branches; edema of the disk is papilledema; the mass of nerve fibers that enter the optic nerve from the central retina is the papillomacular bundle; and the region surrounding the disk is called peripapillary.

The posterior scleral foramen through which the optic nerve leaves the eye is bridged by a sievelike structure, the lamina cribrosa (see Fig 1-3). This is formed by sclera, elastic tissue of the choroid and portions of Bruch membrane, and astroglia derived from the septal framework of the optic nerve. The lamina cribrosa divides the intraocular portion of the optic nerve into prelaminar, laminar, and retrolaminar portions. The prelaminar portion of the optic nerve is not myelinated and contains more glia and fewer collagen septa than the laminar portion.

The laminar portion of the intraocular portion of the optic nerve contains much collagen and many vascular septae. The retrolaminar portion of the optic nerve becomes myelinated by numerous oligodendrocytes that characterize white matter of the brain. The nerve acquires its sheaths of dura mater, arachnoid mater, and pia mater on emerging from the scleral canal.

The *orbital portion* of the optic nerve has an S-shaped curve to permit movements of the eye. It is sheathed with a dense outer dura mater, a middle arachnoid mater, and an innermost pia mater.

The dura mater and the arachnoid mater blend into the sclera anteriorly (Fig 1-49). The dura mater terminates at the optic foramen, whereas the arachnoid mater and pia mater (and the subarachnoid space) are continuous with those of the brain. Near the globe the two long posterior ciliary arteries and the 10 to 20 short posterior ciliary arteries are arranged around the circumference of the optic nerve. From 10 to 15 mm behind the globe, the central artery and vein penetrate the optic nerve. The passage of the central vein through

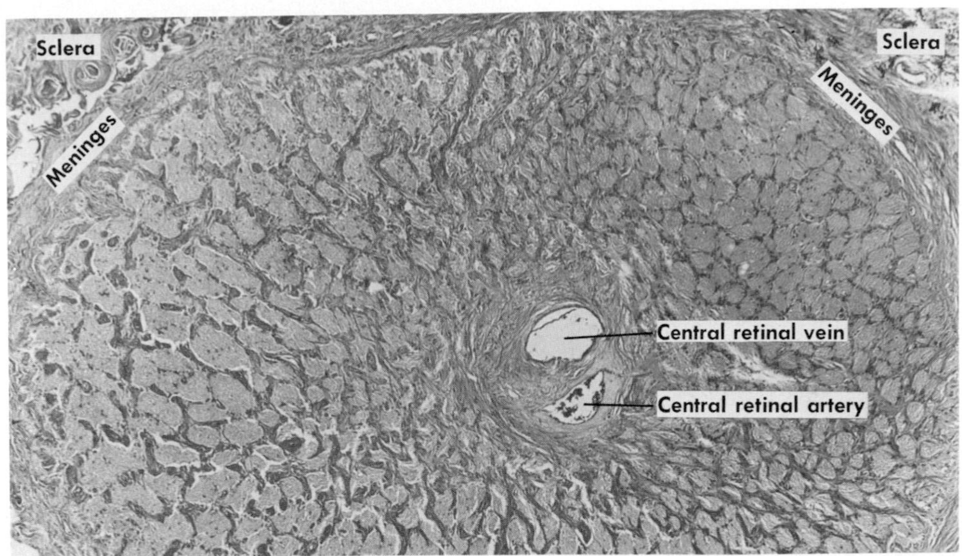

FIG 1-50.
Cross section of the human optic nerve just posterior to the globe. The contribution of the dura mater to the sclera is shown. The central artery and vein share a common adventitial sheath, as they do at points of crossings within the eye. In the nerve the myelinated nerve fibers are divided into septa by delicate, collagenous fibers from the pia. The nerve fiber bundles are separated from the septal system by a layer of astrocytes (×70.) *(Courtesy of Ramesh C. Tripathi, M.D.)*

the subarachnoid space makes it vulnerable to increased intracranial pressure, a factor in papilledema. The intraorbital portion of the optic nerve receives its blood supply from branches of the ophthalmic artery nurturing the pia mater. At the apex of the orbit, the optic nerve is surrounded by the fibrous annulus from which the recti muscles originate, the ligament of Zinn.

In its *intracanalicular portion,* the optic nerve passes through the optic foramen in the small wing of the sphenoid bone. The nerve is accompanied by the ophthalmic artery and the sympathetic nerves that accompany the artery. At the anterior margin of the optic foramen, the dura mater covering the nerve divides so that one portion continues as the periosteum of the orbit and the other continues as the dural sheath of the optic nerve. Within the optic canal, the dura mater is adherent to bone, arachnoid, and pia mater, which firmly fix the nerve.

Within the skull, the intracranial portion of the nerve passes medially where the nasal fibers form the chiasm. The temporal fibers join with the crossed nasal fibers from the opposite side to form the optic tract.

Structure.—The optic nerve contains between 1.1 and 1.3 million afferent axons of ganglion cells. Some 90% of the axons in the optic nerve may originate with ganglion cells that have their cone outer segments in the fovea centralis.

The nerve is composed of bundles of nerve fibers separated by septa that are continuous with the pia mater and carry minute blood vessels to the nerve (Fig 1-50). As in the brain, the nerve fibers are supported by astroglia and oligodendroglia derived from the neural ectoderm and by mesenchymal microglia that have a phagocytic function. Myelinization of the optic nerve begins at the chiasm at about the 24th week of fetal life and, at birth, has reached a point just behind the lamina cribrosa. Oligodendrocytes are associated with the synthesis and metabolism of myelin; these cells are most numerous behind the lamina cribrosa. Astrocytes provide a skeletal framework on the intraocular surface of the optic nerve and are important in providing mechanical support as nerve fibers make the right-angle turn from the retina to the optic nerve.

Blood supply.—The blood supply of the optic nerve is derived from several sources.

Much attention has been directed to the blood supply of the intraocular portion of the optic nerve because of atrophy of the optic nerve, which occurs in glaucoma. Within the relatively rigid wall of the scleral canal, the optic nerve and the intraneural central retinal artery and vein are tightly confined. The blood supply by the pia mater terminates at the sclera, and the optic nerve within the scleral canal is mainly dependent upon the terminal branches of minute arterioles. Because the optic nerve measures less than 1.5 mm in diameter and its intrascleral portion is less than 1.0 mm in length, there is considerable variation in its vasculature. Since the optic nerve is composed of the axons of retinal ganglion cells, many of the abnormalities described as optic atrophy may originate in the retina rather than with the nerve.

The surface of the optic disk receives capillaries from the central retinal artery. The prelaminar portion of the optic nerve (that portion between the lamina cribrosa and the optic disk) receives capillaries from the choroidal arterioles (not from the choriocapillaris). The laminar optic nerve, that portion of the optic nerve within the lamina cribrosa, is supplied by short posterior ciliary arteries that, as they penetrate the sclera, give off branches to form the anastomotic circle (partial) of Haller-Zinn. The region posterior to the lamina cribrosa is supplied by the vascular network of the pia mater, as is the remainder of the orbital portion of the optic nerve.

The intraorbital portion of the nerve has a peripheral and possibly an axial blood supply. The peripheral vessels originate from those of the pia mater and are derived from the neighboring blood vessels. Some axial vessels may be derived from the central retinal artery. The axial vascular system nurtures the central retinal fibers.

The intracanalicular and intracranial portions of the optic nerve are nurtured by the pial fibrovascular meshwork from branches of the internal carotid artery.

Optic chiasm

The optic chiasm is about 13 mm wide. It is attached by the pia mater and the arachnoid to the dorsal surface of the diencephalon, and it forms a portion of the floor of the third ventricle. Its posterior surface is in close contact with the tuber cinereum from which extends the infundibulum or stalk of the pituitary gland (hypophysis cerebri). The chiasm is superior to the tuberculum sellae turcicae and the diaphragma sellae. The chiasm is usually posterior to the optic groove of the sphenoid bone. It is closely related to the internal carotid arteries laterally and to the anterior cerebral arteries and anterior communicating artery anteriorly.

Optic tract

The optic tract extends from the chiasm to the lateral geniculate body. It is composed of axons from ganglion cells of the nasal retina of the opposite side and the temporal retina of the same side. The optic tract sweeps laterally, encircles the hypothalamus posteriorly (in the ventral wall of the third ventricle), and winds around the ventrolateral aspect of the pes pedunculi (the ventral portion of the midbrain). The majority of axons terminate in the lateral geniculate body. A smaller number continue in the superior quadrigeminal brachium to the superior colliculi (reflex ocular movements) and to the pretectal nuclei (pupillary constriction). Other fibers enter the hypothalamus and terminate in the supraoptic nucleus and the medial nuclei of the tuber cinereum. The superior colliculi are sensitive to moving visual stimuli and may direct the eyes and the head toward a visual stimulus.

Lateral geniculate body

The axons of retinal ganglion cells that carry retinal impulses synapse in the lateral geniculate body (Fig 1-51), which is located in the diencephalon lateral to the medial geniculate body. It consists of a dorsal and inconspicuous (in humans) ventral nucleus. In primates the dorsal nucleus is composed of six cellular layers, numbered 1 to 6, beginning at the hilus and continuing toward the dorsal portion of the nucleus. Cells in ventral layers 1 and 2 (magnocellular laminae) are larger and more uniform in size and shape than cells in the remaining four layers (parvocellular laminae). Axons from the temporal retina (uncrossed) on the same side synapse in layers 2, 3, and 5. Axons from the nasal one half of the retina of the opposite eye decussate in the chiasm and terminate in layers 1, 4, and 6. The axons from the lower one half of the retina

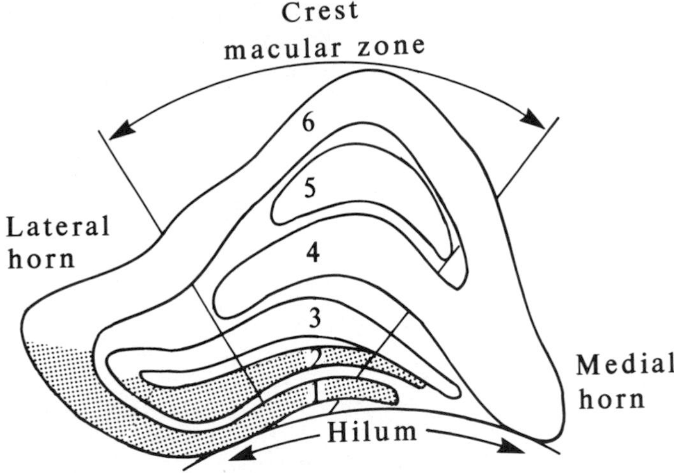

FIG 1-51.
Schema of a coronal section through the lateral geniculate body viewed from its posterior aspect. Uncrossed axons from the terminal retina synapse in layers *2, 3,* and *5.* Crossed axons from the contralateral nasal retina synapse in layers *1, 4,* and *6.* Layers *1* and *2* are magnocellular (motion and flicker), and its axons originate in the ganglion cells in the retinal periphery of each eye. Layers *3* to *6* are parvocellular (color, texture, shape, and stereopsis), and its axons originate mainly in retinal ganglion cells of cones located in and near the fovea centralis of each eye. (*Redrawn from Miller NR:* Walsh and Hoyt's clinical neuro-ophthalmology, *ed 4, vol 1, Baltimore, 1982, Williams & Wilkins.*)

synapse in the lateral portion of the lateral geniculate body, those from the upper one half in the medial portion. Foveal axons are located posteriorly. Central visual fibers are represented in all six layers, whereas peripheral axons are represented in the two magnocellular layers and in two parvocellular layers.

In addition to visual fibers, the lateral geniculate body receives input from the visual cortex, oculomotor centers in the brain stem, and the brainstem reticular formation. The parvocellular laminae (3 to 6) appear to carry the signals that mainly sustain perception of color, texture, shape, and fine stereopsis. The magnocellular laminae (1 and 2) signals sustain the detection of movement and flicker.

Optic radiation

The optic radiation (geniculocalcarine tract) extends from the lateral geniculate body to the superior and inferior lips of the calcarine fissure (area 17; area striata) of the occipital lobe (Fig 1-52). The axons of ganglion cells that have their nuclei in the inferior nasal quadrant of one eye and the inferior temporal quadrant of the opposite eye synapse in the lateral aspect of the lateral geniculate body. (Because light travels in a straight line these fibers carry nerve impulses from light that originates in the visual field of the superior temporal quadrant on the same side [see Chapter 5].) The axons of ganglion cells that have their nuclei in the superior nasal quadrant of one eye and the superior temporal quadrant of the opposite eye synapse in the medial aspect of the lateral geniculate body. (These fibers carry light impulses that originate in the visual field of the inferior temporal quadrant on the same side.)

Damage (trauma, stroke) to the axons in the geniculocalcarine tract that carry nervous impulses from these areas causes a visual field defect (see Chapter 5), which is the same in each eye (homonymous).

The axons in the optic radiation with cell bodies located in the lateral aspect of the lateral geniculate body pass anteriorly around the tip of the temporal horn of the lateral ventricle to form the temporal loop of Flechsig-Archambault-Meyer. Damage to the axons in this loop produces superior homonymous quadrantic field defects. The axons of the temporal loop continue posterior to terminate in the ventral (inferior) lip of the calcarine fissure. Axons from cells located in the medial portion

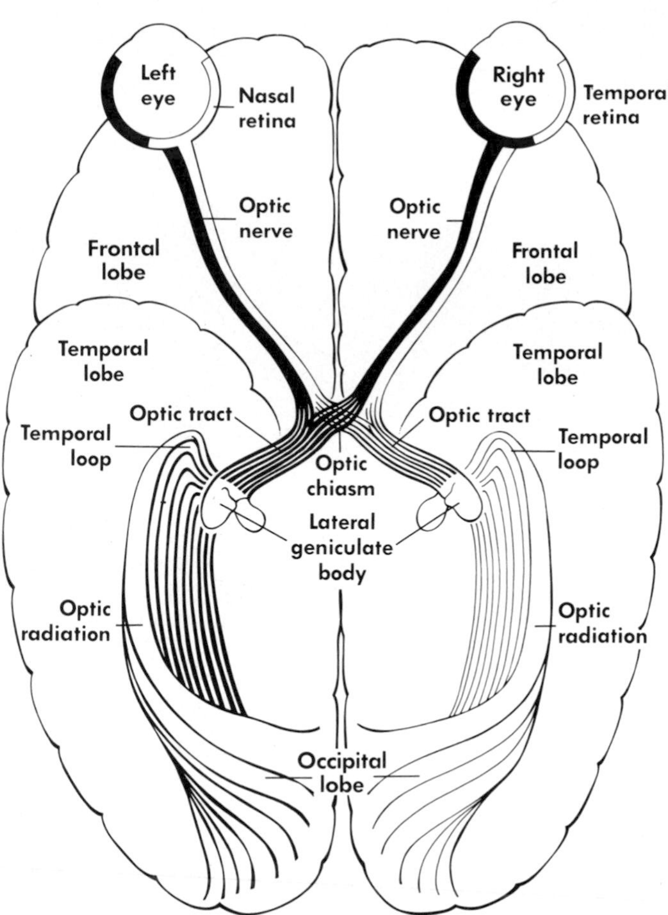

FIG 1-52.
The optic pathways projected onto the base of the brain. All axons that originate from ganglion cells located on the nasal side of a line passing through the center of the fovea centralis decussate (cross) at the optic chiasm. The nasal fibers join uncrossed axons from the temporal half of each retina to form the optic tract. Axons carrying visual impulses synapse in the lateral geniculate bodies with cells whose axons form the optic radiation. Axons carrying impulses related to the pupillary light reflex do not enter the lateral geniculate body but pass to the pretectal nuclei in the midbrain.

of the lateral geniculate body, representing the superior retinal quadrants (inferior visual field quadrants), pass nearly directly posterior through the parietal lobe to terminate in the dorsal (superior) lip of the calcarine fissure.

Visual cortex

The axons of cells located in the lateral geniculate body terminate along the superior and inferior lips of the calcarine fissure. This area is often called the striate cortex (area 17 of Brodmann) because of the prominent band of geniculocalcarine fibers (striae of Gennari). The upper one half of each retina is represented on the dorsal (superior) part of each occipital cortex, and the lower one half covers the ventral (inferior) part. Fibers representing the central retina terminate at the tip of the posterior pole, and more peripheral portions of the retina are represented more anteriorly (Fig 1-53). The visual cortex is composed of six cell layers typical of cortex; most axons from the lateral geniculate body terminate in layer IV (lamina granularis interna of Brodmann) that is divided (in monkeys) into three major layers.

Optic pathways

The retina is divided anatomically into nasal and temporal portions by a vertical line that passes through the exact center of the fovea centralis. All retinal axons that originate from ganglion cells located to the nasal side of this line decussate in the optic chiasm. Retinal axons from ganglion cells temporal to this line synapse in the lateral geniculate body on the same side. A horizontal line that passes through the center of the fovea divides the retina into superior and inferior portions. Thus, each retina is divided into superior temporal, inferior temporal, superior nasal, and inferior nasal quadrants. (Note that the fovea centralis and not the optic nerve is the dividing structure.)

Localization in the visual pathways.—As nerve fibers enter the optic nerve, the axons from

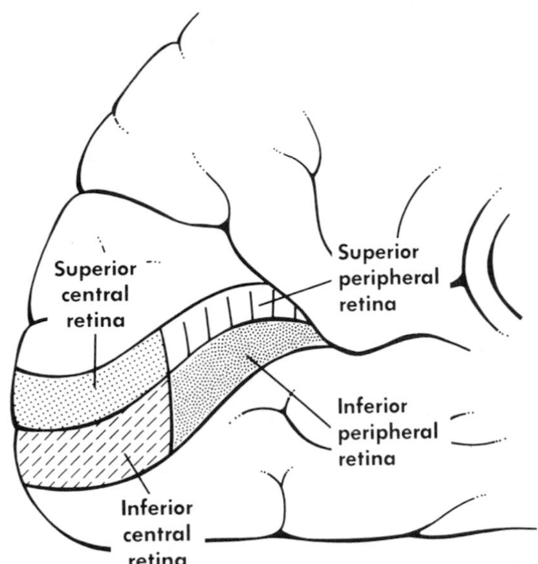

FIG 1-53.
Striate area of left occipital lobe with calcarine fissure widely opened. The central retina is represented posteriorly and is relatively large; the peripheral retina is represented anteriorly and is relatively small.

the fovea centralis and adjacent retina (possibly 90% of the entire optic nerve) occupy the temporal portion. Within 6 mm of the optic disk these central axons are surrounded by axons from the peripheral retina.

The visual field is composed of the total perception resulting from retinal stimulation at one moment. When the eyes are directed straight ahead and fixating a distant object they are described as being in the primary position. While the eyes are in this position, a visual stimulus located below and to the right will stimulate retinal receptors in the superior, nasal quadrant of the right eye and the superior, temporal quadrant of the left eye. The stimuli from the right superior nasal quadrant will pass to the optic nerve, decussate at the optic chiasm, and synapse in the lateral geniculate body. The stimuli from the left superior temporal quadrant will pass without decussation in the optic nerve to synapse in the lateral geniculate body in the same cells as did the corresponding cells of the right eye. Lesions at various sites in the optic tracts produce typical visual field defects (Fig 1-54).

Axons of ganglion cells from the nasal portion of both the central and peripheral retina decussate in the optic chiasm. Axons from the inferior nasal retina are located in the anterior and inferior surfaces of the chiasm (closest to the pituitary gland). Axons from the inferior nasal retina, after decussating, loop forward slightly in the opposite optic nerve before passing into the optic tract. The anterior loop in the contralateral optic nerve is responsible for the rare involvement of the visual field of both eyes in lesions affecting the optic nerve just anterior to the chiasm. The position of inferior nasal axons in the inferior portion of the chiasm makes them vulnerable in pituitary enlargement, so that the initial visual field defect in pituitary tumors is loss of the superior temporal visual field.

The superior nasal axons cross in the superior portion of the chiasm in its posterior aspect. They first pass posteriorly in the optic tract on the same side and then loop forward to decussate.

The distribution of axons in the anterior portion of the optic tract is similar to that in the optic nerve, except that the nasal axons are those that have crossed from the opposite side. The axons are rapidly redistributed so that those from corresponding parts of each retina become associated. Thus, axons from the inferior nasal retina become related to inferior temporal retinal axons of the opposite eye, and superior nasal retinal axons become related to uncrossed superior temporal retinal axons of the opposite eye. Transmission defects in the optic tracts produce homonymous (same side, both eyes) visual field defects, because axons from corresponding parts of each retina are involved in a single lesion (hemianopsia is half-blindness; the reference is to the blind portion of the field).

In the lateral geniculate body, uncrossed (temporal) retinal axons synapse in layers 2, 3, and 5; crossed (nasal) retinal axons synapse in layers 1, 4, and 6.

The axons emerging from the cells of the lateral geniculate body have exact correspondence in each eye so that a lesion in them causes exactly similar visual field defects in each eye (homonymous congruous defects). Lesions in the axons that carry stimuli from the inferior retinas pass around the temporal horn of the lateral ventricle and cause a superior homonymous quadrantanopsia (often a sign of a vascular lesion). Lesions from the superior retinas pass more directly to the cortical striate area and cause an inferior quadrantanopsia.

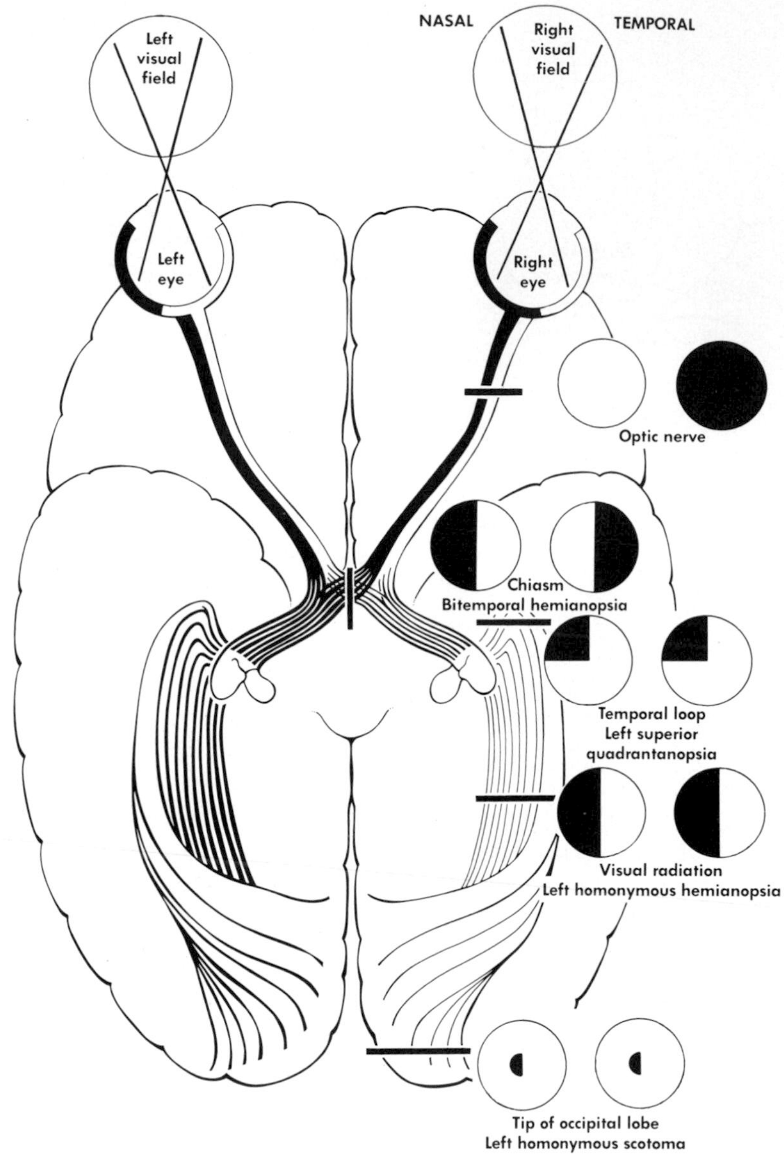

FIG 1-54.

Typical visual field defects that occur with damage to different regions of the optic pathways. The visual fields are diagrammed to reflect the source of the light that stimulates the retina. Light from the temporal side stimulates the nasal portion of the retina, light from above stimulates the lower portion, and so on. Thus, the visual field defect caused by a lesion affecting fibers arising from the nasal half of the retina is diagrammed as a temporal field defect. (The visual pathways are projected onto the base of the brain.)

Fibers that represent corresponding portions of the fovea centralis of each eye and the immediately surrounding retina occupy a relatively large area in the striate area of the visual cortex of the occipital lobe (Brodmann area 17). More peripheral portions of the retina are represented anteriorly. The superior areas of the two retinas (inferior visual fields) are represented on the upper lip of the calcarine fissure; inferior binocular areas (superior visual fields) are on the lower lip. All nasal axons from the fovea decussate completely. The "sparing of the macula," in which destruction of the occipital lobe on one side does not seem to affect all of the central retinal fibers, may be the result of incomplete destruction inasmuch as many arteries supply

TABLE 1-9.
Primordia of the Ocular Structures

I. Surface ectoderm
  A. Lens
  B. Corneal epithelium
  C. Conjunctival epithelium
  D. Cilia
  E. Epithelium, tarsal glands
  F. Epithelium, glands of Zeis and Moll
  G. Epithelium, lacrimal and accessory lacrimal
  H. Epithelium, lacrimal passages
II. Neural crest cells
  A. Corneal stroma
  B. Corneal endothelium (mesothelium) and Descemet membrane
  C. Scleral fibroblasts
  D. Iris stroma and melanophores (not pigmented epithelium)
  E. Iridocorneal angle (trabecular meshwork)
  F. Choroid melanophores, pericytes, and stroma
  G. Orbital bones
  H. Optic nerve meninges
  I. Nerves
III. Neural ectoderm
  A. Sensory retina
  B. Retinal pigment epithelium
  C. Iris pigment epithelium
  D. Sphincter pupillae muscle, dilatator pupillae muscle
  E. Neural portions of optic nerve
IV. Mesoderm
  A. Conjunctival stroma
  B. Episclera
  C. Tenon capsule
  D. Extrinsic ocular muscles
  E. Ciliary muscles
  F. Choroidal endothelium
  G. Vitrous
V. Mixed
  A. Surface ectoderm and mesoderm
    1. Eyelid from ectoderm, mesoderm, and neural crest
    2. Zonule (tertiary vitreous)
  B. Neural ectoderm and mesoderm
    1. Bruch membrane

the region. Alternatively, "central retinal sparing" may be the result of minute changes in visual fixation.

EMBRYOLOGY

The eye and its appendages originate from neural and surface ectoderm, mesoderm, and the neural crest. The sensory retina, retinal pigment epithelium, and neural portion of the optic nerve develop from the neural ectoderm. The neural ectoderm also forms the embryonic optic cup, the anterior portion of which gives rise to the epithelium of the ciliary body, the pigment layer of the iris, and the sphincter pupillae and dilatator pupillae muscles.

The primordial surface ectoderm forms the lens, the corneal epithelium, the conjunctiva and the eyelid epithelium, together with the epithelium of their glandular structures, and the lacrimal gland. Primordial neural crest cells form the corneal stroma, endothelium (mesothelium), Descemet membrane, the iris stroma, the structures of the iridocorneal angle, the fibroblasts of the sclera, the vascular pericytes, the connective tissue of the choroid, and all pigment cells except those in the retinal and iris pigment epithelium (but including those in the iris stroma). Neural crest cells form the bones of the orbit, the meninges, Schwann cells, and the autonomic nervous system and peripheral sensory nerves. Mesoderm provides the striated extrinsic muscles of the eye and the endothelium of blood vessels. The eyelids form from surface ectoderm, mesoderm, and neural crest cells. The tertiary vitreous (zonule) forms from surface ectoderm and mesoderm. The Bruch membrane originates from mesoderm and neural ectoderm (Table 1-9).

The neural crest is the sole source of all pigment cells of the body except those of the retina and iris pigment epithelium, which are derived from the embryonic optic cup. Neural crest cells form all of the skeletal and connective tissues adjacent to the medial and lateral parts of the eye, including the corneal endothelium and stroma and much of the orbit. The extraocular muscles are of mesodermal origin and have but a small contribution from neural crest-derived cells. The connective tissue associated with the extraocular muscles is of neural crest origin, as are the ciliary muscles.

Homeobox (box) genes encode regulatory proteins in early embryonic life. These genes in turn control the expression of hundreds or thousands of genes required to differentiate parts of the body or the eyes. A mutation in a homeobox gene can result in loss of a particular ocular structure, such as the iris (aniridia), or absence of the entire eye (anophthalmia). The homeobox gene Pax-6 is essential for formation of the eye.

THE EYE

Outer coat

The sclera.—The sclera originates as a condensation of secondary mesenchyme (neural crest cells mainly combined with mesodermal cells) that circle the anterior portion of the optic cup and then extend posteriorly. During the fourth month, collagenous fibers extend posteriorly, and by the fifth month the fibrous coat reaches the posterior pole.

The cornea.—The corneal epithelium is formed by the surface ectoderm, from which the lens placode detaches itself. Neural crest cells form the corneal stroma and later the corneal mesothelium (endothelium) and the Descemet membrane. The cells of the corneal stroma provide the primary pupillary membrane, which is then vascularized by mesodermal cells.

Medial coat

The choroid.—The choroid has a complex origin from the secondary mesenchyme surrounding the primary optic vesicle. Its blood vessels are of mesodermal origin, whereas the melanophores, pericytes, and connective tissue originate from the neural crest derivatives. All of its layers can be recognized by the fifth month. Pigment develops relatively late, first near the entrance of branches of the posterior ciliary arteries and then extending forward. At 6 weeks it is highly vascular, and the tissue is spongy. The choroid corresponds to the pia mater and arachnoid of the brain; anteriorly the neural crest derivatives differentiate into the connective tissue of the ciliary body, while the ciliary muscle is of mesodermal origin.

At the anterior edge of the secondary optic cup, the inner sensory and the outer pigmentary layers fuse together to form the following structures: (1) the ciliary epithelium (pars ciliaris retinae), with an inner nonpigmented layer that is a continuation of the retinal sensory layer and a pigmentary layer that is the continuation of retinal pigment epithelium; and (2) further anteriorly, the iris epithelium (pars iridica retinae) together with the sphincter pupillae and dilatator pupillae muscles.

The ciliary body.—The ciliary body is formed by a fusion of the optic cup and the adjacent secondary mesenchyme. The ciliary processes are derived from the pigmented and nonpigmented epithelium of the primitive retina, and the capillaries are derived from mesoderm. The ciliary muscle grows in from mesoderm located between the sclera and the ciliary ectoderm. Longitudinal fibers are formed about the fourth month, and the circular muscle is formed at the end of the sixth month. The attachment of the longitudinal fibers to the scleral spur establishes an anterior chamber angle. Secretion by the ciliary epithelium and outflow through the trabecular meshwork begin about the sixth or seventh month.

The iris and pupil.—The pigment epithelium of the iris, the sphincter pupillae muscle, and the dilatator pupillae muscle are derived from the neural ectoderm of the optic cup. The iris stroma and its melanophores originate with neural crest cells. The surface pattern of the iris in postnatal life closely reflects its embryologic origin. The most anterior extremity of the optic cup is visible as the pupillary frill. The sphincter pupillae muscle and dilatator pupillae muscle are derived from neural ectoderm and, with the arrectores pilorum muscles, are the sole muscles in the body of ectodermal origin. Cells of neural crest origin first grow over the surface of the optic cup to form the anterior stromal layers of the iris. Until the third month of embryonic life, the margin of the optic cup extends only a short distance beyond the equator of the lens. About the fourth month the cup grows forward with an attachment to the mesenchyme. The mesenchyme in the pupillary area then atrophies as far back as this attachment, which forms the collarette. The collarette is concentric with the pupillary margin and marks the position of the minor vascular circle of the iris.

Inner coat

Retinal pigment epithelium.—The outer layer of the optic cup forms the retinal pigment epithelium. Initially, it is some four to six cells thick (32 postovulation days), but with cytolysis of these cells the pigment epithelium becomes deeply pigmented and a single cell layer thick. This cytolysis may influence the stratification of the sensory retina. Because the sensory retina grows at a different rate, the two layers are not in apposition until the stratification of the sensory retina is complete.

Sensory retina.—The sensory portion of the retina develops from the inner portion of the optic cup. It consists, as does the neural tube, of three zones (ependymal, mantle, and marginal) limited by a terminal bar net on the side of the retinal pigment epithelium, and by a basement membrane on the inner side. Because of invagination of the optic cup, the basement membrane is on the surface closest to the vitreous cavity and the terminal bars of Müller fibers on the surface closest to the retinal pigment epithelium. The basement membrane provides the internal limiting lamina of the retina.

The ependymal zone develops cilia that project into the vesicle between the inner and outer walls of the optic cup; these develop into cone and rod outer segments. The central mantle layer develops into the primitive neuroepithelium, which is divided into an outer and inner neuroblastic layer. The outer neuroblastic layer contains nuclei of rods and cones and bipolar and horizontal cells. The inner neuroblastic layer contains ganglion cells, amacrine cells, and Müller cells. The marginal zone develops into the nerve fiber layer (and a transient, nonnucleated layer of Chievitz).

Development proceeds from the posterior pole toward the periphery. The specialized area, the fovea centralis, is identifiable at 22 weeks, but its development proceeds slowly. Anatomic differentiation continues after birth, and the human fovea reaches maturity between 15 and 45 months after birth. It is evident that functional differentiation lags behind anatomic differentiation.

LENS

The tip of the optic vesicle, as it extends laterally, is covered by surface (head) ectoderm. During a brief interval, the ectodermal and vesicular basement membranes adhere to each other. This adherence is followed by elongation of ectodermal cells over the zone of contact to form a lens placode. As the optic vesicle invaginates to form an optic cup, the lens placode invaginates to form a lens cup, the lumen of which is continuous with the surface of the embryo through the lens pore. The lens pore decreases in size until the residual surface ectoderm (the presumptive corneal epithelium) becomes smooth and the lens cup is connected to the surface ectoderm by a solid lens stalk. The stalk attenuates so that the lens cup separates from the surface ectoderm and the basement membrane surrounding the lens cup (anlage of lens capsule) closes completely to envelop the lens cup.

Further maturation of the lens requires a healthy developing neural retina with appropriate positioning of the lens and the rim of the optic cup (presumptive ciliary epithelium). Elongation of the cells on the wall of the lens cup adjacent to the vitreous cavity side of the lens obliterates the lumen of the lens cup. As the apices of the elongating cells (primary lens fibers) approach the presumptive lens epithelial cells on the wall of the lens adjacent to the anterior chamber, they send out processes that are followed by gap junctions between apposed surfaces.

Subsequent fibers (secondary lens fibers) are formed by cells located anteriorly, while the primary lens fibers lose their nuclei when the base of the lens fiber loses contact with the posterior capsule. As secondary fibers form their lateral surfaces, they associate with adjacent fibers by gap junctions, desmosomes, and ball-and-socket interdigitations. As additional lens fibers are laid down and then displaced from contact with the posterior capsule, they meet base to base near the posterior pole to form the inverted Y-shaped posterior suture and apex to apex to form the erect Y-shaped anterior suture.

The nuclei migrate to the equator where secondary lens fibers continue to develop throughout life.

With the development of the ciliary processes, zonular fibers are deposited between the ciliary epithelium and the capsule at the lens equator (12 weeks after ovulation).

VITREOUS HUMOR

The vitreous humor consists of primary or hyaloid vitreous, secondary or definitive vitreous, and tertiary vitreous of the suspensory zonule of Zinn. The primary vitreous begins with protein-rich, PAS-positive material that forms between the lens placode and optic vesicle about the 36th postovulation day. Vascularized mesoderm enters the optic fissure, and by the seventh week the hyaloid artery is developed and reaches the lens. By the ninth week the hyaloid system is fully developed. The hyaloid system begins to resorb about the fifth month, no longer carries blood after the seventh month, and is absent after birth except for its remnant, the canal of Cloquet.

The secondary or definitive vitreous appears about the seventh week as the retinal fissure closes and gradually fills the vitreous cavity as the hyaloid system resorbs. It is apparently of neuroectodermal origin.

The tertiary vitreous, the zonule of Zinn, begins to form in the sixth month. Eventually fibers insert into the basement membrane of the ciliary epithelium and the lens capsule.

BLOOD SUPPLY

The retinal fissure extends to about the anterior one third of the optic stalk. About the end of the first month (when the fetus is 7 to 8 mm), an arterial plexus below the optic cup consolidates into (1) a hyaloid artery that enters the optic nerve and cup through the fissure, and (2) a small annular vessel that ramifies on the rim of the cup and eventually becomes the choroid.

The hyaloid artery forms a network of vessels covering the back of the lens (tunica vasculosa lentis) and filling the vitreous body (vasa hyaloidea propria). The hyaloid system begins to resorb after the fifth month.

The vascular return of the entire hyaloid system is by the capsulopupillary membrane that covers the lens from the equator to the edge of the pupil. As the hyaloid system atrophies, the pupillary membrane is supplied by the long posterior arteries. It continues to develop until early in the sixth month, when the arteries begin to atrophy and disappear.

At about 14 to 15 weeks of gestational life (70 to 110 mm), mesenchymal cells appear in the vicinity of the hyaloid artery. They proliferate into the optic disk and subsequently invade the nerve fiber layer of the retina. The mesenchymal cells differentiate into endothelial cells that form solid cords, which gradually canalize to become capillaries. Thus, arteries and veins originate from capillaries and not the reverse. The growth progresses from the optic disk, and blood vessels reach the ora serrata 39 weeks after gestation, an important factor in retinopathy of prematurity.

A wide variation in orbital blood vessels occurs, mainly because of failure of early branches to disappear. Portions of the pupillary membrane commonly persist over the pupillary aperture, and persistence of the hyaloid artery is common. It extends a variable distance from the optic disk into the vitreous cavity, sometimes as far as the lens. It may form a small opacity (the Mittendorf dot) on the posterior lens capsule. The Bergmeister papilla is a glial sheath that surrounds the first one third of the hyaloid artery. It may persist in the adult as a small tuft of tissue replacing the physiologic optic cup of the optic disk.

The optic stalk provides the neuroglial supporting structures of the optic nerve. The nerve fibers consist of axons of ganglion cells located in the inner layer of the retina together with fibers extending from the brain to the retina. The sheaths and septa of the optic nerve develop from mesoderm.

THE EYELIDS

The eyelids are derived from both the surface ectoderm and the mesoderm. The upper eyelid develops from the frontonasal process in medial and lateral portions. The mesodermal portion of the lower eyelid originates from an upgrowth of the maxillary process. The surface ectoderm provides both the exterior skin and the internal conjunctiva. The eyelids grow together and fuse at approximately 9 weeks, and they do not reopen until the seventh month. The tarsal plate, muscles, and connective tissues of the eyelids are derived from mesoderm. The glands and the cilia originate from the ectoderm.

LACRIMAL APPARATUS

The lacrimal gland develops from the ectoderm forming the conjunctival surface of the eyeball. Once formed, it receives connective tissue septa and supporting structures from the mesoderm.

The lacrimal passages develop in a cleft between the lateral nasal and maxillary processes. This cleft is converted into a tube by canalization of a solid rod of ectodermal tissue cells found beneath the surface, and these epithelial cells form the lacrimal passages. The lacrimal puncta do not open into the eyelid margins until just before the eyelids separate during the seventh month. The lower ends of the nasolacrimal ducts frequently do not open into the nose until birth or shortly thereafter.

BIBLIOGRAPHY

Books

Cogan DG: *Neurology of the visual system,* Springfield, Ill, 1980, Charles C Thomas.

Daw NW: *Visual development,* New York, 1995, Plenum Press.

Dutton JJ: *Atlas of clinical and surgical orbital anatomy,* Philadelphia, 1994, WB Saunders.

Hargrave PA, editor: *Photoreceptor cells. Methods in neurosciences,* vol 15, San Diego, 1993, Academic Press.

Platzer W, editor: *Pernkopf anatomy. Atlas of topographic and applied human anatomy, vol 1, Head and neck,* Baltimore, 1989, Urban & Schwarzenberg.

Rohen JW, Yokochi C: *Color atlas of anatomy. A photographic study of the human body,* ed 3, New York, 1995, Igaku-Shoin Medical Publishers.

Rootman J, Stewart B, Goldberg RA: *Orbital surgery,* Philadelphia, 1995, Lippincott-Raven.

Articles

Matsuo T: The genes involved in the morphogenesis of the eye, *Jpn J Ophthalmol* 37:215-251, 1993.

Mets MB, Smith VC, Pokorny J, Pass A: Postnatal retinal development as measured by the electroretinogram in premature infants, *Doc Ophthalmol* 90:111-127, 1995.

Natori Y, Rhoton AL Jr: Microsurgical anatomy of the superior orbital fissure, *Neurosurgery* 36:762-775, 1995.

Onda E, Cioffi GA, Bacon DR, Van Buskirk EM: Microvasculature of the human optic nerve, *Am J Ophthalmol* 120:92-102, 1995.

Strek W, Strek P, Nowogrodzka-Zagorska M, Litwin JA, Pitynski K, Modonski AJ: Hyaloid vessels of the human fetal eye. A scanning electron microscopic study of corrosion casts, *Arch Ophthalmol* 111: 1573-1577, 1993.

Traboulsi EI: Developmental genes and ocular malformation syndromes, *Am J Ophthalmol* 115:105-107, 1993.

Wirtschafter JD, Lander T, Baker RH, Stevanoviç M, Kirsch J, Kirschen McLoon L: Heterogeneous length and in-series arrangement of orbicularis oculi muscle: individual myofibers do not extend the length of the eyelid, *Trans Am Ophthalmol Soc* 92:71-90, 1994.

2

PHYSIOLOGY AND BIOCHEMISTRY OF THE EYE

Vision is the process initiated when the outer segments of the retina convert the portion of the electromagnetic spectrum that constitutes visible light (400 to 700 nm) to an electrical signal. The electrical signal is elaborately processed by the retina and the brain to create images of the external world, useful to the viewer. This definition conceals enormously complex reactions. The light may be absorbed by more than 110 million rods and 6 million cones that transmit both excitatory and inhibitory nervous impulses, which may be modified some 10 billion times before the signal reaches the 10 million nerve fibers that form each optic nerve. The signal that reaches the brain is processed by more than 30 visual centers that interact with more than 300 centers in the cerebral cortex to create the constantly changing visual images of the external world. The two-dimensional image of each eye is fused to the three-dimensional world with its richness of detail, color, and movement.

The human eye is not equal to those of many species in specific functions. Nonetheless, it provides a wide spectrum of functions that are not duplicated in many orders. The change in shape of the lens in accommodation allows clear images of objects at different distances. The three different pigments of the outer segment disks of the cones initiate excellent color vision. The rhodopsin of the rod outer segments adapts the eye to decreased light intensity over a range of 1 to 100,000 times. The location of the eyes in humans in the front of the head and the decussation of axons from the nasal one half of each retina permit retinal correspondence (see Chapter 24) so that an object may be viewed with depth and solidity (stereopsis).

THE CORNEA

The cornea is a transparent tissue composed mainly of stroma (90%) that is covered externally with a regularly arranged stratified squamous epithelium and lined with a single layer of endothelial cells. The anterior epithelium is bathed by the tears, whereas the apices of the endothelial cells are bathed by the aqueous humor.

The anterior surface of the cornea is composed of stratified squamous epithelium five to six cell layers thick. It is divided into an anterior or squamous cell layer, a middle or wing cell layer, and a posterior basal or germinative cell layer. Cells in the basal cell layer are constantly reformed by mitotic division and move forward to be shed into the tear film 7 days later. The squamous cells are joined by tight junctions that exclude water and water-soluble substances. The microvilli of their anterior surface are coated with the mucin of the tear film.

The basal cells of the corneal epithelium are attached to a basement membrane that consists of a basal lamina and a reticular lamina. The basal lamina consists of a lamina lucida adjacent to the base of the epithelial cells and a lamina densa adjacent to the reticular lamina, or the Bowman zone of the substantia propria. The basal cells are attached to the basement membrane by hemidesmosomes, anchoring filaments, which terminate in the reticular lamina, and the adhesive glycoproteins laminin and fibronectin. The lamina densa is composed of type IV collagen and the anchoring filaments of the type VII collagen. The basement membrane is essential in attaching the epithelial layer to the underlying stroma. It does not regenerate after injury.

The corneal stroma in humans is composed of type I collagen (50% to 55%), type VI collagen (30% to 40%), and type V collagen (5% to 10%). Type III collagen may be present in the human fetal cornea and after injury. The stroma is composed of collagen fibers of uniform diameter gathered together in bundles (lamellae) arranged at right angles to each other. The lamellae are enmeshed in macromolecules, the proteoglycans in which high-molecular-weight glycosaminoglycans are linked to a core protein. Acetylglucosaminoglycan, in which keratan sulfate is the amino sugar, and acetylgalactosaminoglycan, in which chondroitin 4 (6) sulfate (dermatan/chondroitin sulfate) is the amino sugar, act as anions and bind cations and water.

The Descemet membrane, which separates the corneal stroma from the endothelium, is composed of (1) granular basement membrane adjacent to the stroma; (2) wide-spaced collagen at the middle zone; and (3) granular basement membrane adjacent to the endothelium. The major collagen is type VIII (endothelial collagen) with a trace of type IV collagen.

The endothelium is a single layer of cells that rests on Descemet membrane and lines the cornea. It regulates the flow of electrolytes and fluid between the cornea and the anterior chamber. It constitutes the principal mechanism of corneal dehydration (deturgescence).

The central cornea is avascular and derives oxygen from the atmosphere and metabolic materials by diffusion from the tears and aqueous humor. Only the peripheral cornea receives adequate nutrients from the pericorneal capillaries.

Transparency

The cornea transmits electromagnetic radiation having a wavelength* of between 365 nm in the ultraviolet and 2,500 nm in the infrared. Transmission is about 80% at 400 nm and 100% at 500 to 1,200 nm. There are two areas of absorption beyond 1,200 nm, but transmission of long wavelengths is otherwise high. Electromagnetic radiation of wavelengths of more than 700 nm does not stimulate the retinal receptors and is dissipated as heat by the retinal pigment epithelium. Ultraviolet radiation below 365 nm is mainly absorbed by the cornea; the transmitted portion is absorbed by the lens and does not reach the retina unless the intensity is very high (lasers can deliver energy at this high intensity).

The transparency of the cornea is the result of the following: (1) its regular anatomic structure; (2) the tight junctions of the epithelial cells that are not permeable to aqueous solutions; and (3) the dynamic balance between ions and water in the stroma that is maintained by an endothelial pump mechanism that provides corneal dehydration (deturgescence).

The anatomic factors include the absence of blood vessels and pigment in the cornea, the regular arrangement of the epithelial and endothelial cells, and the scarcity of cell nuclei in the stroma. Additionally, the epithelial cells are not keratinized, and the anterior surface of the tear film forms a regular refracting surface. The epithelial and endothelial cells do not reflect light at their interfaces because they have the same index of refraction.

The collagen fibrils of the corneal stroma have an index of refraction of 1.47; that of the surrounding proteoglycans is about 1.34. This difference should produce considerable scattering of light, causing the cornea to be more translucent than transparent. The collagen fibers are, however, oriented in a two-dimensional lattice, with the distance between each fiber approximately equal. Each fibril has a diameter of less than one wavelength of light, so that the lattice is transparent in the direction of an incident beam. The portion of the light that strikes the lattice itself is eliminated by destructive interference.

Relative dehydration (deturgescence) of the stroma is necessary for transparency. Each corneal lamella contains about 75% of the water it is capable of binding. A button of cornea with the stroma exposed swells to about three times its normal thickness and becomes trans-

*The wavelength of electromagnetic energy is designated as nanometers (one billionth of a meter; $m \times 10^{-9}$). Old units included Angstrom units (one ten-billionth of a meter; $m \times 10^{-10}$) and millimicrons, which are the same as nanometers.

lucent. If the endothelium is poisoned with ouabain, cyanide, or iodoacetate, similar swelling occurs. Disease or injury of the epithelium or endothelium causes a corneal edema. The epithelium rapidly replicates itself, and the swelling is transient. The endothelium in humans does not replicate, but the cells increase in size to cover defects. After endothelial damage or in endothelial dystrophy, severe swelling of the stroma and epithelium (bullous keratopathy) occurs (see Chapter 11). The endothelium constantly removes water and ions from the stroma and balances the entry of fluid and ions from the aqueous humor. Additionally, fluid leaks from the stroma into the aqueous humor, predominantly across the endothelium itself.

The blood-ocular barriers

The eye has two barriers that prevent the entry of macromolecules, chiefly proteins, into the eye: (1) the blood-aqueous barrier and (2) the blood-retina barrier.

The blood-aqueous barrier is formed by the nonpigmented layer of the epithelium of the ciliary body and the endothelium of the blood vessels of the iris. The apices of the cells of the nonpigmented epithelium of the ciliary body are joined by zonulae occludentes (tight junctions), which fuse adjacent cells together. The junctions prevent the passage of large molecules, but ions and solutes of low molecular weight pass freely ("leaky" tight junctions). The endothelium of blood vessels of the iris have similar tight junctions. After injury and during inflammation, the blood-aqueous barrier breaks down and protein enters the eye freely.

The blood-retina barrier is formed by the retinal pigment epithelium and the endothelium of the retinal blood vessels. Adjacent cells of each are joined by tight junctions (zonulae occludentes).

Permeability

The metabolic needs of the peripheral cornea are met by the capillary network of the corneoscleral limbus. The nutrition of the central cornea, however, depends on substances that enter through either the endothelium or the epithelium. To penetrate the epithelium a substance must be water-soluble to penetrate the film of tears covering the cornea. The epithelium constitutes the principal barrier of the cornea to ions. The zonulae occludentes and adherentes and maculae occludentes and adherentes of the epithelium make it impermeable to ions and other lipid-insoluble substances. The corneal epithelium is readily permeable to lipid-soluble substances because the cell membranes are composed of a lipoprotein. To pass through the stroma and endothelium the compounds must be water-soluble. Thus, topical medications must be both water- and lipid-soluble to penetrate the normal cornea.

Metabolism

The cornea requires energy (1) to supply its metabolic needs, (2) for continued mitotic activity of the epithelium, and (3) to regulate the flow of fluid and ions through the endothelium. The epithelium, with 15 to 20 times more cells than the remainder of the cornea, is the major site of metabolic activity. The few cells of the endothelium, however, are considerably more active than the more numerous cells of the epithelium. The central cornea derives glucose from the aqueous humor and oxygen from the atmosphere, while the peripheral cornea is nurtured by the corneoscleral capillaries.

Glucose is first phosphorylated to glucose-6-phosphate by the enzyme hexokinase, which uses energy from adenosine triphosphate (Fig 2-1). Glucose-6-phosphate may be metabolized in one of several pathways: (1) glycolysis (Embden-Meyerhof), which yields pyruvate; (2) pentose phosphate pathway; and (3) glycogen synthesis, a storage form that may be found in the basal cells. Pyruvate, in the absence of oxygen, is converted by lactate dehydrogenase to lactic acid and excreted into the tears. When oxygen is present, pyruvate is converted to coenzyme A, which is used in the tricarboxylic acid (Krebs) cycle. Excessive amounts of glucose may enter the sorbitol pathway, an important cause of cataract in diabetes mellitus and of increasing significance in disorders of the corneal epithelium in patients with diabetes mellitus.

The glycolysis pathway requires no oxygen and converts 1 mol of glucose-6-phosphate to 2 mol of pyruvate and yields 2 mol of adenosine triphosphate. In the presence of oxygen, the pyruvate is decarboxylated to acetylcoenzyme A

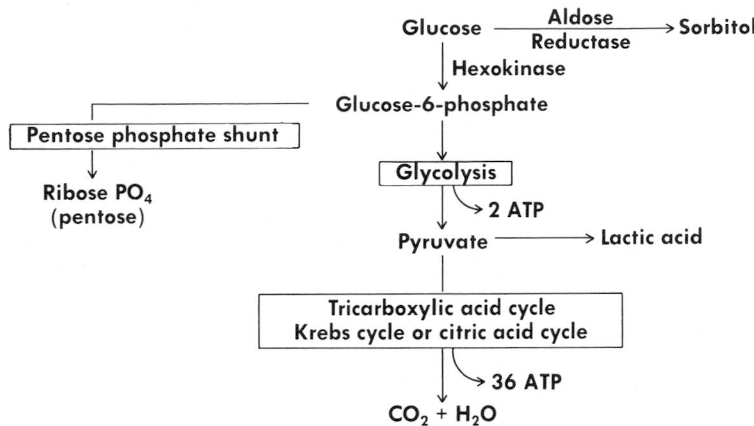

FIG 2-1.

A simplified schema of the metabolism of glucose in tissues. The aldose reductase pathway that forms sorbitol (an alcohol) from glucose (an aldehyde) is active only when an excess of glucose is present. This pathway is important in the retinopathy and the neuropathy of diabetes mellitus and in the formation of "sugar cataract." Glycolysis (Embden-Meyerhof) does not utilize oxygen and is the major metabolic pathway of lens epithelium, which is the major source of lactate in the aqueous humor. The pentose phosphate shunt provides the ribose-6-phosphate for nucleic acid synthesis and reduced nicotinamide adenine dinucleotide phosphate (NADPH) for which both hexokinase and aldose reductase compete. The major energy-producing pathway is the tricarboxylic acid cycle, which requires oxygen. The major metabolism of the cornea is in the epithelium, which has 15 to 20 times more cells than the stroma and endothelium.

and, in a series of reactions in the tricarboxylic acid cycles, is converted to carbon dioxide and water. It provides 36 mol of adenosine triphosphate from each 1 mol of glucose and is the main energy source of the cornea.

The pentose phosphate pathway provides a five-carbon sugar essential to the mitotic activity of the equatorial cells of the lens fibrils and supplies reduced nicotinamide adenine dinucleotide phosphate (NADPH). The pathway maintains ascorbate and glutathione in the reduced state and protects the cells from the oxidative effects of free radicals (molecules containing an unpaired electron, such as the superoxide anion [O_{2-}] and peroxides).

TEARS

The exposed surface of the eye is moistened by the precorneal tear film and the conjunctival tear film. The tear film functions to (1) lubricate the eyelids; (2) cover the irregular corneal surface with a smooth optical surface; (3) supply antibacterial protection; (4) transfer nutrients to the corneal epithelium; and (5) dilute and eliminate irritants. When the cornea is infected, the tears transport granulocytes to the cornea.

The normal eye is moistened mainly by tears secreted by the accessory lacrimal glands of Krause (65%) and Wolfring (35%). These constitute some 10% of the lacrimal gland mass. The glands contain many plasma cells that are independent of antigenic stimulation, as is the lymphoid tissue in the gut. The orbital and palpebral lobes of the lacrimal glands secrete mainly in crying (psychic stimulation), after injury or other stimulation of the trigeminal nerve, and in disease (reflex tearing). Tears flow mainly in the conjunctival cul-de-sac and along the margin of the eyelids (marginal tear strip). Periodic blinking spreads the tears over the surface of the globe and creates a slight suction at the lacrimal puncta.

Orbicularis oculi muscle fibers (N VII) surround the lacrimal puncta and insert into the periosteum of the anterior and posterior lacrimal crests. Blinking draws the puncta nasally, shortens the canaliculi, and forces tears into the lacrimal sac. Contraction of the orbicularis oculi muscle expands the lacrimal sac, creating a

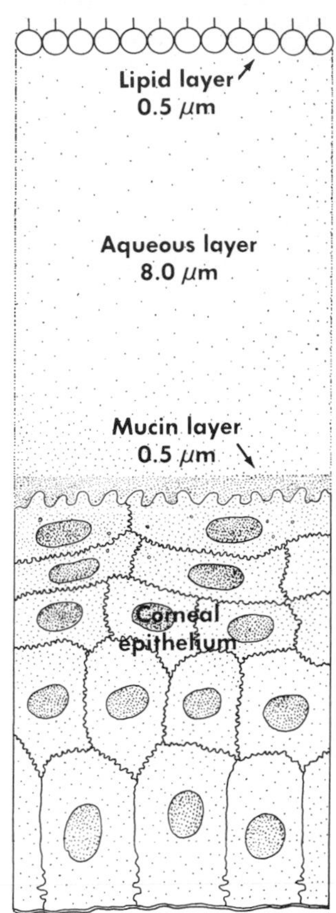

FIG 2-2.
Schema of the precorneal tear film. The mucin layer wets the microvilli of the corneal epithelium.

partial negative pressure to draw in tears. The pumping action of the orbicularis oculi muscle is essential for normal tear drainage.

The corneal epithelium is covered by a relatively stagnant layer of tears, the precorneal tear film. The precorneal tear film is composed of three layers (Fig 2-2): (1) a thin (0.9 to 0.2 μm), anterior lipid layer derived from the meibomian glands, sebaceous glands of Zeis, and sweat glands of Moll; (2) a thick (6.5 to 7.5 μm), middle aqueous layer derived from the accessory lacrimal glands of Krause and Wolfring; and (3) a thin mucin layer derived from conjunctival goblet cells and minimally from lacrimal gland cells. The lipid layer retards the evaporation of tears and provides a smooth and regular anterior optical surface. The mucin layer wets the microvilli of the corneal epithelium and must be intact to retain the precorneal film. A deficiency of mucin occurs in avitaminosis A and scarring of the conjunctiva. An excess of mucin occurs in hyperthyroidism and excessive tearing. The normally acidic glycosoaminoglycans become neutral in corneal inflammation secondary to drying (keratitis sicca; see Chapter 13).

The average normal secretion of tears is between 0.9 and 2.2 μL/min. The maximum capacity of the cul-de-sac is about 30 μL, so that tears overflow if the rate of drainage does not increase with the rate of secretion. Once the rate of tear secretion exceeds 100 μL/min, tearing occurs.

With the eyes open and the precorneal oily film intact, a maximum of 0.85 μL of tears evaporates each minute, and the remainder passes through the lacrimal passages. The evaporation causes the tears to become slightly hypertonic, so that there is a minute osmotic flow of water from the anterior chamber, through the cornea, to the tear film. In sleep the precorneal tear film is in osmotic equilibrium with the aqueous humor, no osmotic flow occurs, and the corneal stroma thickens.

The collection of tears to determine their composition is complicated by evaporation and the dilution that follows stimulation. The anterior lipid layer probably reflects the composition of the meibomian gland secretion and includes mainly wax esters, cholesterol esters, and phospholipids. The aqueous phase is 98% water and 2.0% solids. Sodium and bicarbonate levels parallel the plasma levels, whereas potassium and chloride levels exceed plasma levels. Urea, amino acids, and other small molecules parallel the plasma levels, whereas the glucose content is markedly lower. There is a large amount of protein, averaging approximately 7 mg/mL. The concentration decreases in aging. The protein includes a unique tear-specific prealbumin that buffers the tear system. Additionally, lactoferrin and lysozyme are secreted by the lacrimal gland.

Immunoglobulin A (IgA) and secretory (exocrine) IgA1 and IgA2 are the major immunoglobulins of the tears. Secretory IgA is composed of two IgA molecules synthesized by plasma cells in the main and accessory lacrimal glands and bound together by a secretory piece produced within the epithelial cells of lacrimal glands. IgA neutralizes viruses and inhibits bacterial adherence to the conjunctival surface. IgG is the second major immunoglobulin of tears and probably diffuses through conjunctival capillaries. It promotes phagocytosis and complement-mediated bacterial lysis. Both increase in conjunctival inflammations. Immunoglobulin E increases in allergic inflammations.

Lactoferrin occurs in tears, many mucosal secretions, bile, and human (and bovine) milk. It chelates iron and may deprive microorganisms of iron. It is bactericidal to *Bacillus subtilis, Staphylococcus aureus* and *S. epidermidis,* and *Pseudomonas aeruginosa.* Lactoferrin may extend the lytic action of lysozyme to otherwise insensitive bacteria. Additionally, it may react with specific antibody to produce an antimicrobial system more powerful than lactoferrin or specific antibody does singly. It modulates complement activity in vitro.

Lysozyme (muramidase) is an antibacterial enzyme that is widely distributed in nature (hen's eggs are the commercial source). It causes lysis of the glycosaminoglycan coating of a few nonpathogenic gram-positive bacteria. In the presence of complement, it facilitates IgA bacteriolysis.

Periodic blinking and the tear flow provide barriers to microbial colonization of the external eye. Many protective substances are present in tears, including immunoglobulins, lymphocytes, and complement. Nonspecific factors include phagocytic cells, lactoferrin, lysozyme (muramidase), nonlysozyme antibacterial factor, anticomplement factor, and interferon.

Basic tear formation has no apparent stimulus or specific innervation. Reflex tearing occurs in response to psychic stimuli (crying) and reflex stimulation of fibers of the ophthalmic division of the trigeminal nerve (N V_1). Application of heat to the tongue and mouth and uncomfortable retinal stimulation by bright lights cause reflex tearing. Normal moisture of the eye is maintained entirely by the basic secretion of accessory lacrimal glands; reflex secretion of tears constitutes an emergency or a psychic response.

Clinically, tear formation is measured by folding (see Fig 13-1) a strip of filter paper 5 mm wide over the middle portion of the lower eyelid. The amount of wetting that occurs in 5 minutes, as measured from the fold, indicates the volume of tears. Basic secretion is that which occurs after the eye is anesthetized with a topical anesthetic. Reflex secretion is measured without the use of a local anesthetic (there is no reflex wetting with general anesthesia). There is less tear formation after 50 years of age.

AQUEOUS HUMOR

The aqueous humor, the clear liquid of the anterior and posterior chambers, helps to maintain the intraocular pressure and to provide the metabolic needs of the avascular posterior cornea, the crystalline lens, and the trabecular meshwork. It is formed by the nonpigmented epithelium of the ciliary body by active transport (secretion) and by a diffusional exchange (movement of a substance across a membrane along its concentration gradient). Large protein molecules and blood cells are excluded by the blood-aqueous barrier. Specific transport systems of the nonpigmented ciliary epithelium remove organic ions from the aqueous humor of the posterior chamber.

Aqueous humor passes from the posterior chamber through the pupil into the anterior chamber. It leaves the eye chiefly through the trabecular meshwork, passing into the canal of Schlemm, and then into the deep scleral vascular plexus (Fig 2-3). In humans some 20% drains into the ciliary muscle spaces at the root of the iris and into the suprachoroidal space (the uveoscleral route).

Sodium, chloride, and bicarbonate are secreted across the nonpigmented epithelium of the ciliary body, possibly by an unknown linkage. The osmotic forces of these ions in the eye attract water. The nonpigmented epithelium of the ciliary body in many species contains membrane-bound Na, K-ATPase that facilitates the transport of potassium into cells and sodium out of cells. Inhibition of Na, K-ATPase by ouabain or vanadate decreases the secretion of aqueous humor. Metabolic poisoning of the nonpigmented epithelium of the ciliary body or reduction of its temperature to 19° C also decreases secretory activity.

An excess of bicarbonate is present in newly formed posterior chamber aqueous humor, but it is rapidly metabolized and diffuses into the surrounding ocular tissues. Bicarbonate is apparently deficient in anterior chamber aqueous humor of many species. The cell membranes and cytoplasm of the nonpigmented epithelium of the ciliary body contain carbonic anhydrase type II. Carbonic anhydrase inhibitors are used

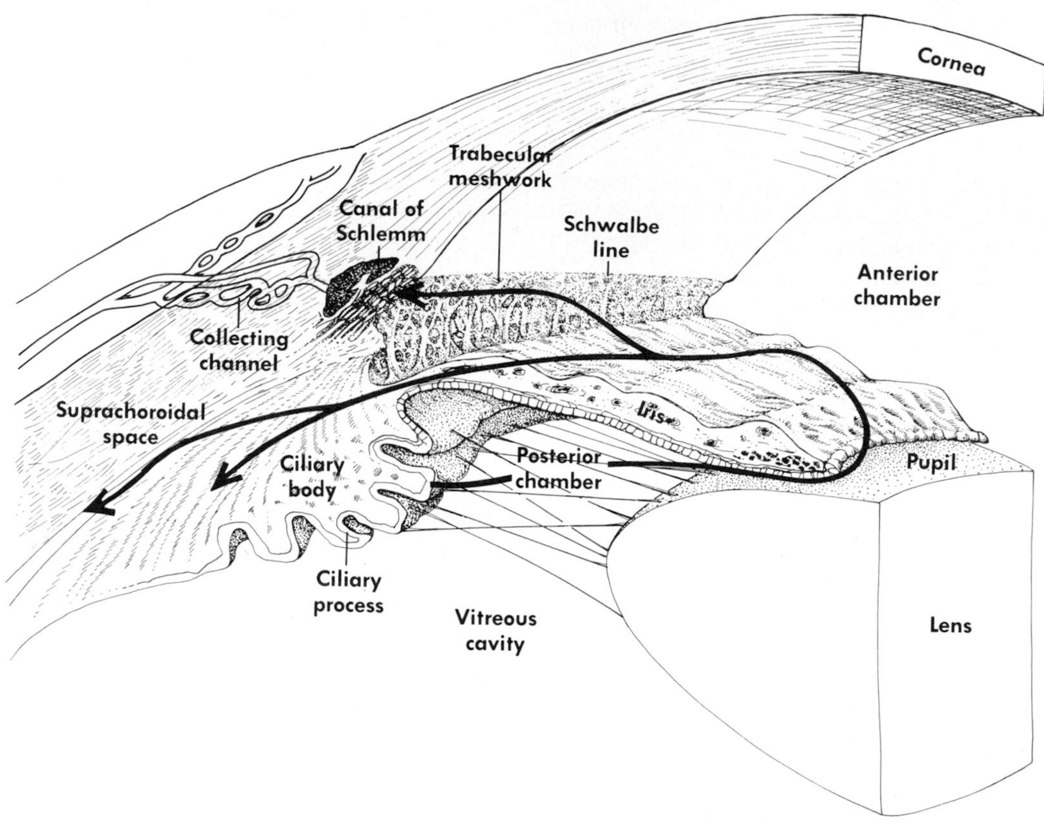

FIG 2-3.
Aqueous humor is secreted by the nonpigmented ciliary epithelium into the posterior chamber. It flows through the pupil into the anterior chamber and leaves the anterior chamber through the trabecular meshwork, which opens into the canal of Schlemm. In humans, about 20% of the aqueous humor leaves the eye through the suprachoroidal space and ciliary muscle spaces.

in glaucoma (see Chapter 22) therapy to lower the intraocular pressure and decrease the rate of entry of bicarbonate and water into the posterior chamber.

Glucose, potassium, oxygen, and some amino acids enter the posterior chamber aqueous humor by diffusional exchange. Lactate, pyruvate, and carbon dioxide are removed by the same route. Ascorbate, some sugars, and some amino acids are actively transported into the posterior chamber aqueous humor.

Two transport systems of the nonpigmented epithelium of the ciliary body actively remove substances from the posterior chamber aqueous humor. A hippuran system, similar to the organic anion system of the renal tubule, transports large anions such as fluorescein, penicillin, prostaglandins, and sulfates from the posterior chamber aqueous humor. Another system transports iodide compounds from the posterior chamber aqueous humor.

Ultrafiltration (dialysis under an applied pressure) favors the movement of water from the plasma into the stroma of the nonpigmented epithelium of the ciliary body, but inhibits the movement of water from the stroma into the posterior chamber. Possibly, ultrafiltration into the posterior chamber occurs in tandem with active transport, but, if so, the mechanism is obscure.

The blood-aqueous barrier is formed by the tight junctions of the nonpigmented epithelium of the iris and ciliary body combined with the tight junctions of the vascular endothelium of the iris. Lipid-soluble substances such as oxygen and carbon dioxide penetrate the barrier at a high rate. Sodium, larger water-soluble ions, proteins, and other large and medium-sized molecules are restricted. The aqueous humor of humans contains about 0.25 mg/mL of protein, mainly orosomucoid, transferrin, albumin, and IgG. The concentration of protein in the aqueous humor varies with the size of the protein molecule; thus, the blood-aqueous barrier is thought to have a pore size of about 104 nm. Injury or metabolic poisoning of the nonpigmented epithelium of the ciliary body or the blood vessels of the iris results in the aqueous humor having the same composition as plasma.

In humans, goats, and horses, the chloride content of the aqueous humor is higher than that of the plasma and the bicarbonate concentration is lower. In monkeys and dogs, both the chloride and bicarbonate concentrations are higher. In rabbits, the chloride content is lower and the bicarbonate is higher than in the plasma. The higher bicarbonate concentrations presumably buffer metabolic lactic acid, the end product of glycolysis, in eyes with a low rate of flow of aqueous humor and a large crystalline lens.

The concentration of ascorbate is 10 to 50 times higher in the aqueous humor than in the plasma. Glutathione concentration is higher than in the plasma, but not higher than in whole blood, where nearly all glutathione is contained in the erythrocytes. The ascorbate and glutathione protect against injury by the oxidative effects of free radicals and peroxides, which are enhanced by light.

The normal rate of flow of aqueous humor in humans is 2 to 3 μL/min. Many drugs depress the secretion. Beta-adrenergic antagonists reduce the rate by 17% to 47%. Carbonic anhydrase inhibitors reduce aqueous formation by about 40% and decrease the rate of appearance of bicarbonate and water in the posterior chamber. Sedatives and anesthetics depress the formation of aqueous humor. Systemic ouabain, an Na, K-ATPase (sodium, potassium-adenosine, triphosphate) inhibitor, also decreases its formation.

INTRAOCULAR PRESSURE

The pressure within the eye must exceed that of the surrounding atmosphere to prevent collapse of the eye. Normal intraocular pressure is between 10 and 20 mm Hg greater than atmospheric pressure. There is a variation of 1 to 3 mm Hg with each cardiac cycle, caused by fluctuation in the intraocular vascular volume, and there are slower variations with respiration. The intraocular pressure normally fluctuates by 2 to 5 mm Hg daily.

The three main factors concerned with the maintenance of intraocular pressure are the rate of formation of the aqueous humor, the ease with which the aqueous humor exits through the trabecular meshwork into the canal of Schlemm, and the pressure in the episcleral veins into which the canal of Schlemm empties.

Most (80%) aqueous humor drains from the anterior chamber through the trabecular meshwork and the endothelium of the canal of Schlemm. The trabecular meshwork functions as a one-way valve that permits bulk flow out of the eye but prevents flow into the eye. The site of the major resistance to outflow is debated. The channels in the trabecular meshwork are too large and too numerous to account for the resistance to outflow. The channels, however, are filled with glycosaminoglycans that might affect ion and fluid movement. In nonprimate eyes, perfusion with hyaluronidase decreases resistance, as does removal of the hyaluronidase-sensitive material by prolonged perfusion. Many studies suggest the major site of resistance to outflow is in the tight junctions of the endothelium of the canal of Schlemm. The aqueous humor may then traverse the endothelium through transcellular channels in the endothelial cells.

In addition to drainage through the canal of Schlemm and eventually into the episcleral veins, aqueous also drains from the eye near the root of the iris, into the anterior portion of the ciliary muscle, and into the space between the sclera and the ciliary body–choroid (the uveoscleral route). The aqueous humor then leaves the eye through the openings in the sclera for blood vessels and nerves and through the substance of the sclera itself. In humans some 5% to 20% of outflow is through this route. This outflow is increased by topical instillation of pilocarpine and decreased by atropine.

The pressure in the episcleral veins connected to the canal of Schlemm is approximately 10 mm Hg. If this pressure markedly increases, or if the pressure of the eye falls, there is a reflux of blood into the canal of Schlemm and increased resistance to outflow. Normally, however, the intraocular arterial and venous pressure and the volume of the arteries remain constant. Markedly increased venous pressure, as occurs in the Valsalva maneuver, is accompanied by a marked increase in intraocular pressure because of the dilation of intraocular veins. The intraocular pressure rapidly returns to normal when the Valsalva maneuver is stopped. Increased osmotic pressure of the blood brought about by administration of glycerol, mannitol, or urea decreases the intraocular pressure. Decreased osmotic pressure of the blood induced by rapid intravenous infusion of saline solution or by drinking a large quantity of water on an empty stomach causes a modest increase in intraocular pressure.

The intraocular pressure may be measured directly by a tonometer or by a pressure-sensitive membrane connected to the anterior chamber by a cannula that does not leak or disturb the flow of aqueous humor and the ocular vasculature. This type of measurement is done in humans only before enucleation of the eye.

Clinically the ocular tension is measured by determining the resistance of the eye to an applied force. Two main types of tonometer are used: (1) applanation instruments that determine the force required to flatten a standard area of the cornea and (2) indentation instruments that measure the indentation of the cornea in response to a weight applied to the cornea. The standard applanation instrument is the Goldmann tonometer, which uses a prism to flatten the cornea and requires a biomicroscope. The Perkins and the Draeger instruments are similar in principles to the Goldmann tonometer and are portable. The standard indentation instrument is the Schiøtz tonometer, which estimates the intraocular pressure by measuring the indentation of the cornea produced by a standard weight. (See Chapter 22, The Glaucomas.)

THE CRYSTALLINE LENS

The lens is derived from surface ectoderm. It is surrounded by a typical basement membrane, the capsule, that is secreted anteriorly by epithelial cells and posteriorly by lens fiber cells that have their nuclei in the nuclear bow. It is continuously renewed by the underlying epithelium and lens fibrils. The lens capsule is permeable to water and to small molecules, including horseradish peroxidase (40,000 daltons) but not ferritin (500,000 daltons). The capsule has no metabolic or enzymatic activity.

The anterior lens epithelial cells are firmly attached to the anterior lens capsule. The normal posterior capsule contains no anterior epithelial cells, and the nuclei of its cells are in the equatorial region. Epithelial cells originate in the anterior subcapsular region adjacent to the lens equator in the germinative zone. These cells migrate mainly to the equatorial region and then to the nuclear bow, where they increase in size and form lens fibrils. Lens fibers are arranged in onionlike layers, with the most recently formed lens fibers located in the peripheral layers near the equator and the oldest located centrally. Thus, the most central lens fibers (embryonic nucleus) are formed in early embryonic life. As the lens fibers age, they lose their cell nuclei and their attachment to the posterior capsule (their basement membrane), and are displaced toward the center of the lens by newly formed cells. This process continues throughout life, and the central portion of the lens (the nucleus of the crystalline lens) becomes increasingly compact.

The fully differentiated lens cell (fibril) has anterior and posterior processes. The processes consist of a protein matrix surrounded by a lipid bilayer membrane that interdigitates with adjacent processes through tongue-and-groove and ball-and-socket structures. The most recently formed lens fibers remain attached to their basement membrane, the posterior capsule.

The lens is held in position behind the pupil by means of zonular fibers. These attach to the anterior and posterior lens capsule in the equatorial region and to the valleys between ciliary processes. The fibers relax with contraction of the ciliary muscle, causing the refractive power of the lens to increase as its inherent elasticity causes it to become more spherical (accommodation).

Transparency.—The lens transmits almost 80% of electromagnetic energy between 400 and 1,400 nm. Small-angle x-ray and light-scattering techniques demonstrate that the spatial correlations between protein molecules of the lens crystallins account for the lens transparency. The nuclei of the single layer of epithelial cells beneath the anterior capsule are not numerous enough to impair transparency.

Despite the homogeneity of the lens structure, its total index of refraction is greater than any single portion. The increased index of refraction results from a concentric structure of layers in which the older central layers have a greater index of refraction than the surrounding younger layers.

The total refractive power of the lens is thus much greater than one would anticipate from its external curvature, thickness, and the index of refraction of individual layers. In a simplifying assumption in physiologic optics, the lens is considered to be composed of a central core with a high index of refraction that has a layer with a lower index of refraction on either side.

Metabolism.—The crystalline lenses of many different species are used to study metabolism, enzyme systems, protein synthesis, and cataract formation. It is difficult to relate the many studies of animals, birds, reptiles, and other species to humans because of the different sizes of the eye, the relative size of the lens to the eye, and their different life spans. The bovine, rabbit, and rat lenses initially grow rapidly, but growth slows in maturity; thus, there is little increase in weight in the second half of life. In contrast, the human lens grows slowly throughout life. The lens changes its shape and thickness for near and far vision (accommodation) only in humans and a few primates. The concentric layers of the human lens, called "zones of discontinuity," have no counterpart in other mammalian lenses. In middle life the color of the human lens slowly yellows, thus decreasing the amount of blue and violet light transmitted. Some of the yellow color may originate from low-molecular-weight derivatives of tryptophan found only in the human and primate lens. These pigments are fluorescent and absorb ultraviolet light maximally at the 360- to 368-nm wavelengths. The bovine, rabbit, and rat lenses do not metabolize tryptophan.

The periphery of the human lens is in close apposition to the tips of the ciliary processes and to the posterior aqueous humor, which has a composition that can only be inferred from animal studies. In fetal life the lens is surrounded by blood vessels, and its metabolism is mainly aerobic. These enzyme systems persist but are presumably inactive.

The proteins of the lens are divided into a water-soluble fraction, the crystallins, and a water-insoluble fraction. Three major crystallins occur in humans: alpha, beta, and gamma. The alpha molecule is the largest and first appears in embryonic life. It constitutes the embryonic nucleus of adult life. The alpha crystallins are composed of related proteins with similar properties but different molecular masses (600 to 900 kD), designated alpha A_1, alpha A_2, and alpha B_2. The beta crystallins compose the majority of human water-soluble crystallins. Their structures suggest that they have developed over eons of vertebrate evolution. Eight basic beta crystallins are divided into beta acidic and beta basic. The gamma crystallins are the smallest and least abundant of the water-soluble proteins. There are some six closely related gamma crystallins. They are possibly more important than the alpha and beta crystallins in maintaining the transparency of the lens.

Glucose penetrates the lens capsule through a carrier system of facilitated diffusion that constantly provides additional glucose. The glucose is converted to glucose-6-phosphate in a reaction catalyzed by hexokinase (see Fig 2-1). The hexokinase is present in a small amount that limits the phosphorylation of glucose. About 85% of the glucose-6-phosphate is metabolized in anaerobic glycolysis in which each molecule is converted to two molecules of pyruvate and two molecules of adenosine triphosphate. The remaining glucose-6-phosphate is metabolized through an aerobic pathway (pentose phosphate or hexose monophosphate shunt) that generates two reducing equivalents of reduced nicotinamide adenine dinucleotide phosphate (NADPH) per mole of glucose. NADPH is used to maintain glutathione in a reduced state, to maintain the supply of pentoses for nucleic acid synthesis, and in the conversion of glucose to sorbitol by aldose reductase.

In many respects the lens behaves as a large erythrocyte. Thus, it maintains a high intracellular potassium content although surrounded by aqueous humor and vitreous humor, both of which have high sodium contents. The lens epithelium of the anterior capsule maintains this gradient and actively transports sodium out of the lens by an Na, K-ATPase pump. The lens transports and accumulates potassium, amino acids, and ascorbic acid. It synthesizes inositol (a completely hydroxylated cyclohexane) and glutathione. With impairment of lens metabolism, sodium and water accumulate in the lens, and it loses potassium, glutathione, amino acids, and inositol.

Aging.—In humans the lens fibers are continuously displaced inward to become increasingly compact in the lens nucleus, which gradually increases in size. The central portion of the nucleus contains the proteins formed during embryonic life. After the age of 40 years, insoluble proteins continuously increase in the lens nucleus. Yellow pigment increases, the lipid composition changes, and the lens fiber membrane protein splits. The crystallin proteins lose sulfhydryl groups, form disulfide bridges, and accumulate high-molecular-weight aggregates. Free radicals are generated, glutamine and asparagine residues are deaminated, and there are many other changes. In many respects the normal changes of aging are identical to the changes of cataract.

Cataract.—Any loss of transparency of the lens is called a cataract. Cataracts are described as nuclear (central) and cortical (peripheral or anterior or posterior subcapsular). The capsule itself remains transparent except when lacerated or in some congenital abnormalities. Nuclear and cortical cataract may be the result of different mechanisms.

When the glucose (or galactose) concentration of the aqueous humor increases, the sugar content of the lens remains unchanged until the external content reaches 175 mg/mL, when control breaks down. The excess sugar is reduced by aldose reductase, an NADPH-dependent enzyme that catalyzes the first step in the pathway to form sorbitol, a polyol derived from glucose (and galactitol [dulcitol], a polyol derived from galactose). The second step is the oxidation of sorbitol to fructose by the enzyme polyol dehydrogenase, which uses oxidized nicotinamide adenine dinucleotide (NAD+) as a cofactor. Galactitol, unlike sorbitol, is not further metabolized.

Polyols do not penetrate membranes well and accumulate within the lens, attracting water that causes swelling of the lens fibers. The lens capsule stretches with a secondary electrolyte imbalance and the loss of amino acids. Aldose reductase is inhibited by many compounds, and it is often studied in experimental cataract. Aldose reductase is concentrated in the Schwann cells of peripheral nerves, the kidney papillae, and the retinal blood vessels. Some aldose reductase inhibitors have been used, without success, in the treatment of the neuropathy, nephropathy, and retinopathy of human diabetes mellitus.

Two types of cataract occur in human galactosemia: (1) hexose 1-phosphate uridyl transferase deficiency, the usual type; and (2) galactokinase deficiency, an uncommon type (see Chapter 21). These cataracts occur during the first 6 months of life as autosomal recessive conditions. Some cataracts in individuals 20 to 40 years of age may reflect a heterozygosity for one of these enzymes.

THE VITREOUS HUMOR

The vitreous humor is a transparent extracellular matrix that fills the posterior (vitreous) cavity of the eye. It is composed mainly of water (98% to 99.7%).

Collagen provides a framework, and hyaluronic acid (one molecule of glucuronic acid and one molecule of acetyl glucosamine) fills the interfibrillar space and provides viscoelastic properties. The vitreous base is firmly attached to the pars plana of the ciliary body and the peripheral retina in the region of the ora serrata. Posteriorly it attaches to the peripheral circumference of the optic disk. In some humans, it is attached to the sensory retina and to retinal blood vessels. Its anterior condensation, the anterior hyaloid, forms the lenticular fossa, a depression for the crystalline lens. The peripheral portion of the anterior hyaloid is attached to the periphery of the posterior lens capsule to form the annular hyaloideocapsular ligament (of Weigert). The attachment usually disappears by the age of 50 years.

The vitreous humor is composed of the following: (1) a cortical tissue layer, whose surfaces are condensed to form an anterior hyaloid adjacent to the lens and the posterior chamber and a posterior hyaloid adjacent to the inner limiting membrane of the retina; and (2) a central vitreous humor proper.

The *cortical tissue* is approximately 100 μm thick and surrounds the central vitreous humor proper. It contains fine fibrils composed of collagen, an accumulation of proteins, a high concentration of hyaluronic acid, and a few migrating monocytes from the blood. The collagen fibrils run approximately parallel to the surface of the vitreous humor. Until age 20 years, they attach to the internal limiting lamina of the retina and the ciliary body. After 20 years of age, such attachments occur only in the anterior one third of the vitreous cavity.

The *vitreous humor proper* is a true biologic and chemical gel. Its framework is composed of fine collagen fibrils. The spaces between the fibrils (the interfibrillar spaces) are filled with hyaluronic acid, which occurs in tissues with a high water content and forms a molecular network in the vitreous.

THE RETINA

The optic cup differentiates as two layers: (1) an outer layer, the retinal pigment epithelium, which at birth is one cell layer thick; and (2) an inner layer, the sensory retina, that consists of the photoreceptor cells, their synaptic connections, and the supporting glia. The terminal ends of the rods and cones and the apices of the cells of the retinal pigment epithelium are enmeshed in the interphotoreceptor matrix, which contains the interphotoreceptor retinoid-binding protein. This is synthesized by the photoreceptors and contains lysosomes from the pigment epithelium. It maintains contact between the two layers of the primitive optic cup and may function in visual transduction. All metabolites from the outer (nearest the sclera) portion of the sensory retina pass through the retinal pigment epithelial cells that are tightly adherent at their apices. These tight junctions (and those of the retinal blood vessels) provide the blood-retinal barrier. The bases of the cells of the retinal pigment epithelium have binding sites for retinol-binding protein (pro-albumin) that transports vitamin A from the choriocapillaris. The dendrites in the outer plexiform layer of the sensory retina mark the approximate division between metabolic support from the choriocapillaris through the retinal pigment epithelium and support by the branches of the central retinal artery.

Physiologically and biochemically the retina may be divided into (1) a light-detecting portion and (2) a signal-processing portion. The light-detecting portion functionally includes the retinal pigment epithelium and the layer of photoreceptor cells. The signal-processing portion consists of the inner layers of the retina that synapse with the axons of photoreceptors and propagate the nervous impulse. The light-detecting portion is nurtured by the choriocapillaris and uses two to three times more oxygen than the signal-processing portion. The signal-processing portion of the retina is nurtured by the capillary branches of the central retinal artery.

Metabolism.—The glucose and oxygen required by the inner layers of the sensory retina are derived from the retinal circulation, while the choriocapillaris nurtures the retinal pigment epithelium and photoreceptor cells. Glucose from the choriocapillaris is converted into glucose-6-phosphate through hexokinase in the pigment epithelium and diffuses to the ellipsoid of the photoreceptor cell. The mitochondria of the ellipsoid cells convert the glucose-6-phosphate rapidly to two molecules of glyceraldehyde (glycolysis), which is converted to two molecules of pyruvic acid. Oxygen is used mainly in the mitochondria of the ellipsoid in the tricarboxylic acid cycle, by which pyruvic acid is converted to carbon dioxide and water and produces adenosine triphosphate (ATP). Glycolysis provides so much pyruvic acid that some is converted to lactic acid even in the presence of adequate oxygen. The ATP provides the energy required to extrude sodium ions from the inner segment through an Na, K-ATPase pump. The ATP also provides energy for axonal transport, outer segment renewal, and biosynthesis of cell membranes.

The enzymes of the phosphogluconic acid pathway are concentrated in the rod and cone nuclei and provide the ribose required for ribonucleic acid synthesis. Müller cells store glycogen, but the quantity is not adequate to support retinal function more than briefly.

The rods and cones.—The rods and cones are the light-sensitive elements of the sensory retina. The rods function at lower levels of illumination (scotopic vision), whereas the cones are functional at medium and high levels of illumination (photopic vision) and in color vision. The cones are concentrated in the fovea centralis, where rods are absent (Fig 2-4). Rods are the main photoreceptors in the peripheral retina, which also contains scattered cones.

The human sensory retina contains about 110 million rods and 6 million cones. The optic disk has no photoreceptors and is a blind spot in

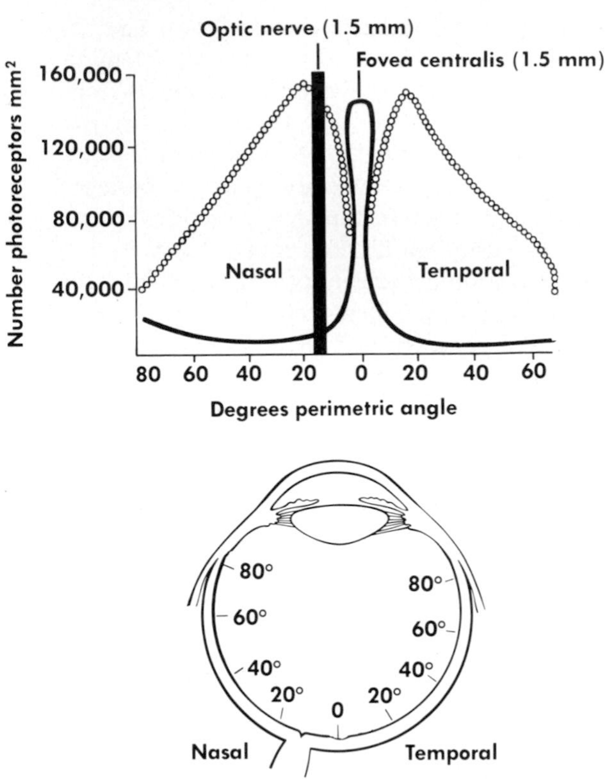

FIG 2-4.
The density of retinal rods and cones as a function of retinal location. The cones are concentrated in the fovea centralis (0°). The rod density peaks at about 20° from the fovea contralis and gradually diminishes to the retinal periphery. There are no rods at the fovea centralis.

the field of vision. The fovea centralis contains approximately 200,000 cones/mm^2. The remaining retina contains about 5,000 cones/mm^2. The rod density peaks about 3 mm (20°) from the fovea centralis at about 150,000 rods/mm^2 and then falls off less abruptly than the cone population to about 35,000 rods/mm^2 at the temporal periphery and 60,000 at the nasal periphery.

The outer segment of each rod and cone cell contains some 700 to 1,000 plasma membrane disks that contain the photopigments. The rod disks float in the cytoplasm and are surrounded by the cell plasma membrane. The cone disks are continuous with the surrounding plasma membrane (Fig 2-5). The inner segment of each photoreceptor cell contains intracellular organelles that synthesize new outer segment disks and a dense concentration of mitochondria.

The distal portions of the outer segments of rods and cones are removed diurnally by the phagocytic action of the pigment epithelium. Thus, the inner segment must constantly synthesize fresh outer segments. The turnover rate of rod outer segments is far more active than that of cone outer segments. Cone disks are shed shortly after the retina is darkened and synthesized during dark, whereas rod disks are shed shortly after the retina is illuminated and synthesized during light.

The axons of rods and cones synapse with horizontal cells and bipolar cells in the retinal outer plexiform layer. Horizontal cells connect photoreceptors (mainly rods) to each other. The axons of the bipolar cells synapse with amacrine cells and with dendrites of the ganglion cells in the inner plexiform layer. Amacrine cells, which have no axons, synapse with bipolar cell processes, dendrites of ganglion cells, and other amacrine cells. The nerve fibers of the retina are the axons of ganglion cells, which join at the optic disk to form the optic nerve.

The ratio of photoreceptors to ganglion cell axons and optic nerve fibers is not uniform. In the foveola, the approximately 150,000 cones are connected to twice that many ganglion cells. In the far periphery, there may be as many as 10,000 rods connected in clusters to a single nerve fiber. There is considerable overlap, so

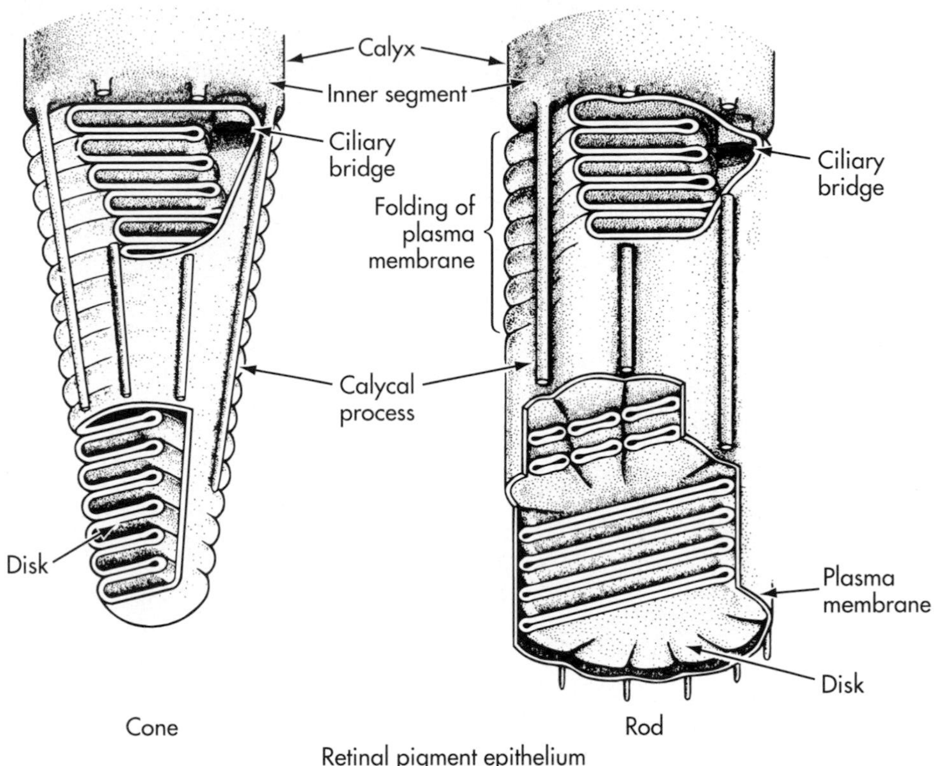

FIG 2-5.
The outer segment of the rod cell and the cone cell. Rod cells (or rods) provide for colorless (achromatic) vision in dim light and produce a measurable electrical signal in response to a single photon. Cone cells (or cones) serve for perception of color and fine detail and require fairly bright light. The rod disks are surrounded by a plasma membrane and the cone disks are continuous with their plasma membrane. They appear to operate on similar principles. (*After Fein A, Szuts EZ:* Photoreceptors: their role in vision, *New York, 1982, Cambridge University Press. Used by permission.*)

that a point of light may stimulate several clusters at once.

The retinal pigment epithelium.—The retinal pigment epithelium extends from the periphery of the optic nerve to the ora serrata, where it fuses with the sensory retina to form the pigment epithelium of the ciliary body. The base of each cell is adjacent to the cuticular layer of Bruch membrane, and the microvilli of its apices invest the outer segments of the rods and the cones. The terminal bars at the apex of each cell constitute the blood-retinal barrier between the freely permeable choriocapillaris and the sensory retina.

The retinal pigment epithelium has a major role in light signal perception: (1) it converts the shedded disks of the outer segments to residual bodies; (2) located at the base of the retinal pigment cell are retinol-binding protein sites, which transfer vitamin A from the blood to the cell where it is stored; (3) in phototransduction the retinal pigment epithelium isomerizes the conversion of all-*trans* retinal to 11-*cis* retinal; and (4) its melanin absorbs light energy and minimizes light scatter.

The retinal pigment epithelium exchanges metabolites and nutrients between the choriocapillaris and the outer layers of the sensory retina. It detoxifies drugs. The transport of fluids to the choriocapillaris contributes to the apposition of the retinal pigment epithelium to the sensory retina. It secretes the extracellular interphotoreceptor matrix, which contains as its major component the interphotoreceptor retinol-binding protein, which is synthesized by the retinal photoreceptor cells. Additionally, the retinal

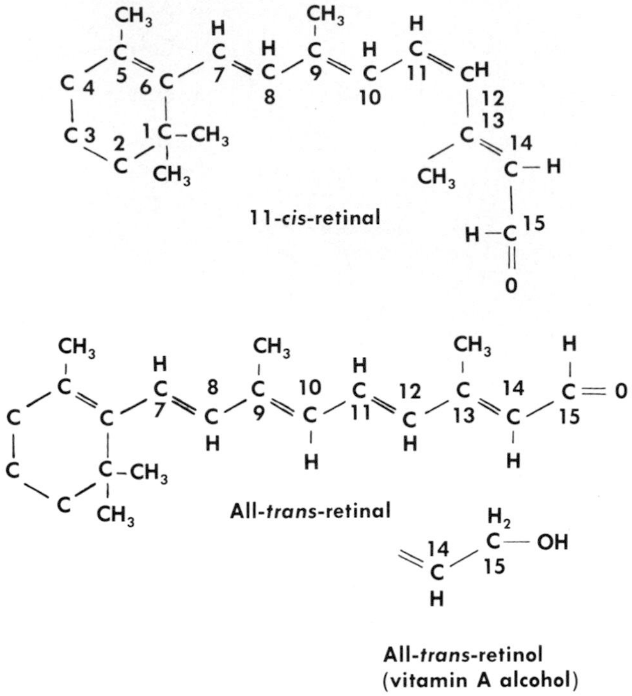

11-*cis*-retinal

All-*trans*-retinal

All-*trans*-retinol
(vitamin A alcohol)

FIG 2-6.
The 11-*cis* isomer of retinal (vitamin A aldehyde). The stereotoxic change from the 11-*cis* isomer to the all-*trans* isomer by light initiates the visual impulse. Vitamin A is an alcohol.

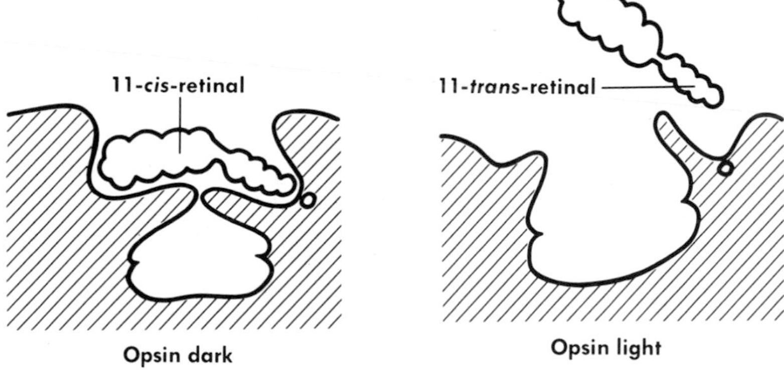

FIG 2-7.
The change in configuration of the rhodopsin molecule as it is activated by absorption of a photon of light.

pigment epithelium synthesizes the extracellular matrix that is located between it and Bruch membrane. After injury and inflammation the retinal pigment epithelium may proliferate.

Photochemistry of vision.—The visual impulse is initiated when a quantum of electromagnetic energy (a photon) transfers its oscillation to a molecule of a photopigment of a rod or a cone with which it shares the same natural frequency. The chromophore of the photopigment, 11-*cis* retinal, is changed to all-*trans* retinal with a substantial change in shape (Fig 2-6), which initiates a cascade of chemical reactions. The plasma membrane of the photoreceptor is hyperpolarized, which reduces the rate of release of the neurotransmitter (glutamate) by the synaptic vesicle of the photoreceptor cell. This reduced rate of neurotransmitter release either polarizes or hyperpolarizes the postsynaptic neurons of the retina, and an electrical signal is propagated to the brain where it is perceived as light.

Human photoreceptor disks contain four different photopigments (opsins), each tightly bound to 11-*cis* retinal, which is the aldehyde of vitamin A, an alcohol (retinol). Vitamin A com-

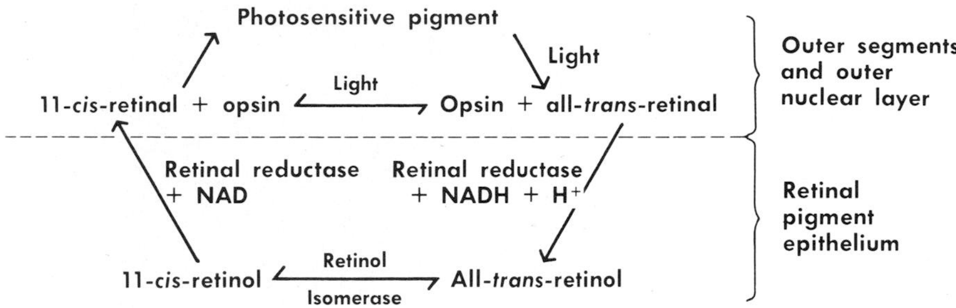

FIG 2-8.
Light absorption by the photoreceptor outer segments isomerizes 11-*cis* retinal to all-*trans* retinal, which disassociates it from opsin. New photosensitive pigment requires isomerization of all-*trans* retinal to 11-*cis* retinal. This occurs by further exposure to light or by a sequence of reactions in the retinal pigment epithelium. Initially, the all-*trans* retinal is reduced to all-*trans* retinol (an alcohol) by the action of retinal reductase and reduced nicotinamide adenine dinucleotide (+NADH + H). The all-*trans* retinol is converted to 11-*cis* retinol by the enzyme retinol isomerase. The 11-*cis* retinol is converted to the 11-*cis* retinal (aldehyde) by reductase and nicotinamide adenine dinucleotide (+NADH).

pounds have four carbon-carbon double bonds. The photopigments (opsins) can bind retinal only when the 11-12 position of the carbon atoms is in *cis* (on this side) position, and the other positions of the carbon atoms are all *trans* (across), the opposite of *cis* (Fig 2-7).

When a photon energizes a photopigment, the 11-*cis* retinal is isomerized to all-*trans* retinal, in a reaction that ultimately results in free opsin and all-*trans* retinal (Fig 2-8). For additional photopigment to be synthesized, the all-*trans* retinal must be isomerized to 11-*cis* retinal. The reaction follows (1) exposure to light in the photoreceptors or (2) a sequence of reactions catalyzed by two enzymes in the retinal pigment epithelium.

All-*trans* retinal (vitamin A_1) and retinol (vitamin A) are transported in the blood bound to a specific retinol-binding protein (proalbumin). The bases of the retinal pigment epithelium cells have specific protein receptor sites where the vitamin A is released to the cell and the carrier protein excluded. Dietary sources of vitamin A are from both the vitamin and carotenoids, particularly carotene, which are converted into vitamin A by enzymatic reactions in the intestinal mucosa and liver.

Human photoreceptor outer segment disks contain four different opsins (light-absorbing proteins). Rhodopsin, the photopigment of rods, has a maximum absorption at 496 nm, an absorption spectrum similar to that of the retina in dim illumination. The outer segments of cone disks contain one of three photopigments: (1) short-wavelength–sensitive (blue) with a maximum absorption of 419 nm; (2) middle-wavelength–sensitive (green) with a maximum absorption of 531 nm; and (3) long-wavelength–sensitive (red) with a maximum absorption of 559 nm.

Phototransduction.—The conversion of light energy to a nervous impulse has been studied mainly in rod rhodopsin, because it is the most abundant and easily available photopigment. The conversion mechanism in cone photopigments is likely similar. The initial step is the absorption of a photon of light by rhodopsin, which isomerizes 11-*cis* retinal to all-*trans* retinal and activates the rhodopsin molecule (Fig 2-9). The activated rhodopsin then activates transducin, a trimeric protein composed of alpha, beta, and gamma subunits. The activated rhodopsin binds to transducin-alpha inducing the exchange of its guanosine diphosphate for guanosine triphosphate and their separation from the inhibitory beta and gamma subunits.

The activated rhodopsin-transducin-alpha-guanosine triphosphate molecule then disassociates and frees the activated rhodopsin to activate additional transducin molecules.

The activated transducin-alpha-guanosine triphosphate molecule then activates the enzyme phosphodiesterase by binding to its two inhibitory gamma units. Phosphodiesterase-alpha-beta then hydrolyzes many molecules of cyclic-guanine-monophosphate, which keep

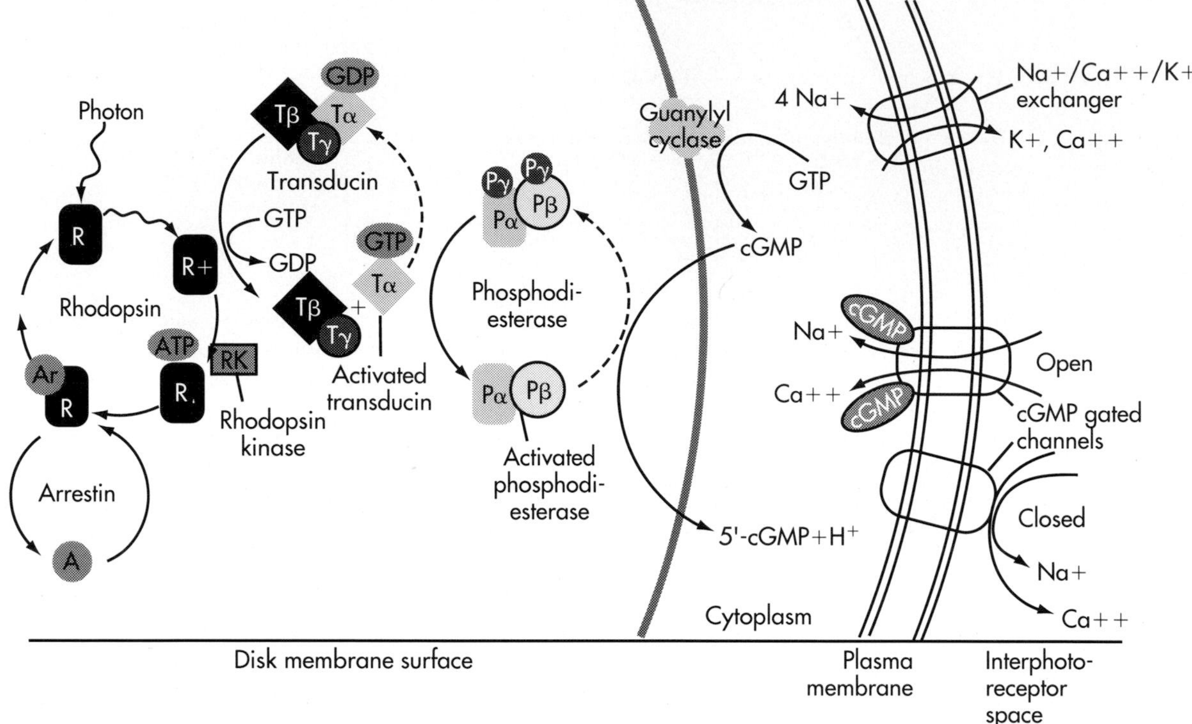

FIG 2-9.
The activation of rhodopsin by light and the biochemical cascade that results in hyperpolarization of the plasma membrane of the outer segment of the retina and a nervous signal. (*Adapted from Farber DB: From mice to men: the cyclic GMP phosphodiesterase gene in vision and disease,* Invest Ophthalmol Vis Sci *36:263-275, 1995.*)

gated-channels in the plasma membrane open in the dark. The cyclic-guanine-monophosphate gated-channels then close, which causes hyperpolarization of the plasma membrane and a change in the electrical signal sent to the inner segment. Closure of the ion channels causes a decrease in the ionic calcium (Ca2+) concentration in the outer segment cytoplasm because ionic calcium cannot enter but continues to be lost through the ionic sodium-calcium exchanger in the plasma membrane. The change in the electrical charge of the plasma membrane is transmitted to the inner segment and initiates the electrical signal interpreted by the brain as light.

Recovery requires that the channels in the plasma membrane reopen and that the cyclic-guanosine-monophosphate levels in the cytoplasm be restored. Recovery is initiated by inactivation of the energized rhodopsin molecule through phosphorylation by a rhodopsin kinase. The phosphorylation creates a binding site for the protein, arrestin (previously called S antigen), which inactivates the light-activated rhodopsin into its opsin and all-*trans* retinal. The activated transducin-alpha-guanosine triphosphate is inactivated by its endogenous GTPase activity, which hydrolyzes guanosine triphosphate to guanosine diphosphate. The quenched transducin molecules disassociate from the phosphodiesterase gamma subunits, which reunite with alpha, beta phosphodiesterase. The cyclic-guanine-monophosphate level of the cytoplasm is restored to its original level by the enzyme guanylate cyclase, the activity of which is enhanced by light stimulation and the reduced amount of intracellular ionic calcium. The ionic calcium concentration falls because of the closure of the plasma membrane cation channel combined with a continued efflux through the ionic sodium-calcium-potassium exchanger in the plasma membrane.

Synaptic transmission.—Synaptic transmission in the retina is both by direct contact and neural transmitters released by axons that react with receptors on the outside of the cell membrane of dendrites. These change the electrical potential of the membrane. Among the neural transmitters in the retina, dopamine, γ-aminobutyric acid, glycine, and taurine exert a depressant action on retinal neurons, whereas glutamate and aspartate excite or depress retinal neurons, depending on their concentration.

Axoplasmic transport.—Axoplasmic transport is the flow of metabolic substances from the nerve cell body through its axon. There are two components of axoplasmic transport: a slow component at a rate of approximately 1 mm a day, and a component 100 times faster. Most materials travel at both rapid and slow rates. Glycoproteins and sulfated glycosaminoglycans are transported almost completely by the rapid component. Rapidly transported material is largely in the membrane or particulate form that includes synaptic vesicles, mitochondria, and smooth endoplasmic reticulum. The slow component consists mainly of soluble protein.

The eyes of birds and goldfish have been used for study because a radioactive amino acid may be injected into the vitreous cavity in proximity to ganglion cells and because there is a complete decussation of optic fibers at the chiasm. Thus, after injection, radioactive-labeled material can be demonstrated in the contralateral optic tract and tectum. Rapid transport is in the circumferential portion of the axons, whereas slow flow progresses within the core of the axon. Rapid transport may be responsible for the movement of substances required at synaptic terminals, including the enzymes necessary for synthesis or destruction of transmitter substances. Slow components maintain and replenish material required for structural integrity of the axon.

Rapid axoplasmic transport is inhibited by anoxia, local anesthetics, and metabolic inhibitors such as sodium cyanide and dinitrophenol. Increased intraocular pressure may impede axonal flow, particularly the slow transport.

The retinal cotton-wool patch (histologically, a cytoid body) follows focal retinal ischemia, which causes localized edema of the axons of ganglion cells. The cotton-wool patch (see Chapter 17) contains aggregations of mitochondria, dense bodies, vesicles, and granules, which indicates interrupted axonal transport in the retinal nerve fiber layer. Papilledema (see Chapter 20) reflects impaired axonal flow at the optic disk.

Neural activity.—Vision is divided into surround (or ambient) vision and focal vision. Surround vision is mediated primarily by the peripheral retina and provides information concerning spatial localization. Focal vision is mediated primarily by the fovea centralis and subserves form perception, identification, and color vision.

The neural circuitry within the retina is complex. The signal from rods is received by rod bipolar cells and by horizontal cells. Cones stimulate two types of bipolar cells—flat and invaginating—and also *a* and *b* horizontal cells. Amacrine cells possibly serve bipolar and ganglion cells (Fig 2-10).

In lower species, neural function is mediated by at least three, and perhaps more, classes of ganglion cells. The X cells have sustained responses to stimuli, have axon conduction velocities of 9 to 14 m/sec, and are concentrated in the fovea centralis. X cells transmit luminance as well as color information. A separate neural channel for red-green information probably does not exist. The Y cells have transient responses to stimuli, have axon conduction velocities of 29 to 39 m/sec, and respond to rapid motions. The W cells appear to respond both to the beginning and to the ending of a flash of light throughout their entire receptive field. Other ganglion cells stimulate pupillary constriction.

Cats achieve spatial orientation with large ganglion cells (mainly Y and transient cells) and Y nerve fibers, which are connected not only with the visual cortex but also with the superior colliculus. Focal vision is sustained through the fovea centralis, using cones, small ganglion cells, and neurons (mainly X cells and sustained cells) that mainly extend to the lateral geniculate body and then to the visual cortex.

Additionally ganglion cells may be divided into two types on the basis of their response to a receptive field. A receptive field consists of the information gathered by a group of photoreceptors as transmitted to the ganglion cells. Receptive fields are organized in a concentric manner. They have a central region surrounded by a ring-shaped outer zone.

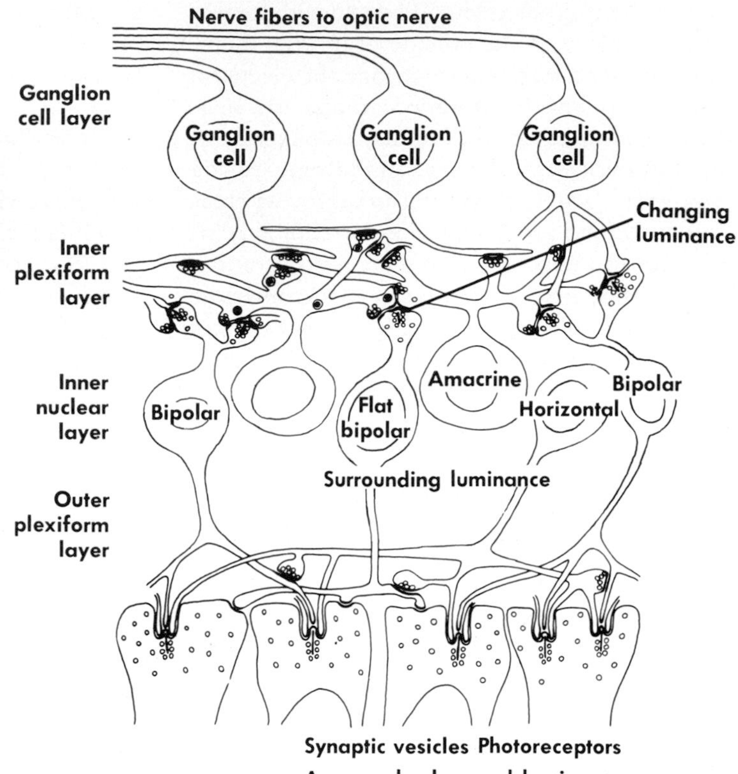

FIG 2-10.
Synaptic contacts found in vertebrate retinas. In the outer plexiform layer, processes from bipolar and horizontal cells penetrate into invaginations in the receptor terminals. The processes of flat bipolar cells make superficial contacts on the bases of some receptor terminals. Horizontal cells make conventional synaptic contacts on bipolar dendrites and other horizontal cell processes. In the inner plexiform layer, bipolar terminals may contact one ganglion cell dendrite and one amacrine process at a ribbon synapse or may contact amacrine cell processes. Amacrine processes in all retinas make synapses of the conventional type back onto bipolar terminals (reciprocal synapse). (*From Dowling J: Organization of vertebrate retinas,* Invest Ophthalmol Vis Sci *9:655, 1970. Used by permission.*)

There are two types of spatial receptive fields: (1) those in which illumination of the center stimulates the ganglion cells and illumination of the periphery inhibits ganglion cells (an on-center, depolarizing type of receptive field); and (2) a reverse type of receptive field in which illumination of the periphery stimulates ganglion cells (an off-center, hyperpolarizing receptive field). In some receptive fields, the "on" and "off" zones are not concentric but are coincidental. There are additional and different receptive fields for color reception. Some receptive fields are most sensitive to moving targets.

Receptive fields are not constant in size, and they are larger in the dark-adapted eye than in the light-adapted eye. They are larger in the peripheral than in the central retina. They change in size and shape and alter in their stimulatory and inhibitory components with the state of light adaptation.

The spiked discharges from retinal ganglion cells are further integrated in the lateral geniculate body. The images from the two eyes may be reinforced in binocularity to cause a more vigorous response or may be inhibited with a diminished response in the absence of binocular vision.

CORTICAL FUNCTION

The nervous impulse that originates in the retina passes in the optic nerves, the optic chiasm, and the optic tract to the lateral geniculate body (see Chapter 1) of the thalamus. Here axons carrying visual impulse synapse with axons that terminate in the visual cortex. Other neurons of unknown function extend to the hypothalamus and midbrain nuclei that belong to the accessory optic tract system.

The complexity and capacity of the human visual cortex in the occipital lobe are emphasized by its size: $3 \times 5{,}000$ mm if flattened out. The major portion of the striate cortex is concerned with form vision.

Form-sensitive cortical cells are described as "simple," "complex," and "hypercomplex." Simple cells are arranged into excitatory and inhibitory regions separated by boundaries that are straight and parallel, and they are related to the X (simple) system. Their fields may be mapped with stationary retinal stimuli. Complex cells (related mainly to the Y system) appear to be combinations of simple cells that respond particularly to moving edges on the retina with directional sensitivity. Hypercomplex cells respond only to moving stimuli on the retina and are most potently stimulated by the ends of lines, line segments, and corners. Again the signal may be inhibited or reinforced. Unlike the retinal receptive fields, which are round, the cortical fields are linear.

Functional magnetic resonance imaging and positron emission tomography indicate a highly complex integration of the visual signals. Different regions of the brain are involved in the initial storage of a visual image and the subsequent recall of a previous image.

The lateral geniculate body receives a massive back projection from the visual cortex of the occipital lobe. This feedback loop functions to synchronize those signals most appropriate for subsequent cortical processing. The neuronal responses evoked by the same object are selected and mapped to each other so as not to be confounded with those of nearby objects or background. The associations are mapped to at least 30 higher cortical centers that interact with several hundred additional centers that integrate the visual impulse into sensory representations and motor responses.

VISUAL MECHANISMS

Electromagnetic radiation.—Energy is transferred through space by means of electrical and magnetic fields in waves that are perpendicular to each other and to the direction of propagation. In a vacuum, electromagnetic radiation has a velocity of 3×10^8 m/sec (186,000 miles/sec). It is characterized by a wavelength and a frequency (the number of vibrations of a wave per unit time). Electromagnetic waves exhibit the properties of wave motion, and processes such as reflection and refraction are best understood by geometric principles.

Electromagnetic energy may be considered as a discrete bundle or quantum that has an energy equal to its frequency, ν, multiplied by Planck's constant, h. A quantum of electromagnetic energy is a photon. Processes such as absorption and emission of electromagnetic radiation are most easily explained in terms of photons.

The arrangement of electromagnetic radiation according to its wavelength or frequency is called the electromagnetic spectrum. The wavelength varies from a minute fraction of a meter (3×10^{-20} m) for cosmic waves to many thousand meters for long radio waves (3×10^6 m). The energy varies inversely with the wavelength so that the energy of a cosmic ray photon is high (4×10^{17} electron volts) while a radio wave photon has minimal energy (4×10^{-13} electron volts).

Light is that portion of electromagnetic radiation that, when absorbed by the photopigment of the photoreceptor disks of the outer segment of the retina, changes the shape of the pigment molecule to initiate a nervous impulse. Light has a wavelength of 380 nm (nm = one-billionth meter) to 770 nm. Electromagnetic radiation with wavelengths greater or less than that of visible radiation either is absorbed by the cornea or passes through the eye without absorption. Cosmic rays stimulate photoreceptors and cause flashes of light (in astronauts), while x-rays stimulate rods in the dark-adapted eye. Laser-generated energy stimulates the retina at extremes of 100 nm (ultraviolet) and 1,000 nm (infrared).

Action of light on the eye.—When that portion of the electromagnetic spectrum known as visible light (400 to 700 nm) is absorbed by the visual pigment in the rods and cones, a nervous impulse is transmitted to the brain and causes a subjective sensation.

Equal amounts of radiant energy that have different wavelengths do not produce equal visual sensations. Thus, 0.001 W of green light appears bright to the observers, while 0.001 W of blue light appears dim. Luminous units express the amount of radiant light energy in terms of the subjective sensation of brightness in the observer. Luminous energy is radiant energy corrected for the sensitivity of the retina to different wavelengths. Since individual visual sensations differ, luminous units are expressed in terms of the average of many observers (the standard observer). Photopic, or cone, luminosity function (V_V) indicates the sensitivity of a light-adapted human eye. It has a maximum sensitivity at 555 nm. Scotopic luminosity function ($V^1\gamma$) indicates the sensitivity of the dark-

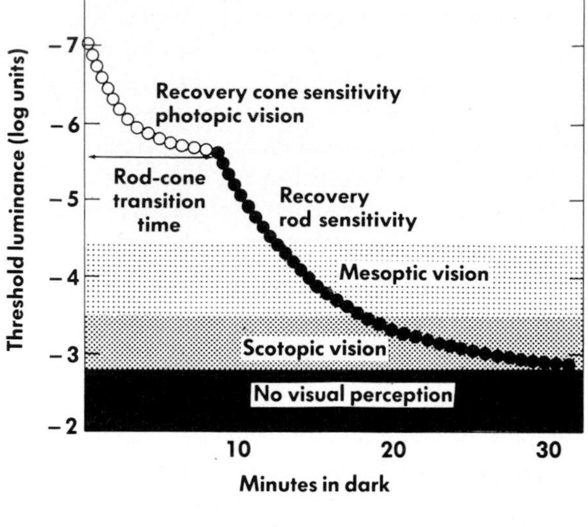

FIG 2-11.
The dark-adaptation curve. There is a plateau between 5 and 9 minutes. The initial portion of the curve indicates the smallest light intensity that will stimulate cones. Rods attain their maximum sensitivity after 30 to 45 minutes. The luminance at −7 is that of sunlight. The luminance at −5 is that of good reading luminance for white paper. The luminance at −4 log units is that at night with city street lighting. The luminance at −3 is mean ground luminance in full moon.

adapted human eye and has a maximum sensitivity at 507 nm. When viewed in dim illumination, a colored object appears to have no color. As illumination is increased, the color of the object appears. This change from achromatic to chromatic vision reflects the change from scotopic (rod) vision to photopic (cone) vision. The change in luminosity function is called the Purkinje shift.

Dark adaptation.—The increased sensitivity of the eye to the detection of light that occurs in reduced illumination is called "dark adaptation." The pupil dilates, and there are both neural (largely unknown) and biochemical changes in the retina. In dark adaptation, after exposure to bright light that bleaches the visual photopigments, there is an initial hundredfold increase in sensitivity following an exponential time course that reaches a plateau after 5 to 9 minutes. This initial phase is attributed to regeneration of photopigments in the cones. Thereafter, there is a 10^3 to 10^5 increase in sensitivity that follows a slower exponential time course, which reaches a plateau in 30 to 45 minutes (Fig 2-11). This second phase is attributed to regeneration of rhodopsin in the rods. In addition to rhodopsin regeneration, changes in the retinal summation and inhibition increase sensitivity further. Dark adaptation is delayed by prolonged exposure to bright light (thus the increased danger of driving at night after a day in bright sunshine). When fully dark-adapted, the retina is about 100,000 times more sensitive than when bleached by light.

The dark-adapted retina is most sensitive in the region of maximum rod density, which is about 2.5 mm from the fovea centralis. In the fully dark-adapted eye, a visual sensation can be evoked by the activity of approximately seven rods, each being stimulated by the oscillation of a single photon. A variation in sensitivity in different parts of the retina probably reflects differences in the number of photoreceptors and their neural summation mechanism rather than a difference in the sensitivity of the photoreceptor itself.

Light adaptation.—Exposure of the dark-adapted eye to bright light results in a marked decrease in sensitivity involving two changes: (1) a neural process that is completed in about 0.05 second and (2) a slower process, apparently involving the uncoupling of 11-*cis* retinal and the opsin of rhodopsin, that occurs in about 1 minute. The neural mechanism occurs regardless of the area of the retina stimulated, whereas the photochemical mechanism involves only the region of stimulation. In the light-adapted eye the rhodopsin is bleached, the pupil is constricted, there is a shift of luminosity to the yellow-red end of the spectrum, and hydrogen ion concentration (pH) of the retina shifts from 7.3 to 7.0.

Color perception.—This complicated topic involves physical, physiologic, and psychologic mechanisms. That portion of the electromagnetic spectrum with wavelengths between 400 and 700 nm is the stimulus for vision. The electromagnetic spectrum has no color, but in humans it is absorbed by the photopigments in the disks of the outer segments of the rods and cones. That portion of the electromagnetic spectrum absorbed by the rhodopsin of the rods initiates the colorless night vision. That portion of the electromagnetic spectrum absorbed by the three different photopigments of the outer segments of cones stimulates the perception of color. The nature of the perception depends upon the level of adaptation of the retina, combined with the wavelength and intensity of the light stimulus.

Trichromatic color vision is initiated by the absorption of light by three different photopigments in the disks of the outer segments of human cone cells. Long-wavelength–sensitive cones (L-cones or red cones) have a maximum sensitivity at 563 nm. Middle-wavelength–sensitive cones (M-cones or green cones) have a maximum sensitivity at 535 nm. Short-wavelength–sensitive cones (S-cones or blue cones) have a maximum sensitivity at 420 nm. Each cone cell contains but one photopigment, and the electrical signal initiated by a light stimulus interacts with those of other cones in the retina and brain. Only 7% to 10% of the cones are S-cones.

Stimuli from cones are recombined by horizontal cells, bipolar cells, and retinal ganglion cells to yield two opponent color pathways (channels). One pathway transmits red-green signals. The second pathway transmits blue to yellow signals. (Yellow is a mixture of the wavelengths [not the pigments] of blue and red.) These signals are transmitted by axons of the ganglion cells, which constitute the optic nerve, to the brain, where they are further refined by the lateral geniculate body and the occipital lobe. The red-green pathway computes the difference in signals from L-cones and from M-cones. Colors described as "red" and "green" are encoded so that redness is signalled by an increase in electrical activity and green is signalled by a decrease. Signals from S-cones oppose the combined signal from L- and M-cones to form the blue-yellow pathway (channel).

Signals from cones are transmitted to two types of horizontal cells, H1 and H2. The dendrites of H1 horizontal cells innervate the majority of cone cells and the red-green pathway. The dendrites of H2 horizontal cells connect to about 8% of cones, which have few if any connections with cones of the red-green pathway.

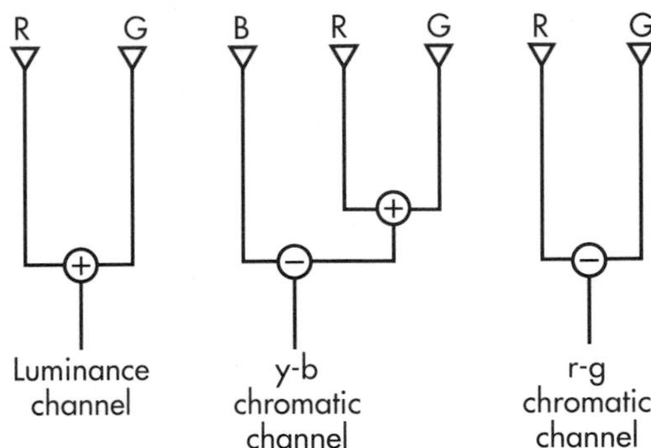

FIG 2-12.
An example of the opponent color model of human color vision. The top row shows the three types of cone cells in the retina. The middle row shows the interaction of cone signals that results in the two chromatic opponent channels. The y-b channel signals yellow and blue, and the r-g channel signals red and green.

It is postulated that the two chromatic pathways are initiated at the level of ganglion cells. Most ganglion cells (midget cells) receive inputs from bipolar cells, and transmit signals for red and green. Some 10% of ganglion cells (small bistratified cells) receive inputs from bipolar cells, which transmit signals from S-cones. These ganglion cells receive a minimal "opponent" input from bipolar cells connected to red-green cones (Fig 2-12) to create the blue-yellow pathway.

Luminance is signalled by the red-green pathway.

Defective color vision.—Defective color vision is mainly transmitted as a hereditary characteristic (Table 2-1) and is but uncommonly secondary to acquired systemic or ocular abnormalities. Hereditary defects of color vision occur because an abnormal photopigment protein (opsin) of the retinal cones is encoded by a faulty gene. In humans the opsin genes that code the photopigments for red and green are located in tandem on the long arm of the X chromosome. Thus, most genetic deficiencies of red-green color vision involve men (8%), and women are affected rarely (0.5%). The gene that codes for the blue-sensitive photopigment is located on chromosome 3. A person with nor-

TABLE 2-1.
Types of Defective Color Perception

I. Hereditary defects
   A. Anomalous trichromatism (abnormality of one photosensitive pigment)
      1. Protanomaly (red)
      2. Deuteranomaly (green)
   B. Dichromatism
      1. Protanopsia (absence of red photopigment)
      2. Deuteranopsia (absence of green photopigment)
      3. Tritanopsia (absence of blue photopigment; ganglion cell deficiency?)
   C. Achromatopsia
      1. Typical (reduced visual acuity and nystagmus)
         a. Complete (rod monochromacy)
         b. Incomplete
            (1) Autosomal recessive
            (2) X chromosome–linked (blue cone monochromacy)
      2. Atypical (normal visual acuity)
         a. Complete (cone monochromacy)
            (1) Protanoid
            (2) Deuteranoid (red cone monochromacy)
         b. Incomplete (pseudomonochromacy)
II. Developmental abnormalities
   A. Progressive cone degenerations
   B. Generalized cone-rod dystrophies
   C. Generalized rod-cone dystrophies

mal color vision has three photopigments in a normal proportion (a trichromat). If only two photopigments are functional, the person is a dichromat; if only one photopigment is present, the individual is a monochromat.

X chromosome–transmitted color deficiencies involve the genes that encode for red and green photopigments. They may be divided into the following: (1) a type in which one of the cone photopigments is abnormal but not entirely absent (anomalous trichromacy); (2) a type in which one of the cone photopigments is entirely absent (dichromacy); and (3) a type in which both L-cones and M-cones lack functional photopigments. The defect is present at birth and does not progress. The visual acuity is normal if only one of the photopigments is abnormal but is markedly reduced if both L-cone and M-cone photopigments are absent (there are apparently no S-cones in the fovea). The defects are designated according to the deficient photopigment: protan (first) long-wavelength–sensitive photopigment and deutan (second) middle-wavelength–sensitive photopigment. In protanomaly there is poor red-green discrimination, and the long-wavelength end of the spectrum appears dimmer than it does with unaffected individuals. In deuteranomaly there is also poor red-green discrimination, but the long-wavelength end of the spectrum appears as bright as it does to unaffected individuals.

Dichromacy is an abnormality in which either the L-cone or the M-cone photopigment is absent. If the L-cone photopigment is absent the condition is protanopsia; if the M-cone photopigment is absent the condition is deuteranopsia. These conditions are clinically differentiated from anomalous trichromacy by color and brightness matching. (Children should be tested for color defects before entering school, both to ease schooling and to prevent the choice of an inappropriate career.)

A dichromatic individual with an X chromosome–linked defect has only two cone pigments. If the long-wavelength–sensitive pigment is absent, the defect is protanopsia. If the middle-wavelength–sensitive pigment is absent, the defect is deuteranopsia. These are differentiated from anomalous trichromacy by color and brightness matching.

Tritan defects are transmitted as an autosomal dominant defect and possibly do not involve cone pigments.

The term “achromatopsia” describes individuals born with severely deficient color perception. Two types may be present at birth: (1) typical, associated with reduced visual acuity and nystagmus, and (2) atypical, associated with normal visual acuity. Either type may be complete or incomplete (see Table 2-1).

Monochromacy (achromatopsia) is a much rarer form of X chromosome–linked color deficiency in which the subjects lack both long- and medium-wavelength cone photopigments. They are completely color deficient and often have a pendular nystagmus and reduced visual acuity.

In humans the genes that encode for the opsins of the photopigments for L-cones and M-cones have closely similar nucleotide sequences. The extensive homology that occurs between the adjacent genes promotes misalignment of gene sequences and unequal crossing-over, with gene duplication and deletion, and the production of hybrid loci. Both genes are composed of six encoding regions or exons. Exons 1 and 6 are identical, and the gene sequence in one color-deficient individual indicated that the difference in the genes encoding the two opsins resides in exons 4 and 5. Individuals with protanopsia have exon 5 for L-cones derived from the gene for M-cones. In individuals with deuteranopsia, exon 5 for M-cones is derived from the gene for the L-cone. Anomalous trichromacy depends on one or two amino acid substitutions in exon 4 (the only two exons on chromosome 4 that are not homologous). In monochromacy the abnormality resides in one of the two following locations: (1) a regulatory region located between L-cone and M-cone photopigment genes and (2) a point mutation in a single remaining L-cone or M-cone photopigment gene that renders its protein product nonfunctional.

Electroretinography.—When the retina is stimulated with light, an action potential is superimposed on the resting potential. A record is made by placing an active electrode on the cornea, usually one embedded in a corneal contact lens, with saline solution bridging the gap between the electrode and the cornea, and placing an indifferent electrode on the forehead. The entire retina is stimulated with light and the small voltage is amplified and usually photographed from the face of an oscilloscope (electroretinogram [ERG] (Fig 2-13). The retina is stimulated with light after either dark (scotopic) or light (photopic) adaptation. After the stimulus, there is a latent period and then an initial negative deflection known as the a-wave, followed by a positive deflection designated as the b-wave. The a-wave reflects mainly cone activity. The b-wave originates from cells in the inner nuclear layer, most likely from cells that undergo depolarization when the retina is stimulated with light. The intracellularly recorded responses of Müller (glial) cells most closely match the b-wave.

The b-wave usually exceeds the largest amplitude of the a-wave by a factor of 1.5 or more. The duration of the entire response is usually less than 250 msec. The value for the b-waves is generally between 75 and 200 mV for photopic response and between 250 and 450 mV for scotopic response.

The ERG is indicative of a mass response of the outer layers of the retina. The record varies with the state of adaptation of the retina, the color of the light used in adaptation, and the intensity and color of the light used for stimulation. In disorders limited to the ganglion cell layer, the nerve fiber layer, or the optic nerve, the ERG is normal. Pathologic responses are described as supernormal, subnormal, or nonrecordable. When a large area of the retina is damaged or diseased, the ERG is subnormal. When the entire retina is affected, the ERG is nonrecordable.

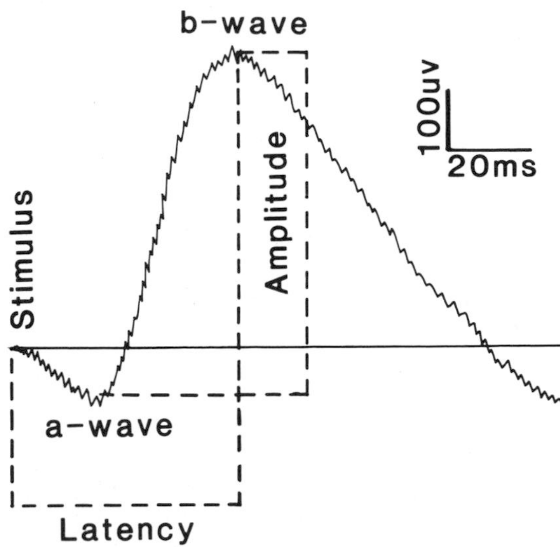

FIG 2-13.
The human electroretinogram. The negative deflection, the a-wave, reflects photoreceptor activity. The positive deflection, the b-wave, originates in the inner nuclear layer.

Intraretinal microelectrodes, in experimental animals, record additional electrical potentials that are not recorded clinically: (1) a steady retinal resting potential from the junction of the photoreceptors and retinal pigment epithelium; (2) an early receptor potential (R_1) from the outer segments of photoreceptor cells, corresponding to the isomerization of photopigments; (3) a later receptor potential (R_2) at the inner portion of photoreceptors, corresponding to the a-wave of the ERG; (4) a slow, widespread S-potential at the level of horizontal cells; (5) a well-defined positive potential at Müller cells, corresponding to the b-wave of the ERG; and (6) an oscillating potential from amacrine cells.

Visual-evoked potential.—Stimulation of the retina with light changes the electrical activity of the cerebral cortex. The visual-evoked potential (VEP) (or response [VER]) is the electroencephalogram recorded at the occipital

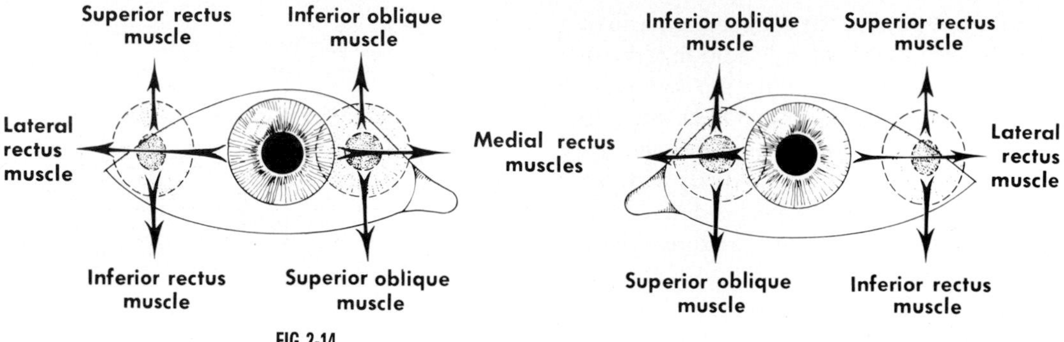

FIG 2-14.
Action of the six extraocular muscles of each eye.

pole. Because the evoked potential is too small to be separated from other cerebral electrical activity, several successive responses are averaged on a computer. Cerebral activity not related to the stimulus occurs randomly and is canceled out in the course of averaging. Electrical activity that is synchronized with a visual stimulus is summed and shown as a measurable electrical wave.

The only consistent recordable response is a large positive deflection occurring about 120 msec after stimulation when a pattern is used and about 100 msec when a flash is used. Pattern VEP is related to visual acuity and to stimulation of foveal cones, since the amplitude decreases when the pattern is not in focus. Flash VEP reflects transmission of light from the entire retina, including fast-conducting axons from the retinal periphery.

The amplitude is reduced and the latency increased in patients who have optic neuritis. In patients who have demyelinating disease, there is often decreased amplitude and delayed peak response even though each retina and optic nerve is clinically normal.

Resting potential.—The electrical potential of the cornea in humans is positive in relation to the back of the eye, and there is a difference in potential of several millivolts. The resting potential is bipolar with the cornea positive. The resting potential is dependent on the retinal pigment epithelium, and it is approximately two times greater in the light-adapted eye than in the dark-adapted eye.

Electro-oculography.—Electro-oculography evaluates the function of the retinal pigment epithelium by measuring the increase in standing (resting) potential that occurs in light adaptation. Electrodes are placed at each canthus, and the changes in the potential between these electrodes are recorded as the eyes move. The average amplitude of the potential in light and dark adaptation is measured as the eyes turn a standard distance to the right and the left. If the light intensity and the period of dark adaptation are adequate, the ratio of the maximum amplitude obtained in the light (light peak) to the minimum amplitude obtained in the dark (dark trough) is normally greater than 2, whereas the ratio is less than 2 in patients with disorders of the retinal pigment epithelium.

EXTRAOCULAR MUSCLES

Each eye is moved by six extraocular muscles. Normally their action is so sensitively adjusted that each eye is directed simultaneously to the same object in space.

When the eye is directed straight ahead, it is said to be in the primary position. If it is directed upward, downward, laterally, or medially, it is said to be in a secondary position. If it is directed in an oblique position, either up and in, down and in, up and out, or down and out, the eye is said to be in a tertiary position.

The medial rectus muscle (N III) has the single action of rotating the eye inward (adduction) (Fig 2-14). The lateral muscle (N VI) has the single action of rotating the eye outward (abduction). The remaining four extraocular muscles, the cyclovertical muscles, have different actions depending on the position of the globe (Table 2-2). Thus, if the eye is rotated downward from the straight ahead position, the superior oblique muscle rotates the globe around an anteroposterior axis so that a point at

TABLE 2-2.
Action of Ocular Muscles

Adduction (in)
  Medial rectus muscle
    Superior rectus muscle
    Inferior rectus muscle
Elevation in adduction
  Inferior oblique muscle
    Medial rectus muscle
Depression in adduction
  Superior oblique muscle
    Medial rectus muscle
Abduction (out)
  Lateral rectus muscle
    Superior oblique muscle
    Inferior oblique muscle
  Elevation in abduction
    Superior rectus muscle
      Lateral rectus muscle
  Depression in adduction
    Inferior rectus muscle
      Lateral rectus muscle
Intorsion
  Superior oblique muscle
  Superior rectus muscle
Extorsion
  Inferior oblique muscle
  Inferior rectus muscle

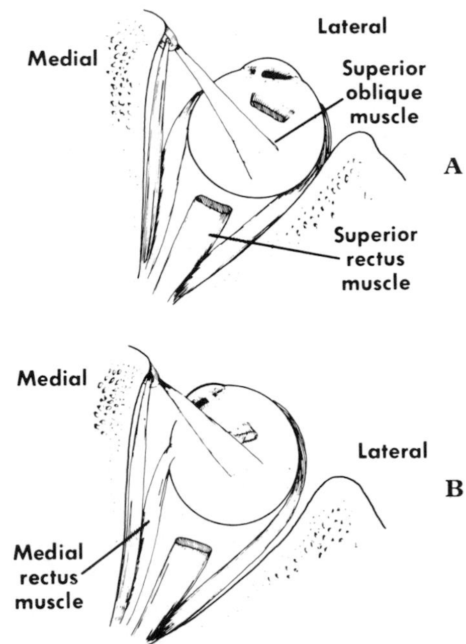

FIG 2-15.
The superior rectus muscle is removed to expose the reflected portion of the superior oblique muscle. **A,** With the eye directed straight ahead (primary position), the main action of the superior oblique muscle is intorsion. **B,** When the eye is turned medially, the main action of the superior oblique muscle is to turn the eye downward (the reading position). When the eye is turned laterally (not shown), the superior oblique muscle aids in the abduction.

the 12 o'clock meridian of the corneoscleral limbus rotates medially (intorsion [Fig 2-15, *A*]). If the lateral rectus muscle abducts the eye, the superior oblique and inferior oblique muscles steady the globe in this position. If the eye is directed medially, the superior oblique muscle depresses the eye (Fig 2-15; see Table 1-5).

Duction.—The rotation of one eye from one position to another is called duction (Fig 2-16). The muscles of one eye that work together in duction are called synergists in that function. In adduction the medial rectus muscle is aided by the superior and inferior recti muscles, whereas in abduction the superior and inferior oblique muscles are synergists of the lateral rectus muscle. In elevation the superior rectus and the inferior oblique muscles are synergistic, and in depression the inferior rectus and the superior oblique muscles are synergistic. In intorsion the superior oblique and superior rectus muscles are synergists, and in extorsion the inferior rectus and inferior oblique muscles are synergists. Each extraocular muscle is opposed by an antagonist that has the opposite action in a particular position. Thus, the antagonist of the medial rectus muscle is the lateral rectus muscle. When the eye is elevated by the superior rectus muscle, its antagonist is the inferior rectus muscle.

An innervational impulse flows to the active muscle while the innervational impulse is inhibited to the muscle's antagonist (Sherrington's principle of reciprocal innervation).

Version.—The simultaneous rotation of both eyes from the primary position to a secondary position is called version. These are: (1) eyes right—dextroversion; (2) eyes left—levoversion; (3) eyes up—sursumversion; and (4) eyes down—deorsumversion. The muscles of each eye primarily responsible for directing the eyes in version movements are yoke muscles. Thus, in turning the eyes to the right, the right lateral rectus muscle is yoked to the left medial rectus muscle. Each superior rectus muscle is yoked to the contralateral inferior oblique muscle, and each inferior rectus muscle is yoked to the contralateral superior oblique muscle.

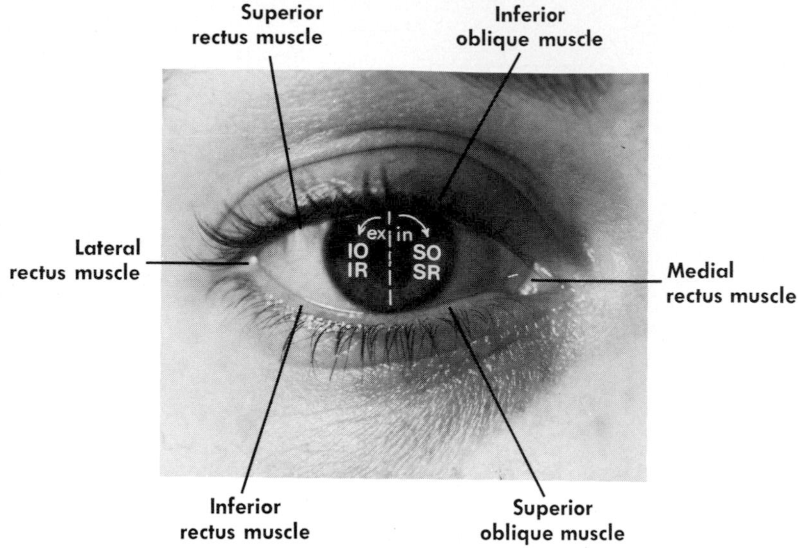

FIG 2-16.
Ductions of the eye showing the main muscle involved in each action. *In* refers to intorsion by superior oblique *(SO)* and superior recti *(SR)* muscles. *Ex* refers to extorsion by the inferior oblique *(IO)* and inferior recti *(IR)* muscles.

In version movements, an equal innervational impulse flows from the cerebral oculogyric centers to each muscle involved in the action (Hering's law). Thus, with both eyes turned to the right, the right lateral rectus and the left medial rectus muscles receive equal innervational stimulus.

This equal innervation is important in the diagnosis of a paretic muscle. Thus, if a paretic muscle is on the right side and the right eye is used for fixing (as occurs when the left eye is covered), the nerve impulse required to hold the right eye in position is greater than would be required if its innervation was normal. Since the nerve impulse is directed equally to the left eye, the left eye yoke muscle receives an excessive innervational impulse and the eye will deviate. The deviation (secondary) of the left eye will thus be greater when the paretic right eye is used for fixation. If the nonparetic left eye fixes, a normal innervation impulse is relayed to the paretic right eye and its deviation (primary) is minimal.

Vergence.—Vergence is the term applied to simultaneous ocular movements in which the eyes are directed simultaneously to an object in the midbody plane, that is, somewhere in front of the nose. The term is applied to convergence, in which the eyes rotate inward toward each other, or to divergence, in which they rotate outward simultaneously. Vertical (sursumvergence) and torsional vergences are minimal.

The locations of convergence and divergence centers in the brain are not known, although convergence and divergence paresis is observed clinically. It is assumed that the nucleus of Perlia (N III) is the center for convergence. Convergence palsy occurs in midbrain disease, and the convergence center is assumed to be located in this region. Divergence paresis may occur after head injury associated with perceptual deafness. The center is postulated to be located in the midbrain near the acoustic nerve nucleus.

Ocular movements.—The two basic types of ocular movements are (1) fast eye movements, or saccades, and (2) slow eye movements (Table 2-3).

Fast eye movements may be reflex, voluntary, or both. They are designed to bring a visual stimulus in the retinal periphery to the fovea centralis. Often the head moves also. Saccades reach an angular velocity of 700° of arc/sec after a latency of 200 msec. Saccadic movements occur in reading, in the fast phases of evoked and pathologic nystagmus, and in the rapid eye movements (REMs) of sleep.

Slow eye movements are smooth rotations designed to maintain the fovea centralis on a moving target. The maximum velocity is 30° to

TABLE 2-3.
Types of Eye Movements

Fast Eye Movements (Version)	Slow Eye Movements	
	Version	Vergence
Saccade		
Refixation	Pursuit (tracking)	Refixation
Reflex		
Voluntary	Voluntary	Tracking (pursuit)
Corrective saccade		
Saccadic pursuit (cogwheel)	Compensatory	Voluntary
Fast phase of nystagmus (pendular)	Slow phase of nystagmus	
Square wave jerk		
Sleep	Afterimage induced	

50° of arc/sec after a latency of 125 msec. If the fovea centralis is fixed on a moving target with an angular velocity of less than 30°/sec, the eye follows the target almost exactly (pursuit or tracking movement). With greater velocity, an irregular type of saccadic movement results, with overcorrection and correction. Slow eye movements (vergence movements) aim to maintain the fixation of the fovea centralis of each eye on an object of attention located approximately in front of the eyes.

The eyes maintain a horizontal position, despite movements of the head, by means of postural reflexes originating in the neck muscles and in each labyrinth. Thus, when the chin is depressed on the chest, an innervational impulse stimulates the elevators of the two eyes and inhibits the depressors, and the eyes remain directed ahead. Elevation of the chin causes the opposite reaction (the depressors are stimulated and the elevators inhibited). If the head is tilted to either shoulder, torsion occurs so that the 12 o'clock meridian rotates and the vertical meridian of the cornea remains vertical, assuming the tilting of the head is less than 20°.

If the fovea centralis is fixed on a *steady target,* three types of movement occur: (1) those with a frequency of 30 to 70/sec and an amplitude of 20 seconds; (2) those with an irregular frequency of about one every second and an amplitude of 3 minutes (saccades, or flick movements); and (3) irregular drifts of about 6 minutes. The fine high-frequency movements permit new retinal receptors to be stimulated during the latent period so that the image does not disappear.

The saccadic or flick movements tend to correct either drift or a previous saccade. During each saccade the retinal image is rapidly displaced but movements are not perceived. (Thus, observe the edge of the pupil of one eye in a mirror. Then direct attention to the pupil of the fellow eye, and note that there is no motion.) During saccades, such as in reading this page, movement is selectively suppressed in the magnocellular pathway from peripheral retinal ganglion cells that have large receptive fields. The pathway carrying the perception of the printed word has no motion detectors.

Fusional movements are slow (vergence) eye movements directed toward the maintenance of a single perception by keeping the retinal image on receptors that have the same visual direction. The near reaction is related to convergence involving the visual response to the awareness of the nearness of an object.

Electrical phenomena.—There is continuous electrical activity in the extraocular muscles during a waking state. Moving the eye into the major field of action of a muscle causes a marked increase in the number and frequency of electrical discharges of the muscle involved. Accompanying this is a reduction in activity of the antagonistic muscle (Sherrington's principle).

The ocular muscles do not exhibit the electrical phenomena of fatigue. Sleep eliminates the electrical activity of the extraocular muscles. During dreaming there are bursts of electrical activity and ocular movements (REMs). During sleep and forced eyelid closure the eyes are usually directed upward and outward in the Bell phenomenon. During general anesthesia, anatomic-mechanical factors position the eyes in the anatomic position of rest in which there is no muscle tone, so that the eyes are divergent.

BIBLIOGRAPHY

Books

Berman ER: *Biochemistry of the eye,* New York, 1991, Plenum Press.

Buser P, Imbert M: *Vision,* Cambridge, Mass, 1992, The MIT Press.

Carr RE, Siegel IM: *Electrodiagnostic testing of the visual system. A clinical guide,* Philadelphia, 1990, FA Davis.

Davson H: *Davson's physiology of the eye,* ed 5, New York, 1990, Pergamon Press.

Hart WM: *Adler's physiology of the eye: clinical application,* St Louis, 1992, Mosby–Year Book.

Scriver CR, Beaudet AL, Sly WS, Valle D, editors: *The metabolic and molecular bases of inherited disease,* vols I to III, New York, 1995, McGraw-Hill.

Wandall BA: *Foundations of vision,* Sunderland, Mass, 1995, Sinauer.

Whikehart DR: *Biochemistry of the eye,* Newton, Mass, 1994, Butterworth-Heinemann.

Articles

Dacey DM, Lee BB, Stafford DK, Pokorny J, Smith VC: Horizontal cells of the primate retina: cone specificity without spectral opponency, *Science* 271:656-659, 1996. Commentary: RH Masland, *Science* 271:516-617, 1996.

Farber DB: From mice to men: the cyclic GMP phosphodiesterase gene in vision and disease, *Invest Ophthalmol Vis Sci* 36:263-275, 1995.

Koutalos Y, Yau K-W: A rich complexity emerges in phototransduction, *Curr Opin Neurobiol* 3:513-519, 1993.

Pugh EN Jr, Lamb TD: Amplification and kinetics of the activation steps in phototransduction, *Biochim Biophys Acta* 1141:111-149, 1993.

3

PHARMACOLOGY

Medications instilled in the conjunctival cul-de-sac enter the anterior chamber mainly through the cornea and, when the crystalline lens is present, their actions are limited to the anterior segment. When the crystalline lens is absent (aphakia), drug diffusion through the vitreous humor is sometimes so marked as to result in edema of the fovea centralis (see Chapter 17), which causes reduced visual acuity. The ocular tissue concentration of drugs administered systemically parallels that of other vascularized tissues, with the important exception that the central cornea, the crystalline lens, and the vitreous humor do not have blood vessels. Additionally, the blood-retina and blood-aqueous barriers limit the entry of drugs into the noninflamed eye.

The blood-aqueous barrier is formed by the nonpigmented layer of the ciliary epithelium and by the endothelium of the iris vessels. Both of these tissues have tight junctions that are selectively permeable to water and ions ("leaky" tight junctions). The blood-aqueous barrier is permeable through both transport mechanisms and pressure-dependent osmotic flow (ultrafiltration).

The blood-retina barrier is located in the retinal pigment epithelium and the endothelium of the retinal blood vessels. Both tissues have tight junctions. Their permeability to water and solubles is determined by the active and passive transport mechanisms of their cells. Drugs enter the eye in proportion to their lipid solubility. Ionized or lipid-insoluble drugs are mainly excluded from the intraocular intracellular space, whether administered topically or systemically. The tight junctions of the endothelium of the retinal and iris blood vessels limit the diffusion of lipid-insoluble substances. The fenestrated choriocapillaris and ciliary body capillaries permit the passage of large molecules, but the tight junctions of the retinal pigment epithelium and its anterior extension, the pigment epithelium of the ciliary body, limit further intraocular penetration. Severe inflammation or trauma damages the blood-aqueous barrier, and compounds that do not penetrate the normal eye penetrate easily under these conditions and are distributed as in other body tissues and fluids.

The ciliary body epithelium transports organic ions from the aqueous humor of the posterior chamber into the blood by a mechanism similar to those in the renal tubule and choroid plexus. Uric acid and drugs such as the penicillins are actively transported out of the posterior chamber by the nonpigmented ciliary epithelium. This transport is inhibited by probenecid.

The sensory retina may be damaged by high levels of phenothiazine concentrated in cells containing melanin, particularly the retinal pigment epithelium. Alternatively, phenothiazine stabilizes lysosomes, which may impair the phagocytosis of retinal outer segments by the retinal pigment epithelium.

TOPICAL ADMINISTRATION

Drugs may be applied to the eyelids or instilled in the conjunctival sac in aqueous or viscous solutions or suspensions, in ointments, as fine powders, on cotton pledgets, by drug-impregnated contact lenses, by injection, by mechanical pumps, or by membrane release systems. In contrast to systemic administration, the ocular concentration after topical administration is high. Dilution of the drug by tears, overflow onto the face, and excretion through the nasolacrimal system limit tissue concentration. Placing the drug beneath a contact lens, applying a cotton pledget, or applying a collagen shield saturated with the drug to the eye ensures a more prolonged contact and enhances ocular penetration.

Subconjunctival or subtenon retrobulbar injections are used for the administration of antibiotics and corticosteroids. Before injection, the conjunctiva is anesthetized with topical 4% cocaine solution or subconjunctival lidocaine. A high tissue concentration is maintained for a long period. Some surgeons inject an antibiotic subconjunctivally at the end of an intraocular operation to ensure a high concentration of antibiotic in the aqueous humor. Injection through the pars plana into the anterior portion of the vitreous body is mainly reserved for the treatment of suppurative infections of the inner eye (panophthalmitis and endophthalmitis [see Chapter 19]).

Proper instillation is required for eyedrops to be effective. For maximal effectiveness in treating inflammations of the conjunctiva, the patient is instructed to look upward, and the skin of the lower eyelid is drawn away from the globe to create a pouch between the eye and the inside of the eyelid. The drug is instilled in this pouch without touching the eyelids or the globe with the tip of the container (Fig 3-1). The patient is instructed to close the eye without squeezing. Pressure by the thumb and index finger to the inner corner of each eye occludes the lacrimal puncta, prevents passage of the drug into the nose, and prolongs corneal and conjunctival contact with the medication. Practitioners should be assured that patients for whom eyedrops are prescribed know how to instill them.

In corneal disease and in the treatment of glaucoma, it is desirable that there be maximal contact with the cornea, which is either the site of the inflammation or the major route of entry of drugs into the anterior chamber. Maximal corneal penetration is best achieved by creating a pocket between the globe and the eyelid as described above, but by having the patient look downward, retracting the upper eyelid, and allowing the drop to flow across the cornea.

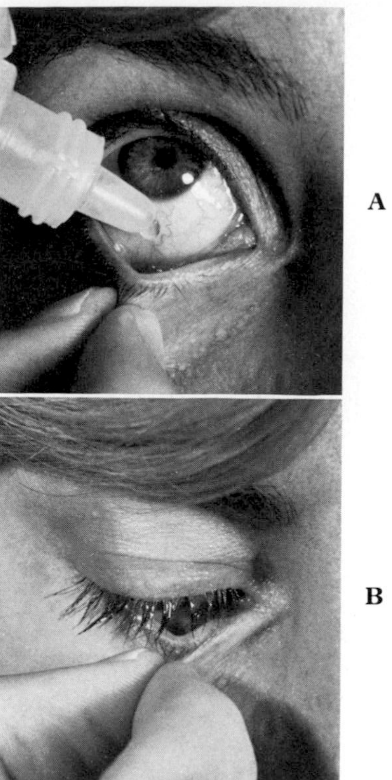

FIG 3-1.
A, The proper method of instilling eyedrops in the eye. The lower eyelid is drawn away from the globe, the patient is instructed to look upward, and the drop is delivered into the pouch. **B,** The patient is then instructed to look downward, and the skin of the eyelid is slowly released. The patient should be warned not to squeeze the eye. The eyelids may then be gently closed for 2 minutes. To prevent systemic absorption through the lacrimal puncta the patient should occlude the inner corner of the eyelids with the thumb and index finger for 2 minutes after the instillation of eyedrops. Adrenergic beta-receptor antagonists (beta-blockers) used in the treatment of glaucoma are particularly liable to cause systemic reactions, especially in the elderly.

In children and infants, it is often easier to apply an ointment to the tightly squeezed eyelids than to attempt to instill an ophthalmic solution. In the prophylaxis of ophthalmia neonatorum, erythromycin or tetracycline ointment may be applied to the closed eyelids at the lash margin with effective results. Silver nitrate eyedrops must be applied to the conjunctival surface.

Medications may be prescribed in oils, ointments, methylcellulose, and other viscous vehicles. The medication must have a greater affinity for the cornea than for the vehicle. If the medication has a greater affinity for the vehicle, it will not be released and will remain in the vehicle rather than being absorbed into the eye.

Corneal penetration.—To enter the anterior chamber, topically applied drugs must be lipid-soluble to penetrate the intact corneal epithelium and water-soluble to penetrate the corneal stroma. The highest concentration in the anterior chamber follows instillation of drugs that are both lipid- and water-soluble. If the corneal epithelium is absent, diseased, or damaged, then water-soluble, polar compounds enter the anterior chamber more readily. Ocular massage or the topical instillation of a local anesthetic or a wetting agent enhances intraocular penetration.

Topical preparations.—Many factors relate to the effectiveness, safety, and comfort of eyedrops and ointments: sterility, hydrogen ion concentration, tonicity, physiologic activity, stability, toxicity, surface tension, and compatibility. Most commonly used medications are prepared commercially and require Food and Drug Administration–approved quality control to ensure sterility.

Ocular medications in interstate commerce are sterile when sold. Once the container is opened the solution is easily contaminated. All solutions in open containers must be regarded as contaminated.

The adenovirus that causes keratoconjunctivitis may be transmitted by means of contaminated ocular anesthetic solutions. Fluorescein solution is susceptible to contamination by *Pseudomonas aeruginosa,* and it may introduce the organism when used in the diagnosis of a corneal abrasion. To avoid infection, fluorescein should be instilled only from a sterile individual container or should be applied by means of a filter paper strip that has been saturated with fluorescein and then sterilized. It must never be used from a stock bottle. Many of the solutions used by wearers of contact lenses are contaminated, as are lens carrying cases. In the event of corneal infection, these containers as well as the eye should be cultured for organisms.

Eyedroppers are easily contaminated by touching the eyelids or the conjunctiva, and then may contaminate a stock bottle. Plastic "squeeze" bottles, in which many commercially available medications are dispensed, are more difficult to contaminate than bottles with eyedroppers. Eyecups are usually contaminated and may be a source of recurrent infection. Contact lens containers are often contaminated. Provided the contents are initially sterile, ophthalmic ointments are rarely contaminated.

Ophthalmic ointments are dispensed in 3.5- or 4.0-g tubes. Medications in larger tubes have not been prepared for ophthalmic use.

ANTI-INFECTIVE AGENTS

Frequent topical instillation of antibiotics or sulfonamides provides unusually high concentrations in the superficial tissues. Compounds that have severe adverse effects when administered systemically often may be useful when instilled locally. Heavy metals such as zinc sulfate are still used in astringent eyedrops, and silver nitrate is used in the prophylaxis of gonorrheal ophthalmia.

Many compounds instilled in the conjunctival sac cause either an irritant or hypersensitive contact dermatoconjunctivitis. Prolonged use of antibiotics combined with corticosteroids predisposes to superinfection, particularly with fungi. A fungal invader must be considered in any persistent conjunctival or corneal inflammation. Local anti-infective agents are diluted rapidly by tears, and they must be instilled at 1- or 2-hour intervals to ensure adequate local tissue concentration.

The blood-ocular barriers limit the intraocular penetration of many anti-infective agents from the systemic circulation. Intraocular inflammation impairs the blood-ocular barriers so that increased amounts of these agents enter the eye from the blood. When an inflammation begins to subside, the blood-ocular barriers regain their integrity, although viable microorganisms may persist in the eye. Drug dosage should therefore not be reduced until the intraocular tissues and fluids are free of organisms.

The injection of the anti-infective agent into the subconjunctival space, subtenon space, or retrobulbar space is generally limited to those instances in which high local concentration is required. Intravitreal injection of antibiotics is limited to endophthalmitis, in which the possible damage caused by the anti-infective agent is balanced by the damage caused by the intraocular infection.

Effective management of endophthalmitis, orbital cellulitis, or ulcers that affect the central cornea requires prompt diagnosis and treatment. Corneal exudate or vitreous humor should be inoculated into culture media before antibiotic treatment so that the causative organism may be identified in the event that initial therapy is not successful. Before the results of culture are known, the therapy is based on the results of the Gram stain. Delaying the culture and Gram stain until it is evident that a change in treatment is required often results in an inability to identify the causative organism.

Local hypersensitivity reactions restrict the usefulness of topical antibiotics, and only a few are commercially available (Table 3-1). In contrast, an enormous variety of artificial tear preparations, eye washes, and contact lens solutions are used. Nearly all become contaminated after use. Many contain preservatives and other compounds that may cause local hypersensitivity reactions.

The local protective mechanisms of the eye are exceptionally efficient, and the miscellaneous minor injuries tolerated by the globe and eyelids are remarkable. Many patients insert contaminated contact lenses or eyedrops without harm. Minor abrasions of the cornea are tolerated with minimal discomfort and rapid healing. The water in swimming pools may be contaminated with chemicals or infectious microorganisms, yet relatively few individuals are adversely affected.

TABLE 3-1.
Topical Anti-Infective Agents Commercially Available

Name	Concentration
Commercially available in solution or ointment	
Gentamicin*	Sol & oint: 0.3%
Chloramphenicol*	Sol: 0.5%; oint: 1%
Sulfacetamide*	Sol: 10%; 15%; 30%; oint: 10%
Sulfisoxazole	Sol & oint: 4.0%
Tobramycin*	Sol & oint: 0.3%
Available as ointment only (3.5 or 4.0 g)	
Bacitracin	500 U/g
Erythromycin	0.5%
Available as solution only (5.0 mL usual)	
Ciprofloxacin (Ciloxan)	0.3%
Norfloxacin (Chibroxin)	0.3%
Ofloxacin (Ocuflox)	0.3%
Polymyxin B mixtures	
With bacitracin (ointment only)	
With bacitracin and neomycin (ointment only)*	
With oxytetracycline (ointment only)	
With neomycin (ointment and solution)*	
With neomycin and gramicidin (solution only)	
With trimethoprim (solution only)	
Antiviral compounds	
Solution only	
Idoxuridine (Herplex)	0.1%
Trifluridine (Viroptic)	1.0%
Ointment only	
Acyclovir (Zovirax)	3.0%
Vidarabine (Vira-A)	3.0%
Intravenous	
Foscarnet sodium (Foscavir)	
Ganciclovir sodium (Cytovene)	
Antifungal (oral after intravenous induction)	
Solution only	
Amphotericin B	0.1%-0.5%
Flucytosine (Ancobon)	1.0%
Natamycin (Natacyn)	5.0% (susp)
Miconazole (Monistat)	1.0% (sol)
Ophthalmic ointments: 3.5- or 4.0-g tubes (never use a larger tube)	
Ophthalmic solutions: 5.0 mL usual but also 2.5 mL, 10 mL, and 15 mL	

*Also marketed with added corticosteroid.

SULFONAMIDES

The sulfonamides are bacteriostatic agents that prevent susceptible microorganisms (*Escherichia coli, Staphylococcus aureus, Streptococcus pneumoniae, Pseudomonas* species, *Haemophilus influenzae, Klebsiella* species, and *Enterobacter* species) from synthesizing folic acid from para-aminobenzoic acid.

Two sulfonamides are used topically in the treatment of conjunctivitis and blepharitis: sulfacetamide sodium and sulfisoxazole. Sulfacetamide is often combined with a corticosteroid, and the topical use of this combination may aggravate keratitis caused by the herpes simplex virus.

Sulfacetamide.—Sulfacetamide is used in 10% and 30% solutions and 10% ointment. It is the most useful of the sulfonamide compounds for local use. It is minimally antigenetic, and it rarely induces hypersensitivity reactions.

Sulfisoxazole.—Sulfisoxazole is used locally in a 4% solution or ointment. A white suspension of the drug may gather at the canthus.

ANTIBIOTICS

Antibiotics are compounds produced by some microorganisms or prepared synthetically, which in dilute solutions suppress the growth of (bacteriostatic effect) or destroy (bactericidal effect) microorganisms. They are effective through one of several mechanisms.

They may (1) inhibit the biosynthesis of the bacterial cell wall of rapidly growing organisms by binding to enzymes that synthesize the cell wall or by inhibiting cross-linkages between peptidoglycan polymers with disruption of cell wall integrity (penicillins, cephalosporins, cycloserine, vancomycin, and bacitracin); (2) bind to the 30 ribosome subunits of bacteria to block access to the mRNA-ribosome complex, and to alter protein synthesis by the organism (tetracycline, aminoglycosides, erythromycin, chloramphenicol, and clindamycin); (3) impair the action of DNA gyrase (topoisomerase II) in DNA replication (quinolones, isoniazid, streptomycin, and ethambutol); (4) bind to ergosterol in the bacterial cell wall to impair cellular permeability with leakage of electrolytes (particularly potassium) and other cellular contents through the cell wall (detergents, polymyxin, amphotericin B, and nystatin); (5) act as nucleic acid analogues to bind to enzymes essential to DNA synthesis (acyclovir, ganciclovir, zidovudine, vidarabine, trifluorothymidine, and idoxuridine); (6) inhibit bacterial RNA synthesis (rifampin); (7) inhibit folic acid synthesis (dapsone); and (8) inhibit thymidylate synthetase to deprive the bacterial cell of an essential DNA component (flucytosine).

The systemic use of antibiotics is complicated by bacterial resistance, hypersensitivity reactions, toxicity, alteration of normal microorganismal flora, peripheral neuritis, and hematologic complications. Staphylococcic beta-lactamase hydrolyzes and inactivates the beta-lactam antibiotic. In some instances, spontaneous mutations cause enzymatic changes that permit microbial resistance. Many gram-negative bacteria contain a resistance transfer factor that may transmit resistance to other bacteria.

Cutaneous hypersensitivity varies in severity from contact dermatitis to purpura, erythema multiforme, and exfoliative dermatitis. Systemic hypersensitivity may be manifested by fever, serum sickness, and (rarely) anaphylactic shock (mainly with penicillin).

Renal toxicity may be produced by a variety of systemic antibiotics (cephaloridine, neomycin, colistin, gentamicin, tobramycin, kanamycin, vancomycin, and amphotericin). Decreased renal excretion may result in exceptionally high blood levels of the antibiotic. Eighth nerve damage has occurred after systemic administration of streptomycin, vancomycin, kanamycin, neomycin, and gentamicin.

Alteration of normal bacterial flora is particularly common after the use of tetracyclines. Topical antibiotic and corticosteroid combinations are factors in superinfection of the cornea with fungi. Systemic administration may be associated with overgrowth of *Candida albicans* in the mouth, pharynx, and bowel, and there may be tetracycline-resistant *Proteus, Pseudomonas,* and *Staphylococcus* organisms in the bowel. Tetracyclines stain developing teeth and are contraindicated before emergence of second dentition in children and in pregnant and nursing women.

Failure of antimicrobial agents results from (1) their use in conditions not caused by microorganisms; (2) the failure to identify the causative organism and to use an appropriate antimicrobial agent in proper dosage; (3) their continued use after bacterial resistance or toxic or allergic reactions have developed, or superinfection has occurred; and (4) the use of inappropriate combinations.

The ocular use of topical antibiotics is complicated by several factors. Many antibiotics are not available for topical administration because they induce a cutaneous hypersensitivity. Often, superficial ocular infections are treated with antibiotics empirically and, when the inflammation does not respond to treatment, bacterial cultures often show no growth and it is not possible to identify the causative organism. In keratitis that involves the central cornea, this may lead to exceptionally serious sequelae, and empiric therapy must always be preceded by

Gram stain and bacterial culture of the exudate. Most external inflammations respond favorably within 48 hours after the initiation of treatment, and failure to improve must lead to more extensive diagnostic studies.

Because endophthalmitis may destroy the eye within hours it requires prompt diagnosis and treatment. Gram staining and culture of the vitreous humor and blood are required. The usual initial therapy is vancomycin for gram-positive infection (the most common) and gentamicin or an aminoglycoside for gram-negative organisms. Further therapy is based on the results of the bacterial cultures. The aminoglycosides induce retinal degeneration and their use is reserved for proven gram-negative organisms.

Beta-lactam antibiotics (including penicillins)

The beta-lactam antibiotics impair bacterial cell wall synthesis in many organisms. They commonly cause hypersensitivity reactions and are never used topically. Many preparations are degraded by gastric acid and are not effective when used orally. The staphylococci produce a beta-lactamase enzyme that hydrolyzes and inactivates many beta-lactams. Nonetheless, they constitute one of the most effective groups of antibiotics and are widely used. The major groups are as follows: (1) the penicillins and (2) the cephalosporins, which are divided into four generations. They are widely used systemically, and many are effective when administered orally.

The beta-lactams are actively secreted out of the eye by the ciliary epithelium and do not cross the intact blood-aqueous or blood-retina barriers. All bind to blood proteins and enter the central nervous system poorly. Methicillin and ampicillin are the least protein-bound.

Penicillins.—All of the penicillins cause hypersensitivity reactions that may range in severity from urticaria to anaphylaxis to delayed hypersensitivity reactions. The penicillins are all cross-reactive, and a patient sensitive to one will be sensitive to other penicillins, although not always to the same extent. Individuals are more sensitive to the natural penicillins than to the semisynthetic derivatives.

A history of adverse reactions to penicillin may be more important than the results of various tests to anticipate allergic reactions. Skin testing may be hazardous, but test material is available to learn if anaphylactic-type allergy is present. If the results are positive, penicillin should be used cautiously, if at all. Additionally, there may be cross-allergy to the penicillins and the cephalosporins.

Penicillin G is the penicillin of choice in the treatment of syphilis and infections caused by streptococci (including the pneumococci), meningococci, gonococci, anthrax, and actinomycetes. It is available in a crystalline form for intramuscular or intravenous use and in a repository form (procaine penicillin G or penicillin G benzathine). Penicillin V is absorbed more readily from the gastrointestinal tract than is penicillin G.

The beta-lactamase–resistant penicillins available for parenteral use include methicillin, oxacillin, cloxacillin, dicloxacillin, floxacillin, and nafcillin. Cloxacillin is absorbed well after oral administration, whereas nafcillin has variable absorption after oral administration. Oxacillin and nafcillin are most active, but methicillin is less bound to serum protein so that more of the drug may be available to enter the eye. Methicillin may cause reversible bone marrow depression and interstitial nephritis. In severe systemic infection, such as orbital cellulitis, a combination of antibiotics provides broad-spectrum coverage pending identification and susceptibility testing of the microbe.

In hospitals where methicillin-resistant strains of *S. aureus* are prevalent, vancomycin, vancomycin and rifampin, or a quinolone antibiotic may be substituted.

Ampicillin and amoxicillin are not resistant to beta-lactamase, but are active against *H. influenzae, Proteus mirabilis,* and *Neisseria* species. Amoxicillin may be combined with a beta-lactamase inhibitor to enhance its activity. Some strains of *H. influenzae* are resistant to ampicillin, and in life-threatening conditions chloramphenicol is substituted. Carbenicillin, carbenicillin indanyl, and ticarcillin are active against the same organisms as well as *Pseudomonas* species, *Enterobacter* species, and indole-positive *Proteus.* Azlocillin is active against *Pseudomonas* and species of *Klebsiella.* Gentamicin, which is also used in *Pseudomonas* infections, should never be mixed in the same bottle with carbenicillin, which inactivates aminoglycosides.

Cephalosporins.—The cephalosporins are beta-lactams classified as first, second, third, or fourth generation, mainly on the basis of the sensitivity of bacteria and the resistance of the antibiotic to beta-lactamases. Many are active after oral administration. The first generation (cephalothin [Keflin], cefazolin [Keflex], cephapirin [Cefadyl], cefadroxil [Duricef], and others) are strongly active against gram-positive bacteria and are active against *P. mirabilis, E. coli,* and *Klebsiella pneumoniae.* They are not active against methicillin-resistant *S. aureus* and *S. epidermidis.*

Second-generation cephalosporins (cefaclor [Ceclor], cefamandole [Mandol], cefonicid [Monocid], ceforanide [Precef], and others) have greater activity against the same gram-negative bacteria as the first generation but somewhat less against the gram-positive organisms. They are active against *H. influenzae, Neisseria* species, and some *Enterobacter aerogenes.*

Third-generation cephalosporins (ceftriaxone [Rocephin], cefoperazone [Cefobid], cefotaxime [Claforan], and others) are inferior to the first-generation cephalosporins in activity against gram-positive organisms but far superior in activity against gram-negative organisms, including those described above. Ceftriaxone and cefoperazone are excreted in the bile and the feces and may be used in patients with renal insufficiency.

Fourth-generation cephalosporins include cefpirone, cefepime, and others that may be more cost-effective or clinically superior to combinations of cephalosporins and aminoglycosides in gram-negative infections.

Cephalosporins are often drugs of choice for patients sensitive to penicillin, although they too may cause sensitivity reactions and cross-reactions with penicillin. Cephalosporins may cause a positive Coombs test for erythrocyte antibodies. Concurrent administration of cephalothin (Keflin) and gentamicin or tobramycin synergistically causes nephrotoxicity.

Cephalosporins are effective systemic therapeutic and prophylactic agents. Many penetrate the blood-ocular barriers and are used in the treatment of endophthalmitis. First-generation cephalosporins are used prophylactically before and after intraocular surgery. Third-generation cephalosporins may be useful in infections caused by nosocomial infections by organisms resistant to some aminoglycosides and first-generation cephalosporins.

Other beta-lactam antibiotics.—Imipenem is strongly resistant to beta-lactamase and is active against a broad range of gram-positive and gram-negative organisms. It is rapidly hydrolyzed by the kidney and is commercially available with cilastatin (Primaxin), an inhibitor of renal dehydropeptidase. There is cross-sensitivity with other beta-lactam antibiotics.

Aztreonam (Azactam) is a beta-lactam compound with an antimicrobial activity that closely resembles that of the aminoglycosides. It is exceptionally active against *P. aeruginosa,* Enterobacteriaceae, *H. influenzae,* and *Neisseria gonorrhoea.* There is no cross-sensitivity with the penicillins or the cephalosporins.

Beta-lactamase inhibitors.—These compounds hydrolyze beta-lactamases and inactivate them, thereby protecting the antibiotics that are the substrates for these enzymes. Beta-lactamase inhibitors are nearly devoid of antibacterial activity. Clavulanic acid has been combined with amoxicillin as an oral antibiotic (Augmentin) and with ticarcillin (Timentin) as a parenteral preparation. A recently isolated beta-lactamase protein inhibitor may be superior to current agents.

Other antibiotics that inhibit bacterial cell wall synthesis

Vancomycin and bacitracin are unrelated to the beta-lactam antibiotics but have a similar action on the bacterial cell wall.

Vancomycin.—This drug is active against gram-positive bacteria that are resistant to most other antibiotics, including methicillin. Additionally, it is synergistic with gentamicin and tobramycin. Gram-negative bacteria are resistant. It is often injected intravitreally in endophthalmitis.

Bacitracin.—Bacitracin has an antibacterial spectrum similar to that of the penicillins, with which it is markedly synergistic. Bacterial resistance is rare, and its potency is not reduced by blood or pus. It is used topically in an ointment particularly in the treatment of staphylococcal blepharoconjunctivitis. It may be combined with neomycin and polymyxin in topical preparations (see Table 3-1). Bacitracin rarely causes hypersensitivity.

Aminoglycosides

This group of antibiotics includes gentamicin, neomycin, tobramycin, amikacin, kanamycin, netilmicin, and streptomycin. Aminoglycosides are important agents in the treatment of gram-negative infections and as synergistic agents in the systemic treatment of staphylococcal and streptococcal infections. They act on the bacterial ribosomes of aerobic gram-negative organisms. They are poorly absorbed after oral administration, do not penetrate the blood-ocular barrier, and may cause auditory nerve (N VIII) and renal toxicity. Gentamicin- and tobramycin-resistant strains of *Enterobacter, Klebsiella, Proteus,* and *Pseudomonas,* particularly in burn units and intensive care units, limit their usefulness. Netilmicin may be active against such organisms.

Gentamicin.—Gentamicin (Garamycin) is bactericidal against most strains of *Pseudomonas, Klebsiella, Aerobacter, Proteus, Staphylococcus,* and *E. coli.* It is used topically in ophthalmology in a 0.3% solution or ointment.

Tobramycin.—Tobramycin has a bactericidal activity similar to that of gentamicin, but it is more active than gentamicin against many, though not all, strains of *P. aeruginosa.* It should be used concurrently with an antipseudomonal cephalosporin for ocular *Pseudomonas* infection. It is used in a 0.3% ointment or ophthalmic solution.

Neomycin.—Neomycin is bactericidal against staphylococci and gram-negative bacteria, but not most *Pseudomonas* species. It is used topically in ophthalmology, often combined with polymyxin B. It is a common cause of contact dermatitis (see Chapter 9).

Tetracyclines

The tetracyclines are bacteriostatic agents that inhibit microbial ribosomal protein synthesis in a broad range of gram-negative and gram-positive bacteria. Additionally, they are active against *Rickettsia, Mycoplasma, Chlamydia,* some atypical mycobacteria, and protozoa. They are the preferred agents in chlamydial infections. In patients intolerant of penicillin, tetracyclines may be used to treat syphilis. *Pseudomonas, Proteus,* and many strains of *Staphylococcus* are resistant to tetracyclines. A variety of compounds are available.

In general, tetracycline (Achromycin) and oxytetracycline (Terramycin) are the least effective, while doxycycline (Vibramycin) and minocycline (Minocin) are the most effective. Milk; antacids containing aluminum, magnesium hydroxide, or silicate; and iron impair gastrointestinal absorption. The compounds penetrate the intact blood-ocular barriers poorly. Resistant strains develop during therapy. After suppression of susceptible microflora, an overgrowth of resistant organisms may cause a superinfection. Demeclocycline (Declomycin) and doxycycline may cause a mild to severe erythema in individuals exposed to bright sunlight.

Tetracyclines are usually administered orally and may cause nausea, vomiting, and diarrhea. Outdated tetracycline may cause reversible renal tubular dysfunction indistinguishable from the Fanconi syndrome. Developing, unerupted teeth may be discolored. The compounds should not be given to pregnant or nursing women or to children before the eruption of all secondary dentition. Demeclocycline causes photosensitivity in some individuals. Pseudotumor cerebri may occur in adults. All tetracyclines potentiate the effects of dicumarol-type anticoagulants. Systemic tetracyclines are particularly useful in the treatment of inclusion conjunctivitis and trachoma.

The quinolones

Replication of the double helix of DNA requires that the strands unwind, a process that requires the enzyme DNA gyrase (topoisomerase II). The quinolones impair the action of the gyrase and inhibit DNA supercoiling. The newer quinolones have broad antibacterial activity and minimal cross-resistance with the beta-lactam antibiotics and the aminoglycosides. They are well tolerated and are used topically and systemically.

Ciprofloxacin.—This is a fluorinated 4-quinolone with broad antibacterial activity and minimal microbial resistance. It is active against *Chlamydia, Pseudomonas,* staphylococci, and streptococci. It is used topically in a 0.3% solution.

Ofloxacin.—This is a fluorinated 4-quinolone with antibacterial activity against a wide range of gram-negative and gram-positive organisms. It is used topically in a 0.3% solution.

Miscellaneous antibiotics

Members of this group include the following: erythromycin, clindamycin, and chloramphenicol.

Erythromycin.—Erythromycin is a well-tolerated systemic antibiotic that has excellent activity against streptococci and *N. gonorrhoeae* and moderate activity against *H. influenzae.* Staphylococci are often resistant. Systemically, in patients sensitive to the penicillins, it is used in the prophylaxis of rheumatic fever. In patients sensitive to the tetracyclines, erythromycin is substituted in the treatment of *Chlamydia trachomatis* infections. It is available in a 0.5% ophthalmic ointment.

Clindamycin.—Clindamycin is active against gram-positive cocci and gram-positive and gram-negative anaerobic pathogens except *Clostridium* species. It is used orally coupled with sulfadiazine and pyrimethamine in the treatment of active toxoplasmosis retinochoroiditis. It frequently causes diarrhea and, in some patients, a severe pseudomembranous colitis (antibiotic-associated colitis). When this occurs, the drug must be stopped at once.

Chloramphenicol.—Chloramphenicol has a wide spectrum of bacteriostatic activity that includes gram-negative bacteria, all anaerobic bacteria, gram-positive cocci, *Clostridium* species, and gram-negative rods. It is rapidly and completely absorbed from the gastrointestinal tract and is not impaired by simultaneous administration of food or antacids. It penetrates well into all tissues, including the brain, cerebrospinal fluid, and aqueous humor. High intraocular concentrations follow systemic administration.

Bone marrow toxicity limits its use to infections in which no other antibiotic may be used. Persistent bone marrow hypoplasia has been described after prolonged local application of eyedrops or ointment. Retrobulbar neuritis, peripheral neuritis or acute encephalopathy has occurred in patients with cystic fibrosis who receive long-term systemic chloramphenicol.

Concentrated antibiotics

In serious disorders, such as suppurative corneal ulcers, endophthalmitis, and orbital cellulitis, concentrated antibiotics are often used topically and subconjunctivally. They are prepared by mixing a parenteral preparation either with sterile artificial tears distributed for topical instillation or with sterile saline for injection. These preparations are much more concentrated than commercially prepared solutions. They are not intended for long-term use because of potential toxicity.

CORTICOSTEROID COMBINATIONS

A variety of antibiotics for topical use are combined with corticosteroids for the treatment of conjunctival and eyelid infections. The antibiotic-corticosteroid preparations are used for the treatment of (1) mixed staphylococcal marginal blepharitis; (2) blepharoconjunctivitis with primary or secondary replicating organisms; (3) marginal corneal ulcers related to staphylococcal infection; and (4) postsurgical trauma.

The use of corticosteroid combinations is often contraindicated. The corticosteroids reduce local tissue immunity and induce increased resistance to the outflow of aqueous humor, which may lead to glaucoma in susceptible eyes. The combination may facilitate the development of a fungal keratoconjunctivitis. Fixed combinations do not permit the administration of the two drugs in different concentrations or at different time intervals. The effects of the antibiotic on the microorganism may also be obscured by the anti-inflammatory action of the corticosteroid.

ANTIVIRAL DRUGS

Viral infections of the eye include herpes simplex keratoconjunctivitis, herpes zoster (varicella-zoster virus), and cytomegalovirus retinitis. Additionally, increased susceptibility of the eye to opportunistic infections, often viral, occurs in the acquired immunodeficiency syndrome (AIDS). All viruses, as obligatory intracellular parasites, replicate by invading the cells of the host and using the biochemical mechanisms of these cells to synthesize viral proteins. Antiviral drugs must, therefore, inhibit viral functions without damaging the host cells. Many different compounds are currently studied for improved activity and favorable pharmacokinetic properties.

Herpes simplex infection of the cornea (see Chapter 12) is treated with topical antivirals, which include trifluridine, vidarabine (which is also used systemically), and idoxuridine. The major drugs available for systemic use include acyclovir, which is used both systemically and topically for herpetic disease, ganciclovir, foscarnet, zidovudine, and interferons.

Trifluridine (Viroptic).—Trifluridine is a synthetic fluorated pyrimidine that inhibits viral DNA polymerase more than DNA synthesis. It is the preferred agent in the treatment of herpes simplex virus types 1 and 2 epithelial keratitis. A 1% solution is instilled every 2 hours for a maximum of nine drops daily. Treatment is continued at a dosage of five drops daily for 5 days after healing.

Vidarabine (Vira-A).—Vidarabine is a purine nucleoside analogue with antiviral activity against several DNA viruses, including herpes simplex virus types 1 and 2, varicella-zoster virus, and vaccinia virus. It inhibits DNA-dependent polymerases 40 times more than host cells. It is incorporated into the terminal positions of herpesvirus DNA and prevents completion of the nucleic acid chain. It is relatively insoluble and requires continuous intravenous infusion.

Vidarabine has been replaced for systemic use by acyclovir, which is less toxic and more effective. A number of analogues and derivatives are used therapeutically in leukemias, lymphomas, and macroglobulinemias.

Herpes simplex epithelial keratitis is treated with a 3% ophthalmic ointment applied topically every 3 hours. Topical therapy of stromal herpes is not practical with vidarabine because the cornea deaminates the compound.

Idoxuridine (Herplex).—Idoxuridine structurally resembles thymidine and is incorporated into DNA during replication. The resultant faulty DNA cannot produce virus particles. Idoxuridine impairs DNA synthesis of the normal corneal epithelium, and punctate epithelial defects develop during treatment. The drug is effective against herpes simplex virus type 1 infections, but not against type 2 or varicella-zoster. It is used in a 0.1% solution every hour during the day and every 2 hours during the night. Therapy is continued for 3 to 5 days after healing is complete. It is commonly used in experimental studies of keratitis.

Acyclovir.—Acyclovir (Zovirax) inhibits viral DNA polymerase after initial activation through phosphorylation by viral thymidine kinase, which is produced only in infected cells. Additionally, it terminates the elongation of the viral DNA strand. It is used orally and intravenously in the treatment of a wide variety of herpes infections including herpes simplex types 1 and 2, herpes zoster, and Epstein-Barr infections. It does not inhibit the cytomegalovirus, adenoviruses, RNA viruses, or the vaccinia virus. Oral administration results in a blood level some 70% to 85% less than that with intravenous administration. It is the drug of choice in the treatment of herpes zoster, but evidence of its efficacy is conflicting. It is most effective when administered within 96 hours of the onset of symptoms.

A 3% ophthalmic ointment (not available commercially in the United States) may be applied topically five times daily in the treatment of herpes simplex infections. Oral acyclovir, 200 mg five times daily, may be substituted. Oral administration may be combined with topical corticosteroids in the treatment of stromal herpes of the cornea associated with iridocyclitis. The acute retinal necrosis syndrome, caused by the herpes simplex or the herpes zoster virus, is treated with intravenous acyclovir, 1,500 mg per day, in three divided doses. After intravenous therapy, oral prophylaxis, 800 mg five times daily, may prevent infection of the fellow eye.

Acyclovir is often used empirically in human immunodeficiency virus (HIV)-seropositive persons treated with zidovudine. The therapy of AIDS is changing rapidly with the introduction of new drugs. Modern therapy often combines several different therapeutic agents.

Ganciclovir.—Ganciclovir is chemically similar to acyclovir but is far more active against cytomegalovirus infections and similarly effective against other herpesviruses. Bone marrow depression limits its use to sight-threatening (retinitis) or life-threatening cytomegalovirus infections in patients with AIDS (see Chapter 25). Initial treatment in retinitis requires intraocular implants, injection, or intravenous administration for 10 to 21 days followed by long-term intravenous suppressive therapy 5 days per week.

Foscarnet.—Foscarnet differs from acyclovir, ganciclovir, vidarabine, and zidovudine (see below) in being a nucleoside pyrophosphate and not a nucleoside analogue. It is active against all herpesviruses and some retroviruses, including HIV. Foscarnet must be administered intravenously in a manner similar to ganciclovir, with initial treatment of 14 to 21 days followed by daily long-term suppressive therapy. Renal impairment is its major toxicity and must be monitored by long-term serum creatinine clearance determinations. Serum ionized calcium levels may be affected, and anemia is common. In AIDS patients the use of foscarnet yields a survival of 12 months compared with 8 months with the use of ganciclovir.

Zidovudine.—Zidovudine (Retrovir) inhibits its RNA-dependent DNA polymerase (reverse transcriptase) of HIV-1 and prevents the production of DNA chains and retroviral RNA and proteins. It is used in the palliation of AIDS and may be of prophylactic value in health workers stuck with needles contaminated with blood from HIV-1 patients.

It is used orally in a dose of 200 mg every 4 hours. Depending on the severity of CD4 lymphocyte reduction at the time the drug is initiated, some 45% of all patients develop anemia 2 to 6 weeks after starting treatment. Granulocytopenia develops after 6 to 8 weeks. Blood transfusions are required in some 30% of the patients. Acetaminophen, aspirin, and probenecid must be avoided. The quality of life is improved, opportunistic infections are reduced, neurologic disease improves, and the median survival of AIDS patients is increased from 8 months to more than 2 years.

Interferons.—Interferons are proteins that induce the synthesis of RNA and protein. Natural interferons are produced in humans by virus infections. Synthetic interferons are compounded by recombinant DNA techniques. There are three major classes, as follows: (1) alpha (leukocyte interferon); (2) beta (fibroblast interferon); and (3) gamma (immune interferon). All frequently cause influenza-like symptoms. They are used in the treatment of AIDS-associated Kaposi sarcoma, early HIV infections, human papilloma viruspapillomas, and hepatitis B, C, or D virus infections. As with zidovudine, systemic use is associated with overgrowth of the eyelashes (hypertrichosis) in some patients.

ANTIFUNGAL AGENTS

Antifungal agents are effective in inhibiting the growth of fungi but are not effective as fungicidal agents. Their penetration into tissue is poor, and chemotherapy of ocular infections is often not effective. The object of treatment is to inhibit growth of the fungus over a long period until it is excluded by the patient's immune mechanisms. Debilitation, trauma, corticosteroid treatment, or immunosuppression each may limit the effectiveness of treatment. Vitrectomy or keratoplasty is often required to remove infected tissue.

Natamycin, which is mainly effective against *Fusarium solani,* is the only antifungal ophthalmic product that is available commercially. Topical, periocular, and intravitreal routes of administration are not approved by the Food and Drug Administration for any other antifungal agent.

Three groups of agents are used in antifungal therapy: (1) polyenes (amphotericin B, nystatin, and natamycin); (2) imidazoles and triazoles (ketoconazole, fluconazole, and miconazole); and (3) pyrimidines (flucytosine).

Amphotericin B binds the ergosterol and increases the permeability of the cell membrane of sensitive fungi. It has clinical activity against *Histoplasma capsulatum, Blastomyces dermatitidis, Coccidioides immitis, Cryptococcus neoformans, C. albicans* and other *Candida* species, *Torulopsis glabrata, Aspergillus fumigatus,* and other species of *Aspergillus* and *Coccidioides.*

Amphotericin B is not absorbed from the gastrointestinal tract and must be repeatedly infused intravenously. Most patients (80%) develop an azotemia that often requires a reduction in dosage or cessation of the drug. It is used topically (0.1% solution) in the treatment of some fungal inflammations of the cornea.

Nystatin (Mycostatin).—Nystatin is administered topically in a concentration of 100,000 units/mL of commercial diluent in demonstrated fungal infections of the anterior ocular segment. Its main value is in the treatment of superficial *Candida* infection. It is ineffective in cutaneous dermatophyte infections. It is not absorbed from the gastrointestinal tract, and its toxicity is such that it cannot be used intravenously. It is insoluble in saline solution and is prepared as a suspension.

Natamycin (Natacyn).—This drug is used topically as a 5% suspension in propylene glycol or as an ointment. It has a fairly broad spectrum and is more useful than amphotericin B in superficial fungal infections. It is the drug of choice in the treatment of infections caused by *F. solani.*

Flucytosine (Ancobon).—Flucytosine is related to 5-fluorouracil, to which it is converted within the cells of sensitive fungi. It has a narrow spectrum of activity, which includes mainly strains of *C. neoformans,* various *Candida* species, and rarely *Aspergillus* species. It penetrates the cornea and the blood-ocular barriers well. It is recommended as an adjunct to systemic treatment with amphotericin B.

Ketoconazole (Nizoral).—Ketoconazole inhibits the synthesis of ergosterol by the cell membrane of susceptible fungi. It is active by oral administration against most dermatophytes, *Candida* species, *Blastomyces dermatitidis, Histoplasma capsulatum, Paracoccidioides brasiliensis,* and *Pseudoallescheria boydii.* It is used orally in a dose of 200 to 400 mg daily. The concentration in the central nervous system and, presumably, in the ocular tissues is low.

HEAVY METALS

All states require prophylaxis of ophthalmia neonatorum (see Chapter 12) within 1 hour of birth, traditionally by the instillation of 1% silver nitrate into each conjunctival cul-de-sac. Silver nitrate precipitates proteins, including those microbes, and prevents gonorrheal ophthalmia neonatorum but not inclusion body conjunctivitis, which is caused by *C. trachomatis.* Erythromycin, which may be substituted for silver nitrate in many states, prevents both. Instillation of tetracycline is permitted by many states and prevents gonorrheal ophthalmia but not inclusion body conjunctivitis.

Only silver nitrate distributed in individual containers should be used. The laws vary in different states and practitioners should be familiar with the local regulations governing the prophylaxis of ophthalmia neonatorum.

Locally applied 1% silver nitrate is also used as a cauterizing agent in superior limbic keratoconjunctivitis. Silver proteinate preparations agglutinate pus so that it is more easily irrigated from the conjunctival sac. The dark brown color of the silver proteinate solutions makes them unpleasant to use. Prolonged topical use of silver compounds may result in the permanent deposition of silver in the tissues (argyrosis).

Mercuric salts are used locally to inhibit sulfhydril enzymes. Nitromersol (Metaphen) is used in a 1:2,500 ointment in the conjunctival sac. Thimerosal (Merthiolate) is used as an antiseptic and as a preservative in eye products. It commonly causes contact hypersensitivity reactions.

Zinc sulfate has been used to treat conjunctivitis caused by the diplobacillus of Morax-Axenfeld (*Haemophilus*), but antibiotics are superior. Zinc sulfate is used as an astringent in many collyria and nonspecific over-the-counter eye preparations.

THE CORTICOSTEROIDS

The adrenal cortex is divided into the medulla and the cortex. The medulla secretes epinephrine and a small amount of norepinephrine. The adrenal cortex is divided into three zones that are stimulated by the adrenocorticotrophic hormone (ACTH) of the pituitary gland, which is stimulated by the corticotropin-releasing factor (CRF) of the hypothalamus. The adrenal cortex secretes three steroids, as follows: (1) mineralocorticoids (aldosterone), which regulates salt and water metabolism; (2) adrenal androgens important in the development of secondary sex characteristics; and (3) the glucocorticoids, cortisol and corticosterone. The glucocorticoids have many actions, as follows: (1) glucose neogenesis, protein catabolism, and lipolysis; (2) resistance to stress by enhancing the affect of adrenergic stimuli on arterioles; (3) anti-inflammatory through inhibition of phospholipase A_2, thereby reducing the production of arachidonic acid, the precursor of leukotrienes and prostaglandins; (4) faulty activation of T cells by antigen-activated macrophages; and (5) stabilization of lysosomal enzymes.

Corticosteroids prevent and suppress edema induced by inflammation, fibrin deposition, capillary dilation and proliferation, leukocyte infiltration, and subsequent scarring. The cause of the inflammatory response is not affected, and an infection may continue to progress in the absence of inflammatory signs. Corticosteroids are thus mainly useful in decreasing inflammation in self-limited disease processes. Long-term administration is associated with many side effects that limit their usefulness. Ocular complications may follow topical, periocular, or systemic administration.

The most common ocular complication of topical administration is secondary open-angle glaucoma, which may cause loss of vision combined with typical excavation of the optic disk and visual field defects. Posterior subcapsular cataracts may occur after topical administration. They are most common in patients with connective tissue disorders who receive systemic corticosteroids for a long period. Patients with rheumatoid arthritis are particularly prone to cataract formation. Cataracts rarely occur in patients with ulcerative colitis or asthma who receive similar doses. Toxoplasmic retinochoroiditis may progress after retrobulbar injection of corticosteroids.

Local tissue immunity usually limits simplex keratitis to the corneal epithelium. Topical corticosteroids reduce local tissue immunity, and the virus infects additional epithelium and may cause stromal necrosis. The anti-inflammatory effect of the corticosteroids is such that the eye is less injected and more comfortable. Unwittingly the patient may use excessive amounts of corticosteroid, which results in eventual rupture of the cornea.

Fungal infections of the cornea may follow the use of topical corticosteroids combined with an antibiotic. A mycotic infection must be considered in any persistent corneal ulceration after long-term treatment with these drugs. Topical instillation of corticosteroids impairs wound healing by delaying fibroblastic regeneration. After systemic administration, the local tissue concentration is usually not sufficient to interfere with wound healing. Topical corticosteroids in small amounts after cataract extraction and corneal transplantation do not appear to affect wound healing adversely. Topical corticosteroids may also cause a mild blepharoptosis and pupillary dilation.

Long-term systemic administration may suppress immunity to *Candida* species, toxoplasmosis, cytomegalic inclusion, and herpesvirus hominis. These organisms may cause widespread intraocular inflammation, necrotizing angiitis, and loss of vision. Similar disorders after immunosuppression are seen in the course of Hodgkin disease, lymphatic leukemia, AIDS, and tumor radiation therapy.

The treatment of ocular disorders with corticosteroids for a long period requires caution. A maintenance dose of 200 mg or less of prednisone every other morning does not seem to have as serious side effects as daily administration. Side effects associated with long-term corticosteroid administration include peptic ulcer, perforation of the stomach and intestine, gastrointestinal hemorrhage, osteoporosis, psychosis, nitrogen depletion, diabetes mellitus, myopathy, sodium retention with edema, vascular hypertension, potassium depletion, and avascular bone necrosis. Side effects also include gain in weight, fat distribution of the cushingoid type, acne, hirsutism, amenorrhea, cutaneous striae, and increased tendency to bruise. Retinal microaneurysms as well as papilledema may occur.

TOPICAL NONSTEROIDAL ANTI-INFLAMMATORY AGENTS

Phospholipids released from cell membranes are converted to arachidonic acid through the action of phospholipase A_2. This enzyme is inhibited by the glucocorticosteroids, and its actions are enhanced by bradykinin and angiotensin. Arachidonic acid may be metabolized by one of two pathways: (1) the 5-lipoxygenase pathway, which leads to the production of leukotrienes; and (2) the cyclo-oxygenase pathway, which leads to the production of prostaglandin 2, prostaglandin H_2, and in turn to prostaglandin E_1, prostaglandin $GF_{2\alpha}$, and thromboxane A_2. The prostaglandins cause inflammation, pain, and fever.

The enzyme cyclo-oxygenase is inhibited by the nonsteroidal anti-inflammatory agents, of which aspirin and its derivatives are the principal members. The different agents differ markedly in their effects on pain, fever, and inflammation. A subclass of cyclo-oxygenase inhibitors, the propionic acid derivatives, are used topically to reduce ocular inflammation and to prevent pupillary constriction in cataract surgery. When the crystalline lens is absent, they penetrate the cornea and diffuse through the vitreous and may reduce the edema in macular lesions. Like aspirin, they may increase bleeding tendencies.

The topical compounds reduce the itching of seasonal ocular allergies and prevent pupillary constriction in cataract extraction. They reduce the discomfort and signs of noninfectious ocular irritation and the inflammation that may follow intraocular surgery. They are often used after excimer laser photoablation of the cornea.

The propionic acid derivatives include many products, of which the following are available in the United States: ibuprofen, naproxen, suprofen, ketorolac, and flurbiprofen. Many others are available.

Ibuprofen.—This is available in a 0.03% solution. It is applied topically at the time of surgery to prevent pupillary constriction during cataract extraction.

Ketorolac.—This is available in a 0.5% ophthalmic solution and is approved to relieve ocular itching in seasonal allergic conjunctivitis.

Diclofenac.—This is available in a 0.1% ophthalmic solution and is approved to minimize ocular discomfort that follows cataract extraction. It has a similar action after excimer laser photoablation and may reduce macular edema.

Suprofen.—This is available in a 1.0% ophthalmic solution. It is used to maintain pupillary dilation during cataract surgery. Five drops are instilled in the conjunctival sac at intervals the day before surgery and three drops the day of surgery.

IMMUNOSUPPRESSION

Immunosuppression agents, particularly cyclosporine, are emerging as major ophthalmic therapeutic agents. Cell-mediated immunity begins with the ingestion and processing of an antigen by macrophages, monocytes, and related phagocytic cells. The activated macrophages secrete interleukin-1, tumor necrosis antigen, and, together with the major histocompatibility antigen, display the processed antigen on the cell surface. Helper T cells, under the influence of interleukin-1, are activated after contact with the processed antigen and the major histocompatibility complex. The helper T cells then secrete interleukin-2 through interleukin-6, gamma interferon, and granulocyte-macrophage colony-stimulating factor. The gamma interferon enhances the processing of antigen by macrophages. The interleukin-2 causes clonal expansion of activated T cells and stimulates cytotoxic (killer) lymphocytes. Interleukin-6 stimulates B cells to produce antibodies against the original antigen.

Corticosteroids inhibit the processing of antigen by macrophages and other phagocytes and impair the release of interleukin-1. Cyclosporin impairs activation of helper T cells. Azathioprine, methotrexate, cyclophosphamide, and corticosteroids impair the production of plasma cells by B cells and activated T cells by cytotoxic T cells.

Cyclosporine.—The exact action of cyclosporine is not known. It inhibits the production of interleukin-2 by helper T cells (CD4) and the production and release of other lymphokines. It reduces glomerular filtration and renal plasma flow in 25% to 75% of patients. Its systemic use must be monitored with serum creatinine levels.

Topical cyclosporine A is used to prevent rejection after corneal transplantation, and in the treatment of patients with atopic and vernal keratoconjunctivitis, Moorens ulcer, and ulcerative keratitis that are not responsive to other therapy. It is used systemically in ocular immune disorders, such as sympathetic ophthalmia, inflammations of the uveal tract, and the Sjögren syndrome.

FK 506 (Tacrolimus).—FK 506 is an immunosuppressive agent with many of the properties (and complications) of cyclosporine. It has been used in organ transplantation and in the treatment of severe, chronic uveitis, such as Behçet disease and Vogt-Koyanagi-Harada syndrome. FK 506 may cause impairment of kidney function, glucose intolerance, and aggravation of neurologic symptoms in Behçet disease. Although its pharmacologic actions are similar to cyclosporine, FK 506 may have different actions on the immune system, so that it may be substituted when cyclosporine is not effective.

Azathioprine.—Azathioprine is used mainly in suppression of organ rejection and is combined with prednisone and cyclosporine. The combination causes frequent infections and malignancies and is reserved for patients in whom the combination of cyclosporine and prednisone has been ineffective.

Cyclophosphamide.—Cyclophosphamide is a nitrogen mustard alkylating agent that interferes with normal mitosis and cell division in rapidly proliferating tissues, particularly those of the bone marrow and lymphocyte tissues. The major effect of cyclophosphamide appears to be on lymphocyte tissue. The drug must be activated by liver enzymes.

In ocular inflammations cyclophosphamide is administered in a dosage of 1 to 2 mg/kg of body weight daily, and the dosage is decreased if the peripheral leukocyte count decreases. Large doses are not used in ocular inflammations because of systemic complications, particularly hemorrhagic cystitis and profound depression of the hematologic system. Cyclophosphamide is teratogenic, and pregnancy is contraindicated during therapy.

INHIBITION OF FIBROBLASTIC PROLIFERATION

The surgical treatment of glaucoma (see Chapter 22) often requires the creation of a filtering cicatrix between the anterior chamber and the subconjunctival space. The procedure may fail if there is excessive proliferation of fibrous tissue from the episclera, Tenon capsule, or conjunctiva. To minimize proliferation of fibrous tissue, mitomycin is applied to the wound bed for 2 to 5 minutes at the time of surgery. In some patients this causes excessive drainage of aqueous humor or a thin conjunctival covering that is prone to secondary infection. Previously, fluorouracil was used, but it required repeated injections after the surgical procedure.

Mitomycin.—Mitomycin is an antibiotic and alkylating agent that inhibits DNA synthesis. Its benefits are limited, and it is rarely used for cancer chemotherapy. It is used in glaucoma surgery to enhance the likelihood of successful filtration of aqueous humor. Usually two or three drops of a 4-mg/mL solution on a minute eye sponge are applied to the sclera and the inner surface of Tenon capsule and kept in position for 2 to 5 minutes. A longer period is used in black patients, patients less than 40 years of age, patients who have conjunctival scarring in the operative area, and patients who have uveitis or rubeosis iridis. Excessive filtration resulting in maculopathy and reduced vision occurs in some 7.0% of the patients.

Topical 0.02% mitomycin is instilled two or three times daily after pterygium resection to inhibit fibroblastic proliferation and recurrence. It must be used no longer than 5 days so as not to induce a necrosis of the sclera.

Fluorouracil.—Fluorouracil (5-fluorouracil, 5-FU) inhibits the synthesis of thymidylate and the functions of RNA. It is used systemically, often in combination with other antineoplastic agents, in the management of metastatic carcinoma of the breast and gastrointestinal tract.

Fluorouracil inhibits fibroblastic proliferation and is injected subconjunctivally to prevent scarring after filtering operations for glaucoma. It is administered daily by subconjunctival injection, in 5-mg dosages after filtering procedures. It may be given the day of surgery and continued for 7 days, or the injections may be started after the anterior chamber has reformed. Mitosis of the corneal epithelium is inhibited, and corneal erosions occur. Controlled studies indicate the compound enhances the formation of filtering blebs in glaucoma surgery.

MAST CELL STABILIZERS

Seasonal allergic keratoconjunctivitis, vernal conjunctivitis, and giant papillary conjunctivitis are type I (immediate) hypersensitivity reactions (see Chapter 25). They result from the binding of an antigen (allergen) to IgE (immune globulin E) on the surface of mast cells, which activates the release of three classes of mediators: (1) histamine; (2) lipid mediators (prostaglandins, leukotrienes, and plasma activating factor); and (3) cytokines (tumor necrosis factor and interleukins). The immediate reaction is vasodilation and increased vascular permeability, mediated mainly by histamine. After 2 to 4 hours, a late phase, mediated mainly by cytokines, promotes a vascular inflammation.

The treatment of immediate allergic reactions of the conjunctiva involves several approaches. Dilution of the antigen by frequent instillation of 0.05% naphazoline (Albalon-A, Naphcon-A, Vasocon-A) minimizes itching, redness, chemosis, eyelid swelling, and tearing.

The nonsteroidal anti-inflammatory agents prevent the arachidonic acid cascade. Topical corticosteroids, never used for more than 7 days, may relieve symptoms.

Levacobastine.—Levacobastine (0.05% suspension) is a topical histamine H1-receptor antagonist. It antagonizes nearly all actions of histamine except those mediated solely by H2 receptors. It is effective after the release of histamine and prevents the released histamine from reacting with the H1 receptor and causing the reactions of allergy.

Lodoxamide.—Lodoxamide stabilizes mast cells and prevents their degranulation with the release of their mediators that occurs when an allergen attaches to the IgE on its surface. It is used in a 0.10% solution four times daily and is highly effective in relieving the signs and symptoms of ocular immediate hypersensitivity.

Cromolyn sodium.—Cromolyn sodium is thought to inhibit the transport of calcium across mast cell membranes and thereby prevent the release of the IgE mediators of the immediate sensitivity reaction. A 4% solution is used topically four to six times a day in the treatment of vernal keratoconjunctivitis, giant papillary conjunctivitis, and allergic keratoconjunctivitis.

THE AUTONOMIC NERVOUS SYSTEM

The autonomic nervous system provides the efferent innervation of all of the structures of the body except skeletal muscle and regulates functions that have no voluntary control. The efferent system may be divided into parasympathetic (craniosacral outflow or cholinergic) and sympathetic (thoracolumbar outflow or adrenergic) (see Chapter 1). It is characterized by peripheral ganglia located outside the cerebrospinal axis, whereas the ganglia of skeletal muscle are located entirely within the cerebrospinal axis. Drugs that bind to receptors of the parasympathetic system to modify their actions are designated cholinergic-stimulating (agonist) or cholinergic-blocking (antagonist) agents. Drugs that bind to receptors of the sympathetic nervous system to modify their actions are designated adrenergic-stimulating (agonist) or adrenergic-blocking (antagonist) agents. The agents are widely used in the treatment of glaucoma (see Chapter 22), in the diagnosis of abnormalities of the pupillary musculature (see Chapter 7), in refraction (see Chapter 24), and for pupillary dilation for intraocular examination.

Acetylcholine is the neurotransmitter of all preganglionic autonomic fibers, all parasympathetic fibers, and a few postganglionic sympathetic fibers (Table 3-2). Norepinephrine (noradrenaline, levarterenol) is the neurotransmitter of nearly all postganglionic sympathetic fibers. Acetylcholine is inactivated by the enzyme acetylcholinesterase (specific or true cholinesterase). Norepinephrine is largely (90%) inactivated by reuptake by the synaptic junction of the axon that released it or by the enzyme catechol-O-methyl transferase. The amount of norepinephrine stored in a synaptic junction is limited by the enzyme monoamine oxidase.

TABLE 3-2.
Acetylcholine Transmission

- Cholinergic synapses
  - Postganglionic parasympathetic innervation
    - Smooth and cardiac muscle
  - Postganglionic sympathetic innervation
    - Sweat glands
    - Arrectores pilorum muscles
  - Preganglionic autonomic fibers
    - Adrenal medulla
    - Parasympathetic ganglia
    - Sympathetic ganglia
  - Some central nervous system synapses
- Acetylcholine receptors
  - Muscarinic (blocked by atropine)
    - Smooth and cardiac muscles
    - Exocrine glands
  - Nicotinic receptors (blocked by *d*-tubocurarine)
    - Autonomic ganglia (blocked by hexamethonium)
    - Motor endplates skeletal muscle (blocked by decamethonium)

The dilatator pupillae muscle is innervated by long ciliary nerve branches of the nasociliary nerve branch of the ophthalmic division of the trigeminal nerve (N V_1) that carry sympathetic fibers that have synapsed in the superior cervical ganglion (see Chapter 1). Vasomotor sympathetic nerves to the blood vessels of the eye pass through the ciliary ganglion, but do not synapse, and are distributed to the choroidal and retinal blood vessels through the short ciliary nerves. The sympathetic nerve fibers destined for the dilatator pupillae muscle do not pass through the ciliary ganglion.

Adrenergic stimulation of the dilatator pupillae muscle causes pupillary dilation. Adrenergic blockade causes pupillary constriction as the result of unopposed action of the sphincter pupillae muscle. Possibly, the ciliary muscle has adrenergic innervation so that stimulation decreases accommodation. The more prominent cholinergic effects obscure any adrenergic effects.

The sphincter pupillae muscle (pupillary constriction) and the ciliary muscle (accommodation) are innervated by parasympathetic autonomic fibers that originate in the Edinger-Westphal portion of the nucleus of the oculomotor nerve (N III). They are distributed to the ciliary ganglion by a short motor branch of the inferior division of the oculomotor nerve. After synapse in the ciliary ganglion, they are distributed to the sphincter pupillae muscle and the ciliary muscle in the short ciliary nerves.

Cholinergic stimulation of the sphincter pupillae muscle causes constriction of the pupil (miosis) and increased accommodation. Cholinergic blockade causes pupillary dilation because of the unopposed action of the dilatator pupillae muscle. Blockade of the ciliary muscle causes decreased accommodation (cycloplegia).

CHOLINERGIC SYSTEM

Acetylcholine is the neurotransmitter substance that stimulates the two major types of cholinergic receptors, nicotinic and muscarinic.

Nicotinic cholinergic receptors, of which there are many subtypes, are located predominantly in the motor endplates of skeletal muscle, in autonomic ganglia, in the adrenal medulla, and in the central nervous system. They are stimulated by small amounts of nicotine and blocked by large amounts. Tubocurarine blocks nicotinic receptors in motor endplates of skeletal muscle but does not penetrate the blood-brain barrier. Hexamethonium blocks nicotinic receptors only in autonomic ganglia. Decamethonium blocks nicotinic receptors only in the motor endplates of skeletal muscle.

Muscarinic cholinergic receptors, of which there are at least five types, are located in smooth muscle, cardiac muscle, the postganglionic nerve endings to sweat glands, the arrectores pilorum muscles, and the central nervous system. Muscarinic cholinergic receptors are blocked by atropine.

Acetylcholine is stored within synaptic vesicles in the nerve and released into the synaptic cleft on depolarization (Fig 3-2). It diffuses across the cleft to activate muscarinic receptors, the predominant receptor of smooth and cardiac muscles and exocrine glands, or nicotinic receptors of autonomic ganglia and skeletal muscle. The acetylcholine depolarizes the postsynaptic membrane, causing transmission of the nervous impulse. The action of the released acetylcholine is terminated within 1 μsec to 1 second by hydrolysis mediated by the enzyme acetylcholinesterase located on the surface of the cholinergic membrane.

Acetylcholinesterase, also called specific cholinesterase, occurs mainly in neurons and at neuromuscular junctions. It is the main cholinesterase of the iris, ciliary muscle, and lens. It inactivates acetylcholine only. Butyrocholinesterase, called serum cholinesterase or nonspecific cholinesterase, occurs in the liver and plasma. It inactivates both acetylcholine and long-chain choline esters. The acetylcholinesterase drugs used clinically inhibit acetylcholinesterase and cause an accumulation of endogenous acetylcholine.

Cholinergic-stimulating drugs mimic the action of acetylcholine on receptor cells or at

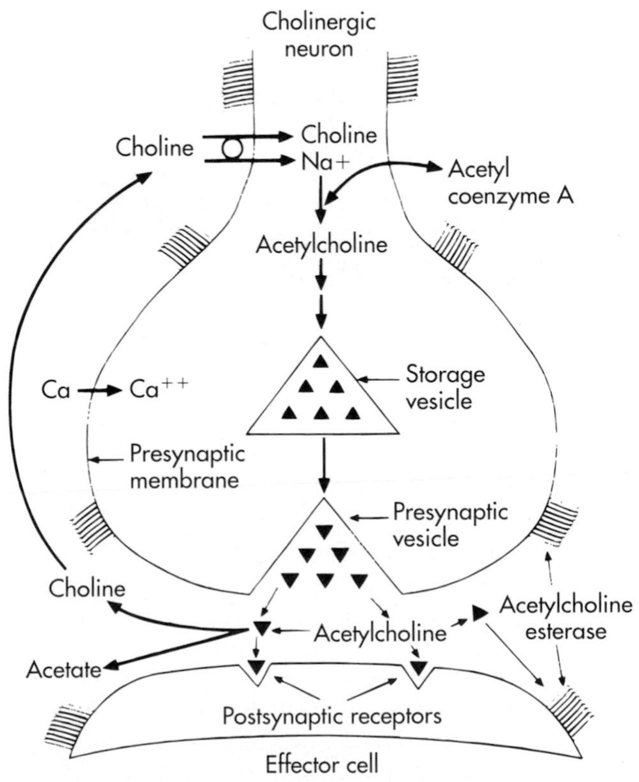

FIG 3-2.
Schema of the cholinergic synapse. Acetylcholine is synthesized from choline and acetyl coenzyme A by the enzyme choline acetyltransferase. The acetylcholine is stored within vesicles in the nerve terminal. When stimulated, calcium gated voltage channels in the presynaptic membrane open and allow calcium to enter the nerve terminal. The excess calcium causes the storage vesicle to fuse with the cell membrane and release acetylcholine into the synaptic cleft. There it fuses with acetylcholine receptors of the effector cell to induce the action of the cell. Acetylcholine is rapidly hydrolyzed by the acetylcholinesterase of the synaptic cleft.

TABLE 3-3.
Cholinergic Agonists Used in Ophthalmology

I. Choline esters
  A. Acetylcholine
  B. Carbachol
II. Cholinomimetic natural alkaloid
  A. Pilocarpine

TABLE 3-4.
Anticholinesterase Agents

I. Physostigmine (eserine)
II. Edrophonium chloride (Tensilon)
III. Organophosphate
  A. Echothiophate iodide (Phospholine Iodide)
  B. Isoflurophate (Floropryl)
  C. Demecarium bromide (Humorsol)
IV. Reactivation of acetyl cholinesterase
  A. Pralidoxime chloride (Protopam Chloride)

synapses. The action may be brought about directly by compounds chemically similar to acetylcholine or by compounds, such as pilocarpine, that act directly on smooth muscle. Indirect stimulation follows the accumulation of acetylcholine when its usual hydrolysis by acetylcholinesterase is blocked. Compounds that block the action of acetylcholinesterase are called anticholinesterases. They are classified as reversible if their action is rapid or irreversible if their action is prolonged.

Cholinergic-stimulating drugs

These compounds (Table 3-3) are not used systemically. When instilled in the conjunctival sac, choline esters dilate the conjunctival and anterior ciliary arteries, constrict the pupil (miosis), and increase the permeability of the blood-aqueous barrier. Most penetrate the intact cornea poorly.

Acetylcholine chloride.—Acetylcholine chloride (1%) in mannitol solution (3%) (Miochol) constricts the pupil when injected into the anterior chamber, usually after cataract extraction. It is rapidly hydrolized by cholinesterase. After topical administration, it is inactivated by corneal cholinesterase so that it does not enter the anterior chamber.

Pilocarpine.—Pilocarpine, like acetylcholine, acts directly on smooth muscle and glandular receptors innervated by postganglionic cholinergic nerves. It stimulates the sphincter pupillae muscle (miosis) and the ciliary muscles (increased accommodation), and increases outflow of aqueous humor through the trabecular meshwork. In some patients, it decreases secretion of aqueous humor. It is used topically in 1% to 4% solution in the treatment of glaucoma (see Chapter 22). It is prescribed in the minimum concentration that will prevent progression of the glaucoma and is seldom instilled more frequently than once every 6 hours. Increased outflow of aqueous humor is its most useful function in open-angle glaucoma, whereas pupillary constriction is its most useful action in angle-closure glaucoma. Systemic toxicity after topical instillation is uncommon, although long-term use may be associated with lens opacities or contact allergy (type IV hypersensitivity) of the skin of the eyelids and conjunctiva. Patients with blue irises are more sensitive to its effects than patients with more pigment in their uveal tract.

Carbachol.—Carbachol, 0.75% to 3.0%, must be combined with a wetting agent to penetrate the cornea. It is not hydrolyzed by cholinesterases and is so potent that it is not used systemically. This drug may be substituted for pilocarpine in patients who have developed a tolerance to pilocarpine. A 0.01% solution (Miostat) is injected into the anterior chamber to produce miosis in intraocular surgery.

Anticholinesterase drugs

Anticholinesterase drugs inactivate acetylcholinesterase, thereby allowing the accumulation of endogenous acetylcholine (Table 3-4). Many anticholinesterase compounds are the active ingredients of insecticides, and accidental human exposure may cause extreme toxicity. They are classified as reversible cholinesterase inhibitors (physostigmine) and irreversible cholinesterase inhibitors (the organophosphates). The reversible inhibitors are short-acting and the irreversible cholinesterase inhibitors are long-acting.

Systemic administration of anticholinesterase compounds causes widespread cholinergic stimulation. There is constriction of gastrointestinal, urinary, and bronchiole muscles. Skeletal muscle is weakened and fibrillates. Salivation, lacrimation, sweating, and pulmonary secretions increase. Central nervous system symptoms range from giddiness to coma and convulsions.

The sphincter pupillae and ciliary muscles contract so that the pupil is miotic and accommodation is increased. Anticholinesterase drugs do not constrict the pupil after retrobulbar anesthesia that blocks the parasympathetic innervation. The organophosphates more markedly dilate the conjunctival and ciliary blood vessels and cause greater permeability of the blood-aqueous barrier than physostigmine.

Physostigmine.—Physostigmine (eserine) was the first miotic used in the treatment of glaucoma (1876). It is used in an aqueous solution in a concentration of 0.25% to 0.5% or as a 0.25% ointment. Usually it is given only at bedtime to supplement the instillation of pilocarpine. After prolonged use, physostigmine becomes less effective in reducing the intraocular pressure (tolerance) and may cause conjunctival irritation and follicular hypertrophy. Solutions that become discolored are less potent.

Edrophonium chloride (Tensilon).— This compound has a systemic action of 2 to 3 minutes. It is used intravenously in the diagnosis of myasthenia gravis, after testing for hypersensitivity to the drug.

Organophosphates.— Organophosphate topical preparations are particularly effective in open-angle glaucoma, glaucoma after cataract extraction, and accommodative esotropia in children. Their use is contraindicated in eyes with shallow anterior chambers and in patients with bronchial asthma, gastrointestinal spasm, vascular hypertension, myocardial infarction, myasthenia gravis, and Parkinson disease. Prolonged topical use may cause iris cysts in children unless applied simultaneously with topical phenylephrine. Topical organophosphates deplete both specific and pseudocholinesterase. They inactivate the Na, K-ATPase of the specific cholinesterase of the lens capsule and may cause fluid vesicles in the anterior portion of the crystalline lens after more than 6 months of use.

Topical administration depletes systemic nonspecific cholinesterases (pseudocholinesterases). Thus, if succinylcholine is used as a muscle relaxant in the induction of general anesthesia, the succinylcholine is not inactivated, and there may be prolonged apnea. Additionally, the compounds may cause intestinal cramping that may be mistaken for an acute surgical abdomen.

Echothiophate iodide (Phospholine Iodide).—This drug is active against both specific cholinesterases and pseudocholinesterases. It is used topically every 12 to 48 hours in open-angle glaucoma in a 0.03% to 0.25% solution. It causes intense miosis and spasm of the ciliary muscle. Because of systemic side effects and the possibility of cataract formation it is used mainly in eyes that have not responded adequately to standard medical measures in glaucoma and in glaucoma in which the lens has been removed.

Demecarium bromide (Humorsol).— This stable, long-acting organophosphate is mainly effective against specific acetylcholinesterase. It is effective in some patients who have not responded to echothiophate but produces tolerance readily. It is applied topically in a 0.12% to 0.25% solution every 12 to 48 hours.

Isoflurophate (DFP; Floropryl).—This is mainly effective against nonspecific cholinesterase rather than acetylcholinesterase. It is administered as a 0.025% ointment or as a 0.01% to 0.10% solution in peanut oil. Hypersensitivity reactions are common, and the drug is easily hydrolyzed and inactivated.

Reactivators of cholinesterase.—Severe toxicity from anticholinesterase compounds in drugs, chemical warfare agents, and insecticides occurs because of the accumulation of systemic acetylcholine. Atropine (2 to 20 mg, intravenously or intramuscularly) blocks acetylcholine at muscarinic receptor sites. Pralidoxime chloride (Protopam Chloride) reactivates acetylcholinesterase, particularly at nicotinic receptors in the motor endplate of skeletal muscle.

Cholinergic blocking drugs

Acetylcholine is the neurohumoral transmitter at two major types of neurohumoral effector sites, the muscarinic and the nicotinic. The muscarinic actions are antagonized by the atropine group of drugs, whereas the nicotinic actions are antagonized by ganglionic blocking agents and neuromuscular blocking agents (Table 3-5).

Atropine group.—These drugs prevent the action of acetylcholine at postganglionic muscarinic receptors in smooth muscle, cardiac muscle, and exocrine glands. Systemic administration increases the heart rate and decreases

TABLE 3-5.
Cholinergic-Blocking Compounds

I. Interference with acetylcholine synthesis
   A. Hemicholinium
II. Prevention of acetylcholine release
   A. Botulinum toxin
III. Blockade of transmitter at postsynaptic receptor
   A. Muscarinic cholinergic receptors
      1. Atropine
      2. Scopolamine
      3. Homatropine
      4. Cyclopentolate
      5. Tropicamide
   B. Nicotinic cholinergic receptors
      1. Competitive antagonist
         a. Nicotine
         b. Tubocurarine
      2. Depolarizing antagonist
         a. Decamethonium
         b. Succinylcholine

sweating, lacrimation, salivary secretion, gastric secretion, gastrointestinal motility, and tone. Many of the compounds depress the central nervous system and may cause confusional psychosis.

These drugs dilate the pupil (mydriasis) through paralysis of the sphincter pupillae muscle, decrease accommodation through paralysis of the ciliary muscle (cycloplegia), and reduce permeability of the blood vessels of the iris and ciliary body when the blood-aqueous barrier is impaired by inflammation.

Systemic administration has less ocular effect than topical instillation because of decreased concentration of the compounds at the effector sites in the eye. Systemically administered atropine has a greater effect on the pupil and ciliary muscle than the atropine-related compounds used for their antispasmodic action on the gastrointestinal tract.

On topical instillation, the atropine-related compounds developed as gastrointestinal antispasmodics have varying degrees of mydriatic and cycloplegic activity. Systemic administration in younger patients may cause an annoying decrease in accommodation. Many patients with ill-defined gastrointestinal complaints for whom such antispasmodics are prescribed also have unsuspected open-angle glaucoma.

Members of the atropine group of drugs used in ophthalmology include atropine, scopolamine, homatropine, cyclopentolate hydrochloride (Cyclogyl), and tropicamide (Mydriacyl).

Atropine.—Atropine is the principal alkaloid of belladonna. It is used in a 0.125% to 2% aqueous solution topically, in an ointment, or in a castor oil base to minimize systemic absorption. It paralyzes the sphincter pupillae muscle and causes pupillary dilation that begins in about 15 minutes, reaches a maximum in 30 to 40 minutes, and persists 7 to 10 days. Paralysis of the ciliary muscle (accommodation) begins 20 to 30 minutes after instillation, reaches a maximum in 1 to 3 hours, and persists 7 to 12 days. Atropine is widely used in the treatment of iridocyclitis and keratitis and for refraction in children, particularly those with esotropia. In keratitis and iridocyclitis, it may be used every 1 to 6 hours. For refraction in children, it is commonly instilled in an ointment base three times daily for 3 days, with examination on the fourth day.

Scopolamine.—This drug is closely related to atropine but has a shorter duration of action (3 to 7 days) on the sphincter pupillae and ciliary muscles. In conditions such as retinal detachment or iridocyclitis, which require prolonged mydriatic and cycloplegic therapy, it is often substituted for topical atropine, which may cause contact hypersensitivity or chronic irritation.

Homatropine.—This synthetic, atropine-like compound is used mainly for refraction. It is used in a 1% to 5% aqueous solution, and it produces mydriasis and cycloplegia that last 24 to 72 hours.

Cyclopentolate (Cyclogyl).—This cholinergic-blocking drug is used almost exclusively for refraction in concentrations of 0.5%, 1%, and 2%. It dilates the pupil and paralyzes accommodation within 25 to 75 minutes; recovery occurs in 6 to 24 hours. Premature and young infants are particularly prone to central nervous system and cardiopulmonary side effects and should have but one instillation of a 0.5% concentration with pressure over the lacrimal sac to minimize systemic absorption. For mydriasis in neonates, a 0.2% solution combined with 1% phenylephrine is commercially available (Cyclomydril).

Tropicamide (Mydriacyl).—Tropicamide causes more rapid mydriasis and cycloplegia and quicker recovery than any other cholinergic-blocking agent. It is used in 0.5% (mydriasis mainly) and 1% (mydriasis and cycloplegia) concentrations. Cycloplegia is maximal 20 to 30 minutes after instillation and disappears within 6 hours. A 0.5% solution is often combined with 2.5% phenylephrine to dilate the pupil for ophthalmoscopy in adults.

***Botulinum* toxin.**—This toxin provides long-lasting interruption of acetylcholine release from individual motor neurons. It is thus a presynaptic blocking agent of cholinergic junctions. It is injected in small amounts (1.25×10^{-5} µg to 6.25×10^{-5} µg) into opposing nonparalyzed muscles in paralytic strabismus and is used in the treatment of blepharospasm.

Ganglionic-blocking drugs.—These agents block the action of acetylcholine at nicotinic receptors in cholinergic autonomic ganglia. They are used systemically in the treatment of hypertensive cardiovascular disease to reduce peripheral resistance by decreasing sympathetic tone to vascular beds. They are also useful in vasospasm therapy and in producing a controlled hypotension in general anesthesia.

The ocular side effects of ganglionic blockade constitute their main ophthalmic interest. The conjunctival blood vessels and the pupil are dilated. The volume of tears and accommodation decrease. The intraocular pressure decreases slightly, apparently because of a decreased secretion of aqueous humor. The decrease is accompanied by an increased resistance to the exit of aqueous humor through the trabecular meshwork. Increased intraocular pressure does not occur because of the reduced secretion of aqueous humor.

Neuromuscular blocking agents.—Pharmacologically the most important effect of these drugs is to block the effects of acetylcholine at the motor endplates of skeletal muscle. There are two types of blocking agents: competitive (stabilizing), of which curare is the classic example; and depolarizing, of which decamethonium is the classic example.

The main ophthalmic application is in general anesthesia. Curare combines with nicotinic receptor sites on motor endplates of skeletal muscle and thereby blocks the uptake of acetylcholine. Succinylcholine and decamethonium depolarize the motor endplate in the same manner as acetylcholine but for a longer period. The initial depolarization contracts the extraocular muscles with an increased intraocular pressure. In patients with lacerations of the eye who require a general anesthetic, succinylcholine is combined with curare and is administered before endotracheal intubation.

Succinylcholine is synergistic with the anticholinesterase agents used in the treatment of glaucoma and accommodative esotropia and may cause prolonged apnea after general anesthesia in patients who use such compounds.

ADRENERGIC SYSTEM

The catecholamines (norepinephrine, dopamine, and epinephrine) are the neurotransmitters responsible for the stimulation of the majority of structures innervated by postganglionic sympathetic nerves. (The arrectores pilorum muscles and sweat glands are exceptional in having postganglionic sympathetic innervation with acetylcholine rather than the catecholamines as the effector substance.) Norepinephrine (noradrenaline or levarterenol) is the major transmitter at most postganglionic sympathetic impulses; dopamine is the major transmitter in the extrapyramidal system; and epinephrine is the major hormone in the adrenal medulla.

The adrenergic receptors are divided into alpha-1, alpha-2, beta-1, and beta-2. Alpha-1 receptor sites predominate in smooth muscles and glands. They are the major adrenergic receptors of the dilatator pupillae muscle. Alpha-2 receptors predominate at presynaptic terminals. Stimulation of alpha-2 receptors inhibits the release of norepinephrine by adrenergic nerve terminals. Beta-1 adrenergic receptors predominate in cardiac muscle. Beta-2 adrenergic receptor sites are present in smooth muscle and glands. The sensitivity of these adrenergic receptors to catecholamines varies considerably. Generally, the effect of sympathomimetic drugs is excitatory on alpha receptors and inhibitory on beta receptors, but isoproterenol is markedly excitatory on both beta-1 and beta-2 receptors.

The norepinephrine released from the sympathetic nerve vesicle is almost completely (90%) inactivated by reuptake by the terminal that released it (Fig 3-3). The norepinephrine that escapes into the circulation is metabolized by the enzyme catechol-O-methyl transferase.

The action of adrenergic compounds in glaucoma is puzzling. Epinephrine, a nonselective adrenergic agonist, and apraclonidine, an alpha-2 agonist, decrease the intraocular pressure, as does timolol, a beta-1 and beta-2 (nonselective) antagonist, and betaxolol, a beta-1

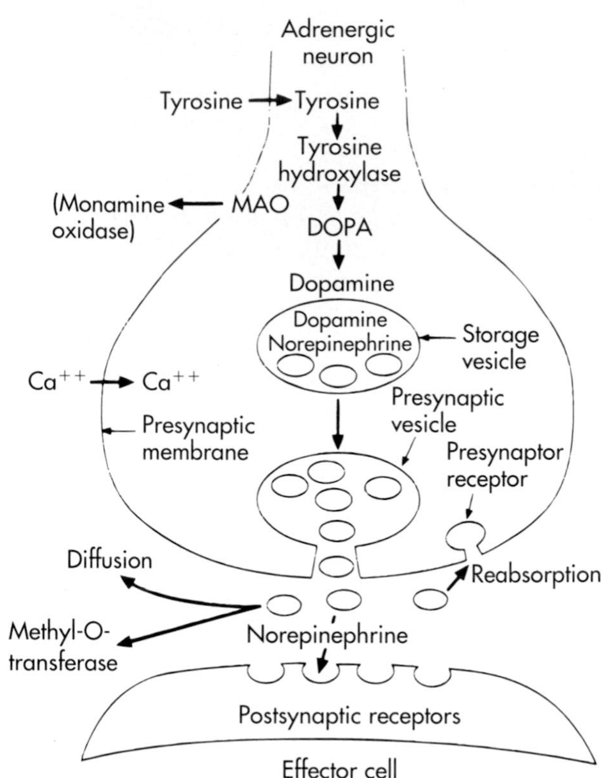

FIG 3-3.
Schema of a postganglionic adrenergic synapse. Norepinephrine is synthesized from tyrosine. Within the neuron, tyrosine is hydrolyzed to DOPA by the enzyme tyrosine hydroxylase. DOPA is converted to dopamine, which is transported to the storage vesicle where it is hydroxylated to norepinephrine. Stimulation of the nerve ending causes an excess of calcium in the cytoplasm of the neuron. The excess calcium causes the storage vesicle to fuse with the cell membrane and release its contents into the synaptic cleft. Norepinephrine fuses with adrenergic receptors of the effector cell resulting in the stimulation of second messengers that results in cell activity. Norepinephrine may be reabsorbed by the adrenergic neuron and again stored, may diffuse into the general circulation, or may be inactivated by methyl-O-transferase.

(selective) antagonist. The synergistic action of epinephrine compounds and beta blockers suggests that the pressure-decreasing mechanism may not be directly mediated through the adrenergic nervous system.

The mechanism of action of adrenergic compounds in glaucoma is not understood. An adrenergic receptor–coupled adenylate cyclase converts extracellular messages to intracellular signals. The receptors are functionally coupled to the enzyme by two proteins, the stimulatory and the inhibitory guanine nucleotide proteins. When the inhibiting protein is absent, the effects of the stimulating protein are modest. When the inhibitory protein is present, the effects of the stimulating protein are much more marked. The inhibitory protein may thus be required both for maximal agonist action and for inhibition of adenylate cyclase. Thus, epinephrine, an adrenergic agonist, has a relatively mild pressure-lowering effect in glaucoma. When administered with an antagonist, such as timolol, betaxolol, or levobunolol, its action is much more marked.

Not all of the adrenergic receptors in the human intraocular musculature have been determined. Both the dilatator pupillae and sphincter pupillae muscles of the monkey eye contain mainly alpha-adrenergic receptors. Thus, stimulation of alpha receptors of the iris musculature produces antagonistic actions, but the larger number of receptors in the dilator muscle causes pupillary dilation. The trabecular meshwork contains mainly alpha receptors, and stimulation increases the facility of outflow. The ciliary epithelium contains mainly beta receptors. Both inhibition and stimulation decrease the secretion of aqueous humor.

Adrenergic-stimulating compounds

Ophthalmic interest in these drugs is concerned with stimulation of alpha- and beta-adrenergic receptors by topical administration. Phenylephrine stimulates alpha receptors, isoproterenol stimulates beta receptors, epinephrine stimulates both alpha and beta receptors, and apraclonidine stimulates alpha-2-adrenergic receptors (Table 3-6). The ocular effects (but not the systemic) are minimal after systemic administration.

Topical instillation of adrenergic-stimulating compounds causes (1) pupillary dilation; (2)

TABLE 3-6.
Ocular Effects of Autonomic Drugs

	Effect on Aqueous Secretion	Effect on Aqueous Outflow	Effect on Intraocular Pressure	Accommodation (Ciliary Muscle)	Sphincter Pupillae Muscle	Dilatator Pupillae Muscle
Cholinergic agonist	±	Increase	Decrease	Increase	Miosis	
Cholinergic antagonist	±	±		Decrease	Mydriasis	
Alpha-adrenergic agonist	±	±	Decrease			Mydriasis
Beta-adrenergic agonist	Decrease	±	Decrease			
Alpha-adrenergic antagonist	±*		Decrease			
Beta-adrenergic antagonist	±†	±	Decrease			Slight mydriasis

*Beta-adrenergic predominance.
†Alpha-adrenergic predominance.

increased facility of outflow of aqueous humor through the trabecular meshwork; (3) decreased secretion of aqueous humor by the ciliary epithelium; and (4) vasoconstriction of the conjunctival blood vessels.

Epinephrine.—Epinephrine (adrenalin) is only slightly lipid-soluble and penetrates the corneal epithelium poorly. In the treatment of glaucoma, 0.25% to 2% epinephrine probably decreases aqueous humor production and increases the outflow of aqueous humor through the trabecular meshwork and the uveoscleral outflow. In glaucoma therapy, epinephrine is often combined with a cholinergic-stimulating drug such as pilocarpine or a beta blocker. In ocular hypertension, topical 1% epinephrine may be used without pilocarpine. In young patients in whom pilocarpine causes a spasm of the ciliary muscle, epinephrine is used alone or combined with timolol.

Pupillary dilation normally does not follow instillation of 1% solution. In denervation hypersensitivity, after the postganglionic sympathetic fibers to the dilatator pupillae muscle have been interrupted, topical instillation of a 0.1% solution will dilate the pupil.

In some individuals, topical instillation of epinephrine produces a black, localized, isolated, subepithelial deposit of adrenochrome in the conjunctiva or corneal epithelium. It is easily removed and may spontaneously peel off. Topical administration of epinephrine after cataract extraction may cause cystoid macular edema because the eye lacks the barrier of the natural crystalline lens or an implanted intraocular lens.

Epinephrine conjugated with two pivalic acid groups yields dipivefrin (Propine), a compound that is 17 times more lipophilic than epinephrine. It easily penetrates the corneal epithelium and is converted to epinephrine by hydrolysis within the eye. It is used topically in a 0.1% solution in the treatment of open-angle glaucoma.

Phenylephrine hydrochloride.—Phenylephrine hydrochloride (Neo-Synephrine), a nearly exclusive alpha-1 receptor agonist, is effective for pupillary dilation. It penetrates the cornea well and is commonly used to dilate the pupil for examination of the ocular fundus. Marked increase in blood pressure may occur in neonates of low weight and adults with orthostatic hypotension. Elderly patients may experience syncope, myocardial infarction, tachycardia, cardiac arrhythmia, and fatal subarachnoid hemorrhage after instillation of a 2.5% solution. A single application of a 2.5% solution in each eye no more than one time each hour is recommended by the manufacturer. Patients using monoamine oxidase inhibitors or tricyclic antidepressants that cause the effects of sympathetic denervation, may be hypersensitive to the alpha-adrenergic stimulation. Phenylephrine is sometimes used in combination with cholinergic-blocking agents to enhance pupillary dilation in the treatment of uveitis. It is available in 1% and 2.5% solutions.

Phenylephrine is the preferred agent for dilating the pupil to study the ocular fundus because it can be easily neutralized with cholinergic drugs. It may prevent the formation of cysts of the pupillary pigmented epithelium in children in whom anticholinesterase preparations are used to minimize accommodation in accommodative esotropia. It is often combined with 0.5% tropicamide for mydriasis.

Apraclonidine.—Apraclonidine is an alpha-2-adrenergic agonist that is used topically 1 hour before and immediately after laser posterior capsulotomy in aphakic eyes. It has a poor affinity for lipids and does not penetrate the cornea or blood-brain barrier. Presumably, it enters the anterior chamber through the sclera, reduces the flow of aqueous humor, and attenuates the incidence and the severity of increase in intraocular pressure that occurs after laser capsulotomy. Patients should have their intraocular pressure measured 1 hour and 24 hours after posterior laser capsulotomy.

Adrenergic blockade

Adrenergic neuron-blocking agents inhibit the synthesis, storage, or release of norepinephrine at the presynaptic vesicle. Adrenergic receptor–blocking agents inhibit the action of norepinephrine and other sympathetic amines on alpha- and beta-adrenergic receptors. Additionally, blockade of adrenergic autonomic ganglia by ganglionic blockade decreases adrenergic stimulation, as do central nervous system depressants.

Adrenergic receptor antagonists.—Agents that block adrenergic receptors are used mainly in the management of vascular hypertension, cardiac arrhythmias, and angina pectoris. Most members of the group block predominantly either alpha- or beta-adrenergic receptors.

Topically administered beta blockers are widely used in the treatment of glaucoma. Timolol, levobunolol, metipranolol, and carteolol are nonselective beta blockers (beta-1 and beta-2) used in glaucoma therapy in the United States. They are absorbed systemically and may adversely affect cardiac and pulmonary function in some patients with heart failure, sinus bradycardia, asthma, or other chronic obstructive pulmonary disease. Postural hypotension induced by topical beta blocker glaucoma medications is a common cause of falls in elderly patients.

Betaxolol is a selective beta-1 blocker used in glaucoma therapy. Carteolol has intrinsic sympathomimetic activity and may be clinically superior to the other nonsympathomimetic beta blockers. Locally, beta blockers cause stinging, burning, redness, itching, tearing, and loss of corneal sensitivity. Betaxolol causes stinging in a third of the patients. Because of the effect of these drugs on lipid metabolism, patients should be instructed to occlude the nasolacrimal puncta after instillation of beta blocker medications.

There may be additive effects in patients receiving catecholamine-depleting drugs such as reserpine. Many side effects are those anticipated from systemic administration of beta-blocking drugs. The twice-daily instillation must not be exceeded. Bradycardia is common, and postural hypotension with syncope may develop in elderly patients. Depression, fatigue, weakness, memory loss, and somnolence occur. Myasthenia gravis may be aggravated or become symptomatic. Superficial punctate keratopathy, keratitis sicca, and corneal anesthesia have been described.

Carteolol.—This is a nonselective beta blocker with intrinsic sympathomimetic activity. Like other beta blockers, it is used topically two times daily. Its most important side effect is related to the action of all beta blockers in decreasing high-density lipoprotein cholesterol levels and theoretically increasing the risk of myocardial infarction. Carteolol either minimally decreases the high-density lipoprotein cholesterol level or increases it. Carteolol (1%) is instilled in the conjunctival sac two times daily.

Timolol.—Timolol is a beta-1 and beta-2 adrenergic receptor–blocking agent (nonselective). It is widely used in chronic open-angle and secondary glaucoma. It is used topically in a concentration of either 0.25% or 0.5% and should never be used more than once every 12 hours. It decreases the formation of aqueous humor through the inhibition of either the synthesis or the action of the adenyl cyclase of the nonpigmented epithelium of the ciliary body.

The pressure-lowering effect of timolol may be lost or decreased over a few days or several months of therapy. The most critical period is within the first 3 days of therapy when, after an initial decrease, the intraocular pressure increases, although rarely to the pretreatment level. Evaluation of timolol treatment after 2 weeks suggests its effectiveness during the subsequent 3 months, at which time its action should again be evaluated.

Timolol and acetazolamide seem to provide additive effects in glaucoma, although both have similar effects in reducing aqueous humor formation. The ocular effects of timolol and epinephrine are poorly additive, although adding timolol to epinephrine therapy may substantially reduce intraocular pressure for several weeks. After patients have been receiving maximum therapy for glaucoma (typically a topical cholinergic agent, epinephrine, and an oral carbonic anhydrase inhibitor), the addition of timolol appears to have a pressure-lowering effect in about 75% of the eyes for more than 1 year.

Betaxolol (Betoptic).—This selective beta-1 adrenergic receptor antagonist reduces intraocular pressure by reducing the secretion of aqueous humor in open-angle glaucoma. It is administered topically every 12 hours in a 0.5% solution. It has a lower potential for compromising pulmonary function than timolol but can exacerbate pulmonary obstruction in susceptible patients.

Levobunolol (Betagen).—Levobunolol is a nonselective beta-1 and beta-2 adrenergic receptor antagonist. Its action and safety are similar to those of timolol.

Metipranolol.—Metipranolol 0.3% (OptiPranolol) is a nonselective beta-adrenergic receptor antagonist for topical use in glaucoma. Its action is similar to that of timolol, but it is effective in some patients resistant to the pressure-lowering effect of timolol. Iritis occurs in some patients, but otherwise its side effects are similar to timolol.

CARBONIC ANHYDRASE INHIBITORS

Carbonic anhydrase is an enzyme that catalyzes the equilibrium between carbonic acid and carbon dioxide. The enzyme is widely distributed in (1) erythrocytes, where it functions in the exchange of carbon dioxide in capillaries; (2) the renal tubule cell, where it functions in the exchange of intracellular hydrogen for tubular sodium; (3) the epithelium of the ciliary body, where it functions in the secretion of aqueous humor; (4) the choroid plexus, where it functions in the secretion of cerebrospinal fluid; and (5) the gastric mucosa and the pancreas.

Inhibitors of carbonic anhydrase were synthesized after it was observed that the systemic administration of sulfonamides caused an acidosis because of loss of sodium bicarbonate to the urine and failure of the exchange of cellular hydrogen for tubular sodium. Despite the widespread distribution of carbonic anhydrase in the tissues of the body, the effects of enzyme inhibition are largely renal. Some of the agents, however, decrease secretion of aqueous humor and cerebrospinal fluid. Decreased secretion of aqueous humor occurs even in the absence of renal effects and is apparently the result of decreased secretion by the ciliary body.

Effective drugs in this group reduce the secretion of aqueous humor by 50% to 60%. There is a concomitant reduction in intraocular pressure. The most commonly used agent is acetazolamide (Diamox). Because of side effects, a number of other compounds have been substituted for acetazolamide.

Until recently, topical carbonic anhydrase inhibitors have not been useful because of their poor penetration through the cornea. A variety of new compounds, mainly conjugates of known carbonic anhydrase inhibitors, have been tested for corneal penetration and the absence of side effects. To be effective they must inhibit the carbonic anhydrase activity of the ciliary body by at least 98% and must not increase the corneal thickness.

Two compounds used topically have been found to lower intraocular pressure in human clinical trials. Many other compounds, mainly substituted sulfonamides, are being studied. Dorzolamide, a sulfonamide, was released for treatment of open-angle glaucoma in 1995. It is often used in conjunction with other topical medications. Ocular discomfort after instillation is common (33%); superficial punctate keratitis occurs in 10% to 15% of patients treated, and ocular allergy in 10%. There is cross-sensitivity with other sulfonamide products.

Acetazolamide.—Acetazolamide (Diamox) is the most widely used carbonic anhydrase inhibitor in ophthalmology. The usual dosage is either 125 or 250 mg orally every 6 hours (not four times daily) or 250 or 500 mg every 12 hours in sustained-release tablets. The ocular effect is observed 1 to 2 hours after oral administration, and the maximum effect persists for 3 to 5 hours. It may be used intravenously in patients with acute angle-closure glaucoma. The secretion of aqueous humor is reduced but never stopped, and it is evident that only mechanisms of secretory activity that involve carbonic anhydrase are concerned. A variety of side effects may occur. Myopia, blood dyscrasias, exfoliative dermatitis, and other reactions observed with sulfonamide derivatives occur rarely. Paresthesia, with numbness and tingling in the extremities and mouth, and anorexia are common. There is a slight tendency to renal lithiasis, gout, and depression; confusion may occur in the elderly.

Ethoxzolamide (Cardrase), dichlorphenamide (Daranide), and methazolamide (Neptazane) are carbonic anhydrase inhibitors that may be substituted for acetazolamide. Their side effects are similar to those caused by acetazolamide, but occasionally one may be substituted to provide equal tension-decreasing effects and fewer side-effects.

HYPEROSMOTIC AGENTS

If the osmolarity of the plasma is increased, fluid is drawn from the vitreous body, and the intraocular pressure is decreased. The increased osmotic pressure of the plasma is usually maintained for only a short time, and within 4 to 6 hours the intraocular pressure returns to its previous level. Osmotic agents are used to decrease the intraocular pressure and volume for a relatively short period, as in the following: (1) in angle-closure glaucoma, to reduce the intraocular pressure to less than 50 mm Hg so that the sphincter pupillae muscle will respond to miotics; (2) immediately before surgery, to reduce intraocular pressure; (3) in retinal detachment surgery, to reduce intraocular volume to aid in scleral wound closure; and (4) in orbital surgery, to reduce orbital volume.

Mannitol.—Mannitol is the alcohol of the sugar mannose and is pharmacologically inert. It is excreted by filtration through the renal glomeruli and is minimally reabsorbed by the tubules. It induces osmotic diuresis. Mannitol is administered intravenously in a 20% solution in a dose of 1.0 to 2.0 g/kg of body weight. Often 500 mL of a 20% solution is used in an average adult. Administration time is 30 to 60 minutes. When mannitol is used before surgery, urinary bladder catheterization is usually required because of diuresis. The maximum decrease in intraocular pressure occurs within 1 hour, and it returns to pretreatment levels after about 4 hours. The rapid expansion of extracellular fluid volume may cause cardiac decompensation in vulnerable persons. Hypersensitivity rarely occurs. Reduction of intracranial pressure may cause headache. It is contraindicated in patients with cardiac decompensation and chronic obstructive pulmonary disease.

Glycerol.—Glycerol is a trivalent alcohol that contributes to glyceride and phosphatide molecules. It is metabolized to carbon dioxide and water by the tricarboxylic acid cycle. (Insulin is not required in its metabolism.) After oral administration of a 50% solution in lemon juice in doses of 1.5 to 3.0 mL/kg of body weight, it decreases intraocular pressure within 10 to 30 minutes. It reaches its maximum effect in 45 to 120 minutes and has a duration of effect of 4 to 5 hours. Side effects are few. Usually headache does not occur, and diuresis is not severe. Nausea and vomiting may prevent its long-term use.

Topical glycerol does not reduce intraocular pressure but reduces corneal edema in glaucoma to make gonioscopy possible.

Isosorbide.—Isosorbide (Ismotic) is a dihydric alcohol formed by the removal of two molecules of water from the glucitol (sorbitol) molecule. It is given orally in a 45% vanilla-mint solution. With an oral dosage of 1.5 to 4.0 mL/kg of body weight, the intraocular pressure reaches a minimal value 1 to 2 hours after administration and remains depressed for 5 to 6 hours.

***Miscellaneous agents.*—**Urea, ascorbate, ethanol, and sucrose produce an osmotic vitreous-blood gradient with reduction of intraocular pressure. Additionally, ethanol inhibits the antidiuretic hormone and induces diuresis. Ingestion of large amounts of ethanol 8 to 12 hours before examination may produce an abnormally low intraocular pressure.

LOCAL ANESTHETICS

The small size of the eye and the accessibility of its nerve supply permit most adult ocular surgery to be done under local anesthesia. The conjunctiva and cornea are readily anesthetized by means of topically instilled agents, of which cocaine, the prototype, has been succeeded by tetracaine (Pontocaine, 0.5%), benoxinate (Dorsacaine, 0.4%), and proparacaine (Ophthaine, 0.5%). Sensory and motor paralysis is readily achieved with skillful infiltration of procaine (Novocain), lidocaine (Xylocaine), bupivacaine (Marcaine), and other agents.

Topical anesthetics are used for procedures such as tonometry or removal of corneal foreign bodies. The severe pain of corneal abrasions, ultraviolet keratitis, and corneal foreign bodies is quickly relieved. Since these agents are potent sensitizers and delay corneal epithelization, they should not be prescribed for analgesia.

Infiltration anesthesia is used mainly in the region of the eyelids for the excision of local lesions. Both motor and sensory block follow injection of the anesthetic agent in the region of the orbital portion of the orbicularis oculi muscle (van Lint technique) to prevent eyelid closure in intraocular surgery.

Blockade of the eyelid musculature is provided by infiltrating fibers of the temporal branch of the facial nerve as they pass anterior to the temporomandibular articulation. Blockade of the motor nerve supply to the extraocular muscles and sensory block of the nerve supply to the globe follow the retrobulbar injection of anesthetic solution posterior to the globe in the region between the lateral rectus muscle and optic nerve. This blocks the nerve supply to all of the extraocular muscles except the superior oblique muscle; it blocks the ciliary ganglion so the pupil dilates; and it anesthetizes the entire globe. Rather than using the retrobulbar route, many surgeons infiltrate the superior subtenon region for extracapsular cataract surgery.

The eyelids and the surrounding tissues receive their major sensory innervation from two sources: the frontal and lacrimal branches of the ophthalmic division of the trigeminal nerve and the infraorbital branch of the maxillary division of the trigeminal nerve. The supraorbital branches of the frontal nerve are commonly blocked by injection at the margin of the orbit just medial to the trochlea. The infraorbital nerve is blocked either in its course along the floor of the orbit, or within the infraorbital foramen.

Epinephrine (1:100,000) induces vasoconstriction, which causes slower absorption of the anesthetic agent and thereby prolongs its action. Epinephrine is contraindicated in patients with coronary artery disease or thyrotoxicosis, and when halothane anesthesia is used.

Hyaluronidase enhances the dispersion of local anesthetic agents and hastens their absorption. Increased dispersion provides a more effective sensory and motor blockade. More rapid absorption reduces the duration of effect of the local anesthetic.

DYES

Sterile sodium fluorescein is used topically (0.25% to 2.0%) to stain areas in which the corneal epithelial cell junctions are disrupted or the cells are absent. It is used intravenously in a 10% to 25% solution to study the retinal circulation and retina. Rose bengal solution (1%) stains cells that lack a tear mucin coating better than fluorescein.

Fluorescein.—Fluorescein has an affinity for the Bowman zone of the cornea, and the corneal stroma stains a bright green in areas where the epithelium is absent. The stain is intensified by the instillation of 2.0% cocaine solution or if the eye is illuminated with a cobalt blue filter to stimulate fluorescence. Because of the possibility of contamination with *Pseudomonas aeruginosa,* fluorescein should be instilled either from a sterile single-dose container or by means of a strip of sterile filter paper saturated with dye. The dye is instilled in the conjunctival sac, and excess fluorescein may be removed by irrigation with sterile saline.

Fluorescein is instilled in the eye to demonstrate the dilution that occurs when anterior aqueous humor escapes from a postoperative fistula, a penetrating wound, or a conjunctival bleb after glaucoma filtration surgery. It is used to demonstrate areas of contact ("touch") between a contact lens and the cornea or sclera in the fitting of lenses. Applanation tonometry is based on the appearance of the fluorescein pattern when pressure is applied to the eye. The rate of disappearance of fluorescein through the nasolacrimal passages is used to estimate their patency.

Intravenous sodium fluorescein is combined with serial fundus photography to study the dynamics of the retinal circulation. Two to five mL of a 10% to 25% solution is injected rapidly into an arm vein, and fundus photographs are taken. Nausea may occur with the injection. Fluorescein is excreted in the urine for the next 24 to 48 hours (and prevents accurate urine testing for sugar). Anaphylactic reactions vary in severity from urticaria to shock. Coma, cardiac arrest, and myocardial infarction have been reported. The drug should not be used in individuals with a history of drug sensitivity. When angiography is performed, an emergency tray and oxygen should be readily available. Administration of the fluorescein through an indwelling catheter permits the intravenous administration of drugs in the event a severe reaction should develop.

Rose bengal.—Rose bengal (1%), a halide derivative of fluorescein, stains epithelial cells of the cornea and conjunctiva that are not protected with tear components such as albumin and mucin. It is superior to fluorescein in demonstrating epithelial defects of the conjunctiva and cornea in keratoconjunctivitis.

Rose bengal binds to the nuclei of viruses and living tissue cells and is toxic on exposure to light or X-irradiation through the production of singlet oxygen and superoxide. This photodynamic action may lead to effective therapy for herpes simplex infections of the cornea and other conditions. Intravenous rose bengal sensitizes corneal blood vessels, which may then be occluded by exposure to argon-green laser irradiation (photothrombosis).

Indocyanine green.—Indocyanine green binds to blood proteins. It absorbs (805 nm) and emits (835 nm) infrared energy beyond the range of sensitivity of the human retina (400 to 700 nm). It is used intravenously to image choroidal new blood vessels. It must be viewed by means of a television monitor or camera film sensitive to infrared energy (see Chapter 6).

OPHTHALMIC SOLUTIONS

A variety of compounds are used for preoperative cleansing preparation of the periocular skin before surgery, for irrigation of the external eye, for maintaining the shape of the cornea during intraocular surgery, and for irrigation of the vitreous cavity during vitreoretinal procedures.

Antiseptic solutions.—Ophthalmic surgeons routinely wash the skin surrounding the eye and usually irrigate the conjunctival sac before surgery. Many of the compounds are toxic to the cornea, although damage is often limited because of the subsequent irrigation. Hibiclens (chlorhexidine gluconate 4% in a detergent vehicle) is toxic to the cornea and binds to proteins of the corneal stroma. Tincture of iodine, hexachlorophene (3%) with detergent (pHisoHex), ethanol (70%), and povidone-iodine (7.5%) with detergent (Betadine Surgical Scrub) may cause conjunctival chemosis, loss of corneal epithelium, and corneal edema in rabbits. Povidone-iodine (10%) without detergent (Betadine Solution) does not cause similar reactions. It has been substituted successfully for silver nitrate in the prophylaxis of ophthalmia neonatorum.

Irrigating solutions.—The conjunctival sac is irrigated immediately before intraocular surgery and during surgery. Irrigation removes blood from the operating field and maintains the contour of the eye and the intraocular pressure. Currently solutions are used that approximate the composition of the normal aqueous humor and contain sodium, chloride, bicarbonate, glucose, and glutathione. The superiority of such solutions over lactated Ringer solution is difficult to quantitate experimentally. Generally, commercially prepared solutions are likely to be free of microbial contamination, improper formulation, or chemical contamination.

Viscoelastic solutions.—These are solutions of sodium hyaluronate (the prototype), chondroitin sulfate, or hydroxypropylmethylcellulose instilled in the anterior chamber during cataract extraction with implantation of an intraocular lens to protect the cornea and maintain its contour. Their high viscosity causes them to block the trabecular meshwork and impair outflow from the eye. They must be irrigated or aspirated from the anterior chamber at the conclusion of surgery to minimize the transient increase in intraocular pressure that occurs, usually within 12 hours. Intraocular carbachol, topical apraclonidine (1%), an alpha-2 agonist, or a systemic carbonic anhydrase inhibitor is used to prevent a pressure increase during the first 24-hour postoperative period.

Artificial tears.—A deficiency of either the aqueous or mucin component of tears causes a drying of the conjunctiva and cornea. A deficiency of the aqueous component is seen in keratoconjunctivitis sicca, while the mucin component is deficient in conditions that cause loss of goblet cells: chemical burns, Stevens-Johnson disease, hypovitaminosis A, and ocular cicatricial pemphigoid.

Many artificial tear preparations are available. Their purpose is to wet the ocular surfaces and to provide moisture and comfort for as long a period as possible. They contain boric acid or saline; a surface polymer to prevent evaporation (often polyvinyl alcohol); and often cellulose compounds, dextran, or dextrose to provide viscosity. Since many patients with dry eyes have hypertonic tears, some preparations are hypotonic. To prevent microbial contamination many contain preservatives such as thimerosal, benzalkonium chloride, chlorobutanol, ethylenediaminetetracetic acid (EDTA), or others. The container tips and caps may be contaminated with bacteria, often gram-negative organisms from the patient's hands. The preservatives maintain the sterility of the solution. Contact hypersensitivity may occur and require another product or one without a preservative. Artificial tears have no pharmacologic action and may be instilled in the conjunctival cul-de-sac as often as necessary for comfort.

Ointments prolong the contact time of a medication but are used mainly at bedtime because they mechanically blur vision. They are exceptionally useful in infants and children, in whom the ointment may be applied to the eyelashes of the closed eyelids. They are composed of white petrolatum combined with mineral oil and lanolin.

Contact lens care.—Soft or hard contact lenses must be cleaned, disinfected, and rinsed before insertion in the eye. More than 100 different products are available for cold or hot disinfection. Mainly they consist of sterile solutions that contain antiseptic agents, hydrogen peroxide, buffers, preservative, and proteolytic enzymes. Faulty care of contact lenses is a frequent source of keratitis. The cases used to store lenses are often contaminated.

COMPLICATIONS OF TOPICAL ADMINISTRATION OF DRUGS

A surprising variety of ocular conditions are either induced, prolonged, or aggravated by excessive use of topical medications. Inasmuch as many eye diseases are self-limited, there is often no indication for the local instillation of medications, particularly without an exact diagnosis.

Local hypersensitivity.—The conjunctiva and the skin of the eyelids may be the sites of atopic inflammation (type I hypersensitivity) or the site of cell-mediated (type IV hypersensitivity) reactions (see Chapter 25). Any drug or cosmetic agent that is repeatedly applied to the ocular tissues (or any other tissue) may be the causative agent.

Contact dermatitis (see Chapter 9) and conjunctivitis occur particularly commonly in patients who use artificial tears and topical glaucoma medication. Artificial tears (and other eyedrops and ointments) often contain benzalkonium chloride, thimerosal, chlorobutanol, phenylmercuric acetate, edetate sodium, and various other compounds as preservatives or buffers. Repeated topical instillation leads to a contact dermatitis, the cause of which is often not immediately evident. Contact dermatitis may also be secondary to cosmetics or products brought in contact with the eyelids by the fingers. Local application of a corticosteroid may provide temporary relief, but exposure to the irritant again causes the inflammation.

Mechanical injury.—Patients and attendants instilling medications into the eye by means of an eyedropper or squeeze bottle should be instructed to place the long axis parallel to the eyelid margin so that if the patient lunges forward, the tip of the dropper will not strike the eye. Patients should be reassured that the conjunctival sac holds but a single drop and the exact measurement of a single drop is not necessary because the excess medication overflows. Physicians must ensure that patients know how to instill topical medications correctly before concluding that a particular drug is not effective.

Pigmentation.—Prolonged instillation of various compounds may cause pigmentation of the conjunctiva and the eyelids. Repeated instillation of silver preparations causes argyrosis. Metallic silver is deposited in the conjunctiva, particularly in the fornices, where it causes a slate-gray color. Microscopically, it results from minute, closely packed dots of gray-black matter of metallic silver. There is no effective treatment.

Long-time use of mercury preparations, such as ammoniated mercury or yellow oxide of mercury, may cause a similar pigmentation from mercury deposition.

Topical epinephrine may cause a black pigmentation of the eyelid margins that resembles eye makeup. More common is a sharply defined, rounded black area of adenochrome pigmentation caused by the oxidation of epinephrine to adrenochrome in the conjunctiva or cornea. There are no symptoms, and the deposits may be wiped off.

Ocular injury.—Many compounds may cause direct ocular injury on instillation. Silver nitrate in concentrations greater than 5% may cause necrosis of the cornea. To be assured of using only 1% silver nitrate in Credé prophylaxis of ophthalmia neonatorum, only the wax ampules distributed for this purpose should be used. Practitioners who cauterize granulation tissue with silver nitrate find silver nitrate sticks safer than strong solutions. Silver nitrate sticks should never be used near the eye.

Many compounds may cause punctate defects of the corneal epithelium, which result in a foreign body sensation. Compounds that denature the protein of the corneal epithelium, such as ethanol and benzalkonium chloride (Zephiran), are common offenders. These may be brought to the eye on instruments used for minor ocular surgery. Local anesthetics are often dispensed in a stronger solution for use on nasal and oral mucous membranes than for the eye. Instillation of these stronger solutions may cause a white precipitate in the superficial corneal epithelium; the precipitate usually disappears when irrigated with sterile water.

Cocaine solutions are markedly hypotonic to the tears and cause desiccation of the corneal epithelium, which may then be removed easily. Cocaine is an excellent local anesthetic, and its use in surgery is sometimes desirable because it produces local vasoconstriction and moderate dilation of the pupil.

Delay of corneal epithelization.—Small defects in the cornea heal by sliding of adjacent epithelium; large defects heal by mitosis and sliding of adjacent epithelium. Many of the compounds used in ocular therapeutics delay mitosis but have no effect on epithelial sliding. Local anesthetics delay corneal wound healing markedly.

Pupillary constriction

Drugs that constrict the pupil also stimulate contraction of the ciliary body muscles, sometimes markedly, and cause a sustained increase in the refractive power of the eye, which induces many symptoms. In patients with minor opacities of the crystalline lens, constriction of the pupil may reduce visual acuity. Conversely, pupillary constriction in some patients may create the effect of a stenopeic opening and permit only parallel rays to enter the eye so that vision is clear at both far and near without the spectacles required when the pupil is of normal size. In young individuals a sustained increase in tone of the ciliary muscle may induce a temporary myopia that is relieved with relaxation of the ciliary muscle.

In patients with a shallow anterior chamber, extreme miosis combined with edema of the ciliary body, particularly that which follows topical instillation of organophosphate miotics, may cause an angle-closure glaucoma. Extreme contraction of the ciliary muscle may cause retinal detachment because of traction by the zonular fibers of the crystalline lens that insert into the anterior retina.

Miotics are used in children in the treatment of accommodative esotropia and may cause pupillary cysts that may be so marked as to occlude the pupil. Instillation of 2.5% phenylephrine immediately after instillation of the miotic prevents the formation of cysts.

Systemic reactions to local instillation.—Atropine, phenylephrine, and glaucoma medications may be absorbed through the conjunctiva or pass through the lacrimal passages to be absorbed by the nasal mucous membranes. They may cause characteristic systemic pharmacologic actions because a single eyedrop (0.15 μL) may exceed the systemic therapeutic dose (Table 3-7). Commercial eyedroppers and squeeze bottles may deliver between 50 and 75 μL, which is two to seven times more than the cul-de-sac can hold. Systemic absorption can be minimized by having the patient close the eyes and compress the lacrimal puncta with a finger for 2 minutes after instillation.

Atropine and scopolamine are often administered either in any oily solution or in an ointment to minimize systemic absorption. Nevertheless, systemic absorption from the conjunctiva and anterior chamber may cause toxicity.

TABLE 3-7.
Therapeutic Dose of Eye Medications

Medication	Dose	
	1 Drop (0.15 μL)	Therapeutic Systemic Dose
1% atropine	1.5 mg	0.6 mg
4% pilocarpine	6.0 mg	5.0 mg
0.25% echothiophate iodide (Phospholine Iodide)	0.375 mg	Too toxic for systemic therapy
2.5% phenylephrine	3.75mg	5.0 mg (intramuscular)

Atropine poisoning develops quickly, causing agitated behavior, hallucinations, and disorientation. The mouth is dry, and speech and swallowing are difficult. The pupils are dilated and accommodation is paralyzed. The skin is dry, red, and hot, and body temperature increases. Treatment is symptomatic: stop the medication and reduce the fever with ice packs or sponging. A cholinergic drug, such as physostigmine, may provide more prompt relief.

Cyclopentolate hydrochloride (Cyclogyl) may cause hallucinations, dysarthria, ataxia, and temporary behavioral changes suggestive of schizophrenia. Only the 0.5% solution should be used in infants and small children.

The topical beta-adrenergic receptor–blocking agents used in glaucoma therapy are particularly liable to cause systemic reactions. They are contraindicated in patients with obstructive pulmonary disease and must be used with caution in patients with cardiac disease. They should be instilled no more than twice daily, and patients should be instructed to apply pressure to the nasolacrimal puncta for 2 minutes after instillation to minimize systemic absorption. The drugs may induce a postural hypotension and cause serious falls in the elderly. Impotence, personality disorders, depression, muscle fatigue, and aggravation of myasthenia gravis have been described. Betaxolol, a selective beta-receptor blocker, may be used in many patients with reactive pulmonary disease and may not aggravate symptoms.

Pilocarpine toxicity may occur after frequent instillation of the drug in patients with angle-closure glaucoma. Some patients are exceptionally sensitive and develop gastrointestinal overactivity and sweating when given small doses. More severe signs include salivation, nausea, tremor, bradycardia, and decreased blood pressure.

Anticholinesterase agents, particularly the organophosphates, significantly depress the erythrocyte cholinesterase levels. Systemic absorption may cause diarrhea, abdominal cramps, and the signs and symptoms of an acute abdominal or other gastrointestinal disturbance. On occasion, these signs have led to unnecessary laparotomy. Children receiving these compounds, particularly echothiophate iodide (Phospholine Iodide), may become irritable and cross; their behavior problems result from chronic cholinesterase poisoning. Children with Down syndrome are particularly sensitive to echothiophate iodide. Patients using organophosphates should be advised to inform their other physicians of the drug they are using. The use of succinylcholine during general anesthesia in a cholinesterase-depleted individual may lead to prolonged apnea.

Phenylephrine is widely used as a nasal decongestant (0.125% to 0.5%), as a mydriatic (2.5%), and in some vasoconstrictor eyedrops. It is a powerful postsynaptic alpha-receptor agonist and increases systolic and diastolic pressure. Cerebrovascular accidents and cardiac arrhythmia with extrasystole occur.

OCULAR REACTIONS TO SYSTEMIC ADMINISTRATION OF DRUGS

The eye may react to many drugs used systemically. Occasionally, ocular reactions do not occur in experimental animals, and severe eye lesions may be produced before the relationship between the eye abnormality and the drug is suspected.

Alcohol.—Alcohol intoxication causes nystagmus, esophoria, and diplopia. Intraocular pressure decreases chiefly through alcohol diuresis. Alcohol amblyopia is a vitamin B deficiency commonly associated with a peripheral neuritis and may cause a toxic optic neuropathy (see Chapter 20). Vision is reduced and there are cecocentral scotomas. Adequate diet and large doses of vitamin B correct the condition, even though alcoholism continues.

Accidental ingestion of methanol causes a severe acidosis, nausea, vomiting, abdominal pain, failing vision, and coma. Those who recover from the coma may have no light perception. These patients initially have edema of the optic nerve and surrounding retina followed by severe optic atrophy. The acidosis must be corrected with alkalyzing therapy. Renal dialysis removes methanol from the blood, and large amounts of systemic ethanol compete successfully with methanol for metabolic sites.

Most central nervous system depressants may cause muscle weakness along with diplopia and, on occasion, blurred vision. In some instances, these compounds aggravate preexisting ocular defects or cause nystagmus. The ocular signs are usually reversible after reduced intake of the medication.

Antimalarials.—Chloroquine is an antimalarial agent commonly used for the treatment of lupus erythematosus, arthritis, and other connective tissue disorders. Chloroquine and hydroxychloroquine have a high affinity for melanin and concentrate in the choroid, ciliary body, and retinal pigment epithelium. Prolonged administration of high doses may cause keratopathy, myopathy, or retinopathy. Generally, the total chloroquine dose must exceed 100 g and the drug must be used for more than a year before a retinopathy develops. The drug may be retained in the body for years after its use has been discontinued, and the retinopathy may develop several years later.

Chloroquine retinopathy is a severe pigmentary degeneration of the retina that may progress to blindness. Initially there is a minute degree of pigment clumping in the central retinal area. A characteristic "doughnut"-shaped retinal lesion develops that may be incomplete. In the end stages there is widespread retinal atrophy, pigment clumping, and threadlike retinal vessels.

Chloroquine keratopathy is a reversible deposition of chloroquine in the cornea. Minute whitish dots distributed in a whorl pattern can be observed with the slit lamp. Patients complain of "glare," ill-defined blurring of vision, and iridescent vision, the halo surrounding lights being identical to that in glaucoma. The condition is entirely reversible on discontinuation of the drug, and it may disappear spontaneously even if the drug is continued.

Quinine.—Quinine in excessive doses has long been known to cause damage to the retinal ganglion cells and constriction of the retinal arterioles. Idiosyncratic reactions may follow administration of even minute amounts of quinine (as little as that contained in quinine water). Constriction of the visual field to a central area 5° to 10° in diameter may also occur. There may be associated deafness and other signs of central nervous system toxicity. Quinine is often mixed with heroin, and drug users may develop typical quinine poisoning. The abnormality is usually reversible, but continued ingestion of quinine may cause irreversible constriction of the visual fields, impaired dark adaptation, and loss of visual acuity.

In rare instances severe atrophy of the pigment epithelium of the iris may follow quinine amblyopia. The sector of the pupil in the region of iris atrophy does not react to light. The condition is presumably caused by ischemia of the anterior uvea.

Ethambutol.—Ethambutol is an oral chemotherapeutic agent used in the treatment of pulmonary tuberculosis. The main ocular complication of long-term use is an optic neuropathy that occurs in about 2% of those treated. Visual acuity should be measured before treatment is started and then monthly during the first months of therapy. Patients must be alerted to note any loss of vision. The optic neuropathy causes reduced visual acuity and color vision as well as a central scotoma. The neuropathy is reversible when the drug is discontinued, and vision improves over a period of weeks. After recovery, the use of the drug may be reinstituted without immediate recurrence of the optic neuropathy.

Digoxin.—Visual symptoms occur in 95% of patients with increased serum levels of digoxin. The classic symptom is xanthopsia, in which objects are tinted a pale yellow. Alternatively, objects may appear to be covered with frost. Blurred vision is more common. There may be disturbed color vision (dyschromatopsia), which may involve colors other than yellow. Photopsia, double vision, or pain on ocular movements may occur. An increased digoxin level must be considered in each patient receiving the drug who has ocular symptoms. Rarely the symptoms occur in patients with therapeutic levels of digoxin.

Xanthopsia is also attributed to the systemic effects of chlorothiazide and to aspidium (male fern).

Oral contraceptives.—The agents most commonly used for oral contraceptive therapy are progesterone and estrogen in combination or in sequence. These may cause occlusive vascular disease in susceptible patients. Women who smoke or who have vascular hypertension, migraine, or vascular disease are thought to be especially vulnerable. Brain infarction may be associated with ocular signs, depending on the area of the brain involved. Papilledema and optic neuropathy appear to occur more commonly in women using oral contraceptives than in others. Retinal hemorrhages may be seen. The indications for using oral contraceptives must be carefully weighed. A patient should not receive them for long periods without medical supervision. They should be discontinued in the event of thromboembolic disease, neurologic disease, or suggestion of liver damage.

Some contact lens wearers develop an intolerance to the contact lenses while using oral contraceptives. Often this is characterized by photophobia, increased irritation caused by the contact lenses, and a prolonged period of recovery from the corneal edema that may occur when wearing the contact lenses.

Induced refractive errors.—Drugs may increase the refractive power of the eye by one of three mechanisms: (1) sustained contraction (spasm) of the ciliary muscle, causing increased refractivity of the lens; (2) increased refractive power of the lens contents as the result of water imbibition; and (3) swelling of the ciliary processes, causing forward displacement of the lens. The sulfonamides and related compounds, particularly acetazolamide (Diamox), may cause edema of the ciliary processes. All of the anticholinesterase compounds may cause ciliary spasm and miosis. Many insecticides are anticholinesterases, and spasm of accommodation combined with pupillary constriction has been described. Increased refractive power of the lens or sustained accommodation reduces hyperopia or increases myopia.

The ganglionic-blocking agents used in the treatment of vascular hypertension decrease accommodation that many patients in the younger age groups find extremely annoying. There may be dilation of the conjunctival blood vessels, giving the appearance of conjunctivitis. The loss of accommodation may have to be corrected by means of bifocal lenses. The conjunctival injection may be alleviated slightly by local instillation of a vasoconstrictor, such as 1:1,000 epinephrine.

Optic atrophy.—Many compounds have been reported to cause optic atrophy. These include chloramphenicol, streptomycin, sulfonamides, and isoniazid. Tryparsamide, a pentavalent arsenical previously used in the therapy of central nervous system syphilis, has a direct toxic effect on the optic nerve.

VITAMIN A

Vitamin A (retinol) and its naturally occurring relatives, retinaldehyde (retinal) and retinoic acid, are members of a class of more than 1,500 naturally occurring and synthetic compounds, the retinoids. Vitamin A is required for vision, reproduction, mucous secretion, and maintenance of differentiated epithelia. Different retinoids exhibit some, but not necessarily all, of the biologic activities of vitamin A. All-*trans* retinoic acid supports normal growth and epithelium but cannot replace vitamin A as a visual pigment precursor and will not support reproduction.

The major natural sources of vitamin A are dietary plant carotenoid pigments, such as beta-carotene, and retinyl esters in meat. They are converted to retinol in the intestine.

The progression of the common forms of retinitis pigmentosa is slowed, but is not prevented, by a daily dietary supplement of 15,000 IU of vitamin A. A daily supplement of 400 IU of vitamin E may have an adverse effect.

Vitamin A deficiency, usually in association with general malnutrition, is a leading cause of blindness in many underdeveloped countries. The array of signs and symptoms grouped under the term xerophthalmia progress from night blindness (XN) to conjunctival xerosis (X1A), to Bitot spots (X1B), to corneal xerosis (X2), and finally to keratomalacia (X3). Hypovitaminosis A in developed countries usually reflects inadequate absorption as the result of small-bowel surgery, malnutrition, alcoholism, or a dietary faddism. Low serum retinol levels may be associated with an increased risk of cancer.

Prolonged intake of dietary carotenes may lead to yellowing of the skin and conjunctiva that resembles jaundice. Long-term intake of 10 to 20 times more vitamin A than required may lead to increased intracranial pressure (with headache, nausea, and papilledema), skeletal pain, and mucocutaneous signs. Isotretinoin, a retinoid, is used in the treatment of cystic acne. Papilledema may develop, particularly when combined with tetracyclines.

Rifampin.—Persons who use systemic rifampin, which is used in the treatment of tuberculosis and in pharyngeal carriers of *Neisseria* meningitis, may have orange, light pink, or red tears (5% to 14% of patients). The tears may stain contact lenses or cause a painful exudative conjunctivitis or blepharoconjunctivitis.

BIBLIOGRAPHY

Books

Burnstock G, Hoyle CHV, editors: *Autonomic neuro-effector mechanisms,* Philadelphia, 1992, Harwood Academic Publishers.

Fraunfelder FT: *Drug-induced ocular side effects and drug interactions,* Philadelphia, 1989, Lea & Febiger.

Fraunfelder FT, Roy FH, editors: *Current ocular therapy 4,* Philadelphia, 1995, WB Saunders.

Grant WM, Schuman JS: *Toxicology of the eye,* ed 4, Springfield, Ill, 1993, Charles C Thomas.

Hardman JG, Limbird LE, editors: *Goodman and Gilman's the pharmacological basis of therapeutics,* ed 9, New York, 1995, McGraw-Hill.

Mauger T, Craig EL: *Mosby's ocular drug handbook,* ed 4, St Louis, 1995, Mosby–Year Book.

Mauger TF, Craig EL: *Havener's ocular pharmacology,* ed 6, St Louis, 1994, Mosby–Year Book.

Mitra AK, editor: *Ophthalmic drug delivery systems,* New York, 1993, Marcel Dekker.

Articles

Christen WG Jr: Antioxidants and eye disease, *Am J Med* 97(suppl 3A):14S-17S, 1994.

de Smet MD, Nussenblatt RB: Clinical use of cyclosporine in ocular disease, *Int Ophthalmol Clin* 33: 31-45, 1993.

PART II

HISTORY TAKING AND EXAMINATION OF THE EYE

4

HISTORY AND INTERPRETATION

Every well-trained practitioner, however specialized, should be able to examine the eyes quickly and competently, to be assured that the widths of the palpebral fissures are equal, the eyes rotate fully and do not cross, the pupils are equal and constrict to stimulation with light, and the optic disks are neither swollen nor atrophic.

Some elementary principles should reassure practitioners (Table 4-1). The eyes are meant to be used and do not wear out. Reading in dim light may be uncomfortable but does not harm the eyes. Organic headaches such as migraine and cluster headaches never originate from the eyes (see Chapter 28). Attention is always directed to the visual acuity with the individual wearing the optical correction required for distinct vision and not to vision without correction.

The eye is remarkably organized. Tears moisten the outer surface efficiently, and it is not necessary to wet the normal eye with collyria (eyedrops or washes). Except in patients with diabetes, annual eye examinations are not necessary once it has been determined that the eyes are healthy. Immediate examination is indicated for symptoms such as severe pain in an eye, loss of vision, double vision, or the sudden appearance of floaters in the field of vision. A variety of symptoms signal the need for immediate attention (Table 4-2).

An enlarged eye or persistent tearing in an infant signals the need for immediate attention. An infant whose eyes cross after 6 months of age should have a complete eye examination with the pupils dilated. The infant's inability to cooperate is not a reason for delay.

With aging every individual loses accommodation (presbyopia; [see Chapter 24]) and the ability to see clearly for both far and near. Those who are nearsighted (myopic) may be able to see near work without correction. Farsighted individuals (hyperopic) will hold material farther from the eye as they age. If an individual develops nuclear sclerosis, there may be a period of being able to see near work without correction as the eye becomes more myopic.

Contact lenses neutralize refractive errors but do not abolish them. The conjunctiva prevents contact lenses from migrating behind the eye, although rarely one slips into the upper conjunctival cul-de-sac and is located only with difficulty. Specially fitted contact lenses may decrease the corneal curvature and provide a temporary period of improved vision without correction. Without the correcting contact lens, the cornea gradually reverts to its original curvature and original visual acuity.

Eyes with open-angle glaucoma, a common cause of loss of vision and blindness, appear normal. In advanced glaucoma, ophthalmoscopic examination discloses the characteristic excavation of the optic disk and primary optic atrophy. Before these changes occur, diagnosis of open-angle glaucoma requires measurement of the intraocular pressure with a tonometer.

Annual professional eye examinations are not necessary. The eyes should be examined if there is severe pain in one or both eyes, if there is loss of both near and far vision, if there is double

TABLE 4-1.
Some Elementary Principles of Eye Care

Chemicals in the eye must be diluted with water immediately.
Reading in dim light does not harm eyes.
Excessive use of eyes does not harm them, and "bad eyes" are not the result of overuse.
Sitting too close to television does not harm eyes.
Too strong, too weak, or wrongly ground glasses do not harm eyes.
Contact lenses neutralize refractive errors but do not correct them.
The eyes clean themselves. Healthy eyes do not require eyedrops.
Organic headaches such as migraine and cluster headaches do not occur because of eye strain.
An eye with open-angle glaucoma does not appear abnormal.
Cataract extraction is indicated only if the opacity interferes with activities.
Persistent watering of an infant's eye suggests either congenital glaucoma or a blocked tear duct.

TABLE 4-2.
Some Serious Ophthalmic Signs and Symptoms

Sudden loss of central or peripheral vision
Sudden occurrence of strings, spots, or shadows before eyes
Colored rays or circles surrounding lights (halos)
Double vision
Intermittent dimming of vision
Marked difference in vision between the two eyes
Pain in the eyes
Redness, discharge, crusting, or excessive tearing of the eye
Curtain or veil blocking vision
Swelling, tumor, or mass of the eyelids, conjunctiva, globe, or orbit
Difference in size of the eyes
Wandering or turning of the eye (strabismus)
Jerky movements of the eye (nystagmus)

vision, or should a sudden shower of floaters occur. Attention is directed to the visual acuity as corrected with lenses, and not to the vision without correction.

Visual impairment refers to limitation of one or more basic functions of the eye: visual acuity, dark adaptation, color vision, or peripheral vision. Visual disability refers to inability of an individual to perform specific visual tasks, such as reading, writing, orientation, or traveling unaided. Visual disability is a socioeconomic indication of an individual's capacity to perform particular tasks. Visual handicap refers to a decrease in the physical, social, and economic function of an individual.

The main symptoms of ocular abnormality include (1) disturbances of vision; (2) pain in one or both eyes or in the head; and (3) abnormal secretion from the eyes.

DISTURBANCES OF VISION

An abnormality of visual function may include decreased central or peripheral vision, deficient color vision, or faulty adaptation to light or dark (Table 4-3). Even if these functions are normal, a patient may complain of abnormal perception that may originate in the eye, in its central connections, or in the higher cortical or motor centers.

Visual defects may originate because of (1) an abnormality in the formation of a clear image on the retina; (2) a defect in the reception or the processing of an image by the retina; (3) interference with the neural transmission between the retina and the occipital cortex; or (4) abnormal visual perceptual centers with faulty processing by the brain. Defects in image formation and abnormalities of retinal processing occur within one or both eyes, although one eye may be more severely affected.

If visual acuity is normal with lenses or improved with a pinhole placed over one eye, the cause of reduced vision is likely a refractive error and not an organic disease. Formation of a clear retinal image requires a clear cornea, lens, and vitreous (the ocular media).

The sensory retina must be intact, must line the interior of the eye regularly, and must be in contact with the retinal pigment epithelium throughout. Its blood supply from the choriocapillaris and retinal vasculature must be intact. Photoreceptors must signal changes in light intensity (adaptation) and wavelength (color) correctly.

The nerve impulse generated in the photoreceptor must be processed correctly by the inner retina and transmitted from the retina to the brain. If transmission of the impulse is interrupted in the retina or optic nerve, only one eye is involved. Interference at the optic chiasm or posterior to the chiasm affects visual processing of both eyes.

TABLE 4-3.
Some Abnormalities of Vision

I. Decreased visual acuity
    A. Distance
    B. Near
II. Diplopia (double vision)
    A. Physiologic
    B. Monocular
        1. Local abnormality of one eye
    C. Near only
        1. Convergence abnormality
    D. Distance only
        1. Divergence abnormality
    E. Severity varies with head or eye movements
        1. Ocular muscle abnormality
III. Abnormal visual field
    A. Monocular
        1. Corneal, lens, vitreous, retina and optic nerve disorders
    B. Bilateral
        1. Disorders of both eyes
        2. Disorders of both optic nerves
        3. Disorders at or posterior to the chiasm
IV. Abnormal color vision
    A. Hereditary: bilateral
    B. Acquired: often monocular
V. Defective dark adaptation
VI. Iridescent vision ("halos")
VII. Vitreous floaters
VIII. Photopsia
    A. Bilateral: visual hallucination
        1. Unformed: occipital lobe origin
        2. Formed: temporal lobe origin
IX. Objects appear smaller (micropsia) or larger (macropsia) than they actually are
    A. Fovea centralis abnormality
X. Cortical blindness
    A. Bilateral lesions of occipital cortex
XI. Perceptual blindness
    A. Lesions of angular gyrus of parieto-occipital fissure

Visual perceptual defects often produce bizarre patterns or inability to recognize or describe objects.

The physician must learn whether any defect involves one or both eyes, if it is corrected with lenses, and if it involves distance or near vision, or both. Additionally, the physician must determine if the visual loss is transient or permanent, if it involves central or peripheral vision, and if the vision itself is normal but abnormalities, such as floaters, are superimposed. If the visual defect disappears when the patient wears corrective lenses, then a refractive error is the most likely cause of symptoms. Many people require corrective lenses but prefer not to use them. These patients describe a variety of unusual, apparently inexplicable, ocular symptoms, all of which would be relieved by corrective lenses. Attempts to provide relief by other means are seldom successful.

Some individuals who have ocular symptoms without an organic basis have accumulated many spectacles, none of which relieve their symptoms. They may be convinced that another pair of glasses will help and firmly refuse to recognize that their symptoms do not originate with a refractive error.

Symptoms that involve near vision when the distance vision is normal (or vice versa) are most suggestive of a refractive error. One or both eyes may be involved.

Diagnosis of the cause of sudden, persistent, unilateral decrease of vision is based on the appearance of the eye. The external eye is abnormal in keratitis, iridocyclitis, and angle-closure glaucoma. With vitreous hemorrhage, retinal artery or vein closure, or optic neuritis, the external eye appears normal. In optic neuritis, the pupillary sensitivity to light stimulation is reduced (see Chapter 20). Periodic visual loss, varying from slight haziness to no light perception and lasting for a few seconds to minutes (amaurosis fugax, transient blindness, transient ischemic attack), may result from spasm of the ophthalmic artery in occlusive disease of the internal carotid artery or from abnormalities of the aortic arch. Gradual unilateral loss of vision occurs with corneal opacities, glaucoma, cataract, vitreous opacities, retinal detachment, central retinal degeneration, or intraocular inflammation.

Sudden loss of vision involving both eyes is uncommon. Inquiry usually indicates that vision failed first in one eye and that the sudden loss described was noted by the patient when vision in the fellow eye decreased. Both eyes may be involved in the diseases that cause sudden unilateral loss of vision, but this occurs rarely. A sudden bilateral decrease of vision is most suggestive of a conversion reaction, the toxic effects of drugs, or poor observation.

Gradual loss of vision in both eyes may result from nearly any ophthalmic disorder. Generally, if visual acuity is decreased and peripheral vision is intact, the disorder is anterior to the chiasm. If

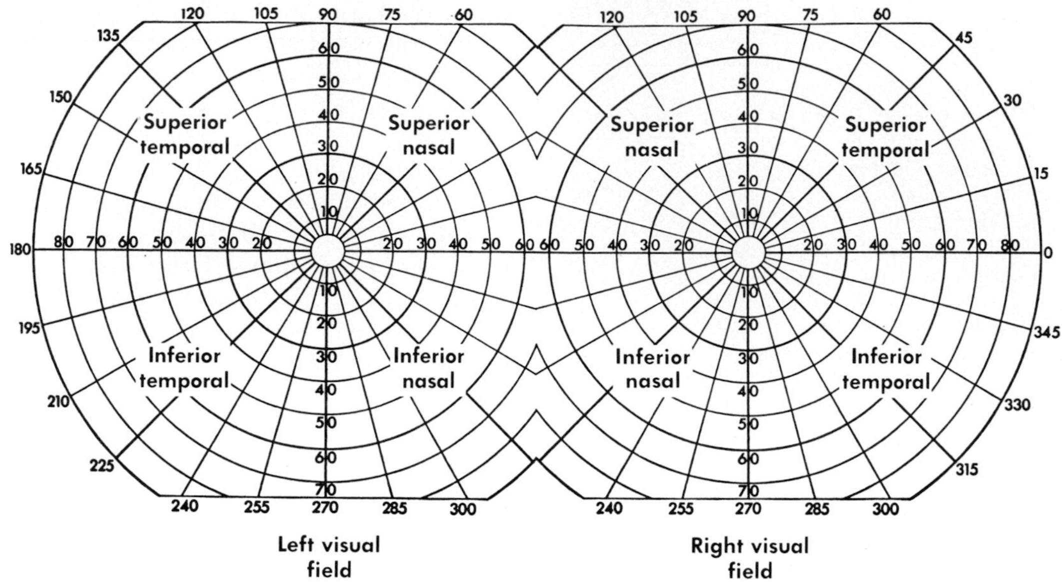

FIG 4-1.
A standard visual field chart. The intersection of the vertical and horizontal lines corresponds to the foveola of the retina and the point of fixation of vision. The concentric circles mark their distance in degrees from the fovea. The temporal quadrants correspond to the nasal retinas, which have axons that decussate at the optic chiasm. The nasal quadrants correspond to the temporal retinas. The superior quadrants correspond to the inferior retinas and the inferior quadrants to the superior retinas.

peripheral vision is decreased in each eye, the disorder may be at or posterior to the chiasm.

Color vision.—Color vision is a cone function. A deficiency in color perception is inherited in approximately 8% of men and 0.5% of women. The most common type is transmitted as an X chromosome–linked abnormality. Visual acuity in these individuals is normal, but color perception is depressed to a varying degree. Acquired unilateral depression of color sense occurs in diseases that affect the cone function of one eye, such as central retinal degeneration (macular degeneration) and optic nerve disease. The decrease in visual acuity parallels the loss of color perception. Bilateral acquired depression in color vision may occur in malnutrition and after the ingestion of toxic drugs. Opacities of the ocular media, particularly those involving the cornea (leukoma) or lens (cataract), may cause depression but not loss of color vision. Color perception is disturbed in a variety of diseases of the optic nerve and fovea centralis as well as in nutritional disturbances.

Peripheral vision.—The retinal periphery contains mainly rods, and cones are scattered throughout. A visual field defect may occur in many abnormalities of the retina, optic nerve, and optic pathways. If the abnormality is anterior to the chiasm, the defect is monocular. Disorders affecting the chiasm or visual pathways involve both eyes. When one eye is involved in retinal or optic nerve disease, the patient frequently describes the sensation of a curtain falling over a portion of the visual field. When both eyes are involved, the patient may be unaware of the defect.

Defects in the visual fields are usually described as central (within 30° of the fixation point) or peripheral. Localized areas of defective vision surrounded by areas of normal vision are called scotomas. Peripheral visual field defects are described as temporal, nasal, superior, or inferior (Fig 4-1). It should be recalled that the visual field reflects the visual function in the opposite areas of the retina involved. A temporal visual field defect reflects light stimulation of the nasal retina. A superior visual field defect involves the inferior retina. Thus, a superotemporal field defect indicates failure to see objects that stimulate the inferonasal retina.

Night blindness.—Patients who have an organic disease that causes night blindness often do not complain of this defect. Conversely, some patients who do not have organic ocular disease may complain about poor vision in reduced illumination. Night blindness is caused by pigmentary degenerations of the retina, optic nerve disease, glaucoma, or vitamin A deficiency that occurs in cirrhosis of the liver or because of inadequate nutrition. It may follow ablation of the peripheral retina by photocoagulation used in the treatment of diabetic retinopathy. The patient may complain of poor recovery of vision during night driving after the headlights of a passing car shine in the eyes. Vision that is poorer in bright illumination than in dim illumination occurs in cone degenerations and in toxic optic neuropathy.

Iridescent vision.—This term is applied to the condition in which colored or luminous rings are seen surrounding lights (halo vision). The most common cause is subepithelial edema of the cornea, which may follow a rapid increase in intraocular pressure. Prolonged wearing of hard contact lenses and swimming in fresh water with the eyes open also cause corneal edema. Pus floating across the cornea in conjunctivitis may cause iridescent vision, which is corrected by rapid blinking. Corneal degeneration (dystrophy) and cataract may also cause the symptom.

Entoptic phenomena.—These originate from visualization of structures within the eye, usually those in the vitreous cavity. Floaters are translucent specks of various shapes and sizes that float across the visual field. They can be seen only when the eye is open. Commonly, the patient observes them when looking at a bright blue sky or a brilliantly illuminated pastel-colored wall. All individuals have small fixed remnants of the hyaloid vascular system in the vitreous humor (muscae volitantes), seen as small dots that dart away as one tries to fix them. Liquefaction (syneresis) of the vitreous humor occurs in aging, in myopia, and after ocular injuries. Leukocytes from inflammation of the retina or uvea may cause floaters, but usually so many are present that vision is severely depressed. A vitreous hemorrhage may cause a sudden shower of floaters in the peripheral visual field. This may be the first symptom of a retinal hole (retinal break) that precedes a retinal detachment. The location of the blood may be helpful in locating the retinal hole. The sudden appearance of a moderately large floater is the main symptom of vitreous detachment. Rarely, a patient learns inadvertently to observe the leukocytes in his or her own capillaries and becomes concerned about disturbing flecks when reading.

Photopsia.—In photopsia visual perceptions are seen in the absence of light stimuli. The term is applied to such visual phenomena as specks, rings, lightning flashes, and luminous bodies that are observed when the eyes are closed. When monocular, photopsia is caused by retinal stimuli other than light (inadequate retinal stimuli). It occurs in traction of the vitreous on the retina or with pressure on the closed eye. Visual hallucinations (bilateral photopsia) are divided into formed and unformed types. Visual hallucinations from the occipital cortex and association areas produce static light and stars, whereas hallucinations from the parastriate area 18 may produce luminous sensations of colored flashes and rings. Hallucinations from the parieto-occipital cortex relate to objects, people, and animals. In addition to photopsia and hallucinations, there may be preservation of the visual image in time (palinopia) or in space (visual illusory spread), impaired visual recognition (visual agnosia), defective visual localization, errors in naming color, or defective perception of color.

Hallucinations that originate in the temporal lobe may be scenes experienced previously, and often consist of landscapes, prairie fires, or seascapes, usually with repetitive activity and a minimum of detail. Visual hallucinations may be associated with auditory hallucinations.

Micropsia and macropsia.—Micropsia, or perceiving images to be smaller than actual size, is caused by an abnormality of image formation at the fovea of the retina or by disorders of the temporal cortex. Edema, tumors, and hemorrhages in the central retina may cause the cones to be spread farther apart and cause micropsia.

Macropsia is an abnormality in which objects appear larger than they actually are. It results from edema, tumors, and hemorrhages in the

TABLE 4-4.
Visual Acuity in Visually Handicapped Persons (Better Eye with Best Possible Correction)

Common Definition	Snellen Index	Practical Test	Legal Significance
No light perception (total blindness)	—	Cannot see light	—
Light perception only	Less than 3/200 (1/60)	Unable to see hand movement at 1 m	Satisfies all criteria for legal blindness*
Form and motion	Less than 3/200 (1/60)	Hand movement visible, but unable to count fingers at 1 m	Total disability for Social Security Administration
Travel vision	Less than 10/200 (3/60)	Unable to read newspaper headlines	Legal blindness
Minimal reading	Less than 20/200 (6/60)	Reads headlines, but not 14-point (4.7-mm) type	Maximum acuity for legal blindness for Internal Revenue Service and most state industrial commissions
Partially seeing (borderline)	More than 20/200 (6/60) but less than 20/70 (6/24)	Cannot read 10-point (3.4-mm) type without marked difficulty	Not legally blind, but eligible for some social services

*Legal blindness also present if visual field is constricted to 20° or less.

foveal region that may cause the cones to be compressed together.

Cortical blindness.—Cortical blindness is an abnormality in vision caused by bilateral impairment of the visual centers of the occipital cortex (area 17). It is characterized by a loss of visual sensation with retention of the pupillary reaction to light. The patient may not be aware of the loss of vision.

Perceptual blindness.—Perceptual blindness is an abnormality caused by lesions in the angular gyrus of the parieto-occipital fissure in which individuals are unable to recognize objects visually (agnosia) but are able to recognize objects by touch. An individual so afflicted will be unable to recognize a key when looking at it but will readily recognize it when touching it. Defects related to this condition include alexia (inability to read), agraphia (inability to write), and dyslexia (disturbance in the ability to read). These abnormalities may be highly selective so that the patient recognizes numbers but not letters, or recognizes printed matter but not written script, and the like.

Blindness.—The definitions of blindness differ, but generally a person is considered legally blind when best visual acuity with corrective lenses in the better eye is 20/200 (6/60) or less or when the peripheral visual field is constricted to within 20° (Table 4-4). The chief causes of blindness in the United States are glaucoma, untreated cataract, and retinal disorders, mainly proliferative diabetic retinopathy and macular (central retinal) degeneration.

The physician treating a blind patient must avoid any hint of condescension and must learn that the patient's interpretation of the physician's voice is the major factor in reassurance. A person talking to a blind individual should identify himself or herself by name, should not shout, and should always give detailed verbal directions and not visual signals. One must never touch the blind patient without warning. Blind persons prefer to grasp the arm of a guide rather than having their own arm held.

Some blind individuals are not aware of the agencies and services available to promote their adjustment and independence. Information may be obtained from the American Foundation for the Blind, 11 Penn Plaza, Suite 300, New York, New York 10001.

DIPLOPIA

Diplopia, or double vision, occurs whenever the visual axes are not directed simultaneously to the same object. Unilateral diplopia is a curiosity in which light rays are split by an opacity in the cornea or lens so that a single object is imaged twice on the retina. Frequently the images are so blurred that the patient notices the defect only under exceptional visual conditions.

Physiologic diplopia is a normal phenomenon in which objects not within the area of fixation are seen double. Usually it does not impinge on the consciousness. It is easily demonstrated by looking at a distant object with attention directed to a near object, which then appears doubled. Such physiologic diplopia contributes to parallax, which enables a person to judge the distance of objects.

Diplopia is a cardinal sign of weakness of one or more of the extraocular muscles. Characteristically, the separation of images increases in the field of action of the extraocular muscle(s) involved. Diplopia can occur only if binocular vision has developed. The absence of diplopia does not guarantee that a paresis of an extraocular muscle is not present. Diplopia may also occur without muscle weakness if there is displacement of the globe, as in proptosis, so that the visual lines cannot be directed simultaneously to the same object.

TABLE 4-5.
Miscellaneous Ocular Symptoms Other Than Visual

- I. Pain in one or both eyes or in the head
  - A. Superficial foreign body sensation
  - B. Deep pain within the eye
  - C. Headache
  - D. Burning, itching, "tired" eyes (asthenopia)
  - E. Photophobia (abnormal ocular sensitivity to light)
- II. Abnormal secretion from eyes
  - A. Lacrimation (excessive tear production)
  - B. Epiphora (defective tear drainage)
  - C. Mucus
  - D. Pus
  - E. Dry eyes
- III. Physical signs described by the patient as symptoms
  - A. Red eye
    1. Conjunctival injection
    2. Ciliary injection
    3. Subconjunctival hemorrhage
  - B. New growths
  - C. Abnormal position of eyes or eyelids
  - D. Protrusion of globe
  - E. Widened palpebral fissure
  - F. Narrowed palpebral fissure
  - G. Pupillary abnormality

PAIN

Pain and aches in the region of the eye or in the head (Table 4-5) may be difficult to interpret and require considerable clinical skill to evaluate accurately. Some patients are phlegmatic about pain, while others would be disabled by pain of the same severity. Moreover, pain is a subjective sensation, and considerable insight into a patient's temperament is required for evaluation.

A superficial foreign body sensation may be caused by several conditions: a lesion in the eyelid, a foreign body on the cornea or the conjunctiva, inflammation of the cornea or the conjunctiva, or loss of conjunctival or corneal epithelium. A local anesthetic instilled in the conjunctival sac usually eliminates the sensation caused by a superficial foreign body but not that caused by inflammation of the conjunctiva and the cornea. If the eyelid is drawn away from the globe, the sensation caused by a foreign body on the tarsal conjunctiva will be eliminated, whereas the sensation caused by a foreign body on the cornea will continue. Patients always localize a foreign body sensation to the outer portion of the upper eyelid irrespective of its location.

Deep, severe pain within the eye may be present in many disorders. The most important causes, since they require immediate attention, are inflammations of the ciliary body and rapid increase in the intraocular pressure, such as that occurring in angle-closure glaucoma. In each of these instances the eye is red and vision is decreased.

Many relatively minor ocular abnormalities manifest themselves by burning, itching, and uncomfortable eyes. These symptoms may originate from an inadequately corrected refractive error, fatigue, keratoconjunctivitis sicca, and chronic conjunctivitis. Mild, nonspecific inflammation of the eyelids or the conjunctiva without obvious signs may cause ocular discomfort, particularly when the eyes are used extensively. Minor ocular irritation caused by prolonged use of the eyes is mainly without significance.

Headache.—The interpretation of headache as a symptom of ocular disease requires familiarity with its causes. Headaches that are relieved by salicylates are usually not caused by serious organic disease. Uncorrected errors of refraction or wearing the wrong corrective lenses do not cause incapacitating headaches. Headaches that are present on awakening in the morning are not caused by excessive use of the eyes the previous night.

One should determine whether a headache is intermittent or continuous, its location in the head, and other associated signs. An aura followed by severe unilateral headache (hemicrania), nausea, and vomiting is suggestive of migraine. A headache aggravated by straining and associated with vomiting without nausea is suggestive of increased intracranial pressure.

Subarachnoid hemorrhage originating from a cerebrovascular aneurysm often causes a severe headache associated with a stiff neck, photophobia, nausea, and vomiting, often with loss of consciousness. About half of such patients experience bleeding episodes days to weeks before they have a major hemorrhage. A warning leak causes a headache so unusual in severity and location that medical advice is sought. There may be nausea and vomiting (anterior communicating artery or anterior cerebral artery aneurysms); retro-orbital pain and oculomotor nerve palsy (internal carotid artery aneurysms); or motor weakness and speech disturbances (middle cerebral artery aneurysms). Generally, ruptured aneurysms that are preceded by a warning leak have a poorer prognosis than those with a single bleeding episode. Lumbar puncture and study of the cerebrospinal fluid for blood or xanthochromic staining are indicated if magnetic resonance imaging has excluded an intracranial mass or intracranial hypertension. Prompt angiography is indicated in those patients with evidence of blood in the cerebrospinal fluid.

Tic douloureux causes a characteristic excruciating pain in the region of distribution of the sensory branches of the trigeminal nerve. Usually the history of episodic pain of a similar type alerts one to the nature of the disorder. In young adults it may be an initial symptom of multiple sclerosis.

Herpes zoster ophthalmicus may cause severe retrobulbar pain, which may precede the cutaneous vesiculation by several days. Often the cause of the pain is not recognized until the typical eruption occurs in the area of distribution of the ophthalmic nerve. Postzoster neuralgia may be extremely disabling in the elderly.

Photophobia is a reflex in which light stimulating the retina causes constriction of the pupil and pain. The term is widely used to indicate any discomfort caused by bright light, such as the reflection of a great amount of light from the sky or an unpleasant contrast between light and dark areas. Glare is the term given to excessive light directed into the eyes from a reflecting surface.

Patients with cone degenerations often have an aversion to bright light that is first noted by the examiner when attempting ophthalmoscopy. Inquiry will then indicate that the patient prefers activities in dim illumination. There may be a reduction in visual acuity as the amount of illumination increases.

ABNORMAL SECRETION

It is sometimes possible to diagnose an ocular disease by observing the nature of an abnormal secretion from the eyes. Pus is found in the conjunctival sac in mucopurulent conjunctivitis. The eyelashes are frequently agglutinated to each other by drying pus, and it may be difficult to open the eyes in the morning. A foamy secretion at the inner canthus is produced by *Corynebacterium xerosis,* which lives solely on desquamated epithelium. A stringy secretion with excoriation of the canthus characterizes the inflammation caused by the diplobacillus of Morax-Axenfeld. A tenacious, stringy secretion occurs in allergic inflammation of the conjunctiva.

A distinction is made between lacrimation, in which there is an excessive production of tears, and epiphora, in which the normal outflow of tears is obstructed. Lacrimation occurs in those diseases that cause reflex secretion of tears, whereas epiphora results from an abnormality of the drainage system. Persistent tearing of one or both eyes of an infant is a cardinal sign of congenital glaucoma. There is an associated corneal edema. Tearing that occurs shortly after birth may be the result of failure of the nasolacrimal duct to open as it normally does about the third week of life. Tearing also occurs in photophobia, in inflammations of the cornea and conjunctiva, and reflexly in inflammations of the ciliary body.

Decreased tear formation causes drying of the eyes (keratoconjunctivitis sicca). This occurs in Sjögren syndrome, in vitamin A deficiency, and in scarring of the conjunctiva that closes the orifices of the lacrimal glands or destroys goblet cells. Erythema multiforme, trachoma, ocular cicatricial pemphigoid, and chemical burns of the eye are the chief causes of such scarring.

DYSLEXIA

Dyslexia is a developmental language disorder in which a basic abnormality of neural processing impairs the ability to process sensory information rapidly (in the millisecond range). Most individuals with a developmental language disorder, possibly 3% to 7% of the general population, appear to have trouble only with spelling and reading, but there are additional widespread perceptual defects. In childhood, reading skills are in the lowest 5% to 10% for their age. There is a history of delay in starting to talk, and a limited memory for verbal material, so there is difficulty in repeating unfamiliar spoken material. Poor readers have difficulty in identifying the number of sounds in the spoken word that allows sounds to be matched with letters. The poor verbal memory impairs learning letter-sound correspondence.

A developmental language disorder is not caused by ocular abnormalities, refractive errors, visual handicaps, emotional disturbance, environmental limitations, or defective intelligence. Reduced vision, ocular muscle imbalance, strabismus, and defective stereopsis have no role except insofar as reduced vision slows the speed with which an individual is able to read but does not limit the comprehension of the printed word. The dyslexic individual not only reads more slowly than normal but does not fully comprehend the material.

Cerebrovascular disease affecting the angular and supramarginal gyri on the opposite side of the dominant hand may cause loss of ability to read in previously competent individuals. If all ability is lost, the condition is classed as alexia; if the difficulty is partial, the condition is classed as neurologic dyslexia or acquired dyslexia. The severity and nature of the defect vary markedly; for example, inability to read letters while retaining ability to read numbers; ability to recognize words in large type but not in small type; and the like. Color perception may be affected (acquired dyschromatopsia). Often there is severe involvement of large areas of the brain, and exact diagnosis is not possible.

PERIODIC EYE EXAMINATION

Examination of the newborn infant should include inspection of the eyelids and the external eye. The pupils should constrict to light, and ophthalmoscopic examination should indicate a red reflex with no opacities of the media. In infants with eyes that are not constantly parallel after 6 months of age or that cross thereafter, a complete eye examination, including refraction with cycloplegia, is indicated.

Vision should be measured in each eye no later than 3 years of age, because strabismic or anisometropic amblyopia may be corrected if detected by this age. A complete eye examination with cycloplegic refraction is desirable before a child begins kindergarten, when in the fourth grade, and before beginning high school, college, and graduate school. If an abnormality is discovered, more frequent examinations may be required. Young adults who are without symptoms and who do not have a refractive error may be examined every 5 years. If corrective lenses are worn, the patient should be examined every 2 years. After 45 years of age, examinations should be done every 2 years.

A complete eye examination should include examination of the eyelids, cornea, sclera, bulbar conjunctiva, anterior chamber, and lens with a biomicroscope. The ocular fundus should be inspected with a direct ophthalmoscope, and the peripheral fundus should be studied with an indirect ophthalmoscope. The intraocular pressure should be measured with a tonometer. The visual fields should be estimated by confrontation, and if there is any question of an abnormality, they must be carefully measured with a perimeter. The ocular rotations and muscle balance for near and far must be measured. The visual acuity should be measured for near and far and the refractive error determined.

Particular attention must be directed to ocular signs of systemic disease. Effective treatment is available for many ocular conditions in their early stages, and it is disheartening to encounter individuals whose ocular abnormalities were not detected in their early stages. Similarly, many systemic diseases are first evident in the eyes. In the Framingham Study, more than 25% of those who were found to have retinal changes characteristic of diabetes had no previous diagnosis of or treatment for diabetes.

BIBLIOGRAPHY

Book

Roy FH: *Ocular differential diagnosis,* ed 4, Philadelphia, 1989, Lea & Febiger.

Article

Hynd GE, Hall J, Novey ES, Eliopulos RT, Black K, Gonzalez MA et al: Dyslexia and corpus callosum morphology, *Arch Neurol* 52:32-38, 1995.

5

FUNCTIONAL EXAMINATION OF THE EYES

The different functions of the eye are evaluated by many tests. The cone function of the fovea centralis is assessed clinically by measurement of the ability to distinguish the shape of symbols such as letters. This function is designated as visual acuity. It is measured for both near and far, with and without the appropriate lenses that correct any refractive error. Because only cones participate in color vision and because they are concentrated in the fovea, the measurement of color recognition also measures foveal function. The function of the peripheral retina, which contains mainly rods, is measured by estimation of the peripheral visual field. Dark adaptation, which is not part of a routine examination, measures recovery of photoreceptor function after exposure to light.

Any reasonably complete physical examination should indicate whether (1) vision when corrected with glasses, if necessary, is normal in each eye for near and far, each eye being measured separately; (2) the peripheral visual field of each eye is intact on gross testing; (3) the ocular movements are normal and the eyes are parallel; (4) each pupil constricts when the retina of each eye is stimulated by light; and (5) the optic disks are flat and of normal color. Such an evaluation is not a complete eye examination, but it can be performed quickly and, when normal, excludes many different disorders.

VISUAL ACUITY

Measurement of visual acuity assesses the function of the fovea centralis and its central connections. The measurement involves several components. Detection measurements consist of recognizing one or two objects, a break of a line, or an opening in a ring. Objectively, one may determine if the eye follows a moving target. Descriptive measurements consist of describing the location of a break in a ring, indicating the direction in which lines point, or drawing what is seen. Interpretive measurements consist of stating what letter, picture, number, or object is seen.

Visual test objects (optotypes) are constructed so that at a particular distance the whole object subtends an angle of 5 minutes of an arc, and different parts of the object are separated by a distance of 1 minute of an arc (Figs 5-1 and 5-2).

Visual acuity is ordinarily designated by two numbers. The first indicates the distance between the test object and the patient. The second indicates the distance at which the test object subtends an angle of 5 minutes. To record visual acuity, both numbers are recorded. Sometimes the two numbers are reduced to their decimal equivalent; thus, 20/100 is 0.2 and 20/40 is 0.5. Such numbers are obviously not as informative as those that indicate both the test distance and the size of the test object.

Letters or numbers are the usual optotypes. Use of test letters requires a literate and cooperative observer. The letters vary in their recognizability. Thus, L is the easiest letter in the alphabet to recognize, and B is the most difficult. The Landolt broken ring (Fig 5-3), in which the break in the ring subtends a 1-minute angle and

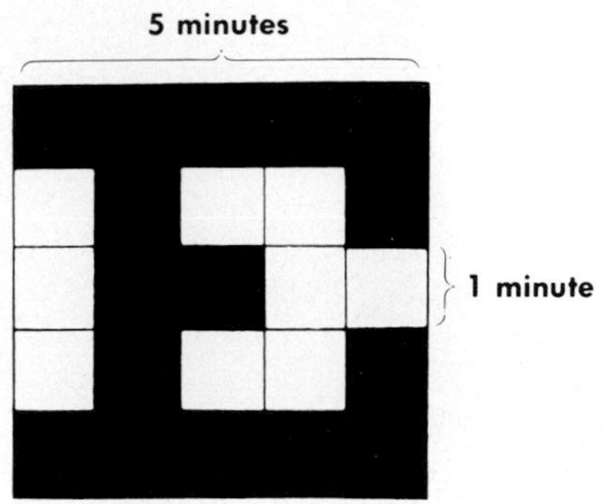

FIG 5-1.
Construction of the Snellen letter to subtend an angle of 5 minutes; each part of the letter subtends an angle of 1 minute. Letters constructed without serifs are recommended. The letter at right measures 1.4375 × 1.4375 inches. It subtends an angle of 5 minutes at a distance of 991.38 inches. The size of the test letter (1.4375 inches) divided by the tangent of 5 minutes (0.00145) equals 991.38 inches (82.61 feet).

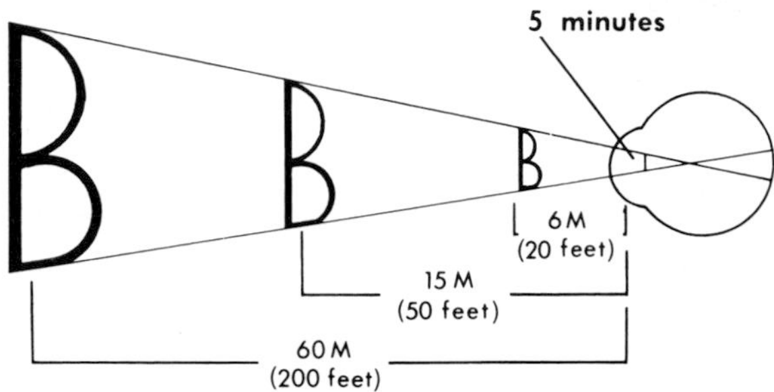

FIG 5-2.
Test letters that subtend an angle of 5 minutes at different distances from the eye. The letter size is equal to the distance from the eye multiplied by the tangent of 5 minutes (50 m × tangent of 5 minutes [0.00145] = 0.0725 m).

the entire ring subtends a 5-minute angle, eliminates this variability. Similarly, the letter E may be arranged so that it faces in different directions (the illiterate E) (see Fig 5-3). The checkerboard design (see Fig 5-3) is arranged so that when the target is too small for the checkerboard to be discriminated, all four squares appear uniformly gray. These test objects may be used to test illiterate individuals and persons not familiar with the Western alphabet. A variety of pictures have been designed for testing children.

The measurement of visual acuity involves many factors not necessarily related to the ability to see test objects. Visual acuity varies with motivation, attention, intelligence, and physical conditions. Lighting, adaptation, contrast, and other factors differ considerably (as does the patience of both the examiner and the patient).

An isolated letter is recognized more easily than a series of letters. This is particularly true in individuals who have an amblyopic eye, who may have a visual acuity as good as 20/50 when measured with isolated letters and as poor as 20/200 when a series of letters is viewed. The visual acuity scores improve if an unlimited time is given in which to recognize the letters; scores decrease when the letters are presented rapidly.

The measurement of visual acuity in a manner that may be consistently reproduced involves attention to a number of complex physical and psychic details that are controlled only in experimental situations. The maximum visual acuity is that in which the individual correctly recognizes 51% of the test symbols within a definite time period. If a portion of the test symbols is not recognized, it is customary to indicate the best vision minus the number of symbols incorrectly identified (for example, 20/30 –2). Well-designed charts have the same number of letters on each line.

Visual acuity for distance should be measured both without lenses and with the most recently prescribed lenses. Distance vision is never measured with the patient wearing the lenses intended for near.

If vision is reduced, a pinhole (discussed later in this chapter) may be used. Normal visual acuity, with or without lenses, indicates that (1) the cornea, lens, and ocular media are relatively clear in the visual axis, permitting an image to be formed on the retina; (2) the fovea centralis is relatively intact, as are its nervous connections to

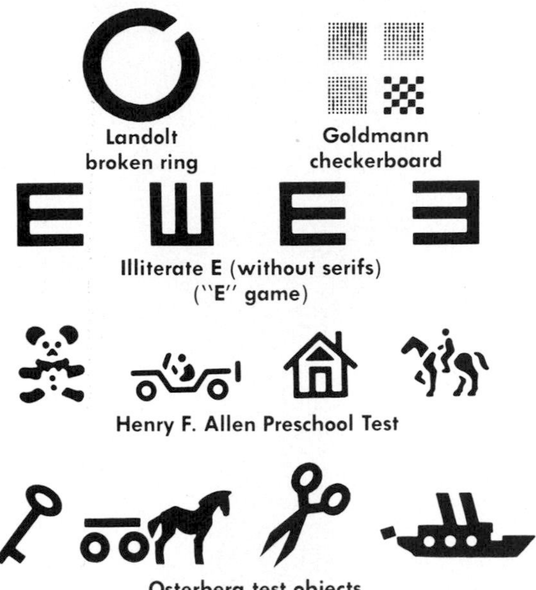

FIG 5-3.
Symbols used in testing distance visual acuity in preschool children and illiterates. The Landolt broken ring and the Goldmann checkerboard are used in research studies.

CM	IN	
353	140	L
176	70	F P
118	47	T O Z
88	35	L P E D
71	28	P E C F D
59	23	E D F C Z P
44	17	F E L O P Z D
35	14	D E F P O T E C

FIG 5-4.
Near vision optotypes designed to subtend an angle of 5 minutes at various distances. Usually the examiner records the smallest optotype seen and does not record the distance of the material from the eye. If distance is recorded, it is measured in inches or centimeters. A patient who reads the smallest optotype, at a reading distance of 14 inches, would have near vision of 14/14.

the brain; and (3) perception by the higher visual centers is intact. Normal visual acuity does not indicate that the eye is free of disease.

The largest test symbol usually used clinically in the United States subtends an angle of 5 minutes at a distance of 200 feet. Smaller symbols subtend a 5-minute angle at distances of 100, 60, 40, 30, 20, and 15 feet (Fig 5-4). If the individual is unable to recognize the largest test symbol, the symbols are brought closer until recognized. If the symbol that subtends a 5-minute angle at 200 feet is recognized when the symbol is 7 feet away, the vision is recorded as 7/200. This is not a fraction but two different values, and both should be recorded.

If no symbols can be recognized, then the examiner learns if the patient can count the examiner's fingers. This is recorded as counting fingers (CF) at a given distance. If the fingers cannot be counted, the examiner determines if the individual can see hand movements (HM). If the patient cannot see hand movements, a small penlight is used to learn if this light can be seen. If the light is seen, the examiner determines whether the patient can recognize its direction (light projection) or whether vision is limited to light perception. (To avoid confusion, the examiner must spell out light perception or projection and not use the abbreviation LP). If the individual cannot see the light, vision is recorded as "no light perception." The word "blind" has so many legal and sociologic implications that it should not be used.

The preceding discussion may suggest that the measurement of visual acuity is a complicated, time-consuming, difficult-to-interpret maneuver. Rather, it is rapidly performed, is simple, and requires minimal equipment.

Measurement of near vision is by no means as accurate as that of distance vision. For the most part, the distance at which near vision is tested is not recorded, and the examiner records the smallest type that can be recognized irrespective of the distance. The standard test distance is considered to be 14 inches (35 cm). Test symbols that subtend a 5-minute angle at various distances, or different size types, are used (see Fig 5-4).

Normal near vision may be recorded as 14/14 (inches), 35/35 (centimeters), or 4-point type at 14 inches (35 cm). Near optotypes (letters of decreasing size) were first described by Jaeger, and thus the designation may be J4.

Many individuals have never had visual acuity measured in each eye separately. Sometimes decreased vision in one eye is first detected when visual acuity is measured after a minor eye injury. If the examiner has not measured the vision before inspecting or manipulating the eye, the patient may mistakenly attribute any reduced vision to the examiner. In an emergency it

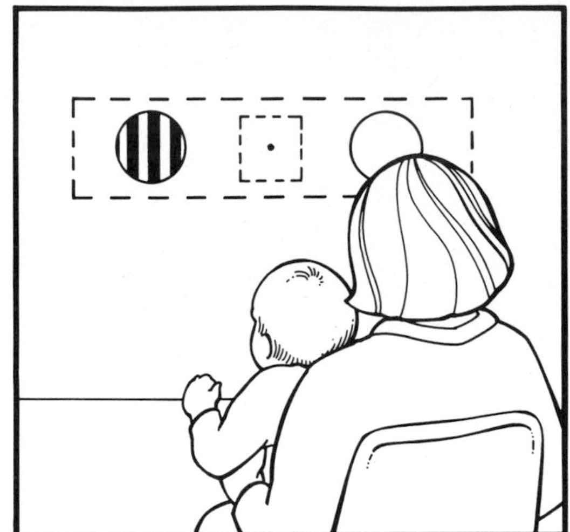

FIG 5-5.
Preferential looking in an infant. The observer is concealed behind the grating target and observes the infant's eyes.

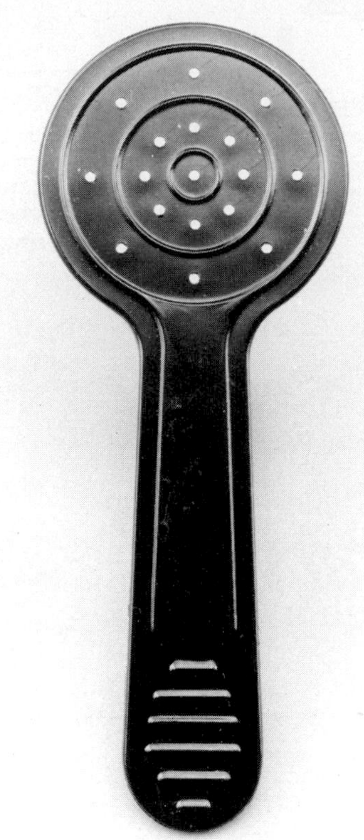

FIG 5-6.
A multiple pinhole shield. Only rays of light that are parallel to the visual axis and are thus not refracted are seen.

is not necessary to have specific testing equipment available. One may gauge the visual acuity by using a telephone book or a newspaper and recording the smallest print that can be recognized with each eye.

It is desirable to measure the visual acuity of children sometime during their third year to detect strabismic or sensory amblyopia and to recognize the presence of severe refractive errors. Picture charts, the illiterate E, or the Landolt broken ring may be used. A rotating drum with alternating strips of black and white that induce rhythmic back-and-forth movement of the eyes (optokinetic nystagmus) is used to measure vision objectively. A strip of cloth 66 by 7 cm may have a series of 5-cm circles of a different color sewn on it. Movement of the strip in front of the eyes induces an optokinetic nystagmus in infants and indicates vision adequate for subsequent normal schooling.

In preferential looking, a calm, alert infant is held in front of two screens of matching luminance, one of which displays a grating pattern (Fig 5-5), the other of which displays a blank field. Infants prefer to look at the pattern rather than the blank field, and visual acuity can be estimated by the stripe width (spatial frequency) seen by the infant.

Pinhole test.—Measurement of visual acuity with the patient viewing test symbols through a small opening in an opaque shield (Fig 5-6) rapidly indicates whether reduced vision is caused by an error of refraction (and is thus correctable with lenses) or by some other abnormality. Vision is improved when a refractive error is present because only rays that are nearly parallel to the visual axis, and thus not refracted, are seen. Usually, if vision is improved with use of a pinhole, a corrective lens will provide even better vision. Exceptionally, visual acuity cannot be duplicated in patients who have keratoconus. The pinhole may reduce vision, rather than improve it, in patients with opacities in the visual axis, such as corneal scars, cataract, or vitreous abnormalities.

Contrast sensitivity.—Contrast is the ratio of brightness to darkness. Black on white has a contrast of 1.0. A uniform all-black or all-white surface has no contrast. The contrast threshold is the minimal amount of contrast required to detect a test pattern. The contrast sensitivity is the reciprocal of the threshold value.

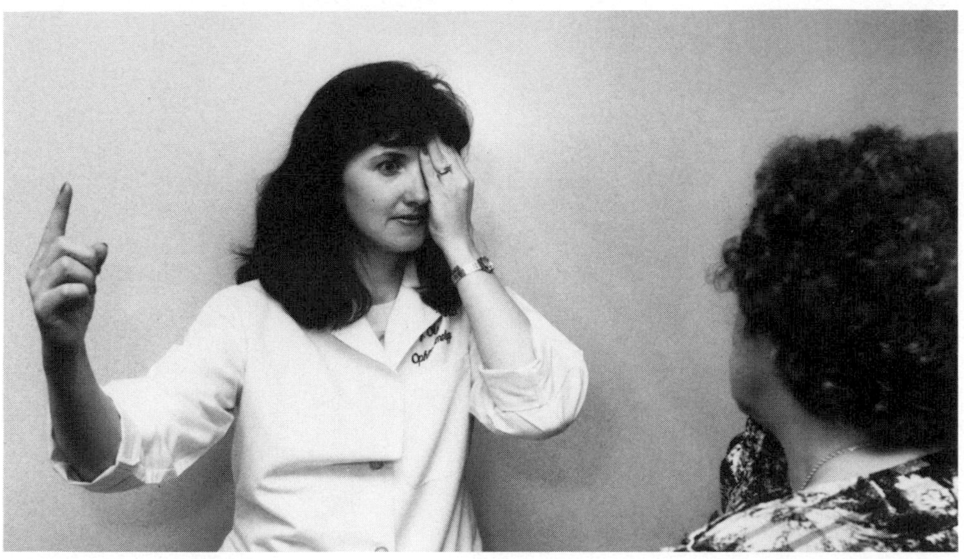

FIG 5-7.
Confrontation fields in which the ability of the subject to see the outstretched fingers is compared with that of the examiner.

An oscilloscope is used in laboratory testing. The screen shows a pattern of alternate bright and dark stripes that can be varied in both width (spatial frequency) and contrast. The number of luminosity variations per degree of visual angle varies from 1.2 to 22 per second. Either the stimuli are switched on and off or the dark and light stripes are quickly reversed (grating contrast alteration). Determination of the spatial frequency with different time intervals and contrast yields the temporal contrast sensitivity. A variety of sophisticated methods have been developed to demonstrate the function of X and Y cells, color recognition, motion detectors, and related properties of the retina and visual pathways.

Contrast sensitivity testing has become popular to demonstrate the deleterious effect of cataract on visual acuity. Cataracts impair contrast sensitivity, but the results mainly parallel those of the usual clinical measurements. The printed charts used clinically consist of test symbols of varying contrast. Their contrast and the spatial frequency cannot be varied simultaneously. Many of the charts have not been validated.

Glare.—Glare is the sensation caused by brightness within the visual field that is greater than the luminosity to which the eye is adapted. It may cause annoyance, discomfort, and decreased visual acuity (disability glare). Attention is directed clinically to the decreased vision encountered by patients with a cataract in which the intraocular scattering of light combined with contraction of the pupil reduces visual acuity. Contrast sensitivity is affected by lesions located anywhere in the visual system. Glare testing is far more sensitive than contrast sensitivity testing to cataract and visual loss secondary to opacities of the anterior segment.

VISUAL FIELDS

The functional capacity of the retina to resolve test symbols decreases rapidly in all directions away from the fovea centralis. The function of the periphery of the retina is assessed by measurement of the visual field, in which the individual detects targets that stimulate the retina at varying distances from the fovea. This function may be measured accurately by one of several instruments, or it may be estimated by means of the confrontation test.

The confrontation test grossly estimates the visual field, and even when the results are normal, a defect may still be detected by more sensitive methods of examination. To determine visual field by confrontation, the examiner faces the patient at a distance of 1 m (Fig 5-7) in an area of good illumination. The patient is asked to

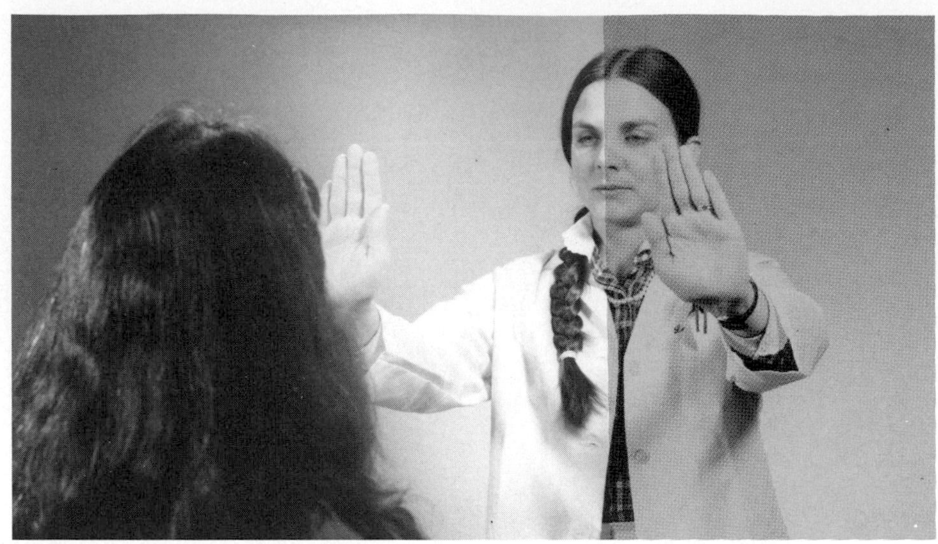

FIG 5-8.
Confrontation fields in which the subject compares the clarity with which the hands are seen in the temporal and nasal visual fields. Each eye is tested separately.

close one eye, usually by holding the eyelids closed with the fingers. The examiner's own eye is the control, and thus the examiner closes the eye directly opposite the patient's closed eye. The patient is then directed to fix attention on the nose of the examiner, whose hand is placed about midway from the patient with one, two, or three fingers extended. The examiner then slowly brings the hand inward and the patient states the number of fingers displayed. When both the patient and the examiner have a normal field of vision, each should see the fingers at about the same distance. Usually the temporal and nasal fields and the superior and inferior fields are tested in turn. Confrontation testing may also be carried out by substituting a hat pin with a 3- or 5-mm white tip. When testing a child, the examiner may stand behind the child, who has one eye occluded, and bring the hand into the nasal and temporal fields from behind the child's head.

Alternatively, the patient, seated 1 m in front of the examiner, closes one eye. The examiner holds one hand on either side of the patient, first above and then below the horizontal plane. The patient is asked if the hands look similar and if they have the same color and distinctness (Fig 5-8).

The patient may be asked to observe two small colored objects (such as the red top of an eyedropper bottle). One is placed centrally and the other to one side. The patient is then asked to describe any difference in color intensity of the two caps (Fig 5-9).

Perimeters and tangent screens.—Visual fields are quantitated by means of kinetic or static perimetry. In kinetic perimetry, a test object of fixed size and illumination is moved from a nonseeing area to an area where it can just be detected by the subject. In static perimetry the test object is of constant size and location, but the light intensity varies and is increased until the subject can just detect it.

Perimeters are constructed so that the eye is at the center of rotation of a hemisphere that has a radius of curvature of 33 cm. Early perimeters consisted of an arc of a circle that was rotated; modern perimeters are constructed as a half-bowl. In the simplest devices, the test object is moved on the end of a wand into the field of view, and in more elaborate perimeters a minute light is projected. The testing distance of 33 cm remains constant.

When recorded, the line that connects the points at which the same object may be recognized is called the "isopter." The size and intensity of the test object are recorded.

Accurate measurement of the visual field requires an attentive and responsive subject. Often the disorder that requires the examination

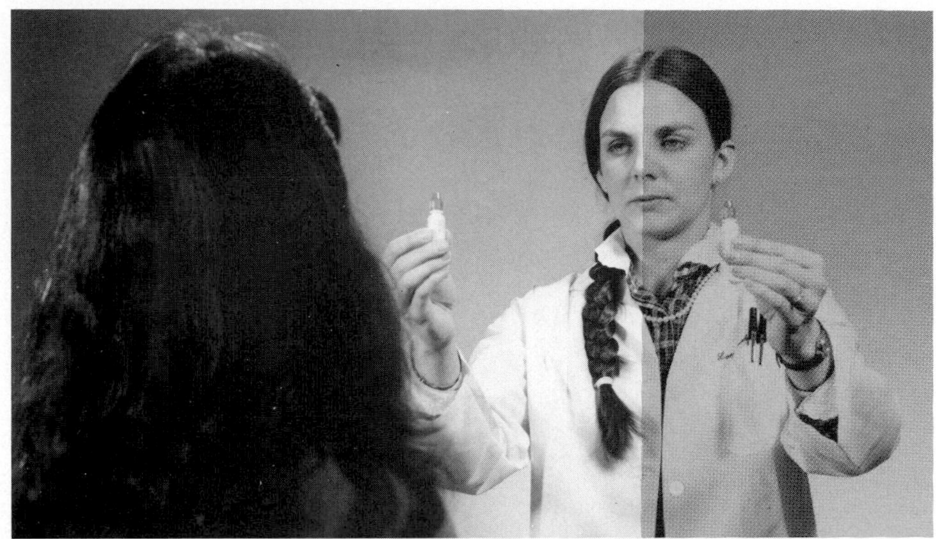

FIG 5-9.
Confrontation test in which the subject compares the brightness of a colored test object used for fixation with the color of a test object in the periphery.

may so impair the patient's awareness that only the grossest responses can be obtained. Computed tomography and magnetic resonance imaging have made perimetry less important than previously in the diagnosis of many intracranial lesions.

Computerized automated perimeters are particularly useful when optic nerve function in glaucoma is evaluated. The instruments minimize errors caused by faulty technique and unskilled examiners but require a high degree of attentiveness and cooperation by the patient. Patients with glaucoma often require repeated testing before reliable measurements are obtained.

Tangent screens.—Because the photoreceptors are concentrated in and near the fovea centralis, determination of field defects within 30° of the fixation point is important. Visual fields within this area may be measured by using a tangent screen (tangent because it is a plane tangent to the arc of a perimeter). A tangent screen is usually covered with black felt, and the test is conducted 1 or 2 m (3 to 6 feet) from the subject. Test objects that vary in size from 1 to 50 mm (0.4 to 2 inches) are used. The peripheral isopter, the blind spot, and various scotomas may be demonstrated (Fig 5-10).

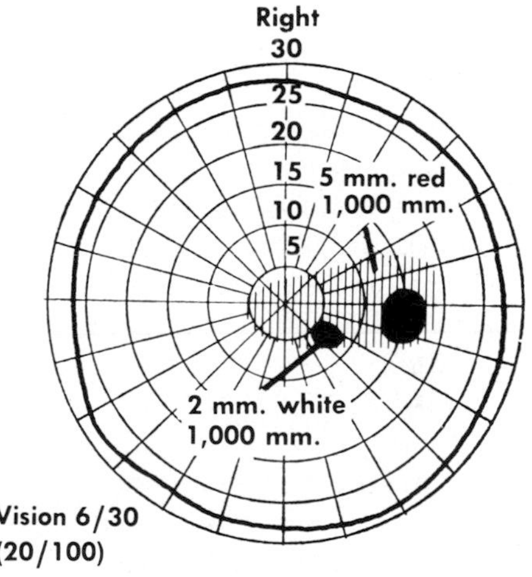

FIG 5-10.
A tangent screen record illustrating a centrocecal (*centro:* the fixation point; *cecal:* a blind spot, the termination of the optic nerve at the optic disk) scotoma. The blind spot demonstrates an absolute scotoma in which there is no perception of light (in black) and is surrounded by a relative scotoma (reduced perception of light [vertical lines]).

The Amsler grid.—This test permits patients to monitor central field defects. It is recommended for individuals with retinal disorders, chiefly age-related macular degeneration, that threaten central vision. The grid consists of 400 squares, each measuring 5 × 5 mm (Fig 5-11), and at the reading distance encompasses the central 20° of the field of vision. The test is performed on each eye separately with the pa-

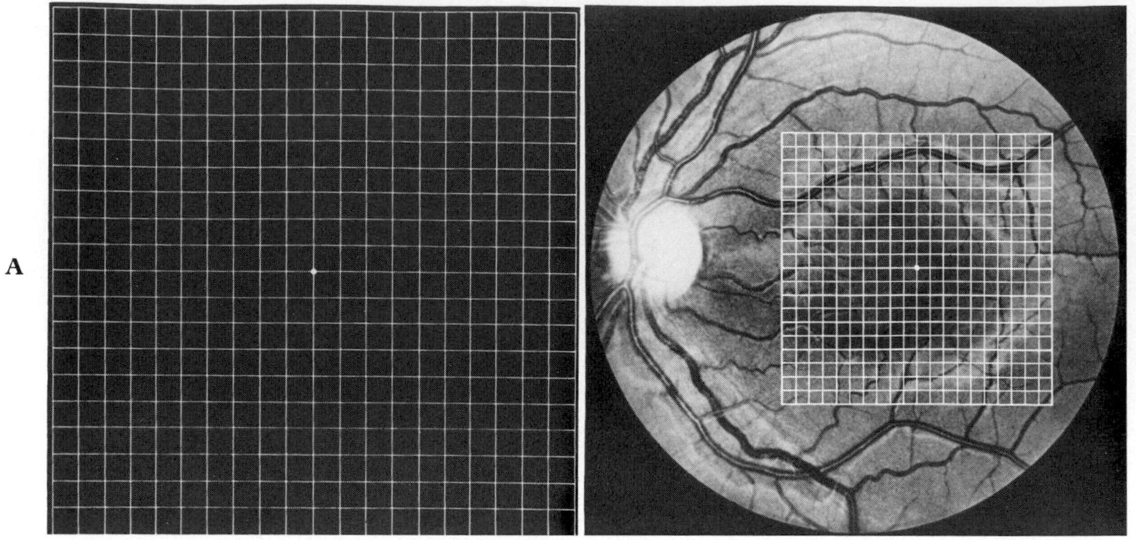

FIG 5-11.
A, The Amsler (1930) grid pattern to enable patients to monitor central field defects. **B,** The Amsler grid superimposed on the area of retina tested.

tient in good light and, if necessary, wearing glasses for near vision. The patient fixes the black dot at the center of the grid and indicates any lines that appear wavy or curved or any squares that appear to be missing. The test is sensitive and should be carried out before pupillary dilation or ophthalmoscopy. In ocular conditions in which subretinal neovascularization may disturb the sensory retina, patients at risk may test themselves daily.

Visual field defects.—Visual fields are charted to represent the visual space as the patient sees it. Thus, the left visual field is charted on the left, and the right visual field is charted on the right side of the viewer. The temporal visual field of each eye reflects stimulation of that portion of the retina located to the nasal side of the fovea centralis and ganglion cell axons that decussate in the optic chiasm. The nasal visual field reflects stimulation of that portion of the retina located to the temporal side of the fovea centralis and retinal ganglion cells that terminate in the lateral geniculate body on the same side. The blind spot (the optic disk, which has no photoreceptors) is located on the temporal side of each visual field.

An imaginary horizontal line that extends from the fovea centralis to the temporal periphery of the retina is the temporal raphe of the anatomic retina. Ganglion cell axons do not extend above or below the horizontal raphe, and it is an important anatomic region in the development of nerve fiber defects in open-angle glaucoma.

Defects in the visual field are usually described as central or peripheral. A defect of the central field, a scotoma, is surrounded by a seeing area. Central scotomas involve the fixation point, and paracentral scotomas involve an area adjacent to the fixation point. Central scotomas characterize diseases involving the fovea centralis and the papillomacular bundle of nerve fibers in the optic nerve. Centrocecal scotomas involve both the physiologic blind spot and the fixation point and are characteristic of toxic diseases of the optic nerve. Annular scotomas form a circular defect around the fixation point and occur in diseases that first manifest themselves at the equator of the eye, particularly retinal pigmentary degenerations. Arcuate (arched) scotomas involve a bundle of nerve fibers and characterize the field defect of glaucoma.

Reference is always made to the blind portion of the visual field. Hemianopsia means half-blindness (Greek, *hemi,* half; *an,* negative; *opsi,* vision). A left hemianopsia indicates a left half-blindness and must involve impulses that originate from the right half of the right or left retina. Homonymous hemianopsia indicates involvement of the right or left portion of each visual field and thus interference with impulse transmission posterior to the optic chiasm.

COLOR VISION TESTING

Good color vision is especially important in industry, school, and vehicle operation, but often color vision testing is neglected in routine clinical testing. The tests used clinically are relatively gross and too insensitive to detect small changes but nonetheless are helpful to the individual. Color vision deficiencies occur as a hereditary defect in about 8% of men and 0.5% of women (see Chapter 2). They are usually transmitted as an X chromosome–linked abnormality.

Autosomal defects in color vision occur in congenital achromatopsias and in cone degenerations. In retrobulbar neuritis, there may be early severe depression of color vision. In foveal degeneration caused by vascular disease, retinal separation, and other acquired disorders, the decrease in color vision parallels the decreased visual acuity. The least accurate test for detecting color deficiency involves the matching of yarns (Holmgren test) or recognizing red and green lanterns. Color plates are available in which numbers are outlined in the primary colors and surrounded by confusion colors. The color-deficient individual cannot discern the figure that is recognized quickly by a person with normal color appreciation. More sensitive tests of color vision involve the use of the Nagel anomaloscope, in which the hue and saturation of yellow are matched by mixtures of red and green. The Farnsworth-Munsell test of hue discrimination consists of 84 chips of color that are matched in terms of increasing hue.

Color perception is disturbed in a variety of diseases of the optic nerve and fovea centralis as well as in nutritional disturbances. Testing has an important role in the diagnosis of total color blindness. Sensitive color vision tests are used routinely in the clinical evaluation of cone degenerations and other foveal disorders.

BIBLIOGRAPHY

Books

Anderson DR: *Perimetry. With and without automation,* ed 2, St Louis, 1987, Mosby–Year Book.

Carr RE, Siegel IM: *Electrodiagnostic testing of the visual system,* Philadelphia, 1990, FA Davis.

Shapley R, Lam D M-K, editors: *Contrast sensitivity,* Cambridge, Mass, 1993, MIT Press.

Article

Kushner BJ, Lucchese NJ, Morton GV: Grating visual acuity with Teller cards compared with Snellen visual acuity in literate patients, *Arch Ophthalmol* 113:485-493, 1995.

6

PHYSICAL EXAMINATION OF THE EYES

The skilled physician studies patients constantly and unobtrusively to learn the physical basis of their symptoms. At their first meeting the examiner should note the size and shape of the patient's head and the position of the eyes. Gross variations in the insertion of the canthal ligaments are observed easily, and the obliquity of the palpebral fissure is readily evident. Simple observation shows wrinkling of the forehead because of photophobia or an attempt to elevate the upper eyelid in blepharoptosis. Good illumination is necessary, but close inspection is not necessary to disclose injection of the conjunctival vessels or jaundice. The position of the eyelid margins in relation to the eye as well as any discomfort in holding the eyes open should be evident.

Entropion or ectropion may be evident without close examination of the eyelid margins. In the course of visiting with the patient, the physician should observe whether the eyes move in unison and whether the movements are full.

More careful inspection may be carried out be means of a small penlight, which provides a concentrated beam of light. Better visualization of details may be obtained if good illumination is combined with inspection through a +20-diopter convex lens (Fig 6-1). This lens may also be used for indirect ophthalmoscopy and for inspection of skin lesions. Better magnification is provided by a binocular loupe that magnifies 1.8 to 5 times.

EXTERNAL EXAMINATION

Examination of the eyes is conducted in a systematic manner that begins with the shape of the head and orbits, moves to the skin of the face and eyelids, and continues inward. The examiner notes the symmetry and width of the palpebral fissures and the position of the eyes. The eyelids normally conceal the corneoscleral limbus in the 12 and 6 o'clock meridians. Proptosis or retraction of the upper eyelid in thyroid ophthalmopathy is often first manifested by exposure of a narrow rim of sclera above or below the corneoscleral limbus. Keratoconus and subtle proptosis are most easily detected by viewing the contact of the cornea with the lower eyelid from above and behind the patient. The examiner stands behind and looks over the brow of the seated patient (Fig 6-2). By drawing the upper eyelids upward, the examiner will easily note any difference in prominence of the two eyes. In keratoconus, the cornea distorts the lower eyelid outward (Munson sign).

Eyelid margin.—The eyelashes (cilia) and the eyelid margin are inspected for the characteristic scaling of squamous blepharitis. Abnormalities in position of the eyelid margin are noted. Intermittent entropion may be demonstrated if the patient squeezes the eyelids closed and then opens them. Particular attention is directed to the position of the lacrimal puncta in relation to the lacrimal lake at the inner canthus. The inferior punctum should be inverted and not visible when the eyes are rotated

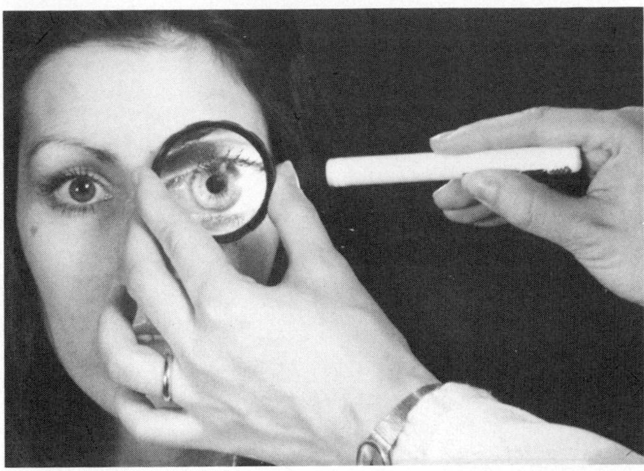

FIG 6-1.
Use of a penlight and a +20-diopter convex lens to study details of the anterior segment.

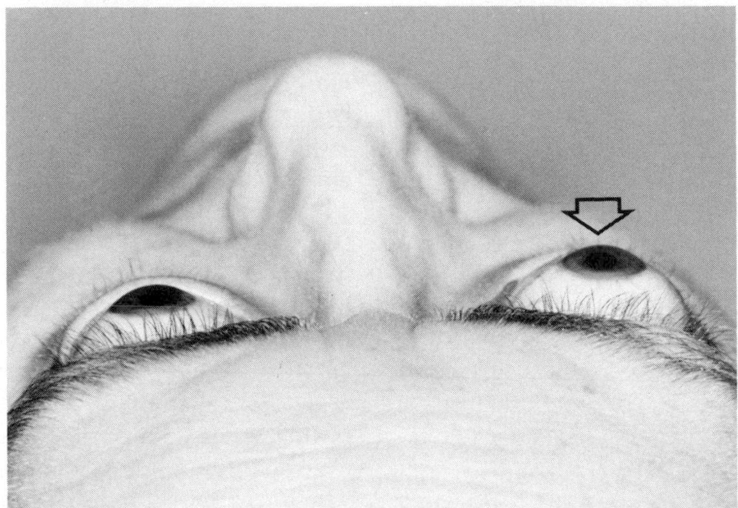

FIG 6-2.
Inspection of prominence of eyes by standing behind the patient, looking over the brow from above and behind, and elevating the upper eyelids. Note the proptosis of the right eye. The abnormal cornea profile in keratoconus may also be demonstrated this way.

upward. Slight eversion of the inferior punctum is a common cause of tearing. Sties involve the eyelid margin, whereas chalazia usually appear as small lumps in the deeper substance of the eyelid.

Conjunctiva.—The bulbar conjunctiva may be inspected directly. The caruncle is evident as a minute pink mass of tissue at the inner canthus. The semilunar fold is not grossly evident unless the conjunctiva is inflamed. The superior and inferior portions of the bulbar conjunctiva are inspected easily by having the patient look upward and downward while the eyelids are drawn apart.

Eversion of the upper eyelid.—Inspection of the upper tarsal conjunctiva requires eversion of the upper eyelid. While the patient looks downward, the lashes of the upper eyelid are grasped by the examiner between the thumb and the index finger. The eyelid is drawn gently outward to break the suction between the eyelid and the globe. The eyelid is then everted on a toothpick or applicator placed on the palpebral sulcus (Fig 6-3). The tarsal conjunctiva is ex-

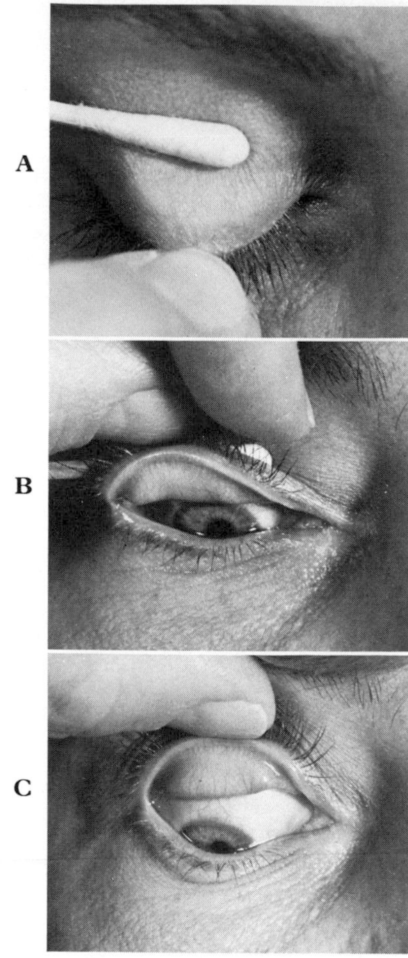

FIG 6-3.
Eversion of the upper eyelid. The patient is instructed to look downward, and the lashes of the upper eyelid are grasped between the thumb and index finger. **A,** A cotton-tipped applicator is placed at the level of the tarsal fold. **B,** The eyelid is then folded back on the cotton-tipped applicator while the patient continues to look downward. **C,** The applicator is then removed, and the details of the tarsal conjunctiva are inspected. The superior conjunctival fornix can be further studied if the eyelid is doubled over a speculum applied to the skin after single eversion.

posed, and the meibomian glands perpendicular to the eyelid margin may be seen through the translucent tarsal conjunctiva. Sometimes the palpebral portion of the main lacrimal gland may be seen at the outer canthus.

Eversion of the lower eyelid.—The inside of the lower eyelid is easily inspected. The patient looks upward, and the eyelid is drawn downward by the examiner's index finger ap-

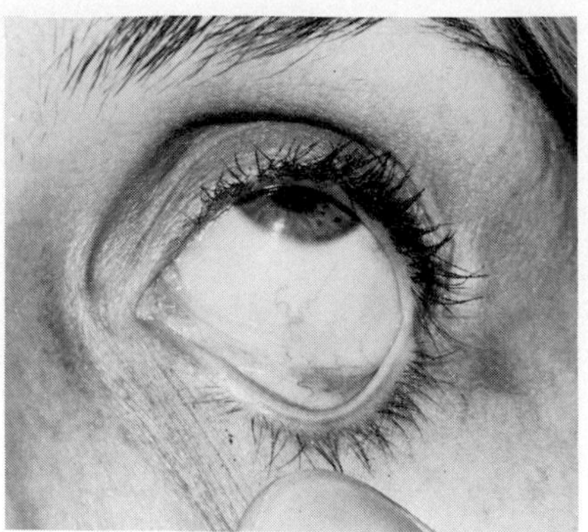

FIG 6-4.
Eversion of the lower eyelid by drawing the margin downward as the subject looks upward.

plied to its orbital portion (Fig 6-4). With the exception of trachoma and vernal catarrh, nearly all conjunctival inflammations are more marked in the inferior fornix than in the superior fornix.

Cornea.—Attention is directed to the diameter and the clarity of the cornea. A cornea with a horizontal diameter of more than 12 mm suggests congenital glaucoma or megalocornea. A horizontal diameter of 9.5 mm or less in an adult suggests a microcornea, in which hyperopia and angle-closure glaucoma may occur.

The evaluation of corneal clarity involves several factors. The anterior surface of the cornea should be smooth, regular, and mirrorlike. The iris pattern should be distinctly seen in all regions. Corneal blood vessels should not be present. When edematous, the cornea has an opalescent appearance. Marked opacities (leukomas) are usually evident, but magnification is required to see less severe defects (maculas). Corneal vascularization may be superficial or deep and may involve the entire cornea or a segment. Stromal vascularization may be manifested solely as a loss of corneal clarity; magnification is required to see the individual blood vessels. The corneoscleral limbus may be involved in corneal arcus, particularly in elderly individuals or in those with lipid disturbances. Staining of the cornea, using a sterile fluorescein strip or a 2% sterile solution, will demonstrate defects in the corneal epithelium.

Anterior chamber.—The normal aqueous humor is acellular and transparent. Even in severe uveal inflammations, good magnification is required to see inflammatory cells and a Tyndall phenomenon (flare) in the anterior chamber. Blood in the anterior chamber (hyphema) usually does not clot and appears bright red, often with a meniscus, and conceals the iris. A severe intraocular inflammation may cause leukocytes to collect in the lower portion of the anterior chamber (hypopyon).

The depth of the anterior chamber is estimated as the distance between the posterior surface of the cornea and the front surface of the iris. Usually it measures 3 mm or more. If the iris appears to be convex and to parallel the posterior corneal surface and if the depth of the anterior chamber is less than 2 mm, there is a danger of angle-closure glaucoma. Directing the beam of a penlight from the temporal side of the eye across the anterior chamber may demonstrate a shallow anterior chamber, since the iris may bow forward and cast a shadow on the opposite nasal side.

If a shallow anterior chamber is present, attention should be directed particularly (1) to a history of episodes of blurring or fogging of vision or severe pain in an eye after watching movies or television or after prolonged darkness; and (2) to occasional halos around lights (iridescent vision). Migraine, a bleeding intracranial aneurysm, or other diseases that cause hemicrania may be erroneously diagnosed in patients who have periodic attacks of angle-closure glaucoma.

Iris and pupil.—The iris crypts and collarette are often clearly visible. In blue eyes, the inability to see them suggests a corneal opacity, erythrocytes or leukocytes in the anterior chamber, or an iritis. A difference in color of the irises of the two eyes (heterochromia iridis) suggests the possibility of uveal inflammation, tumor, or an anomaly in the sympathetic innervation of the dilatator pupillae muscle, as occurs in congenital Horner syndrome. A retained intraocular foreign body containing iron causes the iris to become brown. An absence of some portion of the iris (coloboma) may be surgical (usually a superior portion of the iris) or congenital (usually the inferior portion).

Attention is directed to the shape, size, reaction, and equality of the pupils (see Chapter 7). If the pupil is adherent to the cornea (adherent leukoma) or to the lens (posterior synechiae), it is not round.

Pupillary reactions are observed with surrounding illumination just bright enough to observe the pupils. The patient should fix on a distant target to prevent the pupillary constriction of the near reaction. A flashlight with fresh batteries is used for testing. The pupils are first inspected for size, shape, and symmetry. To observe pupillary constriction to light, the examiner directs the light into one eye for 3 seconds and observes the constriction of the pupil in this eye. The light is then quickly directed into the fellow eye. The pupil of this eye, which is already constricted because of the consensual reaction, should remain constricted and not constrict further or dilate. If the pupil dilates within the 3-second testing interval, an afferent pupillary defect is present (see Chapter 7). If the pupil constricts further when stimulated, then the pupil initially tested has an afferent defect. When the affected eye is stimulated for 3 seconds, the fellow eye receives less consensual stimulus. When the light is quickly directed to the normal eye, the pupil will further constrict. This inequality of pupillary reaction is a valuable sign of extensive, monocular retinal disease or optic nerve disease more advanced or confined to one side.

Lens.—The transparent lens is observed by the image reflected from its anterior surface. Cataract may cause a gray, opaque appearance in the pupillary aperture. The lens is evaluated by means of the biomicroscope, but opacities are evident on ophthalmoscopic examination.

Ocular movements.—The patient is requested to look to the right, left, up, and down. No stimulus to ocular rotation, such as the examiner's finger or a penlight, is used. Full movements indicate integrity of the third, fourth, and sixth cranial nerves. The patient is then directed to look at a penlight held about 33 cm (13 inches) in front of the eyes. Normally the image reflected from the cornea is approximately in the center of the pupil.

The alternate cover-uncover test is used to detect a phoria (a deviation of the eyes compensated for by fusion) or tropia (a deviation of the two eyes that is present despite both eyes being open to permit fusion of the image from each eye). The patient is directed to look at an object located either near (about 13 inches) or far (about 20 feet), and one eye is covered and then uncovered as the fellow eye is covered. Attention is directed to the movement made by the eye as it is uncovered. A recovery movement with the eye rotating nasally indicates an exophoria or exotropia, while a recovery movement with the eye rotating temporally indicates an esophoria or esotropia (see Chapter 23).

Biomicroscopic examination.—The ophthalmic slit lamp consists of a microscope that has approximately the same power as a laboratory dissecting microscope. The light source projects a slit of light that illuminates a thin section of the cornea and lens. When the light source is placed at an acute angle to the microscope, the examiner can recognize the depth at which abnormalities occur.

RED EYE

A red eye is a cardinal sign of ocular inflammation. Dilation of the external blood vessels is customarily divided into ciliary and conjunctival injection (Table 6-1).

Ciliary injection involves branches of the anterior ciliary arteries that become congested in inflammations of the cornea, iris, and ciliary body and in closed-angle glaucoma. Each of these conditions is associated with decreased vision and frequently with pain deep within the eye.

Conjunctival injection affects mainly the posterior conjunctival blood vessels that extend from the peripheral marginal arcade in the eyelid and anastomose with the anterior ciliary arteries at the corneoscleral limbus. The posterior conjunctival vessels are most numerous in the conjunctival fornix and are congested in conjunctival inflammations. There is never a loss of vision, and there is ocular discomfort rather than frank pain. Because the posterior conjunctival blood vessels are superficial, they are more red than the ciliary arteries, which appear to be violet. The posterior conjunctival blood vessels move with the conjunctiva and constrict with topical instillation of 1 : 1,000 epinephrine.

A subconjunctival hemorrhage follows the rupture of a small blood vessel beneath the conjunctiva and causes a bright red blotch of blood beneath the conjunctiva that frequently alarms the patient. The condition is nearly always unilateral, and the hemorrhage absorbs spontaneously within 2 weeks. It has the same causes as a black-and-blue spot elsewhere. A subconjunctival hemorrhage that involves the entire bulbar conjunctiva after head injury is a serious sign and suggests either rupture of the posterior globe or a fracture of one of the bones of the orbital wall.

OPHTHALMOSCOPY

Inspection of the interior of the eye with the pupil dilated is fundamental to diagnosis. Ophthalmoscopy permits visualization of the optic disk, arteries, veins, retina, choroid, and ocular

TABLE 6-1.
Red Eye

Factor	Conjunctival Injection	Ciliary Injection
Blood vessels	Posterior conjunctival arteries	Anterior ciliary arteries
Location	Superficial conjunctiva originating from marginal arcade in eyelids	Deep conjunctiva extends anterior from recti muscle insertions to superficial and deep corneal plexus
Appearance	Vessels superficial, red, removable with conjunctiva, most numerous in fornix, fade toward corneoscleral limbus	Vessels deep, violet, immovable, most numerous at corneoscleral limbus, fade toward fornix
1:1,000 epinephrine	Constricts vessels, "whitens" conjunctiva	No effect
Diseases	Conjunctivitis	Keratitis, iridocyclitis, angle-closure glaucoma
Associated signs	Cornea clear, pupil and iris normal, vision undisturbed, eye uncomfortable	Cornea cloudy, pupil distorted, iris pattern muddy, vision reduced, eye painful

media. There are three methods of viewing the ocular fundus: (1) direct ophthalmoscopy, by which a magnification of about 15 diameters is obtained; (2) indirect ophthalmoscopy, by which a larger field is obtained, but with magnification of 4 to 5 diameters; and (3) biomicroscopy combined with a lens to neutralize corneal refracting power.

Pupillary dilation.—Adequate ophthalmoscopic examination of the ocular fundus requires dilation of the pupils. Without pupillary dilation, the optic disk and surrounding area (about 15% of the fundus) may be visualized (often with difficulty). With pupillary dilation and direct ophthalmoscopy, about half the fundus may be seen. Examination of the entire fundus requires indirect ophthalmoscopy combined with pupillary dilation and scleral indentation.

Selecting drugs to dilate the pupils for examination requires care. Systemic absorption is minimized by pressure over the inner corner of the orbit to occlude the canaliculi. Phenylephrine should not be used in concentrations of more than 2.5%. It should not be used in patients with vascular hypertension or administered simultaneously or within 21 days after the use of monoamine oxidase inhibitors. Tricyclic antidepressants potentiate the vascular response of phenylephrine. In children or infants with cardiac disease, phenylephrine should not be administered. Cyclopentolate drops should not be used in children with a history of seizures. Pupillary dilation in patients with shallow anterior chambers may precipitate an attack of closed-angle glaucoma. There is a greater danger, however, of neglecting significant ocular or systemic disease by failure to dilate the pupils than there is of precipitating glaucoma by dilation of the pupils.

Pupils in brown and deeply pigmented irises are more difficult to dilate than pupils in blue and hazel eyes. Often adequate dilation follows one instillation in patients with fair skin and light hair, while two instillations are required in dark-skinned patients.

The schedule of instillation varies with different physicians. In neonates, 0.1% cyclopentolate is combined with 1% phenylephrine. In infants 1 to 6 months of age, 0.5% cyclopentolate is combined with 2.5% phenylephrine. After 6 months, 1% cyclopentolate is combined with 2.5% phenylephrine. In children over the age of 12 years, often 1% tropicamide is used with 2.5% phenylephrine. In adults older than 40 years, tropicamide drops are instilled one or two times.

Direct ophthalmoscopy.—Direct ophthalmoscopy (Fig 6-5) provides an upright image of the retinal structures that is magnified about 15 times. Maximal pupillary dilation makes it possible to study the ocular fundus as far as an area slightly anterior to the equator; the area between the equator and the ora serrata cannot be seen. The maximum resolving power of the direct ophthalmoscope is about 70 μm, and objects smaller than this, such as capillaries, small hemorrhages, or microaneurysms, are not seen. The illumination by the modern direct ophthalmoscope is so bright that some translucent structures, particularly opacities in the media, may not be seen. Other features, such as copper-wire arteries, are not as yellow with modern ophthalmoscopes as when gas light was used.

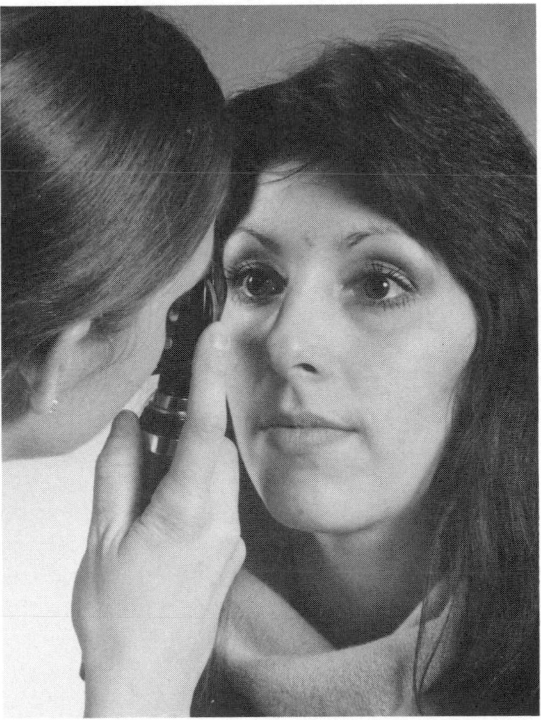

FIG 6-5.
Direct ophthalmoscopy of a patient's right eye. The examiner uses the right eye to study the right eye and the left eye to study the left eye. The ophthalmoscope head is held steady in the bony margin of the examiner's orbit. The index finger of the hand on the side of the ophthalmoscope is used to change the lenses.

Technique.—The patient is examined in a dimly lighted or dark room. The patient fixes on an object other than the ophthalmoscope light. It is preferable to perform the examination while the patient is seated. The examiner who wears corrective lenses constantly should become accustomed to wearing them when learning ophthalmoscopy. Visualization of the fundus of patients with more than 5 diopters of refractive error is easier if they wear their correction.

The examiner examines the patient's right eye with his own right eye and the patient's left eye with his own left eye. The ophthalmoscope is held in the corresponding hand. The examiner sits or stands to the side of the eye to be examined. The head of the ophthalmoscope is steadied in the mediosuperior margin of the examiner's bony orbit. The index finger is used to change lenses. The examiner's free hand rests at the side. Usually it is not necessary to elevate the patient's eyelid for an adequate view of the fundus.

The texture and detail of the retina and the blood vessels are evaluated by constantly focusing the ophthalmoscope lens for superficial and deep views, much as one adjusts a microscope when studying a tissue section.

Initially, a +10-diopter lens is rotated onto the viewing aperture of the ophthalmoscope, and the patient looks at a fixation object. The examiner directs the ophthalmoscopic light into the eye at a distance of about 20 cm. A red fundus reflex will be observed. Any opacities in the ocular media will stand out as black silhouettes against a red background. Keeping attention directed to the red reflex, the examiner gradually approaches the patient's eye while steadily decreasing the power of the ophthalmoscope lens. Once fundus details are seen, a blood vessel is followed to its origin at the optic disk, and the systematic examination usually begins with the optic disk.

Indirect ophthalmoscopy.—Indirect ophthalmoscopy is usually performed by means of a binocular ophthalmoscope that directs light into the patient's eye. The image formed by the emerging rays is observed by means of a convex lens of +14- to +30-diopter power placed in front of this eye. Wearing a binocular indirect ophthalmoscope on the head allows the examiner to use one hand to depress the sclera near the ora serrata to observe the extreme retinal periphery and ciliary body. Thus, the entire retina from the optic disk to the ora serrata may be inspected. The indirect ophthalmoscope has an inverted image that is magnified about five times. The field of observation is much larger than that seen with the direct ophthalmoscope, and a stereoscopic image may be seen with the binocular instrument. The maximum resolving power is about 200 μm, and small hemorrhages or microaneurysms cannot be seen. The stereoscopic image of the binocular instrument permits detection and evaluation of minimal elevations of the sensory retina and retinal pigment epithelium not evident with the direct ophthalmoscope. Because of the bright illumination, this method of ophthalmoscopy is particularly useful when there are opacities in the media.

Biomicroscopy.—The biomicroscope may be combined with a −55-diopter concave contact lens to neutralize the corneal refraction for study of the vitreous and retina. The increased magnification combined with oblique illumination and stereoscopic view allows for more accurate estimation of the depth of the lesion. A contact lens may be fitted with mirrors so that, with adequate pupillary dilation, the retinal periphery may be examined. Alternatively, a +90-diopter hand-held lens may be used and the fundus and vitreous inspected as in indirect ophthalmoscopy.

THE OCULAR FUNDUS

The red background of the ocular fundus results from the blood in the choriocapillaris layer of the choroid, the visibility of which varies with the amount of melanin in the retinal pigment epithelium. The pigment density usually parallels the complexion of the individual. Choroidal veins can be seen in lightly pigmented persons. The arteries supplying the choroid go almost directly to the choriocapillaris, and the major portion of the choroid is composed of freely anastomosing veins. In some patients, the contrast between choroidal pigment and blood vessels causes a tessellated (mosaiclike) or tigroid fundus.

The optic disk is about 1.5 mm in diameter (Fig 6-6). The diameter of the disk is the standard unit of measurement in the fundus.

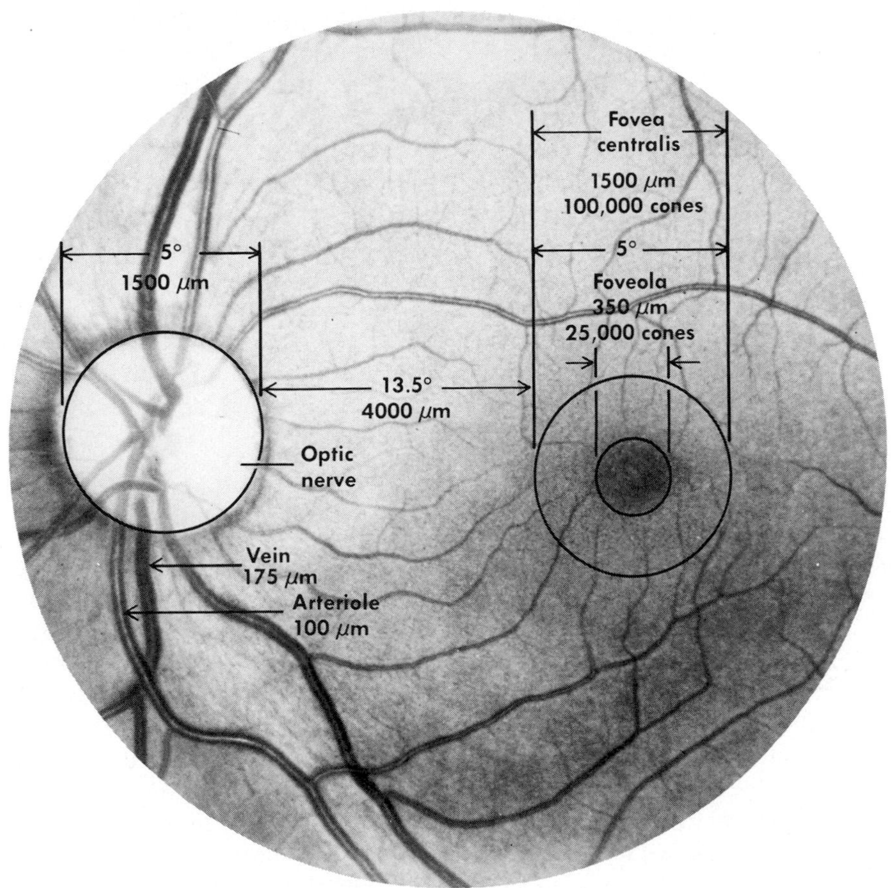

FIG 6-6.
Posterior pole of the left eye. The *optic nerve* and the *fovea centralis* are the same diameter. The macula lutea (yellow spot) is not precisely demonstrated. It extends from the foveola almost to the optic disk and about the same distance in other meridians.

The disk appears to be approximately the same size in most patients. Marked enlargement of the disk is rarely seen, but its occurrence suggests a conus, myopia, or posterior staphyloma. The disk is smaller than normal in hypoplasia of the optic nerve and appears smaller than normal in severe hyperopia and when the crystalline lens is absent (aphakia).

The optic disk is pale pink, except for the physiologic cup, which is nearly white. The edges of the disk are usually flat and sharp, but often the nasal margin is less distinct than the temporal margin. Pigment may be visible, particularly on the temporal side, sometimes as a continuous arc and at other times as linear streaks concentric with the disk. This is called the choroidal ring and is of no pathologic significance. Slightly more uncommon is an arc of stark white tissue on the temporal side of the disk, a scleral ring or conus, which may occur in degenerative myopia. It is often combined with a choroidal ring.

The physiologic cup of the optic disk is a funnel-shaped depression that varies in size and shape. In some eyes it is located almost at the center of the disk, and grayish areas of the lamina cribrosa are evident. In other eyes the cup has a more oblique arrangement and its bottom cannot be seen. The ratio of the horizontal diameter of the cup to the horizontal diameter of the disk is important in glaucoma. In the normal eye, irrespective of the shape of the physiologic cup, there is always a rim of nerve tissue between the cup and the edge of the disk. Occasionally, the region usually occupied by the physiologic cup is filled with glial tissue (Bergmeister papilla) that may extend for a short distance over the arteries and the veins.

The bifurcation of the central retinal artery into its superior and inferior (papillary) branches may be visible within the optic cup. The superior nasal and temporal veins often join at the optic disk or just within the optic nerve to form a superior papillary vein. After a short course it joins an inferior papillary branch, formed by the inferior nasal and temporal veins, and these continue as the central retinal vein. The veins on the surface of the disk often have a pulsation synchronous with the pulse. When this physiologic pulsation is not present, it may be elicited by a slight increase in intraocular pressure induced by pressing the globe with the index finger through the eyelids. In the healthy eye the central retinal artery does not pulsate. Pulsation indicates either an extremely high pulse pressure, as occurs in aortic regurgitation, or an increased intraocular pressure.

The superior and inferior papillary branches of the central artery divide into nasal and temporal branches. The muscular coat and internal lamina of these vessels are incomplete and they are thus arterioles. In the healthy eye the walls of the vessels are never visible. Instead, the column of blood is observed through the transparent vessel wall. The retinal arterioles have a smaller diameter than the venules, the usual ratio of arteriole to venule being 3:4 or 2:3. A broad, bright streak is reflected from the convex surface of arterioles. The reflection from venules is narrower, not nearly as bright, and confined to the major branches near the optic disk. The blood is much brighter red in the arterioles than in the veins.

In an examination of the fundus, the superior and inferior temporal and nasal arteries are followed as far to the periphery as they can be seen.

Final attention is directed to the central retina (macular region) located on the temporal side of the optic disk between the superior and inferior temporal blood vessels. This region surrounds the fovea centralis and is about 5 mm in diameter ($3\frac{1}{3}$ disk diameters) and anatomically corresponds to the retinal region in which the ganglion cell layer contains more than one layer of nuclei. In primates it contains a yellow pigment (xanthophyll) that cannot be seen with the ophthalmoscope and fades quickly after death. The area is called the macula lutea (yellow spot), and the retina of the posterior pole is often called the "macula."

The fovea centralis is situated about 2 disk diameters (3 mm) temporal to the optic disk. Its center is slightly below the center of the optic disk. Usually, pupillary dilation is required for careful examination of this area, since pupillary constriction is marked when the fovea centralis is illuminated. Within the fovea centralis is the foveola, which measures 400 to 500 μm in diameter and corresponds to the capillary-free area of the central retina. The major temporal blood vessels arch above and below the central retina.

FLUORESCEIN ANGIOGRAPHY

Fluorescein angiography plays an important role in ophthalmoscopic diagnosis. Unlike light ophthalmoscopy, in which light is reflected from the column of blood within the blood vessel, the fluorescein emits light so that the entire diameter of a vessel can be seen. After the intravascular injection or oral administration of a solution of sodium fluorescein, ophthalmoscopy with a blue filter to excite the fluorescence (fluorescein angioscopy) is useful in detecting leaking capillaries. The absence of a permanent record limits its value. Photography of the ocular fundus after fluorescein injection (fluorescein angiography) provides much information concerning vascular obstructions, neovascularization, microaneurysms, abnormal capillary permeability, and defects of the retinal pigment epithelium.

For fluorescein angiography, sensitive (usually 400 ASA or higher) black-and-white film is used, and a blue filter is placed in front of the light source to excite fluorescence. The emitted light is green, and a green filter is placed in front of the film carrier. A control photograph is first made to record intrinsic fluorescence of the fundus. Then sodium fluorescein solution is administered. The fluorescein is excreted mainly in the urine during the subsequent 48 hours. It may discolor the skin and conjunctiva, giving a jaundiced appearance, and interfere with urine tests for sugar.

The fluorescein may be seen in the retinal arteries 10 to 13 seconds after intravenous injection (Fig 6-7, *A*). If the patient is lightly pigmented, the filling of the choriocapillaris gives a background mottled appearance except

PART III

DISEASES AND INJURIES OF THE EYE

7

THE PUPIL

Normal pupils are round, regular in shape, and nearly equal in size. There may rarely be a physiologic difference in pupil size (physiologic anisocoria). Each pupil is located with its center a little below and slightly to the nasal side of the center of the cornea.

The pupils are dilated in excitement and in the dark. They are constricted in sleep, in light, and with ocular convergence (not accommodation). Pupils are constricted (miotic) in neonates, reach their maximal diameter at about 21 years of age, and constrict thereafter to become small in old age (involutional miosis). Pupils are considered miotic (constricted) if they are less than 2 mm in diameter and mydriatic (dilated) if they are more than 6 mm in diameter.

The pupillary constriction to light stimulation of the retina regulates the amount of light that enters the eye. The pupil constricts in bright illumination, which increases the depth of focus of the eye, and minimizes chromatic and spherical aberration and the astigmatism caused by pencils of light that enter the eye obliquely. The pupil dilates in dim illumination, which increases the amount of light that enters the eye. Pupillary size is controlled by the opposed action of two smooth muscles, both derived from the neuroectoderm of the secondary optic vesicle: the sphincter pupillae muscle (N III; parasympathetics) and the dilatator pupillae muscle (sympathetics).

The retinal rods and cones are the receptors that control the pupillary constriction to light stimulation (Fig 7-1). Their axons synapse in the retina and the axons of ganglion cells enter the cranial cavity in the optic nerve. The nasal fibers decussate in the optic chiasm. The axons controlling pupillary size do not synapse in the lateral geniculate body as do the visual but pass in the brachium of the superior colliculi to synapse in the pretectal nuclei.

Intercalated neurons from the pretectal nuclei (pretecto-oculomotor tract) then partially decussate and synapse in the Edinger-Westphal nuclei (N III). Preganglionic parasympathetic neurons from the Edinger-Westphal pass with the inferior branch of the oculomotor nerve (N III) into the orbit. The inferior branch of the oculomotor nerve, which terminates in the inferior oblique muscle, gives off a short motor branch to the ciliary ganglion where the pupillary neurons synapse. Postganglionic fibers then pass in three to six short ciliary nerves, which divide into 6 to 20 branches to enter the sclera and pass forward, in the subchoroidal space. About 97% of the fibers are distributed to the ciliary muscle (accommodation) and the remainder to the sphincter pupillae muscle (miosis).

The dilatator pupillae muscle is innervated by sympathetic fibers that originate in the hypothalamus (see Fig 7-4). From here the fibers descend in the lateral columns of the cervical cord and emerge with the eighth cervical and first thoracic ventral nerve roots. The fibers then ascend the sympathetic chain to the superior cervical ganglion, where they synapse. Postganglionic fibers extend cranially along the internal carotid artery, enter the orbit with the optic

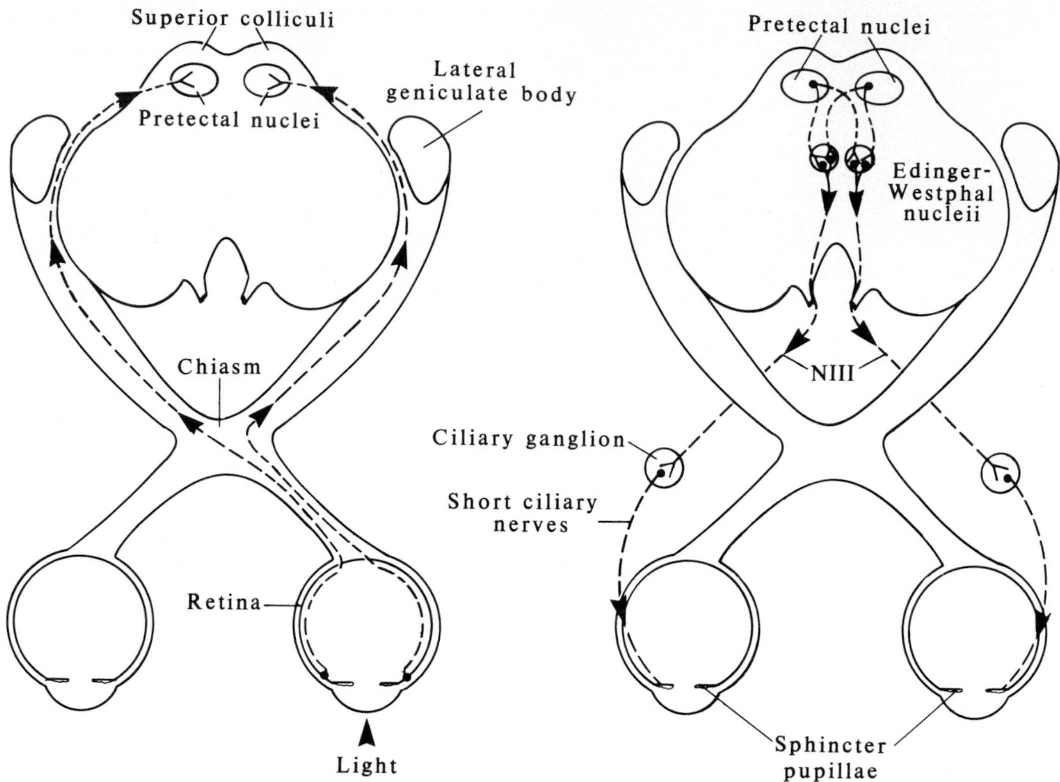

FIG 7-1.
Diagrams of the pupillary light reflex. *Left,* The pupillary impulses originate in the retina. The axons of retinal ganglion cells pass into the optic nerve, decussate in the chiasm, and pass with the optic tract to the midbrain. The pupillary fibers do not synapse with visual fibers in the lateral geniculate body but pass to the pretectal nuclei. *Right,* Pupillary axons synapse in the pretectal nuclei with intercalated neurons that pass to the Edinger-Westphal nuclei of the oculomotor nerve (N III) on each side. Preganglionic pupillary motor axons (parasympathetic) in the inferior branch of the oculomotor nerve synapse in each ciliary ganglion. Postganglionic fibers in the short ciliary nerves are distributed to the sphincter pupillae muscle of each eye.

nerve, and reach the dilatator pupillae muscle mainly with the two long ciliary nerve branches of the nasociliary branch of the fifth (N V_1) cranial nerve. Some sympathetic fibers that pass through but do not synapse in the ciliary ganglion are mainly vasomotor to choroidal arterioles and do not innervate the dilatator pupillae muscle.

Since the sphincter pupillae muscle and the dilatator pupillae muscle are integral parts of the iris, their function may be impaired in iris inflammations, degenerations, and congenital abnormalities. Additionally, the pupil provides the passage between the posterior and anterior chambers for aqueous humor. If the aqueous humor is prevented from passing through the pupil (pupillary block or iris bombé), glaucoma occurs.

Abnormalities of the pupil (Fig 7-2) may be the result of local disease or injury to the iris, or may reflect an abnormality of the afferent or efferent innervation. In anisocoria the pupils are of different sizes. Dyscoria refers to abnormalities in the shape of the pupil. Corectopia refers to displacement of the pupil from its normal position. Polycoria describes additional openings in the iris. Miosis is the condition of excessive constriction of the pupil, generally to a diameter of less than 2 mm. Mydriasis is the condition of excessive dilation of the pupil, generally to a diameter of more than 6 mm. Iridoplegia is the failure of the pupil to constrict to stimulation of

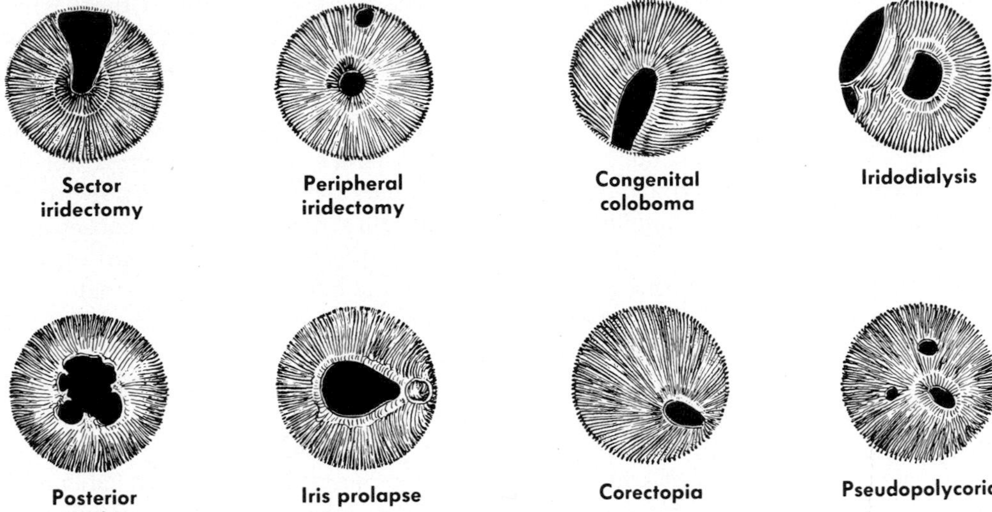

FIG 7-2.
Abnormalities of the pupil in various disorders.

the retina by light or in the near reaction (convergence and accommodation).

SYMPTOMS OF PUPILLARY ABNORMALITIES

The chief symptoms resulting from abnormalities of the pupil relate to its function as a diaphragm in controlling the amount of light that enters the eye. When the pupil is dilated, approximately 50 times more energy enters the eye than when it is constricted. Pupillary dilation and constriction occur constantly in the healthy eye in response to the amount of light that stimulates the retina.

A dilated pupil causes more chromatic and spherical aberration and less depth of focus, as is true of a camera with the diaphragm opened widely (the normal eye is about f 5.6).

Failure of the pupil to dilate in dim light impairs vision. The decreased vision caused by minor opacities of the crystalline lens is markedly aggravated by miosis, which often necessitates that glaucoma be treated with a medication that does not constrict the pupil.

Openings in the iris in addition to the pupil may cause monocular double vision (diplopia). Surgical iridectomies are usually located near the 12 o'clock meridian; they are covered by the upper eyelid and cause no symptoms. In conditions such as polycoria (multiple pupils) or iridodialysis, which is a separation of the base of the iris from the ciliary body, diplopia may be a disabling symptom.

PUPILLARY REFLEXES

Observation of the pupillary reactions to light should follow examination of the eyelids, anterior segment of the eye, and ocular movements. The pupils' reactions to light should be studied in illumination just bright enough to permit observations of the pupils. The patient should be directed to gaze in the distance. Attention should be directed to any difference in size of the pupils (anisocoria), shape (dyscoria), or position (corectopia).

When the amount of light falling on the eye is increased, the pupil constricts. There is a latent period of about 0.18 seconds, and maximum contraction occurs about 1 second after the stimulus begins. Light falling on one eye and causing pupillary constriction also causes the pupil of the other eye to constrict simultaneously and to a similar degree—the *indirect* or *consensual pupillary light reflex*.

To test the pupillary reaction to light, a penlight with fresh batteries is used. The patient is instructed to gaze in the distance to avoid the pupillary reactions of near vision (see below). The light is directed into the eye from below to avoid corneal reflections and the shadow of the nose. Each eye is stimulated for an equal period of time. The examiner first directs attention to the eye stimulated with light and, while continuing this stimulation, observes the size of the pupil of the opposite eye. A normal pupil of the opposite eye constricts equally with the pupil stimulated with light (consensual pupillary reaction). After 1 second to allow the pupils to resume their pretest size, the opposite pupil is stimulated with the penlight. The reaction of the two pupils is exactly the same in normal eyes.

The near vision reaction of pupillary constriction, convergence, and accommodation is not a reflex but an associated reaction of synkinesis. Each or all may be elicited by stimulation of areas 19 and 22 of the anterior occipital cortex. The ciliary muscle responsible for accommodation and the sphincter pupillae muscle responsible for pupillary constriction share a common postganglionic innervation through the short ciliary nerves that originate in the ciliary ganglion. They have different nuclei and different preganglionic nerve fibers, which share the oculomotor nerves. The Edinger-Westphal nuclei are devoted only to the sphincter pupillae muscles, while accommodation impulses reside in an immediately adjacent group, the anteromedian nucleus. The medial recti muscles are responsible for the ocular rotations in convergence. The near reaction is not a reflex but reflects simultaneous associated reactions, and indicates the reason that uncomplicated pupillary reactions should be studied with the individual gazing in the distance.

ABNORMALITIES OF THE LIGHT REFLEX

Abnormalities of the light reflex are divided into lesions that affect one of three portions of the reflex arc, as follows: (1) the afferent pupillary pathway; (2) the intercalated neuron, the pretecto-oculomotor tract; and (3) the efferent pupillary pathway (see Fig 7-1).

The afferent pathway

Retinal abnormalities affect the pupillary light reflex to a varying extent. There is no direct relationship between the visual acuity and the reaction of the pupil to light, and individuals with severe macular lesions or strabismic amblyopia will have a normal direct and consensual pupillary reaction to light. If there is no light perception in one eye, the direct light reaction is lost and the fellow pupil fails to constrict consensually. When the normal eye is stimulated, the pupil of the abnormal eye reacts promptly.

The nature of an optic nerve abnormality determines the pupillary reaction to light. In papilledema the direct and consensual light reflex is normal. In optic neuritis and optic atrophy the light reflex is abnormal.

The afferent pupillary defect (Robert Marcus Gunn) occurs in transmission defects of the optic nerve. It consists of a diminished amplitude of pupillary light reaction, a lengthened latent period, and pupillary dilation (escape) with continuous light stimulus. Patients with an afferent pupillary defect sometimes note that the affected eye is less sensitive to light. Both pupils are of equal size.

When light is directed into the eye on the normal side both pupils constrict promptly to light. When the light is switched to the abnormal side, the pupil, instead of remaining contracted (from the consensual reaction), begins to dilate despite the light stimulation. The reduced or absent conduction in the optic nerve does not transmit an impulse to the pretectal nuclei equal to that from the normal side.

The afferent pupillary defect is highly diagnostic in patients who have sudden decrease of vision in one eye without a large retinal lesion evident on ophthalmoscopy. In cystoid macular edema the pupils react normally. In optic neuritis an afferent pupillary defect is present. Patients with strabismus and amblyopia have normal pupillary reflexes. Patients with conversion reactions or simulated loss of vision have normal pupillary reactions.

In patients who have a hemianopsia caused by a chiasmal or optic tract lesion, light stimulation of the portion of the retina corresponding to the field defect causes a diminished or absent direct light reflex. This is called the hemianopic pupillary reflex. Detection requires a small bundle of light rays so that the uninvolved side is not stimulated by scattered light within the eye. Mainly, only extensive retinal lesions affect the pupillary response. Optic nerve disease causes an afferent pupillary defect.

In patients who have a lesion in nerve fibers carrying visual impulses posterior to the lateral geniculate body, the pupillary reaction to light is intact, because the afferent pupillary fibers are not affected. Thus a patient may be blind from bilateral lesions posterior to the lateral geniculate body and the pupillary reactions will be normal.

The pretecto-oculomotor pathway

Afferent axons of the retinal ganglion cells serving pupillary constriction to light synapse in the pretectal nuclei. Here in the midbrain, intercalated neurons extend to the Edinger-Westphal nuclei of the oculomotor nerve (N III). The neurons may be affected in tumors of the midbrain and in the Argyll Robertson pupils.

Midbrain tumors.—Astrocytomas and meningiomas of the region of the quadrigeminal area and pinealomas cause dilated pupils that do not constrict to light stimulation of the retina. The dilated pupils react promptly with the near reaction. Additionally, pineal gland tumors may cause a vertical gaze palsy, decreased accommodation, and nystagmus during upward gaze (Parinaud syndrome).

The Argyll Robertson pupil.—The Argyll Robertson (Douglas MCL Argyll) pupil is a bilateral abnormality characterized by failure of the pupils to constrict with light but with retention of pupillary constriction with the ocular near reaction. The classic description includes miotic, irregular, and unequal pupils; the retention of some vision in each eye; failure of the pupils to dilate after local scopolamine instillation; and further miosis after eserine instillation. When all signs are present, they characterize tabes dorsalis of central nervous system syphilis.

The efferent pathway

Lesions of the efferent pupillary pathway may affect the parasympathetic or sympathetic system. The lesions of the parasympathetic system may be preganglionic or postganglionic.

Preganglionic parasympathetic lesions.—The Edinger-Westphal nucleus is located in the posteromedial portion of the oculomotor nerve nucleus and may be affected in aneurysms of the posterior communicating artery, subdural hematomas, transtentorial herniations, basal meningitis (tuberculosis or syphilis), neoplasms, and trauma. Accommodation is reduced, pupillary constriction is impaired (internal ophthalmoplegia), and the pupil becomes enlarged and does not constrict with light stimulation of the retina.

Involvement of additional portions of the oculomotor nucleus causes paresis of ocular muscles as well as immediate pupillary dilation of the same side. Head trauma and coma associated with bilateral, dilated fixed pupils often result in death of the patient (85%).

Postganglionic lesions of the parasympathetic pathway.—Postganglionic lesions may affect the ciliary ganglion, the short ciliary nerves, or their branches to the ciliary muscle or the sphincter pupillae muscle. Such lesions result in a dilated pupil, poor or absent light reflexes, slow but persistent pupillary contraction in the near vision reaction, and often minor disturbances in accommodation. The condition is known variously as the tonic pupil, pupillotonic, myotonic pupil, and mydriatic (or nonluetic) Argyll Robertson syndrome. When associated with absent deep-tendon reflexes, it is called the Adie, Holmes, Markus, or Weil-Reyes syndrome.

Tonic pupil.—This is often (75%) characterized by a monocular dilated pupil that is larger than the fellow pupil in ordinary illumination (Fig 7-3). It may show delayed or no constriction to prolonged light stimulation, and a recovery occurs minutes or hours after removal of the stimulus. There is a similar delay in the constriction of the pupil to convergence. The pupillary margin shows segmental, irregular, wormlike undulations. There is supersensitivity to cholinergic stimulation and the pupil constricts with topical instillation of 0.125% pilocarpine solution, to which the normal pupil is not sensitive. Accommodation is less markedly affected, possibly because of the greater number of nerve fibers to the ciliary muscle. Patients usually complain only of the appearance caused by a difference in size of the pupils rather than any visual effects of accommodative abnormalities. A weak solution of pilocarpine instilled in the affected eye may minimize the anisocoria.

Patients of either sex at any age may be affected, but a preponderance of women aged 20 to 40 years is seen. The condition is usually monocular, but the fellow eye may be affected simultaneously or in separate episodes months or years apart. The deep-tendon reflexes, particularly the knee and ankle jerks, may be absent, often with bilateral abnormal pupils.

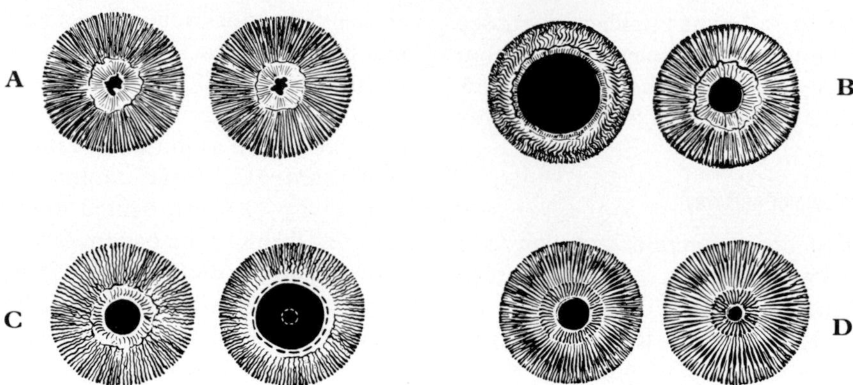

FIG 7-3.
Abnormal pupils secondary to neurologic abnormalities. **A,** Argyll Robertson pupils: miotic, irregular, unreactive to light, but reactive to the near reaction. **B,** Left anisocoria with a dilated pupil that does not react to light. The pupil constricts with the instillation of 1% pilocarpine if the lesion is neurologic (N III) but remains dilated if the dilation is the result of the instillation of a mydriatic or traumatic injury of the sphincter pupillae muscle. **C,** Left Horner syndrome: miosis, blepharoptosis, and sometimes anhidrosis on the side of interruption of the sympathetic innervation. **D,** Tonic pupil: anisocoria with affected pupil either larger or smaller than fellow pupil with slow reaction to light or convergence.

Lesions of the sympathetic innervation.—Any interruption of the sympathetic innervation between the hypothalamus and the dilatator pupillae muscle causes essentially the same physical signs, but a different pharmacologic response to topical 1% hydroxyamphetamine eyedrops (Table 7-1).

Sympathetic pathway lesions (the Horner syndrome).—Interruption of the sympathetic nerves anywhere in their course from the hypothalamus to the orbit results in a constricted pupil and a blepharoptosis, the Horner syndrome (Fig 7-4). The miosis is usually not marked and is often not noticed. In addition to the miosis and the blepharoptosis, there may be anhidrosis of the face as the result of impairment of sympathetic fibers that accompany the external carotid artery. In animals, which have more smooth muscle in the orbit than humans, there may be enophthalmos.

The blepharoptosis is the result of loss of the sympathetic nerve supply to the orbit, particularly the Müller smooth muscle of the upper eyelid, which provides "tone." The loss of sympathetic innervation to the lower eyelid causes it to elevate slightly, which emphasizes the narrowing of the palpebral fissure. The upper eyelid droops only 1 or 2 mm. Enophthalmos is not

TABLE 7-1.
The Pharmacologic Response of the Pupil in Anisocoria

- I. Pupils react to light stimulation equally
  - A. Instill 4% cocaine in each eye
    - 1. Pupils dilate equally
      - (a) Physiologic anisocoria
    - 2. Smaller pupil does not dilate
      - (a) Horner syndrome
        - (1) Instill 1% hydroxyamphetamine
          - i. No effect: postganglionic lesion
          - ii. Pupil dilates: preganglionic lesion
- II. Pupil reaction to light absent or sluggish
  - A. Prompt constriction to near stimulation
    - 1. Large pupil
      - (a) Pinealoma; quadrigeminal tumor
    - 2. Small pupil
      - (a) Argyll Robertson pupils
  - B. Absent reaction to near
    - 1. Large pupil
      - (a) Constricts with 0.125% pilocarpine
        - i. Tonic pupil
      - (b) Does not constrict with 0.125% pilocarpine
        - i. Mydriatic drug
    - 2. Small pupil
      - (a) Constricts with 0.125% pilocarpine
        - i. Tonic pupil
      - (b) Does not constrict with 0.125% pilocarpine
        - i. Abnormal sphincter pupillae muscle

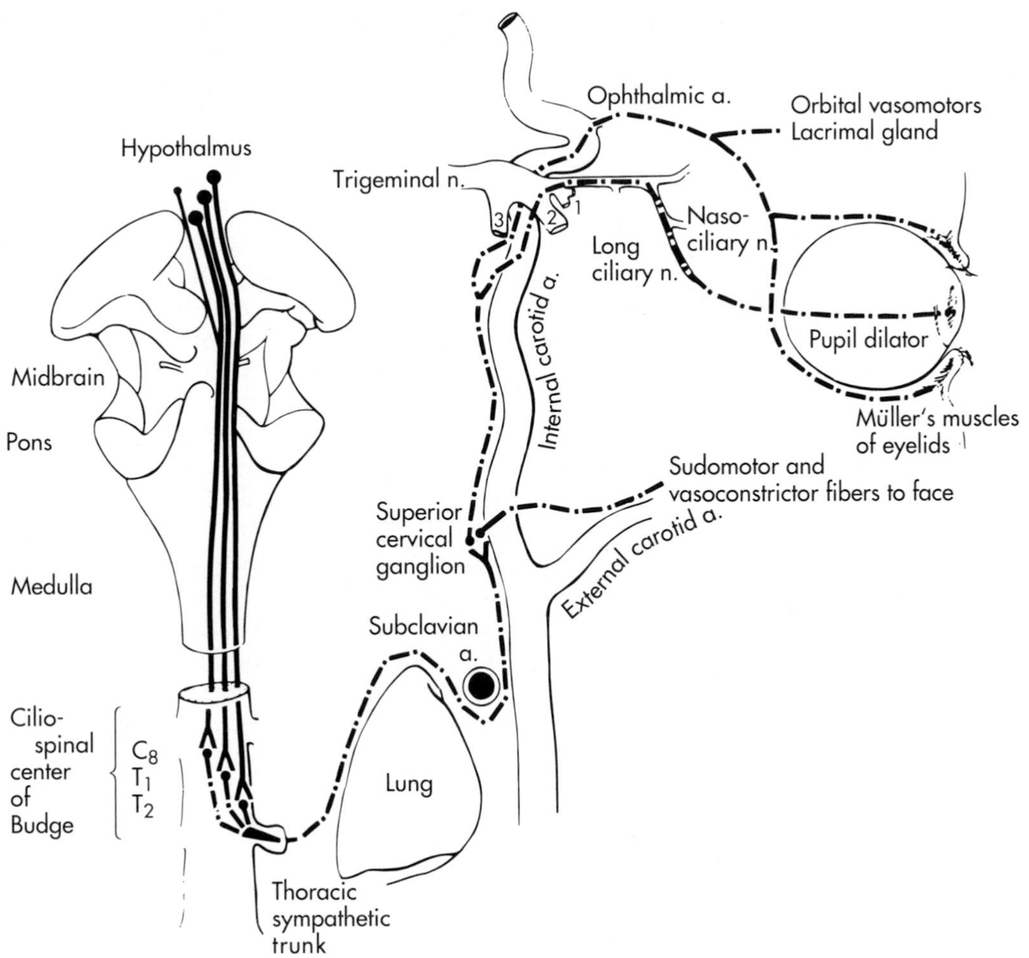

FIG 7-4.
Pathway of the sympathetic nerves to the eye. Sympathetic first order neurons that originate in the hypothalamus descend to the ciliospinal center (of Budge). Second order neurons course through the posterior aspect of the chest and ascend in the neck in close relationship to the carotid artery system. These neurons synapse in the superior cervical ganglion. Some fibers are distributed to the sweat glands and blood vessels of the face in company with the external carotid artery. Other neurons accompany the internal carotid artery and are distributed to the orbit in company with the ophthalmic artery and ophthalmic division of the trigeminal nerve (N V). (*From Glaser JS:* Neuro-ophthalmology, *ed 2, Philadelphia, 1990, JB Lippincott. By permission.*)

present in humans, but the appearance is simulated by the slight blepharoptosis. Anhidrosis occurs only if there is interruption of the sympathetic nerve fibers to the face and neck. The sweating fibers accompany the external carotid artery. In lesions that occur between the bifurcation of the common carotid artery and the orbit, they are not affected.

Horner syndrome is usually caused by interruption of the cervical sympathetic trunk or the lower cervical and upper thoracic anterior spinal roots. Mediastinal tumors are the most common causes, particularly bronchogenic carcinoma, Hodgkin disease, and metastatic tumors. Large adenomas of the thyroid gland and neurofibromatosis may be causes. Surgical and accidental traumas to the neck are the next most common causes. Diseases within the central nervous system that may cause this syndrome include occlusion of the posterior inferior cerebellar artery, multiple sclerosis or syringomyelia involving the reticular substance of the pons, and tumors of the cervical cord. Dissecting aneurysms of the internal carotid artery may cause pain in the ipsilateral forehead, eye, temple, cheek, teeth, and neck, combined with oculosympathetic palsy. A transient Horner syndrome may complicate an obstetric epidural block. Its development signals the need for close monitoring of the anesthesia. Insertion of a central venous catheter by means of percutaneous puncture of the internal jugular vein may produce a permanent Horner syndrome. Congenital and, occasionally, acquired Horner syndrome may be associated with decreased pigment in the iris on the affected side (heterochromia iridis).

The affected pupil does not dilate after instillation of 4% cocaine solution, but the normal pupil does. This occurs because cocaine dilates the pupil by preventing reuptake of norepinephrine at the postganglionic nerve terminal. Because the norepinephrine is absent in the affected eye, instillation of cocaine has little effect. Instillation of 1% hydroxyamphetamine is used to distinguish between preganglionic and postganglionic lesions causing Horner syndrome. In central and preganglionic lesions, the drug causes prompt dilation of the pupils of both eyes. In postganglionic lesions, the drug does not dilate the pupil on the affected side.

CONGENITAL ABNORMALITIES

Since the pupil is an opening in the iris, it is evident that developmental abnormalities of the pupil result because of abnormalities of the structure of the iris or the innervation of its muscles. The most striking change may be the alteration in the size and shape of the pupil. In aniridia the iris is rudimentary and the eye appears to be jet black with no iris present.

A congenital coloboma of the iris may be associated with typical defects in the optic nerve and choroid. Simple coloboma of the iris is more common, in which one or more layers of the iris are absent in a localized area that either extends as far as the ciliary body (total) or affects only the pupillary margin and adjacent iris (partial). The pupil is pear-shaped because of the absence of iris, but the usual layers are retained in the normal sector, and thus the remaining iris musculature shows normal reflexes. Colobomas may be completely surrounded by iris tissue (see Fig 7-2) and appear as additional pupils (pseudopolycoria). The openings lack a sphincter muscle and do not react to light. True polycoria, with multiple pupils each having a sphincter muscle, is extremely rare.

Conspicuous displacement of the pupil from its normal position is corectopia, or ectopic pupil. Relatively minor displacement is common and causes no symptoms. When displacement is severe, the eyes are generally myopic and vision is poor. Marked displacement is often accompanied by subluxation of the lens in the direction opposite the corectopia. Severe corectopia is often an autosomal dominant defect. Rarely, a congenital absence of the dilatator pupillae muscle causes a miosis as the result of unopposed action of the sphincter pupillae muscle.

Small clusters of black pigment may occur at the pupillary margin. They originate from the pigment epithelium of the iris and may be caused by instillation of miotics in children treated for accommodative esotropia. The two layers of secondary optic vesicle fuse to form the pigment layer of the iris, and its most anterior portion at the pupillary margin may form a pigmented pupillary frill, conspicuous in ectropion uveae. The frill is present at the margin of a congenital coloboma and is absent in a surgical coloboma.

Persistent pupillary fibers.—The anterior portion of the tunica vasculosa lentis, which nourishes the lens during embryonic life, is derived from anterior ciliary vessels. These nutritional vessels atrophy about the eighth month and recede to the collarette of the pupil. Occasionally, a delicate strand of fiber remains and extends from the collarette to the anterior lens capsule. Rarely they are sturdy and pigmented, but they do not interfere with vision.

MIOSIS AND MYDRIASIS

MIOSIS

Constriction of the pupil to less than 2.0 mm is called miosis. The pupil is abnormal if it does not dilate in darkness. The most common cause of the condition is the constriction of the sphincter pupillae muscle after the instillation of cholinergic-stimulating drugs in the treatment of glaucoma. Accidental or systemic administration of these compounds may cause miosis, depending on the dose. Morphine causes extreme constriction of the pupil. During sleep the pupils constrict, and the miosis may distinguish true sleep from simulated sleep (as does involuntary fluttering of the eyelids in simulated sleep). Bilateral adhesion of the iris to the lens (posterior synechiae) may cause small, irregular pupils. Congenital absence of the dilatator pupillae muscle results in miosis because of unopposed action of the sphincter pupillae muscle.

Irritation of the conjunctiva, cornea, or iris may cause miosis. Irritative lesions of the efferent parasympathetic pathway, as in meningitis, encephalitis, cavernous sinus thrombosis, and lesions within the superior orbital fissure or orbit, may result in miosis.

MYDRIASIS

Dilation of both pupils to more than 6.0 mm, combined with failure to constrict when stimulated with light, occurs after local instillation of drugs that paralyze the sphincter pupillae muscle (Table 7-2). Pupils dilated with drugs such as atropine do not constrict when 1% pilocarpine solution is instilled. Usually, systemic administration of cholinergic blocking compounds has a minimal pupillary effect. In blindness caused by bilateral lesions anterior to the lateral geniculate body, the pupils are dilated and do not constrict when stimulated with light.

In their course from the Edinger-Westphal nuclei in the midbrain to the eye, paralytic lesions of the parasympathetic efferent pathway of pupillary motor fibers may result in mydriasis. Blunt ocular trauma may rupture the sphincter pupillae muscle, causing mydriasis (traumatic iridoplegia). Increased cerebrospinal pressure, intracranial neoplasms, and aneurysms each may cause mydriasis.

During general anesthesia, the pupils are usually dilated in stages I and II because of excitement, alarm, or adrenergic stimuli. During stage III, the pupils reflect the miosis of coma.

In stage IV, hypoxia of the midbrain and the Edinger-Westphal nuclei causes pupillary dilation. Surprise, fear, and pain cause dilation of the pupil, as does any strong emotion, pleasant or unpleasant, or vestibular stimulation.

The pupil may be dilated in aneurysms of the carotid artery, and after orbital or intracranial trauma to the pupillary fibers in the oculomotor nerve (N III). In acute angle-closure glaucoma the pupil may be semidilated because of hypoxia of the sphincter pupillae muscle. The sphincter is not responsive to topical miotics or mydriatics if the intraocular pressure exceeds 50 mm Hg. In the early stages of Adie syndrome the affected pupil is larger than the fellow and reacts slowly to light.

TABLE 7-2.
Locus of Abnormality Causing a Dilated Pupil That Does Not Constrict to Light

- I. Iris*
  - A. Pharmacologic (cholinergic) blockade of sphincter pupillae muscle
    - 1. Atropine and related compounds
  - B. Inflammatory iris disease (posterior synechiae)
  - C. Ischemia of sphincter pupillae muscle after rapid increase of intraocular pressure
    - 1. Angle-closure glaucoma
  - D. Contused sphincter pupillae muscle
    - 1. Traumatic iridoplegia
- II. Ciliary ganglion or short ciliary nerves†
  - A. Adie syndrome
  - B. Inflammation of ciliary ganglion
    - 1. Viral ganglionitis
      - a. Zoster
  - C. Orbital tumor or trauma
- III. Preganglionic oculomotor nerve (N III)*
  - A. Aneurysm of the circle of Willis
  - B. Herniation of uncus of temporal lobe
  - C. Parasellar tumors
    - 1. Pituitary adenoma
    - 2. Meningioma
    - 3. Craniopharyngioma
    - 4. Nasopharyngeal carcinoma
  - D. Parasellar inflammation†
    - 1. Tolosa-Hunt syndrome
    - 2. Zoster
    - 3. Giant cell arteritis
- IV. Edinger-Westphal nucleus†
  - A. Ventral portion
    - 1. Paralysis oculomotor nerve (N III)
    - 2. Nothnagel, Benedikt, or Weber syndrome
  - B. Dorsal portion (rare)
    - 1. Supranuclear vertical gaze palsy (pupillary constriction of the near reaction retained)

*Pupil does not constrict with topical 0.125% pilocarpine.
†Pupil constricts with topical 0.125% pilocarpine.

IRREGULARITY

Irregularly shaped pupils occur in a variety of disorders. After a corneal laceration, the iris prolapses into the wound, causing a teardrop-shaped pupil. After blunt trauma to the eye, the iris may be torn from its insertion at the scleral spur, causing an iridodialysis. The sector of the pupil corresponding to the iridodialysis is flattened and becomes a chord of the circular pupil.

In uveitis the iris may be bound to the lens by adhesions (posterior synechiae). These may be evident only when the pupil is dilated, but if they formed when the pupil was miotic, the irregularity of the pupillary margin will be marked.

Surgical excision of part of the iris may be recognized by its usual location near the 12 o'clock meridian and by the absence of the iris pigment frill at the edges of the incision. A congenital coloboma involves the inferior nasal iris, and the frill of pupillary pigment lines the margins.

ANISOCORIA

Anisocoria (Table 7-3), or unequal size of the pupils, is a common anatomic variation. The normal difference in diameter, however, is less than 1 or 2 mm and often is not noted. About 20% of apparently healthy individuals have a detectable difference in the size of the pupils, but the pupillary reflexes are normal. The cause is unknown but may be familial. The difference in size persists with variation in lighting, whereas the degree of anisocoria in pathologic abnormalities either increases or decreases with changes in illumination.

Inequality in size of the pupils or a difference in their reflex reactions or responses to locally instilled drugs may indicate serious ocular or neurologic disease, which demands careful study. If the afferent pupillary fibers in one eye are intact, the pupils of both eyes remain equal in size even if there is a lesion of the afferent pupillary axons of the fellow eye. This occurs because the decussation of the efferent outflow innervates the iris sphincter of the involved eye normally. Anisocoria thus mainly reflects an abnormality of the iris musculature of one eye or its efferent parasympathetic or sympathetic motor innervation. The involved pupil may be either smaller or larger than the fellow. Irritative lesions of the parasympathetic pathway cause constriction, whereas paralytic lesions cause dilation. Irritative lesions of the sympathetic pathway cause dilation, whereas paralytic lesions cause constriction.

TABLE 7-3.
Some Causes of Anisocoria (Difference in the Size of the Pupils)

- I. Local ocular causes
  - A. Topically instilled medications
    1. Mydriatic drugs (pupillary dilation)
    2. Miotic drugs (pupillary constriction)
  - B. Ocular injury
    1. Rupture of the iris sphincter muscle (traumatic iridoplegia)
    2. Corneal laceration with adhesions between iris and cornea (adherent leukoma or anterior synechiae)
  - C. Inflammation
    1. Cornea (keratitis) constriction
    2. Iris (acute iridocyclitis: middilation)
    3. Adhesions between iris and crystalline lens (posterior synechiae)
  - D. Disorders of the iris
    1. Ischemia
    2. Iridocorneal syndromes
    3. Aniridia
    4. Congenital variation
  - E. Angle-closure glaucoma
  - F. Ocular surgery
- II. Paralysis of sphincter pupillae muscle
  - A. Intracranial disease
    1. Neoplasm
    2. Aneurysm
    3. Degeneration
  - B. Infection
    1. Herpes zoster ophthalmicus
    2. Meningitis
    3. Encephalitis
    4. Botulism
    5. Syphilis
    6. Diphtheria
  - C. Intracranial vascular disease
    1. Hemorrhage
    2. Cavernous sinus thrombosis
  - D. Toxic polyneuritis
    1. Alcohol
    2. Carbon dioxide
    3. Lead
    4. Arsenic
  - E. Diabetes mellitus
    (Pupil spared in 75% of patients with diabetic ophthalmoplegia)
- III. Paralysis of dilatator pupillae muscle (pupil constricted)
  - A. Horner syndrome
- IV. Lesion of intercalated neuron (pupils constricted)
  - A. Argyll Robertson pupils (tabes dorsalis)

AMAUROTIC PUPIL

The pupil of an eye that is blind as the result of retinal disease or optic nerve disease does not constrict when stimulated by light. The consensual reaction is absent in the fellow eye. When the normal eye is stimulated with light, the pupil in the blind eye constricts promptly. This pupil constricts because the afferent pupillary impulses from the sound eye stimulate the intact efferent innervation of the blind eye. The consensual reaction results in the pupils being equal in size.

BIBLIOGRAPHY

Book

Loewenfeld IE: *The pupil: anatomy, physiology, clinical applications,* Ames, Iowa, 1993, Iowa State University Press; Detroit, 1993, Wayne State University Press.

8

INJURIES OF THE EYE

Prompt and appropriate care of many common eye injuries may prevent much visual disability and, in some instances, the necessity for major corrective surgery. When examining a severely injured patient, the practitioner should determine if the eyes are grossly distorted and, if possible, whether vision is present. Every effort must be made to prevent marked squeezing of the eyes by the patient or pressure on the globes by the examiner.

Except in chemical burns, when immediate dilution is imperative, vision should be measured in each eye as carefully as conditions permit. Many patients do not realize they have defective vision in one eye until there is injury, and they may wrongfully accuse the practitioner of damage that has existed for many years. It is not necessary to use a testing chart—a newspaper or a telephone book will indicate how much vision is present. If the vision is markedly impaired, hand motion and light projection and perception may be tested. The results of testing must be recorded.

If the eye is lacerated, if the pupil is distorted, or if the iris is not visible, both eyes should be covered by a large dressing with no pressure on the globe. The patient should be given parenteral analgesics for pain (aspirin should not be used because it increases the risk of intraocular bleeding). The patient should be moved supine on a litter to a facility for special care.

If the patient is anesthetized for nonocular injuries, the eyelid and conjunctival debris may be carefully irrigated away by using a sterile irrigating solution, preferably Ringer or normal saline solution. This should be followed by the generous topical application of sterile solutions of an ophthalmic antibiotic. Wounds of the face and eyelids should not be debrided.

Administration of tetanus toxoid is indicated: (1) if there has been a delay of more than 6 hours between the time of the injury and definitive treatment; (2) if lacerations are heavily contaminated with dirt and other foreign material; or (3) if there is a deep puncture that favors growth of anaerobic organisms. The highest incidence of tetanus infections occurs in individuals more than 50 years of age, usually from injuries sustained in the garden.

Infants should be actively immunized against tetanus by three injections of tetanus toxoid during infancy. A booster injection should be given 12 months later, when the child enters school, and then at 10-year intervals.

FOREIGN BODIES

CORNEA

Foreign bodies on the surface of the cornea constitute about 25% of all ocular injuries. A history of the injury and the probable character of the foreign body aid in its detection and removal.

The symptoms vary from little or no discomfort to severe pain. Usually there is a sensation of a foreign body that the patient localizes, inaccurately, to the outer portion of the upper eyelid. There may be associated tearing, photophobia, and ciliary injection.

The foreign body may be seen by careful inspection of the cornea, preferably aided by magnification with a loupe or a magnifying glass. Sterile fluorescein strip or solution instilled in the eye stains the corneal stroma and demarcates the foreign body in the cornea. Corneal foreign bodies should be removed entirely to permit reepithelization and to relieve pain. Topical anesthesia must be used to prevent pain and eyelid closure during removal.

An attempt should be made to remove the foreign body by means of irrigation. A bulb-type syringe or a hypodermic syringe without a needle is used with sterile saline solution as the irrigating fluid. Foreign bodies that are not hot when they strike the eye may often be removed by directing a stream of fluid against the foreign body to float it off the cornea. This method is often used by physicians' assistants.

If the foreign body cannot be removed by irrigation, it usually cannot be removed by means of a cotton-tipped applicator, which removes much normal epithelium and is, therefore, undesirable. Minimal injury is caused if the foreign body is lifted gently out of the corneal substance by means of a sharp instrument. Specialists often use a biomicroscope to provide adequate illumination and magnification, but good visualization can be obtained with a binocular loupe. A sterile spud designed for this purpose or, in an emergency, a 25- to 27-gauge hypodermic needle fitted to a syringe may be used. The instrument is held tangent to the cornea so that the cornea will not be perforated if the patient lunges forward. The spud gently elevates the foreign body off the cornea. If a ferrous metal has been embedded for several days, a rust ring may remain after the removal of the main portion of the foreign body; this ring, is removed in the same manner as the foreign body. If it cannot be removed easily at the first attempt, frequently it can be lifted out entirely 24 hours later when leukocytes have softened the surrounding corneal tissue.

After removal of a corneal foreign body, a solution (not ointment) of a sulfonamide such as sulfacetamide or an antibiotic such as gentamicin is instilled. To prevent blinking, which causes discomfort, a dressing is applied to the eye to immobilize the eyelids. The dressing should not be used if it causes discomfort. If there is no keratitis, local medications to cause pupillary dilation are not used. If marked ciliary congestion and photophobia are present or if the removal of the foreign body has been particularly difficult, a cycloplegic such as 5% homatropine is instilled. Atropine causes prolonged pupillary dilation and paralysis of accommodation and is usually not indicated. Since a foreign body may introduce microorganisms into the cornea, the eye should be inspected for infection each day until the area no longer stains with sterile fluorescein. Foreign bodies that damage only the corneal epithelium do not cause a scar. Scarring results from injuries to the Bowman zone.

CONJUNCTIVA

Foreign bodies of the conjunctiva can always be removed with irrigation, a spud, or a cotton-tipped applicator.

Foreign bodies frequently lodge on the upper tarsal conjunctiva. The upper eyelid must be everted to remove them. A foreign body must be removed as soon as the eyelid is everted. If the eyelid is released the foreign body may be dislodged and difficult to locate again.

INTRAOCULAR

Intraocular foreign bodies are present in injuries in which small particles penetrate the cornea or the sclera. Large foreign bodies markedly disrupt the globe and cause so much associated injury that the eye may be disorganized and require eventual enucleation. Wood or plant foreign bodies may introduce infection that causes a severe purulent panophthalmitis within hours. Small metallic foreign bodies are sterilized by the heat created by their high velocity.

Diagnosis and treatment depend on the following factors.

1. *Size of the foreign body.* A foreign body must have a minimal density and size to be demonstrated by means of roentgen-ray examination. Ultrasound or computed tomography will show foreign bodies that are not demonstrable with conventional roentgenography. Magnetic resonance imaging is not used because of the danger of displacing a magnetic foreign body.
2. *Magnetic properties.* Only nickel and iron may be removed by means of a magnet, and for this reason it is important to determine whether the tool or other ma-

terial from which the foreign body originated is magnetic.

3. *Tissue reaction.* Many plastics, stainless steel, and glass do not oxidize, and other materials such as aluminum oxidize slowly and, if retained within the eye, cause minimal damage. Iron slowly oxidizes within the eye and combines with the protein of the intraocular tissues (siderosis) to form an irreversible ferrous compound that results in gradual loss of vision of the eye. The electroretinographic response of the eye is reduced before there is a decrease in visual acuity or a change in the appearance of the retina and foreign body. Unlike siderosis, the tissue reaction caused by retention of copper particles (chalcosis) is reversible if the source is removed. Copper, however, is much more rapidly injurious to the eye than iron. The possibility of an intraocular foreign body must be considered in every patient with uveitis and a history of eye injury. Rarely, a foreign body is enmeshed in fibrous tissue, metallic ions are not released within the eye, and retention of the foreign body causes no further damage.
4. *Location within the eye.* Foreign bodies in the anterior chamber may be directly observed, although gonioscopy is required to see them in the chamber angle recess. Small metallic foreign bodies within the lens may be tolerated for a long period. Severe injury to the lens capsule leads quickly to cataract formation. Foreign bodies in the vitreous humor and retina are often obscured by hemorrhage but sometimes may be seen by ophthalmoscopy, particularly with the indirect ophthalmoscope.

Retained foreign bodies must be suspected in all instances of perforating wounds of the eye. If the point of entry is extremely small, high magnification may be required to see the wound in the cornea or the iris. Transillumination of the iris may demonstrate a small hole. Minute wounds in the sclera are nearly invisible. Computed tomography of the orbit is indicated in such injuries to ensure absence of foreign bodies.

Removal of an intraocular foreign body is indicated unless the surgery would be more traumatic than the damage caused by retention. The foreign body is initially localized by direct visualization, ophthalmoscopy, ultrasonography, soft tissue roentgenography, or computed tomography.

Foreign bodies in the anterior and posterior chambers and the lens are removed through an incision at the corneoscleral limbus. Sometimes foreign bodies in the lens are not removed immediately but are removed with the subsequent cataract extraction. Foreign bodies in the vitreous cavity are removed by a combination of vitrectomy and suction.

Early removal is desirable because foreign bodies may become enmeshed in fibrous tissue and may be difficult to remove after a long period. It is probably better to delay treatment until specialized facilities are available than to attempt removal without the benefit of complete diagnosis.

LACERATIONS

EYELIDS

Lacerations of the eyelids are divided into two groups: (1) those that are parallel to the eyelid margin and hence do not gape and (2) those that involve the eyelid margin and are drawn apart by traction of the fibers of the orbicularis oculi muscle (Fig 8-1). Eyelid margin lacerations that involve the inner one sixth of the eyelid sever the canaliculus and are particularly troublesome to

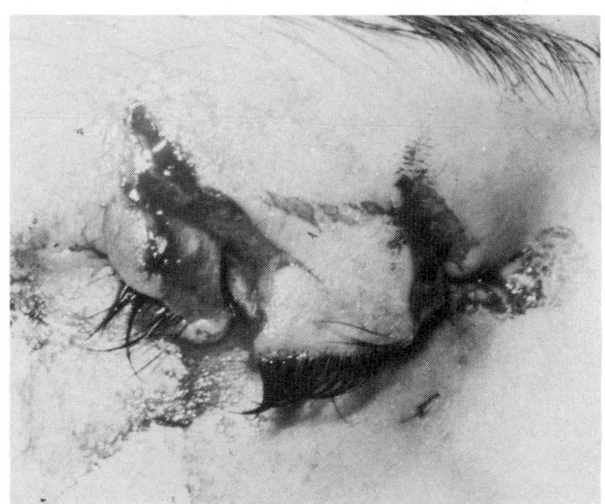

FIG 8-1.
Multiple lacerations of the upper eyelid 3 hours after a dog bite. There was no loss of tissue. Dog bites of the medial portion of the upper eyelid may damage the trochlea, which subsequently results in restriction of the superior oblique muscle.

repair. Children's eyelids are often severely lacerated by dog bites and scratches. If no tissue is missing, surgical correction can be surprisingly effective. Lacerations by dog bites are often contaminated and tetanus prophylaxis is required, together with quarantine of the animal and observation for rabies.

Wounds of the eyelid must be carefully cleaned with soap and water. Care must be taken not to irritate the conjunctiva and the cornea. Even though markedly contused and damaged, skin is not excised from the laceration, because the excellent blood supply ensures survival. Wounds involving the face are never debrided.

Lacerations parallel to eyelid margins require no specialized treatment and are closed with fine sutures. The laceration is parallel to the normal skin folds, and no conspicuous defect results.

Vertical lacerations are divided into those involving the outer five sixths of the eyelid (ciliary) margin and those involving the inner one sixth of the eyelid (lacrimal) margin, which avulse the canaliculi leading to the tear sac.

Ciliary margin.—The key to successful repair of a laceration that involves the outer five sixths of the eyelid margin is the placement of the first suture through the gray line of the eyelid to align the eyelid margin (Fig 8-2). Once the eyelid margin is properly aligned, the remainder of the eyelid can be closed in layers, with catgut sutures used for the tarsus and silk for the skin. The sutures are not tied on the conjunctival surface of the tarsus, where their knots will irritate the cornea. Unless other injuries are so serious that treatment must be delayed, it is better not to procrastinate, for a delay of even 24 hours may be followed by retraction of the wound edges and may require major plastic surgery.

Lacrimal margin.—Lacerations of the inner one sixth of the eyelid that sever a canaliculus require (1) placement of a stent through the canaliculus in the hope that it will remain patent; (2) closure of the laceration; and (3) prevention of traction by the orbicularis oculi muscle located lateral to the laceration. The stent, usually silicone tubing, must be left in place 10 to 21 days. Simple apposition of the laceration causes a typical notched defect of the eyelid margin and constant tearing. Even with highly expert repair, it may not be possible to unite the avulsed ends of a lacerated canaliculus, and additional surgery may be required to correct tearing (epiphora).

Lacerations of the inner one third of the upper eyelid may damage the trochlea of the superior oblique muscle. Damage to the superior oblique muscle (N IV) or the trochlea may impair depression of the eye when adducted (as in reading).

CONJUNCTIVA

Lacerations of the bulbar conjunctiva that do not involve the globe are rarely severe enough to require surgical closure. With such injuries, the physician must be certain there is no associated

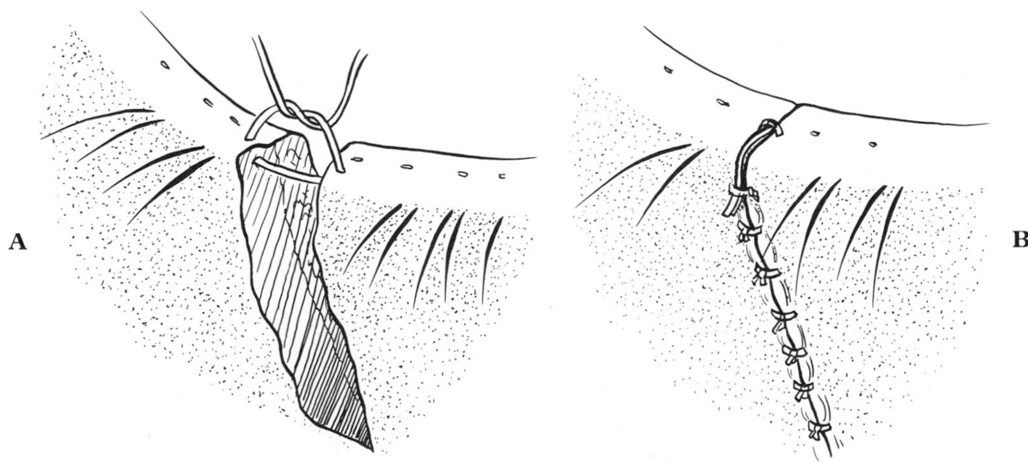

FIG 8-2.

A, The repair of a vertical laceration that involves the margin of the eyelid. The first suture is placed through the gray line. Any interruption in the margin is first sutured. **B,** After alignment of the margin of the eyelid, the skin is closed with interrupted sutures.

laceration of the sclera. Usually the lacerated conjunctiva is surrounded by an area of subconjunctival hemorrhage, and the laceration is evident as a white, crescentic area. The eye is uncomfortable, but there is no loss of vision.

CORNEA

Lacerations of the cornea, unless of a puncture type or beveled, are followed by prolapse of the iris, which closes the wound. A characteristic teardrop distortion of the pupil is present. In severe lacerations, there may be frank prolapse of the iris, ciliary body, lens, vitreous humor, and retina, causing a completely disorganized globe.

If a perforating wound of the globe is diagnosed, further examination should be made only by those responsible for surgical correction. Corneal lacerations are frequently associated with retained intraocular foreign bodies, traumatic cataract, secondary glaucoma, infection, and late complications, so that treatment should be carried out by those able to manage the responsibility of the aftercare. First aid is limited to the diagnosis of the condition. A delay of up to 24 hours is preferable to inexpert examination. A broad-spectrum antibiotic is administered systemically in large doses.

The history of the injury and examination of the eye frequently suggest whether a foreign body has been retained. Local anesthesia is adequate for many injuries. General anesthesia is preferred for extensive trauma. Rapid induction is necessary so that there will be no struggling, which increases the intraocular pressure and enhances prolapse of intraocular contents. Succinylcholine must not be used as a muscle relaxant, because it causes a transient increase in the intraocular pressure.

The method of repair depends on the severity of the injury. Direct appositional sutures are used to close lacerations with well-defined margins. When the wound edges are contused or when there has been a loss of corneal tissue, immediate corneal transplantation is done.

The corneal wound edges are sutured after the prolapsed iris is either excised or replaced in the eye. Because repositioning of the tissue may introduce infection, many surgeons favor iridectomy despite the resulting cosmetic defect. More severe injuries involving the lens and vitreous humor are treated by immediate reconstruction of the anterior segment with lens removal and vitrectomy. The corneal or scleral laceration is then meticulously repaired with fine sutures.

SCLERA

Careful inspection of corneal lacerations is necessary because extension into the sclera may be concealed by an intact conjunctiva. Scleral lacerations are much more likely to produce severe damage to the eye than those that involve the cornea only. For repair, the lacerated area is exposed by dissecting the cut edges of the conjunctiva and Tenon capsule from the scleral laceration. Prolapsed uveal tissue is excised and vitreous removed until the wound is entirely free of prolapsed vitreous. If the lens is damaged, it is removed with a suction-aspirator cutting instrument. The ciliary body is often damaged and the possibility of sympathetic ophthalmia (see below) must be considered. The sclera is closed with interrupted sutures. Diathermy or cryotherapy may be applied to prevent retinal detachment. An inert gas or air may be injected into the vitreous cavity. The conjunctiva is closed separately.

SYMPATHETIC OPHTHALMIA

Sympathetic ophthalmia (sympathetic uveitis) is a bilateral, chronic, diffuse inflammation of the uveal tract. It occurs days, months, or years after injury to the uvea, particularly the ciliary body, by a perforation of the sclera by accidental trauma, intraocular surgery, or an intraocular disease. Neodymium-YAG laser photocoagulation to the ciliary body in an eye operated earlier for glaucoma or cataract may be a precipitating event. The injured eye is the exciting eye and the fellow eye is the sympathizing eye. Most cases (80%) develop within 3 months of the precipitating cause, although onset has been described as early as 7 days and as late as 50 years.

Days to years after the precipitating event a quiet, insidious uveitis affects the exciting eye with ciliary injection, decreased vision, and photophobia. Shortly thereafter the fellow eye is similarly affected. The inflammation varies in severity with remissions and exacerbations. The anterior chamber is clouded with leukocytes that adhere to the corneal endothelium (keratic precipitates). The iris is thickened, dilates poorly, and the pupillary margin is bound to the lens with posterior synechiae (adhesions). Inflammatory cells fill the vitreous, and ophthalmoscopy discloses small yellowish white nodules in the retinal pigment epithelium (Dalen-Fuchs nodules). Fluorescein angiography may show hyperfluorescent dots at the level of the retinal pigment epithelium. A peripheral retinal detachment may occur secondary to vitreous traction, but the sensory retina and choriocapillaris are not inflamed. The uveitis (see Chapter 19) slowly progresses with minor exacerbations and remissions ending in blindness.

The cause is not known. The inflammation appears to be the result of a delayed hypersensitivity reaction (type IV, see Chapter 25) directed against surface membrane antigens shared by retinal rods and cones, the retinal pigment epithelium, and choroidal melanocytes. Approximately one third of the patients have HLA-A11 antigens compared to 7% in healthy persons. An increased serum sialic acid may be diagnostic. Its level is increased and parallels the severity of the intraocular inflammation.

Histologically, there is lymphocytic infiltration of the uveal tract with epithelioid cell nests, phagocytoses of choroidal pigment, and sparing of the choriocapillaris and sensory retina. Dalen-Fuchs nodules composed of histiocytes, lymphocytes, depigmented retinal epithelium cells, and lipofuscin inclusions occur between the retinal pigment epithelium and Bruch membrane.

Removal of a severely injured eye within 7 days after a penetrating injury prevents the development of sympathetic ophthalmia. Emergency enucleation of a damaged eye to prevent sympathetic ophthalmia is never required. Enucleation must be preceded by a skilled evaluation of the extent and nature of the injury, and the possibility of retention of the eye. Once the inflammation has developed, removal of the exciting eye is of no benefit. The exciting eye should be enucleated only if the eye has no light perception. Sympathetic ophthalmia does not occur in eyes with suppurative inflammation (see Chapter 18).

Topical therapy for uveitis is used (see Chapter 19). Systemic prednisone in doses as high as 1.5 mg/kg of body weight is standard. In individuals who cannot tolerate large doses of corticosteroids for many months or years, an immunosuppressive agent, such as cyclosporin (see Chapter 3), is used.

BLUNT TRAUMA

Apparently minor blunt trauma to the eye and orbit may result in surprisingly severe injury. Hemorrhage into the eyelids is in itself usually of little import but may be associated with fractures of the orbital bones. A severe subconjunctival hemorrhage and a persistently soft globe after a severe contusion suggest the possibility of a rupture of the posterior sclera. If the hemorrhage involves the entire conjunctiva with bleeding into the eyelids, there may be a basal skull fracture or ruptured sclera. The small ball used in squash or handball is a common source of serious blunt injury to the eye. Protective spectacles should be worn routinely.

The cornea may be abraded in contusion injuries, and although painful, it heals quickly. The sphincter pupillae muscle may be ruptured, resulting in a semidilated pupil that does not react to light (iridoplegia). In relatively minor contusion injuries there may be minute ruptures of the sphincter so that the pupil is no longer round. In more severe injuries the outer edge of the iris may be torn from its insertion to the scleral spur, causing iridodialysis. This may be so minute as to be visible only with a gonioscope, or it may involve a major portion of the insertion of the iris. An extensive iridodialysis is repaired by suturing the peripheral edge of the iris to the sclera. Correction is indicated when the iridodialysis is extensive or if the additional opening in the iris causes diplopia.

Contusion of the globe may tear a portion of the lens zonule, causing the lens to become subluxated. The vitreous body bulges into the anterior chamber through the ruptured area. The lens is seldom markedly displaced, and it is rarely necessary to remove it. Curiously, lens subluxation is most common after trauma in individuals with syphilis. As years pass, the lens may become opaque. A transient lens opacity may also occur immediately after a blunt injury to the globe.

The injured eye may develop glaucoma 10 to 20 years after the contusion. The glaucoma resembles open-angle glaucoma except that it is monocular. Gonioscopic examination indicates that a sector of the anterior chamber angle is much deeper (angle recession) than other regions. Often the patient does not recall the injury.

Contusion may cause the release of a large amount of pigment into the anterior chamber, which may give the appearance of aqueous flare (cells in the normally clear aqueous humor). There are no keratic precipitates, and posterior synechiae do not form.

TRAUMATIC HYPHEMA

Contusion of the globe is followed frequently by frank bleeding into the anterior chamber. This blood usually does not clot. With bed rest, it settles in the most dependent portion of the anterior chamber, and a red fluid meniscus forms (Fig 8-3). The original hyphema, which is often relatively minute and absorbed in 2 or 3 days, may be followed by more severe bleeding 3 to 5 days after the original injury. A secondary glaucoma may occur immediately. Many years later a monocular glaucoma may develop, which is identical to primary open-angle glaucoma (see Chapter 22), except that a portion of the anterior chamber angle is recessed. Aspirin and related analgesics, which impair blood clotting, should not be used to relieve pain. Acetaminophen may be substituted.

Spontaneous recovery usually occurs if the anterior chamber is not entirely filled with blood.

The injured eye should be protected with a shield for 1 to 2 weeks after injury. Systemic aminocaproic acid (Amicar [100 mg/kg of body weight every 4 hours orally for 5 days]), an inhibitor of fibrinolysis, may prevent early clot retraction within injured intraocular blood vessels and reduces the possibility of secondary hemorrhage. Double-masked prospective studies indicate that the incidence of secondary hemorrhage is not reduced by topical administration of atropine, pilocarpine, estrogens, or corticosteroids.

Secondary glaucoma may cause optic atrophy, corneal blood staining, and adhesions between the peripheral iris and anterior chamber angle (peripheral anterior synechiae). Minor rises of intraocular pressure are treated with topical timolol and systemic acetazolamide. An increase of pressure to more than 50 mm Hg, a persistently (5 to 7 days) high pressure, or early

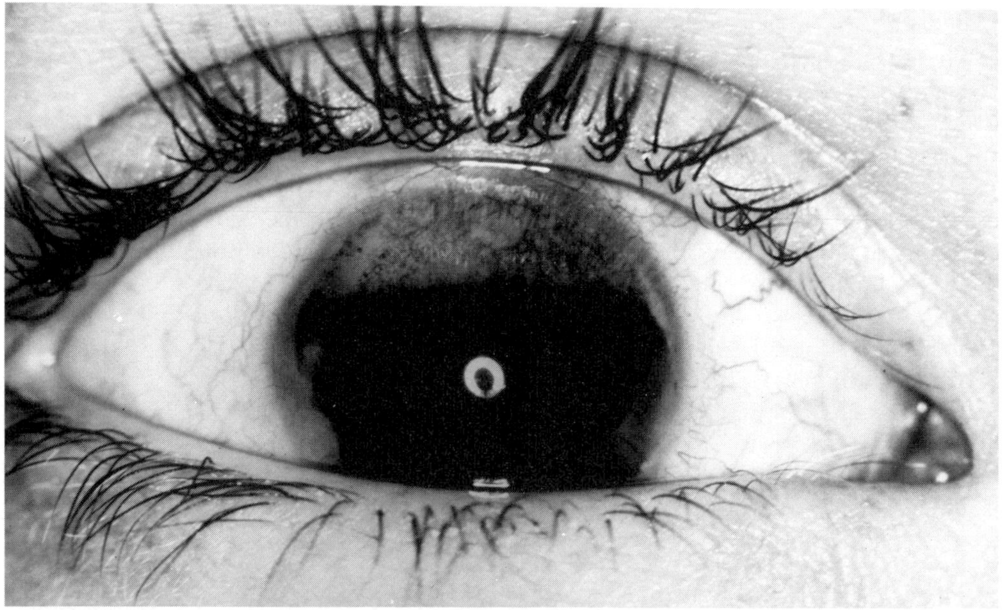

FIG 8-3.
Traumatic hyphema that obscures the iris. The blood in the anterior chamber has not clotted but, during rest, forms a fluid meniscus.

blood staining of the cornea necessitates surgical treatment.

Simple removal of a small amount of aqueous humor (anterior chamber paracentesis) or irrigation of the anterior chamber may be effective. Clots should never be removed by means of forceps because of the difficulty in distinguishing between the clots and iris. A vitrectomy irrigator-aspirator instrument inserted through the corneoscleral limbus may be used to aspirate the blood. Care must be taken not to injure the corneal endothelium, iris, or lens. General anesthesia is usually desirable because of the difficulty in anesthetizing the congested eye. If the intraocular pressure is increased, it is usually reduced by intravenous mannitol before incision into the anterior chamber.

When the anterior chamber is filled with blood, prolonged secondary glaucoma causes blood staining of the cornea. The corneal stroma is infiltrated with hemosiderin, which causes a deep yellowish green opacity of the cornea. Eventually the peripheral cornea clears, but a central opacity remains. Blood in the anterior chamber after cataract extraction may cause corneal blood staining without increased intraocular pressure.

Rarely after a corneoscleral incision for cataract or glaucoma, blood vessels in the wound may bleed and cause a microscopic hyphema with blurring of vision. The blood vessels may be sealed with laser photocoagulation.

FRACTURE DISLOCATION OF ORBITAL BONES

Blunt trauma to the orbital region may cause fractures and dislocations of the walls of the orbit, its margins, or both. Many of these injuries are associated with other fractures, head injury, and severe concussions and lacerations and cannot be treated until shock, coma, and life-threatening injuries have been managed.

Fractures that involve the orbital walls only are termed internal, and those that involve the margins and possibly the walls are external. There may be associated cerebrospinal rhinorrhea resulting from fracture of the cribiform plate or frontal sinus, orbital emphysema, or nosebleed caused by ethmoidal or frontal sinus fractures that require immediate care. Conversely, orbital hemorrhage and soft tissue contusions may simulate bony fractures but improve quickly. An intracranial injury must be considered with any penetrating wound of the orbit. Three-dimensional computed tomography or magnetic resonance imaging may be exceptionally helpful.

Fractures of the medial margin of the orbit are usually associated with nasal fractures. The medial canthal ligament may be severed, causing widening of the medial canthus (telecanthus), relaxation of the eyelids, and ectropion. The lacrimal canaliculi may be lacerated.

Fractures of the bony nasolacrimal canal may sever the lacrimal sac and predispose to dacryocystitis. Infraorbital nerve (N V_2) section or contusion in its canal on the floor of the orbit may cause anesthesia of the lower eyelid and cheek. Fractures of the inferior or lateral orbital margin often include the zygomatic bone. The bony fragments may often be placed in a better position, and depressed fractures may be elevated by means of forceps introduced through a concomitant laceration.

Fracture dislocation of the zygomatic bone and arch is common. The lateral canthus is depressed, and the prominence of the cheekbone disappears. Relatively minor blows may be a cause. The temporal and superior zygomaticofrontal suture and the nasal and inferior zygomaticomaxillary sutures are the weakest portion of the orbital margin and may be fractured simultaneously, a tripod fracture.

Fractures of the supraorbital rim often accompany severe head trauma and intracranial injury. The trochlea of the superior oblique muscle may be selectively involved. This causes the signs of paresis of this muscle and a diplopia that is most marked when the patient is looking down, as in reading. The trochlea tends to reattach itself spontaneously and does not require treatment.

Orbital rim fractures are repaired surgically only if there is a marked functional impairment or severe cosmetic defect. Delayed treatment may result in fibrosis, contracture, and malunion, and early surgery is desirable.

Bony wall fractures.—The walls of the orbit, unlike the margins, are thin. Blunt trauma to the orbit by an object of greater diameter than its anterior dimension may markedly increase the intraorbital pressure and fracture the wall (blowout fracture).

Direct trauma to the medial wall may fracture the thin lamina papyracea of the ethmoid bone and permit air to enter the orbit or the subcutaneous tissue of the eyelid. On palpation there is a peculiar crepitation of the tissues. Violent blowing of the nose forces air into the tissue and, if the orbit is involved, may cause double vision. The condition is self-limited and requires no treatment.

Fracture of the floor of the orbit causes prolapse of the ocular contents into the maxillary sinus, and rarely the entire globe may disappear from sight. The palpebral fissure is narrowed. Most often there is slight enophthalmos, and entrapment of the inferior rectus muscle restricts upward rotation of the eye. In most cases roentgenograms show cloudiness of the maxillary sinus. There is anesthesia in the area of distribution of the infraorbital nerve, including the skin of the lower eyelid, side of the nose, and cheek. A blowout fracture of the orbit should be repaired only if there is a persistent diplopia with restriction of ocular movement, enophthalmos persisting after 2 weeks of injury, or severe prolapse of tissue into the maxillary sinus. The defect may be exposed through a skin incision over the medial or lateral orbital margin, and the fracture opening may be bridged with bone or a plastic plate.

BURNS

CHEMICAL BURNS

Chemical burns of the eye are difficult to manage, and even with good care, vision may be severely impaired and the eye may be unsightly. Alkali burns cause more extensive damage than acid burns. The end result is related to the initial damage to the tissues, the adequacy of the blood supply to the peripheral cornea, the drainage of aqueous humor from the canal of Schlemm, and the epithelialization of the cornea. Deep burns, which give the cornea a marbled appearance and destroy conjunctival and scleral blood vessels, may lead to glaucoma and perforation of the globe.

The immediate treatment is dilution of the chemical with water. There should be no delay in learning the history, examining the eyes, measuring vision, or seeking the appropriate chemical neutralizer. The eye should be copiously irrigated with water. In most industries, employees are routinely taught how to do this. An effective method is to plunge the entire face into a container of water and then to open the eyes under water. Immediate dilution is the most important therapy. The fluid used need not be sterile, at body temperature, or even clean, provided the chemical is diluted promptly.

After dilution and transport to medical care, the irrigation may be repeated with sterile saline or Ringer solution. Irrigation should be continued until litmus paper touched to the inferior fornix indicates neutrality. Solid particles of lime, lye, and other material must be removed from the superior and inferior conjunctival cul-de-sacs. The upper eyelid should be double everted, with the use of a speculum, to make certain all particles are removed. If edema prevents double eversion, the cul-de-sac should be swept with a moistened cotton-tipped applicator. Sodium ethylenediaminetetra-acetic acid may be used to chelate calcium hydroxide. Infection is prevented by use of topical and systemic antibiotics. The associated anterior uveitis is treated with topical atropine to dilate the pupil and paralyze the ciliary muscle.

Topical corticosteroids may be used the first week; thereafter they are contraindicated unless the cornea has been reepithelialized. Symblepharon may be minimized by passing a lubricated probe between the inner surface of the eyelids and the globe. A bandage-type contact lens may prevent apposition of denuded surfaces.

Necrosis of the sclera and the collecting veins of the anterior chamber angle may lead to secondary glaucoma that can be detected by means of a noncontact air tonometer. Timolol, epinephrine, and acetazolamide are used to reduce intraocular pressure.

If epithelialization of the cornea is incomplete after 1 week, there is danger of stromal necrosis. Collagenase and other proteolytic enzymes are inhibited by acetylcysteine, penicillamine, or ethylenediaminetetra-acetic acid instilled hourly. Glued-on hard contact lenses may be helpful in delayed corneal epithelialization.

Chemical burns cause severe scarring and induce marked corneal neovascularization. Keratoplasty or a keratoprosthesis may be required. Visual results after keratoplasty may be poor because of graft rejection of the highly vascularized cornea.

THERMAL BURNS

Thermal burns of the eyelids usually do not involve the globe, since the blinking reflex provides natural protection. Additionally, tightly closed eyelids usually prevent involvement of the eyelid margins themselves.

Burns of the eyelids require prompt care to prevent severe cicatricial contractures. First-aid measures consist of application of sterile dressings and systemic control of pain. Definitive treatment should be carried out within 12 hours of the injury. If dirty, the burned eyelids are cleaned gently with sterile saline solution and a sterile soap. Fluid blebs are left intact. The most important step is suturing the upper to the lower eyelid with fine sutures. A mattress suture is placed through the margin of the lower eyelid and through the margin of the upper eyelid, care being taken not to penetrate the globe. The sutures bring the two eyelids together in the closed position, preventing gross contracture and subsequent ectropion formation. Such sutures, if unnecessary, are easily removed. Early skin grafting in severe second- and third-degree burns may speed convalescence and prevent late deformities. Skin for this purpose may be obtained from behind the ear, the inner side of the forearm, or preferably (provided it is uninjured) from the opposite upper eyelid region.

Severe body burns are often associated with smoke inhalation and carbon monoxide poisoning. There are retinal hemorrhages, hyperemia of the optic disk, and venous and arterial congestion. The ocular changes resemble those seen in altitudinal hypoxemia.

INJURIES CAUSED BY RADIANT ENERGY

Only radiant energy that is absorbed causes a reaction. Electromagnetic energy of extremely short wavelengths (roentgen rays, gamma rays, beta rays) may arrest the progression of actively dividing cells through the cell cycle and stop cell proliferation. Radiation cataract is produced through damage to actively dividing cells at the equator of the crystalline lens. Radiant energy with wavelengths between 400 and 700 nm (visible light) is transmitted by the ocular media, absorbed by the photopigments of the rods and cones, and perceived as light. Excess radiant energy is not absorbed by the photopigments of the sensory retina but is absorbed by the melanin of the retinal pigment epithelium. The energy is dissipated by the blood of the choriocapillaris.

Electromagnetic radiation of longer wavelengths causes changes by the production of heat. Many lasers are available for ocular surgery, and their different effects are related to the different rates of absorption of energy by ocular tissues. Thus, the excimer laser energy (192 nm) is absorbed entirely by the cornea and is used to ablate corneal tissue in photoreactive keratotomy to correct refractive errors. Electromagnetic energy of long wavelengths in the range of radar may cause cataract when focused on the lens. Presumably the changes are caused entirely by increased temperature of the lens and are not specifically related to the type of energy.

Ultraviolet (UV) radiation is divided into three bands: UV-A (320 to 400 nm), which produces tanning of the skin and is almost completely transmitted by the cornea and absorbed by the lens; UV-B (290 to 320 nm), which causes sunburn and tissue blistering and is partially absorbed by the cornea and partially transmitted to be absorbed by the lens; and UV-C (100 to 290 nm), which is entirely absorbed by the ozone and is emitted by the excimer laser, arc welding equipment, and germicidal lamps. It is entirely absorbed by the cornea.

Ultraviolet burns of the cornea occur in arc welders, mountain climbers, persons exposed to snowfields (snow blindness is ultraviolet keratitis), and persons who expose themselves unwisely to sun lamps. Like sunburn, ultraviolet radiation is cumulative; symptoms occur sometime after exposure. A marked foreign body sensation in the eyes, lacrimation, and photophobia are present. Symptoms are entirely relieved by a local anesthetic, which, however, delays epithelialization of the cornea. The condition is entirely self-limited.

There are three main types of retinal injury from radiant energy: (1) mechanical disruption resulting from energy initiated by extremely short pulses of radiation at high power density levels; (2) thermal insult resulting from absorption of energy in the retinal pigment epithelium and choroid that increases ocular tissue temperature more than 10° C; and (3) actinic insult resulting from extended absorption of energy by the photoreceptors to wavelengths between 400 and 500 nm.

Mechanical disruption occurs when the melanosomes of the retinal pigment epithelium absorb radiant energy from Q-switched and mode-locked lasers. The input is so rapid (nanoseconds) and the power so dense (terawatts/ cm^2) that heat dissipation cannot take place and the melanin granules become miniature fireballs.

Thermal insult results from exposure of the retinal pigment epithelium to radiant energy that exceeds the cooling capacity of the choriocapillaris. Wavelengths between 600 and 1,400 nm cause most thermal injury because they are transmitted to the retina with virtually no absorption by the ocular media. With wavelengths below 550 nm, transmission through the ocular media decreases markedly.

The amount of energy absorbed by the retina depends on (1) the duration of exposure; (2) the pupillary size, since pupillary constriction limits the amount of light (and energy) that can enter the eye; and (3) the refractive error, which governs the size of the retinal image. The retina is more sensitive in vitamin A deficiency and may be sensitized by some drugs.

The retina is damaged by increase of the temperature of the retina by more than 10° C. Retinal proteins are coagulated by an increase of temperature to 57° C, the principle underlying photocoagulation therapy with the laser. Accidental damage to the foveola with a photocoagulator reduces vision. Scatter photocoagulation, as required in some instances of diabetic retinopathy, destroys many retinal rods and impairs dark adaptation.

Retinal injury may be caused by the intense light of operating microscopes used in eye surgery or the illumination from intraocular fiberoptics used in surgery of the vitreous. The indirect ophthalmoscope and the slit-lamp biomicroscope used with a convex focusing lens are other possible sources of retinal damage. Laser photocoagulation is used therapeutically, and ophthalmologists using lasers and operating microscopes may damage their color discrimination.

Damage to the eye from sunlight may relate to an increased life span, migration of light-skinned, blue-eyed persons from their traditional settings to sunny tropical climates, photosensitizing drugs such as phenothiazine or psoralens, or diet. Ultraviolet-B is maximally absorbed by the cornea and external eye and may be a factor in pterygia, pinguecula, cataract, and climatic droplet keratopathy. No ultraviolet is transmitted to the retina after age 25, but possibly the retina is injured by sunlight before this age. Patients should be cautioned of the possible cumulative effects of excessive sun exposure during boating, skiing, and sunbathing. Broad-brimmed hats are useful, and sunglasses should block ultraviolet and blue light as well as infrared. Prophylaxis using vitamins C and E and beta carotinoids is unproven but promising.

THE ABUSED CHILD SYNDROME

The abused child syndrome includes nonaccidental trauma as well as other injuries resulting from lack of reasonable care and protection of children by their parents, guardians, or other caregivers. Many cases are first suspected because of an implausible history offered to explain a child's injury, a discrepancy in the history provided by the two parents, or a delay in seeking medical care. Ocular injuries include cigarette burns of the eyelids, hyphema, chemical burns of the eyes, dislocated lenses, and retinal dialysis. Subdural hematomas are often the result of violent shaking and may cause coma and convulsions. Retinal hemorrhages are usually present in these children.

Any child who is a victim of physical abuse requires the protection of admission to a hospital. Further management includes telling those involved the diagnosis, reporting the diagnosis to a protective agency, and seeking social service assistance. The child must not be returned to the caregivers until after adequate intervention.

ALTITUDINAL HYPOXEMIA

Acute mountain sickness occurs within 6 to 12 hours after rapid ascent to altitudes above 8,000 feet. Most individuals show symptoms at elevations of more than 15,000 feet. The symptoms occur within 8 to 24 hours after arrival and clear over a 4- to 8-day period. They include headache, nausea, vomiting, lassitude, insomnia, and peripheral edema. Ocular hemorrhages frequently occur in individuals who ascend to

17,500 feet. There is no association between the retinal hemorrhages and concomitant sickness. A history of migraine as well as rapid ascent, increased physical exertion, and individual susceptibility places the climber at higher risk.

Other ocular changes include increase in the diameter and tortuosity of the retinal arteries and veins together with cyanosis of the vessels. There may be increased retinal blood flow and retinal blood volume while the mean retinal circulation time decreases. The concomitant hypoxia and Valsalva maneuvers required in physical exertion along with the hyperviscosity of the blood occurring at high altitudes may play a role. Similar changes occur in carbon monoxide poisoning in humans. Slow ascent to permit acclimatization as well as ingestion of 250 mg of acetazolamide four times daily for 2 days before ascent to prevent cerebral edema appears to be beneficial.

FETAL ALCOHOL SYNDROME

Maternal alcohol abuse (6 oz of alcohol or more daily) during pregnancy, particularly during the first trimester, is an important cause of mental and physical retardation in infants. It may occur as often as Down syndrome and neural tube defects. Prenatal and postnatal retardation of growth, hypotonia, microcephalus, hyperactivity, mental deficiency, and typical craniofacial malformations occur. The middle part of the face is flattened, the midline groove of the upper lip (philtrum) is poorly developed, the vermillion of the upper lip is thin, the mandibles are short, and the ears are dysplastic. Ocular malformations occur in 90% of the infants. In 20% to 25% of those affected, the eyes are widely separated (telecanthus) and there is blepharoptosis. Vision is reduced with severe myopia or hyperopia, sometimes with optic nerve hypoplasia. There may be strabismus, nystagmus, epicanthus, cataract, tortuous retinal blood vessels, ocular colobomas, and Peters anomaly (iris processes between the collarette and the periphery of a dense central leukoma).

In adulthood the small stature persists, although the weight is normal. The mean intelligence quotient is about 70. Those affected are easily distracted and have poor social interaction. Infants with signs of the fetal alcohol syndrome should have a complete eye examination; systemic defects should be identified and corrected, if possible.

BIBLIOGRAPHY

Books

Cullom RD, Chang B: *The Wills Eye manual. Office and emergency room diagnosis and treatment of disease,* Philadelphia, 1994, JB Lippincott.

Smiddy WE, Chong LP, Frambach DA: *Retinal surgery and ocular trauma,* Philadelphia, 1995, JB Lippincott.

Articles

Alfaro DV, Chaudhry NA, Walonker AF, Runyan T, Saito Y, Liggett PE: Penetrating eye injuries in young children, *Retina* 14:201-205, 1994.

Budenz DL, Farber MG, Mirchandani HG, Park H, Rorke LB: Ocular and optic nerve hemorrhages in abused infants with intracranial injuries, *Ophthalmology* 101:559-565, 1994.

Chan C-C, Roberge FG, Whitcup SM, Nussenblatt RB: 32 cases of sympathetic ophthalmia. A retrospective study at the National Eye Institute, Bethesda, Md, from 1982 to 1992, *Arch Ophthalmol* 113:597-600, 1995.

Endo EG, Mead MD: The management of traumatic hyphema, *Int Ophthalmol Clin* 34:1-7, 1994.

Roh S, Weiter JJ: Light damage to the eye, *J Fla Med Assoc* 81:2-5, 1994.

Sanford JP: Tetanus—forgotten but not gone, *N Engl J Med* 332:812-813, 1995.

Sykes JM, Dugan FM Jr: Evaluation and management of eyelid trauma, *Facial Plast Surg* 10:157-171, 1994.

Young RW: The family of sunlight-related eye diseases, *Optom Vis Sci* 71:125-144, 1994.

9

THE EYELIDS

The eyelids are thin, movable curtains covered with skin on their anterior surfaces and mucous membrane (palpebral conjunctiva) on their posterior surfaces. They protect the eye, distribute tears over its anterior surface, and limit the amount of light that enters the eye. The eyelids contain striated and smooth muscle. Upper and lower tarsal plates composed of noncartilaginous dense connective tissue contain the oil-secreting meibomian glands. The free border of each eyelid contains eyelashes (cilia). The orbitopalpebral ligament divides the eyelids into two portions: (1) a palpebral portion that extends from the margin of the eyelid to the tarsal margin; and (2) an orbital portion that merges into the brow above and the cheek below. The palpebral portion provides reflex blinking, and the orbital portion, forcible closure of the eyelids.

The free margin of each eyelid is about 2 mm wide and has an anterior and a posterior margin. It is divided into two parts: (1) a lateral five sixths, the ciliary portion, which contains the eyelashes; and (2) a medial one sixth, the lacrimal portion, which is without eyelashes and contains the lacrimal puncta, the external openings of the lacrimal drainage system.

The eyelashes extend from the anterior margin of the eyelid. They are darker and more rigid than body hair, do not gray, and are not lost with aging. Glands of Zeis (rudimentary sebaceous [oily, fatty glands]) are attached to each cilium. Glands of Moll (sudoriferous [sweat]) are arranged parallel to the hair bulbs of the cilia and open into the duct of a gland of Zeis. Meibomian glands (oily secretion) are located in the tarsal plate of each eyelid, and their ducts open on the posterior portion of the free margin of the eyelids (Fig 9-1).

The superior and inferior puncta, the openings of the superior and inferior lacrimal canaliculi that drain into the lacrimal sac, are located at the junction of the lateral five sixths and medial one sixth of the eyelid.

The oval openings between the upper and lower eyelids, the palpebral fissures, are normally the same shape, size, and position. The obliquity of the fissure varies with different races and is more slanted in Asians. The inner junction of the eyelids (the medial canthus) is rounded and is normally covered with a fold of skin (the epicanthal fold) in Asians and all newborns. The lateral junction of the eyelids forms an acute angle. The upper eyelid is highest at the junction of the medial one third with the lateral two thirds, while the lower eyelid is lowest at the junction of the medial two thirds with the lateral one third.

The external surface of the eyelids is covered with thin, elastic, easily distensible skin that contains no subcutaneous fat. It is often translucent, and a delicate network of blood vessels may give it a bluish cast. The eyelids are lined with palpebral conjunctiva, and its junction with the skin on the margin of the eyelid is at the level of the meibomian gland openings. At the middle of the free eyelid margin is the intermarginal sulcus (gray line), which is important in eyelid surgery because it divides the eyelid into an inner portion composed of conjunctiva and tarsal

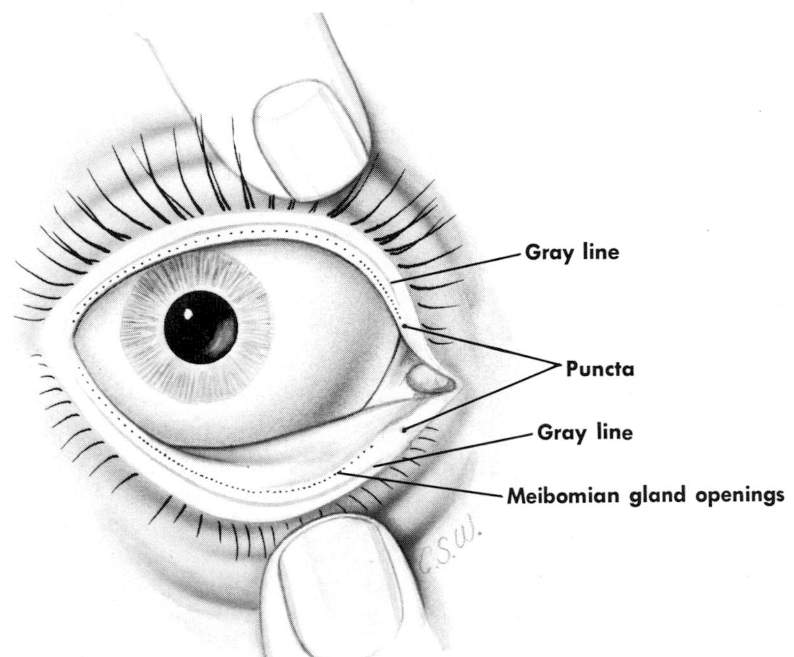

FIG 9-1.
The upper and lower puncta, the openings of the lacrimal canaliculi, divide the eyelids into ciliary and lacrimal portions. The openings of the meibomian glands are visible inside the gray lines. The gray lines mark the anterior surface of the tarsal plates at the eyelid margins.

plate and an outer portion composed of muscle and skin.

The eyelids contain the orbicularis oculi muscle (N VII), a sphincter muscle that surrounds the palpebral fissure. It originates from the medial bony orbit and the medial palpebral ligament and inserts into the lateral orbit and the lateral orbital ligament. Its palpebral portion is responsible for reflex blinking, and its orbital portion, combined with the palpebral portion, for forcible closure of the eye. The upper eyelid is elevated by the levator palpebrae superioris muscle (N III), which originates at the apex of the orbit and is closely associated with the superior rectus muscle. Müller muscle (sympathetic nerves via the ophthalmic artery) provides tone to the upper and lower eyelids.

The eyelids are separated from the contents of the orbit by the dense orbital septum that extends from the anterior margin of the orbit to the tarsal plates. It limits extension of inflammation from the eyelids into the orbit and from the orbit to the eyelids.

SYMPTOMS AND SIGNS OF DISEASE OF THE EYELIDS

The eyelids are composed of skin, mucous membrane, glands, striated muscles, and smooth muscles. They protect and moisten the eye, and characterize the facial appearance and expression. They are subject to a variety of disorders that affect their various parts and functions (Table 9-1). Retraction of the eyelids or protrusion of the globe exposes the normally concealed white sclera above or below the corneoscleral limbus. The eyelid skin is affected in the same disorders as skin elsewhere in the body and may be so severely swollen as to impair the drainage of tears. Seborrheic dermatitis of the scalp and eyebrows may inflame the margins and skin of the eyelids (blepharitis). A sty causes a marked inflammation of the margin of the eyelid. A lipogranuloma of a meibomian gland (chalazion) causes a small tumor deep in the tarsal plate. Abnormalities of the muscles or their innervation may cause conspicuous defects and interfere with vision.

The eyelids normally close simultaneously with blinking and close equally in forcible closure. The palpebral fissures should be equal in shape and size. The eyelid margins should be symmetric and closely adjacent to the globe. The puncta should dip into the lacrimal lake at the medial corner of the palpebral fissure. The eyelashes should be directed outward, and they should be free of seborrheic scales (dandruff), with the adjacent skin free of oily debris. The

TABLE 9-1.
Some Abnormalities of the Eyelids

Abnormality	Definition
Ablepharon	Absence of eyelids
Ankyloblepharon	Adhesion between margins of upper and lower eyelids
Blepharochalasis	Excessive laxity of skin of eyelids
Blepharophimosis	Decreased size of palpebral fissure
Blepharoptosis	Drooping of the upper eyelid
Coloboma	Absence of an ocular tissue
Floppy eyelids	Spontaneous eversion during sleep
Jaw-winking	Paradoxic elevation of eyelid with chewing
Lagophthalmos	Inability to close eye completely
Blepharoclonus	Exaggerated reflex blinking
Blepharospasm	Tonic, spasmodic, eyelid closure
Myokymia	Fascicular tremor of muscle
Distichiasis	Accessory row of eyelashes
Madarosis	Loss of eyelashes
Trichiasis	Misdirected eyelashes
Epiblepharon	Extra fold of skin of lower eyelid
Epicanthus	Extra fold of skin at medial eyelid (palpebranasal fold)
Symblepharon	Adhesions between eyelid and globe
Ectropion	Outward turning of eyelid margin
Entropion	Inward turning of eyelid margin

skin of the eyelids should be free of inflammation. The openings of the meibomian glands on the margin of the eyelid should be barely visible and not occluded with inspissated secretion.

CONGENITAL ABNORMALITIES

Failure of an eye to develop may result in ablepharon, the absence of the eyelid. The eyelid is imperfectly separated from the globe in ankyloblepharon, which results in a horizontally narrowed palpebral fissure. Fetal failure of development of a portion of the eyelid causes a vertical notching defect of its margin, a coloboma of the eyelid.

In blepharoptosis the width of the palpebral fissure is decreased by drooping of the upper eyelid. In blepharophimosis the palpebral fissure is congenitally narrowed both vertically and horizontally. There is often an associated blepharoptosis and an autosomal dominant inheritance.

Epicanthus is by far the most common congenital variation. A vertical skin fold occurs in the medial canthal region that conceals the medial angle and the caruncle (Fig 9-2). It is present in many infants until growth of the nose and face obliterates it. An epicanthal fold may conceal the medial sclera and may simulate the appearance of esotropia (pseudostrabismus). The presence or absence of esotropia is quickly determined by means of the cover-uncover test (see Chapter 24). An epicanthal fold occurs normally in Asians and is often combined with a fold of skin that overhangs the palpebral fissure (mongolian fold), giving it an almond shape.

Distichiasis is a congenital, abnormal, supernumerary row of lashes, which are often directed backward and irritate the cornea.

ABNORMALITIES OF SHAPE AND POSITION

In entropion the eyelid margin, usually the lower, is turned inward, and the eyelashes irritate the eye. In ectropion, the eyelid margin, usually the lower, is turned outward so that the conjunctival surface is exposed and becomes keratinized. In blepharoptosis the upper eyelid is not elevated properly so that the palpebral fissure is narrowed. Blepharoptosis and epicanthal folds may occur simultaneously. In lagophthalmos the eyelids fail to cover the globe.

ENTROPION

Entropion (Fig 9-3) is a condition in which the eyelid margin is turned inward so that the lashes irritate the eye, which causes corneal epithelial defects, injection of conjunctival blood vessels, and tearing, sometimes leading to secondary infection of the cornea (keratitis) or conjunctiva (conjunctivitis). The lower eyelid is usually involved. Entropion occurs in four main forms: (1) atonic (age-related, involutional), the most common type; (2) cicatricial, which may affect the entire upper or lower eyelid; (3) spastic; and (4) congenital.

The atonic type follows atrophy of the lower eyelid retractors (the aponeurosis of the capsulopalpebral head of the inferior rectus muscle and the inferior tarsal muscle, both of which

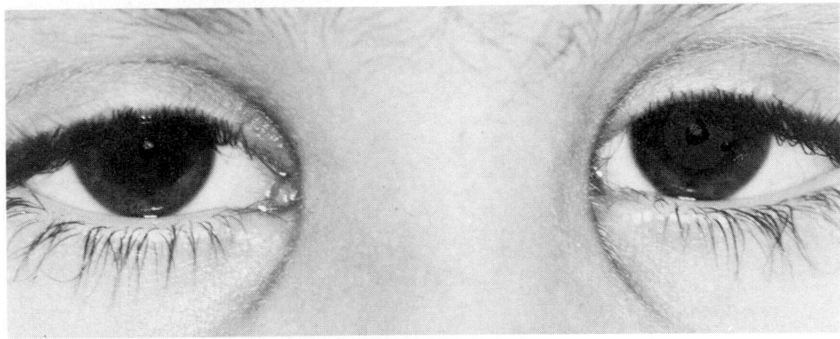

FIG 9-2.
A 5-year-old boy with bilateral epicanthus that is more marked on the left side. The concealment of the left sclera by the fold of skin simulates the appearance of an esotropia (pseudostrabismus).

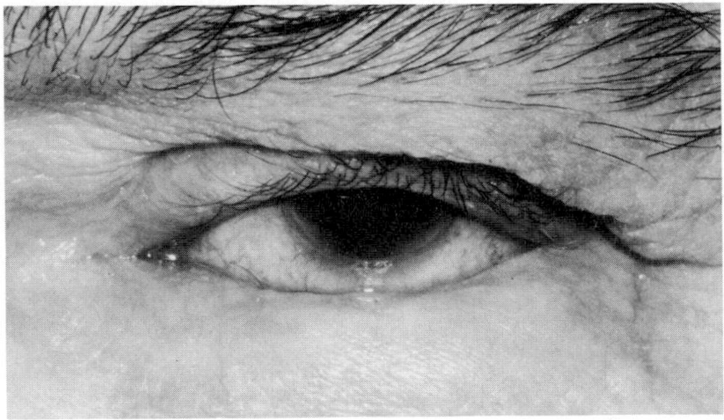

FIG 9-3.
Spastic entropion with the eyelids inverted against the globe.

insert into the lower margin of the tarsal plate). The atrophy reduces the stability of the lower tarsal border and permits contraction of the orbicularis oculi muscle to rotate the eyelid margin inward. Laxity of the orbital septum also contributes. Surgical correction is often required. In minor instances, temporary relief may be obtained by drawing the skin of the outer canthus down and out by means of an adhesive tape strip. The surgical procedures involve a resection of the orbicularis oculi muscle and tarsus to shorten the horizontal length of the eyelid and prevent the inferior margin of the tarsus from rotating outward.

Cicatricial entropion follows scarring of the palpebral conjunctiva, which may be caused by chemical injuries, lacerations, surgical procedures, radiant energy, trachoma, and erythema multiforme. The tarsus is often scarred and distorted. The globe is irritated by the eyelashes. Several surgical procedures have been devised to evert the eyelid margin and the eyelashes. It may be necessary to transplant mucous membrane from the mouth to replace scarred conjunctiva.

Spastic entropion results from excessive contraction of the orbicularis oculi muscle (blepharospasm) combined with atrophy of the eyelid retractors. Ocular irritation from chronic conjunctivitis, keratitis, or ocular surgery is a common cause. Excessive contraction occurring after surgery is sometimes corrected by removing eye dressings. Temporary relief may be provided by alcohol injection into the orbicularis oculi muscle. The surgical correction is the same as that for atonic entropion.

Congenital entropion is usually caused by a deformity of the tarsal plate in which the eyelashes are directed inward and irritate the cornea. Resecting the abnormal portion of the tarsal plate and placing the remainder in its normal position correct the condition.

Epiblepharon may occur with congenital entropion. An abnormal fold of skin, often at the medial one third of the eyelid, turns the eyelid margin inward. Usually the condition disap-

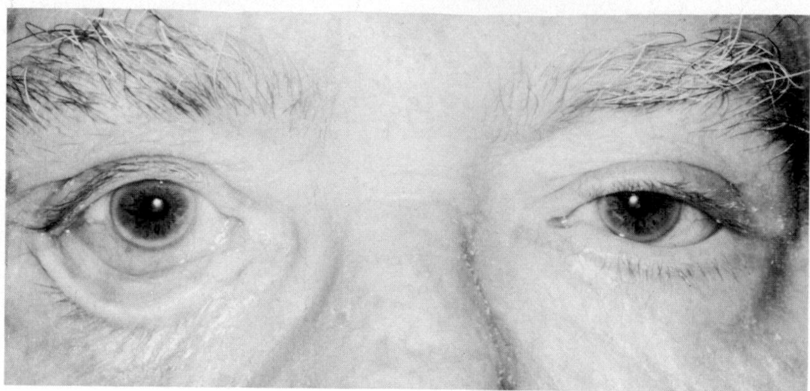

FIG 9-4.
Atonic ectropion in a 74-year-old man.

pears as the face grows. If the condition persists, the capsulopalpebral retractors of the lower eyelid must be surgically united to their normal attachments at the lower border of the tarsal plate and to the eyelid skin fold.

ECTROPION

Ectropion (Fig 9-4) is a condition in which the eyelid margin is turned away from the eye so that the bulbar and the palpebral conjunctivae are exposed. Symptoms result from exposure of the conjunctiva and the cornea. When the lower eyelid is affected, the inferior punctum is not adjacent to the lacrimal lake, and tearing occurs. The exposed palpebral conjunctiva becomes keratinized. Ectropion occurs in several forms: (1) atonic; (2) cicatricial; (3) spastic; and (4) allergic. Only the lower eyelid is involved in the atonic type, but the cicatricial and allergic types may affect either the upper or the lower eyelid or both.

Atonic ectropion is the usual type. Mild types occur in aging and weakening of the orbicularis oculi muscle. Surgical treatment is directed to inverting the lacrimal punctum into its normal position. Severe ectropion follows paralysis of the orbicularis oculi muscle (N VII) in facial nerve palsy (Bell). The medial portion of the eyelid sags outward, and there is marked tearing. Ophthalmic lubricating agents and viscous artificial tears are used initially while spontaneous resolution is anticipated. Persistence of the ectropion after 3 to 6 months requires one of several types of eyelid shortening procedures.

Cicatricial ectropion follows burns, lacerations, and infections of the skin of the eyelids. With most thermal burns, the eyelids close tightly, the eyelid margins are not involved, and an intact margin 1 or 2 mm wide is preserved. Subsequent plastic surgery to correct contracture may often be avoided if the upper and lower eyelid margins are sutured together as early as possible. Early skin grafting is desirable in most burns of the eyelid to prevent ectropion. Skin of the opposite upper eyelid is ideal for this purpose, or skin may be removed from that covering the mastoid region. The plastic surgery required for established cicatricial ectropion is difficult and requires skilled and prolonged care.

BLEPHAROPTOSIS

An abnormality in either the innervation or the structure of the levator palpebrae superioris muscle causes blepharoptosis (Fig 9-5), in which the upper eyelid droops and the palpebral fissure is narrowed.

Blepharoptosis is divided into congenital and acquired types. The congenital type is usually the result of impairment of the superior division of the oculomotor nerve (N III), which innervates the levator palpebrae superioris muscle and the superior rectus muscle. The superior rectus muscle may also be weakened. The superior palpebral sulcus, which marks the insertion of the levator palpebrae superioris aponeurosis into the skin to the upper eyelid, is absent in congenital blepharoptosis but present in acquired blepharoptosis. Both the congenital and the acquired types may be hereditary or occur sporadically.

Congenital blepharoptosis.—Congenital blepharoptosis may involve either one or both upper eyelids. The degree of severity varies. If

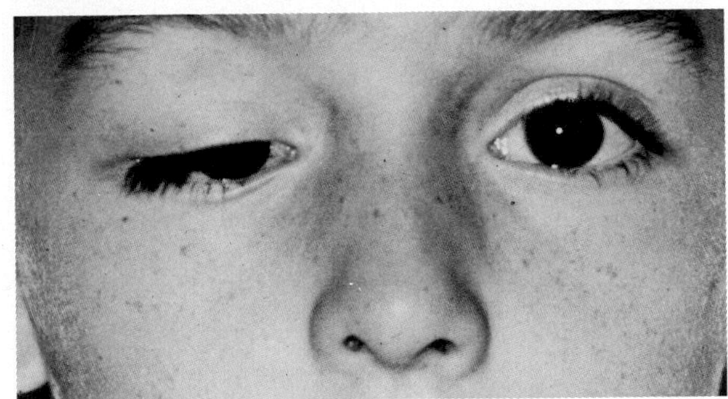

FIG 9-5.
Right blepharoptosis. The absence of a superior palpebral furrow indicates a congenital paralysis of the levator palpebrae superioris muscle.

the visual axes of both eyes are covered by the drooping eyelids, the head is thrown back and the forehead furrowed in a perpetual frown as the child uses the frontalis muscle to elevate the eyelids. If only one eye is affected, the child may develop a sensory amblyopia of the covered eye, so that earlier surgical treatment is required than with bilateral blepharoptosis.

Acquired blepharoptosis.—This may result from any impairment of the nerve supply of the upper eyelid musculature, from disease of the muscles themselves, or from mechanical interference of the elevation of the eyelid by the weight of a tumor. The most common acquired causes of oculomotor nerve impairment are diabetes mellitus neuropathy and intracranial disorders such as aneurysms, neoplasms, injuries, and inflammations. An aneurysm of the internal carotid artery within the cavernous sinus may cause a complete ophthalmoplegia from involvement of nerves III, IV, and VI combined with anesthesia in the area of distribution of the ophthalmic and maxillary divisions of the trigeminal nerve (N V).

Interference with the sympathetic innervation of the smooth muscle (Müller) that provides tone to the upper eyelid causes 1 to 2 mm of drooping, as occurs in Horner syndrome (miosis and blepharoptosis combined with a facial anhidrosis if the portion of the sympathetic nerves distributed with external carotid artery is also interrupted [see Chapter 7]). Acquired blepharoptosis occurs in myasthenia gravis, mitochondrial myopathies, cerebrovascular accidents, fractures of the roof of the orbit, chronic progressive external ophthalmoplegia, and myotonic dystrophy.

It has also been observed in patients who have used topical corticosteroids for long periods. With aging, the loss of tone of the levator palpebrae superioris muscle and Müller muscle, together with loss of eyelid support caused by enophthalmos from atrophy of orbital fat, may cause some eyelid sagging. Injection of a local anesthetic into the eyelid for ocular surgery may cause disinsertion or dehiscence, or both, of the aponeurosis of the levator palpebrae superioris muscle from the tarsus with a narrowed palpebral fissure. A similar blepharoptosis may follow injection of botulinum A toxin into the eyelids in the treatment of essential blepharospasm.

Myasthenia gravis.—Myasthenia gravis is an autoimmune disorder in which autoantibodies against the acetylcholine receptors of the cholinergic nicotinic neuromuscular junctions cause impaired neural transmission. Blepharoptosis is the initial sign in about 50% of the patients, and one half of these never develop generalized signs. Women are affected more frequently than men (3.5:1). Sjögren syndrome is common, and there may be a history of the use of penicillamine for the treatment of arthritis. Diagnosis is based on the demonstration of antiacetylcholine antibodies or on the improvement of muscle function after the administration of anticholinesterase compounds. Myasthenia gravis is treated medically, and it is essential that it be excluded as the cause before attempting surgical correction of acquired blepharoptosis.

Jaw-winking.—Congenital unilateral blepharoptosis may be associated with a paradoxic (synkinetic) retraction of the drooping eyelid when the ipsilateral pterygoid muscle is stimulated, usually as a result of chewing, opening the mouth, or sucking (Robert Marcus Gunn syndrome). Amblyopia (35%) and strabismus (30%) are common; amblyopia occurs in all patients in whom the superior rectus muscle is paretic. The jaw-winking can be corrected only by disinsertion of the levator palpebrae superioris muscle and substitution of a fascial sling. To maintain symmetry, both eyelids must have similar surgery. Spontaneous improvement occurs in many patients, and treatment must be individualized.

Surgical correction of blepharoptosis.—Several procedures may be used to correct blepharoptosis.

1. Resection of the conjunctiva, tarsus, Müller muscle, and aponeurosis of levator palpebrae superioris muscle (Fasanella-Servat) corrects up to 3 mm of blepharoptosis if the levator palpebrae superioris muscle function is good. It is the preferred procedure to correct minor degrees of blepharoptosis, such as that caused by separation of the aponeurosis of the levator palpebrae muscle from the tarsus.
2. For moderate blepharoptosis (3 to 4 mm) with moderate levator palpebrae superioris function, the muscle may be resected through either a skin or a conjunctival incision.
3. When the levator palpebrae superioris muscle function is absent, the upper eyelid is suspended to the frontalis muscle by means of a fascia lata or synthetic material sling. This procedure provides mechanical elevation, but the cosmetic result may be less pleasing than with a levator palpebrae superioris muscle resection. If there is no muscle function, however, the procedure must be used.

Several devices, known as "ptosis crutches," attached to the frame of spectacles elevate the eyelid. They are not particularly well tolerated and, in individuals with unilateral ophthalmoplegia, a drooping eyelid may prevent diplopia.

Blepharophimosis.—Blepharophimosis is a congenital malformation in which the palpebral fissures are vertically and horizontally small. It is often associated with widely separated orbits (telecanthus), blepharoptosis, inverse epicanthus, and a wide and flat nasal bridge. There may be microphthalmia, microcephaly, mental retardation, and many systemic defects. Many instances are associated with interstitial deletion of the long arm of chromosome 3: del (3) (q22.3-23).

LAGOPHTHALMOS

Lagophthalmos is an abnormality in which inadequate closure of the eyelids results in exposure of the eye. It may follow facial nerve (N VII) weakness, proptosis, retraction of the eyelids, or enlargement of the globe. Exposure of the cornea causes drying and secondary infection. Treatment is directed toward the cause. Surgery to prevent exposure keratitis should be carried out as soon as it is evident that exposure of the cornea endangers vision. Permanent or temporary adhesions may be created between the upper and the lower eyelids (tarsorrhaphy). These may be either lateral, medial, or central. In mild lagophthalmos only the central portion of the cornea may be exposed, and the instillation of an ointment base at bedtime may prevent corneal drying during sleep. Plastic wrap held in position with gummed cellophane tape may be used to cover the exposed eye and create a moist chamber. Alternatively, a soft contact lens and artificial tears may prevent corneal drying in a cosmetically more acceptable manner. Craniofacial surgery is required in many bony deformities, whereas orbital decompression may be needed in orbital tumors and thyroid disease.

FLOPPY EYELIDS

This is an abnormality in which one or both upper eyelids lose the elastin and rigidity of their tarsal plates. The exposure causes a chronic papillary conjunctivitis of the upper palpebral conjunctiva. Afflicted individuals are usually obese men between 30 and 50 years of age who may have sleep apnea (25%). The tarsus is rubbery in consistency, and any pressure applied to the upper eyelid causes it to evert. A shield worn over the eyes at night prevents eversion of the eyelid, and the papillary conjunctivitis is relieved within 3 weeks.

DISORDERS OF THE ORBICULARIS OCULI MUSCLE

BLINKING

Blinking spreads tears over the surface of the eye and limits the amount of light entering the eye. It may be involuntary or voluntary. Involuntary blinking occurs as a periodic contraction of the tarsal portion of the orbicularis oculi muscle at a rate peculiar to each individual. It normally occurs about once every 5 seconds and lasts about 0.3 second. Involuntary blinking is absent in infants. Infrequent blinking is seen in progressive supranuclear palsy, parkinsonism, and hyperthyroidism (Stellwag sign; see Chapter 27). Infrequent blinking or incomplete closure of the eyelids may aggravate the symptoms of keratoconjunctivitis sicca.

Reflex blinking may follow peripheral stimulation of the trigeminal, optic, or auditory nerves. Irritation of the cornea, conjunctiva, or eyelashes is followed by eyelid closure. Bright lights or glare may initiate blinking through a reflex arc that begins in the retina. It is mediated by retinal stimuli that pass through the superior colliculi and not the visual cortex. Such reflex blinking is, thus, not a sign that vision is present. A sudden loud noise may cause a reflex closure of the eyelids (acousticopalpebral reflex).

BLEPHAROCLONUS

Blepharoclonus is an exaggerated form of reflex blinking in which either the frequency of blinking is increased or the closure phase is excessively prolonged. There is often marked contraction of the orbital portion of the eyelids. Blepharoclonus may be initiated by irritation or inflammation of the conjunctiva or the cornea and may continue as a tic involving other muscles of the face. When the stimulus cannot be found, effective treatment is difficult. Injection of botulinum toxin into the orbicularis oculi muscle blocks the release of acetylcholine at the neuromuscular junction. It provides relief for up to 100 days but must be repeated.

Children 5 to 10 years of age may develop episodes of rapid blinking. Apparently the child is unaware of blinking, but the parents may be distressed. Almost invariably, examination of the child indicates no ocular abnormality.

BLEPHAROSPASM

Blepharospasm is an involuntary, tonic, spasmodic, bilateral contraction of the orbicularis oculi muscle that may last from several seconds to several minutes. It occurs mainly in individuals over 45 years of age and may be limited to the eyelids or may involve other facial muscles. The levator palpebrae muscle may be normal or participate in the dystonia. The blepharospasm causes a severe cosmetic deformity as well as impaired vision because of persistent eyelid closure. It may occur in postencephalitic states, in hemiplegia from various causes, and after Bell palsy. In such patients the blepharospasm may not disappear during sleep. Injection of botulinum toxin into the affected muscle may be helpful.

ORBICULARIS OCULI MUSCLE TREMOR

Involuntary contraction of a few fibers of the orbicularis oculi muscle (ocular myokymia) causes an annoying twitching of the eyelid, which the patient feels is conspicuous. Examination discloses a barely perceptible contraction of a few fibers of the orbicularis oculi muscle. Often no cause is found, but fatigue, alcohol and coffee consumption, smoking, and ocular irritation are implicated. Reassurance is usually all that is required. Quinine sulfate in doses of 200 to 400 mg increases the latent period of skeletal muscle contraction with relief of symptoms. It may be combined with systemic antihistamines.

MISCELLANEOUS CONDITIONS

BLEPHAROCHALASIS

Blepharochalasis is an abnormality in which atrophy and loss of elasticity of the skin of the eyelids occur. It occurs most commonly in the elderly. There is a loss of skin turgor, and a fold of skin may hang down over the margin of the upper eyelid and impair vision. Treatment is usually not indicated. If the fold of skin interferes with vision, the excess skin may be excised.

ORBITAL FAT HERNIATION

Puffiness or swelling of the eyelids (baggy eyelids) results from localized edema or protrusion of fat from the orbit into the eyelids. Systemic causes of edema include nephrosis and angioneurotic edema. In premenstrual edema,

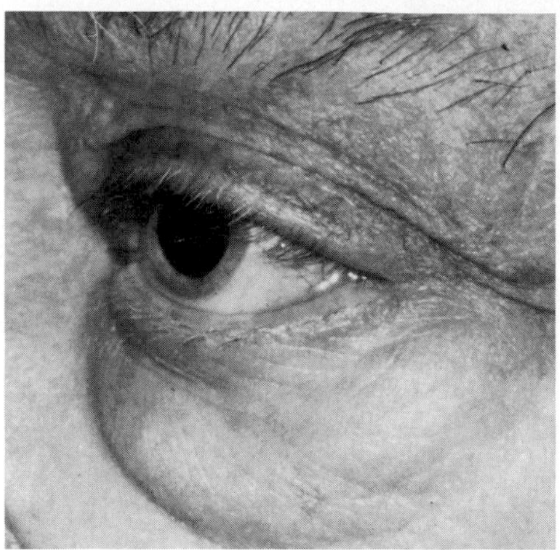

FIG 9-6.
Herniation of orbital far into the lower eyelid.

fluid retention and vasodilation may be conspicuous in this area.

Fat escapes from the orbit into the upper eyelid (Fig 9-6) through the opening in the orbital septum for passage of aponeurosis of the levator palpebrae superioris muscle. Fat herniates into the lower eyelid through the opening for the capsulopalpebral fascia. Fat may also escape through the openings provided for major blood vessels and nerves. Surgical removal of fatty tissue from the eyelid and orbit is a common cosmetic procedure. The incision may be made through the skin or the conjunctiva of the cul-de-sac.

TRICHIASIS

In this condition the eyelashes are directed toward the globe and irritate the cornea and the conjunctiva, causing secondary infection. The condition often complicates blepharitis but may also be associated with trachoma, cicatricial pemphigoid, erythema multiforme, ocular alkali burns, and injuries of the eyelid. The cornea and conjunctiva may be protected by a soft contact lens, but usually the purpose of treatment is redirection of the irritating lashes or destruction of the follicles of the irritating lashes. Eyelashes removed by epilation regrow to full size in 10 weeks. Electrolysis may be used to remove lashes permanently but is seldom practical for more than a few lashes. Reducing the temperature of the hair follicles to −15° C, by means of liquid nitrogen applied to the anesthetized palpebral conjunctiva, may be used to treat extensive trichiasis. Small areas may be treated by direct application to the cilia. The cornea and skin must be protected. Depigmentation of the treated area may contraindicate the process in deeply pigmented individuals. The hair follicle may be destroyed by the argon laser, but repeated treatments are required.

DISTICHIASIS

Distichiasis is an autosomal dominant abnormality in which an additional row of eyelashes together with glands of Zeis and Moll are present on the posterior eyelid margin. Other congenital malformations may be present. If the lashes are numerous and cause irritation of the globe, the area must be excised and replaced with a mucous membrane graft.

HYPERTROPHY OF THE EYELIDS

Immense overgrowth of the eyelids may occur in neurofibromatosis, hemangiomas (particularly in infancy), lymphangioma, and a variety of infections. Treatment is directed toward the cause. Orbital hemangiomas in infancy cause myopia that, if not optically corrected, may result in amblyopia.

INFLAMMATION

The eyelid margins may be involved in inflammations (blepharitis) caused by bacteria, seborrheic dermatitis, or localized hypersensitivity reactions. The skin of the eyelids may be involved in a large variety of inflammations that may be more conspicuous than similar lesions elsewhere on the body because of the looseness of the skin, its exposed position, and secondary involvement of the conjunctiva and cornea. Contact dermatitis and reactions secondary to the application of drugs or cosmetics to the eyelids or conjunctival sac are common.

The glands in the eyelids may be involved in acute suppurative infections such as those occurring with sties that involve the glands of Zeis or Moll. The meibomian glands may be involved in an acute or chronic inflammation called chalazion.

BLEPHARITIS

Blepharitis is a chronic inflammation of the eyelid margins. It begins early in childhood and frequently continues throughout life, becoming more symptomatic in the sixth and seventh decades. Staphylococcal infection and seborrheic dermatitis, often in combination, are its principal causes.

There are two forms of blepharitis: (1) seborrheic blepharitis and (2) ulcerative blepharitis (uncommon). The seborrheic type has hard, brittle fibrinous scales (collarettes) that surround the cilia. The ulcerated type has matted hard crusts that encircle individual cilia, and their removal discloses small ulcers. Both types may be associated with dilated blood vessels on the margins of the eyelids, white eyelashes (poliosis), loss of lashes, and thin, broken, and small lashes. Chalazia and sties may be recurrent. Almost invariably there is an associated chronic papillary conjunctivitis. Keratitis may occur, as may phlyctenulosis. *Pityrosporum ovale* and *Demodex folliculorum* mites may serve as vectors of staphylococci. *Pityrosporum ovale* possibly provokes the inflammation by splitting lipids into irritating fatty acids.

Seborrheic blepharitis.—Simple seborrheic blepharitis is characterized by a hyperemia usually limited to the eyelid margins. It is associated with scaling of the skin that may cause fine flakes and scales surrounding the lashes. In severe cases the eyelid margins may become thickened and everted. Most commonly, however, redness of the eyelid margins is the chief complaint. There may be burning and discomfort of the eyes and an associated chronic conjunctivitis or keratoconjunctivitis sicca that further contributes to discomfort.

The disorder may be infectious (mainly *Staphylococcus aureus*) or secondary to a seborrheic dermatitis of the scalp that may also affect the eyebrows and cause an erythema of the cheeks. Patients with acne rosacea and atopic disease have a greater than normal predisposition. Laxity of the eyelid musculature with aging may decrease expression of meibomian gland contents. Irritation of the eyelid margins by cosmetics, chemical fumes, smoke, and smog may aggravate the hyperemia, as may frequent rubbing of the eyelids. Systemic administration of retinoids in the management of various dermatologic disorders is associated with blepharitis and conjunctivitis in 20% to 45% of patients.

Ulcerative blepharitis.—Ulcerative blepharitis is caused by acute and chronic suppurative inflammation of the follicles of the lashes and the associated glands of Zeis and Moll. *Staphylococcus aureus* is usually the causative organism, but some strains of *S. epidermidis* may be responsible. The eyelid margins are red and inflamed. There are multiple suppurative lesions surrounded by yellow pus that crusts and is removed with difficulty, bringing with it eyelashes. Loss of lashes and the necrotizing inflammation cause distortion of the eyelid margin, leading to ectropion, epiphora, and chronic conjunctivitis.

Treatment of both the seborrheic and ulcerative types is difficult, and recurrences are common. Coexisting seborrheic dermatitis is treated with frequent (daily to twice weekly) selenium sulfide shampooing of the scalp and eyebrows. Excessive meibomian gland secretions are treated with bilateral hot compresses. These may be followed by scrubbing of the eyelids with a moist washcloth. The lid margins are then cleansed with a cotton-tipped applicator moistened with baby shampoo and water to remove scales.

Antibiotic ointment may be applied to the eyelid margins at bedtime or more frequently in severe inflammation. Bacitracin, erythromycin, or sulfisoxazole (Gantrisin) ointments are effective. Systemic tetracycline (erythromycin in children and pregnant women) may be used in acne rosacea and severe inflammation.

Infestation of the eyelids by head lice (phthiriasis palpebrarum) causes a blepharitis and sometimes a dermatitis of the eyelids. The nits and their egg shells are seen adherent to the roots of the eyelashes. Primary treatment is directed to the concomitant infection of the scalp by shampooing with 0.5% malathion (Prioderm) or pyrethrin (NIX). Topical 0.25% physostigmine (eserine) ointment kills the lice through its anticholinesterase action. Shampoos are usually repeated after 10 days to prevent reinfestation. The eyelashes may be treated twice daily with an application of heavy petrolatum or yellow oxide of mercury ointment, which must be continued for some 14 days.

MEIBOMIANITIS

A passive retention of secretion by the meibomian glands may deposit a white, frothy secretion on the eyelid margins and at the canthi. The glands may be massaged to express an oily

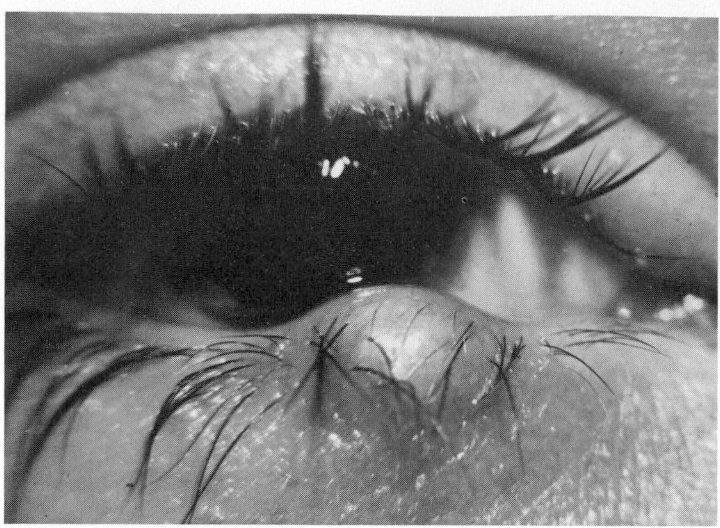

FIG 9-7.
Acute hordeolum of the lower eyelid.

secretion, and eversion of the eyelids may show vertical yellowish streaks shining through the tarsal conjunctiva. Occasionally cellular debris or calcium are deposited in a gland. If this material penetrates the conjunctiva, it causes a foreign body sensation and must be removed.

Meibomianitis is often associated with blepharitis and chronic conjunctivitis and may cause recurrent chalazia. Treatment consists of massage of the eyelids to empty the glands and removal of the secretion with a moist washcloth.

HORDEOLUM

Hordeolum, or sty (Fig 9-7), is an acute suppurative inflammation of the follicle of an eyelash or the associated gland of Zeis (sebaceous) or Moll (special apocrine sweat gland). Like pustules elsewhere, the usual cause is staphylococcal infection. The initial symptom is tenderness of the eyelid that may become severe as the suppuration progresses. The first sign is edema of the eyelid, followed by the development of a red, indurated area on the eyelid margin that may rupture. There is preauricular adenopathy. The main differential diagnosis involves an acute chalazion that tends to point on the conjunctival side of the eyelid and does not affect the margin of the eyelid unless the duct of the meibomian gland, which opens on the eyelid margin, is inflamed. The chalazion is preceded and followed by a minute tumor in the substance of the eyelid that feels like a small buckshot.

Sties tend to occur in crops, because the infecting organism spreads from one hair follicle to another, either directly or by the fingers. Treatment is the same as that for acute suppurative infection elsewhere on the body. Hot compresses applied four or five times daily for 10 minutes hasten resolution of the infection. Frequent instillation of a topic antibiotic prevents extension to adjacent glands. Any associated blepharitis must be treated.

CHALAZION

Chalazion is a chronic inflammatory lipogranuloma of a meibomian gland. It is characterized by a gradual painless swelling of the gland without other external signs of inflammation (Fig 9-8). Palpation indicates a small nodule in the substance of the eyelid, often the only evidence. With increase in size, a chalazion may cause astigmatism by pressure on the globe or it may be evident beneath the skin as a small mass. It may become secondarily infected and cause an acute suppurative inflammation that usually points on the conjunctival surface of the eyelid (internal hordeolum). The lesion is a lipogranuloma that resembles the granuloma seen in sarcoidosis or tuberculosis with giant cells but without caseation.

Asymptomatic chalazia do not require treatment and usually disappear spontaneously

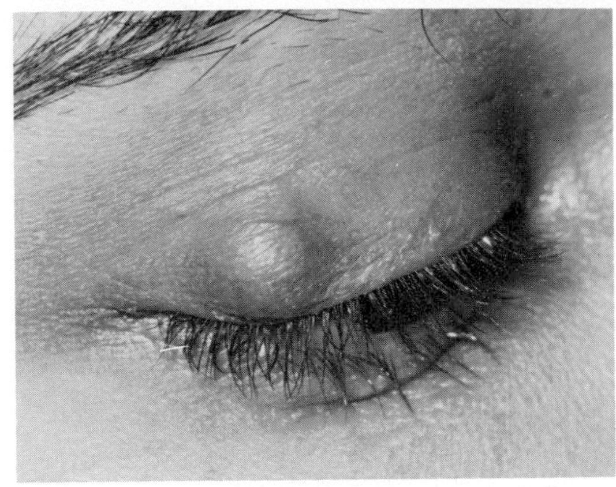

FIG 9-8.
Chronic chalazion (lipogranuloma) of meibomian gland of the upper eyelid.

within a few months. Acute suppuration is treated with local hot compresses and a topical antibiotic or sulfonamide. Local injection from the conjunctival surface (injection through the skin may cause local depigmentation) of 0.5 mL of triamcinolone acetonide into the center of the chalazion may be rapidly effective. Excision, usually through a conjunctival incision, is indicated when persistent or large. Some individuals tend to have a series of chalazia, apparently because of inspissation of the meibomian gland contents in the excretory ducts. If pressure on the eyelid expresses a viscous secretion from the glands, massage of the eyelids, sometimes with a glass rod, may be helpful. Recurrence of what is believed to be a chalazion at the site where it has been excised should make one suspect a meibomian gland carcinoma.

Rarely, a hard contact lens migrates to the supratarsal region of the upper eyelid, becomes embedded, and causes an orbital mass, a blepharoptosis, or a chalazion-like swelling.

DERMATITIS

Infection of the skin of the eyelids may occur with a variety of microbial organisms, and it includes nearly the entire range of dermatitides. The thinness of the skin and its good blood supply allow enormous distention and injection. Secondary infection of the conjunctiva, cornea, and intraocular contents may occur by direct extension from the skin. Conversely, inflammatory skin lesions may originate in the conjunctiva, orbit, nasal accessory sinuses, lacrimal apparatus, or the glands of the eyelids.

Impetigo, erysipelas, anthrax malignant pustule, tuberculosis, chancre, leprosy, yaws, and tularemia may all involve the eyelid on occasion, often with enlargement of the parotid and submaxillary lymph glands.

Herpes zoster ophthalmicus causes a vesicular eruption of the eyelid that is less important than the associated keratitis and uveitis. Verruca vulgaris and molluscum contagiosum infection of the eyelid margins are important because of the resulting viral conjunctivitis and keratitis.

Fungus infections of the eyelid may occur either as a local infection or in the course of widespread systemic disease.

Contact dermatitis.—Contact dermatitis is an inflammatory response of the skin to an external agent. There are two types: (1) primary irritant and (2) immunologic hypersensitivity (see Chapter 25). Immunologic hypersensitivity reactions are divided into immediate and delayed types. The eyelids are particularly vulnerable, even in patients in whom other portions of the skin are not affected. The vulnerability arises in part from the exposure of the eyelids to soaps, cosmetics, perfumes, medications, and contact lens products, and the frequency with which some individuals touch their eyelids. Women are more frequently affected than men and there is often a history of atopy, although hay fever and asthma do not seem to confer a susceptibility.

Primary irritant dermatitis.—This is a nonimmunologic reaction of the skin at the sites of contact of an external agent. Generally, primary irritants elicit a painful response rather than itching. Strong acids and alkalies are obvious causes. The eyelids are often exposed to soaps, cosmetics, detergents, oils, adhesive tape, and different chemicals, which may cause an irritant dermatitis. Topical ophthalmic preparations containing thimerosal or other preservatives have led to the marketing of many preservative-free ophthalmic preparations. Con tact with the calcium oxalate crystals of the *Dieffenbachia* species, a common house plant, may cause an irritant dermatitis of the eyelids. Some of the agents also participate in delayed hypersensitivity reactions (see below).

Immediate contact dermatitis.—These are transient reactions, mediated by immunoglobulin E (IgE), which occurs within minutes to an hour after exposure to an agent to which an individual has become sensitized. There is itching and localized urticaria that frequently affect sensitized eyelids after exposure to cosmetics.

Delayed contact dermatitis.—In type IV hypersensitivity reactions of the skin, an allergen penetrates the skin and reacts with HLA-D region genes on Langerhans cells to form a complex. Circulating T lymphocytes recognize the complex and are activated to proliferate in the regional lymph nodes to produce lymphokines. The expanded T cells are released throughout the body. Three to ten days later there is a release of inflammatory mediators at the site of the original allergen and the inflammation recruits more lymphocytes, which amplifies the inflammatory reaction.

Common ophthalmic sensitizers include ophthalmic eyedrops with names ending in "-caine," atropine, neomycin sulfate, gentamicin, topical antihistamines, artificial tears, contact lens cleaners, and many other compounds. Topical corticosteroids are a rare cause of delayed hypersensitivity reactions. After sensitization, reexposure to the substance, not necessarily at the same site, produces a contact dermatitis at the original site.

The skin reacts with a recurrent, weeping, eczematous lesion. Itching is severe. When the condition is chronic, the skin becomes indurated and brawny with moderate swelling.

Treatment is unsatisfactory until the cause is removed. This may be difficult to determine but is sometimes aided by the patient's keeping a diary to record each day's activities and the severity of the inflammation. Rubbing of the eyes after handling soaps, detergents, garden supplies, or chemicals may cause the reaction. Cosmetics, perfumes, and nail polish may be offenders. The patient should never touch the eyelids. Sometimes only the eyelids on the side of the dominant hand are affected, suggesting that a sensitizer is brought to them by the fingers. All topical medications should be stopped. Perfumed and colored soaps should not be used. Sometimes a bland ointment such as Aquaphor will relieve symptoms. Systemic corticosteroids are not necessary except for severe poison ivy dermatitis.

TUMORS

The eyelids are subject to the usual tumors of the skin. If the eyelid margin is not involved, excision is simple. Involvement of the eyelid margin necessitates skilled surgery to ensure complete excision and satisfactory closure.

CUTANEOUS HORNS

A cutaneous horn is a small, cylindric, protruding, keratic growth of epidermal cells. Its cause is unknown. It may occur near the eyelid margins in middle-aged or older people. It may be solar, seborrheic, inverted follicular keratosis, verucca vulgaris, or, rarely, sebaceous cell carcinoma in origin. Cutaneous horns are easily excised.

MILIA

Milia are small, white, round, slightly elevated cysts of the superficial dermis. They tend to occur in crops localized in a small area of the skin, sometimes on the eyelid. They may be derived from a hair follicle or its associated sebaceous gland. Excision may be desirable for cosmetic reasons.

XANTHELASMA

Xanthelasma is a cutaneous deposition of lipid material that occurs most commonly at the inner portion of the upper or the lower eyelid. The lesion appears as a yellowish, slightly elevated area with sharply demarcated margins tending to be approximately parallel to the eyelid margin. Xanthelasma occurs with primary and secondary systemic anomalies of lipid metabolism, but more commonly occurs spontaneously without evident cause. It produces a cosmetic defect, and treatment is indicated only to remove the defect. The lesion may be excised surgically or destroyed by means of diathermy, laser photocoagulation, or chemical cautery. Recurrence is common.

KERATOACANTHOMA

Keratoacanthoma is a cup-shaped, elevated, benign tumor that has an umbilicated apex. It develops on exposed (usually hairy) areas of the skin of middle-aged and elderly individuals. Sometimes it involves the eyelids. It grows rapidly for 2 to 6 weeks and reaches a maximum size of 1 to 2 cm. It involutes several months after onset, leaving a depressed scar. Histologically, a central crater filled with keratin, acanthosis, and the cellular structure distinguish the whole tumor from a well-differentiated squamous cell carcinoma. This differentiation may be impossible to discern with a partial biopsy specimen. Clinically its initial rapid growth and umbilicated necrotic center distinguish it from squamous cell carcinoma.

CARCINOMA

Basal cell carcinoma is the most common human malignancy of the eyelids, occurring almost 10 times more often than squamous cell carcinoma. Both have a similar nodular appearance with elevated, irregular surfaces and sharply demarcated, pearly margins. The squamous cell tumor produces keratin and may appear more pearly white. The centers may be excavated or ulcerated. Extensive ulceration of basal cell tumors occurs with growth (rodent ulcer). The basal cell tumor may, in about 5% of the cases, be pigmented. Pigmentation, however, may indicate a nevus or a malignant melanoma. Generally, the lower eyelid or the inner canthus and adjacent part of the nose are involved in fair-skinned individuals (Fig 9-9). The patient may neglect the lesion for a long period because there are no symptoms. There is a gradual increase in size of a typical tumor that has pearly margins and an excavated center. If the eyelid margin is not involved, excision in the early stages provides cure. When the eyelid margin is involved, surgical excision may necessitate a major plastic procedure.

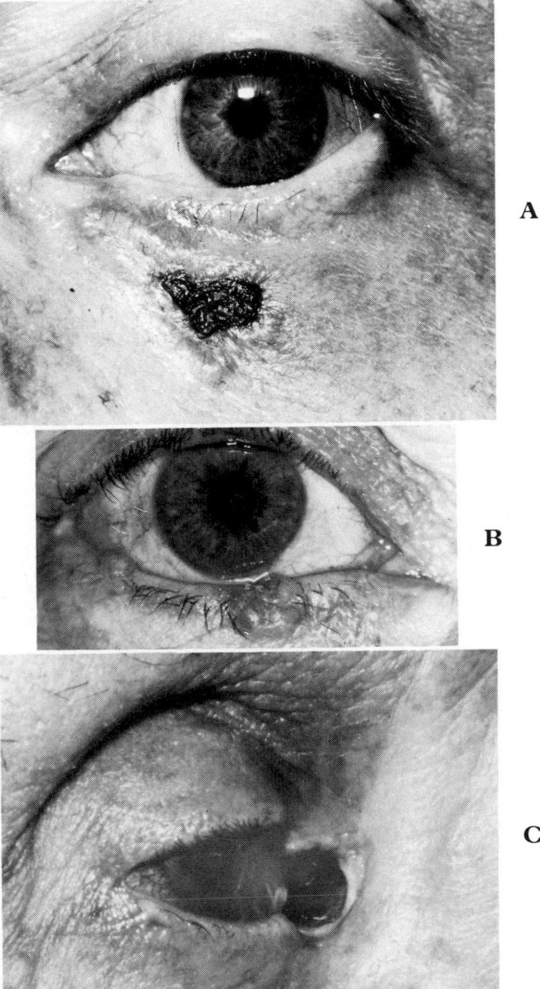

FIG 9-9.
A and **B,** Basal cell carcinomas of the lower eyelid. **C,** Extension of a basal cell carcinoma of the inner canthus into the nose in an 83-year-old man.

Radiation therapy may cause keratinization of the conjunctiva and chronic keratitis. These complications are most likely to occur after treatment of lesions that affect the middle portion of the upper eyelid. When the eyelid margin is involved, surgical excision is preferred to radiation. Excision more fully ensures removal, and inadequate radiation may be followed by metaplasia of basal cell tumors to the squamous cell.

Cryotherapy is indicated in tumors involving the inner canthus because it minimizes damage to the lacrimal drainage apparatus. A thermistor is inserted into the tumor, and liquid nitrogen is sprayed onto the tumor until the temperature within the tumor is reduced to −30° C. Recurrent tumors may have the freeze-thaw cycle repeated several times. Noninfiltrative basal cell tumors of the eyelid that measure less than 10 mm in diameter have a 5-year cure rate of 95%; the rate for infiltrative tumor is 94%. The incidence of periocular tumors can be reduced with long-term use of sunscreens, sunglasses, and broad-brimmed hats. Neglected or mismanaged basal cell carcinoma may invade the orbit and the cranial cavity, causing a widespread destructive lesion.

Squamous cell carcinoma appears as an elevated, indurated plaque that tends to ulcerate.

Like basal cell carcinoma, it tends to involve the lower eyelid. It is the most common epithelial malignancy of the conjunctiva, whereas basal cell carcinoma nearly never occurs. Squamous cell carcinoma affects the upper eyelid and outer canthus more frequently than basal cell carcinoma does. Unlike squamous cell tumors of the bronchus and cervix, squamous cell carcinoma of the eyelid has an excellent prognosis after wide excision.

The sweat glands (of Moll) of the eyelids are apocrine glands and, like such glands elsewhere (axilla, surrounding the nipples, and perianal and perigenital regions), may develop a special type of carcinoma, extramammary Paget disease. The diagnosis is usually based on the histologic appearance of the tissue, which may be resected in the belief that the lesion is a basal cell carcinoma.

Adenocarcinoma may develop in the glandular portion of a meibomian gland. Most commonly, patients are treated for recurrent chalazion before the neoplastic nature of the lesion is evident. Such a delay may permit fatal metastasis. The tissue excised in every recurrent chalazion should be examined histologically.

BIBLIOGRAPHY

Books

Borodic GE, Townsend DJ: *Atlas of eyelid surgery,* Philadelphia, 1994, WB Saunders.

Lisak RP, editor: *Handbook of myasthenia gravis and myasthenic syndromes,* New York, 1994, Marcel Dekker.

Mannis MJ, Macsai MS, Huntley AC: *Eye and skin disease,* Philadelphia, 1996, Lippincott-Raven.

McCord CD Jr, Tannenbaum M, Nunery WR, editors: *Oculoplastic surgery,* ed 3, New York, 1995, Raven Press.

Putterman AM, editor: *Cosmetic oculoplastic surgery,* ed 2, Philadelphia, 1993, WB Saunders.

Rycroft RJG, Menné T, Frosch PJ, Benezra C, editors: *Textbook of contact dermatitis,* New York, 1992, Springer-Verlag.

van der Meulen JC, Gruss JS: *Color atlas & text of ocular plastic surgery,* St Louis, 1995, Mosby–Year Book.

Wolfort FG, Kanter WR: *Aesthetic blepharoplasty,* Boston, 1995, Little, Brown.

Article

Committee on Ophthalmic Procedures Assessment, American Academy of Ophthalmology. Functional indications for upper and lower eyelid blepharoplasty, *Ophthalmology* 102:693-695, 1995.

10

THE CONJUNCTIVA

Conjunctivitis, keratitis, and related inflammatory conditions of the conjunctiva and cornea are discussed in Chapter 12.

The conjunctiva is a thin, translucent mucous membrane that lines the posterior surfaces of the eyelids and covers the scleral portion of the anterior segment of the eye ("the white of the eye"). It is divided into the palpebral and bulbar portions and the regions that connect them, the superior and inferior fornices. It includes the caruncle and the plica semilunaris (semilunar fold) at the medial canthus. Its epithelium is continuous with the epithelium of the cornea, lacrimal glands and passages, and conjunctival glands. Its stratified columnar epithelium varies in thickness from two cell layers over the tarsal plates to five to seven layers at the transitional area at the corneoscleral limbus to the stratified squamous epithelium of the cornea.

Goblet cells are scattered throughout the conjunctiva, and lymphocytes and melanocytes are located in the basal layers. The stroma is closely adherent to the tarsal plates but is thrown into many folds in the fornices and is but loosely adherent to the globe. The stroma is composed of loosely arranged bundles of coarse collagenous tissue containing numerous fibroblasts. Fibroblasts, microphages, mast cells, and leukocytes are found extravascularly in the tissues. Three or four months after birth, the superficial stroma in the fornices contains lymphoid tissue.

Inflammation may result from infection, foreign material, chemicals, or radiant energy. Infection may extend into the conjunctiva from adjacent tissues, be blood-borne as in measles and chickenpox, or be localized to the conjunctiva. Conjunctival allergies may be conspicuous, as in hay fever or vernal conjunctivitis.

SYMPTOMS AND SIGNS OF CONJUNCTIVAL DISORDERS

The main symptoms caused by conjunctival disorders are ocular burning, discomfort, or a foreign body sensation, and sometimes discharge. Severe ocular pain suggests corneal involvement rather than conjunctival disease. Itching is common in allergic reactions. Inflammatory exudates may excoriate the skin, particularly at the outer canthus, or agglutinate the eyelids during sleep. Exudates may float across the cornea and blur vision, or cause halos that surround lights, and disappear with rapid blinking.

The signs of conjunctival disease are mainly related to abnormalities of appearance, vascular changes, and edema (chemosis). The bulbar conjunctiva is easily inspected, but the tarsal conjunctiva can be seen only by eversion of the eyelids. Inspection of the superior fornix requires elevation of the upper eyelid by means of a retractor.

CONJUNCTIVAL BLOOD VESSELS

INJECTION

The normally inconspicuous posterior conjunctival arteries are dilated and engorged in conjunctival inflammations. Conjunctival injection is characterized by superficial bright red blood vessels, which are most conspicuous in the fornices and fade toward the corneoscleral limbus. These blood vessels move with the conjunctiva and are constricted by 1:1,000 epinephrine solution instilled in the conjunctival sac.

Conjunctival hyperemia is a dilation of the conjunctival blood vessels that occurs without exudation or cellular infiltration. Symptoms may be absent, but often a gritty foreign body sensation is aggravated by prolonged near work. Many patients are distressed because of the conjunctival redness, which becomes more severe with insomnia and fatigue.

Both the conjunctival and ciliary vascular beds are usually injected in inflammations of the cornea, iris, and ciliary body, although the ciliary injection is more marked (see Table 6-1). To distinguish conjunctival diseases from deeper diseases of the eye, it is wiser to direct attention to signs of corneal and iris involvement, pupillary reaction to light, and visual acuity than to emphasize the vascular engorgement.

Hyperemia is caused by the following: (1) irritation caused by tobacco smoke, smog, and chemical fumes; (2) exposure to wind and sun; (3) inadequate ocular protection from ultraviolet radiation; (4) uncorrected refractive errors and ocular muscle imbalance; (5) prolonged topical instillation of drugs, including vasoconstrictors; (6) acne rosacea; (7) blepharitis and excessive meibomian gland secretion; and (8) ganglionic blockade in the treatment of hypertension. Scalp or eyelash dandruff may irritate the conjunctiva. Chronic conjunctivitis may be caused by many of the same entities.

Treatment is directed toward removal of the cause. Temporary relief may be obtained by cold compresses or by local instillation of weak solutions of vasoconstrictors. Many over-the-counter preparations that contain epinephrine, phenylephrine, or naphazoline are available and may provide temporary relief. Products containing corticosteroids should not be used because of the danger of inducing infection or glaucoma.

SUBCONJUNCTIVAL HEMORRHAGE

Rupture of a conjunctival blood vessel causes a monocular, bright red, sharply delineated area surrounded by normal-appearing conjunctiva. The blood is located beneath the bulbar conjunctiva and gradually fades in 2 weeks. There are no symptoms, but many patients become alarmed by the conspicuous red appearance. A subconjunctival hemorrhage is caused by the same factors responsible for a black-and-blue spot elsewhere in the body: trauma, hypertension, blood dyscrasias, and the like. Usually no cause is found. Treatment does not hasten the absorption of the blood.

Subconjunctival hemorrhage involving the entire bulbar conjunctiva may follow fracture of one of the orbital bones or rupture of the posterior sclera. Adenovirus conjunctivitis is sometimes associated with severe subconjunctival hemorrhage. Compressive injuries to the chest (traumatic asphyxia) cause vascular engorgement of the head and widespread bleeding, including binocular subconjunctival hemorrhage.

SYSTEMIC DISEASE

Typical abnormalities of the conjunctival blood vessels have been described in (1) hemoglobin SC disease and blood hyperviscosity syndromes; (2) cryoglobulinemia; and (3) diffuse angiokeratoma (Fabry disease) (see Chapter 26). The changes are often evident only with biomicroscopic examination. Since the conjunctival blood vessels often dilate and become tortuous with advancing age, the changes may be difficult to differentiate from those of normal aging.

Conjunctival vascular stasis may be present in hemoglobin SC disease and in hyperviscosity syndromes. Biomicroscopic examination discloses isolated, sharply defined twisted segments of capillaries with both the efferent and afferent connections empty of blood. The vessels of the bulbar conjunctiva near the inferior fornix are the most affected. The blood vessels may also show nonspecific changes of microaneurysms, telangiectasis, and segmental dilation. The typical vascular stasis disappears with the local application of heat and is accentuated by cholinergic blockade or by cold.

Cryoglobulinemia is associated with stasis of blood flow in conjunctival vessels that have a clumping of erythrocytes. Ice water irrigation of the conjunctival sac slows the bloodstream and causes increased segmentation of the blood column. In Fabry disease, aneurysms and tortuous blood vessels are seen in the inferior bulbar conjunctiva. Additionally, there are whorl-shaped opacities of the cornea at the level of Bowman membrane.

Venous congestion, microaneurysms, and venous dilation have been noted in the conjunctival vessels in diabetes mellitus. The changes are nonspecific and may be seen with aging, arteriosclerosis, and vascular hypertension.

PIGMENTATION

The conjunctiva stains with bilirubin in jaundice. (The sclera is stained only after prolonged and severe jaundice.) The normal white appearance of the exposed eye is stained yellow, as is the surrounding skin. A similar yellowish discoloration of the conjunctiva results from an excess of plant pigment (carotene) in food faddists who eat too many carrots.

A dull, grayish discoloration involving the conjunctiva in the lower fornix may occur after repeated instillation of silver or mercury salts. The pigmentation results from the deposition of the metallic ion and cannot be reversed. Prolonged instillation of epinephrine salts may cause deep black subconjunctival deposits of adrenochrome (oxidized epinephrine). Long-standing metallic iron foreign bodies in the conjunctiva may be surrounded by a brown stain. Hemosiderin originating from persistent subconjunctival blood may cause a diffuse conjunctival pigmentation. Abnormalities of the sclera (see Chapter 13) may be mistaken for conjunctival pigmentation: blue sclera, staphyloma, scleromalacia, senile hyaline plaque, and perforating malignant melanoma of the choroid.

In alkaptonuria (ochronosis), oval gray patches of homogentisic acid are deposited in the sclera in the interpalpebral fissure just anterior to the horizontal recti muscles. In Gaucher disease, a brown, triangular mass may occur adjacent to the corneoscleral limbus.

Benign epithelial melanosis.—Benign epithelial melanosis appears as diffuse, flat, brown patches of pigment, produced by normal melanocytes. The patches occur most commonly in deeply pigmented individuals (racial pigmentation) and are rare in lightly pigmented individuals. They are mainly found near the cornea in the interpalpebral space and fade toward the cul-de-sacs. The freckle (ephelis) is the comparable lesion in the skin. Treatment is not indicated.

Primary acquired melanosis.—These are acquired, flat, monocular, golden brown blemishes of the conjunctiva (and skin) that occur, most commonly in whites, after the 40th year. They originate from melanocytes that migrated from the neural crest to the basal layer of the conjunctiva, where they persist in the superficial or deep epithelium. The superficial layer contains dendritic melanocytes and nevocytic melanocytes, while the deep epidermis or subepithelium contains fusiform melanocytes. Dendritic melanocytes cause suntan, freckles, benign epithelial melanosis, and acquired melanosis. Nevocyte melanocytes form nevi. Fusiform melanocytes cause the nevus of Ota, melanosis oculi, and blue nevus. Each may cause benign acquired conjunctival melanosis, and each, particularly dendritic melanocytes, has the potential for malignant melanoma.

All lesions of benign acquired melanosis should be completely excised. The specimen should be examined to determine the presence or absence of atypical cell structure. Hyperpigmentation of the conjunctival epithelium without melanocytic hyperplasia or melanocytic hyperplasia without atypical cells does not progress to malignancy. Lesions that involve the cornea or that are incompletely excised tend to recur. If atypical melanocytes are not arranged along the junction of the epithelium and substantia propria, progression to malignant melanoma is common (90%). When atypical melanocytes are combined with epithelial cells, progression is likely (75%). The problem is difficult inasmuch as skilled pathologists may disagree concerning the nature of the tumor. Large lesions, after diagnosis by excisional biopsy, may be treated by freezing (cryotherapy) after ballooning of the conjunctiva with a local anesthetic to avoid damaging underlying ocular structures. Ablation by means of the excimer laser may prove useful.

OTHER CONJUNCTIVAL DISORDERS

PTERYGIUM

A pterygium is a triangular fibrovascular connective tissue overgrowth that encroaches on the cornea from the conjunctiva in the interpalpebral fissure (Fig 10-1). It usually advances from the nasal side and only rarely from the temporal side of the cornea. The cause is not known, but conjunctival irritations from sun and wind in individuals who spend much time out-

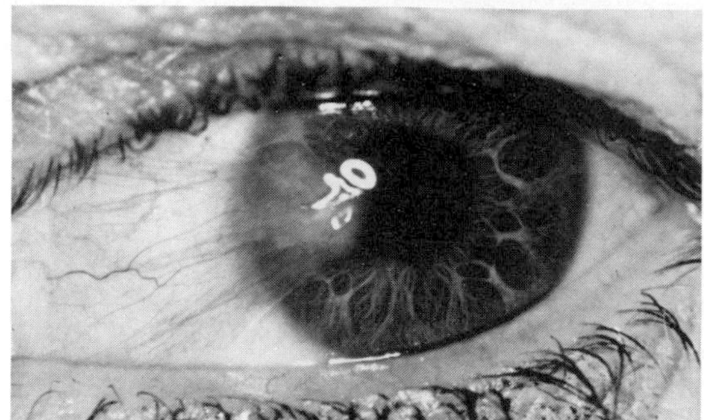

FIG 10-1.
Pterygium extending over the nasal portion of the cornea.

doors are affected. Bilateral pterygia occur in some 40% of patients with xeroderma pigmentosa. Histologically, there is elastotic degeneration (basophilic degeneration) caused by degeneration of subepithelial collagen and replacement with an abnormal material that stains for elastin but is not digested by elastase. There is dissolution of the Bowman zone of the cornea and dyskeratotic epithelial cells overlying the pterygium. The stroma of the pterygium contains lymphocytes, predominantly CD3+, and plasma cells, and immunofluorescent staining shows IgG and IgE.

Initially there may be signs of chronic conjunctivitis, thickening of the conjunctiva, and symptoms of a mild conjunctivitis. The cosmetic appearance is often the only complaint.

In the temperate zone of the United States, pterygia seldom progress rapidly and usually require no treatment, and they rarely recur after excision or transplantation. In tropical areas pterygia progress rapidly, are commonly thick and vascular, and have a pronounced tendency to recur, irrespective of the type of surgery.

A wide variety of surgical methods, including excimer laser photoablation, are used for excision of pterygia. The head of the pterygium is usually dissected from the cornea, and the body of the pterygium is then excised or transplanted beneath the conjunctiva. The conjunctiva is closed or the tissue beneath the body of the pterygium is excised and the sclera is not covered with conjunctiva (bare sclera method). Every effort is made to maintain a smooth corneal contour and avoid depressed areas that will impair the corneal tear film.

Topical 0.02% mitomycin for 5 days after excision minimizes recurrence. Beta and grenz rays have been widely used to prevent recurrence. Beta-ray sources applied to the corneoscleral limbus may cause a sectorial radiation cataract because of damage to cells in the replicative zone of the equatorial portion of the lens. Preoperatively and postoperatively, individuals with pterygia should be protected from ultraviolet light and irritation from wind or dust. A lamellar graft of cornea and sclera after excision of a recurrent pterygium may be effective.

A pseudopterygium is an inflammatory adhesion of the conjunctiva to damaged cornea that occurs after corneal trauma or inflammation. It may occur at any point around the corneoscleral limbus and is not progressive. The pseudopterygium often bridges the corneoscleral limbus so that in this region a probe may be passed between it and the sclera.

PINGUECULA

A pinguecula is a benign degenerative tumor of the bulbar conjunctiva that appears as a yellowish white, slightly elevated, oval elevated tissue mass on either side of the cornea in the palpebral fissure. The lesions are usually bilateral and located nasally. They become more common with advancing age. They cause a cosmetic defect and in some instances appear to precede a pterygium. Treatment is usually unnecessary, but excision is simple. A pinguecula has the same histologic structure as a pterygium but is limited to the conjunctiva. Brown, triangular "pingueculae" may appear in 75% of patients with Gaucher disease (see Chapter 26) and contain Gaucher cells.

LYMPHANGIECTASIS

The lymphatic channels of the conjunctiva may become dilated and cause clear, serous conjunctival cysts. These appear on the bulbar conjunctiva as minute tubules filled with clear fluid. Symptoms are minimal. There is no effective treatment. (Note: There are no lymphatic channels within the orbit posterior to the orbital septum.)

LITHIASIS

Degenerations of the conjunctival epithelium in the elderly or prolonged conjunctivitis may cause yellowish to white concretions in the epithelium. The deposits may be seen as linear streaks in the palpebral conjunctiva or as minute spheres in the inferior fornix. Rarely a dehis-

PLATE 1.

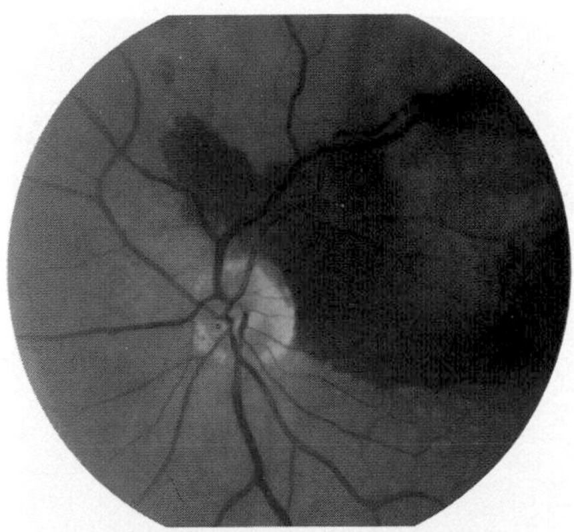

Subretinal (dark) and preretinal (bright) hemorrhages.

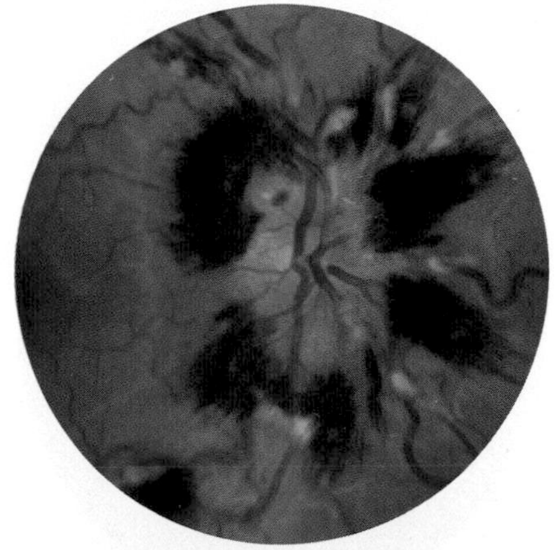

Peripapillary (adjacent to optic disk) hemorrhages and cotton-wool patches (histologic: cytoid bodies) in a woman with lupus erythematosus.

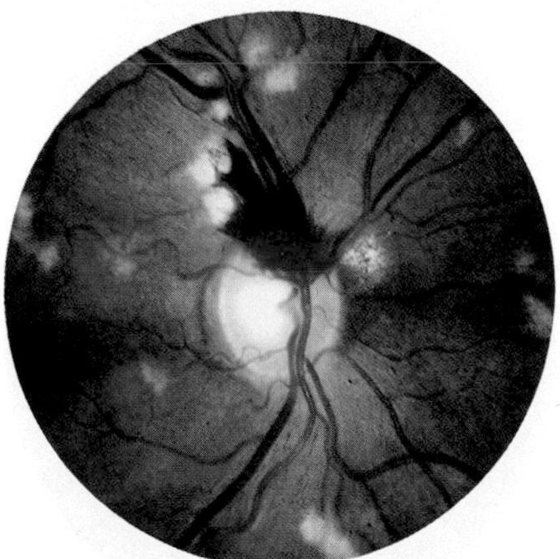

Preretinal hemorrhage above the optic disk and cotton-wool patches in a man with vascular hypertension.

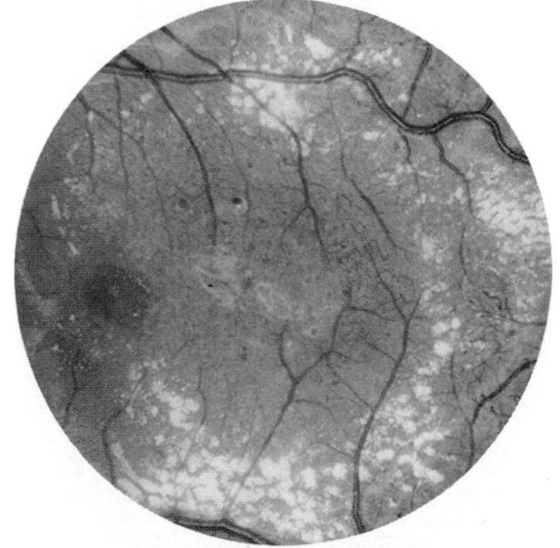

Edema residues (hard deposits or hard exudates) surrounding an area of macular edema in a man with non–insulin-dependent diabetes mellitus. There are microaneurysms above and below the edematous region. The fovea centralis is in the 9 o'clock meridian.

PLATE 2.

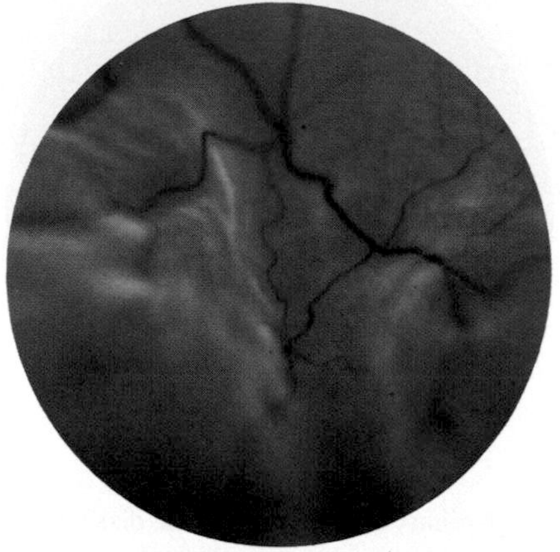

Serous retinal detachment in the sensory retina is not in contact with the underlying retinal pigment epithelium.

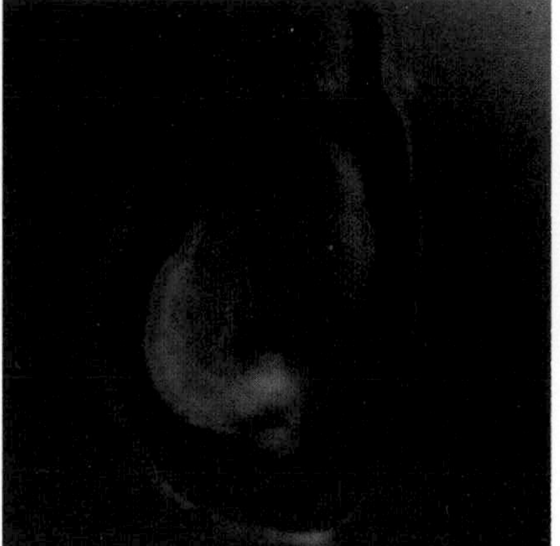

Horseshoe-shaped retinal hole, a common cause of retinal detachment. The portion of the retina between the two sides of the horseshoe is the operculum (Latin: cover). Horseshoe holes are often the result of blunt trauma to the eye.

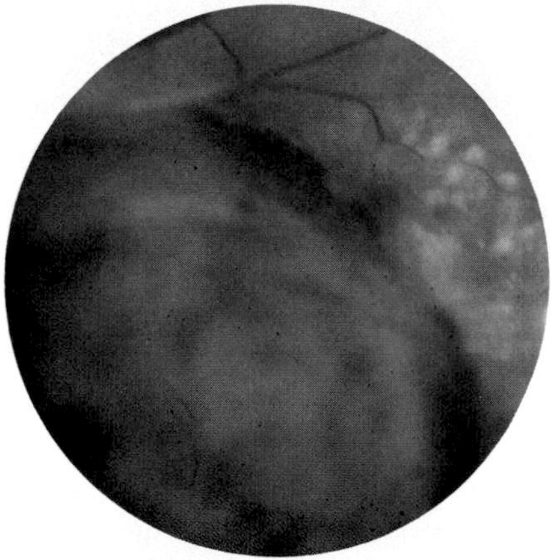

Solid retinal detachment secondary to a malignant melanoma of the choroid. There are hard deposits in the attached retina adjacent to the tumor.

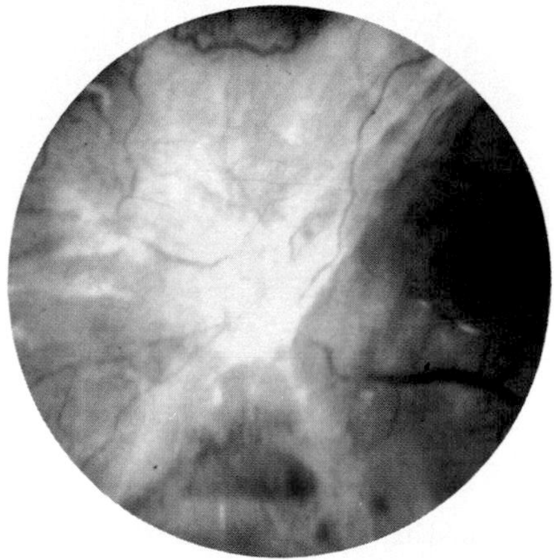

Epiretinal membrane, secondary to blunt ocular trauma, with severe distortion of the underlying sensory retina.

PLATE 3.

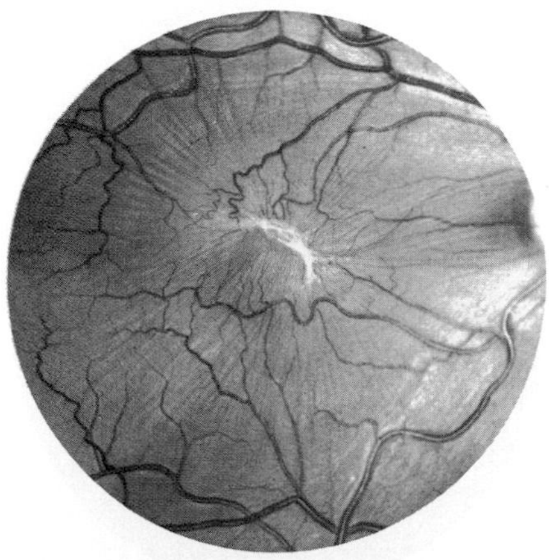

Minute epiretinal membrane involving fovea centralis and causing retinal striae and tortuosity of the retinal blood vessels.

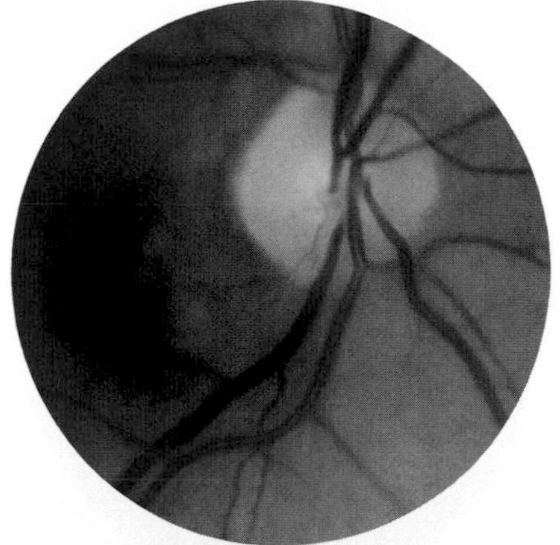

Large nevus of the choroid. Malignant melanomas may occur from preexisting nevi or may occur de novo. Malignant melanomas may also induce the formation of nevuslike structures at their base and periphery.

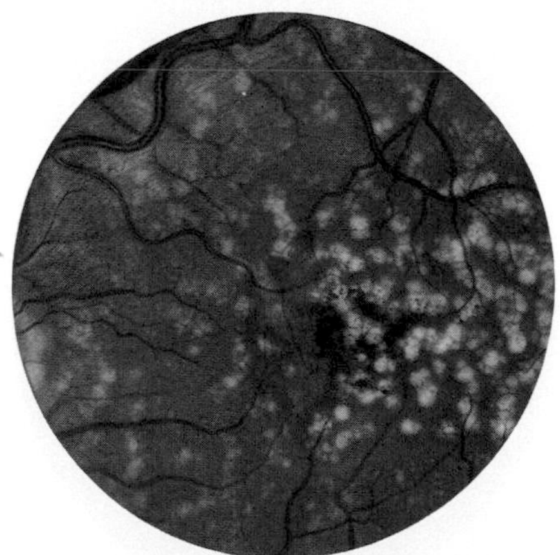

Retinal drusen (German: stony nodules) affecting the posterior retina. They form between the basement membrane and the Bruch membrane of the retinal pigment epithelium and predispose to macular degeneration. This patient retained 20/20 visual acuity.

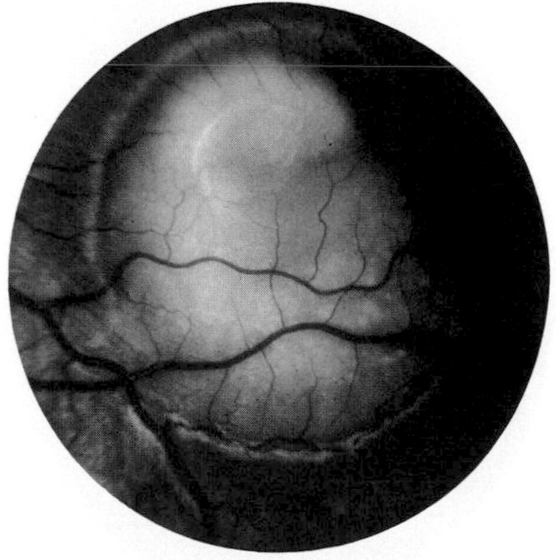

Vitelliform foveal dystrophy (Best disease), the early "egg-yolk" appearance and good central visual acuity. In adolescence the "egg" becomes scrambled and pigmented, the fundus loses its characteristic appearance, and there is loss of central vision with a pigmented scar.

PLATE 4.

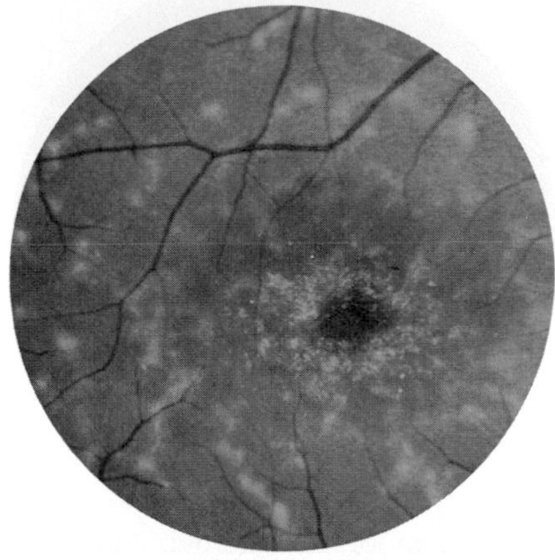

The multiple yellowish flecks of fundus flavimaculatus. Central vision is unaffected unless flecks develop in the fovea centralis.

Retinitis pigmentosa with peripheral pigmentary degeneration often described as "bone corpuscle." The peripheral visual field shrinks and the fovea centralis is affected late in the course of the disorder.

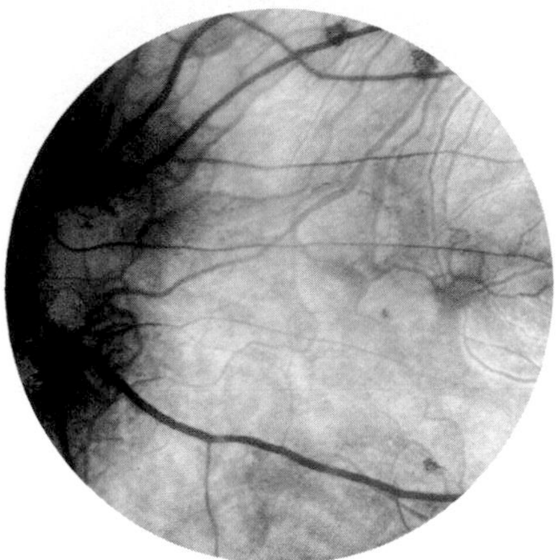

Choroideremia caused by progressive atrophy of the choriocapillaris, which results in atrophy of the retinal pigment epithelium and the outer layers of the sensory retina.

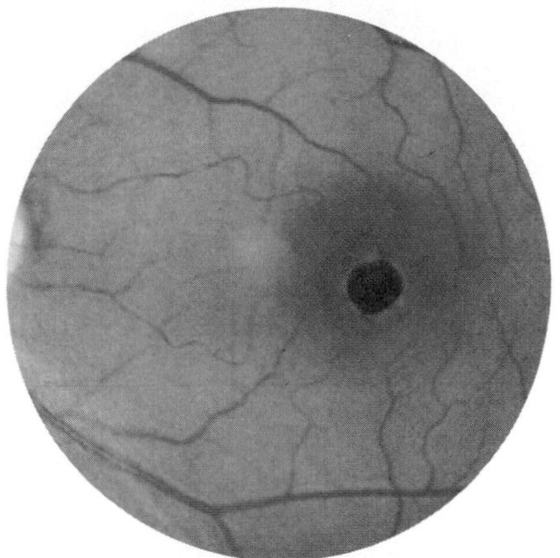

A macular hole that has destroyed the fovea centralis and reduced visual acuity to the 20/200 level. Traction on the sensory retina by contraction of the vitreous humor is the main cause.

PLATE 5.

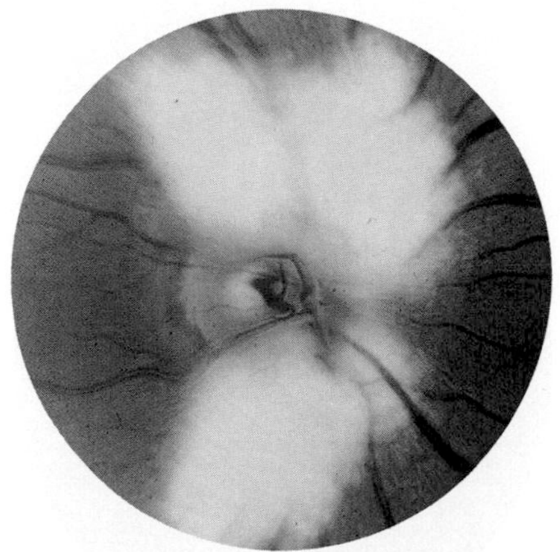

Myelinated (medullated) nerve fibers are usually seen ophthalmoscopically adjacent to the optic nerve. They have a dense white appearance, an arcuate shape, and feathery edges. Any portion of the nerve fiber layer of the retina may be myelinated.

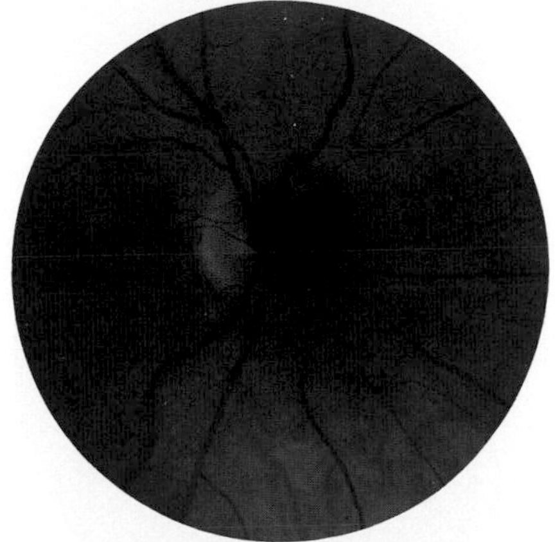

Melanocytoma (magnocellular nevus) of the optic disk located in its usual position on the temporal and inferior side of the disk. It shares with other nevi a low malignant potential.

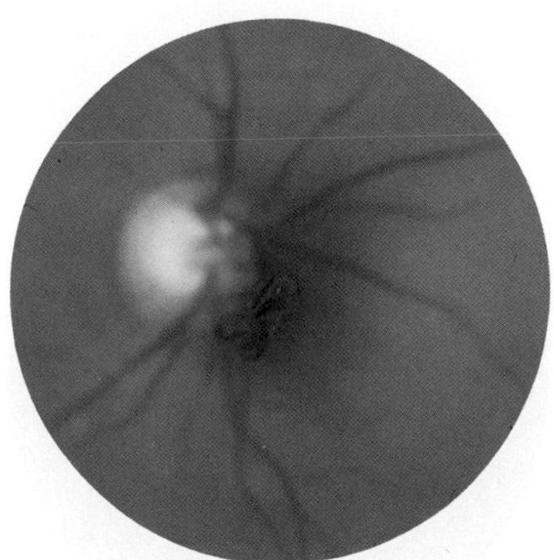

Persistent blood vessels of the fetal hyaloid vascular system on the surface of the optic disk.

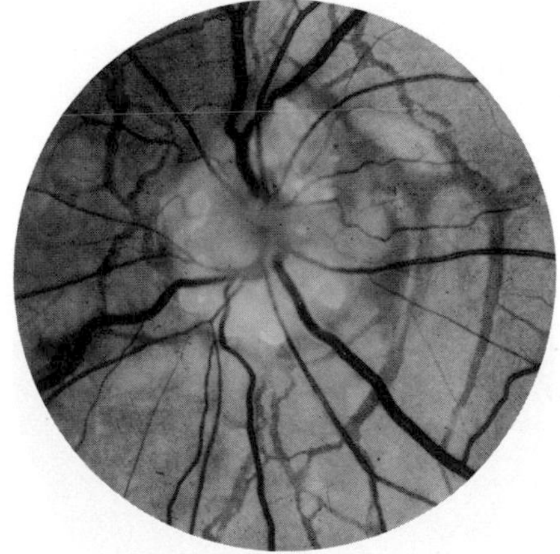

Drusen of the optic nerve are acellular, laminated calcareous bodies that originate in the optic nerve anterior to the lamina cribrosa and enlarge anteriorly. There are breaks in the Bruch membrane, which fill with fibrovascular tissue creating angioid streaks. This patient has pseudoxanthoma elasticum (Grönblad-Strandberg syndrome).

PLATE 6.

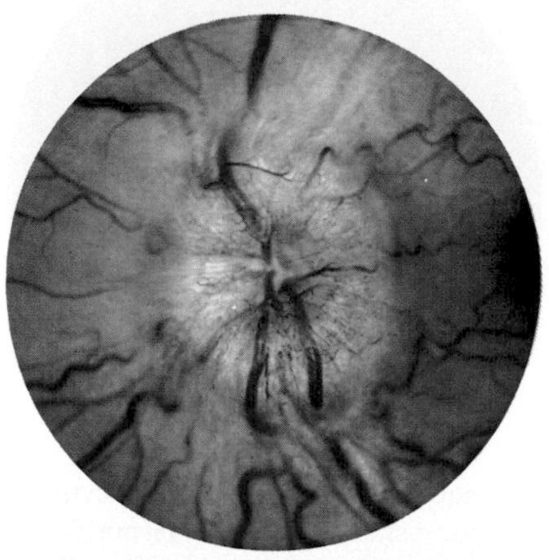

Papilledema with blurred margins of the optic disk, which is elevated above the level of the adjacent retina. The retinal veins are engorged because of impaired venous flow secondary to increased pressure within the subarachnoid space surrounding the optic nerve.

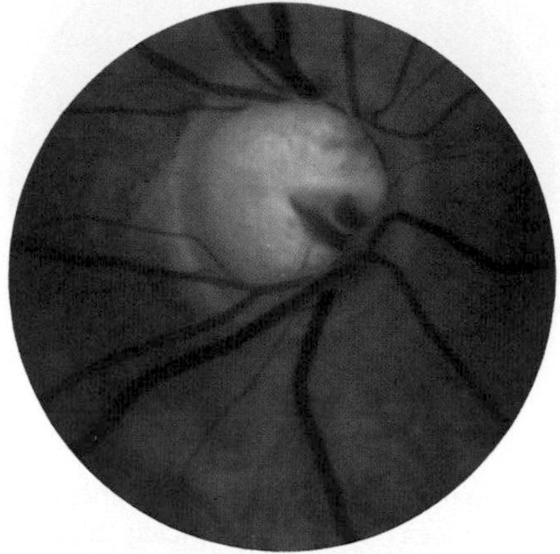

Open-angle glaucoma with advanced optic atrophy, excavation of the optic cup, and nasal displacement of the retinal blood vessels within the optic cup.

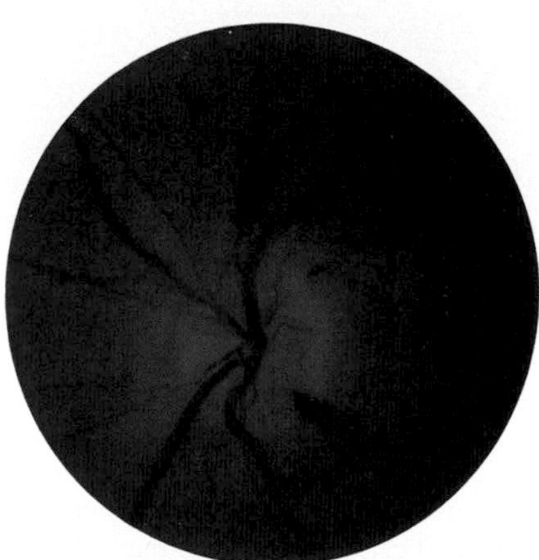

Papillitis in a patient with visual acuity reduced to 20/200. There are flame-shaped ("streak") hemorrhages in the 12 and 5 o'clock meridians.

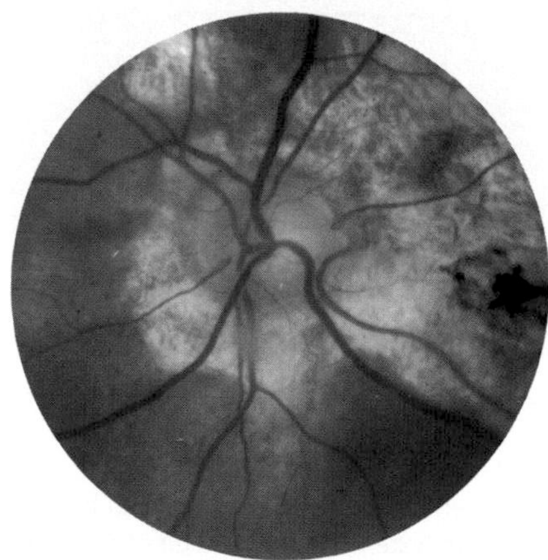

Degenerative myopia with conus of the optic nerve, chorioretinal atrophy, and proliferation of the retinal pigment epithelium.

PLATE 7.

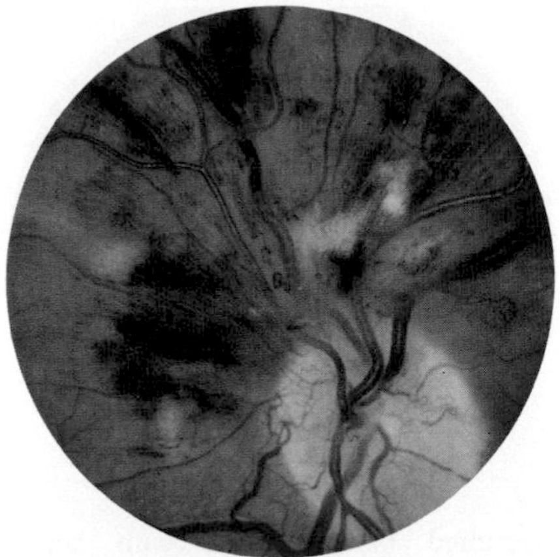

Superior temporal vein occlusion ("apoplexy" of the retina). The vein has likely been occluded with the intraocular portion of the optic nerve.

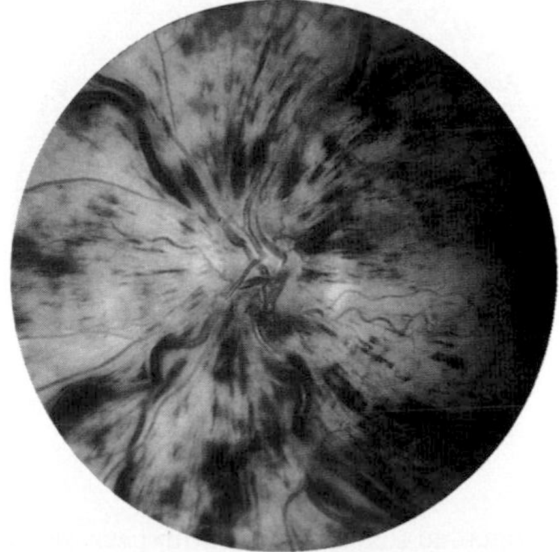

Central retinal vein occlusion. Branch vein occlusion and many central vein occlusions are the result of an atheromatous arterial plaque invading the adjacent vein at a crossing where the blood vessels share an adventitial sheath.

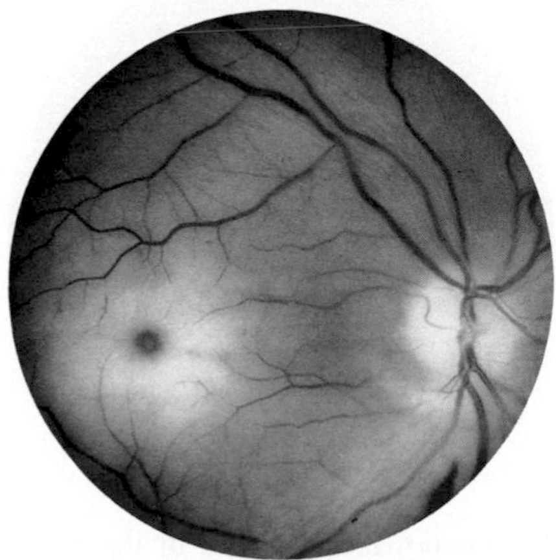

Central retinal artery occlusion with a cherry-red spot at the fovea centralis.

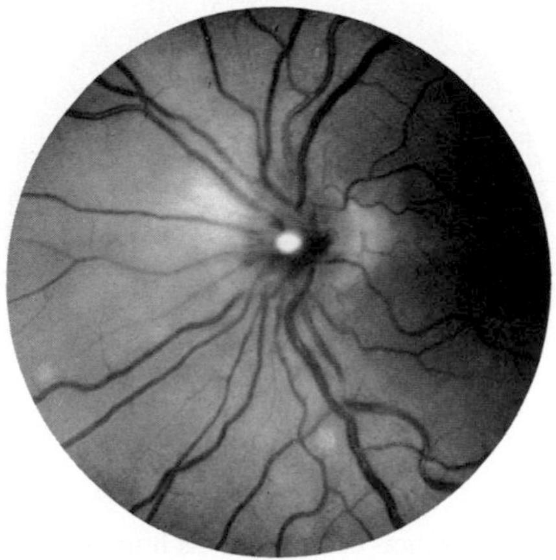

Cholesterol embolus in the central retinal artery.

PLATE 8.

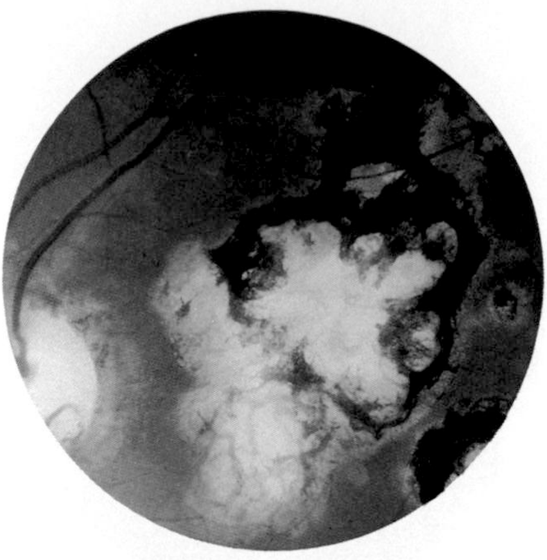

Congenital toxoplasmosis with necrosis of the retina and choroid (the white sclera is visible). In areas in which only the sensory retina has been inflamed the retinal pigment epithelium has proliferated (black regions). The necrosis of the ganglion cells of the fovea centralis caused atrophy of their axons, resulting in optic nerve atrophy.

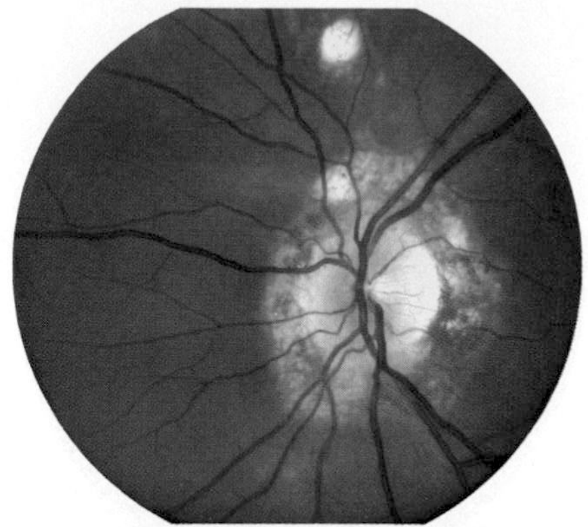

Presumed histoplasmosis with healed chorioretinitis adjacent to the optic disk (peripapillary). Above the disk is a round area of healed chorioretinitis without proliferation of the retinal pigment epithelium ("histo spot").

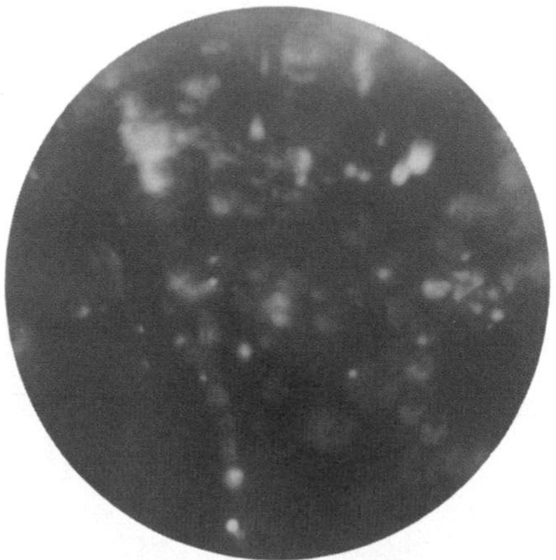

Degeneration of the vitreous humor in asteroid hyalosis in which calcium soaps aggregate on vitreous fibrils. There is rarely any decrease in visual acuity.

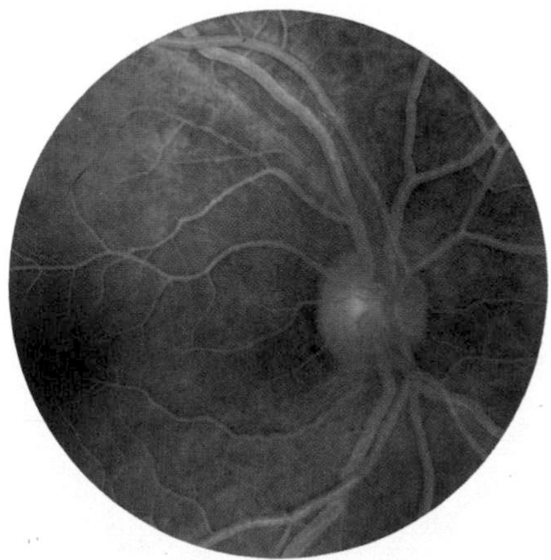

The abnormal appearance of the retinal blood vessels in lipemia retinalis in a patient in whom chylomicrons bound to lipids accumulate in the blood (chylomicronemia).

PLATE 9.

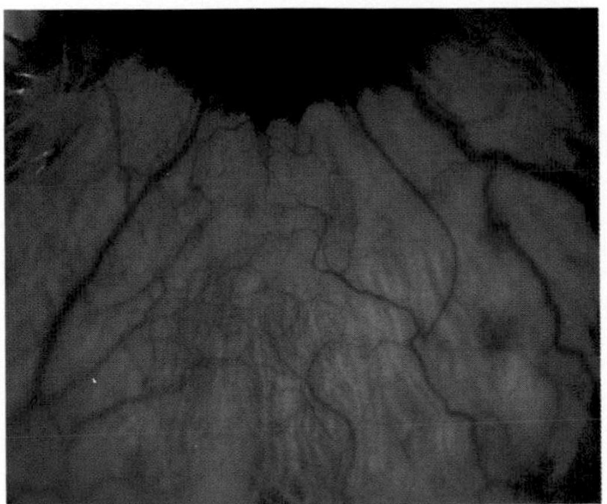

New blood vessels on the surface of the iris in diabetes mellitus (rubeosis iridis). The neovascularization is always associated with an advanced diabetic retinopathy.

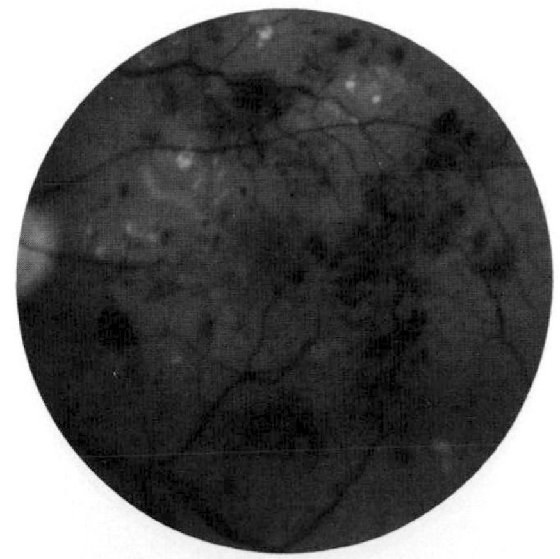

Background retinopathy in insulin-dependent diabetic retinopathy with many large and small hemorrhages and a few hard deposits (above) at the posterior pole of the eye. Fluorescein angiography demonstrates many microaneurysms, which appear with light ophthalmoscopy to be minute round hemorrhages.

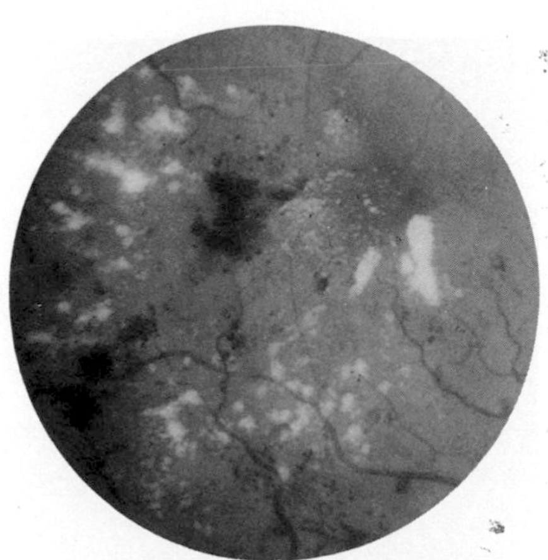

Macular edema with hard deposits surrounding vascular abnormalities at the fovea centralis in a patient with non–insulin-dependent diabetes mellitus.

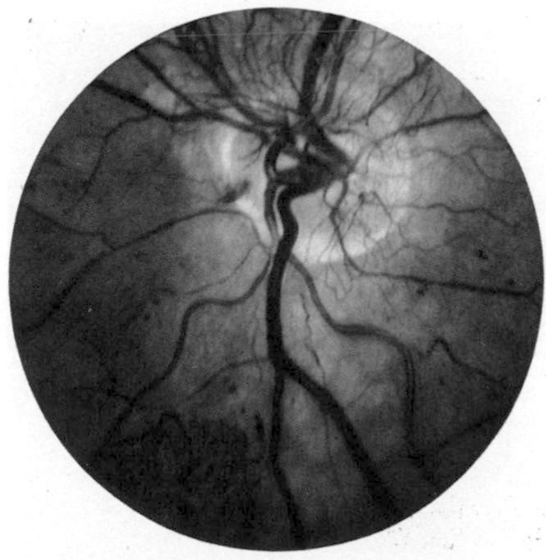

Proliferative retinopathy with conspicuous new blood vessels on the surface of the optic disk and a cluster of new retinal blood vessels at the 7 o'clock meridian.

PLATE 10.

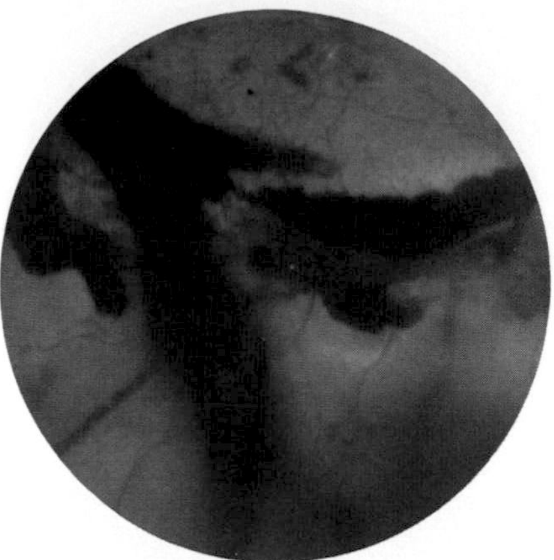

Vitreous hemorrhage in diabetes mellitus.

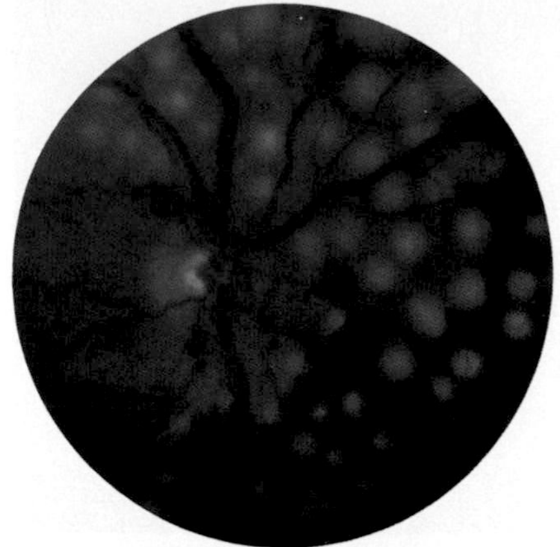

Fundus immediately after scatter photocoagulation of the nasal fundus for progressive retinopathy in diabetes mellitus.

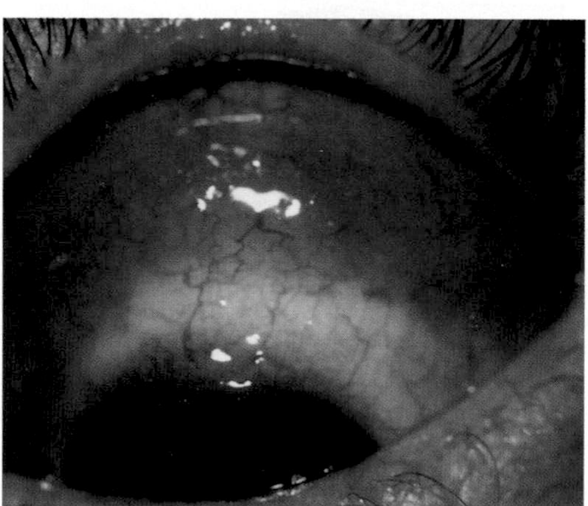

Lymphoma of the orbit evident subconjunctivally in a patient with proptosis.

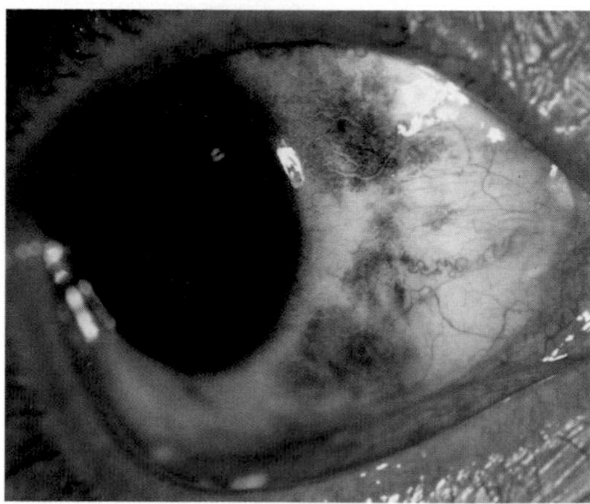

Melanosis bulbi with pigmentation of the sclera associated with a dark brown iris and dark brown fundus.

PLATE 11.

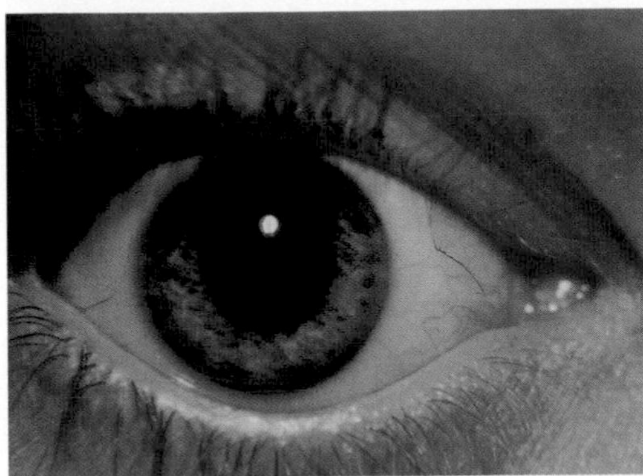

Kayser-Fleischer ring of the cornea in hepaticolenticular degeneration. Often the ring is not complete and can be detected only with high magnification.

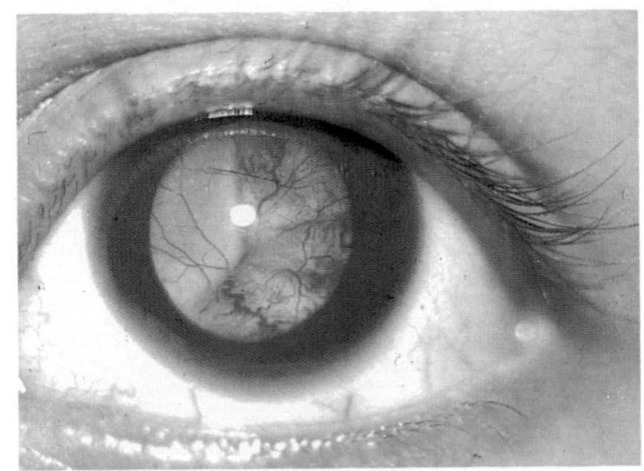

Leukocoria (white pupil; "cat's-eye" pupil) of an advanced retinoblastoma that fills the vitreous cavity adjacent to the crystalline lens. The eye is blind and the pupil does not react to light stimulation of the retina.

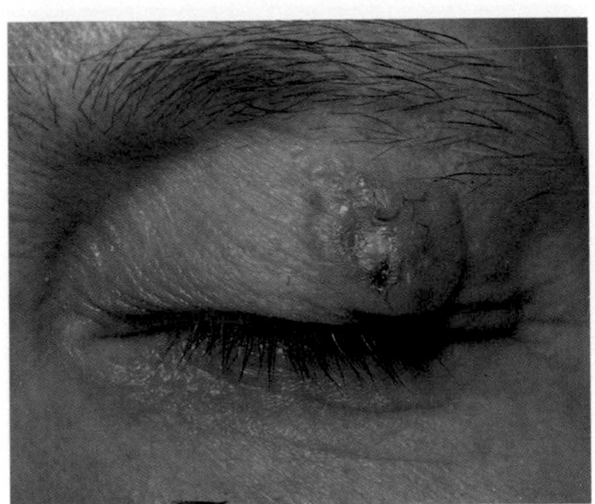

Basal cell carcinoma of the skin of the upper eyelid.

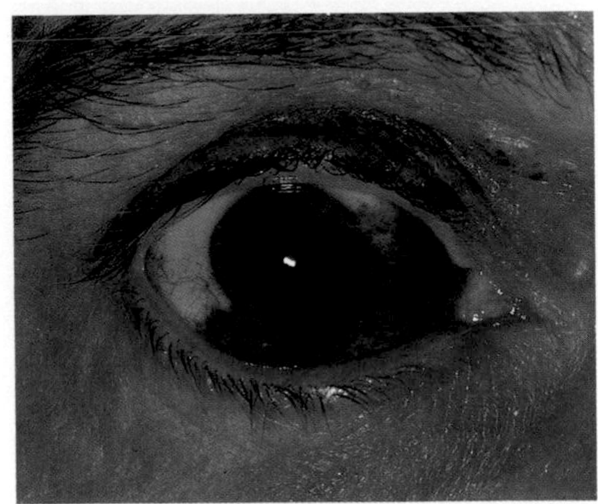

Subconjunctival hemorrhage. Most are spontaneous and require no treatment or diagnostic studies.

PLATE 12.

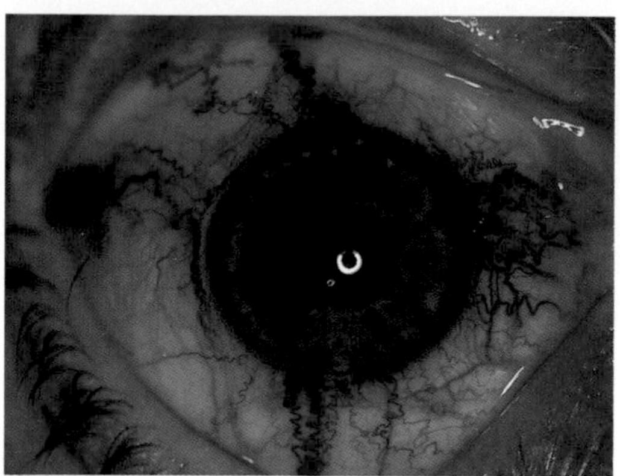

Anterior conjunctival veins that empty into anterior ciliary veins, which are dilated secondary to a fistula of the internal carotid artery into the cavernous sinus, into which the veins ultimately empty. The pattern of dilated veins forms a conjunctival "caput medusae."

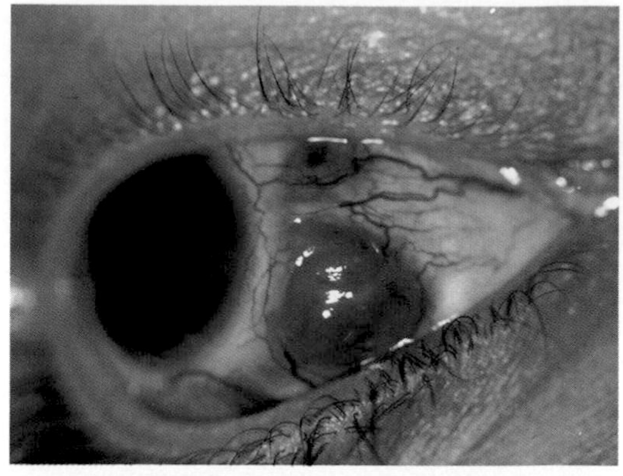

Scleromalacia perforans in a 62-year-old woman with severe rheumatoid arthritis.

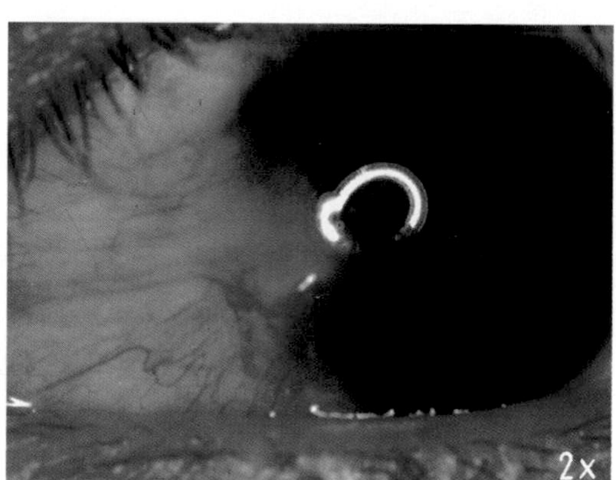

Pterygium encroaching on the cornea from its nasal side.

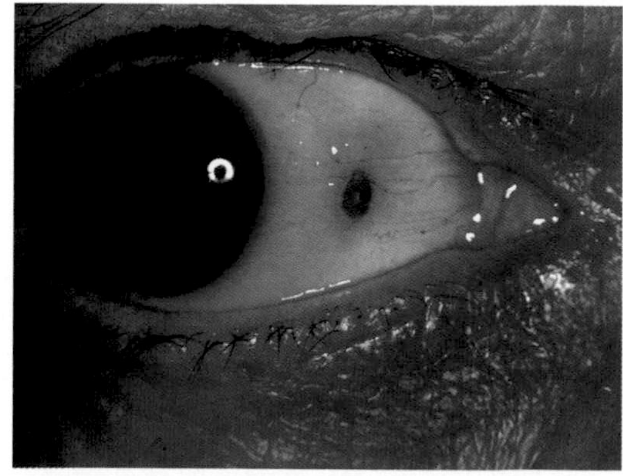

A deposition of calcium phosphate in the sclera of a 66-year-old man. Earlier the condition was mistakenly called a "senile hyaline plaque."

PLATE 13.

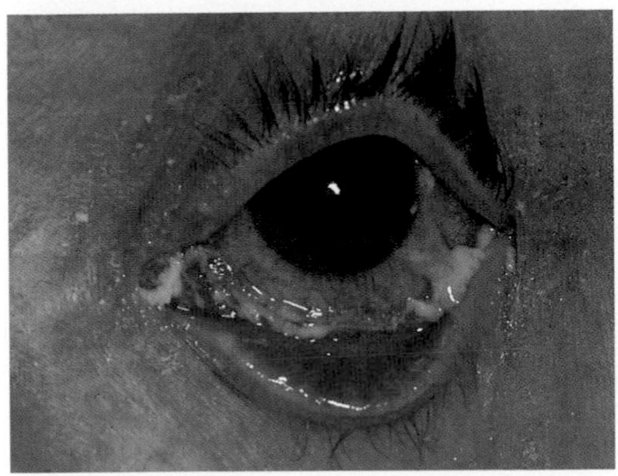

Acute conjunctivitis.

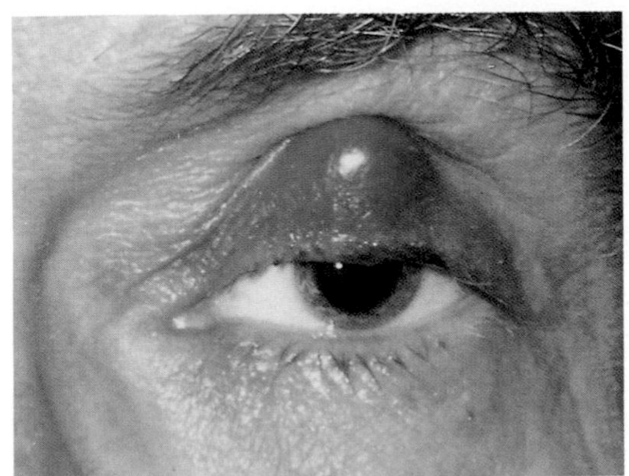

Acute chalazion of the upper eyelid. There is an associated preauricular adenopathy.

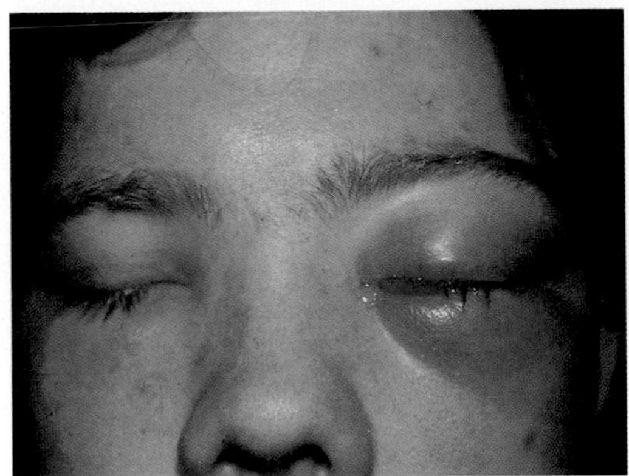

Acute anterior cellulitis.

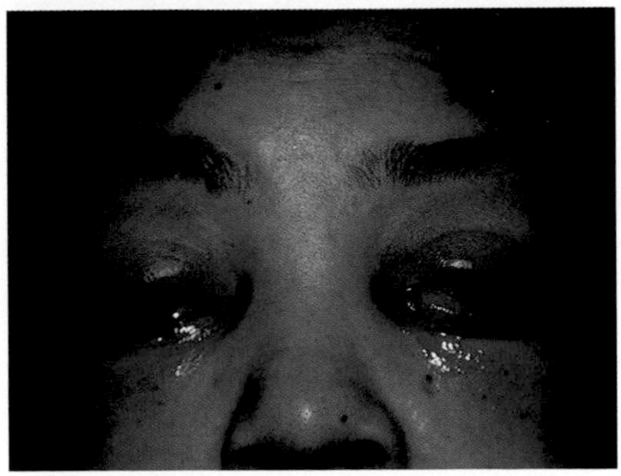

Acute conjunctival chemosis.

PLATE 14.

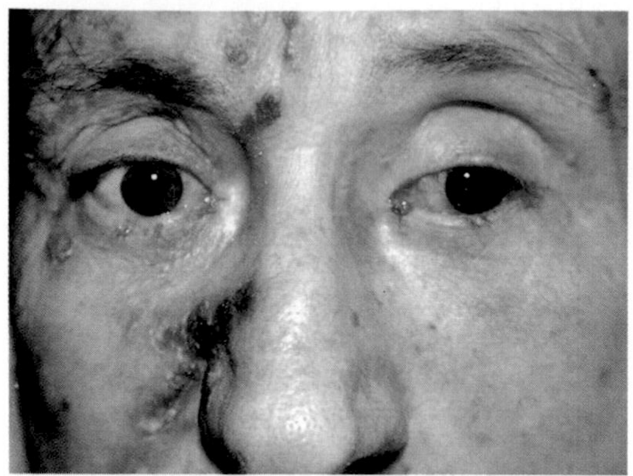

Herpes zoster ophthalmicus caused by replication of the varicella-zoster virus (herpesvirus 3) in the ophthalmic branch of the trigeminal nerve (N V). Usually if the tip of the nose is not affected (nasociliary nerve) in a cutaneous lesion the cornea also escapes inflammation, as in this patient.

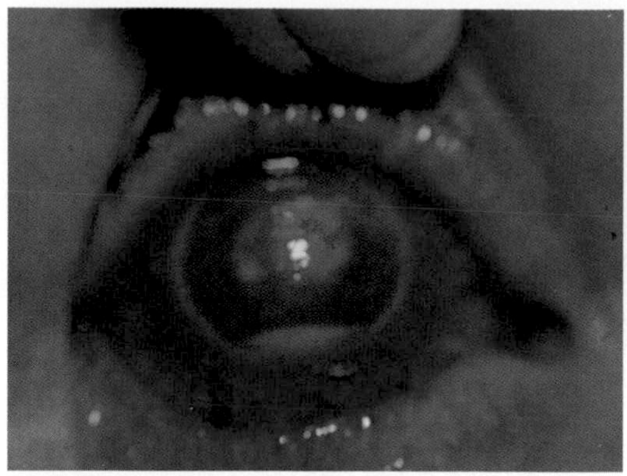

Pus in the inferior portion of the anterior chamber (hypopyon) associated with severe ciliary injection and a corneal ulcer (keratitis).

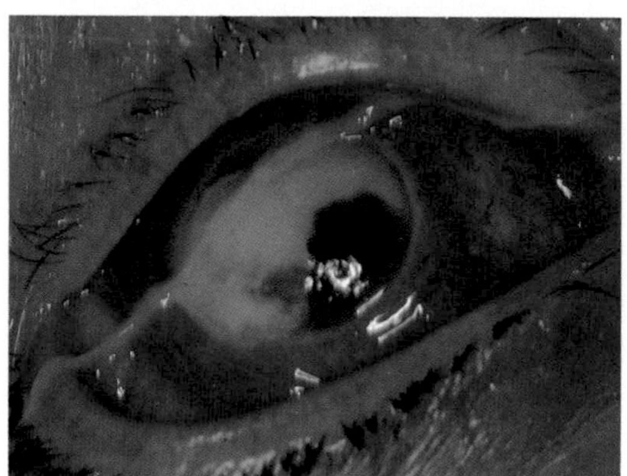

A bacterial corneal ulcer with pus covering much of the infected region. A fundamental principle in the management of corneal ulcers is to irrigate the eye frequently to remove secretions and the engulfed organisms.

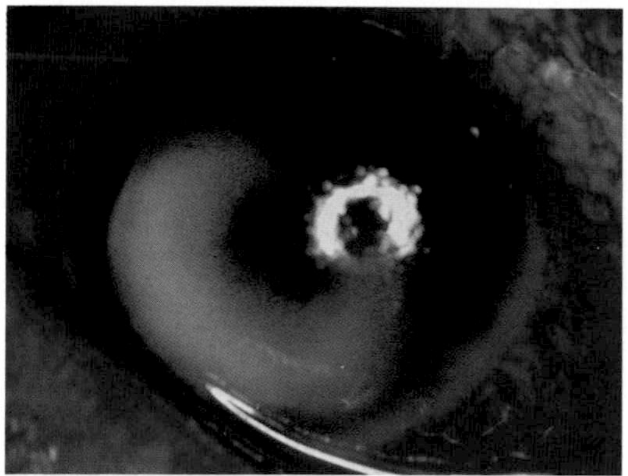

A corneal ulcer caused by a fungus. The cornea is not invaded by blood vessels in fungal infections.

PLATE 15.

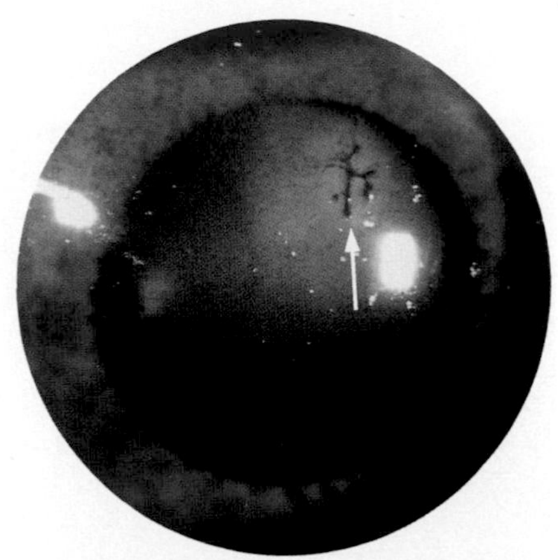

Early dendritic keratitis with the branching linear lesion stained with rose bengal. The patient had an infantile systemic infection with *Herpesvirus hominis* type I with reactivation of the virus causing the keratitis.

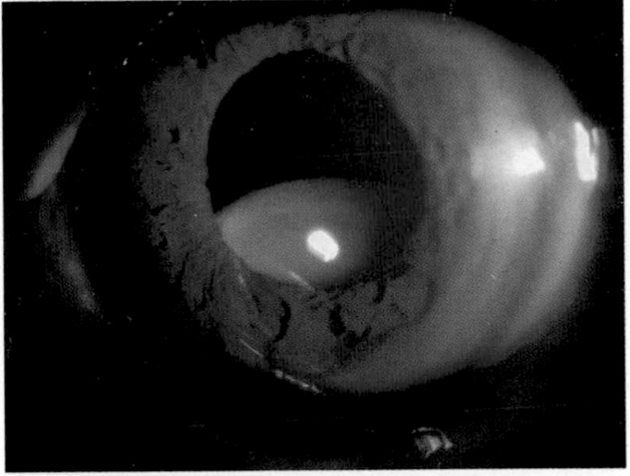

Ectopia lentis (subluxation of the crystalline lens) in Marfan syndrome. Persistent zonular fibers act as a hinge and prevent complete dislocation of the lens.

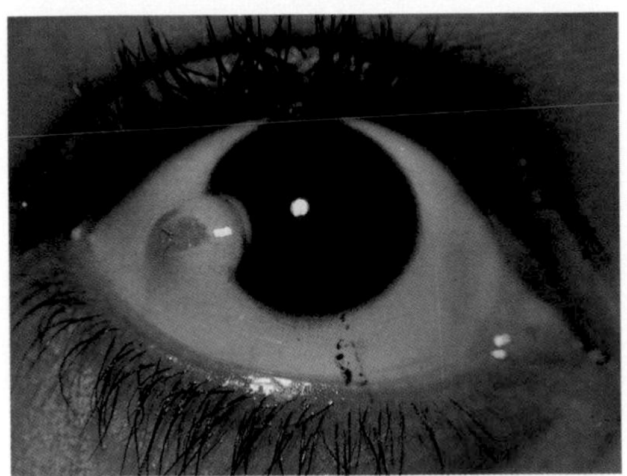

A dermoid of the corneoscleral limbus. It is covered with epithelium (conjunctival and corneal) and contains tissue not normally found in the region (choristomatous tissue).

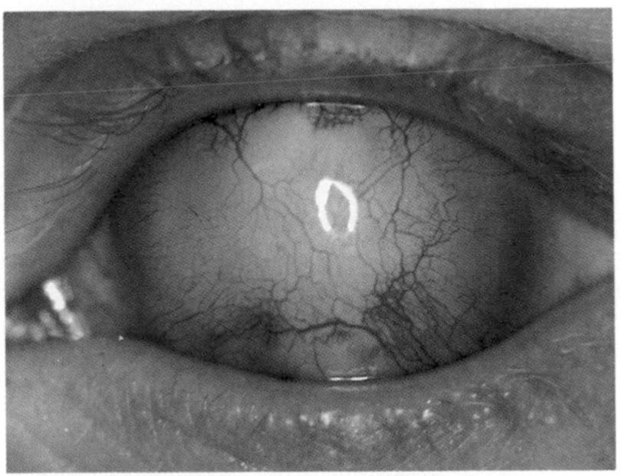

A corneal leukoma in which all layers of the cornea have been converted to fibroblastic tissue with new blood vessel formation inferiorly.

PLATE 16.

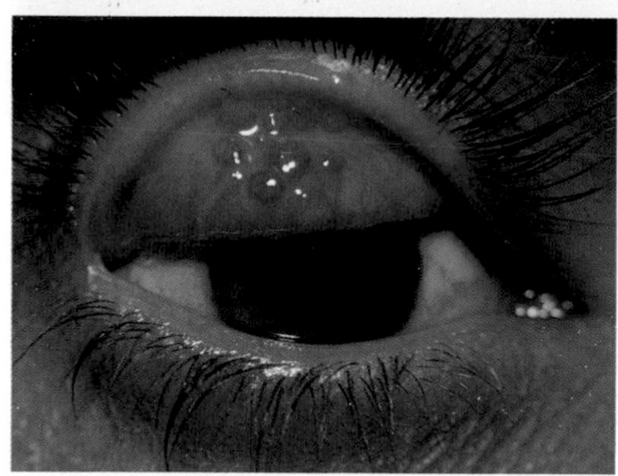

Follicles (lymphoid hyperplasia) of the tarsal conjunctiva of the upper eyelid in a patient with vernal conjunctivitis.

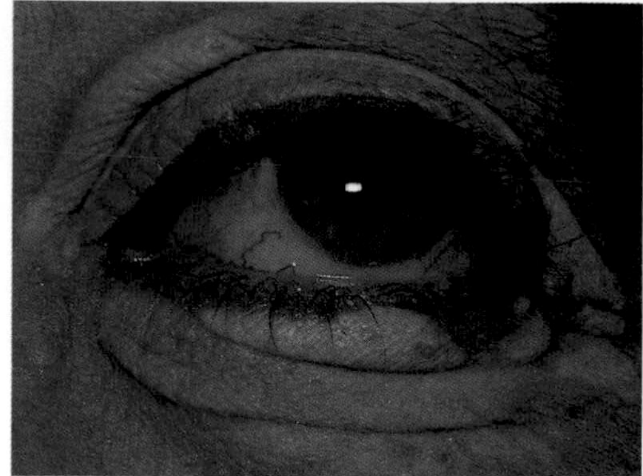

Xanthelasma of the eyelids in an elderly woman. The lesions contain clusters of foam cells, which contain lipids, in the superficial dermis.

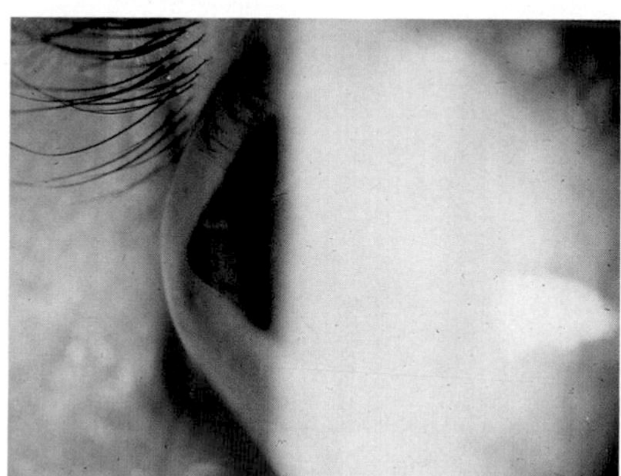

Profile of the cornea in keratoconus. On downward gaze the cone causes the lower eyelid to bulge (Munson sign).

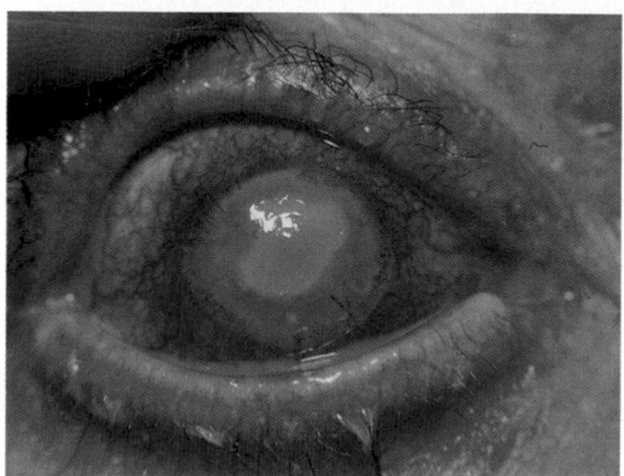

Central corneal ulcer stained with fluorescein. There is marked injection of the ciliary blood vessels.

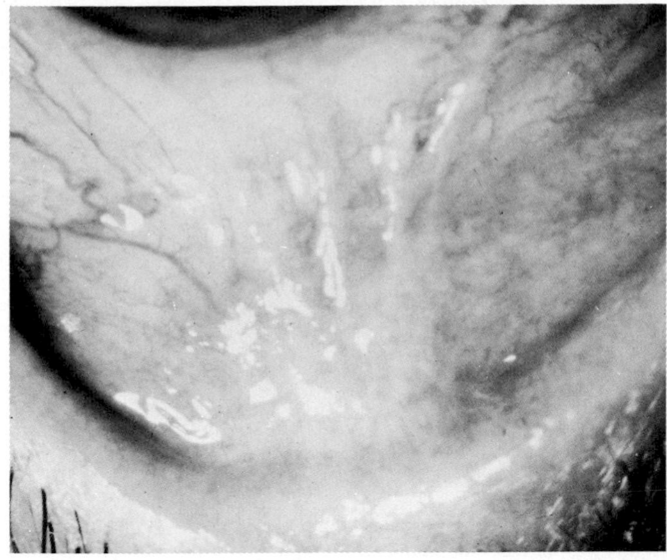

FIG 10-2.
Symblepharon after alkali burn of the bulbar and palpebral conjunctiva.

cence of the overlying epithelium exposes the concretion and causes a foreign body sensation. The deposits may be shelled out of the tissue with a sharp needle after instillation of a topical anesthetic.

GRANULATION TISSUE

Granulation tissue may proliferate after faulty closure of the conjunctival incision in operations for strabismus or retinal detachment. There is a large, red, fungating mass that bleeds readily. Usually simple excision and closure of the conjunctival opening will correct the problem.

SYMBLEPHARON

Symblepharon is a condition in which there are adhesions between the palpebral and bulbar conjunctivae (Fig 10-2). It may obliterate conjunctival cul-de-sacs or form bands of scar tissue. Scarring results from conditions in which apposed areas of the conjunctiva lose their epithelial coverings. The chief causes are chemical burns (particularly caustics), thermal burns, trachoma, erythema multiforme (Stevens-Johnson syndrome), ocular cicatricial pemphigoid, and membranous conjunctivitis. The adhesions cause a mechanical defect, since the eyelids are adherent to the eyeball, and desiccation of the cornea and keratitis occurs because of exposure, loss of conjunctival goblet cells, and atresia of the orifices of accessory and main lacrimal gland ducts.

Treatment frequently is ineffective and disappointing. In the early stages it is directed toward periodic lysis of the adhesions with a glass rod (such as a clinical thermometer) and protection of the cornea with a large, soft corneoconjunctival contact lens. Replacement of the scarred conjunctiva with a mucous membrane graft from the mouth or the inferior nasal turbinate, or conjunctiva from the fellow normal eye, may be required.

TUMORS, CYSTS, AND NEOPLASMS

Choristomas.—Choristomas are congenital tumors composed of tissues that are not normally found in the region.

Dermoid cysts of the conjunctiva may be cystic or solid and contain stratified squamous epithelium, hair follicles, sebaceous glands, hair shafts, brown tissue, teeth, and debris. An epidermal cyst contains stratified squamous epithelium only. A dermatolipoma occurs usually at the superior temporal corneoscleral limbus and appears as a sharply circumscribed, round, slightly yellowish, elevated mass involving the cornea and the sclera. It occurs frequently in mandibulofacial dysostosis. The Goldenhar syndrome (oculoauriculovertebral dysplasia) consists of bilateral epibulbar dermoids combined with appendages and fistulas of the ear and fusion of the cervical spine.

Hamartomas.—Hamartomas are congenital tumors composed of tissues that normally occur in the region, such as hemangiomas, lymphangiomas, and the tumors of the phacomatoses. Hemangiomas and lymphangiomas mainly occur in the orbit and seldom affect the conjunctiva.

Nevi.—Nevi occur commonly, often near the corneoscleral limbus, but may involve the conjunctiva anywhere. They appear as yellowish red areas or deeply pigmented masses and occur usually before the age of 20 years. Sometimes nonpigmented nevi cause alarm when they become pigmented, usually at puberty. Nevi are usually not excised unless cosmetically undesirable or if they enlarge enough to irritate the eye or suggest malignant degeneration.

Telangiectasis.—Telangiectasis of the conjunctiva occurs in all cases of ataxia telangiectasia (Louis-Bar syndrome). There is nystagmus, progressive cerebellar ataxia, deficiency in IgA, and impaired lymphocyte transformation (see Chapter 26).

Conjunctival intraepithelial epithelioma (carcinoma in situ).—This is a slow-growing, dysplastic, squamous cell tumor that usually involves the bulbar conjunctiva in the interpalpebral space in men. The tumor is usually solitary and consists of a sharply demarcated, slightly elevated, reddish gray, gelatinous-appearing mass that may develop a dense white appearance (leukoplakia) secondary to keratinization of its surface. The tumor cells may remain precancerous or undergo malignant transformation to squamous cell carcinoma, which may metastasize. Complete excision is followed by radiation therapy to prevent recurrence.

Squamous cell carcinoma.—Squamous cell carcinoma (Fig 10-3) may be confined to the superficial conjunctiva, or it may invade the adjacent tissues, such as the eye or orbit. The tumor is extremely sensitive to radiation, which should be used if excisional biopsy fails. Basal cell carcinoma rarely affects the conjunctiva.

Malignant melanoma.—Malignant melanoma of the conjunctiva most commonly originates from benign conjunctival melanosis (75%), from degeneration of a nevus (20%), or as a primary tumor (5%). Malignant degeneration in primary melanosis is suggested by nodular thickening of the conjunctiva, bleeding, or fixation of the pigmented area to the underlying tissue. Malignant degeneration of a nevus is suggested by growth or bleeding. Primary tumors without preexisting lesions most commonly occur at the corneoscleral limbus. Regional lymphatics (preauricular, submandibular, and cervical) should be palpated for possible extension. Tumors of the fornices, palpebral conjunctiva, or caruncle have a poor prognosis. Exenteration of the orbit or dissection of the neck does not improve the prognosis.

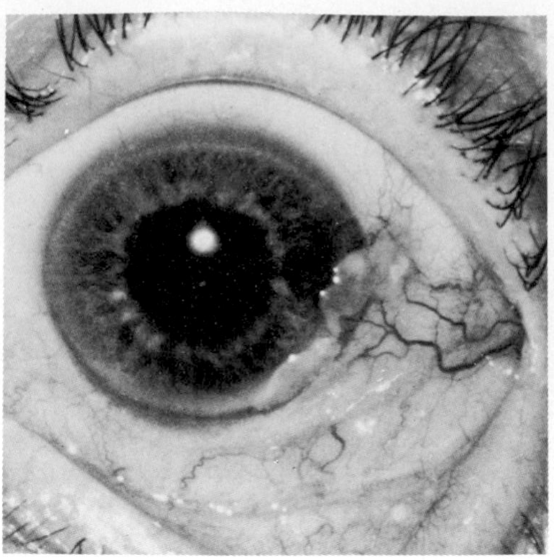

FIG 10-3.
Squamous cell carcinoma of the conjunctiva at the corneoscleral limbus. These tumors occur particularly in compromised hosts, and this 76-year-old patient had a pulmonary mass that could not be diagnosed.

Kaposi sarcoma.—Kaposi sarcoma occurs in about 10% of patients with acquired immunodeficiency syndrome (AIDS) (see Chapter 25). A diffuse or nodular, reddish or bluish tumor may involve the conjunctiva. The tumor responds readily to radiation.

BIBLIOGRAPHY

Book

Fraunfelder FT, Roy FH: *Current ocular therapy 4*, Philadelphia, 1994, WB Saunders.

Articles

Bernauer W, Broadway DC, Wright P: Chronic progressive conjunctival cicatrisation, *Eye* 7:371-378, 1993.

Liesegang TJ: Pigmented conjunctival and scleral lesions, *Mayo Clin Proc* 69:151-161, 1994.

Yunis JJ, Mobini N, Yunis EJ, Alper CA, Deulofeut R, Rodriguez A et al: Common major histocompatibility complex class II markers in clinical variants of cicatricial pemphigoid, *Proc Natl Acad Sci USA* 91:7747-7751, 1994.

11

THE CORNEA

The cornea is the transparent, avascular structure that forms the anterior one sixth of the outer coat of the eye. Through it the iris pattern and the black pupil are clearly visible. At its junction with the sclera is a transitional zone, the corneoscleral limbus. Here the corneal epithelium is continuous with that of the conjunctiva. The corneal stroma terminates, and its endothelium becomes discontinuous and merges with the trabecular endothelium.

The precorneal tear film (see Chapter 2), the most anterior layer of the cornea, covers a constantly renewed epithelium whose basement membrane is attached to the corneal stroma. The substantia proporia or stroma constitutes 90% of the cornea; its anterior condensation, to which the basement membrane of the epithelium attaches, is the Bowman zone. The cornea is lined by a single endothelial cell layer adjacent to the aqueous humor of the anterior chamber. Descemet membrane, the basement membrane of the endothelium, separates the endothelium from the corneal stroma. The central cornea requires atmospheric oxygen for its aerobic metabolism; the peripheral cornea is nurtured by the superficial and deep corneal plexuses derived from the anterior ciliary arteries. The cornea is innervated by nonmedullated sensory nerve fibers that mainly pass to the long and short ciliary nerves of the ophthalmic branch of the trigeminal nerve (N V_1). The sensory nerves of the inferior portion of the cornea pass to the infraorbital branch of the maxillary division of the trigeminal nerve (N V_2).

The cornea, with its +42-diopter refractive power, is the principal refractive surface of the eye because it separates air, with an index of refraction of 1.0, and aqueous humor, with an index of refraction of 1.34. The regular arrangement of the 200 corneal lamellae, the scarcity of keratocytes, the absence of blood vessels, and deturgescence (dehydration) make the cornea transparent. Corneal transparency requires integrity of both the epithelium and the endothelium.

The corneal epithelium consists of stratified squamous epithelium, five to six cell layers thick. Toward the corneal periphery the number of layers increases to eight to ten and the corneal epithelium merges with the epithelium of the conjunctiva; thus, the conjunctiva and cornea are often simultaneously inflamed. The basement membrane of the corneal epithelium is attached to the underlying anterior condensation of the stroma (Bowman zone). The corneal epithelium is constantly renewed, with cells replicating in the basal zone and exfoliated from the superficial zone some 5 to 7 days later. Injury to the corneal epithelium resulting in exposed nerve endings causes severe pain. There may be subepithelial edema, but the anterior condensation of the corneal stroma (Bowman zone) prevents swelling of the stroma. When the cornea is deprived of atmospheric oxygen, as, for example, by a contact lens that is not permeable to air, a subepithelial edema develops (Sattler veil). The edema disappears rapidly when the cornea is in contact with the atmosphere.

The substantia propria or stroma consists of 200 collagenous lamellae arranged nearly parallel to the corneal surface. There are no blood vessels; scattered throughout are keratocytes and occasional leukocytes.

The endothelial layer is of neural crest origin. It is composed of a single layer of five- and six-sided cells that separate the corneal stroma from the anterior chamber. The basement membrane of the endothelium is Descemet membrane, which stops abruptly at the corneoscleral limbus. The endothelium prevents aqueous humor from entering the cornea and pumps fluid from the corneal stroma to the anterior chamber. The corneal endothelial cells in adult humans do not replicate. When they are damaged, the uninjured surrounding cells increase in size to cover the areas. If the area cannot be covered, a generalized edema of the corneal stroma (bullous keratopathy) follows.

SYMPTOMS AND SIGNS OF CORNEAL DISEASE

The three main symptoms of corneal disease are (1) reduced vision, (2) pain, and (3) iridescent vision. Connective tissue scarring, hereditary opacification (dystrophy), blood vessels, stromal edema, accumulations of leukocytes, and irregularities of the surfaces each may interfere with clear image formation and reduce vision.

The corneal epithelium is innervated by sensory nerves that do not have Schwann sheaths. Epithelial defects cause discomfort that may be described as a foreign body sensation, burning of the eyes, or pain so severe that it incapacitates the individual. Reflex lacrimation may occur.

Iridescent vision results from edema of the corneal epithelium, which causes a prismatic effect in which white light is divided into its component parts with blue in the center and red on the outside. The iridescence combined with the round pupil creates a halo in which lights are surrounded by a shimmering rainbow.

The exposed position of the cornea and the lamination of the tissue allow easy observation and precise localization of defects. Inspection through a +20-diopter condensing lens combined with penlight illumination often provides adequate magnification. Attention is directed to the diameter of the cornea, its curvature, and the presence or absence of opacities in the normally transparent tissue. The normal cornea reflects a clear image from its surface. The abnormal cornea reflects a dull, distorted image. Corneal opacities or aqueous humor opacities may obscure the pattern of the iris and prevent observation of the normally black pupil. Fluorescein strips or a sterile 2% solution stain areas of absent corneal epithelium bright green. Corneal sensation is measured by touching the cornea with a wisp of cotton and observing the eyelid closure reflex. Many conjunctival abnormalities, lacrimal disorders, and eyelid disorders may result in corneal disease.

OPACITIES

Opacities in the cornea may be central or peripheral. When located in the visual axis they may impair vision. A minor scar may severely distort vision because it alters the smooth curvature of the corneal refractive surface (irregular astigmatism). Three types of opacities affect the cornea:

1. Leukoma, in which the involved portion of the cornea is totally opaque. Localized leukoma appears as a whitish scar surrounded by normal cornea. In generalized leukoma the entire cornea is white, often with conspicuous blood vessels coursing across its surface.
2. Macula, in which the opacity is more transparent than in leukoma.
3. Nebula, which is a minor decrease in transparency.

Epithelial defects heal without scarring, but defects of the Bowman zone and the stroma heal with permanent opacification. The human endothelium does not replicate, and if there are too few endothelial cells to cover a defect, stromal edema occurs. A corneal scar to which the iris is adherent is called an adherent leukoma.

Congenital leukomas (opacities).—The embryologic formation of the cornea is complex. The epithelium is derived from surface ectoderm. The keratocytes of the stroma, Descemet membrane, and the endothelium are derived from neural crest cells (mesenchyme). (Most of

TABLE 11-1.
Some Congenital Corneal Opacities (Skeletal Malformations May Occur with All)

Axenfeld anomaly (posterior embryotoxon)
Opacity of posterior peripheral cornea with iris processes extending from peripheral iris to the opacity
Congenital corneal staphyloma
Severe Peters anomaly (see below)
Cornea plana
Flat, thin cornea sometimes occurring with scleroderma
Peters anomaly
Iris processes extend from collarette to margin of central leukoma
Posterior keratoconus
Dome-shaped posterior corneal defect
Rieger anomaly
Thickening of peripheral termination of Descemet membrane (Schwalbe line) to which iris processes from hypoplastic iris adhere
Sclerocornea
Peripheral or diffuse corneal opacification with widespread intraocular malformation: trisomy 18

the periocular mesenchyme is of neural crest origin, as there are no mesodermal somites in the head and neck region.) Opacification of the cornea (Table 11-1) may be the result of several mechanisms, either singly or in combination: (1) the lens vesicle may not fully separate from the surface ectoderm; (2) the endothelium may fail to form; (3) the cornea and the sclera may not differentiate (sclerocornea); or (4) the corneal stroma may be thinned. Embryogenesis of the cornea and anterior chamber angle is closely related, and congenital corneal opacities are often associated with abnormalities of the iridocorneal angle and abnormal iris processes between the peripheral iris and cornea.

Neurocristopathies.—The neural crest cells that cap the primitive neural tube migrate and differentiate to evolve into many structures. Neural crest cells either form or contribute to the formation of pigment cells (except those of the optic cup), parasympathetic and sympathetic ganglia, oligodendroglia, Schwann sheath cells, cranial nerves, membranous bones of the head, vascular pericytes, sclera, corneal stroma and endothelium, and the anterior chamber recess. Many developmental abnormalities of neural crest origin (neurocristopathies) involve either the head or eye (Table 11-2) or other systems.

TABLE 11-2.
Some Ocular Disorders of Neural Crest Origin

Deficient neural crest formation
Brain-face-eye malformations: cyclopia, facial hemiatrophy
Abnormal migration of neural crest cells
Congenital glaucoma
Posterior embryotoxon
Axenfeld anomaly
Rieger anomaly
Sclerocornea
Peters anomaly
Treacher Collins syndrome
Abnormal proliferation of neural crest cells
Iridocorneal-endothelial syndromes
Waardenburg syndrome
Abnormal terminal differentiation of neural crest cells
Hereditary endothelial dystrophy
Posterior polymorphous dystrophy
Fuchs endothelial dystrophy
Generalized neurocristopathies with ocular signs
Pheochromocytoma
Neuroblastoma
Medullary carcinoma of the thyroid
Hirschsprung disease (heterochromia iridis)
Neurofibromatosis type 1 (Von Recklinghausen)
Neurofibromatosis type 2 (acoustic neuroma)
Multiple endocrine neoplasia type IIb (III)
Neurocutaneous melanomas

CORNEAL VASCULARIZATION

The central cornea has no blood vessels but requires atmospheric oxygen for its aerobic metabolism. The peripheral cornea is nurtured by superficial and deep arteries at the corneoscleral limbus. The superficial corneal vascular plexus is the source of new subepithelial blood vessels. Interstitial (anterior stromal) neovascularization originates from the deep corneal plexus. Apposition of the major arterial circle of the iris or radial vessels of the iris to the cornea results in neovascularization of the posterior corneal stroma. Blood vessels may extend centrally from the entire corneal circumference or radially from a portion of the corneal margin (fascicular). Subepithelial neovascularization combined with fibroblastic proliferation is called pannus; it often involves the superior portion of the cornea.

In the acute stage of corneal neovascularization, the new blood vessels are easily visible.

After the disease causing neovascularization subsides, the vessels may appear as a grayish bloodless network (ghost vessels) in a relatively clear cornea. Corneal neovascularization is part of the normal inflammatory response, and many corneal inflammations and infections resolve quickly after vascularization. The most serious consequence of corneal vascularization is the loss of corneal transparency combined with a biochemical modification of the corneal tissue, which is converted from an avascular tissue that does not fully participate in the body's tissue immunity to one that has a direct blood supply and partakes of antigen-antibody reactions.

CORNEAL EDEMA

To maintain the cornea in its relatively deturgesced (dehydrated) state requires an intact and functional corneal epithelium and endothelium. The desmosomes of the superficial layer of epithelial cells provide a barrier to external fluids, and the endothelium removes fluid from the corneal stroma. Damage to either of these structures may result in corneal edema. (Drugs must be lipid-soluble to penetrate the epithelium and water-soluble to penetrate the stroma and endothelium [see Chapter 3].)

If the corneal epithelium is deprived of atmospheric oxygen, as for example with a hard contact lens, or if the intraocular pressure rapidly increases to more than 50 mm Hg, an epithelial and a subepithelial edema develops. The compact structure of the Bowman zone prevents edema from extending to the stroma. The cornea appears dull and hazy. The patient has decreased visual acuity and iridescent vision. The edema rapidly disappears when the cause is removed.

Edema of the corneal stroma indicates the failure of the corneal endothelium to transport fluid adequately from the stroma to the aqueous humor. With minor degrees of edema, the cornea is thickened and has a dull appearance. In severe instances, the epithelium may be edematous; the condition is called bullous keratopathy. Vision is severely depressed.

Pseudophakic bullous keratopathy follows cataract extraction in which there are too few corneal endothelial cells to maintain corneal deturgescence (dehydration). Injury to the endothelium in intraocular surgery is its cause. To protect the corneal endothelium during cataract extraction, the anterior chamber is filled with a viscoelastic solution that is irrigated from the eye at the conclusion of the operation.

Endothelial-epithelial dystrophy is the chief cause of nonsurgical bullous keratopathy (see Corneal Dystrophies).

PIGMENTATION

Blood staining of the cornea is caused by blood in the anterior chamber combined with glaucoma, damage to the endothelium, or a corneoscleral incision. The anterior layers of the corneal stroma are transparent, but hemoglobin products in the posterior portion create a rusty to yellow-green colored opacity.

A brownish subepithelial line occurs in normal eyes (Hudson-Stähli line: horizontal), at the base of the cone in keratoconus (Fleischer ring: circular), at the head of a pterygium (Stocker line: vertical arc), immediately anterior to a filtering bleb (Ferry line: horizontal), and after disturbances of the corneal epithelium. Pigmented subepithelial scars occur in about 10% of patients who have a radial keratotomy to correct refractive errors. Pigment lines are composed of ferritin deposited in widened intracellular spaces and within intracytoplasmic vacuoles of the corneal epithelium. Ferritin has a protein shell (apoferritin) and a core of ferric hydroxide. The mechanism of its deposition in the cornea is not known.

In hepatolenticular degeneration (Wilson), deposition of a copper-containing material in the inner layers of the cornea extends as far as the trabecular meshwork of the anterior chamber recess (Kayser-Fleischer ring). It ends abruptly at the posterior edge of the meshwork. The ring is often incomplete—it may be concealed in its early stages by the corneoscleral limbus and can be seen only by using a gonioscope.

The Krukenberg spindle is a vertical pigment deposit on the endothelial surface of the cornea, probably derived from uveal pigment. It is deposited by convection currents in the anterior chamber and is usually arranged in an approximately triangular pattern with the apex near the center of the cornea and the base in the 6 o'clock meridian. In the pigment dispersion syndrome, patchy areas of iris depigmentation appear as defects by iris transillumination combined with pigment accumulation in the trabecular meshwork. Glaucoma may occur.

Melanin lines may extend into the cornea from the periphery in heavily pigmented individuals, particularly after injury. These lines are composed of ectopic melanocytes and are usually the result of trauma.

Keratic precipitates are inflammatory cells adherent to the endothelium in inflammations of the anterior ocular segment. They may occasionally be pigmented.

Heavy metals such as silver (argyria), iron (siderosis), gold (chrysiasis), copper (chalcosis), and mercury may be deposited in the stroma adjacent to the Descemet membrane. Metals are introduced by local medication (silver), intraocular foreign bodies (iron or copper), intraocular blood (iron), systemic therapy (gold), toxic vapors (mercury), or a disordered metabolism (copper in hepatolenticular degeneration) (see Chapter 26).

SUPERFICIAL CORNEAL LINES

Microscopically thin parallel lines arranged in whorls and other concentric patterns originate in the epithelium and subepithelial tissue. The most common type, called fingerprint lines, may be associated with recurrent corneal erosion. When they are bilateral, they may constitute a subepithelial corneal dystrophy that occurs because of a disorder of the epithelial basement membrane.

ABNORMAL DEPOSITS IN SYSTEMIC DISEASE

The cornea is often the site of deposition of abnormal metabolic products circulating in the blood. Often the deposition is not grossly evident and may be overlooked if special magnification is not used.

In corneal arcus (arcus senilis, gerontoxon), there is an extracellular lipid infiltration (neutral fats, phospholipids, and sterols) at the corneal periphery. It first appears inferiorly, then superiorly, and eventually encircles the cornea; it often may involve only a sector of the cornea. It appears as a grayish white infiltrate separated from the white sclera by a clear interval of 1 mm. It occurs almost universally in humans over 60 years of age (see Chapter 26).

Corneal arcus tends to develop more commonly and earlier in life in blacks than in whites. Both races show a tendency to develop the lesion with increasing age. Myocardial infarction is twice as likely to occur in an individual 39 to 49 years of age who has corneal arcus than in one who does not. Additionally, young patients with corneal arcus are likely to have high serum cholesterol levels and to smoke. A corneal arcus does not invariably occur in familial hypercholesterolemia, and there is no relationship between corneal arcus and secondary types of hypercholesterolemia that occur in diabetes mellitus, lipoid nephrosis, and myxedema.

Previous vascularization of the cornea leads to the deposition of lipid adjacent to the blood vessel in some patients with hypercholesterolemia and may occur in association with megalocornea. The optical zone of the cornea is not involved, there are no symptoms, and treatment of the cornea is not indicated.

In posterior embryotoxon, the termination of Descemet membrane (Schwalbe line or ring) at the periphery of the cornea is markedly thickened and located more centrally than normal so that it is visible through the clear cornea. It appears similar to a corneal arcus but on the posterior surface of the cornea. It varies in normal eyes (15%) and is seen in aniridia, megalocornea, and corectopia. It is also seen in arteriohepatic dysplasia, an autosomal dominant condition of failure of hepatocytes to secrete bile, in which strabismus and retinal pigmentary degeneration also occur. In Axenfeld anomaly and Rieger anomaly, strands of the peripheral iris adhere to the posterior embryotoxon.

Jet-black patches of adrenochrome may be seen in the cornea and conjunctiva after long-term use of epinephrine salts in the treatment of glaucomas.

Calcium is deposited in the cornea in two forms: (1) diffuse subepithelial deposition of crystals and (2) band keratopathy in which a horizontal grayish band is interspersed with round dark areas that appear as holes. The first type of deposition is seen in the milk-alkali syndrome (ingestion of milk and calcium carbonate) and is associated with glistening crystals deposited in the diffusely hyperemic conjunctiva. In hypophosphatemia, in which the tissues do not metabolize calcium because of a deficiency in the parathyroid hormone, the cornea, but not the conjunctiva, contains calcium crystals.

Band keratopathy results from the deposition of noncrystalline phosphate and carbonate calcium salts in the epithelium, in the subepithelial tissue, and between the stromal lamellae. In juvenile rheumatoid arthritis (Still disease), band keratopathy may complicate an indolent chronic iridocyclitis. Other causes include hyperparathyroidism, vitamin D poisoning, sarcoidosis, multiple myeloma, renal disorders, and keratoconjunctivitis sicca. It occurs in diseases associated with hypercalcemia, in association with ocular inflammation, and after repeated topical instillation of drugs that have calcium in the vehicle.

In some lysosomal storage diseases (see Chapter 26), the cornea, among other tissues, accumulates an abnormal amount of the storage substances. The cornea is cloudy, not unlike its appearance in corneal edema, and the iris is difficult to visualize.

In cystine storage disease, cystine crystals in the conjunctiva and cornea appear as tinsel-like, fine refractile crystals uniformly scattered throughout the tissue.

In dysproteinemias, particularly multiple myeloma, iridescent crystals may be scattered throughout the cornea and conjunctiva. Deep deposits similar to those in corneal dystrophy may be present in cryoglobulinemia.

Multiple endocrine neoplasia type IIb (III) (see Chapter 27), a neurocristopathy, is characterized by the association of medullary thyroid carcinoma, multiple mucosal neuromas, pheochromocytoma, marfanoid habitus, characteristic facies with large lips, intestinal ganglioneuromatosis, and skeletal anomalies. Prominent corneal nerves occur in a clear corneal stroma. Additionally, conjunctival and eyelid neuromas are present, combined with keratoconjunctivitis sicca. Prompt identification of affected individuals facilitates early treatment of associated medullary carcinoma of the thyroid and pheochromocytoma.

ABNORMALITIES OF SIZE

MICROCORNEA

In microcornea (anterior microphthalmos) the corneal diameter is less than 10 mm and the radius of curvature is decreased (Fig 11-1). The eyes are usually hyperopic and often develop glaucoma in later years. The term "microcornea" is reserved for eyes in which the small corneal diameter is the sole abnormality. When the entire eye is small, the condition is called microphthalmia. Vision is reduced, and ocular nystagmus and strabismus may occur. Usually there are numerous associated developmental abnormalities, and sometimes only cystic remnants of the eye are present (anophthalmos).

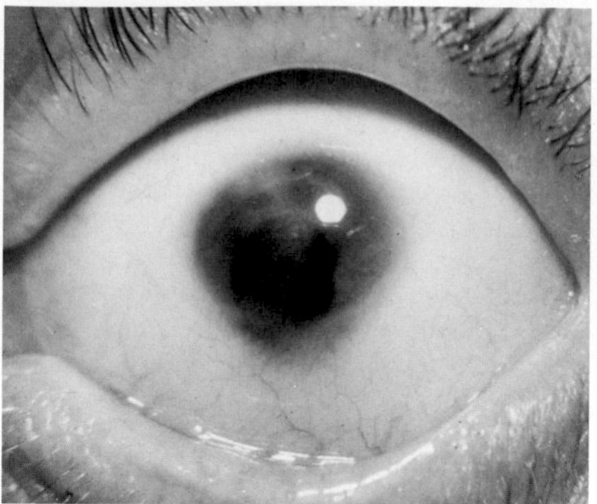

FIG 11-1.
Micrcornea (anterior microphthalmos) in which there is also a corneal nebula (opacity) and an iris coloboma. Visual acuity was 3/200.

Nanophthalmos is the condition in which the eye is exceptionally small but otherwise normal. There is severe hyperopia (up to 20 diopters), a thickened sclera, and a tendency to angle-closure glaucoma as the lens grows. Uveal effusion may occur, presumably as the result of impaired choroidal venous drainage caused by the thickened sclera. It is usually inherited as an X chromosome–linked recessive condition.

MEGALOCORNEA

Megalocornea (anterior megalophthalmos) is a bilateral abnormality in which the diameter of each cornea is more than 14 mm (Fig 11-2). The anterior chamber is deep, the iris stroma atrophic, and the iris tremulous. Posterior subcapsular cataract occurs between the ages of 30 and 50 years. Megalocornea must be differentiated from the enlarged eye in congenital glaucoma, which is not X chromosome–linked and is

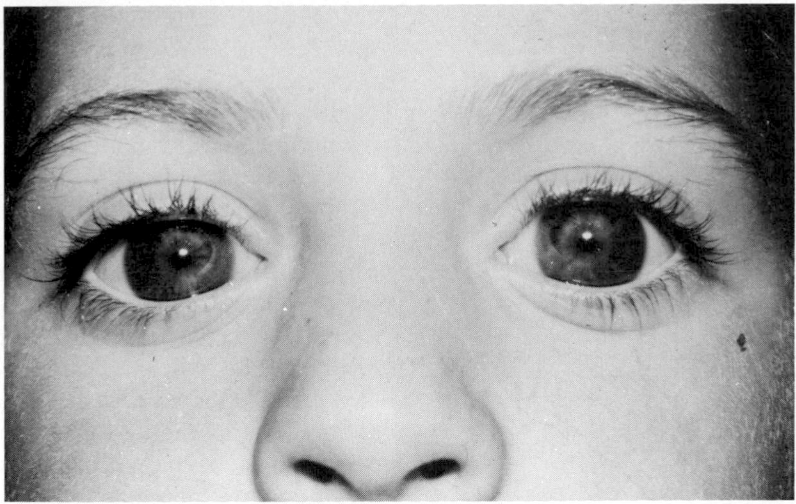

FIG 11-2.
Megalocornea in an 11-year-old boy who also had the Rieger anomaly: bilateral posterior embryotoxon (opacification of the peripheral cornea), iris atrophy, and prominent iris processes. The patient subsequently developed peripheral anterior synechiae (iris adhesions) and secondary glaucoma.

associated with tears in Descemet membrane and increased intraocular pressure early in life.

STAPHYLOMA

An anterior staphyloma is an ectasia or bulging of the cornea that is lined with uveal tissue. It occurs mainly in degenerated eyes after perforation of a corneal ulcer with iris prolapse. The anterior chamber is obliterated, and a secondary glaucoma is present. Often enucleation is required.

Kerectasia is a bulging thinned corneal scar that usually is caused by severe corneal ulceration, which results in a thinned, protruding cornea. It differs from a staphyloma in that it is not lined with uveal tissue.

A descemetocele is a herniation of Descemet membrane through the base of a corneal ulcer.

CORNEAL DYSTROPHIES

Corneal dystrophies (Table 11-3) are bilateral primary hereditary disorders of the cornea that are not associated with previous inflammation or systemic disease. They are occasionally evident at birth but more frequently develop during adolescence and slowly progress throughout life. They are often described on the basis of their appearance or the layer of the cornea involved. Many do not interfere with vision but create interesting abnormal patterns of opacities in the usually transparent cornea. Most are transmitted as autosomal dominant disorders, but central macular dystrophy (Groenouw type II) is transmitted as an autosomal recessive defect. Congenital hereditary endothelial dystrophy is transmitted as a recessive disorder that is manifest at birth or as an autosomal dominant disorder evident in early to late childhood.

EPITHELIAL DYSTROPHIES

The epithelial dystrophies are disorders of the epithelial basement membrane that result in the formation of a variety of abnormal epithelial cells. In Meesman dystrophy and recurrent corneal erosion, there are recurrent episodes of pain when epithelium is lost. In map-dot-fingerprint dystrophy, there are bilateral lines, dots, or blebs that form a changing pattern in the anterior surface of the cornea.

Juvenile epithelial dystrophy (of Meesman).—This is a rare disorder that consists of clear dots or cysts in the corneal epithelium that occasionally rupture. It consists of aggregates of an amorphous electron-dense material that causes marked irregularities in the epithelium. Treatment is solely symptomatic.

Recurrent corneal erosion.—Recurrent corneal erosion often follows an uncomplicated corneal abrasion in which the regenerated basal epithelial cells do not adhere to their basement

TABLE 11-3.
Corneal Dystrophies

- Basement membrane of epithelium
  - Juvenile epithelial (Meesman)
  - Recurrent corneal erosion
  - Epithelial basement membrane (map-lot or fingerprint: Cogan)
- Stromal
  - Bowman zone
    - Subepithelial reticular (Reis-Bücklers)
    - Anterior crocodile shagreen (Vogt)
    - Mosaic
    - Honeycomb
    - Hereditary band keratopathy
  - Central
    - Granular ("bread-crumb"): (Groenouw type I)
    - Crystalline (Schnyder)
  - Central and peripheral
    - Macular ("ground-glass"): (Groenouw type II)
    - Lattice
    - Crystalline (Schnyder)
    - François
  - Pre-Descemet
    - Posterior polymorphous
    - Farinata
- Endothelial
  - Guttata
  - Fuchs
  - Congenital, hereditary stromal
- Ectatic
  - Anterior
    - Keratoconus
    - Terrien marginal
    - Keratoglobus
  - Posterior
    - Keratoglobus

membrane. Thereafter, on awakening the patient experiences a severe, sharp ocular pain, similar to that which occurred with the initial abrasion. It may occur in bullous keratopathy, in which the extracellular matrix proteins, fibronectin, type IV collagen, and laminin are absent in regions of erosion. Some 20% of those affected have an autosomal dominant corneal epithelial basement membrane dystrophy.

Examination indicates a corneal area denuded of epithelium that stains with fluorescein. Between attacks this area shows minute opacities when examined with high magnification. The disorder is disabling because of the painful episodes but there is no loss of vision.

Treatment is difficult. The acute episode is treated with patching, and often adjoining cells cover the area within hours. Instillation of a petrolatum ointment in the eye will prevent the eyelid from adhering to the epithelium and flicking it off when the eyes are opened. A soft contact lens sometimes prevents recurrences. Multiple minute punctures of the basement membrane with a fine curved needle or an excimer or Nd:YAG laser may be followed by synthesis of normal matrix proteins and cure.

Epithelial basement membrane dystrophy.—In epithelial basement membrane dystrophy, the corneal epithelial cells form an ever-changing, subtle pattern of minor opacities described as map-dot-fingerprint, map-like, bleblike, or microcystic. Most patients are asymptomatic unless recurrent corneal erosion occurs. The changes are the result of basement membrane proliferating into the layer of basal cells. The condition is an autosomal dominant disorder transmitted with a variable penetrance. Similar changes are common as an acquired disorder in which only one eye is affected.

STROMAL DYSTROPHIES

Reis-Bücklers central corneal dystrophy.—This is an anterior corneal dystrophy that affects the Bowman zone and adjacent stroma. It is an autosomal dominant condition that begins in early childhood with a ring-shaped, superficial reticular opacity in the central cornea. Painful corneal erosions may occur that gradually cease as the center of the cornea at the level of the Bowman zone thickens and clouds with degenerated type III (fetal or repair) collagen and type IV (mature) collagen. In later life, irregular astigmatism combined with corneal opacification may necessitate corneal transplantation. The opacities show the immunoglobulins IgG, kappa, and lambda. Paraproteinemic crystalline keratopathy occurring in leukemia with an M component in the serum proteins shows identical corneal opacities. In some families, amyloid (see Lattice Dystrophy below) is superimposed on the granular deposits.

Central macular dystrophy (Groenouw type II).—This dystrophy begins in childhood as a diffuse clouding and progresses until, by middle age, the entire thickness of the cornea contains gray confluent spots. Mature keratan sulfate is absent from the cornea and bloodstream. Unlike most corneal dystrophies it is transmitted as an autosomal recessive trait.

Lattice dystrophy.—Lattice dystrophy is an autosomal dominant amyloidosis of the corneal stroma. There are fine, randomly scattered, linear opacities mainly in the central portion of the anterior corneal stroma. There are three types: (1) type 1, the most common, which has onset in childhood; (2) type 2, which is associated with familial amyloid polyneuropathy (Finnish type), which affects skeletal and cranial nerves; and (3) type 3, which affects older individuals than in either type 1 or type 2. The corneal lattice pattern in type 3 is composed of thicker opacities than the other types, and they may extend to the corneoscleral limbus. In all types, painful corneal erosions and reduced vision may require corneal surgery. The opacities may be ablated with the excimer laser or a corneal transplant may be indicated. The gene for type 1 lattice dystrophy and for granular dystrophy maps to chromosome 5q.

The amyloid is composed of protein AA that occurs in secondary amyloidosis, combined with a structural protein AP (amyloid-plasma). Protein AA does not occur in primary familial amyloidosis of the cornea. Gelsolin, a regulatory protein of actin, is found only in type 2.

ENDOTHELIAL DYSTROPHIES

Human corneal endothelium does not regenerate, but when cells are lost, the adjoining cells enlarge to cover the defect. If the defect is not covered, Descemet membrane develops circular, wartlike excrescences that dip into the anterior chamber. These normally occur as a degenerative change with aging, are located at the periphery of the cornea, and are called Hassall-Henle bodies or corneal guttata (Latin *guttae:* drops). They are of no clinical significance except as an indication of aging or previous ocular trauma.

Fuchs endothelial dystrophy.—Fuchs endothelial (sometimes endothelial-epithelial) dystrophy is a bilateral, often asymmetric, slowly progressive endothelial abnormality that leads to edema of the corneal epithelium and stroma and causes pain and reduced vision. In middle life the Descemet membrane develops wartlike excrescences similar to those seen in aging, except for their central location. They may be few or many, but when the deposits become extensive, vision is reduced. The endothelium loses its function in maintaining corneal dehydration (deturgescence) and the cornea becomes edematous. The edema causes a diffraction of light so that the patient sees halos surrounding lights (iridescent vision).

The edema occurs spontaneously or may follow cataract extraction, corneal trauma, or prolonged contact lens wear. The substantia propria is thickened and opacified. Epithelial edema is followed by erosion and bullae (bullous keratopathy or a combined epithelial-endothelial dystrophy). Vision is markedly reduced. The bullae may rupture and expose corneal nerve endings, resulting in severe pain. Soft contact lenses may relieve discomfort. Hypertonic saline or glucose solutions dehydrate the edematous cornea and may improve vision. Early endothelial and epithelial dystrophy responds well to penetrating corneal transplant, provided all of the diseased tissue is removed.

Posterior polymorphous deep dystrophy.—This is characterized by a thickened Descemet membrane with localized excrescences that project into the anterior chamber or form lines that result in white patches that line the cornea. The endothelial cells may resemble fibroblasts or epithelial cells both morphologically and immunologically. The overlying stroma and epithelium are clear, and vision is seldom affected. It is mainly, but not always, transmitted as an autosomal dominant condition with high penetrance. There may be associated defects of the iris and anterior chamber angle. There is often an associated glaucoma. If the opacity impairs vision, penetrating corneal transplantation may be indicated.

KERATOCONUS

Keratoconus (conical cornea) is a noninflammatory abnormality in which the symmetric curvature of the cornea is distorted by an abnormal thinning and forward bulging of its central portion (ectasia) (Fig 11-3). The condition is usually bilateral, but one eye may be involved long before its fellow. Onset is usually at the time of puberty. Women are affected more frequently than men. Keratoconus progresses slowly over many years but may become stationary at any time. The chief symptom is decreased visual acuity for far and near as the result of severe astigmatism, which, as the disease progresses, becomes irregular and cannot be improved with spectacles. Contact lenses provide a regular anterior curvature and usually provide visual improvement. Eventually the

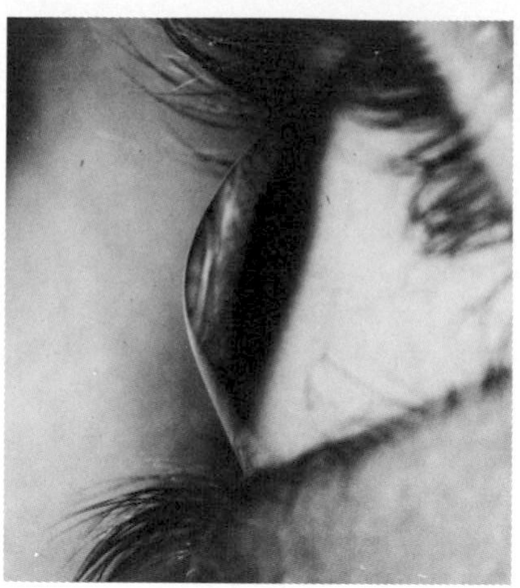

FIG 11-3.
Abnormal corneal profile in keratoconus.

cornea is so distorted that contact lenses cannot be retained.

Diagnosis may be difficult in the early stages. Viewing the cornea from above by looking down from behind the patient and over the brow, as is done in the diagnosis of proptosis, may indicate the corneal cone. The corneal cone distorts the pattern of the Placido disk, a flat disk that has concentric black and white circles and a central opening to observe their corneal reflection. The light reflex in retinoscopy is irregular. The epithelium at the base of the cone may be infiltrated with a ferritin pigment, causing a Fleisher ring. Breaks in the Descemet membrane allow aqueous humor to enter the stroma and cause a severe corneal edema, hydrops of the cornea, a common complication of Down syndrome. Eye rubbing may be a factor.

Vision is usually maintained at a useful level by wearing hard contact lenses. Reduction of the intraocular pressure by use of an antiglaucoma medication such as timolol 0.5% twice daily may prevent progression. If contact lenses cannot be used, a penetrating corneal transplant restores useful vision with a 95% success rate.

Keratoconus may be associated with a variety of other ocular disorders, such as retinitis pigmentosa, retrolental fibroplasia, ectopia lentis, congenital cataract, microcornea, blue sclera, and vernal catarrh. Systemic disorders associated with ocular disorders include the following syndromes: osteogenesis imperfecta, Down, Marfan, Ehlers-Danlos, Crouzon, Laurence-Moon-Biedl, and van der Hoeve.

CORNEAL DEGENERATIONS

Degenerative conditions that may affect the cornea are keratoconjunctivitis sicca, spheroid keratitis, corneal arcus, pterygium, gutter degeneration, band keratopathy, amyloidosis, and dellen. Persistent epithelial defects may develop in an eye that has a preexisting abnormality of the ocular surface. Herpes keratitis, ocular cicatricial pemphigoid, radiation keratitis, or chemical injury may result in chronic epithelial defects of the central stroma. Soft contact lenses, patching, and tarsorrhaphy may be helpful, but recurrence is common.

Spheroid keratitis (climatic droplet keratitis [Labrador keratitis]).—This acquired degenerative corneal disease occurs mainly in elderly patients as subepithelial, spherical, golden, droplet-shaped opacities of various sizes in the superficial corneal stroma. It results from exposure to extreme heat or cold, dust, snow, ice particles, and ultraviolet radiation. The material is deposited in a horizontal fashion in the exposed portion of the conjunctiva and cornea that corresponds to the palpebral aperture with an appearance that resembles band keratopathy.

Marginal ectasia (Terrien).—This is a slow, progressive thinning of the peripheral cornea that results in ectasia and severe astigmatism. Corneal rupture may occur with minor trauma. Excising the ectatic corneal stroma and suturing the stroma of normal thickness together alleviates the astigmatism.

BANDAGE LENSES

Thin (0.1 to 0.2 mm), hemispherical (corneoscleral), gas-permeable shells that cover the cornea and a portion of the sclera (13.5 to 15 mm in diameter), composed of silicon, collagen, or soft contact lens polymer, are useful in the treatment of many corneal disorders. They are widely used in the treatment of bullous keratopathy, recurrent corneal erosion, persistent epithelial defects, trichiasis, and neurotropic keratitis. They are commonly used after keratoplasty and repair of lacerations of the cornea.

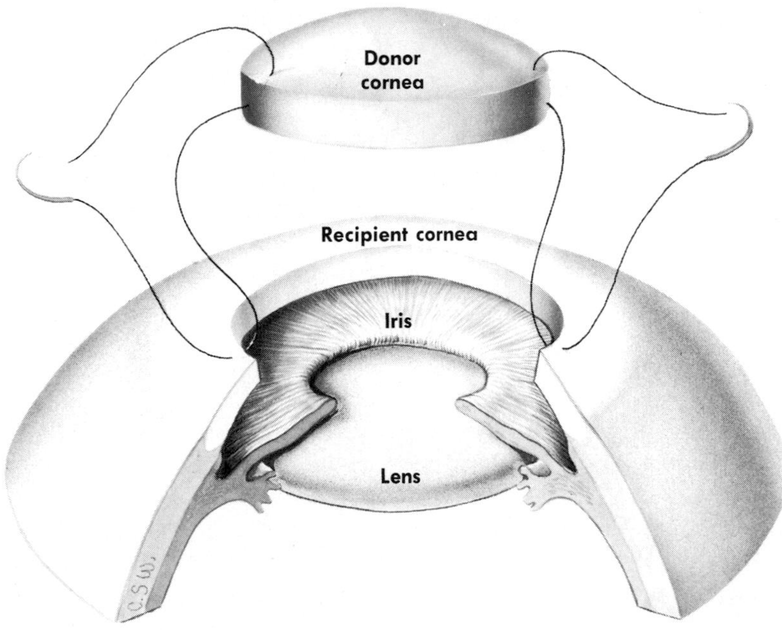

FIG 11-4.
The excised central portion of the cornea is being replaced with a clear donor cornea in a partial penetrating keratoplasty.

Bandage lenses are less useful in conditions in which there are too few tears.

Medicated collagen shields, made of porcine sclera, may be used to deliver high drug concentrations to the cornea. Since the lenses require tears for wetting, they are less useful in dry eye disorders. Nonmedicated shields should not be used in corneal infections.

CORNEAL TRANSPLANT

A major change in diagnostic and surgical methods will markedly modify the indications, methods, and results achieved in the management of corneal disorders in the next decade. Topographic evaluation of the curvatures of the cornea will permit a more accurate correction of keratoconus. The use of the excimer laser and other ultraviolet lasers with an output near 200 nm will make possible the removal of minute amounts of tissue and precise modeling of the donor and recipient in keratoplasty. Refractive surgery promises to be extraordinarily popular and new methods to ensure its accuracy and clarity of vision will emerge.

Corneal transplantation, or keratoplasty, is the excision of corneal tissue and its replacement by a cornea from a human donor. One of several techniques may be used. The two most common are (1) the penetrating graft (Fig 11-4), in which the entire thickness of cornea is removed and replaced by donor tissue; and (2) the nonpenetrating, or lamellar, keratoplasty, in which a superficial layer is removed and replaced without entering the anterior chamber. The diameter of the graft may vary in size from one that replaces the entire cornea (total keratoplasty) to one in which a portion of the cornea is excised (partial).

Because of improved surgical techniques, better selection of donor material, and effective medical treatment of graft rejection, the indications for transplantation relate mainly to the disorder requiring the procedure rather than to the preoperative visual acuity. In every patient, light perception and light projection must be retained. In disorders such as keratoconus, in which there is no corneal neovascularization, the visual prognosis is excellent. The prognosis in corneal dystrophies varies with the type and extent of the disorder. The graft may subsequently develop the same primary dystrophy. Some corneal dystrophies are treated successfully with ablation of the opacities by means of the excimer laser (photoablation), so that a corneal transplant is not required.

In conditions in which the corneal and conjunctival tissues have been replaced with a fibrovascular scar and the conjunctival fornices have been obliterated, the prognosis is poor. Poorly controlled glaucoma or conditions in which the anterior chamber has been lost complicate the operative procedure and impair the visual results.

The absence of blood vessels and lymphatics in the normal cornea prevents the donor cornea from sensitizing the recipient. Clear grafts follow transplantation in minimally vascularized corneas, but less frequently in severely vascularized corneas.

Corneal graft rejection is the chief cause of failure of a technically successful transplant. It proceeds over a period of weeks and affects each layer separately with infiltration by T cells and macrophages. It may begin 3 weeks to many years after the transplantation and may be induced by routine immunization or skin transplantation. ABO blood matching may be effective in reducing the rate of graft rejection, but HLA-A, -B, or -DR antigen matching does not influence the rate. The corneal endothelium appears to be the most antigenic portion of the transplanted tissue, and lamellar corneal transplants are not rejected. There is initial decrease in vision and increased cells and protein in the anterior chamber (flare).

Keratic precipitates accumulate on the graft and extend centrally. New blood vessels invade the graft, and the entire graft becomes opaque but is never extruded. Treatment consists of frequent instillation of corticosteroid (prednisolone) and cyclosporine eyedrops. Severe reactions require systemic corticosteroids. With prompt treatment, the prognosis for a clear graft is good.

Donor material is obtained from a noninfected person, preferably between 5 and 60 years of age, who has died of an acute noninfectious disease or an injury. Cornea from a youthful donor is the more desirable, because the density of corneal cells decreases with aging. The corneas of infants and children less than 5 years old are thin, soft, and difficult to manage. The corneas of those ill for a long period before death are not suitable. Corneas may not be used from patients with the following: terminal septicemia, Creutzfeldt-Jakob disease, or possible other slow virus disease, acquired immunodeficiency syndrome (AIDS), hepatitis, leukemia, or tumors of the anterior portion of the eye. The donor ELISA test for AIDS must be negative.

The donor eye should be enucleated within an hour after death by using sterile instruments and a sterile technique. If the donor eyelids are closed and a small icebag is placed over each eye, delays up to 5 hours are permissible. An ocular prosthesis (artificial eye) should be inserted in the socket to replace the enucleated eye.

Many eye banks store donor corneal tissues as whole eyes in refrigerated, moist chambers for periods of 24 to 48 hours. Corneas may be stored for longer periods by carefully removing the cornea with a 3-mm rim of scleral tissue attached. The corneas must not be folded to prevent damage to the endothelium. The cornea may be stored in a modified tissue-culture medium (M-K medium) and stored at 4° C.

There are always fewer donor corneas (and other organs) than required. Many families will find solace after the death of a loved one, particularly the sudden accidental death of a young person, in knowing that the donation of the eyes and other organs will provide sight and life to others.

PENETRATING KERATOPLASTY

The excision of all layers of the central cornea with retention of a central rim (partial penetrating) and replacement with a clear donor cornea is the traditional type of corneal transplantation. In a complete penetrating transplantation, the entire cornea is removed and replaced. Currently a partial penetrating keratoplasty is mainly performed because of the bullous keratopathy that follows cataract extraction in which an anterior chamber intraocular lens has been used.

In cooperative patients, the operation is usually performed with the use of local anesthesia. The donor graft is prepared first with a trephine. The same trephine or one slightly larger is used to remove the diseased corneal tissue from the recipient eye. A metal mask may be used and the recipient cornea excised with an excimer laser. If necessary, a cataract or intraocular lens is removed. A replacement intraocular lens may be used. The donor tissue is then sutured into position, usually with 10-0 monofilament nylon. Sutures may remain in position indefinitely.

LAMELLAR KERATOPLASTY

In nonpenetrating or lamellar keratoplasty, the entire thickness of the cornea is not removed and the diseased tissue is replaced with a partial-thickness donor cornea. Opacification occurring at the donor-recipient interface may prevent as good a visual result as that obtained with a penetrating graft. The procedure often precedes a penetrating graft required to restore vision. The excimer laser gives promise of improved visual results with lamellar keratoplasty in allowing precise removal of corneal tissue and shaping of the donor tissue. In eyes in which the Bowman zone is not affected, a thin lamellar flap of epithelium and Bowman zone is dissected with a small hinge to the recipient cornea. The excimer laser is then used to remove the diseased stroma, the tissue is replaced with donor stroma, and the hinged flap is reattached with sutures.

Neoplasms, recurrent pterygia, and other peripheral corneal lesions may be excised and the tissue replaced with an excimer-shaped or freehand lamellar transplant in which the incision and suture tracts avoid the optical portion of the central cornea.

KERATOREFRACTIVE SURGERY

The convex anterior surface of the cornea is the major refractive curvature of the eye, and its radius of curvature mainly determines the refractive power of the eye. (Note that refractive errors are determined by the relationship between the refractive power of the anterior segment of the eye, the cornea and the lens, and the length of the eye [see Chapter 24].)

The central 3.0 mm of the cornea, the optical zone, through which the visual axis passes, determines its refractive power. An increased curvature increases the refractive power and a decreased curvature decreases the refractive power. Thus, increasing the refractive power of the cornea will lessen hyperopia. Decreasing the refractive power will lessen myopia. In keratoconus (see Keratoconus), the cone shape of the optical zone of the cornea induces a variable, irregular refractive surface of the optical zone and decreases visual acuity. A penetrating corneal transplant substitutes a cornea with a uniform curvature of the anterior surface of its optical zone.

A variety of surgical procedures have been used to modify the curvature, and thus the refractive power, of the optical zone of the cornea. In keratomileusis, keratophakia, and epikeratophakia, the anterior portion of the cornea is replaced (lamellar corneal transplant). An artificial cornea is a plastic insert in the optical zone to substitute for a severely scarred cornea.

A radial keratotomy seeks to modify the refractive power of the cornea by a series of incisions partially through the thickness of the cornea peripheral to the optical zone. Photorefractive keratoplasty seeks to reduce the refractive power of the optical zone by removing (ablating) some of the corneal tissue in the optical zone by means of an argon-fluoride excimer laser that has an emission in the ultraviolet range (193 nm).

Keratomileusis and keratophakia.—In keratomileusis (Fig 11-5), the refractive power of the eye is increased by increasing the radius of curvature of the anterior surface of the cornea and thus neutralizing or decreasing hypermetropia, particularly that which follows cataract extraction. A disk of tissue 8.5 to 9.0 mm in diameter is resected from the patient's anterior corneal stroma, frozen, and reshaped on a computer-assisted lathe or an excimer laser. The tissue is then reinserted in the cornea to provide an increased radius of curvature. The procedure is the most technically difficult of all the refractive surgical procedures.

In keratophakia, donor cornea rather than the corneal tissue of the patient is reshaped and transplanted. The procedure is used to correct myopia of more than 6 diopters and severe hypermetropia, particularly that following cataract extraction.

Intraocular lenses inserted at the time of cataract extraction or after cataract extraction (secondary implant) and the use of contact lenses have minimized the need for keratomileusis and keratophakia.

Epikeratophakia.—This procedure (Fig 11-5) is similar to keratophakia except that no corneal stroma is removed from the eye. A thin disk of donor corneal stroma is sutured to the patient's cornea from which the epithelium has been removed. In 4 to 10 days the recipient's

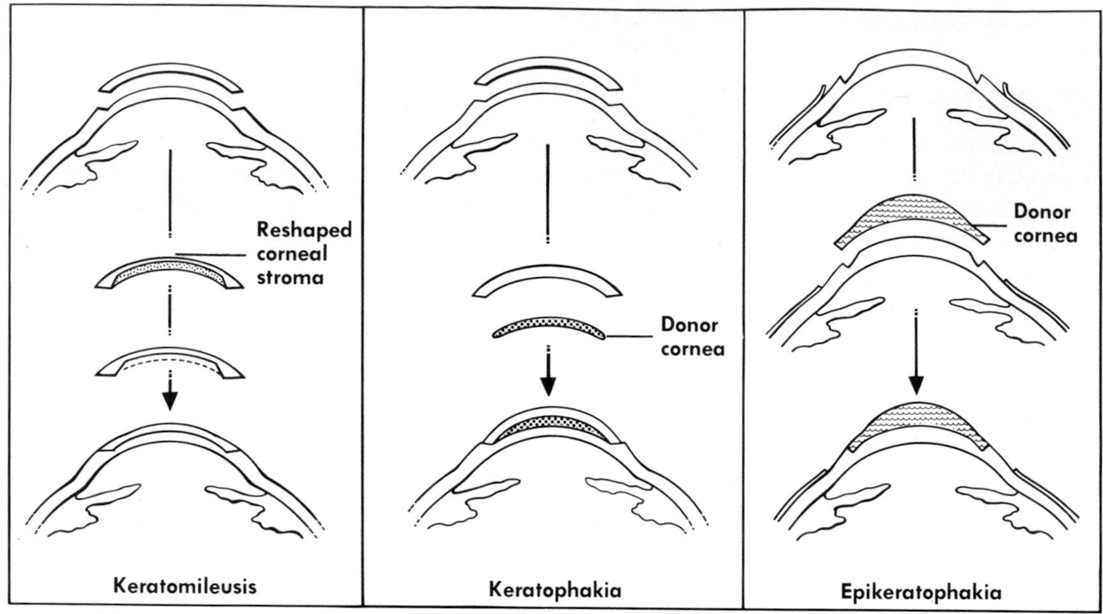

FIG 11-5.
Various types of corneal refractive surgery. In keratomileusis, a portion of the patient's cornea is reshaped to provide a different curvature; in keratophakia, donor cornea or a synthetic lens material is used; in epikeratophakia, the donor cornea is placed over the patient's cornea from which the epithelium has been removed.

epithelium covers the tissue, and in 1 to 2 months the recipient's keratocytes repopulate the donor tissue. The donor tissue is easily removed if necessary.

Artificial cornea.—Persistent epithelial defects of the cornea may complicate chemical burns of the eye and corneal disease. Loss of the epithelium leads to gradual necrosis of the corneal stroma (corneal melting). Hard contact lenses glued to the corneal stroma may permit epithelialization of the cornea. The lenses may be required for as long as a year. They are helpful only in chemical burns confined to the cornea, in which early keratoplasty is not indicated.

Corneal implants made of artificial nonreactive material (keratoprostheses) are used in individuals in whom repeated corneal transplants have been unsuccessful or those in whom excessive corneal scarring, corneal vascularization, or glaucoma contraindicates conventional surgery. Many ingenious devices have been designed but they mainly fail because of extrusion of the implant, aqueous humor leakage, or membrane formation that occludes the optical segment of the implant.

Radial keratotomy.—The refractive power of the cornea is reduced by incisions partially through the thickness of the cornea that extend between the edge of the optical zone and the peripheral cornea (Fig 11-6). The reduced refractive power reduces myopia by 2 to 6 diopters. Modern techniques require accurate measurement of the corneal thickness (pachymetry), precise calibration of the depth of each incision, and the use of an ultrathin, gemstone-quality diamond knife.

Four, six, or eight radial incisions are made in the clear cornea. Surgeons aim to undercorrect the myopia, as a conversion to hyperopia is undesirable. Best results are produced with myopia of less than 6 diopters. The results are less predictable with myopia of 6 to 10 diopters, although many patients are pleased with reduction in the severity of their myopia.

Patients should have a stable myopia that is not actively progressing. Hard contact lenses should not be worn for 2 weeks before the surgical procedure, and soft contact lenses should be avoided for 3 days. Topographic corneal analysis is desirable to identify patients with irregular curvatures of the cornea. Undesirable risks in patients include connective-tissue disorders, blepharitis, rosacea, and ocular diseases that require topical corticosteroids.

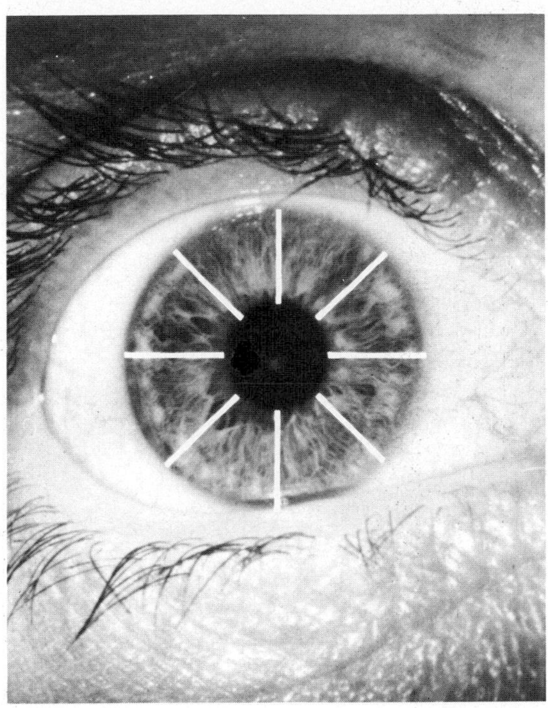

FIG 11-6.
The location of the incisions in radial keratotomy. The central 3- to 4-mm optical zone of the cornea is not incised, and the incisions do not extend beyond the corneoscleral limbus. Four, eight, or sixteen radial incisions are made.

Postoperatively there may be glare, diurnal variation in refraction, and inability to improve visual acuity to the 20/20 level with spectacles or contact lenses. Some 90% of patients with current procedures attain a refractive error within 1 diopter of emmetropia.

Photoreactive keratectomy.—The excimer laser emits molecules that rupture covalent bonds of the molecules of irradiated material, particularly carbon-nitrogen-peptide bonds. When a minute region of the cornea is irradiated by means of the argon-fluoride excimer laser (193 nm), the tissue is ablated (evaporated) without injury to or an increase in temperature of adjacent cells.

The usefulness of the excimer laser is still under study, but the instrument has been approved for use by the Food and Drug Administration. Most attention is directed to removal of a portion of the corneal stroma within the optical zone to reduce the curvature of the anterior surface. The most troubling complication is a haze of the ablated area, which may persist for up to 6 months. Patients who have had a radial keratotomy in one eye and photorefractive keratectomy in the fellow eye prefer the radial keratotomy. To minimize damage to the layer, some surgeons have first removed the corneal epithelium and the Bowman zone surgically and then ablated the exposed corneal stroma and reattached the dissected Bowman zone and epithelium.

INJURIES

CHEMICAL BURNS

Every practitioner and lay person should know that every chemical injury of the eye and face should be diluted as quickly as possible with water. There should be no delay to learn the history, seek an appropriate chemical neutralizer, or summon specialized assistance; rather, the eye and face should be irrigated at once. The fluid need not be sterile, at body temperature, or even clean provided the chemical is promptly diluted.

FOREIGN BODIES

Every practitioner should know how to evert the upper eyelid to remove a foreign body. Foreign bodies on the cornea cause symptoms of discomfort localized (usually incorrectly) to the upper outer cornea. Often the foreign body may be removed by directing a fine stream of sterile saline from a hypodermic syringe or bulb-type syringe to the base of the foreign body.

RADIANT ENERGY

Ultraviolet energy is almost entirely absorbed by the cornea and, like sunburn, the radiation damage is cumulative. Ultraviolet burns of the cornea occur in arc welders, mountain climbers, skiers, and after unprotected exposure to sun lamps. There is a severe foreign body sensation with tearing, and the individual may be unable to open the eyes. Curiously, many patients do not volunteer the information concerning the exposure. The symptoms are entirely relieved with a topical anesthetic, which, however, delays epithelial regeneration. Patching of the eyes to prevent blinking is followed by prompt recovery.

Accidental removal of the corneal epithelium exposes nerve endings and causes much pain and lacrimation. The usual causes are a superficial scratch or excessive exposure to ultraviolet light ("snowblindness"). The abraded area stains with fluorescein (2% sterile solution or a fluorescein strip) and in mechanical trauma is seen as a bright green patch and in ultraviolet exposure as stippled dots. The epithelium heals quickly with patching of the eye, and the lesion is of little importance unless infection occurs. Local anesthetics relieve pain but delay healing. If infection is feared, sulfacetamide solution (10%) is preferred to broadspectrum antibiotics. Fingernail scratches of the cornea, often in a mother scratched by an infant, are particularly likely to be followed by recurrent erosion of the corneal epithelium.

LACERATIONS

Corneal lacerations are particularly serious, because the interior of the eye is opened to infection and there is the likelihood of injury to intraocular structures. Initial treatment is directed toward prevention of infection by administration of an antibiotic and avoidance of prolapse of intraocular contents that may occur with repeated examinations. The laceration is closed with sutures after excision of prolapsed intraocular tissue. If the lens is lacerated, it is removed at the time the corneal laceration is repaired.

BIBLIOGRAPHY

Books

Chandler JWS, Sugar J, Edelhauser H: *External diseases: cornea, conjunctiva, sclera, eyelids, lacrimal system,* St Louis, 1994, Mosby–Year Book.

Karlin DB, editor: *Lasers in ophthalmic surgery,* Cambridge, Mass, 1995, Blackwell Scientific Publications.

Krachmer JH, Palay DA: *Cornea color atlas,* St Louis, 1995, Mosby–Year Book.

Salz JJ, editor: *Corneal laser surgery,* St Louis, 1995, Mosby–Year Book.

Smolin G, Thoft RA, editors: *The cornea: scientific foundations and clinical practice,* ed 3, Boston, 1994, Little, Brown.

Zierhut M, Pleyer U, Theil H-J: *Immunology of corneal transplantation,* Newton, Mass, 1994, Butterworth-Heinemann.

Articles

McDonnell PJ: Excimer laser corneal surgery: new strategies and old enemies, *Invest Ophthalmol Vis Sci* 36:4-8, 1995.

Tuft SJ, Moodaley LC, Gregory WM, Davison CR, Buckley RJ: Prognostic factors for the progression of keratoconus, *Ophthalmology* 101:439-447, 1994.

Zhao J-C, Jin X-Y: Local therapy of corneal allograft rejection with cyclosporine, *Am J Ophthalmol* 119: 189-194, 1995.

12

CONJUNCTIVITIS AND KERATITIS

The epithelium of the cornea and conjunctiva is continuous, and superficial inflammations often affect both tissues. The transparency of the cornea is essential to clear vision; thus, corneal inflammations are particularly serious and are often aggravated by the avascularity of its central portion.

The normal eye is protected by eyelids that periodically open and close to distribute tears over the surface of the conjunctiva and cornea. Located on the margins of the eyelids are the opening of glands that provide the oily outer surface of the precorneal tear film. The conjunctiva, a thin translucent mucous membrane, is divided into a palpebral portion that lines the eyelids, a bulbar portion that covers the anterior sclera, and a superior and inferior fornix that connects the two. The conjunctival epithelium, unlike the corneal epithelium, contains lymphatics and goblet cells. The conjunctiva contains the accessory lacrimal glands that are mainly responsible for the normal lubrication and wetting of the cornea. (The tears of the lacrimal gland are secreted in response to emotion or injury.)

The cornea is the grossly transparent structure that forms the anterior one sixth of the eyeball, through which the colored iris surrounding the black pupil can be seen. Its most anterior layer, the precorneal tear film, covers an epithelial layer five cells thick. The corneal stroma constitutes 90% of the cornea. Its anterior surface is adjacent to the basement membrane of the epithelium and its posterior surface is adjacent to the basement membrane (Descemet) of the corneal endothelium. The posterior surface of the cornea is covered with the corneal endothelium, which is mainly responsible for maintaining a relatively dehydrated corneal stroma.

SYMPTOMS AND SIGNS OF CONJUNCTIVITIS AND KERATITIS

Conjunctivitis causes ocular discomfort and burning rather than frank pain. There is no loss of vision, although pus floating across the cornea may distort vision. There may be chemosis (edema) of the conjunctiva. There is an excessive secretion, and the eyelids may stick together in sleep. The normally inconspicuous posterior conjunctival arteries and veins are dilated and engorged. The blood vessels are bright red, most conspicuous in the fornices, and fade toward the corneoscleral limbus. These blood vessels move with the conjunctiva and are constricted by a 1:1,000 epinephrine solution instilled in the conjunctival sac.

The most serious symptoms of conjunctivitis originate from secondary corneal involvement. This may occur by extension of inflammation from the conjunctiva or by irritation of the cornea because of continued contact with keratinized epithelium of the tarsal conjunctiva. Corneal inflammation may be secondary to exposure in cicatricial conditions that limit eyelid mobility, or it may be caused by loss of mucin secreted by goblet cells, which results in an abnormal tear film.

Inflammation of the cornea (keratitis) causes discomfort that varies from the sensation of a cinder in the eye to incapacitating pain. Inflammatory cells invade the cornea and appear as a grayish infiltrate in the clear tissue. The ciliary blood vessels beneath the conjunctiva are dilated and appear dark red or purplish through the overlying tissue. They are most evident at the corneoscleral limbus and fade toward the fornices. They do not move with the conjunctiva and do not constrict with topical instillation of epinephrine. Areas in which the epithelium is absent stain with topical fluorescein (2% sterile solution or a fluorescein strip). Corneal scarring is a common cause of loss of vision. Trachoma, a chlamydial infection that initially involves the conjunctiva, is the major cause of blindness in tropical regions.

CONJUNCTIVITIS

Conjunctivitis, an inflammation of the conjunctiva, is characterized by cellular infiltration and exudation. Classification is not satisfactory but is often based on the cause (bacterial, allergic, viral, fungal, or lacrimal), the age of occurrence (ophthalmia neonatorum), the type of exudate (purulent, mucopurulent, membranous, pseudomembranous, or catarrhal), or duration (acute, subacute, or chronic). There may be an associated corneal inflammation (keratoconjunctivitis).

DIAGNOSIS

The diagnosis of conjunctivitis is based on (1) the history and clinical examination; (2) Gram and Wright stains of conjunctival scrapings; and (3) culture of conjunctival scrapings to identify a microbial cause.

The history of the inflammation may be helpful. Infectious disease is often bilateral and may involve other members of the family or community. Unilateral disease suggests a toxic, chemical, mechanical, or lacrimal origin. A copious exudate suggests a bacterial inflammation. A stringy, sparse exudate suggests an allergy or a viral infection. A preauricular adenopathy suggests an adenovirus infection. Meibomianitis and chronic blepharitis with an associated conjunctivitis are common.

Clinical examination requires good illumination and magnification. Attention should be directed to the possibility of preauricular adenopathy, involvement of the eyelid margins, patency of the lacrimal system, severity and nature of the conjunctival injection, follicle formation or papillary hypertrophy, and the nature of the secretion (Table 12-1).

Staining and culture.—Initial treatment is based on the Gram stain of smears of the conjunctival exudate. Intraepithelial gram-negative diplococci of gonorrheal ophthalmia may be demonstrated by Gram stain 48 hours before their demonstration in culture. The conjunctiva is the portal of entry for meningitis in about half of the cases of *Neisseria meningitidis* conjunctivitis.

Exudate for culture is collected with a calcium alginate swab moistened with sterile saline or broth. The material is collected from the lower conjunctival fornix without prior topical anesthesia. Sheep blood and mannitol agar plates are used routinely. If *Haemophilus* or *Neisseria* species are suspected, chocolate agar is used; Sabouraud agar is used for suspected fungi. A transport medium should not be used. Viral material for culture is collected in a sterile swab and transferred immediately to a tissue culture medium. The *Chlamydia* group may be cultured in HeLa 229 or pretreated McCoy cells.

Conjunctival scrapings are preferred for cytologic examination. The conjunctiva is anesthetized, the site of maximum involvement is lightly scraped with a sterile spatula, and the material is spread on a glass slide to cover an area approximately 1 cm in diameter. The Gram stain demonstrates most bacteria and fungi. A microimmunofluorescent assay detects IgG or IgM antibodies to *Chlamydia.* A variety of enzyme immunoassays use a spectrophotometer to detect antigens. Giemsa-stained material is read for the predominant cell type present (Table 12-2). Direct microscopic examination of Giemsa-stained material for inclusion bodies has a low yield, except in neonatal inclusion conjunctivitis.

Frequently patients with conjunctivitis are prescribed an antibiotic empirically without a Gram stain or culture of the exudate. Often this suffices, for most instances of conjunctivitis are self-limited. In those instances in which the conjunctivitis does not respond to simple therapeutic measures subsequent bacterial and viral cultures often show no growth and the opportunity for specific treatment is lost. This failure

TABLE 12-1.
Clinical Findings in Conjunctivitis

I. Preauricular adenopathy
   A. Palpable: inclusion conjunctivitis, most adenoviruses, herpes simplex, sties, acute suppurative chalazion
   B. Gross enlargement with suppuration: Parinaud oculoglandular syndrome
II. Blepharitis and meibomiantis: *Staphylococcus* sp.
III. Excoriation of skin of medial and lateral cantus: *Staphylococcus* sp., diplobacillus of Morax-Axenfeld
IV. Conjunctival injection
   A. Red: infectious disease
      1. Intense with petechial hemorrhages: *Streptococcus pneumoniae* or *Haemophilus aegyptius* (Koch-Weeks)
      2. Subconjunctival hemorrhage: adenovirus or acute hemorrhagic conjunctivitis (picornavirus)
   B. Pale whitish: allergy
V. Chemosis: gonococcus, trichinosis, orbital infections, atopic disorders
VI. Exudate
   A. Stringy, white: allergy
   B. Purulent: gonococcus, meningococcus
   C. Mucopurulent: pyogenic bacteria
   D. Scanty: virus
   E. Foamy, whitish secretion: *Corynebacterium xerosis*
   F. Pseudomembrane: *Corynebacterium diphtheriae, Streptococcus* sp., erythema multiforme, APC type 8, vernal conjunctivitis
VII. Follicle formation (lymphatic hypertrophy)
   A. Lower eyelid: follicular conjunctivitis, APC viruses, inclusion conjunctivitis, molluscum contagiosum, hypersensitivity to pilocarpine, eserine, and other topical medications
   B. Upper eyelid: trachoma
VIII. Papillary hyperplasia: vernal conjunctivitis (neovascularization with lymphocyte infiltration)
IX. Conjunctival scarring
   A. Upper eyelid; trachoma
   B. Lower eyelid; erythema multiforme, alkali burns, radiation burns, cicatricial conjunctivitis
   C. General: diphtheria, infectious membranous conjunctivitis (herpes simplex, adenovirus, *Streptococcus* sp.)
X. Corneal involvement
   A. Purulent: gonococcus, *Pseudomonas aeruginosa*
   B. Marginal infiltrates: *Staphylococcus,* diplobacillus of Morax-Axenfeld (*Haemophilus* sp.)
   C. Punctate epithelial defects: *Staphylococcus* (lower half), trachoma (upper half)
   D. Generalized epithelial defects: Sjögren syndrome
   E. Superior vascularization: pannus of trachoma, phlyctenular disease
XI. Unilateral inflammation: Parinaud syndrome, adult gonococcus, contact allergy, lacrimal occlusion, viral infection

is particularly serious in cases of corneal ulcers that involve the central cornea.

CLINICAL TYPES

The clinical types of conjunctivitis vary with the cause. The onset is often insidious. The patient notices a fullness of the eyelids and a diffuse, gritty, foreign body sensation. Examination indicates diffuse conjunctival injection, a clear cornea, a distinct iris pattern, and normal pupillary reaction. Within several hours of the onset, there is exudation. There may be swelling of the eyelids and edema (chemosis) of the conjunctiva.

To determine if papillary hypertrophy or follicles are present, the tarsal border must be examined. Papillary hypertrophy is characterized by folds or projections of hypertrophic epithelium that contain a core of blood vessels surrounded by edematous stroma infiltrated with lymphocytes and plasma cells. It is basically a vascular response with secondary monocytic infiltration. All conjunctival inflammations have some degree of papillary hypertrophy. Large papillae occur characteristically in vernal conjunctivitis and in exceptionally severe or prolonged conjunctival inflammation.

Follicular hypertrophy is characterized by small follicles that are smaller and paler than papillae and lack the central core of blood vessels.

TABLE 12-2.
Cytologic Findings in Conjunctivitis

I. Polymorphonuclear leukocytes
   A. Neutrophils
      1. Bacterial and mycotic infections
      2. Erythema multiforme
      3. Chlamydial infections
   B. Basophils and eosinophils
      1. Allergies
         a. Vernal conjunctivitis (often fragmented)
         b. Hay fever
         c. Sensitivity to drugs, cosmetics, etc.
II. Monocytes
   A. Lymphocytes
      1. Virus infections
   B. Plasma cells
      1. Trachoma
   C. Phagocytes (Leber cells)
      1. Trachoma
III. Inclusion bodies
   A. Basophilic
      1. Upper tarsal: trachoma
      2. Lower tarsal: inclusion conjunctivitis
   B. Acidophilis
      1. Molluseum contagiosum
      2. Herpes simplex
IV. Epithelial cells
   A. Keratinized
      1. Sjögren syndrome
   B. Multinucleated
      1. Virus infection

Basically a follicle is a lymphoid hyperplasia and occurs in some normal children, chlamydial infections, and T cell–mediated reactions (type IV hypersensitivity).

Mucopurulent conjunctivitis.—Bacterial organisms causing mucopurulent conjunctivitis in the United States include gram-positive cocci *(Staphylococcus aureus, Staphylococcus epidermidis, Streptococcus pyogenes,* and *Streptococcus pneumoniae),* gram-negative cocci *(Neisseria meningitidis, Moraxella lacunata* [of Morax-Axenfeld]), and gram-negative rods (genus *Haemophilus,* family Enterobacteriaceae [genera *Proteus* and *Klebsiella*]). Almost any bacteria may be involved. Moreover, the causative organism may be one of a number of bacteria or fungi intermediate between saprophytes and pathogens. They may be recovered in culture or found in Gram-stained epithelial scrapings.

The onset is acute, and both eyes are involved with a mucopurulent exudate. Drying of inspissated pus during sleep may cause the eyelids to be agglutinated on awakening.

Physicians and other medical personnel must wash their hands thoroughly and use eyedrops in individual containers to avoid transmitting infection. Contaminated multiple-use containers of anesthetic solutions or fluorescein solutions together with contaminated tonometers have been the source of endemics of conjunctivitis (see Chapter 25) affecting patients and clinical personnel in several large ophthalmic clinics. The patients should be instructed concerning the danger of infecting family members and should not share towels or eye makeup. Eyedrops containing corticosteroids are contraindicated. An inflamed eye should not be patched.

Most bacterial infections of the conjunctiva are self-limited. Treatment with topical sulfacetamide, sulfisoxazole, or antibiotics may limit its duration. Initial treatment may consist of hourly instillation of sulfonamides, erythromycin, or gentamicin eyedrops. Instillation of an ointment at bedtime may prevent the eyelids from adhering together during sleep. A poor clinical response after 72 hours suggests either that the causative bacteria are not sensitive to the medications or that the cause is not bacterial. Further therapy should be based on the results of culture. Conjunctivitis caused by gonococci, *Chlamydia trachomatis,* or *Pseudomonas* organisms may require systemic as well as topical treatment. Gram-negative cocci may be *Neisseria meningitidis* and require systemic antibiotics to prevent meningitis.

Purulent conjunctivitis.—This is a severe, acute, purulent inflammation caused by *Neisseria gonorrhoeae.* It has an incubation period of 2 to 5 days. It occurs in newborn infants who are infected during passage through the birth canal, and in older individuals as a result of contamination from acute gonorrheal urethritis. Any ocular discharge in the newborn is suggestive of infection because tears are generally absent before the age of 3 weeks.

The inflammation may have a relatively mild onset but progresses rapidly. Marked swelling and redness of the eyelids and severe chemosis of the conjunctiva occur. The exudate is first serous and then purulent. The disease is well established after 2 days, reaches its height in 4 or 5 days, and then regresses over a 4- to 6-week period. Inflammation of the central cornea is common, and perforation of the eye may occur. The gram-negative intracellular organism may be demonstrated in conjunctival scrapings at the time of onset of the disease and in cultures 48 hours later.

Ideally the infected mother should be treated with penicillin or a penicillin derivative before delivery. Regardless of prophylaxis with silver nitrate, erythromycin, or tetracycline, the infant of an infected mother should be treated with a single injection of aqueous procaine penicillin G (50,000 units for full-term infants and 20,000 units for low-birth-weight infants). An intramuscular injection of ceftriaxone may be used.

Purulent conjunctivitis without keratitis in both children and adults may be treated with intramuscular administration of 1 g of ceftriaxone. In adults this dosage is followed by a 1-week course of oral tetracyline or doxycycline. Children should be treated with systemic erythromycin. Purulent conjunctivitis with corneal involvement or disseminated gonococcal infection requires admission to a hospital, and precautions must be taken with wound, skin, and secretions. In adults intravenous ceftriaxone is used daily for 3 to 5 days and intramuscular injections are used in infants. Hourly irrigation of the eyes with normal saline or tetracycline solution may be necessary if the secretion is copious.

Gonococcal urethritis is sometimes complicated by a bacteremia that causes an acute migratory polyarthritis or a tenosynovitis. A sterile catarrhal conjunctivitis occurs in about 10% of those affected. The condition must be differentiated from Reiter syndrome, which causes a sterile urethritis, arthritis, and iridocyclitis.

Ophthalmia neonatorum.—Ophthalmia neonatorum is a purulent conjunctival inflammation that occurs within the first 10 days of life. In most states it is a reportable infectious disease. The most serious cause is *Neisseria gonorrhoeae.* The most common causes today are inclusion body conjunctivitis *(Chlamydia trachomatis)* and bacteria, mainly *Staphylococcus* species and *Streptococcus pneumoniae.* Diagnosis is based on epithelial scrapings stained with Gram stain, on fluorescent antibody staining, on culture, and on cytology of the exudate. Treatment with systemic and local antibiotics is effective in bacterial disease. Inclusion conjunctivitis in the newborn must be treated by means of systemic and topical erythromycin (see below).

Credé prophylaxis.—Credé prophylaxis for gonorrheal ophthalmia is the instillation of one drop of 1% silver nitrate solution into the lower conjunctival cul-de-sac of each eye immediately after birth. Only a single-dose ampule should be used. Alternatively, an ophthalmic ointment containing 1% tetracycline or 0.5% erythromycin from single-use tubes may be used in each eye within 1 hour after birth. The agent should not be flushed from the eyes. Infants born by cesarean section should also be treated. Prophylaxis with erythromycin ointment may prevent chlamydial infection, which is not prevented with either silver nitrate or tetracycline.

Trachoma and inclusion conjunctivitis (TRIC).—The genus *Chlamydia* contains two species: *Chlamydia trachomatis* and *Chlamydia psittaci. Chlamydia trachomatis* is parasitic, principally in humans, and causes a variety of oculourogenital diseases: trachoma, inclusion conjunctivitis, lymphogranuloma venereum, urethritis, and proctitis. Pneumonitis occurs in the newborn. *Chlamydia psittaci* is an intracellular parasite of vertebrates and causes a variety of nonocular disorders in birds and mammals; rarely, pet parakeets transmit a chronic chlamydial conjunctivitis (see Chapter 25).

Inclusion conjunctivitis.—Inclusion conjunctivitis is an acute ocular inflammation caused by *Chlamydia trachomatis.* Newborns are infected in the birth canal (inclusion blennorrhea) and develop an acute mucopurulent conjunctivitis after an incubation period of 5 to 14 days. Adult inclusion conjunctivitis is transmitted venereally and by contaminated eye cosmetics. About 90% of adult women who have chlamydial eye infection have an associated chlamydial genital infection.

Inclusion conjunctivitis is one cause of ophthalmia neonatorum. After a variable period of 5 to 14 days, an acute conjunctivitis occurs with a profuse discharge. A chlamydial pneumonitis occurs up to 6 months later in 10% to 20% of those who develop a conjunctivitis. The newborn does not have subconjunctival lymphoid tissue until 4 to 6 weeks of age and there is no follicular reaction. Epithelial scrapings stained with Giemsa stain demonstrate many basophilic inclusion bodies combined with elementary bodies. Other laboratory procedures may include the highly sensitive and widely available enzyme-linked immunosorbent assay (ELISA), direct fluorescent monoclonal antibodies (DFA), microimmunofluorescent (MIF) testing, and complement fixation.

If the inflammation is not treated, the acute phase lasts 10 to 20 days and then subsides into a gradually diminishing chronic follicular conjunctivitis that persists 3 to 12 months. Infants should be treated systemically with daily administration of 40 mg/kg of erythromycin in four divided doses. Systemic tetracyclines are contraindicated in pregnant women and infants because of yellowing of the permanent teeth.

Gonorrheal conjunctivitis may be differentiated by a shorter incubation period (1 to 3 days), by involvement of both the superior and inferior fornices, by cytology, and demonstration of the causative organism.

Adult inclusion conjunctivitis begins as an acute follicular conjunctivitis that persists 3 to 12 months. There may be an associated preauricular adenopathy, epithelial keratitis, and sometimes peripheral corneal focal infiltrates. There is follicular and papillary hypertrophy. The disease may be distinguished from adenovirus infections by the polymorphonuclear cytologic response and the basophilic intracytoplasmic inclusion bodies, in contrast to the mononuclear response seen in adenoviral infections. Other sexually transmitted diseases must be excluded. Serologic tests for syphilis should be routine. Adult patients and their sexual partners must be treated with systemic tetracycline (1 to 2 g daily in four divided doses), doxycycline (200 mg daily in two divided doses), or erythromycin (1 to 1.5 g daily in four divided doses) for 3 weeks. Topical ocular therapy is not required. Infants, children, pregnant women, and nursing mothers should be treated with erythromycin.

Virus inflammations.—Invasions of the conjunctiva by a variety of viruses can cause conjunctivitis. Many mild, nonincapacitating conjunctival inflammations in which microorganisms are not demonstrated are probably caused by viruses. Conjunctival involvement may be part of a systemic infection, or the disease may be limited to the epithelium of the cornea and conjunctiva.

Adenovirus.—This is a group of at least 50 different virus serotypes with several different genotypes within serotypes. They cause diarrhea and upper respiratory tract infections primarily in infants, children, and military recruits. Some strains cause a conjunctivitis combined with a preauricular adenopathy, fever, and pharyngitis (acute pharyngeal fever). Other strains cause epidemic keratoconjunctivitis, which has been so widespread as to necessitate temporary closure of major eye centers.

Acute pharyngoconjunctival fever.—This is one of a spectrum of infections caused by the adenoviruses and characterized by fever, pharyngitis, cervical adenopathy, and acute follicular conjunctivitis. The conjunctivitis is often first monocular; the fellow eye is involved within a week. There is often intense hyperemia, particularly in the lower cul-de-sac, a preauricular adenopathy, a scanty secretion, and often a pseudomembrane. Adenovirus type 4 is associated with a pharyngitis in about one third of the patients. Adenovirus types 3 and 7 cause a particularly severe conjunctival inflammation.

The parents of children with acute pharyngoconjunctival fever may develop a monocular conjunctivitis with follicle formation, preauricular adenopathy, and fever.

Epidemic keratoconjunctivitis.—This is an acute inflammation of the conjunctiva and cornea often caused by adenovirus serotype 8 and less commonly by serotype 19, a pathogen of the uterine cervix. Serotypes 11 and 37 are rare causes. Young adults aged 20 to 40 years are most often affected. The incubation period ranges between 2 and 14 days, usually 7 to 9 days. The infection starts unilaterally with hyperemia and swelling of the conjunctiva (chemosis). There is a thin watery discharge and a tender preauricular adenopathy. Unlike pharyngoconjunctival fever, there are no constitutional symptoms and often only one eye is affected (66%). If the fellow eye is affected, inflammation occurs about 5 days after the first and is less severe. Conjunctival hemorrhages may occur, and there is papillary and follicular hypertrophy. Papillary hypertrophy affects mainly the upper tarsal conjunctiva, while follicular hypertrophy affects the conjunctiva of the upper and lower fornices. Pseudomembranes may occur. About 1 week after the onset of the conjunctivitis, a punctate corneal epitheliitis begins with discomfort and lesions that stain with fluorescein. These lesions progress to nonstaining, large, dense, well-marked subepithelial whitish patches 1 to 2 mm in diameter, which involve the central cornea and reduce vision. Vision may be impaired for many months, but the infiltrates gradually disappear. No specific treatment is available. Frequent instillation of antimicrobial eyedrops may sooth the eye and prevent secondary infection.

The infection occurs among individuals exposed to others with the infection, such as patients in nursing homes and hospitals, school children, or family members. Swimming pools may be a source. There may be a history of visits to eye practitioners, the use of contact lenses, testing of conjunctival specimens, or treatment of patients with the disorder. Contaminated anesthetic solutions used before tonometry are a cause, as are contaminated eye instruments, particularly tonometers.

Acute hemorrhagic conjunctivitis.— This is a specific violent inflammatory conjunctivitis caused by a picornavirus type 70. The disorder is endemic and appears to be selflimited, without sequelae. It was first seen in Africa in 1969 and has appeared in west and north Africa, the Orient, Latin America, and Florida. There is an explosive onset of conjunctivitis with eyelid edema, tearing, serous discharge, and conjunctival hemorrhages. Conjunctival follicles and enlarged preauricular lymph nodes occur. Reticulomyelitis has been reported. Acute and convalescent serum samples indicate increasing titers of picornavirus type 70 antibodies, but the virus is seldom recovered from the eye.

Acute bacterial conjunctivitis caused by *Streptococcus pneumoniae, Haemophilus influenzae,* other bacterial pathogens, or adenovirus infections may produce conjunctival hemorrhages without follicular reaction. By contrast, acute hemorrhagic conjunctivitis is explosive at onset, bilateral, and characterized by eyelid edema, chemosis, follicles, and hemorrhages; the signs peak at 48 hours and rapidly regress.

Lacrimal conjunctivitis.—Lacrimal conjunctivitis is a monocular conjunctivitis secondary to infections caused by microorganisms in the lacrimal sac in which drainage into the nose is blocked. The inflammation persists until lacrimal drainage is established. Usually dacryocystitis does not involve the conjunctiva. Pneumococcus infection of the lacrimal sac may cause keratitis. Fungal occlusion of the canaliculi can sometimes be recognized by a scraping sound when the lacrimal system is probed.

Parinaud oculoglandular syndrome.— This is a traditional ophthalmic eponym, but the condition is rarely seen. It consists of a monocular, granulomatous, necrotic conjunctival lesion associated with a suppurative preauricular adenopathy. The name must be differentiated from Parinaud sign, which is the inability to rotate the eyes upward because of a midbrain neoplasm, principally pinealoma. The chief causes of Parinaud oculoglandular syndrome include chancre, tuberculosis, lymphogranuloma venereum, oculoglandular tularemia, infectious mononucleosis, cat-scratch disease, and fungal infections.

CHRONIC CONJUNCTIVITIS

Chronic conjunctivitis is a general term applied to persistent conjunctival inflammation characterized by injection, scanty exudation, and periodic exacerbations and remissions. It may be caused by many agents. Symptoms vary from mild grittiness or foreign body sensation, with heaviness of the eyelids, to burning, photophobia, and irritation. The symptoms may be severe enough to handicap the patient and are often disproportionately severe for the clinical signs of disease. Examination indicates hyperemia, microscopic papillae, thickening of the conjunctiva in the fornices, mucous secretion, and sometimes epithelial keratitis. Causes include the following:

1. *Staphylococcus aureus* infection is usually associated with a chronic blepharitis and an epithelial keratitis involving the lower half of the cornea. Both *Moraxella* species and *Staphylococcus aureus* may cause inflammation of the temporal conjunctiva (angular conjunctivitis). There may be a follicular reaction in patients with *Moraxella* infections.
2. A variety of microorganisms often considered nonpathogenic, such as demodex mites, have been implicated. These organisms often reside on body surfaces but may be found in almost pure culture. Presumably, when appropriate predisposing conditions are present, they may produce inflammation.
3. Molluscum contagiosum skin nodules and verruca vulgaris (warts) of the eyelid

margin may cause a chronic conjunctivitis with epithelial keratitis. Molluscum contagiosum nodules must be removed to relieve the conjunctivitis; excision of warts may lead to seeding. Cryotherapy is effective.

4. Chemical and physical irritants and unsuspected foreign bodies may be a cause. The use of sun lamps without ocular protection may cause an actinic keratoconjunctivitis. Chemical irritation from the chlorine in swimming pools is an obvious cause. Drugs used to treat ocular disease may cause irritant or contact conjunctivitis.
5. Excessive meibomian secretion is characterized by a frothy secretion at the inner and outer angles of the eyelids and may either cause or complicate chronic conjunctivitis.
6. Chronic conjunctival inflammation in acne rosacea may precede acne rosacea corneal vascularization.

Treatment of chronic conjunctivitis is difficult. Careful diagnosis is essential, and the cause must be eliminated if possible. Lesions of the eyelids and eyelid margins, such as cysts, warts, and nodules of molluscum contagiosum, must be eliminated. Keratoconjunctivitis sicca must be excluded, and the tear ducts must be tested for patency. Allergy and irritations caused by chemicals, smoke, and cosmetics must be minimized. Many of the same symptoms result from abnormalities of the precorneal tear film.

Trachoma.—Trachoma is a chronic, bilateral, cicatrizing keratoconjunctivitis caused by *Chlamydia trachomatis.* There are three main serotypes, and the disease varies considerably in severity. It is endemic, often associated with conjunctivitis, and is the chief cause of blindness in the world. It is estimated that 500 million people have trachoma and that 5 million are blind because of its complications. Basophilic inclusion bodies may be found, particularly in the acute stage, in epithelial scrapings stained with Giemsa stain. Antibodies to *Chlamydia* may be present both in eye secretions and in the serum. The severity of the disease varies markedly, and there are unexplained regional differences. In the United States trachoma is largely confined to Native Americans in the Southwest. Entire populations in regions of poverty, flies, dryness, and poor hygiene may be infected. Scarring of the tarsal conjunctiva leads to entropion and trichiasis. The scarring occludes the orifices of goblet cells and accessory and main lacrimal glands with mucous deficiency and ocular drying. Corneal vascularization with superimposed infection by *Neisseria gonorrhoeae* or *Haemophilus aegyptius* (Koch-Weeks bacilli) further complicates the disease.

Chlamydia organisms are sensitive to sulfonamides, tetracyclines, and erythromycin. Topical therapy with tetracycline or erythromycin eye ointment three times daily for 6 weeks or 10% sulfacetamide eyedrops three times daily for 8 weeks are effective in the acute stages. Corrective surgery of deformed eyelids may prevent blinding complications. Flies must be eliminated and hygiene improved, a major problem in regions with neither running water nor plumbing. Active immunization by inoculation is complicated by the several strains, poor cross-immunity, and weak antigenicity. Surgery is required for cicatricial distortion of the eyelids.

IMMUNE RESPONSES OF HYPERSENSITIVITY

An immune response is a beneficial reaction of the tissues to a specific protein or material that is foreign to the organism (antigen). Hypersensitivity is an exaggerated or inappropriate immune response that causes inflammatory reactions and tissue damage. The first contact with an antigen does not cause a hypersensitivity reaction but results in the formation of antibodies on cell surfaces. Four types of hypersensitivity reactions are described (types I, II, III, and IV) (see Chapter 25). These may occur in isolation or occur simultaneously.

Type I hypersensitivity (immediate hypersensitivity) occurs when a mast cell sensitized by immunoglobulin E (IgE) encounters an antigen to which it is sensitive and releases histamine and the mediators of inflammation. Type II hypersensitivity (antibody-dependent cytotoxic hypersensitivity) develops when antibody binds to either an individual's self-surface antigen or to a foreign antigen on the cell surfaces and leads to phagocytosis, killer cell activity, or complement-mediated lysis of target cells. Type III hypersensitivity (immune complex mediated) develops when antigen-antibody immune complexes form in such excessive quantities that they cannot be cleared adequately by the reticuloendothelial system. Type IV hypersensitivity (delayed hypersensitivity) develops when macrophages do not properly degrade an antigen and subsequently encounter T cells sensitized by the same antigen. The T cells elaborate lymphokines, which attract and activate additional macrophages to release inflammatory mediators.

Type I hypersensitivity reactions of the eye include hay fever conjunctivitis, acute and chronic conjunctivitis, atopic keratoconjunctivitis, vernal conjunctivitis, giant papillary conjunctivitis, and the reactions to insect stings. Type II hypersensitivity may mediate cicatricial conjunctivitis (conjunctival pemphigoid). Type III hypersensitivity may play a role in Stevens-Johnson syndrome, Sjögren syndrome, Reiter syndrome, anterior uveitis, and retinal vasculitis. Type IV hypersensitivity occurs in corneal graft rejection, sympathetic ophthalmia, posterior uveitis, Vogt-Koyanagi-Harada syndrome, and ocular tuberculosis.

TYPE I HYPERSENSITIVITY

Hay fever conjunctivitis.—This is a mild, recurrent, seasonal hypersensitivity that is usually associated with allergic rhinitis. There is sneezing, rhinorrhea, nasal obstruction, and conjunctival and pharyngeal itching. The conjunctiva and eyelids are swollen and the conjunctiva is milky or pale pink in color. A clear, watery exudate in the acute phase becomes thick and stringy in the chronic phase.

Airborne allergens such as pollen, molds, dust, and animal dander trigger a type I hypersensitivity. The allergens react with specific IgE immunoglobulins bound to mast cells and basal cells located on the nasal mucosa and conjunctival epithelium. This reaction releases inflammatory mediators of the arachidonic acid cascade and the degranulation of mast cells with the release of histamine.

Treatment is directed toward minimizing exposure to the responsible allergens. Vasoconstrictive eyedrops, cold compresses to the eyes, and systemic antihistamines provide symptomatic relief. Mast cell stabilizers applied topically four times daily reduce symptoms. Topical corticosteroids provide prompt relief but cannot be used for the prolonged periods required.

Atopic keratoconjunctivitis.—Male teenagers with a history of childhood atopic dermatitis (often before the age of 2 years) may develop a bilateral conjunctival inflammation that resembles vernal conjunctivitis but is not seasonal. There may be erythematous and exanthematous inflammation of the skin of the eyelids and a seborrheic blepharitis. The conjunctiva is pale with papillary hypertrophy of the palpebral conjunctiva that is more marked on the lower eyelids. In vernal conjunctivitis, which may resemble atopic keratoconjunctivitis, the papillary hypertrophy affects the upper eyelids. There may be corneal staining with fluorescein and vascularization of the cornea. Keratoconus is common. A cataract may affect the anterior cortex (anterior shieldlike). The personal and family history of atopic dermatitis, and the wheal-and-flare reaction to many common antigens, help differentiate the condition from vernal conjunctivitis.

Treatment is difficult. Patients should avoid irritating soaps, excessive sweating, rough-textured clothing, scratching, and emotional stress. Topical corticosteroids may be helpful for skin lesions but, generally, administration of systemic corticosteroids should be minimized. Oral antihistamines may control itching. Topical mast cell stabilizers instilled four times daily may be helpful.

Giant papillary conjunctivitis.—Hard and soft (rarely) contact lenses, an ocular prosthesis (artificial eye), or the exposed tip of a buried suture may sometimes stimulate giant papillae on the upper tarsal conjunctiva. The papillae are similar to those of vernal conjunctivitis, but there is less itching. Conjunctival mucus production impairs vision and is unsightly. If contact lenses are the cause, the wearing time is reduced, followed by inability to tolerate the lenses. A lens of a different polymer, a change from soft to hard lenses (or vice versa), or a substitution of hot sterilizers for cold may be helpful. Preservatives in eye solutions may be the cause, and single-unit eyedrops that do not contain preservatives are commercially available.

A new ocular prosthesis may be helpful in patients who have had an enucleation. Irritating sutures may be removed. All symptoms and signs stop if the exciting agent is removed. Topical mast cell stabilizers may help, but often contact lens wearers find no relief and require corneal surgery to correct the refractive error.

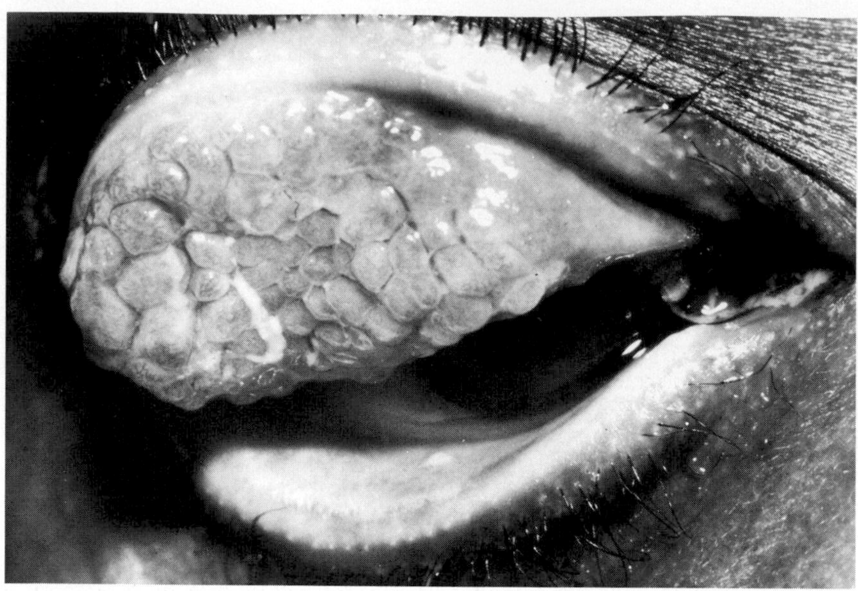

FIG 12-1.
Palpebral form of vernal conjunctivitis with marked papillary proliferation of the tarsal conjunctiva.

Insect bites and stings.—These cause both a toxic inflammatory response and an immunologic IgE-mediated response. Hypersensitivity reactions vary from simple urticaria to anaphylactic shock. Mild symptoms of pruritus and urticaria can be controlled by subcutaneous administration of 0.2 to 0.5 mL of 1:1,000 epinephrine. Severe symptoms require intravenous infusions, tracheostomy, and early supportive management to prevent death.

Vernal conjunctivitis.—Vernal conjunctivitis is a bilateral recurrent hypersensitivity that occurs during the warm months of the year, particularly in hot climates. Boys are more commonly affected until puberty; thereafter, both sexes are affected equally. Three forms occur: (1) palpebral (Fig 12-1), which involves the tarsal conjunctiva of the upper eyelid with the formation of typical thickened gelatinous vegetations; (2) limbal, the most common form in blacks, associated with the formation of a gelatinous, elevated area about 4 mm wide at the corneoscleral limbus; and (3) mixed. There is often a personal or family history of hay fever, asthma, or atopic eczema.

The principal symptom is itching, which may be nearly intolerable. It is aggravated by sweating, ocular irritation, and rubbing the eyes. Papillary hyperplasia of the upper tarsal conjunctiva appears as large, grayish pink, vegetating masses. Limbal nodules appear as small, semitransparent elevations. There is a thin, ropy, white secretion. Conjunctival scrapings contain numerous eosinophils, plasma cells, and mast cells. Tear IgG and histamine levels are increased.

The disorder gradually subsides over a 5- to 10-year period. Residence in a cool climate and air conditioning of sleeping areas may be helpful. Removal of the thick, ropy secretion with a 10% solution of acetylcysteine may be helpful. Topical corticosteroids or topical mast cell stabilizer eyedrops are used. Radiation therapy is contraindicated. Topical cyclosporine may be helpful.

TYPE II HYPERSENSITIVITY

Chronic cicatricial conjunctivitis.—Chronic cicatricial conjunctivitis (benign mucous membrane pemphigoid, ocular cicatricial pemphigoid, essential shrinkage of the conjunctiva) is a chronic, autoimmune, systemic, progressive disorder that particularly affects women more than 60 years of age. The deposition of anti-basement membrane zone antibodies, particularly in the subepithelium of the conjunctiva and oral mucosa, causes subepithelial fibrosis. The mucous membranes of the esophagus, pharynx, and nose and, more rarely, the vaginal and anal mucosa may be affected.

Initially there are conjunctival erosions that stain with 1% rose bengal solution and a mucoid discharge. There is an associated subconjunctival fibrosis. The conjunctiva shrinks with obliteration of the fornices, ectropion, and trichiasis. Destruction of the goblet cells with loss of mucin leads to dryness of the eye with keratinization of the conjunctiva and cornea. The progressive scarring may obliterate the conjunctival fornices, fuse the eyelids together, and cover the cornea with a leathery membrane.

The lesions appear to be the result of a type II hypersensitivity reaction in which antibodies against the lamina lucida of the basement membrane of stratified squamous epithelium bind to all of the body's epithelium. The antibodies may be demonstrated in about 25% of the patients and their titers may parallel the clinical course of the disorder.

Immunofluorescent studies show deposition of immunoglobulins, chiefly IgG, but also IgA, IgM, and complement 3, in the basement membrane of the skin, conjunctiva, and other mucous tissues. Levels of tumor necrosis factor alpha are increased and those of interleukin 6 are markedly depressed. There may be a 30-fold increase in T cells, with more CD8-positive cells than CD4. (CD refers to cluster of differentiation. CD8-positive cells are cytolytic and CD4-positive cells are helper.)

Treatment is not satisfactory. Artificial tears (without preservatives) and ointments are used for lubrication. Local mucus production may be reduced by instillation of a 10% acetylcysteine solution. Aberrant eyelashes should be removed, and if cryotherapy for epilation is used, care must be taken to avoid freezing the conjunctiva. Systemic azathioprine and transplantation of nasal mucosa from the inferior turbinate to the conjunctiva ameliorates pain. Early use of systemic corticosteroids in large doses sometimes combined with cyclophosphamide or azathioprine may help, but one fourth of the patients are blinded by the disease.

Similar conjunctival inflammation may occur in erythema multiforme (Stevens-Johnson syndrome), epidermolysis bullosa, toxic epidermal necrolysis, linear IgA disease, and alkali burns of the eye. Topical application of pilocarpine, echothiophate, epinephrine-containing compounds, and idoxuridine may produce scarring of the conjunctiva that resembles chronic cicatricial conjunctivitis.

TYPE III HYPERSENSITIVITY

The Sjögren syndrome is the major ocular condition attributed to intolerance of the patient's own tissue antigens. It causes dry eyes (keratoconjunctivitis sicca) (see Chapter 13). Rheumatoid arthritis is the most prevalent systemic disorder related to type III hypersensitivity.

TYPE IV HYPERSENSITIVITY

Delayed hypersensitivity is a frequent cause of many conditions that include chronic microbial infections, transplant rejection, neoplasms, and reactions to simple chemicals. This mechanism affects the conjunctiva in phlyctenulosis and hypersensitive contact conjunctivitis.

Phlyctenulosis.—This is a monocular, localized, cell-mediated type of conjunctival hypersensitivity. Hypersensitivity to tuberculoprotein and staphylococcal antigen are common causes. *Candida albicans, Coccidioides immitis, Leishmania* species, and the agent of lymphogranuloma venereum are also causes. Phlyctenulosis is most common during the first two decades of life, when there is a particularly high degree of responsiveness to cell-mediated hypersensitivity. Usually the bulbar conjunctiva is affected with a nodule 0.5 to 3 mm in size that follows a 10-day course of elevation, infiltration, ulceration, and resolution. There is severe photophobia if the cornea is involved, but otherwise symptoms are minimal. Corneal phlyctenules attract a stalk of new blood vessels from the corneoscleral limbus and may cause loss of vision, requiring keratoplasty. Phlyctenules caused by tuberculoprotein hypersensitivity respond quickly to topical corticosteroids. The *Staphylococcus* type requires treatment of the associated blepharitis.

Phlyctenular keratoconjunctivitis.—This is a cell-mediated immune response of the cornea and conjunctiva. It is a common cause of decreased vision among Eskimos, presumably because of their increased sensitivity to tuberculin.

Contact conjunctivitis.—This occurs in one of two forms: (1) irritant (the most common) and (2) hypersensitive. Hypersensitive contact conjunctivitis (and dermatitis) is nearly always caused by tissue sensitization as the result of topical administration of ophthalmic drugs. Those most likely to induce sensitization are neomycin, atropine, idoxuridine, gentamicin, and thimerosal. Other medications include chloramphenicol, penicillin, topical anesthetics, antihistamines, homatropine, scopolamine, benzalkonium, and silver and zinc salts. Other substances include mascara, eye shadow, eyebrow pencil, soap, hair dye, nail polish, perfumes, cosmetics, shampoo, hair spray, eye makeup, and eyeglass cleaning fluid. The pattern of an eyelid reaction may suggest the cause. Adhesive tape and nickel (eyeglass nasal pads) cause sharply demarcated lesions; linear streaks are caused by plants; spreading lesions may be caused by cosmetics, poison oak, or poison ivy; and monocular lesions are caused by eyedrops and contamination by the patient's fingers. The condition is marked by itching, chemosis of the conjunctiva, and eosinophils in the scrapings.

Primary irritant contact conjunctivitis is a follicular type of conjunctivitis that is particularly marked in the lower cul-de-sac. Symptoms are minimal, and the disease is often considered a chronic conjunctivitis. Eosinophils are not found in conjunctival scrapings. Almost any topical medication or its vehicle may be a source of such irritation. The conjunctivitis disappears when the medication is stopped, and once it has improved, the drugs may sometimes be reinstituted without recurrence. The irritation may constitute an untoward reaction to the vehicle or a preservative rather than the active principle of the medication.

Contact with the offending agent must be eliminated. Corticosteroids may aggravate contact conjunctivitis, and the preservative in corticosteroid eyedrops may cause the condition.

KERATITIS

Corneal inflammation may be caused by microorganisms, tear deficiency, denervation, exposure, drying, immune reactions, ischemia, and mechanical, photic, or chemical trauma. There may be associated lesions of the eyelids (nodules, vesicles, ulcers) or conjunctiva (follicles, papillae, inflammation, fibrosis), and these structures must be evaluated in every instance of corneal inflammation.

Corneal inflammations cause ocular discomfort that ranges in severity from a foreign body sensation to incapacitating pain. Bowman membrane beneath an epithelial defect stains a bright green with topical fluorescein solution (sterile 2% or a fluorescein strip). The cornea through which the iris pattern and pupil are normally clearly visible is clouded with edema, inflammatory cells, and sometimes new blood vessels. The ciliary blood vessels are injected.

The cornea and conjunctiva are protected by the periodic closure of the eyelids; the Bell phenomenon, in which the eyes turn up and out in closure; the sensory innervation; the flow of tears; the antimicrobial action of tears; and the tight junctions of the corneal epithelium. The many nonpathogenic microorganisms normally present on the ocular surface may suppress the growth of pathogenic bacteria. Inflammations of the peripheral cornea are often secondary to conjunctivitis, drying, or a localized ischemia. Central corneal ulceration is often preceded by a break in the corneal epithelium, which allows introduction of organisms. Corneal inflammations may be ulcerative with loss of tissue or nonulcerative. They may be central, peripheral, superficial, or stromal. They may be infectious or noninfectious.

Ulcerative inflammations affect the epithelium, stroma, or both in a progressive necrosis with loss of corneal tissue. Corneal necrosis adjacent to the corneoscleral limbus stimulates early neovascularization from the corneal vascular arcade that often results in rapid repair. Central ulcerative lesions tend to have more tissue destruction than those in the periphery, possibly secondary to the absence of blood vessels or a collagenase stimulated by, or provided by, neutrophils.

Nonulcerative inflammations affect the epithelium, subepithelium, or stroma in a generalized or nodular lymphocytic infiltration. There is no tissue necrosis, but corneal opacification, neovascularization, or both, may impair vision.

ULCERATIVE KERATITIS

Ulcerative keratitis may involve all layers of the cornea and may be central or peripheral. There is an outpouring of polymorphonuclear leukocytes that is often combined with extensive necrosis of the corneal stroma. Healing results in scarring (leukoma). In severe necrosis, the Des-

TABLE 12-3.
Microbial Inflammation (Keratitis)

Type	Cause
Bacterial	
Keratoconjunctivitis	Extension of conjunctivitis to corneal margin, staphylococci, streptococci
Keratitis	Enterobacteriaceae, fecal contamination
Necrotizing keratitis	*Pseudomonas aeruginosa* and trauma, contaminated eyedrops
Acute hypopyon ulcer (pus in anterior chamber)	Trauma combined with *Streptococcus pneumoniae* or hemolytic streptococci
Indolent ulcer	*Haemophilus* sp., *Moraxella liquefaciens*
Pannus (vascularized scar)	*Chlamydia trachomatis*
Interstitial keratitis	Spirochaetaceae, *Treponema* sp., congenital syphilis (rare in acquired)
Fungal	
Keratomycosis	Injury by plant material, prolonged topical antibiotics and corticosteroids, compromised host
Viral	
Dendritic keratitis epitheliitis	Herpes simplex (*Herpesvirus hominis* type I)
Adenovirus keratitis	Any adenovirus
Epidemic keratoconjunctivitis	Adenovirus 8 or 19
Zoster keratitits: epitheliitis (early); mucous plaques (late)	Varicella-zoster virus involving the ophthalmic branch of trigeminal nerve (N V)

cemet membrane may thicken and bulge through the base of an ulcer, a descemetocele. The cornea may perforate with a subsequent endophthalmitis. A staphyloma or kerectasia may follow healing.

The major causes of central ulcerative keratitis are microbial invasion, corneal anesthesia, exposure, and vitamin A deficiency. The corneal stroma requires an epithelial covering, and a persistent epithelial defect results in stromal thinning ("melting"). All bacteria except *Neisseria gonorrhoeae* require a break in the epithelium to infect the cornea. The organisms may be introduced by a corneal foreign body, may be present in the lacrimal system, conjunctiva, or eyelids, or may enter the cornea through contaminated fingers or contact lenses (Table 12-3).

The major bacterial families (see Chapter 25) that cause keratitis are (1) Micrococcaceae (*Staphylococcus aureus, Staphylococcus epidermidis,* and *Micrococcus* species); (2) Streptococcaceae (hemolytic *Streptococcus* species and *Streptococcus pneumoniae*); (3) Pseudomonadaceae *(Pseudomonas aeruginosa);* and (4) Enterobacteriaceae. Less common bacterial causes include *Moraxella* species and *Serrata marcescens.*

Many "nonpathogenic" fungi cause keratitis, particularly in eyes treated with corticosteroids and after immune suppression. The most common fungi that cause corneal ulcers are *Aspergillus fumigatus, Candida albicans, Fusarium solani,* and *Curvularia* species.

Protozoa of the genus *Acanthamoeba* are free-living amebas that are found in water, soil, and sewage. They may contaminate contact lens solutions and infect the cornea after minor injury to the epithelium by the lens. Immunofluorescent staining of excised corneal tissue may be required to demonstrate the organism, which is often resistant to treatment.

Treatment of infectious ulcerative keratitis requires preliminary identification of the likely organism followed by specific identification after appropriate microbial studies. Often, treatment is initially empiric, and appropriate diagnostic steps are initiated only after the ulcer has progressed. Identification of the microbial cause may then be impossible.

The first step in treatment is to collect material by scraping the ulcer with a platinum spatula under magnification. Scraped material should be stained with Gram stain for bacteria and fungi, Giemsa for cytology, and Grocott methenamine silver stain for fungi. The limulus lysate assay detects gram-negative endotoxin. Scrapings are often plated on the following media: rabbit blood agar at 37° C; sheep blood agar at 25° C; chocolate blood agar at 37° C under increased CO_2 tension, Sabouraud dextrose-peptone agar with yeast extract, and 50 μg/mL of gentamicin, maintained on a ro-

TABLE 12-4.
Treatment of Microbial Corneal Ulcers Based on Gram Stain

Gram Stain	Topical	Subconjunctival if Central or Peripheral (More Than 5 mm in Diameter)	Systemic if Perforation Threatened
Gram-positive cocci: Micrococcaceae, Streptococcaceae, *Sarcina* sp.	Cefazolin, 50 mg/mL, and tobramycin, 11 mg/mL	Cefazolin, 100 mg, and tobramycin, 40 mg	Methicillin, 200 mg/kg/day
Gram-positive rods: *Corynebacterium* sp., Bacillaceae, *Propionibacterium* sp.	Gentamicin, 14 mg/mL; or tobramycin, 11 mg/mL, and cefazolin, 50 mg/mL	Penicillin G, 500,000 units; gentamicin, 20-40 mg	Penicillin G, 2-6 kg/4 hr; gentamicin, 5 mg/kg/day
Gram-negative cocci: *Moraxella* sp., *Neisseria* sp. (diplococci)	Gentamicin, tetracycline, or erythromycin	Penicillin G, 500,000 units/mL	Penicillin G, 2-6 g/kg/4 hr
Gram-negative rods: Pseudomonadaceae, Enterobacteriaceae *(Escherichia coli, Proteus* sp., *Klebsiella pneumoniae)*	Tobramycin, 11 mg/mL, and carbenicillin, 4 mg/mL	Tobramycin, 40 mg, and carbenicillin, 25 mg	Carbenicillin, 46 kg/4 hr
No organisms stained	Tobramycin, 11 mg/mL, and cefazolin, 50 mg/mL	Cefazolin, 100 mg, and tobramycin, 40 mg	Methicillin
Possible fungi	Natamycin, 50 mg/mL; or miconazole, 10 mg/mL; or amphotericin B, 2.5-10 mg/mL	Amphotericin, 750 μg	Amophotericin Ketoconazole, 200-400 mg/day
	Nystatin ointment, 100,000 units		Flucytosine, 150 mg/day

tary shaker at 25° C; and thioglycolate broth at 37° C. Usually virus infections are not cultured unless a superinfection is suspected; however, blood is drawn for measurement of antibodies.

The contact lenses and the lens storage cases of patients who wear contact lenses should also be cultured. Attention should be directed to prolonged or repeated use of the same disposable contact lens.

Initial treatment with concentrated antibiotic eyedrops (Table 12-4) is based on the results of the Gram stain. Local experience determines the choice of antibiotic. After isolation of the causative organism, determination of its antibiotic sensitivity may indicate specific therapy. Concentrated eyedrops are prepared by mixing antibiotics formulated for intravenous administration (Table 12-5) in a small volume of sterile artificial tears (a method not described by the Food and Drug Administration). Collagen shields saturated with the appropriate medication give promise of delivering a high concentration of antibiotic.

Patients with ulcers smaller than 2 mm that involve the anterior one third of the cornea may be treated as outpatients. Larger and deeper ulcers should be treated in a hospital. A 1% atropine solution is instilled two or three times daily. If there is severe corneal necrosis, a temporary gas-permeable bandage contact lens may be used.

TABLE 12-5.
Initial Treatment of Corneal Ulcer before Examination of Scrapings

	Topical	Subconjunctival
Cefazolin	50 mg/mL	100 mg
Tobramycin	11 mg/mL	40 mg
Bacitracin	10,000 units/mL	—
Gentamicin	15 mg/mL	40 mg
Methicillin	—	100 mg

Ulcerative inflammations of the peripheral cornea are often associated with conjunctivitis. Initially there is a marginal corneal infiltrate at the corneoscleral limbus. Patients complain of tearing, redness, and photophobia. There is marked ciliary and conjunctival vascular congestion in the affected quadrant. The infiltration extends to form an arc-shaped ulcer par-

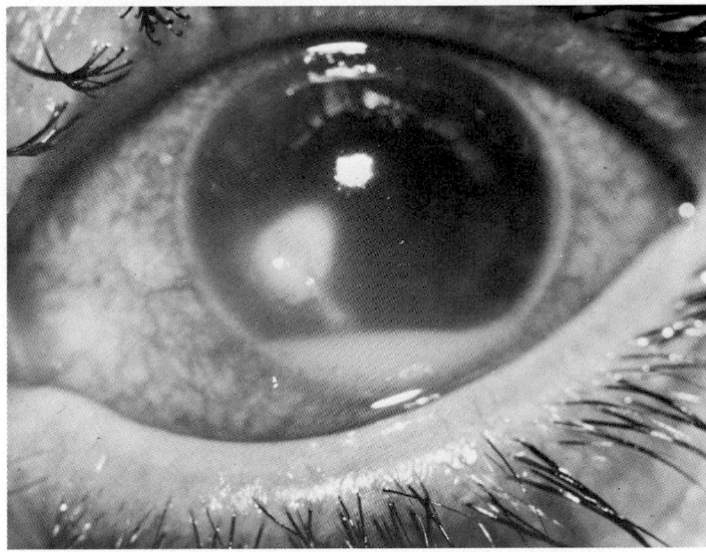

FIG 12-2.
An acute hypopyon ulcerative keratitis caused by a *Streptococcus* infection in a 69-year-old patient with facial nerve paralysis that prevented adequate closure of the eyelid. Leukocytes in the anterior chamber form a hypopyon.

allel to the corneal margin. The most common cause is hypersensitivity to *Staphylococcus* exotoxin or antigen in blepharitis or conjunctivitis. Such ulcers respond favorably to corticosteroids combined with erythromycin or bacitracin ointments. An associated acne rosacea requires the addition of tetracycline systemically.

Peripheral ulcers as the result of microbial conjunctivitis may extend centrally and require the same treatment as central ulcerative keratitis.

MICROBIAL KERATITIS

Bacterial infections

Acute hypopyon ulcer.—An acute hypopyon ulcer (once considered the classic type of central ulcerative keratitis) is a severe bacterial inflammation of the cornea associated with pus in the anterior chamber (hypopyon) and a severe iridocyclitis (Fig 12-2). *Streptococcus pneumoniae* (pneumococcus) is the usual cause; the organism often originates in an infected lacrimal system. Other bacterial causes are *Staphylococcus aureus* and *Moraxella* (in the homeless). Often the keratitis is preceded by mild trauma and loss of corneal epithelium, which allows entry of the organism. The ulcer is a dirty gray color, with overhanging margins. The cornea is thinned, and the conjunctiva is violently injected. If untreated, the cornea may perforate and the eye may be lost because of a purulent inflammation.

The bacteria are sensitive to many antibiotics, and the ulcer responds quickly to treatment. A concurrent pneumococcal dacryocystitis may necessitate dacryocystorhinostomy or temporary occlusion of the canaliculi.

Pus in the anterior chamber, in the absence of keratitis, is a cardinal sign of endophthalmitis. It may occur months after uncomplicated cataract surgery with an intraocular lens implant or indicate a bleb infection after glaucoma filtering surgery. Rarely, it complicates fungal keratitis. It may be a sign of leukemia in the absence of intraocular infection.

***Pseudomonas aeruginosa* central ulcer.**—*Pseudomonas aeruginosa* ulcer is caused by a common gram-negative aerobic bacillus found in the normal skin and intestinal tracts of humans. The organism produces an extracellular protease that enzymatically degrades corneal proteoglycans. Additionally, the invading polymorphonuclear leukocytes and the cornea itself produce collagenases that degrade corneal collagen.

Pseudomonas keratitis is more common in men than in women. A history of corneal trauma, contact lens wear, previous inflammatory eye disease, or concurrent serious systemic

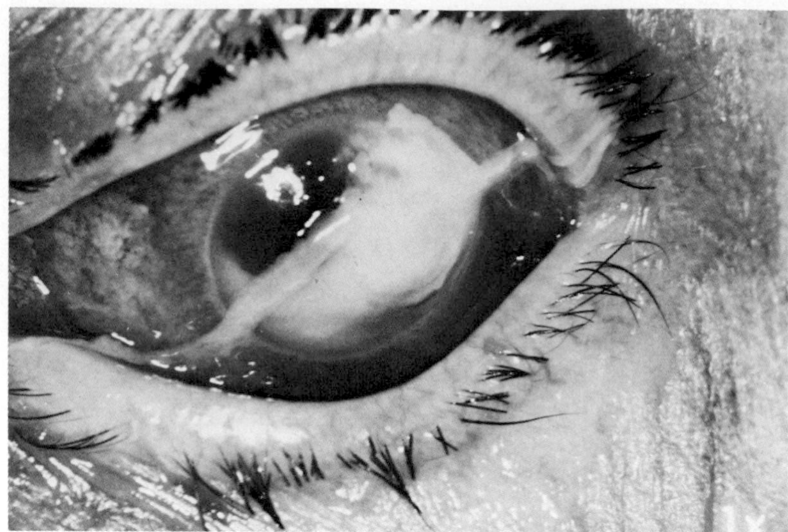

FIG 12-3.
Pseudomonas aeruginosa infection of 3 days' duration that developed during the topical treatment of uveitis with atropine and prednisolone.

disease is common. The ulcer (Fig 12-3) usually begins centrally. It quickly broadens and deepens and has a fulminating course. The cornea may perforate within 48 hours of onset.

Treatment is by subconjunctival injection of tobramycin or ciprofloxacin together with topical instillation of concentrated ciprofloxacin or tobramycin every 30 minutes.

A corneal abrasion caused by a contact lens is more likely to cause a *Pseudomonas* keratitis than one caused by a fingernail. The abrasion should not be treated with occlusion of the eye with an eye patch or with any topical medication that contains corticosteroids.

Protozoan infections

***Acanthamoeba* keratitis.**—A severe persistent keratitis may be caused by members of the genus *Acanthamoeba*. These are small, ubiquitous, free-living protozoa that feed on bacteria and are found in contaminated water and material. The organisms may be introduced into the cornea by minor trauma.

Many instances of *Acanthamoeba* keratitis occur in contact lens users who wear disposable lenses for prolonged periods or do not discard them after a single use. The use of tap water to make solutions for use with contact lenses, or to clean contact lenses or their carrying cases, may lead to *Acanthamoeba* infection. The inflammation often becomes resistant to medical treatment. Infections that are present for more than 4 weeks usually require keratoplasty.

Bacteria are often present on culture, but the causative *Acanthamoeba* is never demonstrated on culture. Corneal examination using a tandem scanning corneal microscope discloses bright, ovoid to round objects in the epithelium that measure between 5 and 30 μ in diameter. The diagnosis is confirmed by cytologic analysis of the infected epithelium. The absence of bacteria, which the ameba requires for nutrition, minimizes ameba in the corneal stroma. Topical anti-ameba medications, such as chlorhexidine digluconate (0.02%), sometimes combined with oral itraconazole, may be effective in infections of less than 4 weeks' duration.

Fungal infections

Infection of the cornea by fungi has increased 15-fold since the introduction of topical administration of corticosteroids and antibiotics. The disorder is common in subtropical climates during dry, windy months. Except for *Candida* infections, which often occur (55%) in women with severe debilitating disease, most fungal infections occur in otherwise healthy men, often farmers who have a history of a recent ocular injury. There may be a history of contact lens wear or prolonged topical corticosteroid and antibiotic therapy.

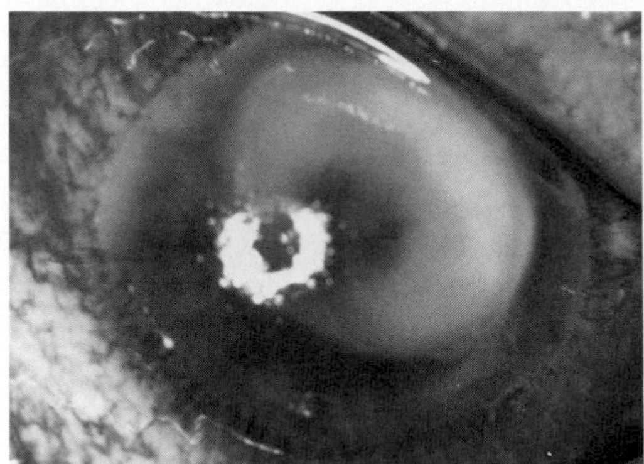

FIG 12-4.
Fungus ulcer of cornea with deep infiltrate and severe ciliary injection. There is no corneal vascularization.

Clinically the fungal ulcer (Fig 12-4) appears as a fluffy, grayish white elevation, having a dry rough texture and feathery margins. It may be surrounded by a grayish, sharply demarcated halo that persists for months. The central lesion may have satellite lesions or pseudopods. Corneal vascularization is minimal but a hypopyon is common. The ciliary injection may be disproportionately severe for the amount of keratitis present.

The mycotic ulcer has a rapid onset and resembles ulcers caused by bacteria. A specimen obtained by scraping the base and edges of the ulcer is essential to the diagnosis. Treatment is difficult, and a conjunctival flap or a penetrating keratoplasty combined with antifungal therapy may be required. Topical atropine cycloplegia is used. Initial treatment is topical 5% natamycin once every waking hour. Topical 1% solutions of miconazole, clotrimazole, econazole, or ketoconazole have broad antifungal activities except against *Fusarium,* which requires natamycin. Ketoconazole may be given orally in daily doses of 200 to 400 mg. Amphotericin B may be used topically in concentrations of 0.15%, but systemic administration is not effective against keratomycosis. Corticosteroid administration is always contraindicated even when a graft rejection follows keratoplasty. The selection of treatment is complex and must be guided by identification of the causative organism in scrapings or culture.

Many eyes do not heal until a conjunctival flap is drawn over the cornea surgically. Mechanical removal of the fungi by curettage may be beneficial. Rapidly progressive deep ulcers with descemetocele or perforation require a penetrating transplant with a diameter that encompasses all of the pseudopods to remove as much of the fungi as possible. A lamellar corneal transplant may not be effective because of failure to remove all fungi.

TABLE 12-6.
Herpesvirus Hominis Disease

Type 1: Lips, skin, eye, and genitalia
Type 2: Genitalia, lips, skin, and eye
Primary herpes infection
Recurrent herpes infection
  Epithelial infectious keratitis
    Dendritic
    Geographic
Herpes-induced ocular abnormalities (noninfectious)
  Viral interstitial keratitis (antigen-antibody response to live virus)
  Disciform keratitis (T cell–mediated response to herpes simplex virus antigens fixed to epithelial cells)
  Epithelial trophic keratitis (metaherpetica; secondary basement membrane defects)
  Sterile stromal ulceration (failure of corneal collagen synthesis, secondary to persistent absence of epithelium)
  Iridocyclitis

Viral infections

Herpesvirus hominis infections of the cornea (Table 12-6) are initially limited to the epithelium but, with recurrence, involve the corneal stroma (disciform keratitis) in a central ulcerative keratitis. Conjunctival scrapings generally show a mononuclear leukocyte response; the virus may be isolated in tissue culture. Fluorescent antibody staining of corneal scrapings are often more reliable and rapid than culture.

There are two types of *Herpesvirus hominis:* type 1, the usual cause of facial, oral, or ocular lesions; and type 2, associated mainly, but not exclusively, with genital infections (see Chapter 25). Herpes simplex type 1 is nearly as common a cause of genital infection as type 2.

Primary infection affects about 80% of the population who usually do not recall an earlier infection. Clinical signs occur in less than 10% of those with primary infection, but all become carriers and are subject to recurrent infections. Primary infection is usually transmitted by an individual with an acute recurrent inflammation of the lips or mouth (cold sore). After primary infection, the virus persists in a latent form in ganglia, and recurrent infection occurs throughout life. Replication of the virus may be triggered in some persons by fever, ultraviolet light, immunosuppression, trauma, stress, or menstruation. Most individuals have no specific initiating factor.

When the primary infection causes clinical signs (10%), there may be vesiculation of the lips, mouth, genitalia, or skin, or a severe systemic disorder (0.1%). Primary herpes infection of the eye is rare. Initial herpes vesicles of the eyelids are followed by unilateral, ulcerated blepharitis with preauricular adenopathy. Follicular or pseudomembranous conjunctivitis may occur with preauricular lymphadenopathy. The rare corneal involvement resembles small phlyctenular spicules.

Neonatal infection may follow prolonged labor or premature rupture of the membranes in mothers with genital herpes. Babies may also be infected from maternal nongenital lesions, from other infants in a nursery, and by professional staff. Neonatal ocular infection with herpesvirus type 1 or type 2 causes a severe inflammation with conjunctivitis, keratitis, cataract, necrotizing retinitis, optic neuritis, and encephalitis.

Dendritic keratitis.—Dendritic keratitis (Greek *dendron:* tree) is an acute or chronic corneal inflammation that occurs in an individual who has had a primary infection with *Herpesvirus hominis* type 1. The latent virus (or the virus genome) persists in the trigeminal or ciliary ganglia.

Epithelial keratitis (Fig 12-5) begins with punctate epithelial opacities that become vesicular and coalesce in a branching linear pattern, which stains with fluorescein. Corneal sensitivity is markedly diminished. The epithelium between the dendrites is lost; the result is a sharply demarcated, irregularly shaped geographic (ameboid) ulcer. Both eyes are infected in fewer than 10% of patients and rarely simultaneously. Symptoms include foreign body sensation, lacrimation, and reduction of vision if the optical area of the cornea is involved. After frequent attacks, the patient is aware of recurrence even before signs of inflammation are present.

Initial treatment consists of mechanical removal of the virus-laden epithelial cells. After topical anesthesia (4% cocaine solution loosens epithelial cells) the cells are removed with a moist cotton-tipped applicator or scalpel blade. The basement membrane must not be injured. Trifluridine (1%) is instilled topically every waking hour for 14 days, or vidarabine ointment (3%) is instilled five times daily. Topical acyclovir (3%) heals dendritic ulcers more rapidly than trifluridine but is not available for topical ophthalmic use in the United States.

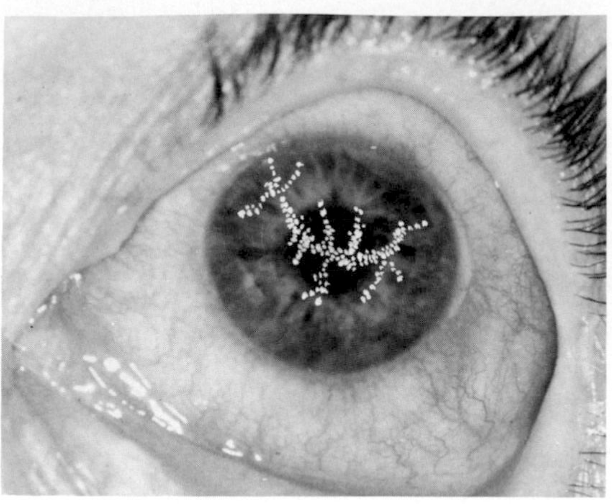

FIG 12-5.
The branching pattern of dendritic keratitis.

Stromal inflammation occurs in several forms. The most common, disciform keratitis, consists of a disk-shaped, localized grayish area of stromal edema, with localized keratic precipitates. The edema may be limited to the stroma adjacent to the epithelium or involve the full thickness of the cornea.

Disciform keratitis is a CD4 cell (helper)–mediated immune reaction against herpesvirus antigens, HLA-DR, and intercellular adhesion molecules fixed to corneal cells. The HLA-DR–dependent immune response is inhibited by the cytokine interleukin 10, which does not affect those responses initiated by the intercellular adhesion molecule. Treatment is individualized, depending on involvement of the visual axis and severity of the disease. Ophthalmic ointments prevent epithelial disruption, and cycloplegics combat the iritis. If the inflammation progresses or the visual axis is affected, a corticosteroid may be instilled every 2 to 4 hours. Antivirals must be instilled prophylactically at full dosage. Patients readily become dependent on the relief of corticosteroids, and the corneal stroma may

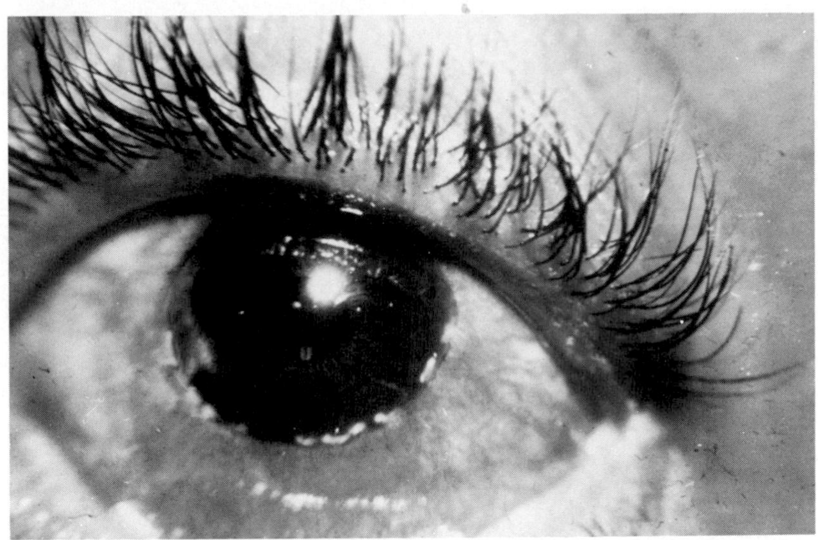

FIG 12-6.
Acute *Staphylococcus aureus* conjunctivitis with marginal corneal infiltrates caused by sensitivity to the exotoxin of the bacteria.

slowly thin, with eventual corneal perforation. A full-thickness corneal transplant may be required.

Peripheral ulcerative keratitis

The peripheral cornea is nurtured by the corneal capillary arcade so that this portion of the cornea is less vulnerable to progressive infection than the central cornea. Additionally, any opacities are not in the visual axis. Conversely, the blood vessels of the conjunctiva may deposit immune complexes as well as Langerhans cells with their inflammatory mediators and histocompatibility antigens in the peripheral cornea. Loss of the normal conjunctival blood supply causes an ischemia of the peripheral cornea. Progressive necrosis, loss of tissue, and inflammation of the peripheral cornea occur less commonly than in central ulcerative keratitis. The inflammation may be secondary to a collagen disease, infection, bacterial hypersensitivity, or phlyctenular keratoconjunctivitis.

Marginal catarrhal ulcers.—Marginal catarrhal ulcers (Fig 12-6) complicate longstanding staphylococcal blepharoconjunctivitis. The ulcer is not a corneal infection but an antigen-antibody immune complex reaction in a tissue sensitized to the staphylococcus. The reaction activates complement, which attracts neutrophils. The treatment must be directed to the blepharoconjunctivitis with eyelid scrubs and topical erythromycin. The corneal inflammation improves with topical corticosteroids.

Mooren ulcer.—This is a chronic, painful, progressive, nonpurulent ulceration that originates in the superficial layers of the peripheral cornea of elderly people. It may be bilateral (25%). A similar ulceration may develop in the Wegener granulomatosis, Vogt-Koyanagi-Harada disease, and periarteritis nodosa. The ulcer has a gray, overhanging margin that may be elevated. It extends circumlimbally or centrally and may cover the entire cornea with scar tissue. The ulceration may be caused by an autoimmune response of the corneal stroma to corneal or conjunctival epithelium. There are circulating antibodies to conjunctival epithelium but not to corneal epithelium.

Mooren ulcers in younger persons and bilateral ulcers are less responsive to treatment. Systemic immunosuppressive therapy is indicated, as is excision of the conjunctiva at the corneoscleral limbus adjacent to the ulcer. A corneoscleral homograft is useful.

CENTRAL ULCERATIVE KERATITIS

Anesthesia of the cornea, failure of the eyelids to cover the eye, continued corneal irritation by the eyelashes or eyelid, dryness of the eye, or vitamin A deficiency may lead to a central ulcerative keratitis (Table 12-7).

TABLE 12-7.
Central Corneal Inflammation

Immunologic abnormalities
- Anaphylactic: vernal keratoconjunctivitis
- Cytotoxic: Mooren ulcer
- Immune complex: marginal catarrhal ulcer
- Cell mediated: phlyctenular keratitis

Vascular disease
- Arteritis: interstitial keratitis and N VIII (Cogan)
- Ischemia: surgical, systemic disease; collagen disease

Nutritional deficiency
- Vitamin A and protein: keratomalacia
- Acne rosacea

Innervational
- Neurotropic keratitis (section N V and N VIII)

Tear film abnormality
- Keratoconjunctivitis sicca
  - Loss of aqueous portion: Sjögren
  - Loss of mucin: erythema multiforme, ocular cicatricial pemphigoid
  - Local drying (delle; *pl.* dellen)
  - Superior limbic (failure to wet epithelium)

Eyelid abnormalities
- Entropion or ectropion
- Trichiasis and eyelid margin abnormalities
- Corneal exposure: lagophthalmos, exophthalmos
- Faulty blinking

Trauma
- Radiation: ultraviolet exposure, "snow blindness," laser
- Mechanical
- Chemical
- Climatic droplet keratopathy, spheroid degeneration (wind, sand, snow)

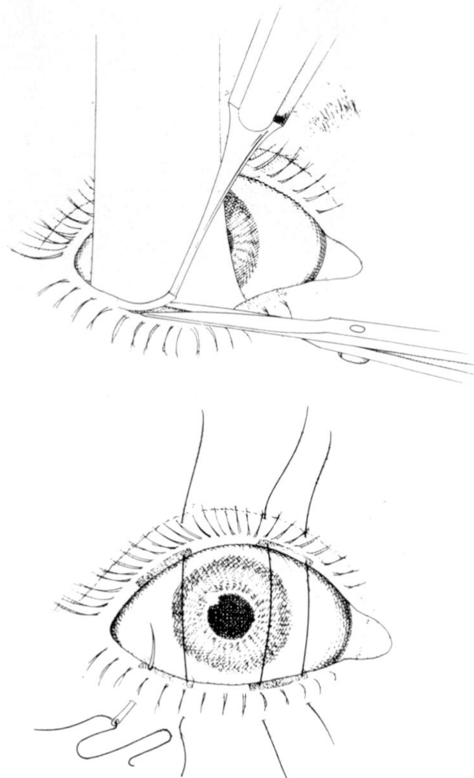

FIG 12-7.
Temporary tarsorrhaphy in which posterior portions of the upper and lower eyelid margin are denuded and brought together with sutures to prevent exposure of the cornea.

Neuroparalytic keratitis.—This is a corneal inflammation that results from anesthesia of the cornea, which permits trauma and desiccation of the corneal epithelium, which has lost its reflex protection. Additionally, the trigeminal nerve may play a role in the metabolism of the cornea. Because the cornea is anesthetic, there is no pain, but the conjunctiva is inflamed. The lesion begins inferiorly with exfoliation and ulceration, and it may progress until there is loss of the eye. Suturing the upper to the lower eyelid (tarsorrhaphy; Fig 12-7) is the usual method of treatment.

If a neurosurgical procedure requires section of both the trigeminal and facial nerves, a neuroparalytic keratitis should be anticipated and a tarsorrhaphy performed before the cornea ulcerates. Other causes include surgery for trigeminal neuralgia, herpes zoster ophthalmicus, familial dysautonomia, and corneal anesthesia as the result of trigeminal nerve impairment.

Exposure keratitis.—Exposure keratitis, sometimes called keratitis e lagophthalmos, is an inflammation caused by the failure of the eyelids to cover the globe. There is exfoliation of the corneal epithelium followed by secondary infection. The condition is most commonly associated with facial nerve (N VII) disorders in which the orbicularis oculi muscle is paralyzed. The cornea may be similarly exposed after blepharoptosis surgery or in severe proptosis.

Keratitis e lagophthalmos causes pain and ciliary injection. It is evident on examination that the cornea is not protected by closure of the eyelids. Treatment is directed toward prevention of corneal drying. In mild cases, the instillation of an ointment at bedtime and protection of the globe are all that is required. In facial nerve paralysis, a temporary blepharoplasty may be carried out. Soft contact lenses may be effective. If the paralysis is permanent and there is no likelihood of restoration of the facial nerve function, a permanent type of blepharoplasty is done. Proptosis with exposure keratitis requires a central tarsorrhaphy and correction of the proptosis.

Keratomalacia.—Vitamin A deficiency is a major cause of childhood blindness in many developing countries. Vitamin A is a fat-soluble vitamin derived either from conversion of carotene or from preformed vitamin in the diet. Carotene is present in many plants, particularly leafy greens and yellow vegetables. Preformed vitamin A is derived from butterfat, cheese, and liver. Failure to ingest adequate vitamin A or its precursors is commonly associated with other dietary deficiencies, notably inadequate protein. Secondary deficiency occurs because of inadequate saponification of vitamin A in the gut. The deficiency is observed in sprue, in celiac disease, after extensive resection of the small intestine, and in cystic fibrosis of the pancreas. Failure to store vitamin A occurs in cirrhosis of the liver.

Vitamin A deficiency in the retina has been studied carefully, particularly in animals in which nutrition can be supported by administration of vitamin A acid, which is not converted to retinal. In humans, vitamin A deficiency causes blindness by (1) destruction of the cornea in xerophthalmia (dry eye) and keratomalacia (cornea softening); (2) loss of 11-*cis* retinal of the photopigments of the retina; (3) faulty growth of bone causing optic nerve compression in the optic canal; and (4) faulty fetal development in a vitamin-deficient mother.

Impression cytology of the bulbar conjunctiva detects early absence of goblet cells and enlarged epithelial cells in early vitamin A deficiency. In children with acute deficiency, dryness of the conjunctiva (xerosis conjunctivae) is the initial clinical sign of the deficiency. It is paralleled by night blindness, which may not be evident. Bitot spot is present, particularly in boys. It occurs on the exposed bulbar conjunctiva, usually in the palpebral fissure on the temporal side. It appears as a highly refractile mass with a silvery gray hue and a foamy surface. It is superficial, and the foam may be rubbed off, leaving a roughened conjunctival surface that fills with foam again in several days.

The keratomalacia, or softening of the cornea, may be generalized or localized. It may lead to destruction of the eye if infection occurs. It is particularly common with an associated protein deficiency. Generally, it occurs in infants and not in adults.

Mild vitamin A deficiency caused by improper nutrition may be reversed by a diet that contains protein and carotene. Severe disease requires supplemental vitamin A.

NONULCERATIVE KERATITIS

Nonulcerative keratitis is a corneal inflammation that may be self-limited and temporary or progressive and prolonged. Unlike ulcerative keratitis, it is not associated with tissue loss or tissue necrosis. It may involve the corneal epithelium, the subepithelium, or the corneal stroma. Epithelial keratitis occurs in conditions in which basal corneal cells are separated from their basement membrane, causing either punctate defects in the epithelium or large erosions. Subepithelial keratitis involves both the epithelium and its basement membrane in a punctate inflammation, which is caused by trauma, ultraviolet burns, and adenovirus infection, but may also occur with spheroidal degeneration, acne rosacea, and onchocerciasis. Stromal keratitis, particularly of the deeper layer of the cornea, is seen in syphilis, onchocerciasis, sarcoidosis, and tuberculosis, and with vestibuloauditory symptoms (of Cogan).

Epithelial keratitis.—In epithelial keratitis, separation of basal cells from their basement membrane causes either punctate epithelial defects or large erosions. Epithelial keratitis occurs in viral infection with the herpesvirus and adenovirus and ultraviolet burns of the eye. In stromal keratitis there is infiltration of edematous corneal tissue with lymphocytes and plasma cells, often accompanied by an iritis. Stromal inflammation occurs in the interstitial keratitis in herpes zoster ophthalmicus, tuberculosis, leprosy, and onchocerciasis.

Superficial punctate keratitis.—Superficial punctate keratitis (Thygeson) is a chronic, bilateral, possibly viral disorder, in which numerous, irregular, randomly distributed, epithelial corneal opacities occur in both eyes intermittently over a 3- or 4-year period. The lesions stain variably with fluorescein.

There are many remissions and exacerbations and eventual healing without corneal opacities. Patients complain of intermittent burning, irritation, tearing, and blurred vision. Under magnification, from 1 to 50 (usually about 20) minute, oval, corneal opacities are visible. They are composed of a conglomeration of minute dots. New lesions appear as old ones heal so that their distribution varies from examination to examination. Hyperemia of the conjunctiva is present in the 12 o'clock meridian.

Topical corticosteroids relieve the irritation and sometimes resolve the epithelial lesions. Soft therapeutic contact lenses may provide relief, but the lesions may recur when the use of the lenses is discontinued.

Superior limbic keratoconjunctivitis.— This is a bilateral chronic keratinization of the superior bulbar conjunctiva, which results in a papillary reaction of the tarsal conjunctiva and punctate staining of the superior cornea, sometimes (25%) with filaments. It occurs more often in women than in men. It is usually but not always bilateral and occurs at all ages. There is burning, a foreign body sensation, and sometimes tearing. The superior cornea and adjacent epithelium stain with rose bengal solution. The symptoms may originate with inadequate wetting of the superior cornea and may be relieved by resection of the adjacent conjunctiva. Topical corticosteroids are not effective. Therapeutic contact lenses may be helpful, but their use may be precluded by inadequate tearing.

Syphilitic interstitial keratitis.—Syphilitic interstitial keratitis is mainly a complication of congenital syphilis that affects predominantly boys, 5 to 20 years after birth. There is associated anterior uveitis followed by endothelial edema and then a generalized corneal edema. The cornea is then invaded by peripheral blood vessels that appear to push a faint opacity in front of them. The blood vessels meet to form a "salmon patch" and the inflammation subsides. Years later the empty corneal blood vessels (ghost vessels) appear as faint gray lines.

Onchocerciasis.—Infection with the nematode *Onchocerca volvulus* results in deposition of the adult worm in subcutaneous fibrous nodules. The adult worms produce microfilariae that evoke a severe localized inflammation of the corneal stroma. There is an anterior uveitis and a progressive opacification of the corneal stroma. Ivermectin reduces the number of systemic microfilariae.

Viral keratitis.—Nonulcerative keratitis occurs in many viral infections and may or may not be associated with prominent systemic abnormalities. Many of the adenoviruses cause corneal inflammation (epidemic keratoconjunctivitis). Herpes zoster ophthalmicus, which is caused by varicella-zoster, may cause severe anterior uveitis and keratitis. The photophobia observed in measles is caused by a keratoconjunctivitis that is frequently not diagnosed. Mumps may cause a transient corneal edema. Mononucleosis may be associated with deep corneal infiltrates.

Molluscum contagiosum.—This is a mildly contagious skin disease caused by a virus of the pox group that is characterized by the occurrence of small, smooth, waxy, umbilicated papules. When they occur on the eyelids, a follicular conjunctivitis and epithelial keratitis may occur. Effective treatment requires removal of each papule, usually by lightly freezing it and removing its core with a curette.

Verruca (wart).—Verrucae of the eyelid margin or surface of the eye caused by the human papilloma virus (wart virus) generally disappear spontaneously and are usually not treated. Shedding of the virus into the conjunctival sac may cause inflammation that requires excision of the wart. Excision of warts may cause seeding; cryotherapy or electrodesiccation may be used. The excimer laser is useful.

BIBLIOGRAPHY

Books

Pepose JS, Holland GN, Wilhelmus KR: *Ocular infection and immunity,* St Louis, 1995, Mosby–Year Book.

Smolin G, Thoft RA, editors: *The cornea: scientific foundations and clinical practice,* Boston, 1994, Little, Brown.

Articles

Donshik PC: Giant papillary conjunctivitis, *Trans Am Ophthalmol Soc* 92:687-744, 1994.

Tugal-Tutkun I, Akova YA, Foster CS: Penetrating keratoplasty in cicatrizing conjunctival diseases, *Ophthalmology* 102:576-585, 1995.

13

THE LACRIMAL SYSTEM

The lacrimal system consists of glands that secrete tears and a drainage system that collects them. The glands include the lacrimal gland in the upper outer portion of the orbit and the basic tear secretors, located in the conjunctiva and in the margins of the eyelids. The drainage system is composed of tubes (the canaliculi) that extend from openings (the puncta) located at the inner corners of the upper and lower eyelids to the lacrimal sac that opens into the nose.

The tears (see Chapter 2) consist of a relatively stagnant layer, the precorneal tear film, and an aqueous layer that flows in the inferior conjunctival cul-de-sac to the inferior punctum. The precorneal tear film provides the smooth and regular anterior refracting surface of the eye. It has three layers: (1) a superficial oily layer that prevents evaporation that originates from the meibomian glands and the sebaceous glands of Zeis, located in the margins of the eyelids; (2) a middle aqueous layer that originates from the conjunctival glands of Krause and Wolfring; and (3) an inner mucin layer that originates from conjunctival goblet cells (mainly), glands of Manz, and crypts of Henle and that wets the hydrophobic corneal epithelium. The glands in the conjunctiva and eyelids are the basic secretors. They produce tears at a constant rate and are not controlled by the nervous system or by emotion. The lacrimal gland secretes both aqueous and mucous components in response to trigeminal nerve (N V) stimulation and to psychic stimulation (crying).

SYMPTOMS AND SIGNS OF LACRIMAL SYSTEM DISEASE

Diseases of the lacrimal system cause either abnormalities of tear secretion or faulty drainage of tears. Excessive tear formation indicates either reflex stimulation of the lacrimal gland (lacrimation) or occlusion in the lacrimal drainage system (epiphora). Decreased tear formation usually indicates either atrophy of the basic secretors of the conjunctiva and eyelids or conjunctival abnormalities, particularly scarring, that occlude their orifices. Neoplasms or inflammation of the lacrimal gland cause a characteristic local swelling and an S-shaped curve of the upper eyelid. Neoplasms of the lacrimal drainage system are uncommon. Acute inflammation of the lacrimal sac (dacryocystitis) causes a cellulitis of the inner canthus. Chronic inflammation mainly results in a painless swelling of the lacrimal sac and pus expressed from the puncta when pressure is applied to the sac.

The main symptoms of diseases of the lacrimal system are related to an excess or a deficiency of tears or to swelling of the lacrimal gland or lacrimal sac. Excessive tear formation or poor drainage is a nuisance, since vision is blurred by tears that overflow onto the face. Deficient tear secretion, however, may be associated with keratinization of the conjunctiva and cornea. It may cause nearly intolerable symptoms of burning and dryness of the eyes.

TEARING AND DRY EYES

Excessive tear formation (lacrimation) or defective drainage of tears (epiphora) is associated with blurring of vision and constant discomfort caused by tears running down the cheek. In every instance it is necessary to learn whether there is excessive production or defective drainage of tears.

MEASUREMENTS OF TEARS

The volume of tears is measured clinically (Table 13-1) by means of a 35 × 5.0-mm strip of Whatman 41 filter paper (available commercially as Iso-Sol strips) that is folded 5 mm from one end. The folded end is hooked over the lateral portion of the lower eyelid (Fig 13-1). The extent to which the filter paper beyond the fold is wet by tears is measured after 5 minutes. The test is conducted in a dimly lit room to diminish reflex stimulation.

Reflex secretion of tears by the lacrimal gland is measured without conjunctival anesthesia (Schirmer I). Reflex tear secretion is considered normal if 10 mm or more of the paper from the fold is moistened. In the absence of psychic tearing and excessive ocular irritation (the filter paper itself causes some irritation), more than 25 mm of wetting indicates excessive tear formation.

The basic tear secretion by the accessory lacrimal glands occurs at a constant rate and is not controlled by the nervous system. It is the sole supply of tears during sleep and in the newborn. Basic tear secretion is measured with filter paper in the same way as reflex secretion, but the conjunctiva and cornea are first anesthetized with a topical anesthetic solution. Basic secretion is considered normal if 8 to 15 mm of the filter paper measured from the fold is moistened.

If the basic test is combined with irritation of the nasal mucosa with a cotton-tipped applicator used to stimulate reflex tearing, both basic and reflex reaction is measured (Schirmer II). Less than 15 mm of wetting of the filter paper 2 minutes after hooking over the eyelid indicates a deficiency of tear formation.

A drop of 1% rose bengal dye in the conjunctival sac stains dead or damaged conjunctival and corneal cells. Patients with a deficiency of the aqueous portion of tears have punctate staining of the lower two thirds of the cornea, and the bulbar conjunctiva stains bright red in the region corresponding to the palpebral apertures.

TABLE 13-1.
Tests for Secretion of Tears and Patency of Lacrimal Drainage System

- I. Tear secretion
  - A. Reflex tear secretion
    - 1. Schirmer I: Wetting of Whatman filter paper
  - B. Basic tear secretion
    - 1. Wetting of filter paper after topical anesthesia
  - C. Combined reflex and basic secretion
    - 1. Schirmer II: Topical anesthesia plus irritation of nasal mucosa
  - D. Tear film breakup
    - 1. Disappearance of fluorescein from corneal surface
    - 2. Norn: Dilution of fluorescein in the conjunctival cul-de-sac
  - E. Lactoferrin assay
    - 1. Radial immunodiffusion
- II. Lacrimal drainage
  - A. Jones I: Appearance of fluorescein in nose after topical instillation
    - 1. Use cobalt light to excite fluorescence
  - B. Jones II: Irrigate lacrimal sac with fluorescein solution
    - 1. Use cobalt light to excite fluorescence
  - C. Fluorescein disappearance
    - 1. Disappears from conjunctival cul-de-sac within 1 minute
  - D. Dacryocystography
    - 1. Radiography after injection of radiopaque medium in sac
  - E. Taste test (saccharine or quinine)
    - 1. Sweet or bitter taste after instillation of solution in conjunctival cul-de-sac

LACRIMATION

Lacrimation, or the overproduction of tears, is caused by emotional or reflex stimulation of the lacrimal gland (Table 13-2). Prolonged tearing may deplete the lacrimal gland so that the tear testing shows normal or decreased tear formation. Abnormal regeneration of the seventh cranial nerve after facial nerve paralysis may result in tearing during eating (crocodile tears). Hyperthyroidism, tic douloureux, pseudobulbar palsy, or cholinergic stimulation

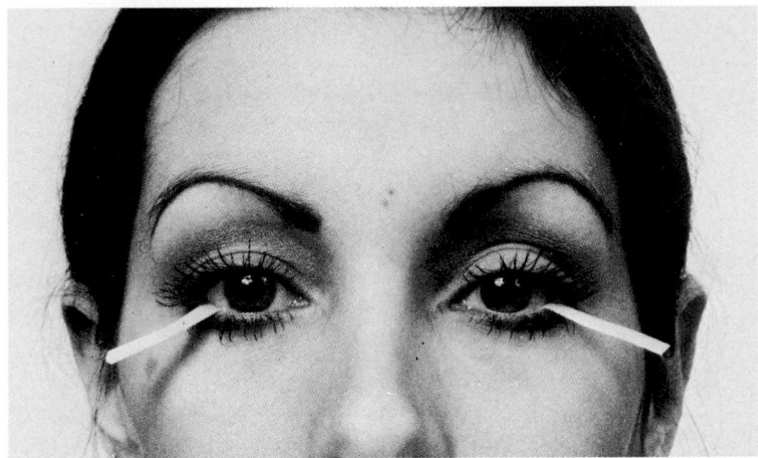

FIG 13-1.
Measurement of the quantity of tears by using strips of filter paper hooked over the lateral portion of the lower eyelid.

TABLE 13-2.
Causes of Lacrimation (Excessive Secretion by Lacrimal Gland)

I. Crying (psychic stimulation)
II. Trigeminal nerve (N V) stimulation
  A. Lesions of eyelids, conjunctiva, cornea, iris
  B. Angle-closure glaucoma
III. Retinal (N II) stimulation
  A. Glare, excessive light
IV. Facial nerve (N VII) abnormalities
  A. Sphenopalatine ganglion
    1. Inflammation
    2. Neoplasm
  B. Misdirected regeneration
    1. With chewing (crocodile tears)
  C. Medications
    1. Cholinergic
    2. Anticholinesterase
V. Lacrimal gland
  A. Inflammation (dacryoadenitis)
  B. Neoplasm

by either cholinergic or anticholinesterase drugs may lead to a pharmacologic type of lacrimation. Often the cause of lacrimation can be easily identified and corrected.

Epiphora

Epiphora is a condition in which there is tearing because of impaired drainage of tears through the lacrimal passages (Table 13-3). It has a variety of causes: entropion or ectropion with faulty apposition of the lacrimal puncta to the lacrimal lake; scarring and occlusion of the puncta; paresis or paralysis of the orbicularis oculi muscle, which impairs the pumping action of the canaliculi; foreign bodies in the canaliculi; occlusion of the canaliculi; and obstructions in the lacrimal sac and the nasolacrimal duct. The accumulation of tears at the inner canthus causes irritation, which by reflex stimulates additional tear formation.

The patency of the lacrimal drainage system may be demonstrated in several ways. Inspection of the eyelids indicates the position of the lacrimal puncta at the inner corner of each eyelid, in contact with the lacrimal lake. When the patient looks upward, the puncta of the lower eyelids turn inward and cannot be seen without everting the eyelids. Forcible closure of the eyelids indicates the adequacy of the orbicularis oculi muscles (N VII) in creating a small suction in the drainage system with normal blinking.

Fluorescein (sterile, 2% solution) instilled in the lower conjunctival cul-de-sac can normally be seen, after 1 minute, beneath the inferior turbinate or in the nasopharynx. If the fluorescein is not seen, normal sterile saline is irrigated through the inferior punctum. If fluorescein is then seen in the nasopharynx, it indicates a functional obstruction in the nasolacrimal duct that opens into the nose (Jones test II). If fluorescein cannot be demonstrated in the nasopharynx after irrigation, it suggests a block in the canaliculi.

Inability to irrigate the lacrimal system through the puncta demonstrates a severe obstruction. If, however, a fold of mucous membrane obstructs the lacrimal sac, the irrigating fluid may force its way into the nose and wrongly indicate a patent lacrimal sac.

TABLE 13-3.
Causes of Epiphora (Impaired Drainage of Tears)

- I. Eyelids
  - A. Puncta
    - 1. Malposition (ectropion)
    - 2. Occlusion
      - a. Scarred
      - b. Congenital absence
      - c. Impacted secretion
  - B. Orbicularis oculi muscle (N VII)
    - 1. Weakness
      - a. Impaired canalicular suction
- II. Canaliculi
  - A. Occlusion
    - 1. Fungal impaction
    - 2. Scarred
    - 3. Inflamed
- III. Lacrimal sac and nasolacrimal duct
  - A. Neoplasm
  - B. Scarred
  - C. Inflamed
- IV. Nasal meatus
  - A. Stenosis
    - 1. Congenital
    - 2. Acquired
      - a. Edema nasal mucous membrane

TABLE 13-4.
Some Causes of Dry Eyes

- I. Lacrimal gland disorders
  - A. Local disorders
    - 1. Atrophy or aplasia
    - 2. Radiation
    - 3. Excision
  - B. Denervation
    - 1. Facial nerve
      - a. Between lacrimal nucleus and geniculate ganglion
      - b. Greater superficial petrosal nerve
      - c. Sphenopalatine ganglion
    - 2. Trigeminal nerve
      - a. Decreased reflex secretion
- II. Systemic disease
  - A. Sjögren disease
  - B. Sarcoidosis
  - C. Connective tissue disease
  - D. Lymphoma
  - E. Adie syndrome
  - F. Familial dysautonomia
- III. Medications
  - A. Cholinergic blockade (atropine-type drugs)
  - B. Antihistamines
  - C. Analgesics
  - D. Glaucoma medications
    - 1. Beta-blockers
- IV. Disorders of accessory tear glands
  - A. Meibomianitis
  - B. Conjunctival scarring
    - 1. Trauma (chemical, radiation, thermal, surgical)
    - 2. Cicatricial conjunctival pemphigoid
    - 3. Erythema multiforme
    - 4. Trachoma
- V. Eyelid abnormalities
  - A. Infrequent blinking
  - B. Exophthalmos
- VI. Abnormal ocular surfaces
  - A. Pterygium
  - B. Dellen
- VII. Excessive evaporation of tears
  - A. Air conditioning
  - B. Low humidity
  - C. Excess tear lipids
    - 1. Blepharitis
    - 2. Acne

The management of epiphora depends on its cause. Surgery of the eyelid is indicated when the punctum is not in contact with the lacrimal lake. Obstruction in the lacrimal sac may require repeated probing with successively larger probes or a dacryocystorhinostomy. Atresia of the canaliculi may be difficult to correct. If the lacrimal sac has been obliterated, a glass tube extending from the conjunctival cul-de-sac into the nose or maxillary sinus will provide drainage.

DRY (SICCA) EYE

A tearing eye is a nuisance and may blur vision, but it never causes blindness. The absence of tears, however, may cause keratinization of the corneal and conjunctival epithelium and may result in blindness (Table 13-4). Removal of the lacrimal gland is not associated with drying of the eye, although reflex and psychic tearing is lost. The accessory lacrimal glands maintain normal moistening of the eye in most but not every person.

Decreased tear secretion is particularly associated with conjunctival scarring that occludes the orifices of the glands of the conjunctiva and margins of the eyelids that moisten the eye. Decreased tear secretion occurs predominantly in keratoconjunctivitis sicca and may occur in Sjögren syndrome, amyotrophic sclerosis, and some bulbar palsies. There is less than 10 mm of wetting of filter paper (Schirmer I test; see Fig 13-1) in a 5-minute period even after irritation of the nasal mucosa. The eyes burn, feel dry, and have a constant foreign body sensation. Symptoms are aggravated by warmth and conditions that cause rapid evaporation of tears. There may be punctate epithelial erosions of the cornea and the conjunctiva, which stain with rose bengal solution.

Keratoconjunctivitis sicca.—Keratoconjunctivitis sicca is a common symptom complex, particularly in the elderly. Disturbances in the stability of the precorneal tear film (see Chapter 2) causes dry spots to form on the corneal epithelium. The cornea loses its usual luster and mucus floats as strands or sheets in the tear film or may adhere to the epithelium. Filamentary strands of epithelium may be present. Chronic conjunctivitis and seborrheic blepharitis are common. The cornea and the conjunctiva stain with 1% rose bengal solution.

Patients complain of gritty, sandy, foreign body sensations in the eye or irritation and itching, all of which are worsened by a hot, dry atmosphere and tobacco smoke. Symptoms may be aggravated by reading or by infrequent or incomplete blinking.

Four types of keratoconjunctivitis occur:

1. In the fluid deficiency type, there is atrophy of the main or accessory lacrimal glands, and the aqueous portion of the tear film is thinned and deficient. This is the classic type seen in Sjögren syndrome. A decreased amount of lacrimal gland tissue occurs in collagen diseases. In the Riley-Day syndrome, there is deficient lacrimal gland innervation that may also be pharmacologically induced by ganglionic blockade.
2. Mucin secreted by conjunctival goblet cells is required to wet the hydrophobic corneal epithelium. Mucin deficiency occurs in ocular cicatricial pemphigoid (see Chapter 12), and erythema multiforme. These disorders ultimately reduce the aqueous portion of tears through scarring of the secretory ducts of the accessory lacrimal glands of Krause and Wolfring. Mucin deficiency also occurs in vitamin A deficiency and chemical burns of the conjunctiva.
3. Elevated lesions of the cornea or conjunctiva may cause the tear film to break up at the apex of the lesion as occurs in pterygium, trachoma, herpes simplex, and similar disorders that induce irregularities of the ocular surface. A similar mechanism may cause a relatively depressed area adjacent to an elevated area to dry, which causes a failure of synthesis of corneal stroma with a corneal pit (German *dellen:* pits or depressions).
4. Failure to blink or infrequent or incomplete blinking may cause inadequate distribution of normal tears, as occurs in neuroparalytic keratitis. Localized dry spots occur next to dellen and pterygium because their elevation prevents tears from wetting depressed regions of the conjunctiva in blinking. Any abnormality of the eyelids in which the globe is not covered may cause inadequate wetting of the ocular surface.

The treatment of dry eyes is often difficult. Any medical or mechanical cause must be corrected. Patients should avoid tobacco smoke and smog, which irritate the eyes. Hot and dry atmosphere encourages evaporation of tears and should be avoided. The superior and inferior puncta may be occluded to reduce the drainage of tears by using either punctum plugs or surgical closure. Punctal closure may result in a reflex diminution of tear secretion and must be used with much caution. Airtight covering of the eyes with swimming goggles may conserve tears. If the parotid gland secretion is adequate, transplantation of the Stenson duct may moisten the eye with a generous salivary secretion.

A number of artificial tear products are available, and patients often experiment until they find one that is satisfactory. Physiologic saline provides only momentary relief. Artificial tears containing methyl cellulose, polyvinyl alcohol, or 0.2% sodium hyaluronate solution provide more prolonged wetting. Ointments should not be used during waking hours because they tend to dry the eyes and blur vision. The preservatives used to prevent contamination of artificial tears may cause hypersensitivity reactions of the conjunctiva and eyelids. If solutions that do not contain preservatives are used, they must be changed frequently to avoid secondary infection. Hypotonic and alkaline eyedrops may provide the greatest relief.

Sjögren syndrome.—Sjögren syndrome is an autoimmune, slowly progressive disorder, which mainly affects middle-aged women, but which affects all ages and both sexes. It is characterized by dry eyes (keratoconjunctivitis sicca), a dry mouth (xerostomia), and lymphocytic infiltration of the lacrimal and salivary glands. Interleukin 10, a cytokine usually produced by T cells (see Chapter 25) is produced in large amounts by activated B lymphocytes and mononuclear leukocytes.

The deficient tear production causes red, dry, burning, itching eyes, and photophobia. There may be an accumulation of thick strings of mucus at the inner canthus. The conjunctiva and cornea stain with 1.0% rose bengal solution in regions of detached epithelium and the Schirmer I test discloses markedly reduced tear secretion.

The dry mouth makes it difficult to swallow dry food, to speak continuously, and to wear full dentures. The oral mucosa is red and dry and there is atrophy of the fuliform papillae of the tongue. Salivary gland scintigraphy is the most reliable test of salivary function in Sjögren syndrome. In primary Sjögren syndrome the salivary and lacrimal glands may be enlarged with lymphocyte infiltration, whereas these changes are not common in the secondary types.

Secondary Sjögren syndrome complicates rheumatoid arthritis, systemic lupus erythematosus, and scleroderma. Some 60% of the patients with the primary syndrome develop arthritis and arthralgias. Some 60% of the patients with primary Sjögren syndrome develop rheumatoid arthritis. B cell lymphoma and Waldenström macroglobulinemia may occur.

HLA-B8, -DR8, -DR3, and Drw52 are prevalent in Sjögren syndrome. A condition identical to the primary Sjögren syndrome occurs in AIDS.

DISORDERS OF THE COLLECTING SYSTEM

CANALICULITIS

Canaliculitis is an inflammation of the canaliculi, the ducts that extend between the lacrimal puncta in the upper and lower margins of the eyelids and the lacrimal sac. It is secondary to an obstruction in the lumen of the canaliculi.

Most attention has been directed to the inflammation associated with obstruction by *Actinomyces* species. Canaliculitis causes tearing and inflammation of the adjacent conjunctiva. Recovery of the organism from the canaliculus and a gritty foreign body sensation during probing in the canaliculus establish the diagnosis.

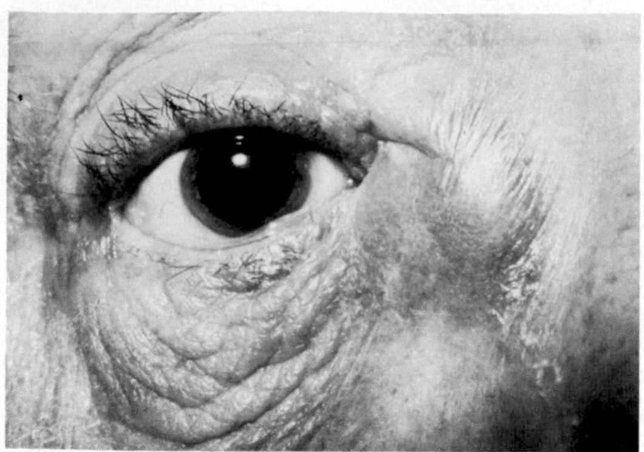

FIG 13-2.
Acute dacryocystitis in a 71-year-old woman.

DACRYOCYSTITIS

Dacryocystitis is an acute or chronic inflammation of the lacrimal sac. It is caused by an obstruction of the lacrimal sac or the nasolacrimal duct into the nose that prevents normal drainage followed by microbial infection.

Acute dacryocystitis.—Acute dacryocystitis is a suppurative inflammation of the lacrimal tissues (Fig 13-2). The onset is rapid, and a painful cellulitis affects the tissues overlying the lacrimal sac. Exquisite tenderness in the region is often combined with widespread swelling. The main differential diagnosis involves other causes of cellulitis in the region. Local hot compresses and systemic antibiotics are used in treatment. Incision and drainage are required if there is abscess formation.

Chronic dacryocystitis.—Chronic dacryocystitis occurs because of obstruction of the nasolacrimal duct, and it is seen most frequently shortly after birth and in middle life. The chief symptoms are epiphora and regurgitation of pus through the puncta when the lacrimal sac is compressed.

Infantile stenosis.—Dacryocystitis in infants occurs because of failure of the nasolacrimal duct to open into the inferior meatus, as normally occurs about the third week of life. The initial symptom is constant tearing. The tearing is distinguished from that in congenital glaucoma by the clear and transparent cornea and the absence of blepharospasm. Tearing is followed by regurgitation of pus through the puncta. Acute dacryocystitis is exceptional.

There is a strong tendency toward spontaneous establishment of normal patency of the lacrimal system by the age of 6 months. Often a topical medication such as sulfacetamide is instilled topically to prevent lacrimal conjunctivitis. While awaiting spontaneous correction, the parents are instructed to massage the lacrimal sac daily to keep it empty of pus. Sometimes pressure over the sac while the puncta are simultaneously occluded will establish normal patency.

If the obstruction persists after 12 months of age, lacrimal probing is indicated. The patient is mummified in a blanket, and a local anesthetic is instilled into the conjunctival sac. General anesthesia may be used. A lacrimal probe is inserted into the upper punctum, directed medially and into the lacrimal sac, and then turned at right angles into the nasolacrimal canal and the inferior meatus. The nose is inspected to be certain that the tip of the probe is not covered by mucous membrane. Rarely, more than one probing must be done.

Exceptionally, the nasolacrimal duct fails to canalize, and a dacryocystorhinostomy is necessary. Such surgery is wisely deferred until the child is 3 or 4 years of age. Because of the softness of the bone, it is an uncomplicated procedure in the young.

Adult chronic dacryocystitis.—Adult chronic dacryocystitis results from occlusion in the lacrimal sac, which may occur spontaneously, after injury, or because of nasal disease. Spontaneous atresia is more common in women in middle life. An annoying epiphora occurs initially, and, as the occlusion continues, pus regurgitates from the lacrimal sac. If the condition is neglected, marked dilation and thinning of the walls of the lacrimal sac occur—a mucocele or hydrops of the lacrimal sac. Acute suppuration is unusual. Differential diagnosis involves mainly the various causes of tearing and granulomatous infections of the lacrimal sac.

Surgery is the only satisfactory treatment. When mild, instillation of zinc and epinephrine collyria may be helpful in the elderly. Probing of the lacrimal passages with probes of successively greater size may be useful, but for the most part relief is transient and the procedure is painful.

The surgical procedure of choice if the canaliculi are patent is a dacryocystorhinostomy, in which a connection is established between the lacrimal sac and the nose. Many procedures have been recommended. If the bony opening into the nose is large enough, most patients improve. Extirpation of the sac (dacryocystectomy) is not done, except in elderly patients who require intraocular surgery. The lacrimal sac is removed to eliminate the regurgitation of pus into the conjunctival sac.

LACRIMAL SAC TUMORS

The lacrimal sac is lined with pseudostratified columnar epithelium, and the uncommon tumors are similar to those that involve the similar tissue of the upper respiratory tract. Squamous cell papillomas, carcinoma, transitional cell carcinoma, and adenocarcinoma are described.

Epiphora is the initial symptom and may be followed by a chronic dacryocystitis. Regurgitation of blood suggests a malignant tumor. A painless, nonreducible swelling occurs in the region of the lacrimal sac, and eventually the tumor extends outside the lacrimal fascia. The tumor may be demonstrated by computed tomography or magnetic resonance imaging. Excision is the treatment of choice.

DISEASES OF THE LACRIMAL GLANDS

The lacrimal glands are tubuloracemose, similar in structure to the salivary glands. In general, they are subject to the same inflammations, diseases, and tumors. The two groups of glands are often involved in the same inflammatory and degenerative diseases.

INFLAMMATION

Acute dacryoadenitis.—Acute dacryoadenitis is an uncommon inflammation of the lacrimal gland that usually accompanies systemic diseases. Mumps and infectious mononucleosis are the usual systemic causes of an acute inflammation. A purulent infection may be secondary to extension of inflammation from the eyelids or the conjunctiva.

Pain and discomfort in the upper outer portion of the orbit are the chief symptoms. Swelling and redness of the lacrimal gland cause a mechanical blepharoptosis of the upper eyelid and an S-shaped curve of the eyelid margin. Other causes of cellulitis of the skin and orbit must be considered in the differential diagnosis. Eversion of the upper eyelid indicates a swollen, reddened gland.

Treatment is directed to the cause. If a purulent infection is present, antibiotics and local hot compresses, possibly combined with incision and drainage, are indicated. Dacryoadenitis is usually self-limited, and therapy is directed toward preventing the extension of infection.

Chronic dacryoadenitis.—Chronic dacryoadenitis is a proliferative inflammation of the lacrimal gland that occurs in a variety of disorders: sarcoidosis, Sjögren syndrome, leukemia, lymphoma, amyloidosis, tuberculosis, syphilis, eosinophilic granuloma, and foreign body granuloma. Clinically it is characterized by painless enlargement of the lacrimal glands (Fig 13-3), most evident when the upper eyelid is everted. Treatment must be directed toward the cause.

Sarcoidosis (see Chapter 25) may cause chronic dacryoadenitis without enlargement of the gland. Dry eyes are the only symptom, but the gland accumulates radioactive gallium and has the histologic changes of sarcoid.

Mikulicz syndrome is the term applied to chronic bilateral swelling of the lacrimal and salivary glands. It may occur in reticuloendothelial disease, leukemias, Hodgkin disease, and sarcoidosis. It is not a specific entity.

TUMORS OF THE LACRIMAL GLAND

Tumors of the lacrimal gland may be benign, as occur in reactive lymphoid or plasma cell hyperplasia, chronic dacryoadenitis, and benign epithelial mixed tumor. Malignant tumors occur in malignant degeneration of benign mixed tumor, adenoid cystic carcinoma, and a variety of other carcinomas (adenocarcinoma, mucinous carcinoma, mucoepidermoid carcinoma, and undifferentiated carcinomas). Malignant tumors may metastasize to the lacrimal gland or extend from adjacent structures.

The tumors cause swelling of the upper outer portion of the upper eyelid, which may give the appearance of a blepharoptosis. The eye may be proptosed downward and inward with diplopia and loss of vision. Eversion of the upper eyelid discloses the tumor mass.

About 75% of the tumors of the lacrimal gland are inflammatory pseudotumors or benign epithelial mixed tumors. The remainder are malignant. An inflammatory pseudotumor or lymphoma may affect the lacrimal gland solely, the orbit solely, or involve both. Pseudotumors of the lacrimal gland are similar to those of the orbit (see Chapter 15). Benign mixed tumor (pleomorphic adenoma) is the most common epithelial tumor of both the lacrimal gland and the salivary glands.

Inflammatory, malignant, and lymphoid lesions usually cause symptoms within 12 months

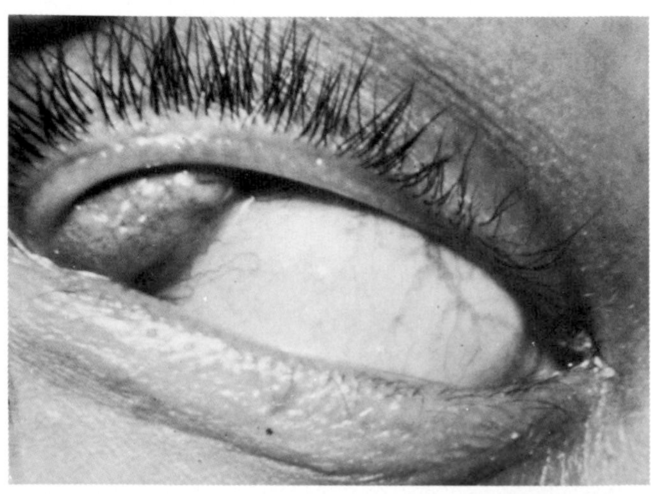

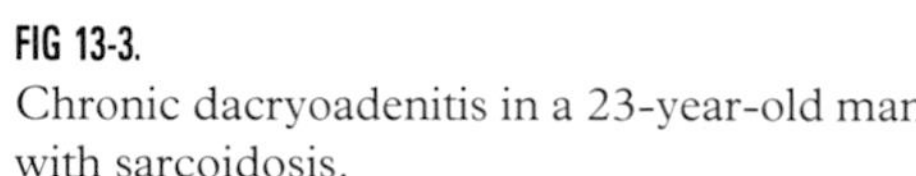

FIG 13-3.
Chronic dacryoadenitis in a 23-year-old man with sarcoidosis.

of their onset, whereas benign mixed tumors grow slowly and may cause marked proptosis with such gradual and painless growth that there is no diplopia or loss of vision. Orbital pain suggests a malignancy or an inflammatory lesion. A rounded or globular configuration on computed tomography suggests an epithelial neoplasm, whereas inflammatory and lymphoid lesions have a diffuse configuration that accentuates the normal oblong shape of the lacrimal gland. Erosion of the bony orbit suggests an epithelial malignancy. Inflammatory and lymphoid lesions affect predominantly the palpebral lobe, whereas benign mixed tumors and malignant tumors affect the orbital portion of the gland. Benign mixed tumors occur at about 35 years of age; other tumors have an onset after 50 years, but all may occur in both youth and old age.

Benign mixed tumor (pleomorphic adenoma) is the most common epithelial tumor of the lacrimal gland. It contains mesenchymal elements (myxoid, chondroid, and osteoid) and double-layered, tubular epithelial units. It is slowly progressive, predominantly involves men (2:1), and begins at a median age of 35 years. There is often a long history (1 to 4 years) of painless fullness of the upper, outer orbit and moderate proptosis with displacement of the globe downward and inward. Exceptionally, there may be radiographic signs of erosion of the bone of the lacrimal fossa. The tumor should be removed through a lateral orbitotomy within its capsule. If there is bony erosion, the bone must be resected. Incomplete excision results in recurrence.

A malignant mixed tumor originates as a benign mixed tumor but, through seeding at the time of removal or nontreatment, undergoes malignant degeneration into an adenocarcinoma or adenoid cystic carcinoma. It has no sex predilection and occurs most commonly after 50 years of age. There is sudden onset of pain, with rapid tumor growth, in a patient with a history of a recurrent benign mixed tumor or in a patient with a lacrimal tumor present for several years. Erosion of the lacrimal fossa may occur.

The adenoid cystic carcinoma (malignant cylindroma) is the most common malignant epithelial tumor of the lacrimal gland. It occurs in both sexes. Median age at onset is 38 years. It is notorious for slow, relentless spread, despite multiple radical excisions. It has the most unfavorable prognosis of all lacrimal gland malignancies. The most common symptom is proptosis with pain, diplopia, decreased visual acuity, blepharoptosis, and lacrimation. Histologically it is composed of aggregates of small undifferentiated neoplastic cells separated by small and large cystoid spaces containing mucin ("Swiss cheese"). The onset is relatively rapid—always less than a year. Unlike patients with benign mixed tumor, patients have pain and diplopia. Radiographic studies may show bone erosion.

Adenocarcinoma occurs at a median age of 53 years, predominantly in men (3:1), and has a longer duration of symptoms than adenoid cystic carcinoma. It is more likely than adenoid cystic carcinoma to metastasize.

Older patients may develop squamous cell carcinomas, undifferentiated carcinomas, or mucoepidermoid carcinomas. These patients are from 50 to 70 years of age and have histories of recent onset and often bone destruction.

Management of tumors of the lacrimal gland is not standardized. Possibly half of the tumors are inflammatory or lymphomatous and responsive to systemic corticosteroids or radiation therapy. These tumors do not cause erosion of the bone. Thus, removal of a small piece of tissue for histologic diagnosis is tempting. Such an excision is associated with repeated recurrences of benign mixed tumors and impairs the survival rate in patients with malignant tumors. A 2-week trial of systemic corticosteroids may result in a marked regression (50% or more) of a reactive lymphoid hyperplasia and may have little effect on other tumors.

Removal of any lacrimal tumor through an intracranial approach is contraindicated because of the danger of direct intracranial seeding. Radiation therapy of benign mixed tumors increases the possibility of malignant change. Surgery requires that every tumor be excised within its capsule. An en bloc resection including the bony lacrimal gland fossa and adjacent tissue and eyelids is indicated in malignant tumors. The prognosis is poor and therapy is not standardized.

BIBLIOGRAPHY

Book

Hurwitz JJ: *The lacrimal system,* Philadelphia, 1995, Lippincott-Raven.

Article

Vitali C, Moutsopoulos HM, Bombarideri S: The European Community Study Group on diagnostic criteria for Sjögren's syndrome. Sensitivity and specificity of tests for ocular and oral involvement in Sjögren's syndrome, *Ann Rheum Dis* 53:637-647, 1994.

14

THE SCLERA

The sclera is a dense, connective tissue structure composed of bundles of collagen of varying diameters. It constitutes the posterior five sixths of the globe. Its anterior portion is visible beneath the translucent conjunctiva as the white of the eye. Careful examination shows a fine network of blood vessels located in the anterior portion of the globe between the conjunctiva and the sclera. Inflammations, often associated with immune-mediated diseases, are its main disorders. Additionally, the sclera may change in shape, size, or translucency in a variety of systemic disorders. The corneoscleral limbus is the site of incision for cataract extraction and for filtering operations in glaucoma. The sclera overlying the pars plana of the ciliary body is the site of incisions to introduce surgical instruments into the vitreous cavity. Strips of plastic encircle the posterior sclera in retinal detachment surgery. Rarely, during a retrobulbar injection, the needle perforates the posterior sclera, often through a localized scleral protuberance (staphyloma or ectasia).

SYMPTOMS AND SIGNS OF SCLERAL DISEASE

Inflammations of the sclera cause a deep, dull ocular discomfort that is aggravated by ocular movements if the inflamed region is near the insertion of an ocular muscle. If the inflammation affects the posterior portion of the sclera, there may be no external signs, but the deep aching ocular pain without obvious cause suggests the diagnosis. Vision is lost only if the inflammation extends to the underlying choroid and retina.

Inflammation of the anterior portion of the sclera induces generalized or localized areas of deep reddish injection of the episcleral tissues. These areas may be painful on palpation. In thinning or necrosis of the sclera, the bluish black choroidal pigment may be exposed.

PIGMENTATION OF THE SCLERA

The sclera is normally dull white. When thin, it appears blue because of visualization of the pigment of the underlying uveal tract. A blue sclera may be seen in premature babies, in white newborns, and sometimes in degenerative myopia, keratoconus, osteogenesis imperfecta, Ehlers-Danlos syndrome, pseudoxanthoma elasticum, and Marfan syndrome. An iron deficiency anemia may impair collagen synthesis by the sclera and cause it to thin.

Localized discolorations of the sclera occur in an intrascleral nerve loop, in alkaptonuria and in scleral hyaline plaques. A blue nevus may be associated with an underlying choroidal nevus or a melanocytoma with an underlying melanocytosis. The most serious abnormality is extension of a malignant melanoma of the choroid through the sclera, often at the site of one of the small openings that transmit nerves or blood vessels. The differential diagnosis of a black elevated mass in the sclera includes staphyloma with an extremely thin sclera, as occurs in necrotizing scleritis, or extraocular extension of an intraocular malignant melanoma. The yellowish appearance of the globe in jaundice is caused by

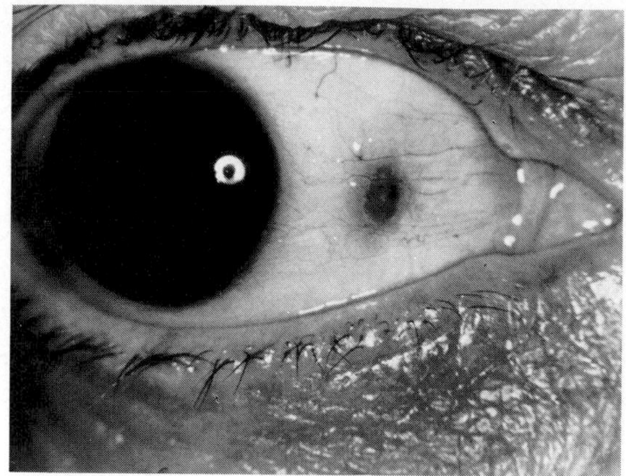

FIG 14-1.
Senile hyaline plaque located immediately in front of the insertion of the lateral rectus muscle in a 65-year-old man. The plaque shells out of the sclera easily and contains calcium sulfate (gypsum).

bilirubin in the conjunctiva. In severe jaundice of long duration, the sclera may be stained, rarely monocularly.

Intrascleral nerve loop.—An intrascleral nerve loop (of Axenfeld) is an anatomic variation in which an anomalous loop of a short ciliary nerve, often accompanied by a blood vessel, partially or completely perforates the sclera in the region of the ciliary body and then returns to the inner surface of the sclera. It appears as a 1- to 2-mm black dot on the sclera, about 4 to 5 mm from the corneoscleral limbus. Its unchanging appearance and location suggest its nature. Treatment is not indicated.

Scleral hyaline plaque.—A scleral hyaline plaque (once called senile) is a painless, nonprogressive, dark-colored oval patch that has a translucent center, located in the sclera immediately anterior to the insertion of the medial and lateral recti muscles (Fig 14-1). It is often surrounded by a yellowish halo. It occurs in both sexes in individuals aged 60 years or more. The plaque is easily shelled out of the slightly thinned sclera and contains fragments of scleral fibers, degenerated hyaline, and calcium phosphate. It is symptomless and requires no treatment.

STAPHYLOMA AND ECTASIA

Staphylomas and ectasias are localized protuberances or enlargements of the sclera secondary to embryonic defects of the sclera, localized areas of degeneration, or increased intraocular pressure. If only the sclera bulges, the condition is called an ectasia, whereas if the uvea lines the bulging sclera, it is called a staphyloma.

Ectasias are usually associated with abnormalities in closure of the optic vesicle; thus, colobomas of the uveal tract and retina often occur. Failure of the scleral mesoderm to contribute to the lamina cribrosa creates an ophthalmoscopic appearance of a large but normal optic disk at the bottom of a deep hole (see Chapter 20). In myopia a localized bulging of sclera may develop between the insertions of the recti muscles and may be associated with retinal detachment. In adult glaucoma, the sclera (and cornea) is resistant to the increased intraocular pressure, but a partial ectasia at the lamina cribrosa creates the characteristic glaucomatous excavation (cupping) of the optic disk.

Staphylomas may be total or partial. In congenital glaucoma, a uniform stretching of the sclera occurs before the scleral and corneal collagen fibers have matured. The result is the total staphyloma of buphthalmos (Greek, ox eye).

Localized staphylomas are divided into anterior and posterior types. Anterior staphylomas occur anterior to the equator; ciliary staphylomas occur over the ciliary body; and intercalary staphylomas occur between the ciliary body and the corneoscleral limbus. These bulges frequently follow either inflammation of the anterior uveal tract or laceration of the sclera combined with increased intraocular pressure. The staphyloma appears as a region of scleral thinning lined with the dark pigment of the uveal tract.

Staphylomas posterior to the ocular equator occur in Marfan and Ehlers-Danlos syndromes, and in degenerative myopia in which there are thinning and stretching of the posterior pole as the axial length of the globe increases. Vision is decreased. Ophthalmoscopic examination often shows macular degeneration. Indirect ophthalmoscopic examination demonstrates the sharp, well-defined edge of the anterior scleral protuberance.

Equatorial staphylomas and ectasias occur near the points of exit of the vortex veins from the eye. Either may be a factor in retinal detach-

TABLE 14-1.
Inflammation of the Sclera

- I. Episcleritis
  - A. Diffuse
  - B. Nodular
- II. Anterior scleritis
  - A. Diffuse
  - B. Nodular
  - C. Necrotizing
    - 1. With uveitis
    - 2. With no inflammation
      - a. Scleromalacia perforans
- III. Posterior scleritis

ment and are often detected only after surgical exposure of the site.

INFLAMMATIONS

The sclera proper has a modest blood supply and an inactive metabolism, but the episclera has a rich vascular network. Scleral inflammations tend to be noninfectious, torpid, and unresponsive to treatment. There is often an associated rheumatoid arthritis or other immune-mediated disorder. Two types of scleral inflammation occur: episcleritis and scleritis (Table 14-1). A causative factor is not found in most cases of episcleritis, whereas scleritis is often associated with an immune-mediated disorder.

EPISCLERITIS

Episcleritis (Fig 14-2) is a benign, recurrent, mainly noninfectious inflammation of the episcleral tissue in the region between the insertion of the recti muscles and the corneoscleral limbus. There are two types: simple and nodular. Women are mainly affected (75%), and it has a peak incidence between 40 and 50 years of age. The onset is sudden, with intense redness affecting one or more quadrants of the globe. There are minimal ocular symptoms. The inflammation usually disappears in 7 to 10 days without treatment. Inflammations that persist longer are often associated with a connective tissue disorder, which, however, is less severe than that which occurs in scleritis.

In nodular episcleritis there is intense engorgement of the episcleral blood vessels that surround a localized subconjunctival, slightly tender, dark red, movable swelling. There are recurrent attacks, sometimes over a period of years, that affect the same area or different quadrants of the same eye or the fellow eye. In about one third of the patients a systemic cause is found. Of these, about one half have a connective tissue disorder, and the remaining have either rosacea or a hypersensitivity disorder.

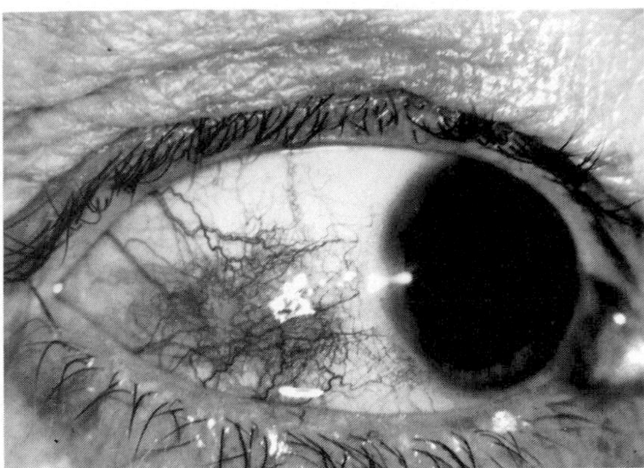

FIG 14-2.
Localized area of acute episcleritis on the temporal side of the sclera in a 35-year-old woman.

SCLERITIS

Scleritis is a severe, progressive, serious inflammation that can lead to loss of vision or even to loss of the eye. It may be the initial sign of a potentially fatal disorder. There is more severe pain than that associated with episcleritis, and both eyes may be affected simultaneously.

Diffuse anterior scleritis causes a deep ache within the orbit that radiates to the jaw and cheek. The superficial and deep episcleral vascular plexuses appear as deep, multiple, small radial blood vessels, surrounded by dilated capillaries and swollen subconjunctival tissue. The blood vessels do not blanch with topical instillation of epinephrine. Treatment consists of topical instillation of corticosteroids and systemic nonsteroidal anti-inflammatory drugs.

Anterior nodular scleritis is intensely painful, with an extremely tender, firm, immobile nodule composed of inflamed scleral tissue near the corneoscleral limbus. The nodule is not attached to the overlying conjunctiva, and there may be multiple nodules. Progression of the nodule around the corneoscleral circumference or avascularity suggests a conversion to necrotizing scleritis. Nonsteroidal anti-inflammatory drugs are used together with topical corticosteroids.

There are two types of necrotizing anterior scleritis. In one there is severe ocular pain and many ocular complications, including keratitis, uveitis, glaucoma, cataract, retinal detachment, and macular edema. Every effort must be made to identify any systemic disease and treat it effectively. The necrotizing scleritis associated with polyarteritis nodosa or Wegener granulomatosis requires immunosuppressive chemotherapy.

In the second type of necrotizing anterior scleritis, painless rheumatoid nodules in the sclera (scleromalacia perforans) create large defects through which the choroid bulges. Treatment is directed to the rheumatoid arthritis, relying mainly on nonsteroidal anti-inflammatory drugs and the use of systemic corticosteroids if necessary.

Posterior scleritis affects the sclera posterior to the ora serrata and may involve the adjacent choroid, uvea, and retina. It may be confused with an inflammation or tumor of the orbit. It may be a posterior extension of anterior scleritis or may be confined to the posterior sclera. Vision is decreased; there is retrobulbar pain; there may be choroidal folds; and a posterior uveitis. Ultrasonography is the most useful diagnostic test.

INJURIES

Lacerations of the sclera invariably involve the underlying uvea and often the retina. An associated vitreous hemorrhage impairs the ophthalmoscopic view. Blunt trauma to the eye may rupture the posterior sclera as the result of a contrecoup phenomenon. A history of blunt trauma associated with a severe subconjunctival hemorrhage, reduced vision, and a persistently soft eye suggests a rupture of the posterior sclera.

BIBLIOGRAPHY

Books

Foster CS, de la Maza MS: *The sclera,* New York, 1994, Springer-Verlag.

Watson P, Ortiz JM: *Color atlas of scleritis,* St Louis, 1995, Mosby–Year Book.

Article

Tu EY, Culbertson WW, Pflugfelder SC, Huang A, Chodosh JC: Therapy of nonnecrotizing anterior scleritis with subconjunctival corticosteroid injection, *Ophthalmology* 102:718-724, 1995.

15

THE ORBIT

The orbit is a pear-shaped cavity. The stem is located on the cranial side and the base faces outward. The medial wall extends directly forward from its apex, whereas the lateral wall diverges about 45°. The annulus of Zinn, the circular fibrous origin of the recti muscles, circles the orbital apex that provides the passage for orbital blood vessels and nerves. The apex of the orbit is located almost immediately posterior to the medial canthus and not directly behind the eye. The middle portion of the orbit expands to contain the eye. The base of the orbit forms the thick margins that protect the eye. The maxillary sinus is adjacent to the inferior wall and the ethmoid sinus to the medial wall of the orbit. The temporalis muscle is adjacent to the anterior portion of the lateral wall and the temporal lobe of the brain to the posterior part. Superiorly, the frontal sinus is located anteriorly and the frontal lobe of the brain is located posteriorly (Fig 15-1). The junction of the anterior and middle cranial fossae is located at the apices of the orbits.

Affections of the orbit include a heterogeneous group of abnormalities that originate within a bony cavity, which contains tissue of neural crest, ectodermal, and mesodermal origin. Tumors, inflammations, and normal tissues that originate in the intracranial cavity or the nasal sinuses may extend into the orbit and displace the eye or impair its movement. The superior and inferior orbital veins of the orbit drain into the cavernous sinus, and an aneurysm or fistula of the internal carotid artery within the cavernous sinus may result in a pulsating exophthalmos of one or both eyes.

DEVELOPMENTAL ABNORMALITIES

The orbit and its contents may be affected by congenital abnormalities that involve the bones of the orbit, skull, or face (Table 15-1). Often the skull has a characteristic shape or the facial features are typical of the abnormality. There may be an associated exophthalmos from shallow orbits, optic atrophy, papilledema, and strabismus. Exotropia occurs with widely separated orbits. Esotropia occurs with poor vision. The neural crest contributes to the brachial arches, and abnormalities occur with a wide variety of hereditary, chromosomal, and congenital defects. The first brachial arch subdivides into maxillary and mandibular portions. Abnormalities of the maxillary portion result in downward- and outward-slanting palpebral fissures (antimongoloid) and a sunken upper face with depressed cheek bones. Abnormalities of the mandibular portion result in a receding chin. Abnormalities of the second brachial arch may cause nerve deafness and pterygium colli (a congenital web of skin of the neck).

CRANIOSYNOSTOSIS

Craniosynostosis follows premature union of one or more cranial sutures, which causes a complete arrest of bone growth at right angles to the closed suture. It occurs as an isolated abnormality, with syndactyly, with and without poly-

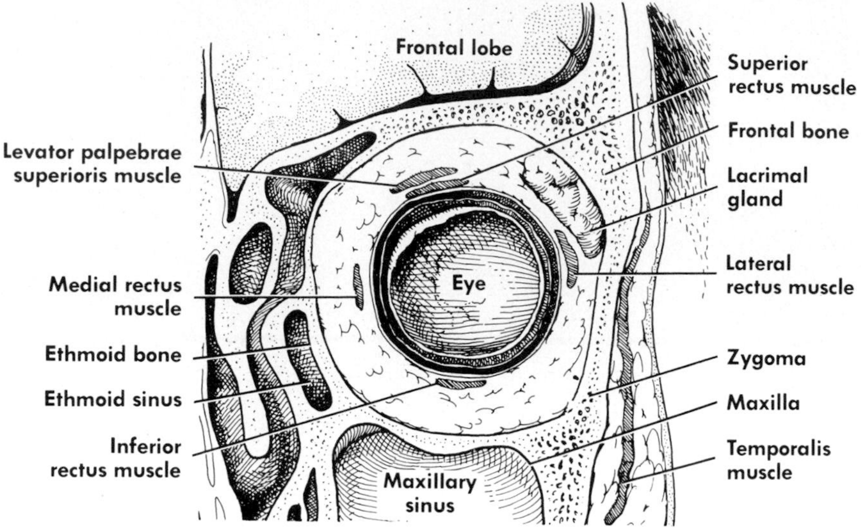

FIG 15-1.
Coronal section of the left orbit about 15 mm from the apex of the cornea. The frontal sinus is adjacent to the orbit in its anterior portion, whereas the frontal lobe is adjacent to the orbit posteriorly. Laterally the temporalis muscle is adjacent to the orbit anteriorly, whereas the temporal lobe of the brain is located posteriorly. The ethmoid sinus is located medially and the maxillary sinus inferiorly.

dactyly, and with other somatic abnormalities. It is an autosomal dominant condition, with incomplete penetrance, and the gene locus is assigned to 5qter. A compensatory growth of the skull in its other diameters causes anomalies in its shape. The deformity progresses until the brain ceases to grow at about 8 years of age.

Increased cerebrospinal fluid pressure is common and may cause papilledema followed by secondary optic atrophy. Pressure on the optic nerve by downward displacement of the base of the brain or because of compression in the optic foramen may result in primary optic atrophy. The orbit may be unusually shallow because of an abnormal growth of the lesser wing of the sphenoid bone and vertical inclination of the orbital apex. Exotropia or, less commonly, esotropia may occur. Esotropia may follow amblyopia as the result of optic atrophy. Exotropia may be the result of the abnormal shape of the orbit.

Increased cerebrospinal fluid pressure, papilledema, and optic atrophy require cranial surgery. Some physicians advocate craniectomy in the early months of life in all instances of craniosynostosis to prevent mental retardation and the cosmetic defect. Others believe that the procedure should be individualized, that a cosmetic defect is not constantly produced, and that mental retardation is not caused by the bony abnormality.

Dysostosis of the upper face and skull

Dysostosis of the upper face and skull is often associated with widely spaced orbits (hypertelorism) with a resultant increase in interpupillary distance so that convergence is impaired. Most cases are associated with widespread abnormalities.

Acrocephalosyndactyly (Apert).—This is an autosomal dominant disorder. The skull is tall (oxycephaly) and the occiput flat. The eyes are protuberant and widely spaced with the palpebral fissures slanting downward and outward. The maxillary bones and nasal bridge are underdeveloped and the cerebral ventricles are dilated. Mentation is normal. In type I there is complete syndactyly of the hands and feet ("mitten hands," "sock feet"); in type II there is partial syndactyly.

Cephalopolysyndactyly (Greig).—This is an autosomal dominant disorder mapped to chromosome 7p13. It is characterized by widely spaced eyes (hypertelorism), a large head, a broad base of the nose, and a prominent forehead. There may be associated defects of the

TABLE 15-1.
Developmental Anomalies of the Skull, Face, and Orbit

I. Dysostosis of the skull
  A. Craniosynostosis
    1. Oxycephaly (tower skull); premature union of coronal suture, often with high forehead (dolichocephaly)
    2. Scaphocephaly (boat skull); premature union of sagittal suture, with a long, narrow skull
    3. Brachycephaly (short skull; cloverleaf skull); premature union of all cranial sutures
II. Craniofacial dysostosis
  A. Upper face and skull
    1. Acrocephalosyndactyly (Apert)
    2. Crouzon
    3. Cephalopolysyndactyly (Greig)
  B. Mandibulofacial dysostosis
    1. First brachial arch
      a. Maxillary
        (1) Palpebral fissures slant downward and outward
        (2) Malar hypoplasia with sunken upper face
      b. Mandibular
        (1) Receding chin
    2. Second brachial arch
      a. N VII
      b. Nerve deafness
      c. Pterygium colli (webbed skin of the neck)
III. Orbital wall defects
  A. Mucocele
  B. Meningocele
  C. Encephalocele
IV. Developmental tumors
  A. Hemangioma
  B. Lymphosarcoma
  C. Dermoid cyst
  D. Lipoma
  E. Choristoma

eyelids that include epicanthal folds, accessory nasal tissue medially with displacement of the inferior lacrimal puncta, and colobomas. Epibulbar dermoid tumors, microphthalmos, and vitreoretinal degeneration with retinal detachment occur. A polysyndactyly of the hands and feet is present; radiographs of the hands and feet are indicated if the thumbs are broad.

Craniofacial dysostosis (Crouzon).— Craniofacial dysostosis is an autosomal dominant condition in which brachycephaly (widened skull) is combined with hypoplasia of the maxillary bones. The forehead is broad, and there is prominence of the anterior forehead region. The eyes are widely separated, and the shallow orbits make them prominent.

Surgical treatment of the abnormalities of the vault of the skull is not effective. The nose is broad and hooked, the upper dentition irregular, and the palate high. The earlobes are often large, and atresia of the external auditory canal is common. Optic atrophy may occur. Exposure keratitis may necessitate a lateral blepharoplasty. The disorder does not involve loci on chromosome 5q or 7p.

Mandibulofacial dysostosis

Mandibulofacial dysostosis abnormalities affect the first and eventually the second brachial arches.

Treacher Collins syndrome.—This is an autosomal dominant abnormality of craniofacial development with hypoplasia of the zygomas and mandible. The palpebral fissures point outward and downward. There may be colobomas of the lower eyelids, absence of eyelashes on the inner one third of the lower eyelids, and absence of the inferior lacrimal puncta. Strabismus and amblyopia occur in about one third of the patients. The external ears may be abnormally small (microtia), and there may be atresia of the external auditory canal. Atrophy of the mandible causes a prognathism of the upper jaw and an open bite. Associated skeletal abnormalities are common, and dermolipomas of the conjunctiva occur. Children must be monitored for impairment of the airway through adolescence. The gene for the condition is mapped to chromosome 5q 31-33.

Dyscephalic syndrome (Hallermann-Streiff).—This is a congenital disorder in which a large nose that resembles a parrot beak is combined with mandibular hypoplasia to give a "birdlike face." The palpebral fissures slant down and out. Microphthalmia may be present. A hypermature cataract with rupture of the lens capsule and secondary glaucoma may occur in the first weeks of life. Several different genetic loci have been described.

SYMPTOMS AND SIGNS OF ORBITAL DISEASE

Abnormalities of the orbit often manifest themselves by displacement of the globe, which is sometimes associated with local pain, redness,

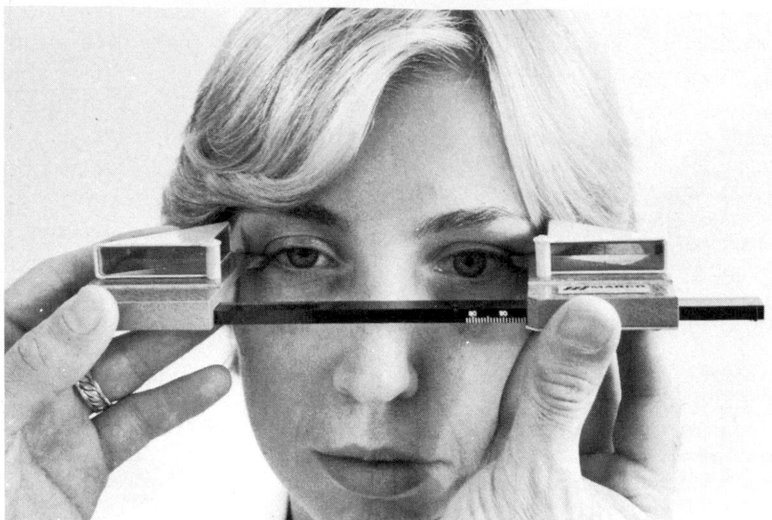

FIG 15-2.
Measurement of exophthalmos with a modified Hertel exophthalmometer. The observer views the position of the eyes in the mirrors. The numbers on the rule refer to the distance separating the two eyepieces and must be the same with repeated measurement.

and swelling. Proptosis often refers to unilateral displacement of an eye and exophthalmos to bilateral displacement.

In proptosis or exophthalmos, the palpebral fissure widens, and a rim of sclera is often visible above and below the cornea. In thyroid disease, retraction of the upper eyelid accentuates this appearance. In enophthalmos, the palpebral aperture is narrower, and the upper eyelid may droop.

Ocular protrusion may be detected by viewing the eyes over the brow of the patient from above and behind. Several instruments (exophthalmometers) will measure the distance between the anterior surface of the cornea and the zygomatic arch on the lateral margin of the orbit (Figs 15-2 and 15-3). The measurements with the usual exophthalmometers are accurate to within 1 to 2 mm. An exophthalmometer may be improvised by holding a ruler against the zygoma and viewing the front surface of the cornea from the side of the patient.

Displacement of the globe is often complicated by decreased vision, double vision, congestion and edema of the eyelids and conjunctiva, a bruit in the head, optic disk swelling, and venous congestion.

Displacement of the globe.—A relatively small mass in the muscle cone causes early forward displacement of the globe. The nerve supply to the extraocular muscles may be affected, causing a paralytic strabismus. Masses outside the muscle cone must be larger to displace the globe, and cause the eye to be deviated up or down, in or out, as well as forward. Tumors of the lacrimal gland may not cause proptosis, or they may displace the globe

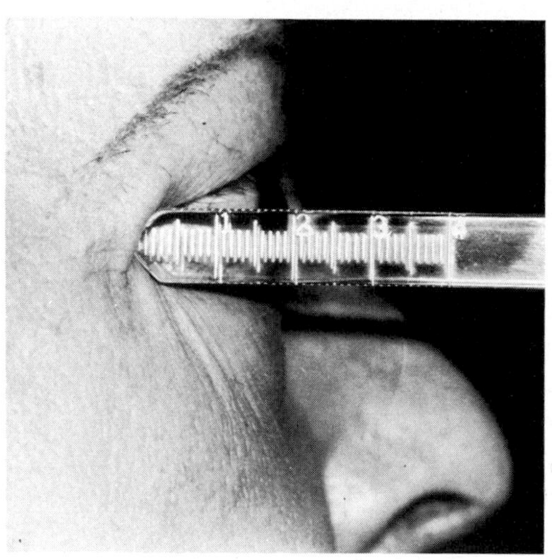

FIG 15-3.
Estimate of degree of proptosis by means of a transparent exophthalmometer (Luedde). Here the anterior surface of the cornea is 19 mm from the zygoma.

downward and inward. The lacrimal gland itself may be proptosed when there is a marked increase in the volume of the orbital contents.

Visual abnormalities.—Diplopia is often an early sign of proptosis and may occur before development of gross displacement of the globe. Decreased vision is generally a late sign. It may indicate corneal clouding from exposure, retinal edema, or optic nerve impairment.

Congestion and edema of the eyelids and conjunctiva.—Marked congestion of the vessels of the globe suggests an infection, a thyroid abnormality with rapid progression of exophthalmos, or a carotid-cavernous sinus fistula.

Bruit in the head.—An abnormal blowing sound heard on auscultation of the head is a classic sign of carotid-cavernous sinus fistula. The patient usually hears noises in the head, such as the sound of running water or the swishing of water. It may be most marked on the side of a carotid-cavernous sinus fistula. The bruit is synchronous with the heart and may disappear when pressure is applied to the carotid artery in the neck. Bruits occur with some orbital and intracranial tumors, and they occur in some healthy infants.

Palpable tumors.—Tumors located in the anterior half of the orbit may be palpated through the eyelids. Often a lateral canthotomy or a conjunctival incision in the lower outer canthus will allow the surgeon to palpate deep in the orbit. Such an incision should never be used in the upper eyelid because of possible damage to the levator palpebrae superioris muscle, causing blepharoptosis. The tendon of the superior oblique muscle, localized fat in the eyelids, and indurated orbital inflammatory tissue all yield the tactile sensation of a tumor.

Choroidal folds.—Orbital tumors, hyperopia, Graves disease, posterior scleritis, and ocular hypotony may cause folds or striae in the posterior fundus (Fig 15-4). These appear as alternating bright and dark lines, with the peaks being bright and the valleys a darker shade of red. They are more common temporally than nasally and may be associated with congestion of the optic disk. Fluorescein angiography causes the peaks to fluoresce brightly, creating a pattern of alternate bright and dark lines. Vision is not affected, although the refraction may be altered because the posterior pole of the eye is displaced forward. With time, the slopes of the folds become pigmented.

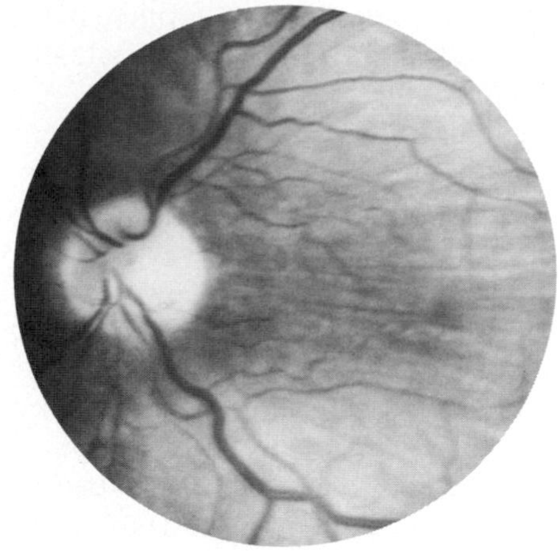

FIG 15-4.
Choroidal folds in a 53-year-old man with a long-standing hemangioma of the orbit.

Miscellaneous signs.—Impairment of venous drainage of the optic nerve may cause a papilledema that may be followed by secondary optic atrophy. Marked congestion of the orbit may severely restrict ocular movements. Failure of the eyelids to cover the eye causes lacrimation, photophobia, and exposure keratitis.

DIAGNOSIS

An initial decision must be made as to whether one or both eyes are displaced or whether the appearance is simulated. Retraction of the upper eyelid causes the eye to appear more prominent, although it is not displaced. Eyelid retraction is a common sign of thyroid disease. A slight blepharoptosis, as occurs in Horner syndrome, may simulate an ocular proptosis of the opposite side. Congenital abnormalities of orbital structure that cause a shallow orbit, as in Crouzon disease, simulate proptosis. Marked enlargement of the eye such as occurs in congenital glaucoma or unilateral severe myopia makes the eye more prominent without displacement.

Physical examination should be directed to possible herniation of the contents of a nasal sinus, or the intracranial cavity. Thyroid ophthalmopathy, orbital inflammation (bacterial cellulitis, acute or chronic pseudotumor, lymphoma, and benign reactive lymphoid hyperplasia) must always be excluded. Evaluation of thyroid hormones may be indicated. A chest roentgenogram may exclude metastatic malignancy. Excision of a localized tumor may provide both a diagnosis and a cure. Lacrimal gland tumors must be completely excised to avoid seeding.

After excisional biopsy or needle biopsy, the diagnosis should be based on the best possible histologic sections and not on frozen sections.

Computed tomography.—Computed tomography has virtually replaced conventional roentgenography in the diagnosis of orbital abnormalities. Better spatial resolution and decreased scanning time of modern equipment make it possible to demonstrate the origin and insertion of ocular muscles, fascial planes, large blood vessels, and bony detail. The computed tomographic image enables one to distinguish fat from solid tissues, and provides visualization of the location of the eye and its intraocular contents in relation to other orbital structures. Three-dimensional reconstruction of thin images allows precise localization for radiation therapy, removal of foreign bodies, and surgical reconstruction of the orbit. Benign tumors are well localized, whereas malignant tumors have irregular margins. Pseudotumors are often molded around orbital structures and demonstrate a ring of increased density. Lymphoid tumors are diffuse and homogeneous and have a relatively high density.

The breakdown of the blood-tissue barriers makes possible contrast enhancement, in which neoplastic and inflammatory tissue become more evident after the intravenous injection of a contrast medium.

Magnetic resonance imaging.—Magnetic resonance imaging provides multiple sagittal and coronal views without requiring positioning of the head as is required for coronal computed tomographic views. It provides a high soft-tissue contrast without exposure to ionizing radiation or the infusion of iodine-containing contrast material. Magnetic resonance imaging requires long exposure times, and relative immobility of the eyes is required for orbital studies. It should not be used in patients who have a cardiac pacemaker and is contraindicated in patients whose bodies may harbor magnetic foreign bodies. It is inferior to computed tomography in demonstrating bony erosion or in detecting tissue calcification. Studies after gadolinium enhancement increase tissue differentiation and are particularly useful in the diagnosis of metastatic tumors, hemangiomas, and optic nerve gliomas and meningiomas. Magnetic resonance imaging is superior to computed tomography in the delineation of intraocular tumors (calcification of retinoblastoma is best demonstrated with computed tomography) and ischemic ocular disease, and for the diagnosis of intracranial diseases, particularly those that involve the posterior fossa or the brain stem.

Ultrasonography.—Ultrasound study of the orbital contents has the advantage of relatively low cost, compared to computed tomography or magnetic resonance imaging, and its availability in many ophthalmic offices. Imaging with a colored Doppler signal superimposed on the conventional gray scale yields dynamic information concerning blood flow. In thyroid ophthalmopathy, A-scan ultrasonography may provide better diagnostic information than computed tomography, but the associated clinical signs and abnormal serum thyroxine values often establish the diagnosis. Ultrasonography will demonstrate many inflammations and tumors, but its diagnostic usefulness is limited.

ORBITAL INFLAMMATION

CELLULITIS

Acute orbital cellulitis is commonly caused by direct bacterial extension from the ethmoid or maxillary sinus, by pyogenic thrombophlebitis from a focus in the skin of the eyelids in regions drained by orbital veins, or by a penetrating orbital trauma. The orbital septum, the dense connective tissue that separates the eyelids from the orbital contents, prevents anterior inflammations, mainly periorbital cellulitis, from extending into the orbit itself. Acute intraorbital inflammations are far more serious than preseptal periorbital cellulitis and may involve both the anterior and posterior orbital contents. Frontoethmoidal sinusitis and maxillary sinusitis are common causes of both intraorbital and preseptal cellulitis. Preseptal cellulitis has a sudden onset, with swelling, redness, and increased warmth of the eyelids. There is conjunctival edema, leukocytosis, and sometimes fever. A fluctuant mass signifies abscess formation. Preseptal inflammations are most common in patients less than 5 years of age.

Orbital cellulitis may have the same signs and symptoms as preseptal cellulitis, but they are more severe. Additionally, proptosis, anesthesia of the area innervated by the ophthalmic and maxillary branches of the trigeminal nerve, impaired ocular rotations, ocular pain aggravated by ocular rotation, and increased intraocular pressure occur. Increased severity of signs and symptoms, decreased visual acuity, an afferent pupillary defect, venous congestion, and papilledema indicate abscess formation. Orbital cellulitis is dangerous to life, particularly in the second decade of life in boys.

Management of both preseptal and orbital cellulitis requires a complete general and ocular examination, combined with imaging studies to learn its site and extent. Fine-needle aspiration biopsy under computed tomographic guidance is exceptionally useful. A complete and differential blood cell count as well as Gram stain and culture of secretions from the conjunctiva, nasopharynx, and any lacerations, abscesses, or fistulas are indicated. If meningeal signs are present, the cerebrospinal fluid is cultured. Initial treatment consists of appropriate intravenous antibiotics based on the results of Gram stain. Continued antibiotic therapy is guided by the result of culture. Abscess drainage with sinus drainage, sinus drainage alone, or incision and drainage of eyelid abscesses may be necessary. Cavernous sinus thrombosis, meningitis, brain abscess, optic nerve atrophy, and death may occur in neglected cases.

Mucormycosis.—Mucormycosis is the most rapidly fatal fungal infection in humans. Rhino-orbital–cerebral infection is the most common clinical type. The infection is characterized by an orbital ischemia with a mild proptosis, total external and internal ophthalmoplegia, and early blindness. A few patients have black eschar of the midface, nasal passages, palate, or orbit. There is a periorbital puffiness that is cool to the touch. Patients may have leukemia, lymphoma, diabetes mellitus, renal failure, or a history of organ transplantation. Systemic amphotericin B combined with surgical debridement may be effective if the infection is confined to the sinuses and orbit.

Cavernous sinus thrombosis.—This is an acute thrombophlebitis that originates from a purulent infection of the face, sinus, ear, or other areas that drain through veins that empty into the cavernous sinus. Ophthalmoplegia occurs; the lateral rectus muscle is usually the first muscle involved. Irritation of the ophthalmic division of the trigeminal nerve causes severe pain. There may be papilledema, visual failure, and other signs of involvement of the nerves passing through the optic foramen and superior orbital fissure. Computed tomography may demonstrate a thrombus in the superior sagittal sinus, cerebral edema, and venous stasis. The disease requires intensive antibiotic chemotherapy combined with anticoagulation.

IDIOPATHIC ORBITAL INFLAMMATION (PSEUDOTUMOR)

This is an acute, subacute, or chronic inflammation of the orbit that mainly affects middle-aged men. The onset is acute, with pain, edema of the eyelids and conjunctiva, and weakness of the extraocular muscles. There is a rapid development of proptosis. At times, the inflammatory signs may be so conspicuous as to suggest an orbital cellulitis. Computed tomography demonstrates inflammation of extraocular muscles, orbital fat, and perineural connective tissue. Histologically, most pseudotumors are nonspecific inflammatory reactions composed of perivascular lymphocytes, plasma cells, and some polymorphonuclear leukocytes. In children there may be a large eosinophilic component often combined with a peripheral eosinophilia. In chronic inflammation collagen is deposited in the orbital fat, within the extraocular muscles around the optic nerve, and within the lacrimal gland. Magnetic resonance imaging may indicate the extent of the granuloma.

The main treatment consists of systemic administration of corticosteroids, often combined with retrobulbar corticosteroids. Resolution is often prompt, but proptosis persists in nonresponsive patients. Treatment is often unsatisfactory, but there may be spontaneous remission. Excision is always incomplete and is often followed by recurrence. A variety of surgical procedures may be used to protect the cornea from exposure and to prevent keratitis e lagophthalmos. The fellow orbit becomes involved in about 25% of the cases.

Benign reactive lymphoid hyperplasia (pseudolymphoma) causes a slowly progressive, painless tumor of the orbit, lacrimal gland, conjunctiva, and, rarely, the uvea. Histologically, mature lymphocytes are arranged in sheetlike, hyperplastic, hypercellular accumulations. Subconjunctival tumors occur in the fornices and are a salmon color. Orbital involvement occurs in middle-aged persons and causes a progressive proptosis. The majority of cells are T lymphocytes and the remainder are polyclonal B lymphocytes. Malignant lymphomas are composed predominantly of monoclonal B lymphocytes. Radiation therapy is the preferred therapy for benign reactive lymphoid hyperplasia.

Burkitt lymphoma is the only lymphosarcoma that affects children. It probably originates in the abdomen and metastasizes to the facial bones and then encroaches on the orbit. Hepatosplenomegaly and central nervous system involvement occur. Chemotherapy is curative if done before central nervous system involvement. Burkitt lymphoma may complicate the late stages of acquired immunodeficiency syndrome (AIDS).

TUMORS AND RELATED CONDITIONS

A large variety of new growths, inflammations, congenital abnormalities, and systemic diseases may manifest themselves by orbital involvement (Table 15-2). Diagnosis is complicated by the frequency with which ocular manifestations of thyroid gland abnormalities and idiopathic orbital inflammation exhibit similar symptoms and signs. The medical history is helpful. A sudden onset and a rapid progression suggest an inflammatory process rather than a neoplasm. Orbital pain results from inflammation and is also caused by an adenoid cystic carcinoma of the lacrimal gland. A history of hyperthyroidism suggests a thyroid abnormality even though the patient may be euthyroid or hypothyroid. A complaint of noise in the head suggests a carotid-cavernous sinus fistula. Intermittent proptosis may be caused by varices of the orbit, and the congestion is aggravated by increased venous pressure induced by coughing or bending over.

Proptosis, the most common sign (50%), is followed by periorbital edema. The most frequent causes of proptosis (Table 15-3) in the adult are thyroid disease, orbital inflammation, hemangioma, and mucocele of the frontal sinus. There is considerable variation in the orbital diseases encountered in different institutions, which may reflect the interests of the staff and the type of patient referred for care.

TABLE 15-2.
Systemic Disorders Affecting the Orbit

- I. Thyroid disease
- II. Osteitis deformans (Paget disease)
  - A. Osteosarcoma after osteitis deformans
- III. Histiocytosis
  - A. Juvenile xanthogranuloma
  - B. Eosinophilic granuloma
  - C. Hand-Schüller-Christian disease
  - D. Letterer-Siwe disease
  - E. Sinus histiocytosis
- IV. Hematopoietic disorders
  - A. Lymphoma
    - 1. Malignant
      - a. Lymphocytic type
        - (1) Nodular
        - (2) Diffuse
        - (3) Well differentiated
        - (4) Poorly differentiated (Burkitt)
      - b. Hodgkin type
  - B. Plasma cell
    - 1. Primary
    - 2. Metastatic
  - C. Granulocytic sarcoma (chloroma)
  - D. Gammopathies
    - 1. Monoclonal
    - 2. Polyclonal
  - E. Multiple myeloma
  - F. Immune vasculitis
    - 1. Wegener granulomatosis
    - 2. Lethal midline granuloma
- V. Vascular abnormalities
  - A. Carotid-cavernous sinus fistula
  - B. Cavernous sinus thrombosis
  - C. Intraorbital aneurysm
  - D. Hemorrhage; hematoma
  - E. Angioneurotic edema
- VI. Metastatic tumor
  - A. Neuroblastoma (infants)
  - B. Lung carcinoma (men, women)
  - C. Breast carcinoma (women)
  - D. Prostate, urinary bladder, thyroid
- VII. Chronic granulomatous inflammation
  - A. Sarcoidosis
  - B. Tuberculosis
  - C. Foreign body
    - 1. Ruptured dermoid cyst
  - D. Lymphogranuloma
  - E. Gumma

Neuroblastomas in infants and children may metastasize (20%) to the orbit. They sometimes

TABLE 15-3.
Orbital Neoplasms and Other Tumors

- I. Choristomas (tissues normally not present)
  - A. Dermoid cyst
  - B. Epidermoid cyst
  - C. Teratoma
- II. Hamartomas (tissues normally present)
  - A. Hemangioma
    - 1. Capillary
    - 2. Cavernous
  - B. Neurofibromatosis
    - 1. Optic nerve glioma (juvenile pilocytic astrocytoma)
    - 2. Plexiform neurofibroma
    - 3. Neurilemmoma (schwannoma)
- III. Systemic disease
- IV. Primary
  - A. Mesenchyme
    - 1. Bone
      - a. Cyst, osteosarcoma, dysplasia
    - 2. Cartilage
      - a. Chlondroma, chondrosarcoma
    - 3. Muscle
      - a. Rhabdomyosarcoma, rhabdomyoma
      - b. Leiomyoma, leiomyosarcoma
    - 4. Vascular
      - a. Kaposi sarcoma, hemangiopericytoma
    - 5. Fat
      - a. Lipoma, liposarcoma
    - 6. Connective tissue
      - a. Meningioma
      - b. Nodular fasciitis, fibroma
  - B. Lacrimal gland
  - C. Optic nerve
- V. Secondary
  - A. Direct extension
    - 1. Eyelid (squamous cell, basal cell)
    - 2. Eye (malignant melanoma, retinoblastoma)
    - 3. Intracranial cavity (meningioma)
    - 4. Nasal accessory sinus (mucocele, osteoma)
  - B. Metastatic
    - 1. Neuroblastoma
    - 2. Granulocytic sarcoma (leukemia)
    - 3. Lymphatic leukemia
    - 4. Carcinoma: breast, lung, prostate
  - C. Inflammatory
    - 1. Pseudotumor
      - a. Chronic granuloma
      - b. Chronic nongranulomatous
        - (1) Inflammatory pseudotumor
        - (2) Benign reactive lymphoid hyperplasia
    - 2. Cellulitis, abscess
    - 3. Periostitis

occur together with periorbital ecchymosis. Neuroblastoma may also cause Horner syndrome. There may be opsoclonus-myoclonus ("dancing eyes").

Gliomas of the optic nerve may occur as an isolated tumor or in association with neurofibromatosis. Children are principally affected during their first 10 years. The prognosis is good if the tumor is confined to the optic nerve but rapidly fatal with posterior extension to the optic chiasm.

Rhabdomyosarcoma occurs more frequently in the orbit than anywhere else and is the most common primary malignancy in the orbit in children.

Superior orbital fissure syndrome.—The superior orbital fissure syndrome is characterized by local pain, proptosis, and paralysis of the oculomotor, trochlear, and abducent cranial nerves. Usually there is loss of sensation only in the area of distribution of the ophthalmic division of the trigeminal nerve (N V_1). Proptosis and loss of corneal sensation distinguish the syndrome from cavernous sinus tumor. Blepharoptosis is present, and the eye is usually turned down and out. The most common cause is a neoplasm that involves the apex of the orbit, but in some instances a pseudotumor may be responsible.

INJURIES

Injuries to the orbit are divided into penetrating, nonpenetrating, and those with indirect damage to the orbit and its contents. Fractures of the facial and orbital bones often complicate blunt trauma. Penetrating injuries may lacerate the globe or perforate the thin posterior walls of the orbit to enter the cranial cavity or a nasal sinus.

Blunt trauma to the orbit may cause severe intraorbital hemorrhage that suffuses readily beneath the conjunctiva and under the eyelids and may markedly limit ocular rotations. Severe hemorrhage may also be a sign of fracture of the wall of the orbit and may be associated with serious brain damage.

The most frequent fracture of the orbit involves the medial portion of its floor (blowout fracture) with a prolapse of orbital contents into the maxillary sinus (Fig 15-5). The palpebral fissure is narrowed and there is a slight enoph-

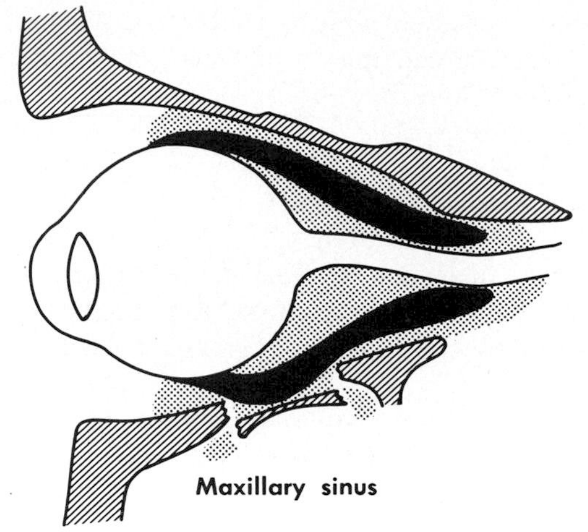

FIG 15-5.
Blowout fracture of the orbit with prolapse of the orbital tissue and the inferior rectus muscle into the maxillary sinus, where the muscle may become entrapped.

thalmos. The area innervated by the infraorbital nerve (the skin of the lower eyelid, the nose, and the cheek) is anesthetic. Entrapment of the inferior rectus muscle results in an inability to rotate the eye upward. Surgical correction of the defect is required if the restricted ocular rotation persists more than 2 weeks, or if there is severe prolapse of orbital tissue into the maxillary sinus. The defect in the floor of the orbit is exposed either through an incision in the inferior conjunctival fornix or through a skin incision. The prolapsed tissues are replaced in the orbit and the bony defect is bridged with a plastic implant.

The most frequent fracture of the orbital rim involves its medial margin and the nose and is particularly likely to occur as a result of automobile accidents, in which the face of the front-seat passenger is struck by a suddenly inflated air bag or strikes the dashboard. Fractures of the superior margin of the orbit may damage the trochlea and may cause the symptoms of a superior oblique muscle paralysis. Fractures of the lateral margin are fairly common and result in depression of the cheekbone. Early surgery to elevate the arch of the zygoma bone can prevent much subsequent surgery. Fractures of the inferior margin are frequently comminuted and associated with fractures of other facial bones.

Trauma may rupture the thin lamina papyracea of the medial wall of the orbit, allowing air to enter the orbit (emphysema of the orbit) and sometimes the eyelids. There may be proptosis and diplopia. The condition may be readily recognized by the peculiar crepitation of the eyelids with palpation. Treatment is usually not necessary, but, if the condition is severe, the orbit may be decompressed.

SURGERY OF THE ORBIT

Procedures involving the orbit include decompression to permit expansion of orbital contents that cannot be removed, excision of orbital tumors, exenteration of all orbital contents, enucleation of the eye, and correction of bony defects.

Orbital decompression is mainly indicated in thyroid disease in which expansion of the orbital contents causes exposure keratitis or optic neuropathy. Expansion of the orbital contents into a nasal sinus or the fossa of the temporalis muscle reduces the forward displacement of the orbital contents.

Often, the initial procedure is removal of one or more walls of the orbit endonasally or through a skin or conjunctival incision. Surgery may be required subsequently to relieve diplopia. Orbital decompression is frequently combined with procedures to decrease the width of the palpebral fissure by joining the lateral margins of the upper and lower eyelids (lateral blepharoplasty).

Tumors of the orbit may be approached from the orbit's anterior margin or its lateral or superior wall. The anterior approach is made through an eyebrow incision and is used solely for palpable tumors. The lateral approach is used for benign tumors of the posterior orbit. A combined anterolateral approach is used for malignant lacrimal gland tumors. A superior approach requires a craniotomy and is indicated mainly in tumors such as meningioma or glioma that involve both the orbital and cranial cavities. The cornea may be protected by adhesions between the upper and lower eyelids (blepharoplasty) or with a conjunctival flap.

Exenteration of the orbital contents is a mutilating procedure indicated mainly for malignancies of the lacrimal gland, for extension of eyelid malignancies into the orbit, for malignant melanoma of the conjunctiva, for malignant melanoma or retinoblastoma that involves the orbit, and for primary intraorbital malignancies such as rhabdomyosarcoma. The procedure may be lifesaving in lacrimal gland tumors in which areas of bony extension must be removed. In malignancies that have extended into adjacent nasal sinuses and the intracranial cavity, the procedure is mainly palliative.

Removal of the eye.—Enucleation of the eye is indicated for a blind and painful eye, in ocular malignancies too large to respond to other treatment, in severe injuries of the globe when restoration of a functional eye is not possible, and in early sympathetic ophthalmia. The conjunctiva is opened as close to the corneoscleral limbus as possible and each muscle is separated from the globe at its insertion. The optic nerve is then severed as far behind the globe as possible.

A number of ingenious procedures have been proposed to provide motility to the ocular prosthesis after enucleation. Most recently a hydroxyapatite (a coral) is implanted in the muscle cone beneath a covering of conjunctiva and Tenon capsule. Its porous composition permits it to become vascularized and to impart satisfactory movement to the artificial eye (ocular prosthesis). Even greater mobility follows connection of the prosthesis by a peg connected to the implant. With careful matching of the normal eye, the cosmetic defect is minimal. The artificial eye should be removed only once or twice a month, and every precaution should be taken to prevent contamination.

Loss of an eye does not cause a 50% loss of visual efficiency (one may estimate the loss by covering one's own eye) but may be accompanied by severe emotional problems.

Bony defects of the orbit.—These may be repaired by means of plastic implants or bone taken from the iliac ridge. Commonly the surgery is indicated because of incarceration of an ocular muscle in an orbital fracture, and considerable judgment is required so as not to overcorrect the defect.

BIBLIOGRAPHY

Books

Dortzbach RK, editor: *Ophthalmic plastic surgery: prevention and management of complications,* New York, 1994, Raven Press.

Henderson JW, editor: *Orbital tumors,* ed 3, New York, 1994, Raven Press.

McCord CD Jr, Tannenbaum M, Nunery WR, editors: *Oculoplastic surgery,* ed 3, New York, 1995, Raven Press.

Rootman J, Stewart B, Goldberg RA: *Orbital surgery, a conceptual approach,* Philadelphia, 1995, Lippincott-Raven.

16

THE MIDDLE COAT: THE UVEA

The middle coat of the eye, the uvea (Latin *uva:* grape), consists of the choroid, the ciliary body, and the iris. The choroid is the vascular layer of the posterior three fifths of the eye, which nurtures the adjacent retinal pigment epithelium and the outer portion of the sensory retina. The ciliary body secretes aqueous humor and contains the smooth muscle (N III) that controls accommodation. The iris, a diaphragm that rests upon the lens, separates the anterior and posterior chambers of the eye. It contains a central opening, the pupil, through which aqueous humor passes from the posterior to the anterior chamber. The iris contains two muscles, the sphincter pupillae (N III, parasympathetics) and the dilator pupillae (sympathetics), which regulate the amount of light entering the eye.

The choroid extends from the margin of the optic disk posteriorly to the ciliary body anteriorly. It consists of the choriocapillaris, an inner layer of specialized, large-diameter (21 μm), fenestrated capillaries (Fig 16-1), which is separated from the retinal pigment epithelium by the lamina basalis choroideae (Bruch membrane). The outer layers of the choroid consist of arteries and veins of successively larger diameter that empty into the vortex veins. The blood supply of the posterior half of the choroid is derived from 10 to 20 short posterior ciliary arteries, while that of the anterior half is derived from the long posterior and anterior ciliary arteries. The blood supply of the iris and ciliary body is similar to that of the anterior choroid.

The ciliary body is composed of a corona ciliaris (pars plicata), which contains ciliary processes, and an orbicularis ciliaris (pars plana), a transitional area with the choroid. The ciliary processes secrete the aqueous humor into the posterior chamber.

Located within the ciliary body is the ciliary muscle, divided into well-defined longitudinal and circular muscle fibers and poorly defined radial muscle fibers. Zonular fibers, which do not have contractile properties, connect the equatorial region of the anterior and posterior lens capsule with the ciliary body. Contraction of the circular fibers of the ciliary muscle relaxes the zonule, causing the lens to become more spherical (accommodation).

The iris contains a variable amount of pigment in its anterior stroma. The anterior stroma is absent in some areas, forming iris crypts. The stroma rests on a layer of pigment epithelium that is continuous with that of the retina. The pigment epithelium contains the dilatator pupillae muscle on its anterior surface. The sphincter pupillae muscle is located near the pupil in the posterior iris stroma. Both muscles originate from neural ectoderm. The iris is divided by the collarette, a remnant of the minor vascular circle of the iris, into a central pupillary zone (concentric with the pupil) and a peripheral ciliary zone. The blood vessels of the iris are arranged in a radial pattern and have a thick adventitia. The blood vessels of the iris and the pigment epithelium of the ciliary processes are not permeable to large molecules (blood-aqueous barrier).

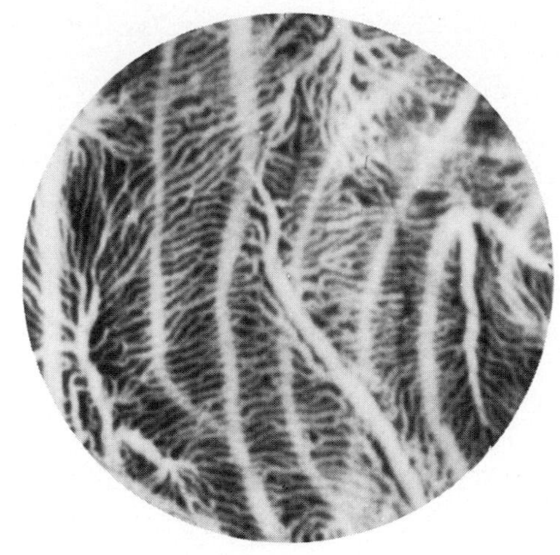

FIG 16-1.
Injected specimen of human choroid showing choriocapillaris and large collecting veins. The choriocapillaris is composed of such large vessels that it resembles vascular sinuses rather than the usual capillaries.

SYMPTOMS AND SIGNS OF UVEAL DISEASE

The symptoms and signs of uveal disease vary with the portion affected. Abnormalities of the iris may distort the shape of the pupil or may impair its dilation and constriction. Inflammations of the iris and the ciliary body cause a ciliary type of injection. Diseases of the ciliary body and the iris may be associated with severe, deep, boring, dull, aching pain within the eye. Inflammation of the posterior choroid occurs without ciliary injection or pain.

In many inflammations of the ciliary body, painful spasm of the ciliary muscle increases accommodation. Impairment of the oculomotor nerve (N III) supply causes pupillary dilation and loss of accommodation. Inflammations of the choroid often extend into the adjacent retina. Vision is reduced because of exudation of inflammatory cells and protein into the vitreous cavity. Reduced blood flow through the choriocapillaris impairs both the visual acuity and the visual field. Inflammations of the ciliary body release cells and protein into both the vitreous cavity and the anterior chamber. Inflammatory products from the iris are confined to the anterior chamber.

The iris may be examined directly. The internal face of the ciliary body can be seen with a gonioscope after maximal pupillary dilation or by using indirect ophthalmoscopy and scleral indentation.

Ophthalmoscopic visualization of choroidal details is obscured by the pigment epithelium of the retina that causes the fundus to appear reddish brown. Often a portion of the choroid is visible at the temporal side of the optic disk as a choroidal crescent. In blond individuals, the large choroidal veins may be seen. A white sclera may be observed between blood vessels that usually belong to the outer vessel layer of the choroid (Haller), which consists of veins that have a considerably larger diameter than the corresponding retinal arteries. Details of the choriocapillaris may be seen with fluorescein or indocyanine green angiography, but ophthalmoscopically it consists of a thin sheet of blood that creates the red fundus reflex. In atrophy of the choriocapillaris, the choroidal veins may be seen as a dense network of white vessels.

The melanin of the choroid is browner than the jet-black retinal pigment. The choroidal pigment cells do not proliferate in inflammatory irritation as do the retinal pigment epithelial cells.

The lamina basalis choroideae (Bruch membrane) is composed of (1) the basement membrane of the endothelium of the choriocapillaris; (2) an elastic tissue layer sandwiched between two collagen layers; and (3) the basement membrane of the retinal pigment epithelium. Deficiencies in the elastic layer cause a variety of fundus abnormalities, such as angioid streaks and rare hereditary diseases. Holes in Bruch membrane precede subretinal neovascularization (new blood vessels from the choriocapillaris), which complicates many retinal disorders.

CONGENITAL AND DEVELOPMENTAL ANOMALIES

OCULAR COLOBOMA

Failure of the optic cup to fuse at the fetal fissure results in an ocular coloboma. Uveal tissue is absent in the lower, nasal quadrant and creates a defect that may extend from the margin of the optic disk to the pupil. The choroid and retinal pigment epithelium are missing, but the sensory retina and its blood vessels are usually present.

The white sclera is seen ophthalmoscopically at the base of choroidal colobomas (Fig 16-2). The sclera may bulge outward (ectasia). A col-

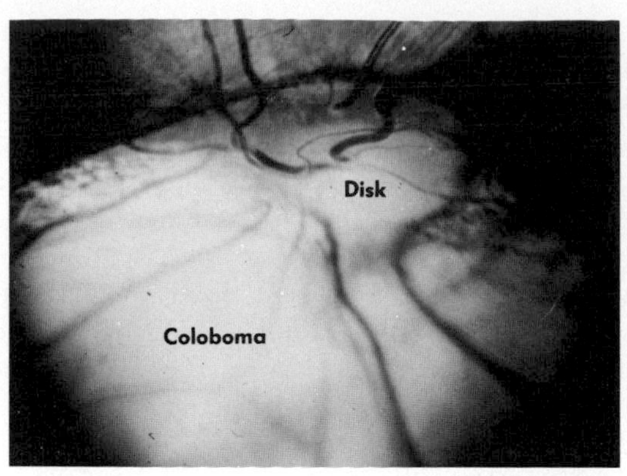

FIG 16-2.
Large coloboma of the inferior choroid. The retinal arteries and veins are present, but the large white area is sclera visible through the transparent sensory retina, which lacks its normal blood supply from the choriocapillaris.

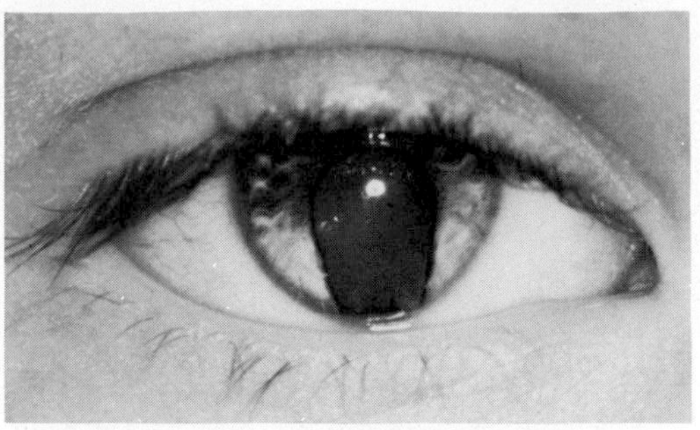

FIG 16-3.
Congenital coloboma of the iris located in the characteristic down and slightly nasal position in the region of the site of closure of the fetal fissure.

oboma of the ciliary body may be associated with a notching defect of the lens that corresponds to the deficient zonule in the area. The appearance of a choroidal coloboma may be simulated by prenatal retinochoroiditis caused by toxoplasmosis. These inflammatory lesions, however, do not usually occur in the inferior nasal quadrant, and there is proliferation of the retinal pigment epithelium.

Typical congenital colobomas of the iris involve the inferior nasal portion and cause a (keyhole) defect in the shape of the pupil (Fig 16-3). The margins of the coloboma show the pupillary frill with pigment epithelium, unlike surgical iridectomies.

Ocular colobomas may occur as an autosomal dominant condition, as a part of recessive syndromes with multiple systemic defects, or as a chromosomal duplication affecting 22pter-22q11.2. When there are systemic abnormalities, slightly more than one half of patients are mentally retarded.

ANIRIDIA

Aniridia (absence of the iris) is a congenital, often hereditary, usually bilateral, failure of growth and differentiation of the anterior portion of the optic cup. The iris is not entirely absent but is more or less rudimentary. When visible, its remnants can be seen by means of gonioscopy behind the corneoscleral limbus.

The PAX genes in mice are developmental control genes (homeobox) that have a key role in the embryonic development of the spinal cord and brain. The PAX 6 gene affects the embryonic development of the cerebellum and eye. Mutation of the PAX 6 gene in mice results in small-eye mice (mSey), and in humans it results in aniridia. Mutation of the PAX 3 gene in humans results in the Waardenburg syndrome (lateral displacement of medial canthi and lacrimal puncta; increased width of the root of the nose; irides of different color [heterochromia]; and cochlear deafness). The parents and siblings of every patient with aniridia should have a complete eye examination, and the patients should have chromosome analysis and DNA analysis to detect deletion of band 11p13, to exclude the risk of developing Wilms tumor.

Clinically the region with an iris coloboma appears black with an enormous pupil and no iris visible. Photophobia is often present, and patients squeeze the eyelids almost closed and furrow the brow. Family members may have hypoplastic irides or iris colobomas. Visual acuity is usually about 20/100 or poorer, but in some kindreds vision is good. Visual acuity may deteriorate because of glaucoma. In the usual phenotype, aniridia is associated with nystagmus, foveal and optic nerve hypoplasia, corneal pannus, cataract, secondary glaucoma, and strabismus. Blood vessels may occur in the normal avascular fovea centralis.

Provision of an artificial pupil by means of an iris painted on a contact lens reduces photophobia but does not improve vision. Glaucoma often develops in adolescence and responds poorly to surgery and medical treatment.

CHARGE is an acronym for an ill-defined group of developmental abnormalities that includes *c*oloboma (ocular), *h*eart disease, *a*tresia

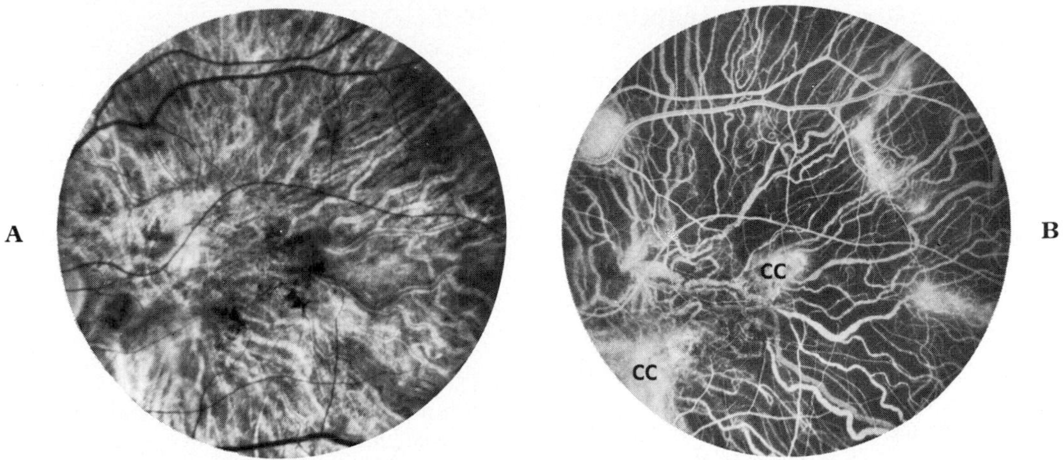

FIG 16-4.
A, Light ophthalmoscopy of atrophy of the choriocapillaris. The choroidal vessels appear as white lines through the atrophic pigment epithelium. **B,** Choroidal circulation in the late phase of fluorescein angiography. There is atrophy of the choriocapillaris, and the choroidal arteries and veins are clearly seen. Some islands of choriocapillaris *(CC)* remain.

choanae, *r*etarded growth and development, *g*enital malformations, and *e*ar malformations. The cause is unknown.

Every patient who has a Wilms tumor and deletion of band 13 of the short arm of chromosome 11 has aniridia. Not all patients with aniridia and 11p13 develop Wilms tumor. Rhabdomyosarcoma, nephroblastoma, adrenal tumors, hepatoblastoma, and gonadoblastoma have also been described. As with some hereditary tumors, such as retinoblastoma, the individual inherits a gene deletion or a mutant gene on one chromosome, and a second abnormality of its allele results in tumor formation.

ATROPHY OF THE CHORIOCAPILLARIS

Atrophy of the choriocapillaris occurs in two forms: (1) a benign type, depigmentation in situ, in which there is no functional impairment; and (2) a degenerative type, which may be either generalized or focal, in which functional impairment is severe. The sole pathologic change in the benign type is attenuated pigment in the retinal pigment epithelium. In the degenerative type, the choriocapillaris is absent, as are the retinal pigment epithelium and the outer layers of the sensory retina in the affected areas. Sclerosis of the choroidal vessels does not occur in either condition.

Depigmentation in situ is seen commonly in simple myopia and less frequently as a change with aging. The choroidal vasculature is conspicuous ophthalmoscopically. Vision and fluorescein angiography are normal.

Degenerative choriocapillary atrophy occurs in a generalized or diffuse form or in a focal form confined to the posterior pole of the eye. The generalized form occurs sporadically (Fig 16-4) in X chromosome–linked choroideremia, gyrate atrophy, and hereditary and toxic retinal pigmentary degeneration. The focal type (also known as central areolar choroidal sclerosis, central progressive areolar choroidal dystrophy, or central choroidal sclerosis) occurs mainly as an autosomal recessive disorder. Central vision is reduced in both types. In the generalized type there is night blindness, loss of the electroretinographic response to light, and a reduced electro-oculographic light-dark ratio.

Degenerative choroidal sclerosis begins in the retinal pigment epithelium and is followed shortly thereafter by impaired filling of the lobules of the choriocapillaris and then atrophy. With atrophy, the retinal pigment epithelium, together with the adjacent outer retina, degenerates, and the major arteries and veins of the choroid become visible. The precapillary arterioles and branches of the short posterior ciliary arteries also atrophy, but to a lesser extent than the choriocapillaris.

Choroideremia.—Choroideremia is an X chromosome disorder secondary to deletion of chromosome Xq21 that results in choroidal atrophy, secondary atrophy of the retina, night blindness, and ultimately loss of all light perception.

In the female carrier, the condition is asymptomatic but is associated with increased pigmentation and depigmentation of the fundus that is most marked in the equatorial region. The pigment granules have an irregular, square appearance similar to chunks of coal and are about 100 μm in diameter (the optic disk is 1,500 μm). Under or adjacent to the clumps of pigment are depigmented areas up to 0.5 disk diameter in size. They may appear paler than the rest of the fundus or have a bright yellow color.

Choroideremia in the hemizygous male has its clinical onset between 10 and 13 years of age. Night blindness, which becomes complete in about 10 years, is the initial symptom. The peripheral field then begins to contract, and finally, after about 35 years, all vision is lost. The earliest fundus lesions resemble the pigmentary changes of the female carriers. Eventually atrophic changes dominate, and the white sclera becomes exposed in the equatorial region. At this time, night blindness occurs and an annular scotoma is present. The atrophy then spreads centrally and peripherally until all vision is lost. The retinal vessels remain normal.

Gyrate atrophy of the choroid.—This is a progressive disorder of the choroid and retina caused by inactivation of the mitochondrial matrix enzyme ornithine aminotransferase. A variety of mutations are most efficiently detected by the polymerase chain reaction amplification of gene sequence, denaturing gradient gel electrophoresis, and direct DNA sequencing. Only the eyes appear to be involved, although the blood levels of ornithine are markedly increased (20x) and those of ammonia, lysine, glutamine, and glutamic acid, metabolic products of ornithine, are low.

Myopia occurs in the first decade, night blindness in the second, severe cataract in the third, and pigmentary changes of the macula with progressive loss of vision in the fourth. The chorioretinal atrophy begins at puberty, in the equatorial region of the fundus, with sharply punched-out oval areas of atrophy, with scalloped borders, obliteration of the choriocapillaris, narrowing of the retinal vessels, and optic nerve atrophy. The chorioretinal atrophy slowly spreads toward the fovea centralis, which is preserved until adulthood. In the late stages of gyrate atrophy, there is fine, velvety pigmentation with glittering crystals that are not seen in choroideremia. Additionally, pigmentation of the central retina conceals the choroid, which is exposed in choroideremia.

Daily administration of 500 to 1,000 mg of pyridoxine hydrochloride decreases plasma ornithine, which slows but does not prevent progression of the choroideremia. Restriction of the dietary intake of arginine, the precursor of ornithine, decreases ornithine levels and increases plasma levels of its metabolites. The results have been equivocal in a small group of patients.

TABLE 16-1.
Heterochromia Iridis

Lighter-colored iris abnormality
Simple heterochromia iridis
Arachnodactyly
Facial hemiatrophy
Mandibulo-oculofacial dyscephaly
Hallerman-Streiff syndrome
Waardenburg-Klein syndrome
Horner syndrome
Heterochromic cyclitis of Fuchs
Glaucomatocyclitic crisis
Amelanotic tumors
Cutaneous xanthomatosis
Reactive lymphoid hyperplasia of uvea
Darker-colored iris abnormality
Retention of intraocular iron foreign body
Malignant melanoma of the iris
Ocular hemosiderosis
Trauma
Microcornea

CONGENITAL ECTROPION UVEAE

The pigmented margin of the pupil marks the anterior border of the secondary optic cup. Rarely, flocculi or cystic dilations of the marginal sinus of the pupillary margin develop into dark brown bodies that may extend on the surface of the iris. They may occasionally break free to appear as movable pigment masses on the iris surface. They have no harmful effects. Treatment of accommodative esotropia with miotics in children causes similar cysts. Concurrent administration of 2.5% phenylephrine eyedrops prevents cyst formation.

HETEROCHROMIA IRIDIS

In heterochromia iridis, the two irides differ in color (Table 16-1). In simple heterochromia iridis, there is relative hypoplasia of the lighter-colored iris combined with a relative hyperplasia of the iris architecture on the side of the darker-colored iris. The abnormality may be transmitted as an autosomal dominant trait.

In hypochromic heterochromia, the eye with the lighter-colored iris is abnormal. The difference between the two eyes may be minimal when both irises are blue. The condition occurs in many different disorders. In Horner syndrome, there is paralysis of the dilatator muscle of the iris. Heterochromia iridis, displacement of the medial canthi, hypertrophy of the nasal bridge, white forelock, and deafness constitute the Waardenburg-Klein syndrome, an abnormality of neural crest cells. In Fuchs heterochromic cyclitis there is a mild inflammation of the iris as well as the ciliary body, often complicated with cataract and sometimes with glaucoma. In glaucomatocyclitic crisis, there is diffuse iris atrophy secondary to inflammation, trauma, and ischemia of the iris. Infiltration of the iris by any nonpigmented tumor causes a hypochromic iris.

In hyperchromia iridis, the iris on the side of the anomaly or disease is darker than its fellow. The condition occurs with retention of an iron foreign body in the eye (siderosis), with malignant melanoma of the iris, in monocular melanosis in which there are excess chromatophores in the iris stroma, after anterior chamber hemorrhage from any cause, after perforating injuries or contusion of the globe before 10 years of age, and in association with microcornea.

IRIS ATROPHY

Normally the pupillary zone of the iris is relatively flat because of an atrophy of the anterior leaf of the stroma during fetal life. The gossamer appearance of the ciliary zone may be lost in conditions in which the blood vessels and fine collagen fibers atrophy and are replaced by a network of connective tissue. Hypochromia iridis causes such an atrophy combined with a loss of chromatophores. The atrophy may be diffuse or localized. Minor degrees of iris atrophy occur with aging, and the atrophy may be severe after ocular inflammation, trauma, ischemia, and glaucoma. It may occur in tabes dorsalis without pupillary abnormalities. Decreasing pigmentation of the iris is a risk factor for the development of macular degeneration.

Iridocorneal endothelial syndrome.— Glaucoma, progressive iris atrophy, abnormal corneal endothelium, extensive peripheral anterior synechiae, multiple iris nodules, and a transparent membrane covering the anterior surface of the iris are seen in varying combinations in three conditions: (1) progressive essential iris atrophy; (2) iris atrophy with corneal edema and glaucoma (Chandler); and (3) iris-nevus syndrome (Cogan and Reese).

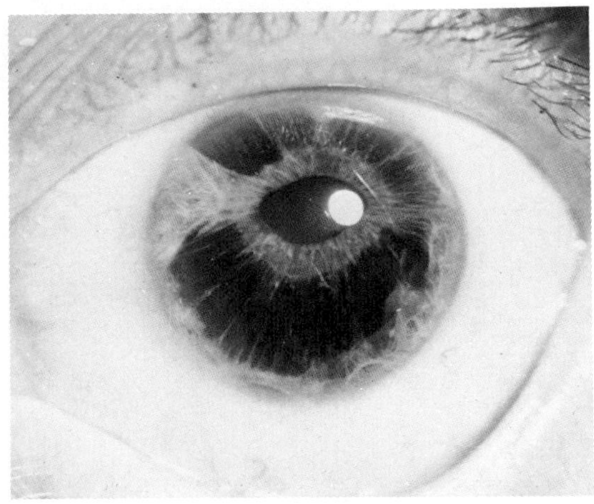

FIG 16-5.
Essential atrophy of the iris with loss of iris stroma below and an opening through all layers of the iris in a 33-year-old woman. Intraocular pressure is easily controlled by instillation of 2% pilocarpine, but when treatment is omitted, pressure increases precipitously, resulting in corneal edema and loss of vision.

The disorders are slowly progressive over a period of 10 or more years. Women are more commonly affected than men. After metaplasia, the corneal endothelium proliferates and is disrupted by loss of cells. Minor increases in intraocular pressure cause severe corneal edema, particularly in the Chandler syndrome. The iris stroma atrophies and develops a matted appearance caused by abnormalities of its basement membrane.

Essential iris atrophy (Fig 16-5) is a rare, progressive, usually unilateral disease predominantly affecting women between 30 and 60 years. It is characterized by a distorted, displaced pupil, corneal endothelial degeneration, patchy atrophy of the iris with partial or complete hole formation, peripheral anterior synechiae, and secondary glaucoma. The onset is gradual, and the patient is aware only of a change in shape or position of the pupil. During the next several years, holes develop in the iris. Second-

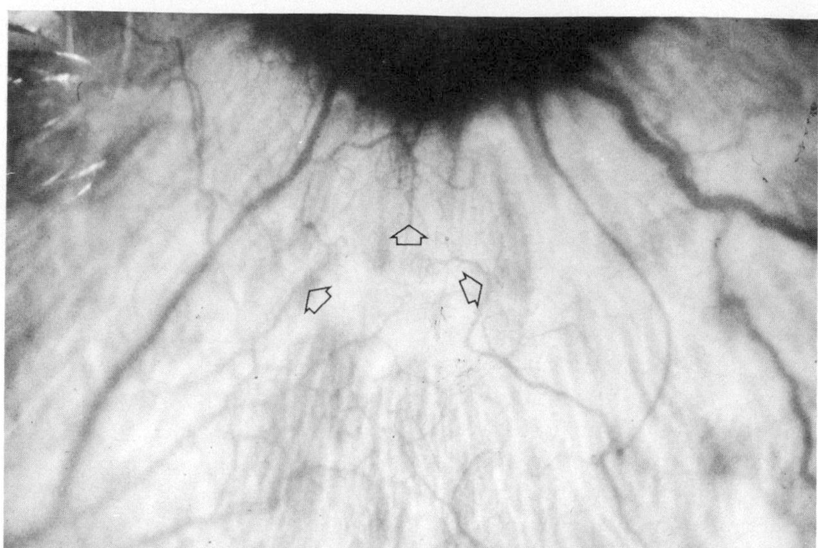

FIG 16-6.
New blood on surface of the iris (*arrows;* rubeosis iridis) in a 48-year-old diabetic patient.

ary glaucoma then ensues from peripheral anterior synechiae and damage to the trabecular meshwork from a cuticular membrane. Direct inspection of the iris indicates the loss of iris tissue and displacement of the pupil. Treatment is directed toward the secondary glaucoma and is often not effective. Visual loss results from either corneal edema or secondary glaucoma.

A less severe form of iris atrophy (Chandler syndrome) is associated with an endothelial disturbance and corneal edema combined with multiple small iris nodules and an ectopic Descemet membrane on the iris surface. Glaucoma may eventually occur secondary to obstruction of outflow by peripheral anterior synechiae. Corneal edema occurs with minor increases in intraocular pressure.

The iris-nevus syndrome begins as a progressive iris atrophy, but after many years light tan, yellow, or dark brown nodules appear as little spheres of tissue in the iris stroma. Similar-appearing nodules may also be seen in the neurofibromatoses (Lish nodules), in melanomas, in flocculi of the iris, and in inflammatory granulomas.

Secondary iris atrophy.—Secondary iris atrophy does not cause the iris holes seen in the essential type. The atrophy may result from anterior uveitis, ocular trauma, or herpes zoster ophthalmicus. The sphincter pupillae muscle may atrophy after an attack of closed-angle glaucoma. Iris atrophy may be caused by ischemia of the iris secondary to closure of the anterior ciliary arteries or long ciliary arteries that may follow carotid artery insufficiency or lupus erythematosus. Local interference with blood supply may follow retinal detachment operations, freezing or cauterizing of the corneoscleral limbus region, or detachment of three or four recti muscles.

RUBEOSIS OF THE IRIS (RUBEOSIS IRIDIS)

Neovascularization of the iris (Fig 16-6) occurs as an irregularly distributed or generalized network of fine, markedly tortuous, anastomosed, tightly meshed new blood vessels on the surface and within the stroma of the iris. It follows occlusion of the capillaries of the iris, and may constitute a harmful compensatory mechanism in response to the loss of the blood supply. The new blood vessels and associated fibrous tissue may cover the trabecular meshwork and cause peripheral anterior synechiae that close the anterior chamber angle and cause an intractable neovascular glaucoma. Hemorrhage into the anterior chamber may occur.

The proliferative retinopathy of diabetes mellitus commonly precedes rubeosis iridis. The disorder often follows central vein closure and, more rarely, central retinal artery closure. It occurs in vascular insufficiency, such as the aortic arch syndrome, carotid artery occlusive disease, carotid artery fistula, giant cell arteritis, anterior ocular segment ischemia, intraocular tumors, and after ocular radiation and intraocular inflammation. It is the most common complication of vitrectomy, particularly if the lens is absent.

Neovascular glaucoma is difficult to treat. Scatter photocoagulation (ablation) of a neovascularized retina may be followed by involution of the iris vessels. Photocoagulation of the iris and anterior chamber angle causes a temporary ischemia that allows a filtering operation or implantation of a filtering valve. Cryotherapy of the ciliary body (cyclocryotherapy) may reduce the secretion of aqueous humor and possibly impair sensory innervation. Retrobulbar alcohol injection relieves pain for up to 3 months. Enucleation may be deferred if the eye is not too unsightly and if ultrasonography confirms the absence of an intraocular tumor.

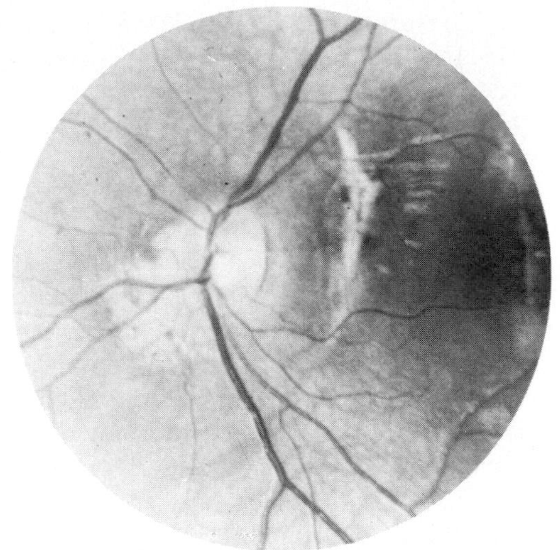

FIG 16-7.
Choroidal tears after blunt trauma to the anterior portion of the eye.

INJURIES

CONTUSIONS

Contusion to the eye may cause a variety of injuries to the uvea: (1) rupture of the sphincter pupillae muscle, with nonresponsive sector of the pupil (iridoplegia); (2) iridodialysis, in which the root of the iris is torn from its insertion, causing an additional opening at the periphery of the iris; the pupil in the sector of the defect to become a chord rather than an arc; (3) hemorrhage into the anterior chamber (hyphema), vitreous, or both; (4) glaucoma; (5) choroidal hemorrhage; and (6) choroidal tears.

Damage to the ciliary body cannot be seen. Many hyphemas probably originate from a tearing of the ciliary body from the scleral spur with bleeding from the major arterial circle of the iris. Gonioscopy indicates a localized deepening (recession) of the anterior chamber angle. Two or three decades after angle recession, a glaucoma, indistinguishable from open-angle glaucoma, may develop.

Hemorrhage into the choroid varies from a small intrachoroidal hemorrhage to massive bleeding. When located in the choroid, the hemorrhagic area is a dark brown elevation with pink to red edges evident in retroillumination. Hemorrhagic areas are frequently absorbed slowly and leave a residue of mottled pigment in the retinal pigment epithelium with areas of hypopigmentation and hyperpigmentation.

Choroidal tears (Fig 16-7) are frequently caused by severe contusions to the anterior segment of the eyeball. They occur most frequently on the temporal side of the fundus, are concentric with the optic disk, and are usually located between the disk and the fovea centralis or temporal to the fovea centralis. They may be single or multiple. They probably result from stretching of the posterior choroid caused by compression of the eye, the temporal side being more vulnerable because of its greater extent and the blow being more commonly directed to the less protected temporal side.

The tears are crescentic, vertical, and of variable length. Hemorrhage into the choroid, subretinal area, or the retina frequently occurs. As the hemorrhage and edema absorb, the yellowish gray lesions become well defined. When the tear is between the optic disk and the fovea centralis, vision is reduced and disruption of the overlying sensory retina causes a nerve fiber bundle visual field defect. Tears of the choroid lateral to the fovea centralis may not affect vision.

CHOROIDAL EFFUSION

Choroidal effusion (choroidal edema, combined retinochoroidal detachment) occurs after intraocular surgery and complicates nanophthalmos. Five to fifteen days after the operation, folds develop in the Descemet membrane, and the choroidal detachment causes a low intraocular pressure. Occasionally, leakage of aqueous humor from the corneoscleral wound causes hypotony. Through a dilated pupil, the detachment of the choroid appears as a dark gray-brown mass. Ophthalmoscopically, the detachment is a smooth, round swelling, extending hemispherically into the vitreous cavity. The detachment may be single or multiple and usually is located in the inferior fundus anterior to the equator. The borders are dark and well defined.

A choroidal detachment requires trauma combined with decreased intraocular pressure (hypotony). The normal pressure relationships within the choroid are disturbed, producing a transudation of fluid in the suprachoroidal space and resulting in choroidal edema. The serous choroidal detachment often slowly recedes after the reaction to surgery subsides. A small wound fistula or an aqueous humor shunting implant that permits loss of aqueous humor is a common cause of a persistent serous choroidal detachment. If this cause can be excluded, the persistence may be caused by an organized hemorrhage, which may take months to absorb.

LACERATIONS

A laceration of the cornea may be followed immediately by prolapse of the iris into the wound. If the wound is small, the pupil is distorted and has a teardrop shape. If extensive, the entire iris may prolapse.

Prolapse of the ciliary body through a scleral or corneal laceration is particularly serious because vitreous humor is lost and the zonule is damaged. Neglected prolapse of the ciliary body is more likely to cause a sympathetic ophthalmia than is prolapse of other portions of the uveal tract.

TUMORS OF THE CHOROID

MALIGNANT MELANOMA

The most common intraocular tumor is malignant melanoma of the choroid (Fig 16-8). It usually occurs after puberty and increases in frequency between the ages of 30 and 70 years. The tumor is rare in blacks and is slightly more common in women than men. Most eyes removed because of malignant melanoma also contain benign nevi along the edges or within the tumor. These cells may reflect the effects of tumor on the cells of the choroid and are not a tumor stimulus.

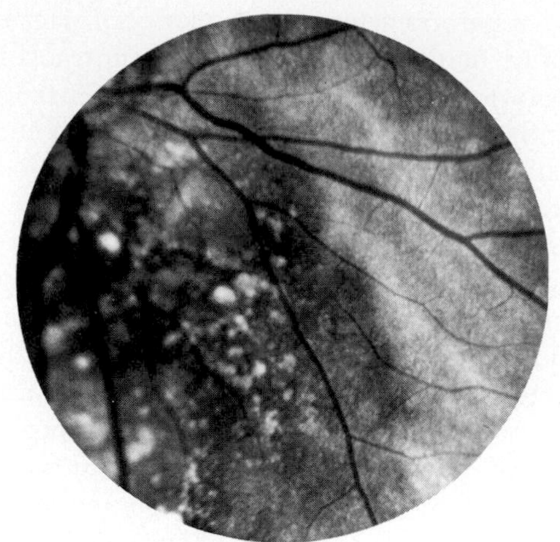

FIG 16-8.
Malignant melanoma of the choroid causing a solid retinal detachment. Numerous drusen are evident over the surface of the tumor.

Most malignant melanomas of the uveal tract develop from preexisting benign melanomas often misdiagnosed as nevi. Most benign melanomas never undergo malignant transformation. Malignant melanomas are found in approximately 10% of eyes blind from injury or inflammation, a finding that suggests irritation may play a role in malignant transformation.

Malignant melanomas originate most frequently in the outer layers of the choroid and may spread carpetlike in the choroid between the sclera and Bruch membrane. Tumors may remain quiescent for long periods and then, without apparent reason, suddenly begin rapid growth. With increase in size, there may be globular growth inward (Fig 16-9). Eventually Bruch membrane perforates, and there is sudden growth of a mushroom or collar-button–shaped tumor.

Symptoms and signs.—The chief symptoms of malignant melanoma result from the solid retinal detachment caused by the increase in the volume of the choroid. Early metamor-

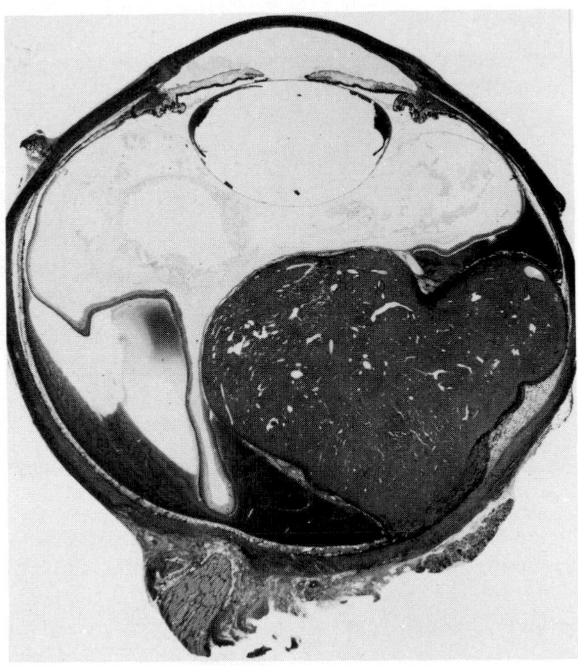

FIG 16-9.
Malignant melanoma of the choroid that has ruptured through the Bruch membrane into the eye. (Hematoxylin and eosin; ×5.)

phopsia may be associated with macropsia or micropsia. A loss of visual field in the area corresponding to the area of the tumor may follow. An associated secondary serous retinal detachment causes more extensive visual field loss than would be anticipated from the size of the tumor. Glaucoma may occur late in the development of the tumor, but initially the tension is low because of decreased secretion of aqueous humor. A malignant melanoma of the choroid must be considered as the cause of obscure intraocular inflammation, particularly when opaque media make it impossible to inspect the fundus with the ophthalmoscope. Ultrasonography and magnetic resonance imaging aid in the diagnosis when the fundus cannot be seen.

Sudden loss of vision or rapid increase in the size of a mass over several days' time suggests that a lesion is not a malignant melanoma. A drawing of the tumor, with emphasis on its relationship to blood vessels, and photography with fluorescein angiography of the lesion may be helpful in making an exact diagnosis. Any increase in size of the tumor is monitored by ultrasonography or magnetic resonance imaging. Physical examination, with particular attention to possible liver metastasis, should be done, but metastatic disease, even when present, is seldom detected by any test. Neovascularization or vasodilation of episcleral vessels in the quadrant of involvement suggests a neoplasm, as does melanosis oculi. A vascularized mass on the sclera suggests an extraocular extension. Anesthesia of the cornea, partial paralysis of the iris, or dilated iris vessels occurring in the sector of tumor involvement and vitreous hemorrhage have been noted in some patients.

Ophthalmoscopy indicates a retinal detachment of grayish brown color. The pigmentation is distinctly lighter than the jet-black color seen in inflammatory retinal proliferation. Spots of light orange pigmentation (lipofuscin) may occur over the solid detachment. Drusen may be scattered superficially. The retina is smoothly elevated, usually without a break, and has little tendency to form traction folds. There may be two areas of detachment, seemingly not connected. With increase in size a malignant melanoma becomes more distinct, but with an intraocular inflammation the lesion becomes less distinct. Bed rest does not reduce the extent of the detachment.

Vessels on the retinal surface not associated with the retinal vasculature are suggestive of

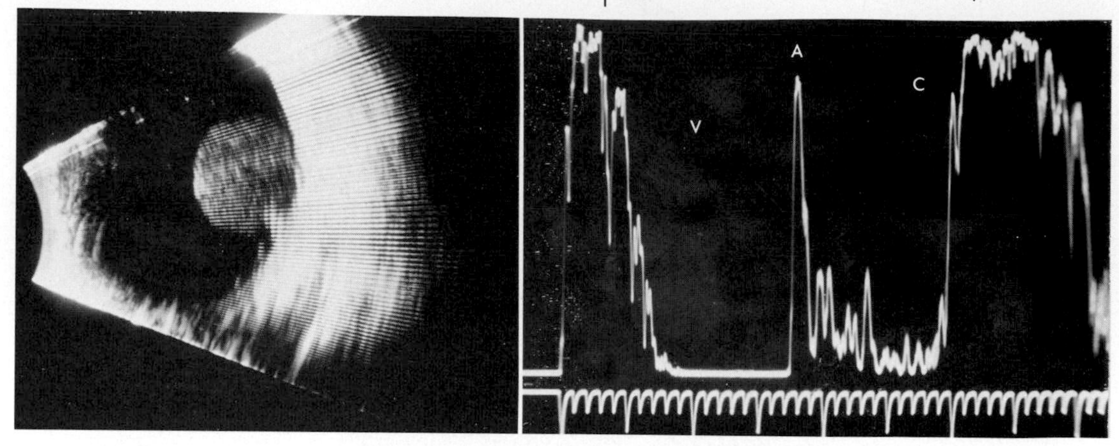

FIG 16-10.
A, B-scan echogram of a melanoma of the choroid. **B,** A-scan of the same melanoma. *I* is the initial spike that corresponds to the surface of the eye opposite the tumor; *V* corresponds to the vitreous; *A* indicates the anterior tumor surface; and *P* indicates the posterior surface on the inner surface of the sclera. The small spike at *C* is the interface between the tumor proper and the infiltrated cornea. *(Courtesy of Prof. Karl C. Ossoinig, M.D., The University of Iowa.)*

tumor. Hemorrhage is uncommon except when large necrotic tumors break through the Bruch membrane.

Biomicroscopy of the fundus by using a Goldmann or Hruby lens with the pupil fully dilated provides details. Cystoid degeneration of the overlying retina suggests a malignant melanoma. Cells in the vitreous humor and an indistinct retina suggest an inflammatory lesion, unless a necrotic tumor has broken through Bruch membrane. Ophthalmoscopic study of the border of an elevated lesion may show a reddish or pink halo, indicating a hemorrhage rather than a tumor.

Visual field studies aid in differentiating between a benign and a malignant melanoma. Usually the choriocapillaris is intact when a benign melanoma is present; either there is no field defect or the defect is proportionate to the size of the lesion. In malignant melanoma, the defect is larger and progressive. A hemangioma causes a sector-shaped field defect.

After intravenous injection of sodium fluorescein, most malignant melanomas of the choroid begin to fluoresce slightly before or during the retinal arterial phase. Their fluorescence increases in intensity, and staining of the tumor may persist for 45 to 60 minutes after injection. Metastatic tumors of the choroid and hemangiomas may have a similar hyperfluorescence. Sometimes hemorrhage or pigment overlying a malignant melanoma will prevent visualization of the fluorescence.

Simultaneous A- and B-scan display (Fig 16-10) is helpful in the diagnosis of choroidal neoplasms. When the A-scan ultrasonic beam strikes the tumor, high-amplitude echoes are reflected from the anterior boundary of the mass. As the beam traverses the tumor, there is a steep decay in the amplitude of the echo. The B-scan display shows a smooth convex tumor surface with an echo-free area appearing within the depth of the melanoma and a characteristic apparent excavation of the tumor and sclera posteriorly.

The single most important clinical prognostic factor is the size of the tumor. If the largest tumor measurement is 10 mm or less (6⅔ disk diameters), the mortality is 13%, but if the size exceeds 12 mm, the mortality is 70%.

Patients with tumors composed of epithelioid cells, or epithelioid cells and spindle cell A or B, or with necrotic tumor have a grave prognosis. Spindle cell A tumors have the best prognosis.

Treatment.—The appropriate treatment of malignant melanoma of the choroid is not known. The treatment is complicated by the inability to provide a histologic diagnosis of eyes that are treated and not removed combined with an inability to detect liver metastasis smaller than 0.5 mm in size. Many published survival studies are retrospective and without random assignment of patients to different treatment groups. The exact cause of death is often not learned, and there is sometimes an excessive loss in follow-up studies.

The current collaborative ocular malignant melanoma study (National Eye Institute) divides patients into three groups, based on the size of the tumor. Large tumors exceed 8 mm in height or 16 mm in the largest basal dimension. Patients with such tumors are randomized to treatment either by enucleation of the eye or by external beam radiation (2,000 cGy) delivered over a 5-day period before removal of the eye.

Patients with medium-size tumors (between 3 and 8 mm in height and less than 16 mm in the largest basal dimension) are randomly assigned to treatment either by enucleation of the eye or by application of an iodine-125 plaque to the sclera adjacent to the tumor.

Patients with small tumors are examined every 6 months for evidence of growth. Ultrasonography is used to measure the height of the tumor, and fluorescein angiography is used to measure the basal dimensions. In the event of growth, the tumor is treated either by external beam radiation or by means of an iodine-125 plaque applied to the sclera.

Generally, tumors located in the anterior choroid are less likely to metastasize than those located in the posterior choroid. Conversely, tumors of the anterior choroid may be without symptoms and undetected until very large. Small malignant melanomas of the anterior choroid may be treated by removing the overlying sclera and the adjacent tumor.

CHOROIDAL NEVI

Nevi of the choroid or ciliary body occur in about 30% of white individuals, are multiple in one eye in about 7%, and bilateral in about 4%. Often (55%) there are iris freckles or nevi in the same eye. Nevi are oval or circular in outline, vary from 0.5 to 4 disk diameters in size, and occur most commonly at the posterior half of the fundus. The lesion is sharply demarcated from the surrounding fundus, but the contrast between the melanoma and the adjacent choroid may be so slight that careful ophthalmoscopic examination is necessary for detection. The lesion usually becomes pigmented between 6 and 10 years of age.

The tumor varies in color from "slate gray" to "blue ointment." The choroidal pattern can easily be seen encircling the tumor. Since nevi do not involve the choriocapillaris layer, there is usually no visual field defect, as there is with malignant melanoma. Treatment is not indicated.

HEMANGIOMAS

Hemangiomas (angiomas) of the choroid are rare and are associated in about one half of individuals affected with skin angioma (nevus flammeus), frequently in the region innervated by the first or second branch of the trigeminal nerve. The Sturge-Weber syndrome consists of intracranial angiomas, nevus flammeus, and glaucoma. A number of variants may occur. Glaucoma develops in some 30% of those affected. The glaucoma may develop before the age of 2 years (60%) with a chamber angle that resembles that seen in congenital glaucoma. The glaucoma develops in the remaining patients (40%) in late childhood and early adulthood and resembles primary open-angle glaucoma. Neurologic signs may occur occasionally; the hemangiomas are then a manifestation of the Sturge-Weber syndrome.

Choroidal hemangiomas vary in size from 2 to 17 mm in diameter and from 1 to 9 mm in thickness. They may increase slowly in thickness, causing a progressive hyperopia when the hemangioma involves the posterior pole. Rarely, both eyes may be involved in a similar process.

METASTATIC CARCINOMA

The breast and lung in women and the lung in men are the most common primary sites of tumors that metastasize to the choroid. Other sites are uncommon in women. In men, tumors in the kidney, testicle, and prostate gland may metastasize to the choroid. Choroidal metastases are common in the terminal stages of malignant disease; patients are so ill, however, that the diagnosis is not made. Both eyes are affected with equal frequency. Me-

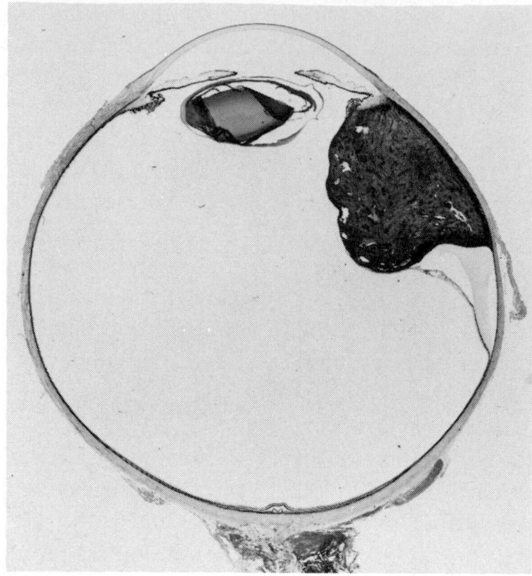

FIG 16-11.
Malignant melanoma of the ciliary body that has detached the peripheral retina. (Hematoxylin and eosin; ×4.)

tastasis to the choroid rather than to the retina may reflect the larger number of blood vessels that go to the choroid from the ophthalmic artery.

Metastasis to the choroid leads to an overlying serous retinal detachment, which causes loss of vision in the area of involvement. The posterior segment is frequently involved, and early loss of central vision occurs. The ophthalmoscopic appearance is characteristic. There is a yellow-orange elevation of the retinal pigment epithelium and an overlying serous retinal detachment with sharp delineation and no retinal breaks.

The diagnosis depends mainly upon an accurate history and careful physical examination. The primary malignancy may have been resected months to years before the onset of symptoms. There may be no evidence of metastasis elsewhere in the body, but often osteolytic or pulmonary lesions can be demonstrated.

Treatment of a metastatic malignancy to the choroid must be directed to the primary disease. In tumors that are not hormone-dependent, the ocular treatment is related to the life expectancy and whether both eyes are involved. Enucleation is not indicated. Radiation therapy with a tumor dose of 25 to 35 Gy may be used, with precautions to protect the lens. The adult lens is relatively resistant to radiation so that cataract formation will probably not be a problem because of the limited life expectancy of the patient. If the metastasis is binocular and the patient is not within the final weeks of life, radiotherapy may be carried out on both eyes.

CILIARY BODY TUMORS

Tumors of the ciliary body may involve the pigmented or nonpigmented epithelium or the stroma. The epithelium may be involved in a variety of uncommon types of hyperplasia or in a neoplastic process, medulloblastoma. The stromal tumors are essentially the same as those of the choroid, and malignant melanoma is the predominating type. A leiomyoma may originate from muscle cells.

MALIGNANT MELANOMAS

Malignant melanoma of the ciliary body (Fig 16-11) is less frequent than malignant melanomas of the choroid. The tumor tends to extend to the choroid, the iris, or both. Ciliary body tumors may follow the course of the major arterial circle of the iris and spread in a ring. Symptoms are minimal, and diagnosis may be delayed until the tumor causes a serous retinal detachment or extends to the anterior chamber. The mass may be seen by indirect ophthalmoscopy or gonioscopy.

Since melanomas of the ciliary body have a low degree of malignancy, resection rather than enucleation is often indicated.

MEDULLOEPITHELIOMA (DIKTYOMA)

Intraocular medulloepitheliomas are embryonal neuroepithelial tumors that originate from the embryonic or developing nonpigmented epithelium of the ciliary body. They are divided into medulloepithelioma and teratoid medulloepithelioma (heteroplasia with hyaline cartilage, cerebral tissue, and skeletal muscle). They are further divided into benign and malignant forms. They are unilateral and nearly always occur in children. Enucleation is done at a median age of 5 years (range, 1 to 43 years). There may be poor vision and pain. There may be a white pupil, a mass in the iris, anterior chamber, or ciliary body, glaucoma, cataract, iritis, and rubeosis iridis. Local excision is preferred, but commonly the tumor reaches large size before producing symptoms and requires enucleation.

LEIOMYOMA OF THE CILIARY MUSCLE

Leiomyoma of the ciliary muscle is an uncommon neoplasm that requires electron microscopy to differentiate it from an amelanotic spindle cell melanoma. It may also originate in the iris musculature.

CILIARY BODY CYSTS

Ciliary body cysts form in the nonpigmented epithelium of the pars plana and pars plicata. Those in the pars plicata contain proliferated nonpigmented epithelium and a watery substance. Cysts of the pars plicata contain hyaluronic acid. In multiple myeloma, cysts may occur in either location and contain IgG.

TUMORS OF THE IRIS

There is considerable variation in the amount of pigment in the anterior stroma of the iris. About one half of lightly pigmented individuals have pigment flecks on the surface of the iris. The flecks are of no clinical importance. They originate from increased pigmentation of melanocytes and do not proliferate.

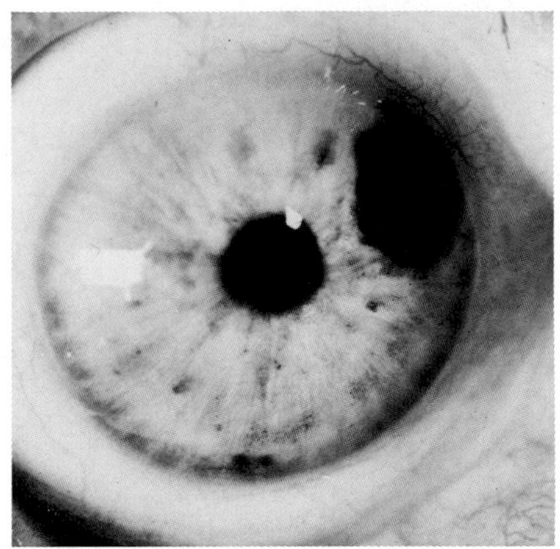

FIG 16-12.
Benign melanoma of the iris. There are freckles in the interior portion of the iris.

An iris nevus consisting of a slightly elevated, localized, discrete, pigmented mass (Fig 16-12) is composed of proliferated melanocytes. It may be associated with peripheral anterior synechiae in the iris-nevus syndrome. Iris nevi are associated with neurofibromatosis and malignant melanoma of the choroid and ciliary body. These nevi (benign melanomas) are not progressive and do not distort the pupil.

Malignant melanomas of the iris are predominantly spindle A type and do not metastasize. Mixed spindle cell and epithelial cell tumors metastasize, a complication that may follow incomplete excision. A pigmented tumor that increases in size may be difficult to diagnose clinically. Inflammatory nodules, iris cysts, metastatic tumors, lymphoid tumors, and iris abscesses have all been mistaken for malignant melanoma. Fluorescein angiography of the iris defines the dimensions of a tumor but does not differentiate between malignant and benign lesions.

Juvenile xanthogranuloma is a skin disorder with yellowish orange accumulations of histiocytes in the dermis layer. Infiltration of the iris causes a glaucoma and spontaneous bleeding into the anterior chamber (hyphema).

BIBLIOGRAPHY

Books

Nussenblatt RB, Whitcup SM, Palestine AG: *Uveitis. Fundamentals and clinical practice,* St Louis, 1996, Mosby–Year Book.

Sanborn GE, Gonder JR, Shields JA: *Atlas of intraocular tumors,* Philadelphia, 1994, WB Saunders.

Article

Shields JA, Shields CL, Kiratli H, De Potter P: Metastatic tumors to the iris in 40 patients, *Am J Ophthalmol* 119:422-430, 1995.

17

THE RETINA

The invagination of the lateral optic vesicles in embryonic life forms the double-walled secondary optic vesicles, or optic cups. The inner wall forms the light-sensitive sensory retina. The outer wall thins to a single layer, the retinal pigment epithelium. The photopigment molecules located in the disks of the rod and cone outer segments absorb light that passes through the transparent inner portion of the sensory retina (*inner,* nearer the vitreous cavity; *outer,* nearer the choriocapillaris). Light activates the molecules in the photopigment of the rods and cones in the retinal outer segments, which initiates a cascade of reactions (see Chapter 2) that are converted to graded electrical potentials. These potentials are modulated and amplified by bipolar, horizontal, and amacrine cells. The axons of ganglion cells transmit the graded potentials to the lateral geniculate body as spike discharges.

The rod and cone disks of the outer segments of the sensory retina are enmeshed in the microvilli of the retinal pigment epithelium. The disks of the outer segments are continuously renewed by their cell bodies, and clumps of the oldest disks are phagocytized by the retinal pigment epithelium. If this phagocytosis stops, the sensory retina degenerates.

The sensory retina may be divided into a central portion (macula), which contains the fovea centralis that functions in photopic vision, and into four peripheral quadrants that function in spatial orientation and in reduced light (scotopic vision). The central retina, the macula, located between the superior and inferior temporal vessels, extends temporally from the optic disk to about 2 disk diameters lateral to the fovea centralis. It contains the fovea centralis, a pit in the retina in which the innermost layers of the sensory retina are displaced so that light falls directly upon the cone photoreceptors without traversing the inner retinal layers. The foveola at the center of the fovea centralis contains only cones (see Fig 1-27). The clinical and anatomic names for these areas are sometimes used interchangeably. The fovea centralis functions in bright illumination (photopic vision), form vision, and color vision. Rod photoreceptors are most common in the peripheral quadrants and function in dim illumination (scotopic vision).

The blood supply to the retina in humans is derived from two sources: (1) the choriocapillaris, which nurtures the retinal pigment epithelium and the outer portion of the sensory retina adjacent to the choroid; and (2) the branches of the central retinal artery, which supply the inner half of the retina. The border between the retinal and choroidal blood supply is at the junction of the outer one third and the middle one third of the outer plexiform layer of the retina. Normal retinal function requires both systems.

The central retinal artery is the first branch of the ophthalmic artery within the orbit. It is a medium-sized artery, 0.20 to 0.30 mm in diameter, which has well-developed intimal, muscularis, and adventitial layers. Within the optic nerve the adventitial layer is augmented by the pia mater. The artery enters the eye through the lamina cribrosa and ascends the nasal portion of the optic cup in company with the central retinal vein that is located temporally. Within the optic nerve the artery divides into superior and inferior papillary branches, and loses the muscularis coat. The vessels within the eye are thus arterioles or capillaries. The papillary branches are divided into nasal and temporal branches that divide dichotomously to the capillary level. The capillaries do not anastomose.

Retinal vessels lack nervous control, and their constriction and dilation are in response to autoregulation (intravascular resistance-pressure and partial pressure of carbon dioxide [PCO_2]). The endothelial cells lining the retinal vessels are not fenestrated and tightly joined. These vessels provide a portion of the blood-retina barrier, which is similar to the blood-brain barrier. The retinal blood vessels are susceptible to the same diseases as blood vessels elsewhere in the body, but because their intravascular pressure must exceed the intraocular pressure to prevent collapse, they form a highly specialized vascular bed without counterpart elsewhere.

Retinal veins follow a course similar to that of the arteries but do not parallel them exactly. Generally the diameter of an artery is about two thirds to three quarters that of the corresponding vein. The veins do not anastomose. At their crossings the arterioles and veins share a common adventitial sheath, a factor in the genesis of venous sclerosis at arteriole-venous crossings.

SYMPTOMS

Visual disturbance without pain is the main symptom of a retinal abnormality. Disorders that affect peripheral retinal function are associated with night blindness (impaired vision in reduced illumination) or visual field defects. Disorders of foveal (cone) function result in reduced visual acuity and impaired color vision. Opacities of the cornea, crystalline lens, or vitreous humor, which impair image formation at the fovea centralis, depress vision generally. Localized disturbances in the fovea centralis, such as hemorrhage, edema, deposits, or tumors, may cause a metamorphopsia, such as micropsia (small images) or macropsia (large images).

Traction on the retina may cause photopsia, which consists of sparks, rings, lightning flashes, or luminous bodies observed when the eyes are closed. Unlike visual hallucinations that originate from lesions in the temporal or occipital lobes of the brain, photopsia does not affect both eyes simultaneously.

Frequently the patient is unaware of retinal disease, and the abnormality is detected by means of functional testing or ophthalmoscopic examination.

FUNCTION

Five measurements indicate the major functions of the sensory retina (see Chapter 5): (1) visual acuity (the form sense); (2) color vision; (3) central and peripheral visual fields; (4) dark adaptation; and (5) electroretinography. The function of the retinal pigment epithelium is inferred from electro-oculography.

To exclude refractive errors as a cause of decreased vision, visual acuity must be measured while the patient is wearing lenses that provide the best possible vision for the distance at which vision is being tested.

The common types of hereditary defects of color perception (see Chapter 2) are transmitted as X chromosome–linked recessive defects, and affected individuals have good visual acuity. In most patients with acquired central retinal lesions, such as central retinal (macular) degeneration, the defect in color perception parallels the reduction in visual acuity. Some individuals may have marked impairment of color vision, decreased visual acuity, and nystagmus transmitted as an autosomal recessive condition (achromatopsia); others may be born with normal color vision but develop hereditary types of cone degenerations heralded by characteristic impairment in color perception and in the photopic electroretinogram. Parietal lobe disorders may impair color-naming ability and sometimes color perception.

Measurement of the central visual field tests the retinal function within 30° from the fixation point. Measurement of the peripheral field is less sensitive and determines the function of the entire retina. Since the optic nerve is composed of axons of the ganglion cells that form the nerve fiber layer of the retina, optic nerve disease may cause many of the same symptoms as retinal disease.

The measurement of dark adaptation sensitively determines the synthesis of retinal photopigments, particularly the rhodopsin of the rods.

Electroretinography measures the action potential evoked by light stimulation of the retina (see Chapter 2). Because this is a mass response, it may be normal when retinal lesions are focal.

Electro-oculography measures the standing potential between the cornea and the retina. A decrease in the ratio between the response in the light- and dark-adapted retina indicates a disorder of the retinal pigment epithelium.

OPHTHALMOSCOPIC FINDINGS

The retina is examined with a direct or indirect ophthalmoscope or with a biomicroscope and a convex lens to neutralize corneal refraction (see Chapter 6). The main abnormalities of the fundus that are visible ophthalmoscopically include the following: (1) disturbances of the blood vessels; (2) opacities of the sensory retina, which include hemorrhages, exudates, edema residues, cotton-wool patches, and proliferated vascular and glial tissue; (3) disturbances in the position of the sensory retina in rhegmatogenous (with hole formation) and nonrhegmatogenous (without hole formation) retinal detachment; (4) derangements of the retinal pigment epithelium; and (5) abnormalities of the Bruch membrane and choroid.

DISTURBANCES OF BLOOD VESSELS

The skilled observer constantly changes the focus of the direct ophthalmoscope to permit better definition of the size, shape, and depth of lesions. When viewed with an ophthalmoscope, the normal sensory retina is transparent, except for the blood vessels. The major retinal vessels are located in the nerve fiber layer, and the capillary plexuses are located in this layer and the inner nuclear layer.

Abnormalities such as vascular hypertension and its sequelae tend to affect capillaries at the level of the nerve fiber layer, whereas disorders such as diabetes affect intraretinal capillaries located in the inner nuclear layer of the retina. New blood vessels form on the inner (vitreal) surface of the retina, the surface of the optic nerve, between the retinal pigment epithelium and the choroid, and between the sensory retina and the pigment epithelium.

The retinal blood vessels are normally transparent tubes through which the contained blood is visible with an ophthalmoscope. The oxygenated blood in the artery is brighter red than the blood in the veins. The muscularis coat of the artery reflects light and causes a white reflex that parallels the axis of the vessel.

Vascular pulsation.—Visible pulsation of arteries or veins occurs when the intraocular pressure equals the pressure within the vessel. The normal pulsation of the central retinal vein is best seen on the surface of the optic disk. It is synchronous with the heartbeat, and originates from transmitted central retinal artery pulsation. If the venous pulsation cannot be seen, gentle pressure on the globe will elicit it. Venous pulsation is absent and cannot be elicited in impending central vein closure; it usually cannot be elicited in papilledema.

Spontaneous arterial pulsation is always abnormal. It occurs when the intraocular pressure is equal to the diastolic blood pressure (in glaucoma) and in aortic regurgitation, in which there is a high pulse pressure. It may be elicited by pressure on the globe as is applied diagnostically in ophthalmodynamometry.

Venous dilation.—Increased venous pressure, markedly decreased intraocular pressure, or hyperviscosity of the blood cause dilated veins. The vessel wall widens in three dimensions and the vessel becomes tortuous. Dilated veins occur in diabetes mellitus at any stage, in papilledema, in impending or partial closure of the central retinal vein, in vascular tumors of the retinal blood vessels, and in hyperviscosity of the blood syndromes.

Neovascularization.—New blood vessels that originate from retinal veins may carpet the inner (vitreal) surface of the sensory retina or optic disk or extend into the vitreous cavity. New blood vessels that originate from the choriocapillaris may extend between the choriocapillaris and the retinal pigment epithelium and between the retinal pigment epithelium and the sensory retina.

New retinal vessels originate mainly on the venous side of the circulation. The stimulus is the vascular endothelial growth factor, which may be the common element in combinations with other growth factors that differ with the primary disease. The vitreous humor is never invaded by new retinal blood vessels. The new vessels consist of fenestrated endothelial tubes that leak protein and tend to bleed. New blood

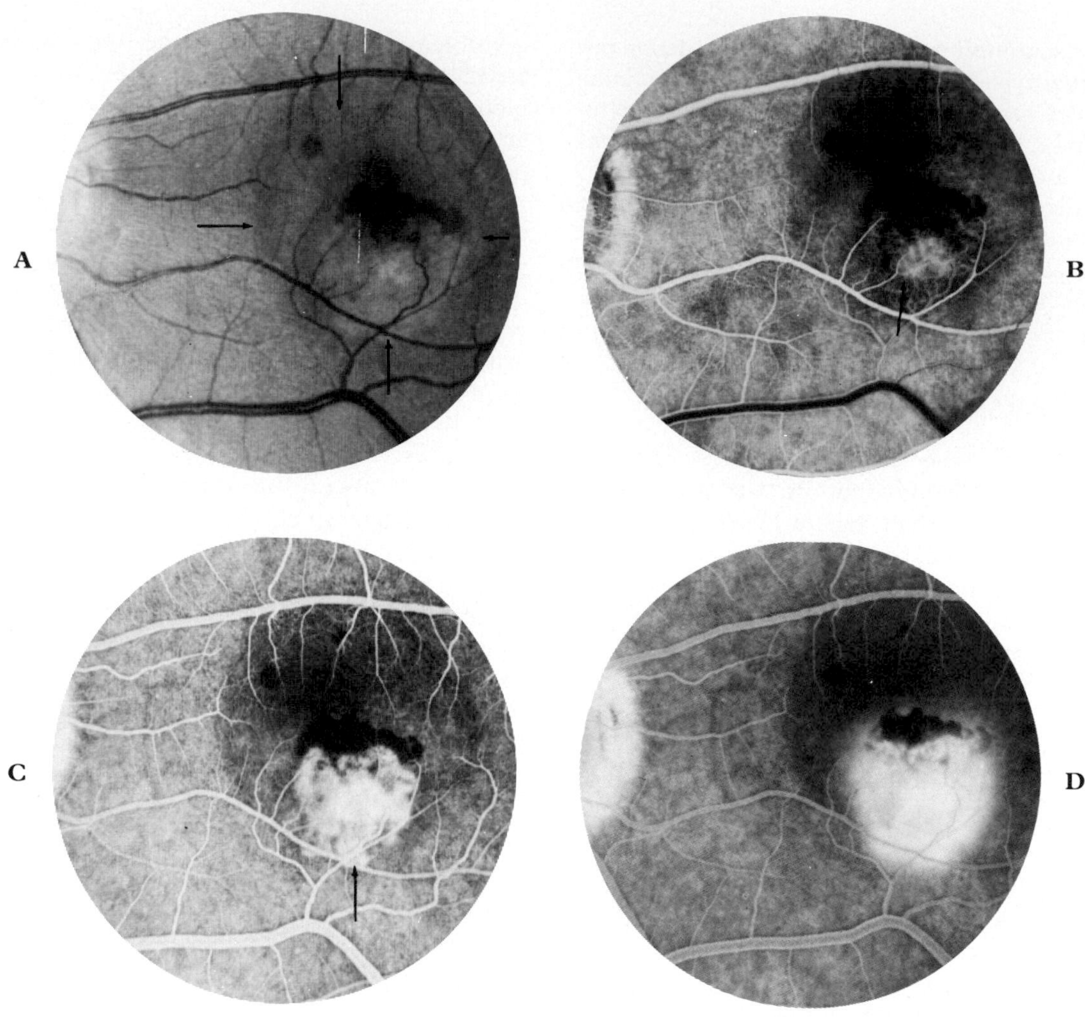

FIG 17-1.
A, Ophthalmoscopic appearance of subretinal neovascular membrane in presumed ocular histoplasmosis. There is hemorrhage into the sensory retina above the membrane and there is marked retinal edema *(arrows)*. **B,** A fine tracery of choroidal blood vessels appears *(arrow)* beneath the sensory retina early in fluorescein angiography. **C,** The blood vessels of the network *(arrow)* are filled with fluorescein. **D,** At 90 seconds, the neovascular membrane leaks fluorescein.

vessels on the iris, optic disk, and retina distant from sites of treatment may disappear after retinal photocoagulation, possibly because of removal of an angiogenic factor. Subretinal new blood vessels that originate from the choriocapillaris proliferate through defects in Bruch membrane.

Neovascularization originating from retinal blood vessels occurs in a variety of conditions in which the circulation is impaired: diabetes mellitus; vascular occlusion, particularly venous closure; stasis caused by decreased blood flow or blood hyperviscosity; the retinopathy of prematurity; sickle cell trait (SC hemoglobin); retinal inflammation; Eales disease; sarcoidosis; familial exudative vitreoretinopathy; and talc emboli. The first arteriovenous crossing in the superior temporal quadrant is the most vulnerable area, followed in turn by the inferior temporal quadrant, the superior nasal quadrant, and the inferior nasal quadrant. New blood vessels may extend along the inner surface of the retina. They may grow into the vitreous cavity as a network of endothelial channels (rete mirabile) with supporting fibrous tissue (proliferative retinopathy).

Subretinal neovascular membranes.— New blood vessels that originate from the choriocapillaris develop between Bruch membrane and the retinal pigment epithelium and subsequently between the retinal pigment epithelium and the sensory retina. They reduce visual acuity in retinal drusen, disciform macular degeneration, angioid streaks, degenerative myopia, and presumed ocular histoplasmosis. These vascular membranes may occur in any part of the fundus, but are particularly common beneath the fovea centralis where a hemorrhage, which occurs in about two thirds of the cases, severely impairs visual acuity.

The initial event is hole formation in Bruch membrane. Plasma from the choriocapillaris results in a separation of Bruch membrane from the retinal pigment epithelium. Capillaries then proliferate from the choriocapillaris in the new space between the Bruch membrane and the retinal pigment epithelium. A hole in the retinal pigment epithelium permits the new blood vessels to proliferate between the pigment epithelium and sensory retina. Hemorrhage into the sensory retina is followed by fibrous metaplasia of the retinal pigment epithelium, which obliterates the choriocapillaris and causes the fibrous scar of disciform degeneration. If the fovea centralis is affected, final visual acuity is 20/200 or less.

The membrane appears as a dark green circular or oval area. There may be a ring of pigment (Fig 17-1, *A*). The overlying retina may be detached, infiltrated with hard yellow deposits, or swollen with cystoid edema. Blood in the sensory retina is bright red, crescent shaped, and located at the outer edge of the neovascular membrane. Fluorescein angiography demonstrates the network of new blood vessels derived from the choriocapillaris and not the retinal blood vessels (Fig 17-1, *B* to *D*). Fluorescein leakage may be marked in the late phases of angiography.

Surgical removal of the subretinal membrane in its early stages, before the new blood vessels have invaded the adjacent sensory retina, may preserve central vision. Closure of the initial hole in the Bruch membrane may prevent the subretinal neovascularization. If the membrane is not adjacent to the fovea centralis, the entire membrane may be photocoagulated. Partial photocoagulation stimulates additional neovascularization. Often, the patient first becomes aware of the disorder only after central vision is affected and treatment is not effective.

Hemorrhage.—The size and shape of hemorrhage within the retina depend on the layer in which the bleeding occurs. Preretinal (subhyaloid) hemorrhages (Fig 17-2) occur between the retina and the vitreous body. They are large and tend to form a meniscus because the blood is not clotted and is but loosely restricted. Flame-shaped hemorrhages (Fig 17-3) occur in the nerve fiber layer and tend to parallel the direction of the nerve fibers in the region of the retina where they occur. Round hemorrhages originate from the deep capillaries of the retina. They are confined by Müller cells to the outer nuclear layer and the fibers of the inner and outer plexiform layers. Because the layers of the sensory retina are transparent, hemorrhages are initially bright red and become yellowish as they are absorbed.

Hemorrhages between the choriocapillaris and retinal pigment epithelium are dark brown and well circumscribed. They are sometimes elevated and may stimulate a neoplasm. The blood may rupture into the sensory retina and appear as a bright red crescent at the margin of the subretinal neovascular membrane.

Retinal and preretinal (subhyaloid) hemorrhages occur in 15% of the adults and almost 70% of the young children with subarachnoid and subdural hemorrhage. The mortality in individuals with intraocular hemorrhages exceeds 50%, in contrast to a mortality of about 20% in those without retinal hemorrhages. Mortality is higher in those with bilateral intraocular hemorrhages (58%) than in those with monocular hemorrhage (48%). Usually the hemorrhages are absorbed without sequelae. If they break into the vitreous, they cause the same complications as other intravitreal bleeding.

Retinal hemorrhages occur because of abnormalities of blood vessel walls, excessive intravascular pressure, fragility of new retinal and subretinal blood vessels, diseases of the blood, or vitreous traction on a blood vessel. Ocular causes include trauma, vascular obstruction, and vasculitis. Systemic causes include diabetes mellitus, hypertension, and blood dyscrasias. A preretinal hemorrhage adjacent to the optic disk

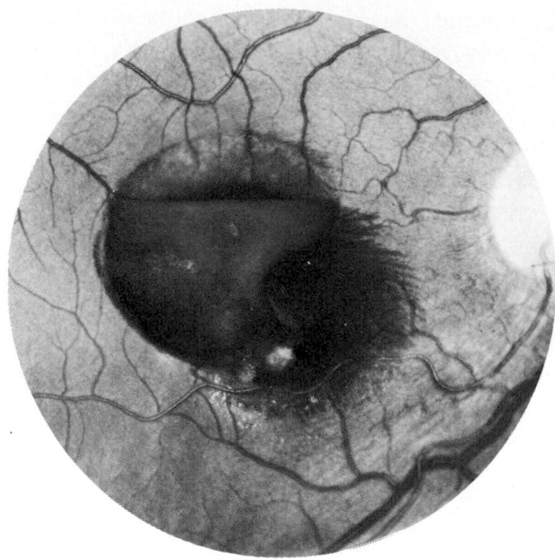

FIG 17-2.
Preretinal hemorrhage in the macular region. A meniscus of blood forms when the head is erect.

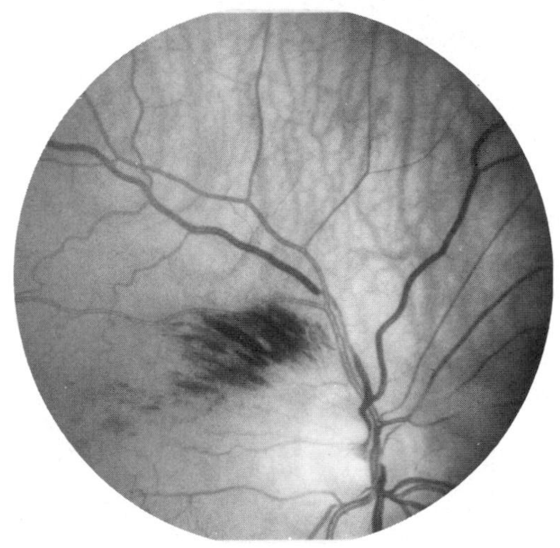

FIG 17-3.
Flame-shaped hemorrhage in the nerve fiber layer of the retina.

may be a sign of subarachnoid hemorrhage. In glaucoma a small flame-shaped hemorrhage sometimes occurs at the disk margin (see Chapter 22).

Microaneurysms.—Microaneurysms are a common retinal abnormality. Many form in diabetes mellitus (see Chapter 27), and these are characteristically on the venous side of the capillary network. Microaneurysms occur in most of the conditions associated with retinal venous stasis: central or branch vein obstruction, Coats disease, periphlebitis, and hyperviscosity of the blood. Microaneurysms are identified with certainty by fluorescein angiography or histologic examination. Ophthalmoscopically they appear as minute red dots of unchanging appearance that are not related to visible blood vessels. They remain unchanged for months but eventually become minute white dots or disappear. Small, deep, round hemorrhages with a similar appearance are absorbed more rapidly and disappear without leaving a residue. Microaneurysms leak plasma and are often surrounded by edema, which gives the retina a hazy appearance. Sometimes hard yellow deposits (edema residues) surround the microaneurysms. Although microaneurysms occur in many conditions, it is only in diabetes mellitus that large numbers occur, and these are mainly at the posterior pole.

The resolving power of the direct ophthalmoscope is about 75 μm. Most retinal microaneurysms are smaller than 75 μm and are invisible ophthalmoscopically. They may be demonstrated by fluorescein angiography or histologically in flat preparations of the retina.

Capillary perfusion.—Fluorescein angiography indicates that poor retinal function in vascular closure and diabetic retinopathy is secondary to inadequate perfusion of the retinal capillaries.

The various abnormalities that decrease capillary perfusion include carotid artery occlusive disease; ophthalmic artery occlusive disease; ischemic neuropathy of the optic nerve; vascular stasis in glaucoma; blood disorders such as leukemia, polycythemia, hemorrhage, hemoglobinopathies, and dysproteinemias; vascular inflammations; diabetes; and vascular hypertension.

OPACITIES OF THE SENSORY RETINA

The sensory retina is transparent. The red background of the fundus results from the blood in the choriocapillaris screened by the pigment in the retinal pigment epithelium. The normal red fundus reflex may be obscured by the following: (1) opacities of the media (cornea, lens, vitreous); (2) inflammatory retinal exudates; (3) deposits (acute or chronic retinal edema); (4) hemorrhages (preretinal, retinal, subretinal); (5) blood vessel malformation (neovasculariza-

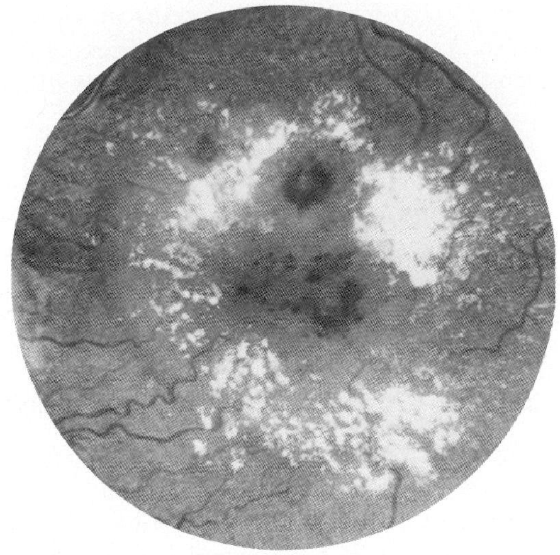

FIG 17-4.
Lipid deposits (edema residues) surrounding area of retinal microangiopathy in a patient with diabetes mellitus.

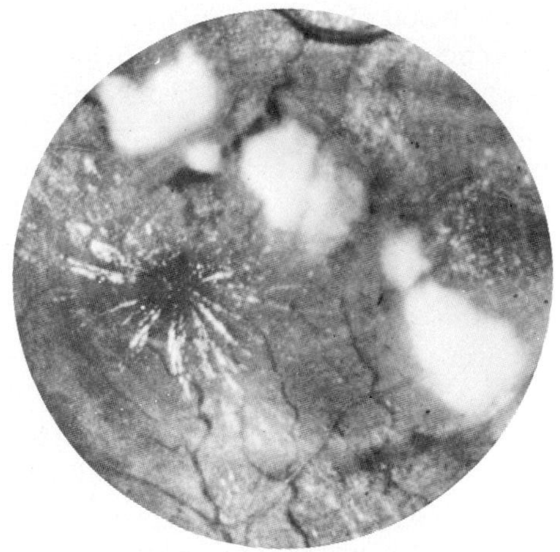

FIG 17-5.
Foveal star of edema in the outer plexiform layer of the retina (Henle layer), which surrounds the foveola. The cotton-wool patches are in the nerve fiber layer. These changes occurred in a 39-year-old man with accelerated vascular hypertension.

tion, aneurysms); (6) epiretinal membranes; and (7) detachment of the sensory retina from the underlying retinal pigment epithelium.

Inflammatory retinal exudates are opacities that result from inflammation of the retina or choroid. They are often obscured by inflammatory cells in the vitreous. They appear as grayish white areas with ill-defined margins. The underlying retinal pigment epithelium and choroid may be destroyed and the cells of the retinal pigment epithelium may proliferate.

Retinal deposits (also called hard exudates, fatty exudates, or chronic edema residues) follow localized areas of retinal edema. They consist of fats and lipid-filled macrophages in the outer plexiform layer of the retina. They are distributed in one of several patterns: (1) a ring or partial ring in circinate retinopathy; (2) a foveal star; or (3) scattered irregular deposits in disorders such as diabetes mellitus or Coats retinal telangiectasis. They occur at the junction between leaking and competent retinal capillaries.

Retinal deposits at the posterior pole may have a circular or arcuate (circinate) pattern that surrounds a permeable blood vessel such as an aneurysm, shunt, or area of neovascularization (Fig 17-4). A circinate pattern may be seen in diabetes mellitus, vascular hypertension, and other retinopathies. Deposits in that portion of the outer plexiform layer that surrounds the fovea centralis (Henle layer) result in a foveal star (Fig 17-5), which appears as broken lines radiating from the fovea centralis. The pattern is visible in accelerated vascular hypertension, papilledema, and papillitis. Diffuse lipid deposits (chronic edema residues) are similar to the deposits of circinate retinopathy but do not have a circular pattern and appear as scattered yellowish to white regions of varying size with sharply defined edges. In Coats disease there is a massive outpouring of lipids, mainly cholesterol, into and beneath the retina.

Cystoid central retinal edema results from a variety of conditions that cause abnormal permeability of the capillaries surrounding the fovea centralis. The retina appears slightly raised and white, with a cystoid pattern of edema that is visible ophthalmoscopically. The loss of vision directs most attention to the condition. Fluorescein angiography provides a typical picture with spokes radiating from the fovea centralis.

Cotton-wool patches (cytoid bodies).— Cotton-wool patches appear ophthalmoscopically as indistinct, white retinal opacities with a hazy, irregular outline ("soft" exudates). They are usually ovoid in shape, variable in size and number, and mainly seen in the posterior fundus. They occur in the nerve fiber layer of the retina as a result of capillary infarction. Cotton-wool patches occur in the retina following retinal trauma and in severe arterial hypertension, severe anemia, papilledema, diabetic retinopathy, generalized carcinomatosis, acute systemic lupus erythematosus, and dermatomyositis. They may be the first clinical sign of the acquired immunodeficiency syndrome (AIDS).

Microscopically, cotton-wool patches occur in axons in the nerve fiber layer of the retina. They consist of an accumulation of cell organelles and reflect obstruction of axonal flow in the nerve fiber layer. In AIDS, they do not contain infective particles.

Epiretinal membranes.—Membranes on the vitreal surface of the retina result from proliferation of one or more of three retinal elements: (1) fibrous astrocytes; (2) fibrocytes; and (3) retinal pigment epithelial cells. Localized epiretinal membranes may occur at the posterior pole of the eye without clinical signs or may cause marked loss of vision as a result of covering, distorting, or detaching the fovea centralis. Epiretinal membranes may cause vascular leakage and secondary retinal edema. In younger individuals some membranes appear to be developmental in origin and occur in otherwise normal eyes. The majority occur in association with retinal holes, ocular concussions, or retinal inflammation, or after ocular surgery. A number of terms are applied: preretinal fibrosis; surface wrinkling retinopathy, when mild; macular pucker, when severe; and massive periretinal proliferation, when extensive. When epiretinal membranes impair vision, they may be removed by vitreoretinal surgery.

DISTURBANCES IN THE POSITION OF THE SENSORY RETINA

The sensory retina normally lines the globe smoothly without elevation or distortion. In retinal detachment (separation), serous fluid or blood separates the sensory retina from the retinal pigment epithelium. Vision is lost in the region of the detachment because the outer layers of the sensory retina depend on the retinal pigment epithelium for metabolism, vertical orientation, and phagocytosis. The entire sensory retina or a localized portion may be involved. The area of detachment loses its sheen and the red reflex of the choroid appears gray.

Retinal detachment may be divided into (1) rhegmatogenous (Greek *rhegma:* breakage + *gen:* producing), in which a hole occurs in the sensory retina; and (2) nonrhegmatogenous, in which there is no break in the continuity of the sensory retina.

In retinoschisis (Greek *schisis:* division) the sensory retina splits into two layers at the level of the inner plexiform layer. It occurs mainly in middle-aged women, presumably as an exaggerated form of peripheral cystoid retinal degeneration. Another form occurs as a recessive X chromosome–linked abnormality.

DERANGEMENTS OF THE RETINAL PIGMENT EPITHELIUM

The retinal pigment epithelium obscures the view of the choriocapillaris, and the amount of melanin in its cells largely determines the degree of redness of the normal ocular fundus. Decreased pigmentation occurs in aging, myopia, and atrophy of the choriocapillaris. Melanin (but not the pigment cell) is absent in albinism. The choroidal blood vessels are clearly visible, and the white sclera may be seen. In destructive inflammatory lesions involving both the choroid and the retina, all retinal and choroidal layers may be destroyed so that the white sclera is visible. Proliferation of the retinal pigment epithelium is stimulated in inflammatory processes, with resultant deep black clumps of pigment that commonly surround an area of chorioretinitis. In tapetoretinal degenerations, the proliferated pigment often has a central density with dendrites (bone-corpuscle pigment) and is most marked at the equator.

In detachment of the retinal pigment epithelium, serous fluid or blood accumulates between the pigment epithelium and Bruch membrane, which elevates the sensory retina in the area.

ABNORMALITIES OF THE BRUCH MEMBRANE (LAMINA BASALIS CHOROIDEAE)

The main abnormalities recognized ophthalmoscopically are breaks in the elastic layer of the Bruch membrane with replacement by fibrous tissue, which results in angioid streaks and drusen. Both conditions favor the formation of a subretinal neovascular membrane.

CONGENITAL AND DEVELOPMENTAL ABNORMALITIES

Myelinated nerve fibers.—Myelination of the optic nerve is completed shortly after birth.

Sometimes the process does not stop at the lamina cribrosa but extends a short distance over the retinal surface (see Fig 20-1).

Rarely, the nerve fiber layer in the peripheral retina may be myelinated. The involved area is translucent, with the blood vessels visible beneath a thin, stark white opacity that is more dense near the disk, follows the distribution of the nerve fiber layer, and has feathery-appearing margins. The visual field is normal.

Melanosis of the retina.—Melanosis of the retina, or grouped retinal pigmentation, is a rare nonfamilial, nonprogressive retinal abnormality characterized by small grayish to black spots scattered throughout the fundus or limited to a single quadrant. They vary in size and sometimes are grouped aggregations that resemble animal footprints ("bear tracks") on the surface of the retina. They consist of densely pigmented accumulations of retinal pigment epithelium cells that have migrated to the region normally occupied by photoreceptors that have failed to develop. There are no symptoms, although minute visual field defects correspond to these areas.

Bilateral, multiple, peripheral patches of congenital hypertrophy of the retinal pigment epithelium occur in familial adenomatous polyposis coli. In affected families, about one third to one half of those with the ocular pigmentation develop polyposis coli, which often progresses to colorectal cancer. The ocular lesions, unlike grouped pigmentation, are located in the peripheral retina and are surrounded by a halo of depigmentation.

Retinal dysplasia.—Retinal dysplasia is a congenital, sometimes hereditary, often bilateral retinal abnormality characterized by outer nuclear retinal cells at various stages of differentiation, arranged in a palisading or radiating pattern that surrounds a central ocular space. The eye is often microphthalmic with a shallow anterior chamber. The retina forms tubes, and one-, two-, or three-layer rosettes form, suggestive of a detached mature retina that has been thrown into folds.

The condition may occur because of separation of the sensory retina from the adjacent retinal pigment epithelium during a critical stage of its differentiation. Retinal dysplasia is associated with trisomy 13-5 and other chromosomal abnormalities, congenital retinal folds, Norrie disease, colobomas or cysts, and cyclopia. A small blind eye with a white mass in the pupil (leukocoria) characterizes the condition.

Pseudoglioma (pseudoretinoblastoma) is an obsolete term used to describe many conditions that cause a white pupillary reflex (leukocoria) or amaurotic "cat's eye reflex." It may be produced by persistent hyperplastic primary vitreous, retinal dysplasia, congenital retinal folds, Norrie disease, chromosome 13 trisomy, retrolental fibroplasia, Coats disease, larval granulomatosis, toxoplasmosis, retinoblastoma, incontinenti pigmenti, massive retinal fibrosis caused by organization of neonatal retinal hemorrhage, metastatic retinitis, secondary retinal detachment, juvenile retinoschisis, and embryonal medulloepithelioma.

Coats disease.—This is a chronic, progressive, vascular abnormality in which telangiectatic retinal vessels leak fluid, which results in an exudative, bullous retinal detachment. It affects boys, predominantly between 18 months and 18 years of age, with peak incidence at about 10 years of age. It is usually unilateral, but when both eyes are involved, one is more affected than the other.

The main symptom is decreased central or peripheral vision. In the very young, attention may be directed to the abnormality because of a white mass behind the lens, suggesting a retinoblastoma, which may lead to enucleation. Microscopically, there are telangiectatic retinal vessels, an eosinophilic transudate predominantly in the outer retinal layer, and a massive subretinal fluid containing foamy macrophages and cholesterol crystals.

Ophthalmoscopic examination discloses yellowish white exudative patches beneath telangiectatic retinal blood vessels. These wax and wane and may disappear in one area while occurring in another. Subretinal hemorrhages are frequent and are usually associated with numerous glistening cholesterol deposits. The retinal vessels may develop a tortuous course, aneurysms, fusiform dilations, and loops. Hemorrhage into the vitreous humor may occur with a subsequent development of proliferative retinopathy. Eventually there may be total retinal detachment, iritis, cataract, and secondary glaucoma. Treatment is often ineffective, but early photocoagulation or cryotherapy may be helpful.

RETINOPATHY OF PREMATURITY

This is a bilateral (usually) failure of normal retinal blood vessels to vascularize the immature sensory retina. It occurs almost exclusively in premature infants who have a birth weight of less than 1,500 g. Before 1970, administration of excessive oxygen to premature infants was probably the major, but not the only, contributing cause. Today, the survival of many premature infants with birth weights of less than 1,000 g suggests that the basic cause is the extrauterine maturation of the peripheral portion of the inner retinal layers. (The outer layers of the sensory retina are nurtured by the choriocapillaris and the inner layers of the sensory retina are nurtured by branches of the central retinal artery.)

The inner layers of the sensory retina are without blood vessels until the fourth gestational month, when blood vessels begin to extend from the optic nerve toward the periphery. The nasal portion of the inner retina is vascularized by the eighth gestational month. The temporal retina, which is more distant from the optic nerve than the nasal retina, is not fully vascularized until shortly after full-term birth. It is, thus, the temporal retina of the premature infant that is most vulnerable to the development of abnormal vascularization.

Indirect ophthalmoscopy of the premature infant discloses a sharp flat junction between the vascular and avascular retina that is most marked in the temporal retina. The initial sign (stage 1) of the retinopathy of prematurity is the development of a flat, white line of demarcation between the normally vascularized and the peripheral avascular retina. At this junction there is an arcade of dilated and extensively branching retinal capillaries. With progression, the line increases in width and height (stage 2) and appears above the level of the retina as a pink ridge with small blood vessels on its surface.

New blood vessels then extend into the vitreous cavity (stage 3) either from the surface of the ridge or from the retinal vessels posterior to the ridge. There may be dilation and tortuosity of the retinal blood vessels posterior to the ridge, a haze of the vitreous humor, dilation of the blood vessels of the iris, and rigidity of the pupil (stage 3 plus ["plus disease"]).

The retina then detaches from the ridge because of exudative effusion, traction, or both (stage 4). The retinal detachment may be extrafoveal (stage 4A) or detach the fovea (stage 4B). In the terminal stage the retina is entirely detached, the pupil is white, and the eye is blind. The end stage (stage 5) of the retinopathy of prematurity is called "retrolental fibroplasia."

Cryotherapy of avascular retina immediately anterior to the retinal ridge is beneficial if used in stage 3 plus disease or early in stage 4. The prognosis is poorer the more posterior the retinopathy extends from the initial ridge, the more quadrants of the globe that are affected, and the more advanced the retinopathy. Laser photocoagulation of the new blood vessels is helpful. The argon laser may damage the crystalline lens; this danger is avoided with the indirect ophthalmoscope endolaser, which may yield results better than those with cryotherapy.

Removal of a disk of cornea, which is replaced at the conclusion of the procedure; vitrectomy; and excision of fibrous retinal membranes to permit the retina to be restored to its normal position restore limited vision in end-stage (stage 5) retinopathy of prematurity.

The diagnosis of fully developed retrolental fibroplasia (the end stage of retinopathy of prematurity) is evident. The eyes are small and sunken with fetal grayish blue irises. A white mass presses against the lens. Glaucoma may be accompanied by tearing and corneal edema, but without enlargement of the eye. The infants often sit rocking back and forth and grinding their eyes with their fists.

Early arrested stages of the retinopathy of prematurity may be associated with a variety of ocular abnormalities. Myopia is common. The blood vessels at the posterior pole may appear to be dragged temporally. The fovea centralis may be displaced temporally (ectopia maculae), causing a divergent strabismus. Minimal degenerative changes in the peripheral retina and abnormal vitreoretinal adhesions may result in a retinal detachment that requires surgical correction.

The idiopathic respiratory distress syndrome affects 10% of all infants who weigh less than 2,500 g at birth. High concentrations of oxygen are required for several days after birth. The cardiac and pulmonary deficiencies may disappear at any time, but the high oxygen concentration of the arterial blood may cause retinal damage.

Premature infants with a gestational age of less than 35 weeks who have received supplemental oxygen and those with a birth weight of less than 1,301 g, irrespective of supplemental oxygen, should have an eye examination between the fifth and sixth weeks of extrauterine life, or before discharge from the hospital. The examination should be conducted by one skilled in neonatal ophthalmology and indirect ophthalmoscopy. The pupils are dilated with topical phenylephrine combined with 0.2% cyclopentolate (Cyclomydril). The eyelids are separated with an infant speculum and particular attention is directed to the peripheral retina, with scleral depression used if necessary. Infants in whom retinal vascularization is not complete and those with early retinopathy of prematurity should be again examined at 1- to 6-week intervals. If there is retinal scarring after the active stage, children should be followed up throughout life, but particularly in childhood, to prevent amblyopia, angle-closure glaucoma, and retinal detachment.

Prevention of the retinopathy of prematurity is difficult because many of the factors required for survival may also contribute to its development. Extremely low birth weight (less than 1,500 g), minimal gestational age (less than 33 weeks), supplemental oxygen with hyperoxia (PaO_2 levels above 100 mm Hg), hypocapnia (PCO_2 levels below 35 mm Hg), and blood transfusions may contribute. Maternal use of beta-blocking drugs immediately before delivery may be a factor. Ambient light in the nursery is considered a factor.

The development of the retinopathy of prematurity does not indicate poor, dangerous, or inept medical care. Rather, it reflects the essential care required for an often fatal condition. Parents and physicians must weigh the risk of survival against the possibility of severe ocular involvement, often with markedly reduced vision and severe neurologic defects. It is not clear whether stage 3 disease requires treatment if it does not extend posterior to the retinal equator.

Familial exudative vitreoretinopathy.— This is an autosomal dominant disorder of high penetrance and variable expressivity that occurs in individuals of normal birth weight, normal gestation, and an uneventful neonatal course. Most patients are asymptomatic. Incomplete vascularization of the periphery of the retina with abnormally straight blood vessels anastomosing along a vascular interface is detected only after the severe disorder in siblings prompts examination. The severe form has its onset between 3 months and 11 years of age and resembles stages 4 and 5 of the retinopathy of prematurity. There is an accumulation of subretinal exudates, progressive traction on the central retina, cicatricial changes in the temporal retina, and peripheral vitreous hemorrhages. Temporal displacement of the fovea centralis causes a pseudostrabismus as the result of an abnormal angle kappa. The condition is distinguished from the retinopathy of prematurity by the normal birth weight, usual absence of myopia, and results of family studies.

VASCULAR DISORDERS

The human retina and optic nerve are nurtured by blood vessels derived from the ophthalmic artery, the first branch of the intracranial portion of the internal carotid artery. Capillaries derived from branches of the central retinal artery nurture the inner layers of the sensory retina. There are capillaries at the level of the nerve fiber layer and in the inner nuclear layer (see Chapter 1). Reduced blood flow through these vessels results in decreased retinal perfusion and loss of function in the affected portion of the retina. Normal perfusion requires that the vascular pressure in the retinal arteries, capillaries, and veins exceed the intraocular pressure. The outer layers of the retina are nurtured by the choriocapillaris, and vascular abnormalities are not common as long as the outer retina is not detached from its blood supply.

RETINAL ARTERY OCCLUSION

Occlusion of the central retinal artery (Fig 17-6) causes sudden, painless loss of vision. Occlusion of a branch of the central retinal artery results in a defect in the field of vision corresponding to the branch affected. The main causes of central retinal artery occlusion are emboli from atherosclerotic plaques of the carotid artery in older patients, emboli from cardiac valves in younger individuals, and thrombosis from arteriosclerosis (Table 17-1). Branch artery occlusions are usually caused by emboli. Other conditions that cause arterial occlusion include atheroma formation complicated by

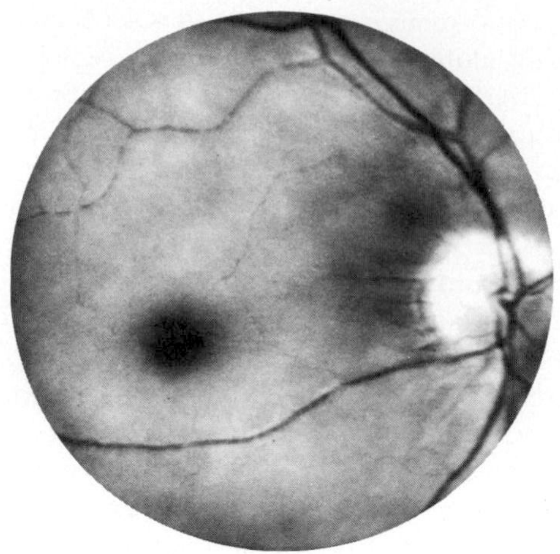

FIG 17-6.
Central retinal artery occlusion in a 19-year-old woman with mitral heart disease. Vision was suddenly lost 24 hours earlier. The sensory retina is edematous, but the normal red reflex is retained at the fovea centralis, causing a cherry-red spot. The blood column is segmented ("box cars") in the superior temporal artery.

subintimal hemorrhage, vascular spasm, and a dissecting aneurysm of the central retinal artery. Arterial emboli may develop in patients with chronic rheumatic heart disease (particularly mitral stenosis) and in myocardial infarction with mural thrombi. Vasospasm is secondary to arteritis in elderly persons or to vasomotor instability in younger individuals.

Occlusion by emboli may be preceded by episodes of flickering vision caused by minute emboli momentarily interrupting blood flow in an arteriole and then disintegrating and passing to the periphery. A large embolus may then cause a sudden loss of vision that is complete if the central artery is affected or partial if a branch is affected.

Vasospastic disease is often preceded by repeated transient episodes of decreased vision or blindness in the affected eye (amaurosis fugax), and finally there is an attack in which vision does not return. The symptom of unilateral periodic blindness must be differentiated from the vascular spasm of internal carotid-basilar occlusive disease, in which ophthalmodynamometry indicates a decreased pressure in the ophthalmic artery. Carotid occlusive disease seldom causes permanent loss of vision even though the carotid artery is completely occluded, provided the central retinal artery remains patent.

TABLE 17-1.
Some Causes of Retinal Artery Occlusion

- I. Embolic obstruction
  - A. Cardiac disease
    - 1. Valvular
      - a. Mitral stenosis, regurgitation, prolapse
      - b. Aortic stenosis
    - 2. Atrial myxoma, thrombus
  - B. Aorta, ipsilateral carotid artery
    - 1. Atheromatous ulceration
    - 2. Dissection
  - C. Trauma
    - 1. Long-bone fracture (fat emboli)
    - 2. Intravenous drug contaminants
  - D. Systemic disease
    - 1. Pancreatitis
    - 2. Sickle cell trait (SC)
- II. Angiospasm
  - A. Migraine
  - B. Raynaud disease
- III. Abnormal intraocular pressure
  - A. Increased
    - 1. Glaucoma
    - 2. Intraocular tumor
    - 3. Orbital compression
      - a. Emphysema
      - b. Tumor
      - c. Hyperthyroidism
      - d. Anesthesia mask
  - B. Decreased
    - 1. Hypotension
      - a. Anesthesia
      - b. Alcohol-drug-induced stupor
      - c. Coma
- IV. Endarteritis
  - A. Giant cell arteritis
  - B. Thromboangiitis obliterans
  - C. Polyarteritis nodosa
  - D. Wegener granulomatosis
  - E. Varicella
- V. Miscellaneous
  - A. Blood hyperviscosity
    - 1. Dysproteinemia
  - B. Oral contraceptives

Ophthalmoscopic examination after central retinal artery occlusion discloses white opacification of the inner layers of the sensory retina as a result of edema. The fovea centralis stands out conspicuously as a cherry-red spot because the inner layers of the retina are absent and the choroidal circulation is visible. Initially, the retinal arteries appear as thin red threads. The blood column may be segmented so that there are segments with blood interspersed with empty segments. On fluorescein angiography, the artery fills with the dye after a delay, but the dye does not perfuse the retinal capillaries. After 1 week, the retina resumes its normal ophthalmoscopic appearance, but vision is permanently reduced. The arteries, however, may remain as thin lines that, in time, may develop parallel sheathing and appear as white threads. The optic nerve becomes atrophic and appears dead white against the normal red fundus background.

Occlusion of the arterial blood supply causes a retinal ischemia with a coagulative necrosis of the inner layers of the retina. The necrosis is followed by autolysis and macrophages loaded with lipids. In the final stages, the outer half of the retina, which is nurtured by the choriocapillaris, is well preserved. The layers of the inner retina become relatively acellular and their boundaries are obliterated.

The prognosis is related to the cause, the degree of obstruction, and the length of time the occlusion has persisted. Relief within 1 hour may restore all vision, whereas relief within 3 or 4 hours may restore peripheral vision with a persistent loss of central vision. After 3 hours or after development of a cherry-red spot, the visual defect is likely to be permanent.

Treatment is directed toward relief of vasospasm or an attempt to dislodge an embolus to a more peripheral and smaller vessel. Immediate intermittent massage of the globe is indicated. Moderate pressure is applied to the globe for a period of 5 seconds, then suddenly released for 5 seconds, and then repeated. Superior results have been achieved with infusion of urokinase or tissue plasminogen activator into the origin of the ophthalmic artery as it branches from the internal carotid artery. The vessel is catheterized with a microcatheter under radiologic control. Urokinase is infused in doses of 200,000 to 1,200,000 units. The best results are obtained with treatment within 6 to 8 hours in eyes that retain some vision and minimal retinal edema. The poorest results follow treatment initiated more than 20 hours after the occlusion. Since many occlusions occur during sleep, it is often impossible to learn the time of the occlusion, and the physician must estimate the severity of the retinal edema.

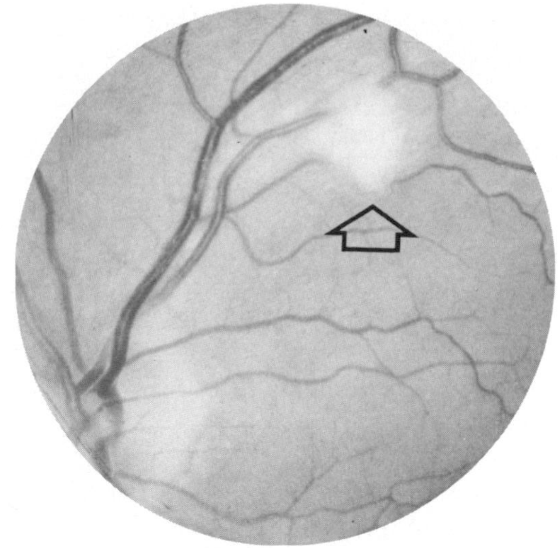

FIG 17-7.
Capillary occlusion by an embolus in a 32-year-old man with mitral valve prolapse. The cotton-wool patch was the sole evidence of the embolus. A permanent paracentral scotoma resulted.

Transient emboli of the retinal arteries may result from atherosclerotic occlusive disease of the carotid arteries or from diseased heart valves. The emboli are of two main types: cholesterol ester flakes from atheromatous ulcers in the carotid artery or platelet-fibrin aggregates from thrombi in the carotid artery or the heart. The embolus causes a transient loss of vision corresponding to the branch in which it lodges. Attacks caused by platelet emboli are brief and frequent and often involve the same vessel. There is no residual abnormality in the retinal blood vessel. Those caused by cholesterol emboli are more variable both in severity and frequency (Fig 17-7). They may be associated with a lasting visual field defect and visible emboli in the retinal blood vessels.

Patients with retinal artery occlusion require careful evaluation of the cardiovascular system, especially the carotid arteries (auscultation for bruits, palpation of facial pulses, ophthalmoscopy for emboli, ophthalmodynamometry, and angiography). Systemic diseases include those associated with atherosclerotic cardiovascular disease and with hypertension. In addition to hematologic and systemic disease studies, patients less than 40 years of age require an echocardiogram or cardiac catheterization, or both, to screen for atrial myxoma or mitral valve prolapse.

RETINAL VEIN OCCLUSION

Retinal vein occlusion may involve the central retinal vein, which causes immediate severe loss of vision, or a branch retinal vein, which results in partial loss of vision, depending on the region of the retina drained by the vein. Three basic mechanisms are involved in both types: (1) external compression of the vein; (2) venous stasis; and (3) degenerative disease of the venous endothelium.

External compression results from arteriosclerosis or arteriolosclerosis of the central retinal artery or its branches that reduces the diameter of the lumen of the central retinal vein within the optic nerve or at arteriovenous retinal crossings. Additionally, a connective tissue strand within the floor of the physiologic cup or from the cribriform plate may compress the central vein.

Venous stasis follows a spasm of the central retinal artery or a retinal arteriole that reduces the perfusion pressure within the corresponding vein, a process aggravated by retinal edema. Other causes include reduced blood pressure in cardiac decompensation or therapy for hypertension, traumatic or surgical shock, carotid artery occlusive disease, and increased blood viscosity in dysproteinemias and obstructive pulmonary disease.

Degenerative disease of the venous endothelium causes intravascular detachment, proliferation, and hydrops. It occurs in severe systemic disease, such as arterial hypertension, cardiac decompensation, and diabetes mellitus. A similar degeneration may follow inflammation of the optic nerve or systemic granulomatous disease. Additional factors include head trauma and, in women, the use of oral contraceptives.

Central retinal vein closure is often preceded by episodes of transient decrease in vision. Visual loss does not occur within seconds, as in central retinal artery closure, but develops over several hours.

Ophthalmoscopic examination indicates engorgement of the venous tree. Physiologic pulsation of the vein is absent and cannot be elicited by pressure on the eye. The involved retina has multiple, scattered, superficial and deep hemorrhages (Fig 17-8). The optic disk may be covered with blood, which may break into the vitreous humor. The veins are enlarged, engorged, tortuous, and dark blue. Segments may be hidden beneath edematous retina. Cotton-wool patches may be present, which indicates concomitant retinal ischemia. Fluorescein angiography shows marked leakage of the dye at the site of the occlusion.

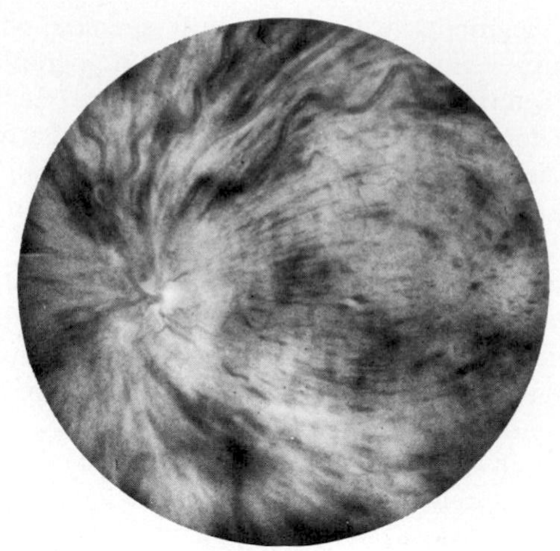

FIG 17-8.
Occlusion of the central vein of the retina. The old term, "retinal apoplexy," is highly descriptive. The disk margins and the arteries are blurred by retinal edema. The veins are dilated. There are retinal hemorrhages that parallel the distribution of the nerve fiber layer of the retina in the central retinal area.

The pathologic changes are dominated by hemorrhage, retinal edema, neovascularization, and glaucoma. There is secondary destruction of the retina, which is replaced with glial tissue. Hemosiderosis of the retina occurs, with most hemosiderin located within macrophages. Some eyes develop neovascularization of the iris (rubeosis iridis), which may cause a painful vascular glaucoma.

An open-angle or secondary glaucoma is more likely to precede central vein closure than a branch vein closure. Additionally, about 20% of patients with central vein occlusion later develop rubeosis iridis and vascular glaucoma (see Chapter 23).

Treatment of central vein occlusion is not satisfactory. Rubeosis iridis may be prevented by ablation of the retina with photocoagulation. Major attention is directed to the prevention of a similar episode in the fellow eye. Glaucoma or ocular hypertension must be treated and in-

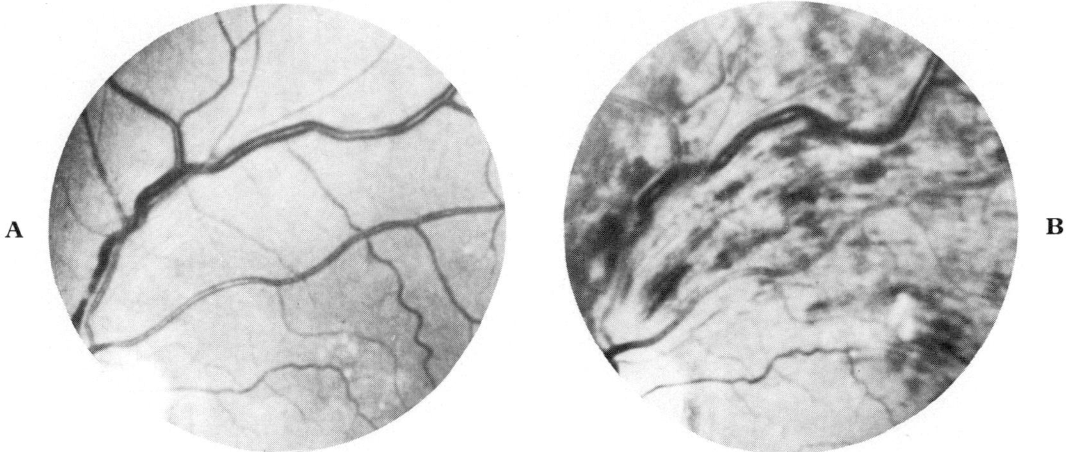

FIG 17-9.
Retinal branch vein closure in a 70-year-old woman. **A,** When the woman was 66 years of age the superior temporal vein was found to have multiple arteriovenous crossings with venous notching and peripheral dilation. There were a few drusen inferiorly. **B,** Four years later a branch vein occlusion occurred with flame-shaped hemorrhages and deposits; visual acuity was reduced to 20/60.

traocular pressure maintained at the lowest possible level. Long-term anticoagulation is indicated if pulsation of the central retinal vein of the uninvolved eye cannot be induced with pressure on the globe. Usually dicumarol is used after initial anticoagulation with heparin. Patients and physicians must be on the alert for transient diminution of vision and signs of venous engorgement, after the fellow eye has been lost from a venous occlusion.

Branch retinal vein occlusion may occur near the optic disk and involve a major quadrant of the retina (Fig 17-9), or it may occur at a peripheral crossing of an artery or vein. If a temporal branch is occluded, vision will be reduced if there is hemorrhage into or edema of the fovea centralis. Occlusion of a nasal branch or a branch temporal to the fovea centralis may cause an inconspicuous loss of visual field that is not noticed by the patient.

The pathogenesis is complex. If capillary perfusion is not impaired, vision often returns to normal. If arteriolar perfusion is impaired, or if there is actual arteriolar insufficiency and retinal ischemia, permanent retinal changes occur. Ophthalmoscopically, retinal hemorrhages, retinal edema, and sometimes cotton-wool patches are visible. The affected vein is dilated and tortuous and may appear segmented. Fluorescein angiography may show diffuse staining and leakage from the involved venous and arterial trees. As the hemorrhage clears, dilated and tortuous collateral vessels may course across the central retina and the median raphe from normal to abnormal retina (Fig 17-10). The capillaries are dilated and leak plasma. Surface neovascularization occurs, and there may be proliferative retinopathy and vitreous bleeding. The leakage of plasma from capillaries causes central retinal edema with reduced vision even after the absorption of the hemorrhage.

The main differential diagnosis, in the prodomal stage, includes those conditions that cause dilation and tortuosity of retinal veins. After frank occlusion has occurred, the same vascular signs persist in combination with loss of vision. The conditions that cause venous dilation include diabetes mellitus, blood dyscrasias (particularly those with associated increased blood viscosity), congenital tortuosity of retinal vessels, arteriovenous aneurysms of the retina, angiomas of the retina, papilledema, and congenital heart disease.

Treatment is directed to correction of the underlying cause if possible. Systemic corticosteroids may be used to minimize retinal edema and phlebitis. Anticoagulation may be used to open collateral venous channels. Aspirin, 300 mg every second day, is sometimes prescribed to inhibit thromboxane A synthesis and to inhibit

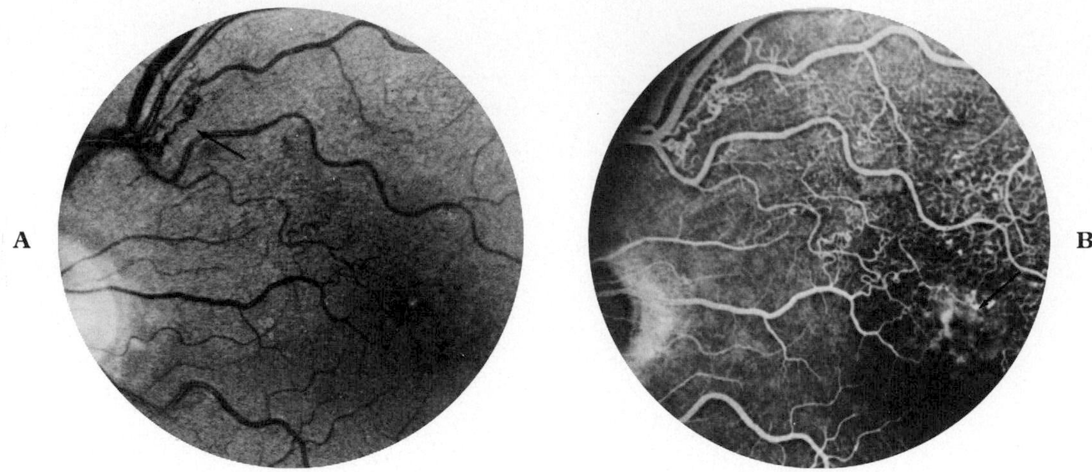

FIG 17-10.
A, Compensated branch vein closure of superior temporal vein of the right eye. New blood vessels direct blood around obstruction. **B,** Late venous angiogram of occlusion showing numerous dilated collateral vessels and many microaneurysms. There is plasma leakage above the fovea centralis that could cause loss of vision.

prostaglandin synthesis by blood vessel walls. Higher doses of aspirin may inhibit prostacyclin synthesis by the blood vessel wall and cause vasoconstriction. Glaucoma, if present, must be vigorously treated. Controlled studies have not been done. Venous stasis and signs of impending vein occlusion in the fellow eye require anticoagulation.

Retinal photocoagulation is indicated to prevent visual loss from macular edema, neovascularization, and vitreous hemorrhage from new blood vessels. Many patients do not develop these complications, and careful evaluation, including fluorescein angiography, is essential. Branch occlusions of nasal veins are usually minor and do not cause macular edema, although neovascularization occurs. Occlusion of the inferior temporal vein is less likely than occlusion of the superior temporal vein to cause macular edema. Occlusions of branches beyond the foveal region are not likely to cause macular edema. Neovascularization is most likely in eyes with large areas (5 or more disk diameters in size) of capillary nonperfusion. Macular edema present within 3 months after branch vein occlusion should be treated with photocoagulation of the region of abnormally permeable blood vessels (Fig 17-11). All areas of neovascularization should be treated. Treatment of areas of capillary nonperfusion in which there is no neovascularization is difficult to evaluate, since many of these eyes do poorly with or without treatment. Generally the prognosis is poorer in eyes with large areas of capillary nonperfusion.

Hyperviscosity syndromes.—Patients with extreme hyperviscosity of the blood ophthalmoscopically show venous dilation and tortuosity, hemorrhages, microaneurysms, exudates, and papilledema. The condition resembles an impending venous closure and may cause frank occlusion. Blood serum abnormalities include macroglobulinemia, hyperglobulinemia, and cryoglobulinemia, whereas the blood cell abnormalities include leukemia and polycythemia. A similar fundus appearance occurs in stasis retinopathy secondary to carotid artery occlusive disease.

RETINAL VASCULITIS

Retinal vasculitis is primarily an inflammation of veins. The most frequent cause is extension of an adjacent chorioretinitis. Other causes include angiitis, multiple sclerosis, tuberculosis, lupus erythematosus, sarcoidosis, syphilis, Behçet disease, and cytomegalic inclusion disease. Inflammation of the capillaries of the central retina may cause a cystoid central macular edema with reduced vision.

Retinal arteriolitis may occur spontaneously or in cases of necrotizing angiitis. Inflammation of both arteries and veins leads to localized

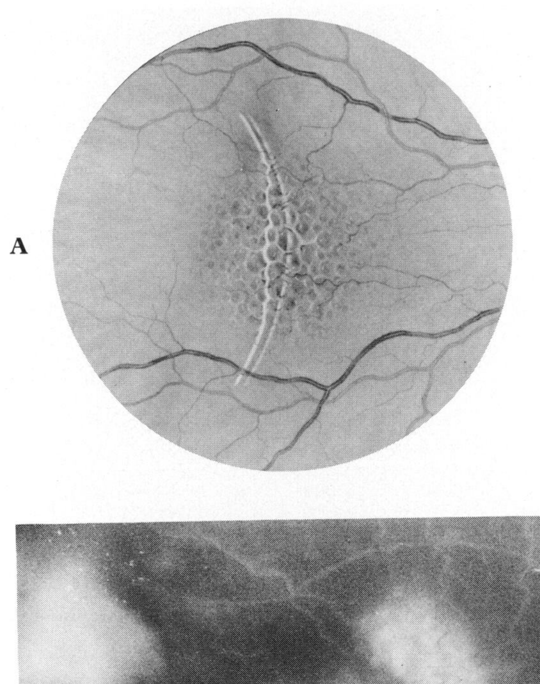

FIG 17-12.

A, The biomicroscopic appearance of cystoid macular (central) edema. *(Courtesy of P. Henkind: Surv Ophthalmol 28 [suppl]: May 1984, cover photograph.)* **B,** Late fluorescein angiogram of cystoid macular edema *(arrows)* that occurred after cataract extraction in a 78-year-old man. Visual acuity was reduced to 20/200 but later improved to 20/60.

athing or exudation, and blood in the vitre-s body and the retina.

Occlusion of the affected vessels by means of otocoagulation, which may have to be re-ated, is effective in preventing progression.

TINAL EDEMA

The blood-retina barrier limits plasma from tering the sensory retina, which has but a nall extracellular space. Failure of the blood-tina barrier results in an increase of the ex-acellular fluid within the sensory retina. Ex-essive flow through the retinal pigment epi-helium causes a central serous choroidopathy. Retinal branch vein occlusion or arterial mac-oaneurysms may cause diffuse retinal edema. Intrinsic capillary endothelial dysfunction in diabetes mellitus may result in edema that appears as "hard exudates." Retinal edema, particularly prominent in the central retina (cystoid macular edema), commonly occurs in chronic mild uveitis as in pars planitis, after cataract extraction, age-related hyalitis, and retinitis pigmentosa.

Central cystoid macular edema.—Central cystoid macular edema is a disorder of the retinal capillary bed that surrounds the fovea centralis. The vessels become abnormally permeable and leak fluid into the sensory retina. The fluid accumulates in the outer plexiform layer (which in this region courses tangentially from the fovea centralis) and causes edema and cysts. Visual acuity is often reduced to 20/200, but ophthalmoscopic signs are minimal. The

A

C

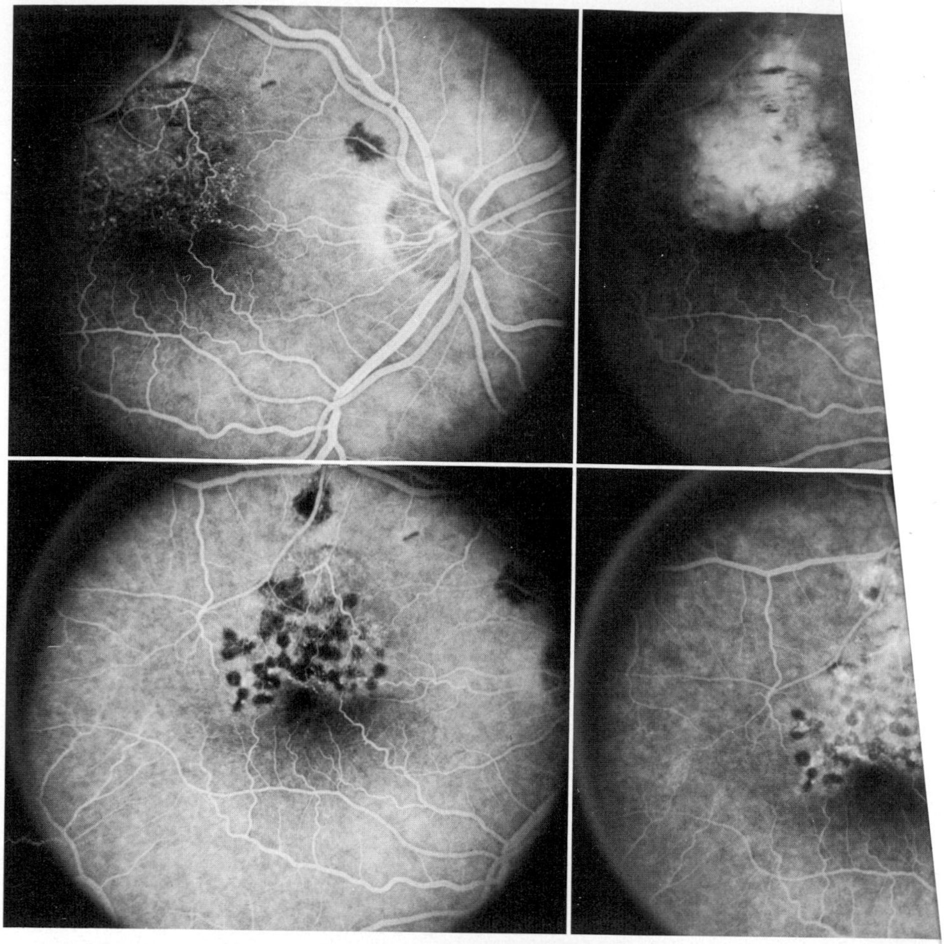

FIG 17-11.

A, Pretreatment fluorescein angiogram, transit phase, showing dilated retinal superior to the fovea centralis. **B,** Pretreatment fluorescein angiogram, late phase, leakage of fluorescein from dilated retinal capillaries. **C,** Posttreatment (6 weeks af laser photocoagulation) fluorescein angiogram, transit phase, showing pattern of pho lation to region of permeable capillaries. **D,** Posttreatment fluorescein angiogram, la demonstrating decrease of edema. (*From the Branch Vein Occlusion Study Group: Ar photocoagulation for macular edema in branch vein occlusion,* Am J Ophthalmol *98:271, 19 by permission.*)

thrombus formation followed by neovascularization.

Retinal phlebitis.—Phlebitis may rarely involve the central retinal vein. Ophthalmoscopically, the disk is swollen as in papillitis, but vision is not reduced. Branch vein phlebitis appears as a branch vein closure, which clears spontaneously. Vaso-obliterative vasculitis may occur in peripheral retinal veins.

Eales disease is a nonspecific peripheral periphlebitis that mainly affects men between 15 and 30 years of age. It is characterized by recurrent retinal hemorrhage ad inflamed veins and by vitreous Both eyes are involved in about h The cause is not known, but the co result from a T cell–mediated vas sensitivity. The chief symptom is lo caused by vitreous hemorrhage. Al hemorrhage tends to absorb rapidl bleeding results in vascularization of t humor, chronic uveitis, and glaucom

Ophthalmoscopic examination indi mental, dilated, beaded, occluded ve

TABLE 17-2.
Major Causes of Leakage of Perifoveal Capillary Network Resulting in Cystoid Macular Edema

Retinal vascular disorders
Diabetic retinopathy
Central retinal vein occlusion
Branch retinal vein occlusion
Retinal telangiectasis (Coats)
Intraocular inflammation
Pars planitis
Retinal vasculitis (Eales, Behçet, sarcoidosis, necrotizing angiitis, multiple sclerosis, cytomegalic inclusion disease)
After cataract extraction
Vitreous traction to corneoscleral incision
Intraocular lens implantation (mechanism?)
Retinal degeneration
Retinal drusen
Epiretinal membranes
Retinitis pigmentosa
Medications
Topical epinephrine after lens extraction
Nicotinic acid
Acetazolamide
Chlorthalidone
Methyldopa

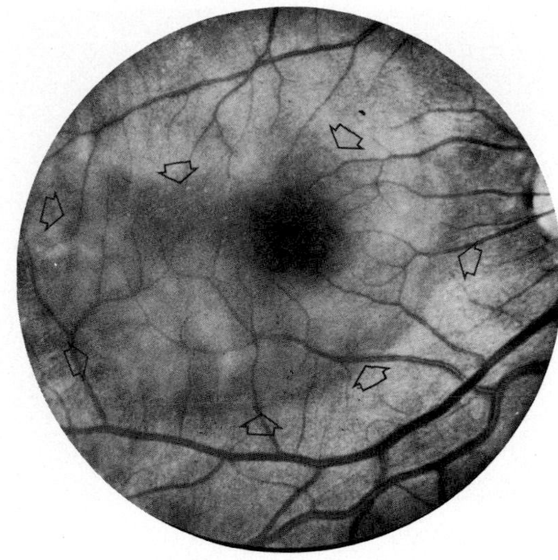

FIG 17-13.
Central serous chorioretinopathy of the right eye. There is elevation of the sensory retina in the region of the central retina. Arrows indicate lower border of the elevation. A fluid level is visible just above the foveal region. Small white dots adjacent to the superior blood vessels are residues of chronic edema.

retina is edematous and wrinkled, and cystic changes are sometimes present. Fluorescein angiography demonstrates leakage of the dye from the perifoveal capillaries and its accumulation within the sensory retina. In the late stages a spoke pattern develops in which the fluorescein surrounds the capillary-free area that marks the foveola, which lacks the inner plexiform layer (Fig 17-12).

There are many causes (Table 17-2). Originally the disorder was described as following cataract extraction (40% to 60%), particularly with vitreous adherent to the wound edges (Irvine-Gass syndrome). The lesion is nonspecific and occurs with a variety of retinal vascular abnormalities, degeneration, and intraocular inflammations as well as intraocular surgery.

The edema is self-limited and there is often spontaneous improvement. Systemic corticosteroids are often used in vascular and inflammatory disorders. In about one third of aphakic eyes that do not contain an intraocular lens, topical epinephrine causes a retinal edema (cystoid macular edema), which is reversible when the medication is stopped.

Central serous retinopathy.—In central serous retinopathy a serous detachment of the macula occurs without obvious cause. The serous fluid originates because of a defect in the tight junctions at the apices of the retinal pigment epithelial cells that normally provide a blood-retina barrier. Damage to the retinal pigment epithelium permits fluid to accumulate between the sensory retina and the retinal pigment epithelium. Men are affected more than women, with the peak incidence occurring at about age 55 years. Both eyes may be affected, but usually only one is affected at one time.

There is reduced visual acuity, metamorphopsia, and increased hyperopia or reduced myopia. Ophthalmoscopically, the fundus lesion is characterized by one or more circumscribed elevations of the pigment epithelium or sensory retina at the posterior pole (Fig 17-13). The lesions tend to remain unchanged for long periods but resolve spontaneously. Histologically, there is dilation and stasis in the orbital and vortex veins and their tributaries, and the lesion is suggestive of a systemic hemodynamic disturbance. There may be active proliferation of the pigment epithelium, producing elevated, pigmented lesions that suggest chorioretinitis. The lesions tend to disappear, leaving a residue of whitish yellow deposits deep to the sensory

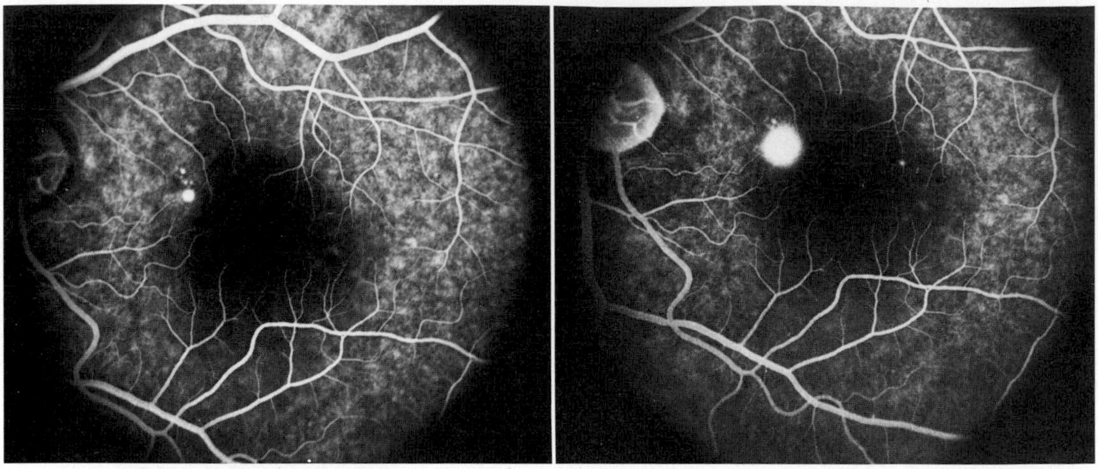

A B

FIG 17-14.
Fluorescein angiograms of serous choroidopathy. **A,** Late phase showing leakage of fluorescein from choriocapillaris through retinal pigment epithelium and under sensory retina. **B,** Late phase (5 minutes) showing increased accumulation of fluorescein.

retina or areas of hypopigmentation and hyperpigmentation.

Fluorescein angiography indicates one or more areas of leakage in the choriocapillaris (Fig 17-14). Photocoagulation of the area is followed by prompt resolution, but spontaneous, although delayed, resolution is usual. Often initial attacks are not treated, but recurrent attacks are promptly photocoagulated.

The cause of the reduced vision may be difficult to establish. If the beam of a small penlight is directed into the eye for 10 seconds, vision may be reduced one line or more for more than 1 minute. Eyes with optic nerve disease recover within 30 seconds. Pupillary constriction to light stimulation is prompt in choroidopathy, whereas an afferent pupillary defect occurs in optic neuritis.

SHUNT VESSELS BETWEEN CHOROIDAL AND RETINAL VASCULAR CIRCULATION

Anastomoses between the retinal and choroidal vascular beds in the peripheral fundus are relatively common. They mainly connect capillaries. Large, anomalous blood vessels on the surface of the optic disk shunt retinal blood into the choroidal circulation in occlusive retinal venous disease, glaucomatous optic atrophy, retinal proliferative vascular syndromes, congenital diseases, and meningiomas of the optic nerve sheaths. When there is interference with the venous outflow in the optic nerve just behind the globe, convoluted dilated channels of preexisting capillaries develop on the surface of the disk. These occur with optic nerve gliomas, chronic atrophic papilledema, orbital cysts, and orbital meningiomas. The triad of shunt vessels, disk pallor, and loss of vision in middle-aged women suggests meningioma of the sheaths of the optic nerve. The outlook for retained vision is poor.

RETINAL DEGENERATIONS

Genetic defects, inflammation, trauma, vascular disease, or aging cause either focal or generalized retinal degeneration. An accurate diagnosis often requires psychophysical, electroretinographic, and ophthalmic evaluations combined with fluorescein angiography of the patient and family members. Many of these disorders have not been studied histologically or they have been studied only in their end stages, when nonspecific changes predominated. Molecular biologic and biochemical studies in the early stages of the disease can provide more precise information concerning the etiology.

Previously the retinal pigment epithelium was called the tapetum (Greek *tapetion:* rug). The term tapetoretinal degeneration describes hereditary disorders of this layer, although the initial involvement is not always in the retinal pigment epithelium. Atrophy of the choriocapillaris can reduce the blood supply to the overlying pigment epithelium and sensory portion of the retina. Many disorders affect the longevity of rods and cones, whereas others cause defects in the synthesis of rod membranes, or abnormal visual pigments. Subretinal neovascularization causes disciform degeneration of the retina in a variety of acquired and hereditary disorders. Many disorders once thought to affect predominantly the central retina are now recognized as involving the entire retina, with attention directed to the fovea centralis because of decreased visual acuity.

Retinal photoreceptors.—Most pigmentary degenerations of the retina predominantly affect the layer of photoreceptors, the rods and cones. Nutrition for this layer must pass through the retinal pigment epithelium, which additionally phagocytizes the outer segments of the rods and cones.

Possibly, in retinal degenerations the lysosomal system of the retinal pigment epithelium may not fully phagocytize outer segments that contain genetically altered proteins. This failure results in the accumulation of cellular debris with pigment proliferation and degeneration of the overlying photoreceptors. Transfer of appropriate genes to the retinal photoreceptors or to the retinal pigment epithelium by means of a viral carrier gives some promise of future treatment of retinal degenerations.

Retinitis pigmentosa.—This is a hereditary group of progressive disorders of the rods and cones secondary to mutations of different genes. The disorder is called by a variety of names: primary, hereditary, pigmentary retinopathy, retinitis pigmentosa, and tapetoretinal degeneration. Initially the retinal rods are affected; eventually all visual cells are impaired. X chromosome–linked forms of the disease (mainly recessive) are rare and the most severe; autosomal dominant forms are the least severe; autosomal recessive forms are moderately severe. (Usually severity is used to designate the visual defects at a particular age and not the progress of the disease.) Retinitis pigmentosa can also be inherited by a digenic mode of transmission, in which gene mutations on two different chromosomes result in the degeneration.

Night blindness during adolescence is the initial sign of the disorder. A ring scotoma develops and then extends peripherally and centrally until only a small contracted visual field remains (tubular vision). Eventually this too is lost. The scotopic electroretinogram is reduced in amplitude and becomes nonrecordable. The amplitude of the electro-oculogram does not increase in light. Eventually all vision is lost—earliest in the X chromosome–linked form and latest in the autosomal dominant form.

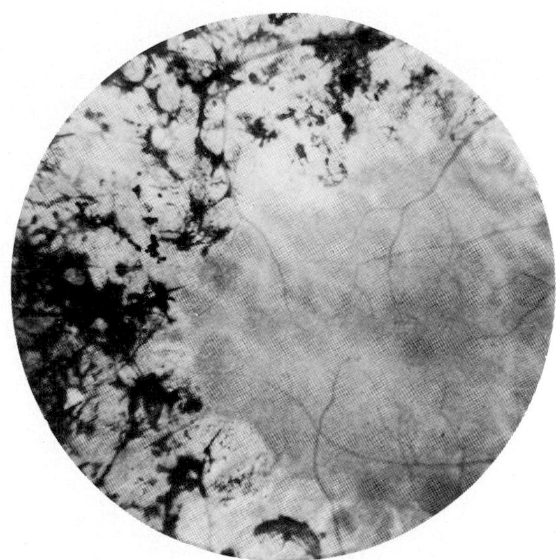

FIG 17-15.
Bone-corpuscle pigment proliferation and attenuated arterioles of primary pigmentary dystrophy of the retina (retinitis pigmentosa).

Ophthalmoscopic examination (Fig 17-15) in advanced cases discloses a waxy yellow optic nerve, secondary to glial proliferation. The retinal blood vessels are markedly attenuated. There is atrophy of the retinal pigment epithelium and later of the choriocapillaris. The retinal pigment epithelium may have a mottled gray appearance, and there are areas of hyperpigmentation and hypopigmentation. There are accumulations of pigment shaped as bone corpuscles. Pigment proliferation often begins in the midperiphery and then extends centrally and peripherally. With atrophy of the choriocapillaris, large vessels of the choroid are exposed and the fundus develops a whitish yellow appearance. A tapetoretinal reflex occurs at some time during the disorder in some patients. It has a metallic yellow refractile appearance, affecting particularly the temporal retina.

Fluorescein angiography shows a mottled hyperfluorescence of the posterior fundus,

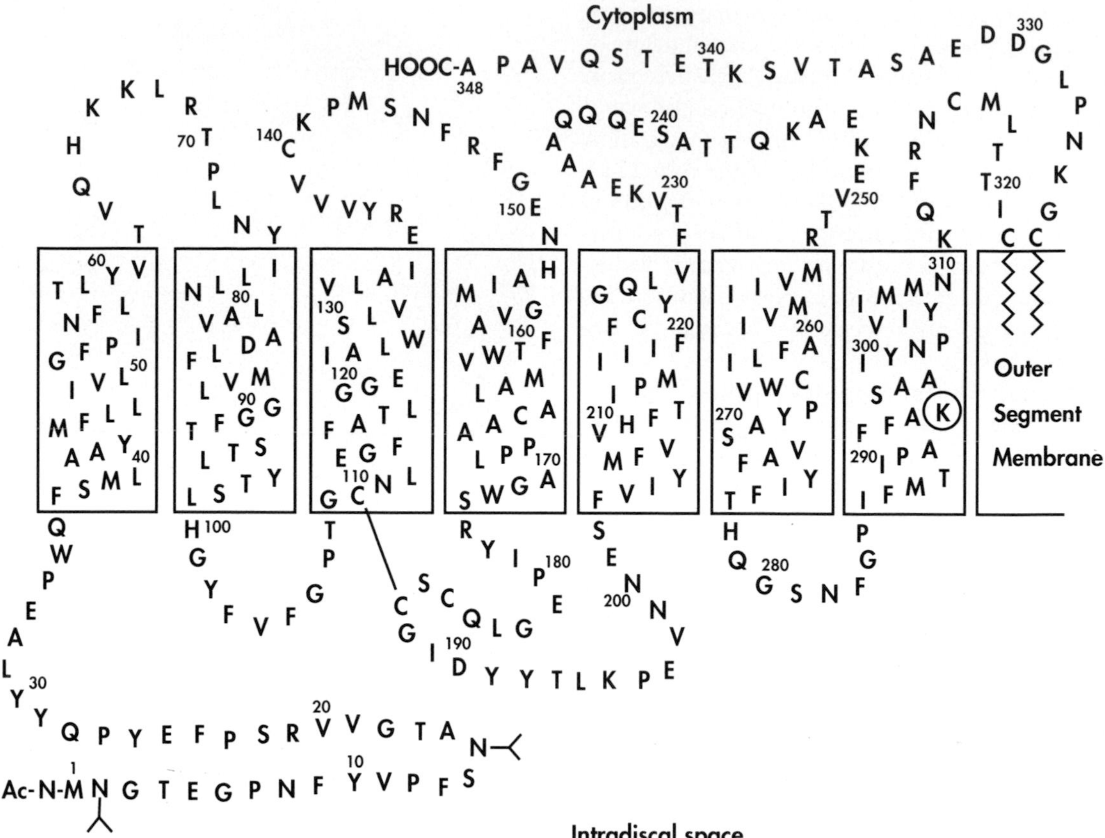

FIG 17-16.
The sequence of the 348 amino acids in the rhodopsin molecule. They are arranged in seven domains (1-7), which are surrounded by an outer segment membrane. More than 70 mutations of the rhodopsin gene have been discovered in families with retinitis pigmentosa. The lysine amino acid residue (K *[circled];* number 296), in the seventh domain, binds 11-*cis* retinal (see Chapter 2). The enzymes transducin, arrestin, and rhodopsin kinase are active in the cytoplasm.

The single letter amino acid code is as follows: *A,* Alanine; *R,* Arginine; *N,* Asparagine; *D,* Aspartic acid; *C,* Cysteine; *E,* Glutamic acid; *Q,* Glutamine; *G,* Glycine; *H,* Histidine; *I,* Isoleucine; *L,* Leucine; *K,* Lysine; *M,* Methionine; *F,* Phenylalanine; *P,* Proline; *S,* Serine; *T,* Threonine; *W,* Tryptophan; *Y,* Tyrosine; *V,* Valine. (*Redrawn from Bird AC: Retinal photoreceptor dystrophies,* Am J Ophthalmol *119:543-562, 1995.*)

sometimes with exposed large choroidal blood vessels. The retinal capillaries perfuse poorly, and there is often low perfusion pressure in the retinal, but not in the choroidal, blood vessels.

Myopia is common. A posterior subcapsular complicated cataract may further reduce vision and require extraction. Cystoid macular degeneration occurs in young individuals. Some cases are associated with drusen of the optic disk or optic disk hamartomas.

Molecular genetic studies have thus far disclosed abnormalities in seven genes that result in this phenotype, which can account for about 15% to 20% of all cases. The seven genes code for (1) rhodopsin; (2) the alpha subunit of rod cGMP phosphodiesterase; (3) the beta subunit of cGMP phosphodiesterase; (4) the alpha subunit of rod cGMP-gated channel protein; (5) peripherin/RDS (retinal degeneration slow); (6) rod outer segment protein 1 (ROM 1); and (7) myosin VIIA. The first four of these genes encode proteins involved in phototransduction (see Chapter 2). The peripherin/RDS gene and the ROM 1 gene encode proteins that maintain the structure of the outer segment membrane. The myosin VIIA gene is the cause of retinitis pigmentosa associated with profound deafness (Usher syndrome, type 1).

More than 70 different dominant rhodopsin gene mutations have been described as causing retinitis pigmentosa (Fig 17-16). The codon Lys296 is the binding site for 11-*cis* retinal. The mutation Lys296Glu (the substitution of glutamine for lysine at amino acid 296) causes retinitis pigmentosa. The same mutation occurs in the same families and results in similar but not identical phenotypes. Patients with Pro23His have, on average, a more severe disease at a similar age than patients with Pro34Leu. The clinical expression varies both within the same family and between different families who have the same mutation, suggesting the possibility that some factor or factors other than the rhodopsin gene defect contribute to the severity of the disease at a given age.

Pigmentary degeneration of the retina occurs with a number of hereditary disorders (see Chapter 26) with widespread systemic defects. These are often loosely diagnosed as retinitis pigmentosa and may seriously depress visual function. Generally, the retinal abnormalities differ from those of true retinitis pigmentosa.

Many different treatments have been suggested: vitamin A in high doses, cataract extraction, various subconjunctival injections, and the like. In 1916 Leber suggested that exposure to light accelerated the process and the degeneration of the retina. Animals deficient in vitamin A develop retinal degeneration only when they are exposed to light. The inability to provide effective treatment has made the victims of the disease and their families easy prey for many nostrums.

The following regimen is suggested for patients afflicted with retinitis pigmentosa:

1. The eyes should be examined annually to determine the progression of the disease.
2. A complete family history and ocular examination of family members should be performed to classify the disorder accurately. The possibility of affected children may be estimated through known family inheritance patterns.
3. Supplementation of the diet with vitamin A (15,000 IU-day) can delay the onset of blindness in adults. Beta-carotene is not a suitable substitute for vitamin A palmitate in this prophylactic treatment. (Women who are pregnant or planning pregnancy should not take high-dose vitamin A supplements.) Dietary supplementation with vitamin E may accelerate the progression of retinitis pigmentosa.

It is probably unwise for individuals with pigmentary degeneration to be exposed to bright sunlight. If such exposure is necessary, extremely dark sunglasses should be worn (lenses with less than 15% transmission).

Vitelliform macular dystrophy (Best disease).—This is an autosomal dominant disorder that is evident at birth or shortly thereafter. The central retinal region is occupied by a bright orange deposit that looks like the yolk of a "sunny-side up" fried egg (Fig 17-17). Vision is normal as long as the "sunny-side up" appearance continues. Between 7 and 15 years of age, the material is dispersed ("scrambled"), and scarring and pigmentary changes occur with depressed vision. In about 75% of the patients visual acuity is at the 20/40 level, but the scarring markedly reduces vision in others.

The light-dark ratio of the electro-oculogram is decreased, and there is a mild disturbance of dark adaptation. Tests indicate a generalized involvement of the retinal pigment epithelium, although the lesion appears to be confined to the central retinal region. The fundus lesion may spare the fovea centralis, and in some family members there are no gross ocular lesions. Although the fundi may appear normal, all affected individuals have a decreased light-dark ratio with electro-oculography. The disease gene is localized to the pericentromeric region of chromosome 11.

Fundus flavimaculatus.—Fundus flavimaculatus (Stargardt disease) consists of multiple, round and linear, pisciform, yellow or yellow-white lesions, usually involving the posterior fundus (Fig 17-18). The flecks vary in size, shape, outline, density, and apparent depth. The abnormality is transmitted as an autosomal recessive disorder and rarely as autosomal dominant.

The disorder has its onset in the first or second decade and may take one of several courses: atrophy of the central retina with development of flecks, cone degeneration with severe

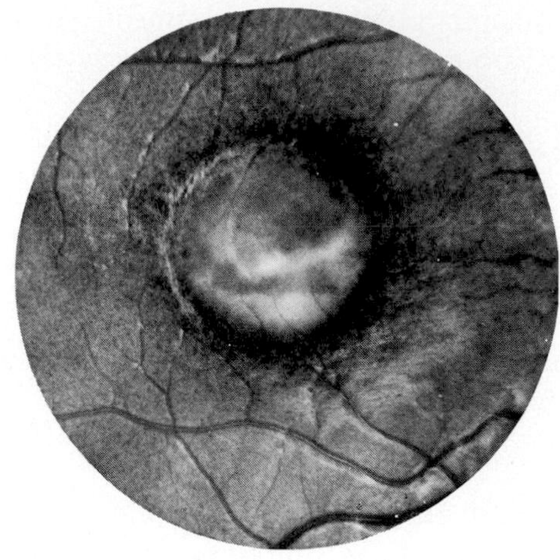

FIG 17-17.
Vitelliruptive degeneration in a 9-year-old girl with normal vision.

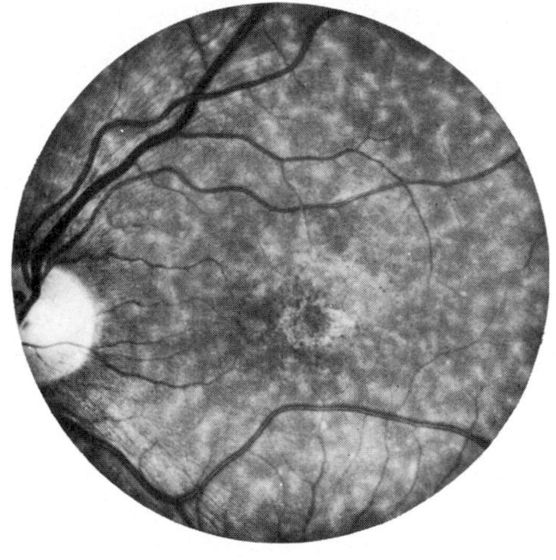

FIG 17-18.
Fundus flavimaculatus with central atrophic lesion (Stargardt disease).

color vision impairment, mild loss of visual acuity followed by flecks, or development of flecks without preceding macular involvement. Rarely, patients lose vision because of a deposit of flecks beneath the fovea centralis, which causes secondary changes in the overlying cones.

The deposits usually first appear in the perimacular area and are isolated with fairly sharp borders and variable shapes, many of them linear and fishtail-like. Clusters of fresh lesions appear from time to time, and older lesions eventually disappear. The older lesions are less sharply demarcated, appear less dense, and show a greater tendency toward confluence. There is considerable familial variation in the size, number, and distribution of the deposits.

Fluorescein angiography does not demonstrate the early lesions. Hyperfluorescence is seen at the sites of old lesions when choroidal fluorescence is viewed through depigmented retinal pigment epithelium. The fuzzy, irregular hyperfluorescent blotches at such sites are entirely different from the discrete, sharply outlined hyperfluorescent areas seen in retinal drusen.

The gene of fundus flavimaculatus has been mapped to chromosome 1p21-13. In another family the gene was mapped to the peripherin-RDS (retinal degeneration slow) on the short arm of chromosome 6. In this family, one member had retinitis pigmentosa, one had pattern dystrophy of the retina, and one had fundus flavimaculatus.

Fundus albipunctatus.—Fundus albipunctatus is a rare autosomal recessive disorder characterized by yellowish white dots of uniform size located in the retinal pigment epithelium and particularly concentrated at the midperiphery of the fundus. The deposits usually increase in number, but occasionally they may decrease or even disappear.

Progressive retinitis albipunctatus begins with a similar ophthalmoscopic picture as the usual type. The electroretinogram is nonrecordable, and there is a markedly increased rod threshold with dark adaptation. Eventually bone spicule pigmentation, vascular attenuation, and optic atrophy develop as in rod-cone dystrophy.

Bruch membrane (lamina basalis choroideae).—The Bruch membrane separates the choriocapillaris from the retinal pigment epithelium. It consists of the basement membrane of the retinal pigment epithelium and the basement membrane of the endothelium of the choriocapillaris. It has inner and outer collagen layers that are separated by a layer of elastic tissue. It is freely permeable. Drusen of the retinal pigment epithelium rest on the Bruch membrane and thus have been incorrectly designated as emerging from it. Ruptures of the elastic layer of the Bruch membrane occur in angioid streaks, subretinal neovascularization, and degenerative myopia.

Angioid streaks.—Angioid streaks consist of an irregular and jagged network of red to green striations, visible through an attenuated

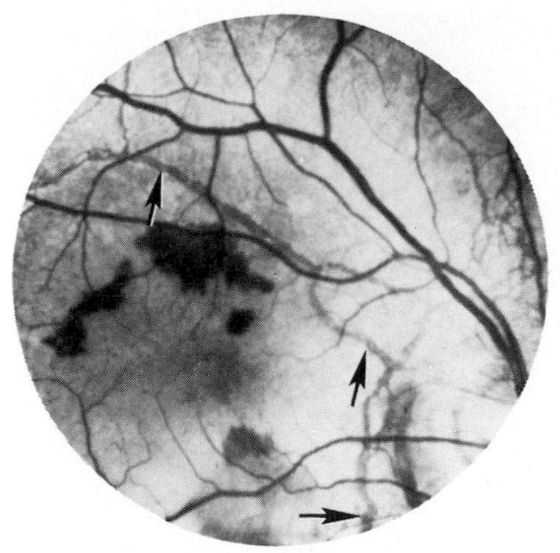

FIG 17-19.
Marked angioid streaks *(arrows)*. There is a subretinal neovascular membrane with bleeding and early development of disciform degeneration.

retinal pigment epithelium. They are produced by linear dehiscences developing as cracks in the collagenous and elastic portion of the Bruch membrane. The condition is bilateral, but ocular involvement is not symmetric. Both sexes are affected equally.

Angioid streaks occur most commonly in pseudoxanthoma elasticum (of Grönblad and Strandberg) and fibrodysplasia hyperelastica (of Ehlers-Danlos). In these diseases there is a degeneration of the elastic tissue portion of the Bruch membrane, which ruptures and secondarily calcifies. Other causes include sickle cell anemia (5%), osteitis deformans (of Paget), and, rarely, acromegaly, hypercalcemia, and lead poisoning. Those conditions with generalized elastic tissue disease may show concurrent vascular hypertension because of involvement of elastic tissue in the walls of arteries.

The optic disk is surrounded by one or more rings with offshoots extending toward the equator in a radial distribution (Fig 17-19). In the early stages, the streaks are red but later become gray, brown, or black. The striations are flat, serrated, and may be several times wider than retinal veins. They gradually taper off toward the periphery of the fundus, where they appear as thin lines. They do not branch dichotomously as do retinal vessels, and they give the appearance of cracks in dry mud.

Ocular changes are asymptomatic unless a subretinal vascular membrane forms. A vascular membrane is often preceded by retinal bleeding, which is followed by subretinal neovascularization.

Drusen.—Retinal drusen are localized deposits that lie between the basement membrane of the retinal pigment epithelium and remnants of the Bruch membrane. They may occur as an autosomal dominant disorder, secondary to a variety of ocular and systemic disorders, and with aging. They reflect an outpouching of the basal cytoplasm and basement membrane of the retinal pigment epithelial cell into the Bruch membrane. The basement membrane subsequently degenerates and the cell fragments separate from the parent cell and in turn degenerate. They are associated with serous detachment of the retinal pigment epithelium, subretinal choroidal neovascularization, and disciform scarring of the macula. (Drusen of the optic disk are a different and unrelated disorder.)

Drusen may be divided into nodular (hard) and granular (soft) types. Nodular drusen ophthalmoscopically appear as discrete, small, round, globular, golden masses, usually no larger than the diameter of a tertiary arteriole. Granular drusen are larger, amorphous, yellow deposits with indistinct margins, irregular shape, and varying size. They tend to change in shape and size and may even disappear. Both types may become calcified, and there are often small flecks of pigment surrounding them. Drusen cause "window defects" on fluorescein angiography (Fig 17-20) in which the fluorescein in the choroidal vasculature is clearly seen. The drusen themselves stain but do not cause fluorescein leakage.

Drusen occur commonly as an aging change and occur in association with other ocular diseases, such as angioid streaks, and systemic diseases, such as recurrent polyserositis, scleroderma, and Rendu-Osler-Weber disease. They occur almost universally with aging, particularly in the peripheral fundi. Secondary drusen often, but not invariably, precede the subretinal neovascularization of disciform degenerations of the retina. Degenerative drusen occur in endophthalmitis and in eyes that are becoming phthisical. Secondary drusen may occur adjacent to areas of choroidal abnormality, such as malignant melanoma. Age-related drusen tend to involve the equatorial to peripheral retina,

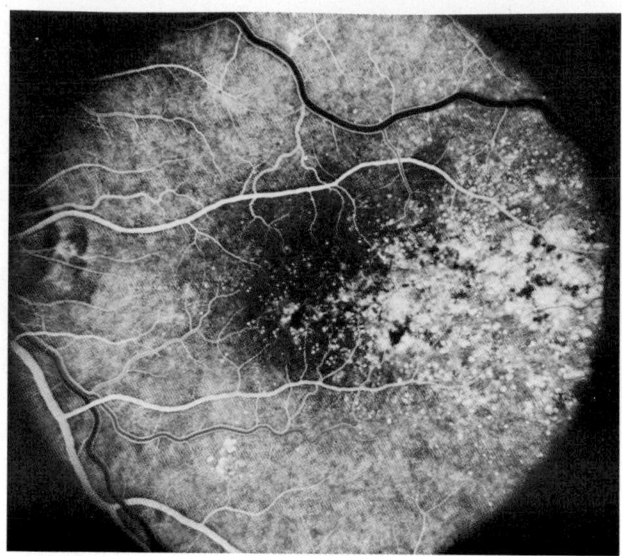

FIG 17-20.
Early venous angiogram of drusen. There is an absence of melanin in the retinal pigment epithelium overlying the summit of drusen that provides windows through which choroidal fluorescence is seen.

whereas familial drusen affect both the posterior pole and the periphery.

In some patients, mainly dark-complected white women, drusen may be preceded by innumerable, small, discrete, round, yellow, subretinal deposits described as "stars in the sky." They are caused by focal nodular thickening of the basement membrane of the retinal pigment epithelium. These may cause a yellow subretinal exudate as well as initiate larger drusen.

Familial drusen occur as an autosomal dominant disorder. They are divided into three stages on the basis of their ophthalmoscopic appearance. During the first to third decades, they appear as small, discrete spots that are slightly pinker than the surrounding fundus. Eventually the dots become bright yellow, and larger ones tend to appear. Later, they tend to calcify and form minute pigment clumps. Eventually familial drusen become confluent and plaque formation occurs, particularly in the macula.

The defects in the retinal pigment epithelium caused by drusen commonly lead to a subretinal fibrovascular membrane and retinal degeneration. Serous elevation of the central retina with hemorrhagic and edematous subretinal areas may be the first sign of neovascularization. If the initial neovascularization is not immediately beneath the fovea centralis, argon laser photocoagulation may be used to obliterate new blood vessels. In the early stages the subretinal membrane can be excised through a transscleral approach and an incision through the choroid temporal to the fovea centralis.

MACULAR DEGENERATIONS

The central retina (macula) is located temporal to the optic disk and surrounds the fovea centralis. The fovea centralis contains the cones mainly responsible for form vision and color vision. The area is involved in the same vascular, inflammatory, and degenerative diseases that affect other areas of the retina and underlying choroidal vasculature. Several factors so modify disease in the central retina that its abnormalities are often considered separately from diseases of the remainder of the retina. A minute lesion that would not affect visual function if located peripherally may cause a severe loss of visual acuity. The spreading of the inner layers of the retina to expose the cones in the fovea centralis is conducive to swelling of the outer plexiform layer of the retina (called the Henle layer in this region). This swelling is seen particularly in neuroretinitis with the formation of a circular area of deposits surrounding the fovea centralis (macular star). The optical system of the eye focuses light energy in this region, so that degeneration of the area may result from excessive exposure to the light of the sun, as occurs in eclipse retinopathy. Additionally, the central retinal area is involved preferentially in a variety of degenerative conditions.

Degeneration of the fovea centralis may be divided into primary and secondary types. The primary type results from a genetically transmitted defect, which is familial, bilateral, and progressive. It includes vitelliform degeneration, fundus flavimaculatus, autosomal dominant drusen, and typical achromatopsia.

Other genetic types include ganglion cell abnormalities that affect both the retina and the brain. Involvement of the central nervous system often leads to early death. In some patients the condition is not accurately diagnosed because the fundi have not been examined.

Age-related macular degeneration.— This is the most common cause of legal blindness in persons older than 60 years in the United States. After the age of 65 years its prevalence increases markedly, and some 28% of individuals between the ages of 75 and 85 years are affected. Smokers have a nearly threefold greater risk than nonsmokers. Age-related macular degeneration is associated with arteriosclerosis, stroke, and transient ischemic attacks. Possibly vascular hypertension and a genetic component are factors.

Two main types of degeneration occur: (1) areolar (geographic; "dry") degeneration and (2) disciform ("wet") degeneration. Areolar macular degeneration may be regarded as a gradual atrophy of the choriocapillaris. Disciform (disk-shaped) degeneration is preceded by subretinal new blood vessels that cause a serous or hemorrhagic separation of the retinal pigment epithelium from the adjacent Bruch membrane. The separation is followed by a fibrous metaplasia of the retinal pigment epithelium that replaces the sensory retina in the foveal and surrounding (macular) region.

Areolar macular degeneration is preceded by nodular ("hard") drusen that sometimes become calcified. There is gradual diminution of central vision. The retinal pigment epithelium beneath the macular region becomes depigmented with exposure of large blood vessels in the choroid. There are scattered small regions of pigment proliferation. About one fourth of those affected develop subretinal new blood vessels and a disciform scar.

Disciform degeneration is often preceded by granular ("soft") drusen that have indistinct borders and a tendency to confluence. Often there is sudden loss of vision combined with metamorphopsia, with apparent bending of straight lines or with objects appearing too small (micropsia). A subretinal neovascular membrane appears as a dark green area deep to the retinal pigment epithelium. Indocyanine green angiography demonstrates blood vessels that cannot be seen ophthalmoscopically. With progression, bright red blood is evident ophthalmoscopically in the sensory retina. It is followed by a white-gray scar with scattered pigment that obliterates the fovea centralis and surrounding retina. Visual acuity is reduced to 3/200 or less.

Treatment of age-related macular degeneration is not satisfactory. I recommend that everyone past 55 years of age take 400 units of vitamin E daily; this prophylaxis is probably ineffective once the changes of macular degeneration have occurred. Every patient with retinal drusen should check the central field of each eye separately with an Amsler chart (see Fig 5-11) each day to detect metamorphopsia. Early detection of new blood vessel formation allows either photocoagulation of blood vessels outside of the foveal region or the excision of the new blood vessels before they have vascularized the fovea.

Every patient with age-related macular degeneration should be assured that peripheral vision will be retained and that the loss of central vision will not result in dependency. Some patients obtain useful vision with telescopic readers, and similar optical aids. Single vision spectacles for reading, which have convex lenses from 5 to 10 diopters more than any distance correction are often most helpful. Although the proportion of patients who obtain satisfaction is small, each patient should try these aids before it is concluded that they are of no use. There are many devices and services of value that many with low vision find useful.

Secondary macular degeneration may follow trauma from mechanical or radiant energy injuries as well as vascular, inflammatory, or degenerative disease. Secondary degeneration is com-

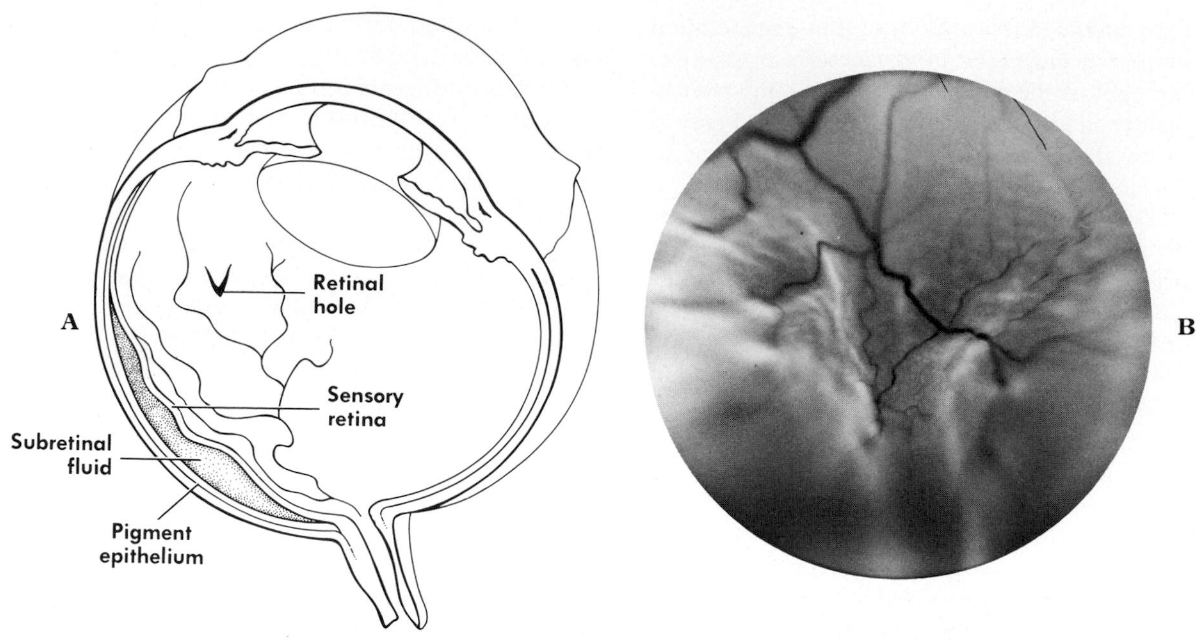

FIG 17-21.
A, Retinal detachment with horseshoe-shaped hole in superior temporal quadrant. **B,** Ophthalmoscopic appearance of a retinal detachment.

monly unilateral and frequently does not progress after the cause has been removed.

RETINAL DETACHMENT AND RETINOSCHISIS

The sensory retina normally lines the interior of the eye with the vitreous humor on its inner side and the retinal pigment epithelium on its outer side. The sensory retina may be drawn away from the retinal pigment epithelium by traction of a shrunken vitreous body. An adhesion between a strand of shrunken vitreous and the sensory retina may cause a hole in the sensory retina and permit fluid to accumulate between the sensory retina and the retinal pigment epithelium. Serous fluid may accumulate between the sensory retina and the retinal pigment epithelium without hole formation. Tumors of the choroid or fluid accumulation within the choroid (effusion) may elevate both the sensory retina and retinal pigment epithelium. A cyst at the level of the outer plexiform layer of the sensory retina may separate the inner retinal layers from the outer layers (retinoschisis).

Retinal detachment

The invagination of the primary optic vesicle (see Chapter 1) forms two layers of retina: the outer retinal pigment epithelium and the inner sensory retina. Traction by either the vitreous humor or an opening in the sensory retina (retinal hole: an opening in the sensory retina caused by retinal atrophy; retinal tear: an opening caused by vitreous traction; or retinal break: an opening adjacent to an area of chorioretinal inflammation, sometimes that secondary to chorioretinal treatment) allows fluid to accumulate between the layers derived from the primary optic vesicle. Retinal detachments (separations) with holes, tears, or breaks are called rhegmatogenous (Greek *rhegma:* break). Those without a defect in the sensory retina are called serous or nonrhegmatogenous.

Rhegmatogenous retinal detachment occurs secondary to the formation of tears, holes, or breaks in the continuity of the sensory layer of the retina (Fig 17-21), or because of separation of this layer at the ora serrata (dialysis). Retinal tears result from vitreous traction on the sensory retina, secondary to vitreoretinal proliferation or degeneration or after laceration or contusion of the eye. Tears caused by vitreous traction are either horseshoe-shaped or round. The vitreous remains attached to the flap (operculum) of a horseshoe-shaped tear and elevates the edges of the tear. Degeneration of the retina causes small round holes without opercula, a purely degenerative or atrophic process without vitreous traction. Detachment of the retina at the ora serrata, a retinal disinsertion, occurs mainly in young individuals either as a congenital defect or after ocular trauma.

Lattice degeneration of the retina is present in about 30% of all rhegmatogenous detachments but occurs far more frequently without causing detachment. There is a sharply demarcated retinal thinning at the ocular equator or anterior to it. Located within this region is a network of fine white lines that are continuous with blood vessels. Pigment accumulates along the white lines. Small white particles lie on the surface of the lines and in the adjacent vitreous. There is liquefaction of the adjacent vitreous humor, and vitreous strands may attach to the margins of the retinal thinning. Both tractional and nontractional tears may develop in this area of retinal thinning.

Retinal detachment occurs more commonly in men than in women, in eyes with degenerative myopia, and in older individuals. Retinal detachment is rare after an uncomplicated cataract extraction, particularly an extraction with implantation of an intraocular lens in which the posterior lens capsule is preserved. Retinal detachment is common after intraocular surgery in which there has been loss of vitreous humor.

An ocular contusion or a penetrating injury commonly causes a retinal detachment in all age groups. Often, however, there is a history of ocular trauma, but the detachment is secondary to degenerative changes of the retina. Lattice degeneration of the retina is a cause at all ages, whereas separation of the sensory retina at the ora serrata (dialysis) tends to involve youthful patients.

Tractional detachments tend to occur secondary to a horseshoe-shaped tractional tear in older patients (see Fig 17-21). The two main premonitory symptoms are (1) photopsia, or flashes of light without retinal stimulation by light caused by vitreous traction on the retina; and (2) a sudden shower of black dots in the peripheral visual field resulting from a ruptured retinal capillary that causes a minute hemorrhage from a ruptured retinal blood vessel into the vitreous humor at the site of tear formation in the sensory retina. Without traction, premonitory symptoms are absent and the first symptoms are decreased vision and a progressive defect in the visual field corresponding to the area of detachment.

The diagnosis of retinal detachment is based on the ophthalmoscopic appearance of the retina. Indirect ophthalmoscopy may be combined with scleral depression, and the examiner may study the retina from the optic disk to the ora serrata. Full pupillary dilation is required. The peripheral retina may be studied with a biomicroscope and a contact lens containing prisms that allow visualization of the periphery or with a +90-diopter lens.

On ophthalmoscopic examination, the detached retina is gray or translucent and the normal choroidal pattern cannot be seen. The retina may be thrown into folds that change in location or shape with shifts in position of the eye or the head. The retinal vessels are dark red in the area of detachment and have an undulating course over its surface. The arteries and veins appear to contain blood of the same color.

Retinal holes are recognized by the bright red choroid shining through the grayish, opaque veil of detached retina. Additional holes may be found in areas of attached retina. Horseshoe-shaped holes are common in the superior temporal quadrant peripheral to the equator. Their operculum (Latin *operculum:* cover) is a flap of retina that is attached to the peripheral retina, which has a detached free edge that floats in the vitreous humor. Small round holes may be found anywhere and are frequently seen anterior to the equator. Retinal dialysis usually occurs in the inferior quadrants. It is most often single, semilunar, and at the extreme retinal periphery.

The most important condition to exclude is a solid detachment caused by tumor, particularly malignant melanoma of the choroid. Failure of the detachment to regress with bed rest, the darker color, yellowish infiltrates, associated drusen, failure to transilluminate, and absence of hole formation suggest a tumor.

The treatment of retinal detachment is surgical and directed toward reestablishing the apposition of the sensory retina to the retinal pigment epithelium. Once the condition is diagnosed, immediate treatment is indicated. The fellow eye must be carefully studied to exclude the early stages of similar retinal and vitreous abnormalities.

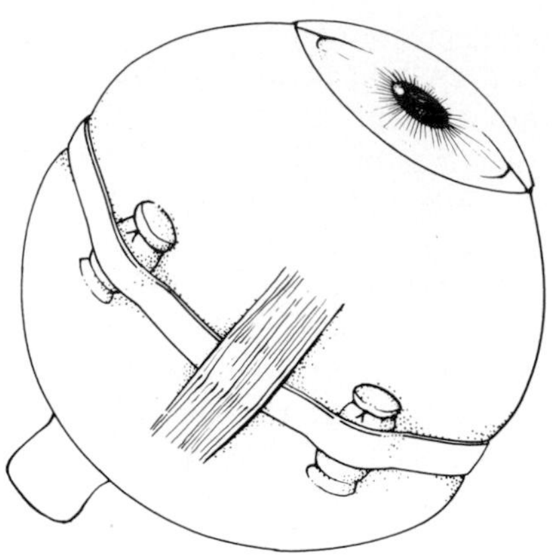

FIG 17-22.
Encircling rod (cerclage) with two radial sponges to indent the choroid to a retinal hole.

A variety of treatments are used. Chorioretinal adhesions are induced in the region of holes, tears, or breaks by inducing a localized choroidal inflammation by the scleral application of intense cold (-80° C), or diathermy. Laser energy may be directed to the region through the pupil or by means of an endolaser introduced through the sclera into the vitreous cavity. The retina must be in contact with the retinal pigment epithelium, which is adjacent to the choroid, to induce a chorioretinal adhesion.

The retina may be brought into apposition with the retinal pigment epithelium. This may be accomplished by indenting the sclera (buckling) or by increasing the volume of vitreous. The sclera is indented (plombage) with a silicone plastic implant secured to the sclera with sutures either segmentally or encircling the eye (cerclage) (Fig 17-22). The vitreous volume is increased by injection of air, an expanding gas, perfluoropropane, or viscoelastic substance. If the retina is too rigid to conform to the shape of the eye, it may be incised (retinotomy).

Proliferative retinopathy is the most important complication of the treatment of retinal detachment. It is characterized by fibrovascular membranes that form on the retinal surface of detached vitreous and the inner and outer surfaces of the sensory retina. The membranes originate with cells of the retinal pigment epithelium that have migrated into the vitreous cavity through the tear, hole, or break in the retina. Glial cells of the sensory retina may also contribute to the membranes. The membranes shrink and form fixed retinal folds so that it cannot be apposed to the retinal pigment epithelium. Treatment is difficult and often requires vitrectomy, stripping of the membranes from the retina, retinotomies, and vitreous tamponade.

Retinoschisis

Retinoschisis (Greek *schisis:* division), a splitting of the sensory retina, occurs in two forms: (1) a degenerative peripheral type that affects both sexes equally and is not hereditary; and (2) an X chromosome–linked type that affects mainly the central retina. Rarely a peripheral type occurs in retrolental fibroplasia or diabetic retinopathy. Patients may complain of light flashes and floaters.

Degenerative retinoschisis.—This usually occurs after 40 years of age. The retina splits into two layers at the level of the outer plexiform layer (rarely the inner nuclear layer). It begins as a cystic degeneration in the extreme retinal periphery, most commonly in the inferior temporal quadrant. The cavity may extend to encompass the entire retinal periphery markedly elevated confluent cysts. Generally, though, the condition is not progressive.

Patients may complain of light flashes and floaters. Ophthalmoscopically, there is a transparent elevation of the retina, which has a smooth, convex, sharply limited surface.

Usually no treatment is indicated. Annual ophthalmoscopic and visual field examinations are advised. Progression may be limited when necessary by photocoagulation, surface diathermy, or cryotherapy of the advancing edge of the retinoschisis.

X chromosome–linked juvenile retinoschisis.—This is an X chromosome recessive disorder, found nearly exclusively in males, in which initially a cystlike structure involves the fovea centralis. It has a spoke pattern with the hub corresponding to the foveola. Later the radial folds disappear and are replaced by a nonspecific atrophic appearance. In about half the patients there is a peripheral retinoschisis, often in the inferior temporal region. There are silver-gray glistening spots scattered throughout the retina in all cases. The vitreous contains veils, most often in the periphery.

Visual acuity may be normal in early childhood and may gradually deteriorate to about

20/200 at puberty. Strabismus and nystagmus may occur, but most commonly the condition is detected when the child fails to pass vision tests on entering school. The electroretinographic b-wave amplitude is reduced with a normal electro-oculogram. There are no signs in carrier females.

INJURIES

Contusions and retinal holes.—Contusion to the eye may cause a variety of injuries, including retinal holes that lead to retinal detachment. A traumatic retinal tear that occurs in an otherwise healthy retina is usually single, often horseshoe-shaped, and located in the superotemporal quadrant of the eye. At 3 and 6 months after a severe ocular contusion, the peripheral fundus of the eye should be studied after maximal pupillary dilation to detect retinal holes. An open-angle glaucoma may occur 20 to 30 years later because of recession of the anterior chamber angle (see Chapter 23).

Macular hole.—Macular holes are circular, red, sharply defined defects of the fovea centralis that measure ¼ to ½ disk diameters in size. They are surrounded by a small rim of detached retina and have yellowish deposits at their base. Often there is a cap of Müller cells and astrocytes, which resemble the operculum that occurs with peripheral horseshoe-shaped retinal holes (this chapter). The macular hole may involve all layers of the sensory retina or it may be partial. Visual acuity is reduced to 20/100 to 20/400 but in exceptional instances visual acuity may be 20/50. Exact diagnosis is difficult and necessitates ophthalmoscopy using a contact lens and biomicroscope or optical coherence tomography. Retinal cysts, partial thickness holes, and pseudoholes, have a similar appearance when viewed with the usual ophthalmoscope.

Most macular holes are secondary to retinal traction by a thin epiretinal membrane or cortical vitreous humor (see Chapter 19). They may also follow blunt trauma to the eye and gazing at a solar eclipse with the eye not protected. Spontaneous macular holes of less than 1 year duration, with visual acuity of 20/50 to 20/100, and a hole of less than ⅓ disk diameter in size may be treated by removal of the vitreous humor adherent to the posterior pole, fluid/gas exchange, excision of any epiretinal membrane, and intraocular instillation of transforming growth factor beta 2.

Commotio retinae.—Commotio retinae is a contrecoup phenomenon in which the retina at the posterior pole develops edema and hemorrhages because of a blunt contusion to the anterior segment. Vision is markedly reduced and often does not improve. Ophthalmoscopically, edema of the sensory retina obscures the retinal pigment epithelium and choroid. Commotio retinae may disappear spontaneously or may be followed by atrophy of the retina and choroid.

Perforations of the retina.—Perforations of the retina are usually associated with loss of vitreous and disorganization of the globe. Retinal detachment may result because the trauma stimulates proliferation of glial or mesodermal tissue, or both, that causes retinal traction.

Purtscher injury.—Purtscher injury is a rare abnormality in which the sudden increase in intravascular pressure associated with crushing injury of the chest causes retinal hemorrhages and edema.

Fat emboli.—Fat emboli of the retinal blood vessels may be seen in fractures of long bones and pancreatitis. They have the same prognosis as emboli from other causes.

Radiant energy.—The cornea and the lens transmit long visible light rays and infrared with nearly 100% efficiency. These rays are usually absorbed by the retinal pigment epithelium, and the energy is dissipated by the choriocapillaris. They may cause injury to the retina if (1) the exposure is of long duration and continuous; (2) the energy is a particular wavelength; (3) the pupil does not constrict to limit the amount of energy entering the eye; (4) the eye is nearly emmetropic so that the rays come to focus on the fovea centralis; (5) the retina is sensitized by vitamin A depletion; or (6) the retina is sensitized by drugs. The classic injury follows observation of a solar eclipse, in which the pupil is dilated because of low light intensity and infrared rays are focused on the fovea centralis. Lasers provide high levels of electromagnetic energy that damage the retina, choroid, and their blood vessels through heating the tissues, protein coagulation, or photodisruption in which the high energy strips atoms of their electrons (see Chapter 8).

Light damage (photic retinopathy) to the retina may occur in those who gaze at the sun as part of sun worship or because of a psychosis. Marked pupillary constriction may prevent sunlight injury. Infants with hemolytic anemia, in whom light oxidizes the bilirubin in the skin, must have their eyes protected during phototherapy. Ocular surgeons routinely protect a patient's retina from injury from operating lights during surgery, particularly after the insertion of an intraocular lens in cataract extraction.

Retinal poisons and toxins.—Chloroquine and the phenothiazines in large doses cause a pigmentary degeneration of the central retina. Topical administration of epinephrine eyedrops in aphakic eyes without intraocular lenses also causes a maculopathy with loss of vision. In susceptible persons, a small amount of quinine may cause severe vasoconstriction of retinal arteries with the central visual field reduced to 5° to 10° in diameter.

TUMORS

RETINOBLASTOMA

A retinoblastoma is a malignant neoplasm of the embryonic sensory retina characterized by proliferation of minimally differentiated retinal cells (retinoblasts). It is the most common intraocular tumor of childhood and has an incidence of 1 : 17,000 live births. It is second only to malignant melanoma of the choroid as the most common intraocular tumor of any age group. Among black individuals, in whom malignant melanoma is not common, it is the most frequent intraocular tumor.

Tumors of both eyes and multiple tumors in one eye are the result of a mutation in the autosomal dominant retinoblastoma tumor suppressor gene (Rb) (see next section). Tumors that affect both eyes and multiple tumors in one eye are mainly familial. Single tumors in one eye are usually not familial, but 15% of those affected transmit a mutated retinoblastoma suppressor gene.

A retinoblastoma is first evident as (1) a white pupil (leukocoria); (2) less frequently as the crossing of an eye (esotropia or exotropia); (3) a red painful eye; (4) a dilated and nonreactive pupil in one eye; or (5) a difference in the color of each iris. The tumor is a pale pink or white mass, with newly formed blood vessels on its surface. There may be several isolated tumors with implantations on the iris and cornea. Dull, white, globular tumor seeds may fill the vitreous cavity. Calcium on the surface of the tumor appears as pearly white, sharply defined regions and as chalky white, poorly defined areas when located deep within the tumor. Calcium is best demonstrated with computed tomography, whereas the tumor is best defined with magnetic resonance imaging.

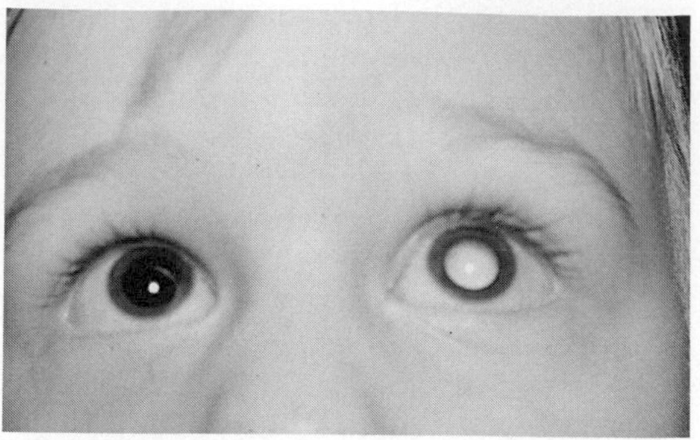

FIG 17-23.
An advanced retinoblastoma in the left eye of a 2-year-old boy. The white pupil ("leukocoria") is often the first sign of retinoblastoma. The fellow eye was not affected.

Often the tumor is first diagnosed when it has protruded far forward, fills the vitreous cavity, and is seen as a grayish white mass behind the lens (Fig 17-23). There is no light perception, and the pupil does not react to direct light stimulation. The major ocular disorders from which a retinoblastoma must be differentiated include persistent hyperplastic primary vitreous (see Chapter 18); retrolental fibroplasia (this chapter); toxocariasis (see Chapter 25); and Coats disease (this chapter). There must be no delay in accurate diagnosis and skilled treatment.

Treatment.—Effective treatment of retinoblastoma is highly individualized and requires lifelong care by skilled practitioners. Both eyes must be studied using general anesthesia, maximal pupillary dilation, and scleral depression. The number, size, and location of each tumor must be mapped so that subsequent progression or regression can be evaluated. Possible vitreous seeding must be determined. Fundus photography, ultrasonography, computed tomography, or magnetic resonance imaging may be used.

Magnetic resonance imaging is particularly valuable in determining the extent of the tumor, including extraocular extension into the optic nerve or through the sclera.

The ocular fundi of both parents and every sibling must be examined for possible retinomas or retinoblastomas. The eyes of every child who has a family history of retinoblastoma should be examined immediately after birth by an ophthalmologist to detect and treat any tumor.

Often one eye is filled with tumor and there is no possibility of restoring vision. The only possible treatment is removal of the eye including a segment of optic nerve at least 10 mm long. The tumor is often less advanced in the fellow eye, and external beam radiation, radioactive scleral plaques, chemotherapy, laser photocoagulation, or a combination of modalities are selected for therapy.

The most unfavorable factors include tumors located anterior to the equator, particularly those that extend to the ora serrata; single or multiple tumors more than 10 disk diameters (15 mm) in size; complete retinal detachment; intraocular hemorrhage; and severe vitreous seeding. Bone marrow aspiration from several sites, usually the iliac crests, and lumbar puncture for cerebrospinal fluid are indicated to exclude metastatic disease.

Survivors of the tumor require lifelong medical vigilance. They are at risk for secondary tumors that include osteosarcoma, Ewing sarcoma, leukemia, and lymphoma.

The parents of an affected child and the child require much psychologic support. The Institute for Families of Blind Children, Mail Stop #111, P.O. Box 54700, Los Angeles, CA 90054-0070 provides a sensitive and helpful newsletter.

Retinoblastoma gene.—The retinoblastoma gene (RB1) is a tumor suppressor gene, which is mapped to chromosome 13q14. The gene product normally inactivates the transcription factors required for cell mitosis. Mutation, loss, or inactivation of the retinoblastoma gene and the failure to transcribe its normal protein is implicated not only in retinoblastoma but in some malignancies of a number of different organs, which include the bones, the breast, and the bladder. Additionally, the tumor suppressor gene p53 appears to have an abnormal gene product in some patients with retinoblastoma.

Both alleles for the retinoblastoma (suppressor) gene must be deleted, mutated, or otherwise inactivated for retinoblastoma to occur. The genetic material of an individual who transmits a hereditary retinoblastoma carries an autosomal recessive gene, which causes an abnormal retinoblastoma tumor suppressor protein. The gene is recessive, however, and an abnormality is not expressed. Loss, mutation, or inactivation of the allele for this gene results in defective control of cell mitosis.

Patients with heritable retinoblastoma are vulnerable to osteosarcoma at the portals of therapeutic radiation and at distant sites. Other family members, without retinoblastoma, are susceptible to the development of other malignant tumors that do not involve the eye. The fathers of patients who have sporadic retinoblastomas tend to be significantly older than most fathers and to have relatives less than 55 years of age who develop malignancies more frequently than expected.

The majority of retinoblastomas (60%) affect one eye only and are not hereditary, and most (85%) survivors do not transmit a defective allele for the retinoblastoma gene. Some 15% of patients with a monocular retinoblastoma, however, transmit an abnormal gene.

BIBLIOGRAPHY

Books

Hollyfield JG, Anderson RE, LaVail MM, editors: *Retinal degeneration. Clinical and laboratory applications,* New York, 1993, Plenum Press.

Ryan SJ, editor: *Retina,* ed 2, vols 1-3, St Louis, 1994, Mosby–Year Book.

Wu G: *Retina: the fundamentals,* Philadelphia, 1995, WB Saunders.

Yannuzzi LA, Guyer DR, Green WR: *The retina atlas,* St Louis, 1995, Mosby–Year Book.

Articles

Berson EL: Retinitis pigmentosa, The Friedenwald Lecture, *Invest Ophthalmol Vis Res* 34:1659-1676, 1994.

D'Amico DJ: Diseases of the retina, *N Engl J Med* 331:95-106, 1994.

Meyers SM: A twin study on age-related macular degeneration, *Trans Am Ophthalmol Soc* 92:775-843, 1994.

18

THE VITREOUS HUMOR

The vitreous humor, a transparent tissue with the physical properties of a gel, fills the largest chamber of the eye, the vitreous cavity. It comprises about two thirds of the volume (4.5 mL) and about three fourths of the weight of the eye. Normally it fills the entire vitreous cavity (Fig 18-1), and its collagen fibers blend with the fibers of the internal limiting membrane of the retina. The vitreous humor, 99% water, is a physiologic and biologic gel. Its collagen meshwork contains long, coiled hyaluronic acid molecules that retain water and provide its viscosity. There are a few large, flat cells, hyalocytes, that function as connective tissue macrophages.

The vitreous humor consists of a peripheral cortex and a central region. The cortex is but 0.1 mm thick and contains many more fibrils than the central vitreous to which it sends a delicate meshwork. The vitreous base, a band of cortex about 4 mm wide, straddles the ora serrata and is attached firmly to the peripheral retina and the ciliary body. Retinal holes, which initiate retinal detachments, are common along the retinal border of the vitreous base. In the young, but not the aged, the cortical vitreous attaches to the posterior lens capsule of the crystalline lens, near the full circumference of the equator (the hyaloid-capsular ligament of Weigert). The posterior cortical vitreous humor is attached to the periphery of the optic disk but not to its surface.

Aging, injury, and retinal disease disturb the suspension of water in the vitreous humor and cause it to contract. The contraction is not uniform, and portions of the cortical vitreous may adhere to the retinal surface and cause a tractional retinal hole. With loss of the gel structure, nearly transparent membranes and fine fibers in the contracted vitreous become visible and annoy the individual. In diabetic retinopathy (see Chapter 27) new blood vessels never invade the normal vitreous humor but readily proliferate in the contracted vitreous.

SYMPTOMS AND SIGNS OF DISEASE

Abnormalities of the vitreous humor are the result of (1) cells, membranes, and protein aggregates being imaged on the retina ("floaters"); (2) loss of the gel structure with the vitreous contracting and a grossly clear fluid filling the space that once contained normal vitreous humor; and (3) traction by vitreous strands on the sensory retina. The surface of the vitreous sometimes provides the skeleton on which retinal glia and blood vessel adventitial cells proliferate (vitreoretinal proliferation). Minute fragments of the hyaloid artery, which nurtured the eye in embryonic life and then atrophied, may be seen darting to and fro (muscae volitantes) when gazing at a bright blue sky. In disease states, blood cells, membranes, and clumps of protein may float across the visual axis and impair vision, sometimes markedly.

Photopsia is an important symptom that results from traction of the vitreous on the sensory retina and may signal actual or impending retinal tear formation. Shrinkage of the vitreous causes a variety of entoptic phenomena that can be seen with the eyes closed or in the dark. As the eyes move, the shrunken vitreous

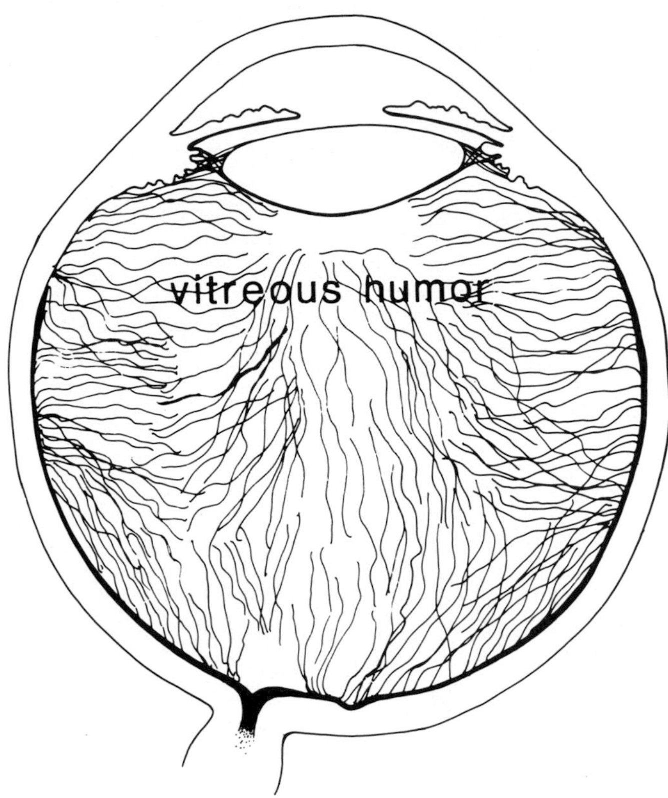

FIG 18-1.
The vitreous humor fills the vitreous cavity of the eye. The vitreous humor is firmly adherent at the pars plana of the ciliary body and the ora serrata of the retina, the vitreous base. It is adherent to the circumference of the optic disk but not to its surface. The surface of the vitreous humor anterior to the vitreous base is the anterior hyaloid, and that portion of its surface adjacent to the sensory retina is the posterior hyaloid.

gently bumps the retina, initiating a nervous impulse and perception of light.

The vitreous humor is studied with an indirect ophthalmoscope and a convex lens so that opacities are visible against the red background of the fundus. It may be studied with a biomicroscope and either a −50- or a −90-diopter contact lens equipped with inclined mirrors to study the ocular periphery. Gross vitreous opacities can be seen with a direct ophthalmoscope.

DEGENERATIONS

Syneresis.—Syneresis describes the physical chemical change in a gel that occurs when it contracts with loss of fluid. Syneresis occurs in the vitreous humor in aging, after injuries, and in inflammations of the eye. The condition is caused by depolymerization of hyaluronic acid and a breakdown of the collagen network of the vitreous humor. The vitreous cavity is partially or completely filled with fluid (Fig 18-2), which creates the ophthalmoscopic appearance of membranes or strands floating in front of the retina. Patients find the appearance of these strands annoying, and occasionally they are so numerous as to reduce vision. Correction of any refractive error will minimize symptoms but will not restore the normal viscosity and structure of the vitreous. Portions of the vitreous may not detach from the sensory retina and retract to cause retinal tears, folds, cystoid edema, and preretinal membranes.

Posterior vitreous detachment.—The vitreous humor is firmly attached to the circumference but not to the surface of the optic disk. With aging, particularly in eyes with more than 3 diopters of myopia (see Chapter 24), syneresis of the central portion of the vitreous humor adjacent to the optic disk causes a fluid-filled space

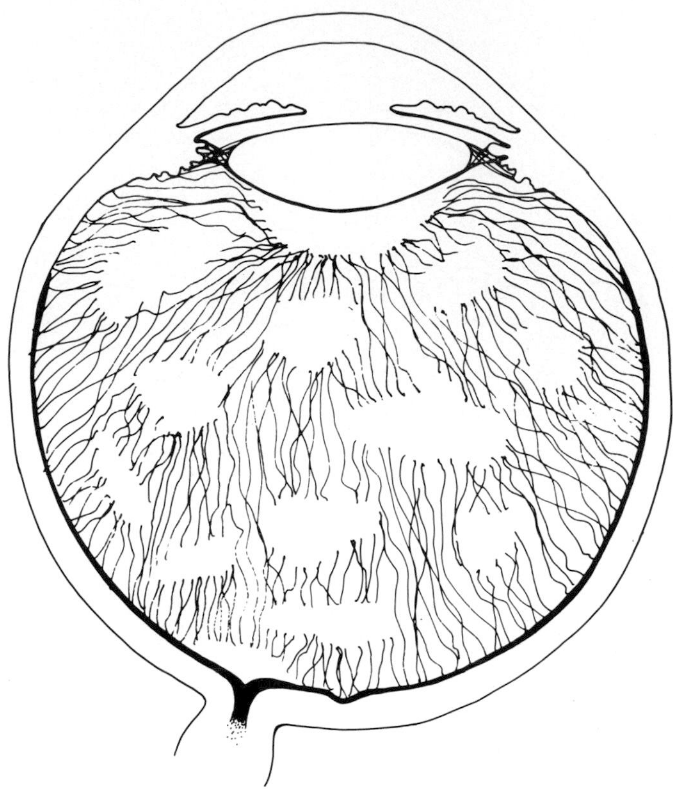

FIG 18-2.
Syneresis with fluid-filled spaces in the vitreous humor.

in front of the disk (Fig 18-3). A ring-shaped opacity is often visible ophthalmoscopically, on the posterior surface of the contracted site of attachment of the vitreous to the margin of the optic disk. Posterior vitreous detachment occurs most commonly in women between 55 and 65 years of age. They suddenly notice a relatively large, fixed floater near the point of fixation. As the individual attempts to fix on the floater, it darts out of the field of vision. There may be subjective light flashes, so that with the eyes closed or in a dark room a sudden movement of the eye causes a flash of light, which is caused either by vitreous traction on the retina or by the detached vitreous bumping the retina. The fellow eye usually becomes involved within a few months. There is no effective treatment, although with time the floater tends to become less apparent to the patient. Traction on a retinal vein may cause a minute hemorrhage and a greater likelihood of subsequent retinal detachments than when floaters or light flashes are the only symptoms.

The disturbance of the vitreoretinal interface may lead to several abnormalities of the retina. Accessory retina astroglia may migrate from the inner retinal layers and proliferate on the posterior surface of the detached vitreous to form an epiretinal membrane. The membranes are clinically subtle and may be symptomless or reduce vision. Surface wrinkling retinopathy likely originates similarly, but the irregularity of the retinal surface dominates the clinical condition.

A more severe group of related conditions includes macular pucker after retinal detachment surgery, preretinal macular fibrosis, and star folds of the retina.

The most severe condition initiated by detachment of the vitreous is massive vitreous retraction or massive periretinal proliferation, which complicates retinal detachment surgery. After surgery the detached retina develops fixed folds, and the vitreous is sprinkled with pigmented cells. Cells from the retinal pigment epithelium proliferate on the inner and outer

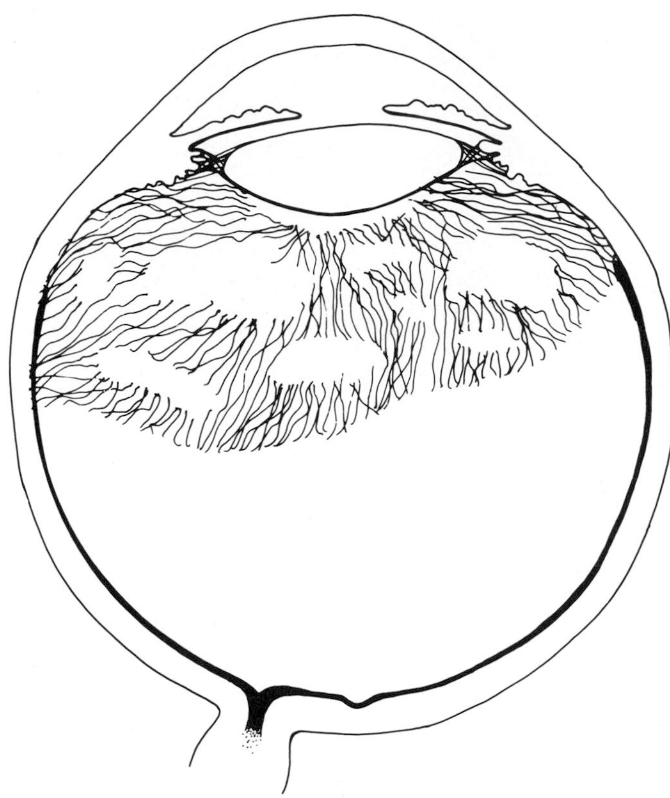

FIG 18-3.
Vitreous detachment with fluid-filled optically empty space between the retina and posterior hyaloid.

surfaces of the sensory retina, and irreversible blindness is a frequent outcome.

Vitreous adhesion is a destructive phenomenon in which contraction of the vitreous causes traction on the retinal areas to which it is normally attached (Fig 18-4). Shrinkage in the peripheral region may cause a horseshoe-shaped tear, with the flap held open by the persistent attachment of vitreous. Traction by the vitreous in the region of the ora serrata may be a factor in the production of peripheral retinal holes or retinal dialysis.

Hereditary vitreous degeneration.—Hereditary degeneration of the vitreous and retina (hyaloideoretinopathy) may occur because of genetic abnormalities of either tissue. The following are discussed elsewhere: recessive X chromosome–linked juvenile retinoschisis; lattice degeneration of the retina; familial exudative vitreoretinopathy; hereditary degenerative myopia; facial clefting syndrome; and familial primary amyloidosis. Other forms of inherited vitreoretinal degeneration include hyaloideotapetoretinal degeneration of Goldmann-Favre, hyaloideoretinopathy of Wagner, and arthro-ophthalmopathy of Sticker.

Hyaloideotapetoretinal dystrophy of Goldmann-Favre is an autosomal recessive progressive disorder that includes a liquid vitreous humor, vitreous veils with central and peripheral retinoschisis, retinitis pigmentosa, and complicated cataracts. Blindness ultimately results.

Dominantly inherited hyaloideoretinopathy of Wagner is associated with liquefaction and destruction of the vitreous humor with grayish white avascular preretinal membranes, myopia, cataracts, and pigmentary degeneration of the retina.

Arthro-ophthalmopathy of Stickler is an autosomal dominant disorder of connective tissue, which shows nearly complete penetrance but markedly variable expressivity. There are 8 to 18 diopters of myopia and a vitreoretinal degeneration that leads to retinal detachment. Retinal

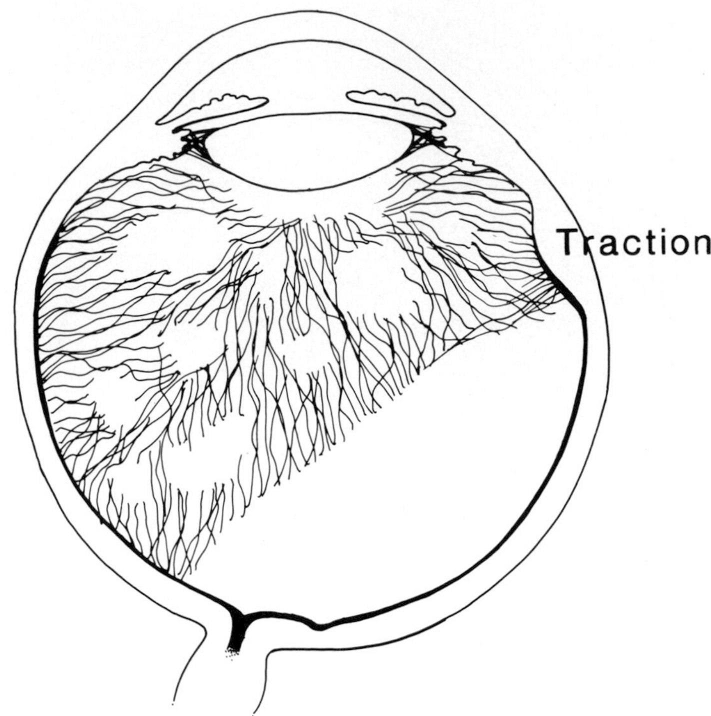

FIG 18-4.
Detachment of the vitreous humor with persistent adhesion on the right side that may cause traction on the retina and a retinal tear.

detachment is prevented by means of an encircling plastic band (see Chapter 17). Prophylactic laser photocoagulation of the peripheral retina is not effective.

Strabismus with amblyopia occurs and cataract is common after age 40 years. The mandible and tongue may be small, with a cleft palate (Pierre Robin syndrome). The skeletal abnormalities vary widely: spondyloepiphyseal dysplasia, hyperextensible joints, abnormalities of pelvic bones, and muscular hypoplasia. Sensorineural deafness and mitral valve prolapse may occur.

VITREOUS OPACITIES

Many foreign substances may be suspended in the vitreous body: (1) exogenous material, such as parasites or foreign bodies; or (2) endogenous substances, such as leukocytes or erythrocytes from the blood, retinal pigment epithelium, tumor cells, cholesterol, or calcium salts. Each causes the symptoms of floaters and may reduce vision. The sudden appearance of a shower of opacities suggests vitreous traction causing rupture of a retinal blood vessel, resulting in a hemorrhage and possible retinal tear. A large opacity of relatively fixed position suggests a less serious abnormality. Whatever the appearance of the opacities, examination of the peripheral fundus with dilation of the pupils and indirect ophthalmoscopy are required to exclude a retinal hole as the cause.

Muscae volitantes.—These physiologic opacities consist of minute residues of the primitive hyaloidal vascular system that begins to atrophy in embryonic life. An individual may image them in bright illumination, against a cloudless sky, or against a pastel-shaded wall. They drift in and out of the visual field and dart from the field of vision on attempts to fixate directly on them. Some patients, after first observing them, require reassurance about their universal occurrence. Correction of ametropia makes the opacities more difficult to see.

Hemorrhage.—The moment that the retina tears may be signaled by a minute hemorrhage into the vitreous body as the vitreous traction tears the sensory retina and ruptures a retinal blood vessel. The sudden appearance of diffusely scattered dots is a signal for immediate examination to locate a possible retinal tear and close it before a retinal detachment occurs.

Bleeding into the vitreous humor results from rupture of newly formed, fragile blood vessels that originate from the optic disk or retina. Neovascularization may be caused by trauma, inflammation, vascular and metabolic disease, tumors, or rupture of a subhyaloid retinal hemorrhage secondary to a subarachnoid hemorrhage (Terson). The blood may be evenly dispersed throughout the vitreous humor, localized, or distributed in sheets. In a young person resorption may be rapid, but persistent or recurrent hemorrhages are followed by yellow or white debris and fibrous membranes in the vitreous humor. The symptoms depend on the location of the vitreous hemorrhage. Blood in the retinal periphery causes floaters, whereas blood in the visual axis reduces vision and may result in reddish, hazy vision. Vitreous hemorrhage may reduce vision because of inflammation, glaucoma, siderosis, or fibrous tissue proliferation that contracts to cause retinal detachment. Vitrectomy through the pars plana removes diseased or opacified vitreous and membranes.

Asteroid hyalosis.—This is an age-related, mainly monocular degeneration that predominantly affects men, in which hundreds to thousands of stellate or discoid ("snowball") opacities are suspended throughout or in a portion of a solid vitreous. They are creamy white when viewed with the ophthalmoscope and sparkle like Christmas ornaments in the illumination of a biomicroscope. The opacities consist of various calcium-containing lipids and apparently result from degeneration of vitreous fibrils. They are suspended in vitreous of normal viscosity. They cause no symptoms and, although they obscure the view of the fundus, they do not indicate disease, cause symptoms, or require treatment.

Cholesterolosis bulbi.—This abnormality was known, inaccurately, during much of the 20th century as synchysis scintillans. The vitreous need not be liquefied, and the crystals may occur in the iris and retina. Cholesterol crystals occur in blind eyes together with retinal detachment or may be secondary to severe ocular disease or injury. They are mainly observed in enucleated eyes. If the lens has been removed, the crystals may be located in both the anterior chamber and in the vitreous cavity.

Persistent hyperplastic primary vitreous.—The primary vitreous is a fibrillar meshwork that bridges the region between the lens vesicle and the inner wall of the optic cup. At the 11-mm stage of gestation, the primary vitreous is invaded by mesoderm and intermingles with the elaborate vasa hyaloidea propria. The hyaloid vascular system begins to atrophy at the 60-mm stage, and by the eighth month of gestation the process is completed, leaving only minute remnants visible as muscae volitantes.

Failure of the hyaloid artery to regress, combined with the hyperplasia of the posterior portion of the vascular meshwork of the embryonic lens (tunica vasculosa lentis), produces persistent hyperplastic primary vitreous. This monocular condition occurs in full-term infants. The eye fails to develop and is smaller than the fellow eye, and the initially clear lens becomes opaque. Immediately behind the lens is a pinkish white fibrous mass that may vary in size from a small plaque to one entirely covering the posterior surface of a shrunken lens. Traction elongates the ciliary processes that extend to the mass. The equator of the lens is smaller than normal. The anterior chamber is shallow. The tissue posterior to the lens is vascular, and the vessels radiate from the center. The posterior capsule may rupture and cause cataract. Buphthalmos may develop.

The elongation of the ciliary processes, the microphthalmos, and the rupture of the posterior lens capsule occurring in one eye of a full-term, normal-weight infant distinguish the condition from microphthalmos, retinoblastoma, retinopathy of prematurity, retinal dysplasia, and congenital cataract. Computed tomography may indicate persistence of intraocular fetal vasculature.

Early removal of the lens is necessary to preserve the eye. Some vision, but usually not normal vision, is retained, but without lens extraction the eye is destined to require removal because of glaucoma. Preferably, the lens is removed together with the retrolenticular membrane by means of a suction-aspiration-cutting instrument. Patients should be operated on as early as possible (1 to 28 days of age). Optical correction with a contact lens immediately thereafter may prevent amblyopia.

Macular holes.—Macular holes are round, sharply defined, red holes of the fovea centralis that measure ¼ to ⅓ disk diameter and reduce visual acuity to 20/200. They may complicate intraocular inflammation or follow blunt ocular trauma, intraocular surgery, or gazing at the sun (solar retinopathy). Most instances are caused by tangential traction of the cortical vitreous on the posterior pole in individuals more than 60 years of age.

In the impending stage, which lasts a few weeks to a few months, there is detachment of the fovea centralis with metamorphopsia and a minimal decrease of vision. In about one half of the patients, the attached vitreous humor spontaneously detaches with recovery. Ultrasonography of the posterior pole of the eye confirms the vitreous traction. Vitrectomy with removal of the attached vitreous prevents progression and relieves the symptoms. The symptoms at this stage are minimal, the surgery is difficult, and many patients with monocular involvement are reluctant to undergo a major surgical procedure for a condition that has a 50% chance of disappearing without treatment. If there is a fully developed hole in the fellow eye, the need for prompt surgery is more evident.

Persistent vitreous traction leads to detachment of the fovea centralis that appears bright red and surrounded by a yellowish ring, a lamellar hole. The hole is hyperfluorescent on angiography, and round white deposits occur on the surface of the retinal pigment epithelium. Within 3 to 6 months the hole affects all layers of the fovea, and visual acuity is reduced to 20/70 to 20/400. An operculum may float in its center. Most holes show no further progression with time, but photoreceptor degeneration occurs in some.

Vitrectomy with removal of the bands of vitreous traction, including excision when adherent, may improve visual acuity. Vitreous tamponade (see Chapter 17) with perfluoropropane gas combined with transforming growth factor beta 2, a chorioretinal adhesive agent, may partially restore central visual acuity.

PROLIFERATIVE VITREORETINOPATHY

Proliferative vitreoretinopathy is the most common complication that causes operations to correct retinal detachments to fail. Cells that originate from the retinal pigment epithelium and glial elements of the sensory retina proliferate within the vitreous cavity and coat the inner and outer surfaces of the sensory retina. Previous uveitis, ocular trauma, and intraocular blood are predisposing factors. The tissue, in minor cases of proliferation, may be too thin to be observed directly but causes folds in the detached retina. The folds remain in a fixed position with ocular rotations. The vitreous may appear hazy, and there may be pigment clumps on the inner surface of the retina. In moderately severe cases the retinal surface is wrinkled, the blood vessels are tortuous, and the posterior edge of a retinal hole may be everted. Fixed folds form in one or more quadrants of the retina in a more advanced condition. In the most severe cases, massive proliferative vitreoretinopathy, all quadrants of the retina contain fixed folds that may contract from a wide funnel to a closed funnel so that the optic nerve cannot be observed.

Treatment is exceptionally difficult, and the visual results, which depend largely on the cause of the proliferative vitreoretinopathy, are often poor. Note that peripheral vision, however limited, is preferable to no light perception. Scleral buckling, relaxing retinotomies, and removal of retinal membranes are often necessary to bring the sensory retina into apposition with the retinal pigment epithelium. Retinal tamponade with gas, silicone oil, or both may be required. Removal of cataract or a clear crystalline lens may be required for visualization of the peripheral retina. A successful apposition of the retina may be subsequently complicated by a secondary glaucoma.

VITRECTOMY

Simultaneous removal and replacement of the vitreous humor with balanced saline solution, which is soon replaced by the body fluids, is indicated in patients with vitreous opacities that cause legal blindness or in patients with complications of intraocular surgery, inflammation, trauma, or complicated retinal separations (Table 18-1). Additionally, vitrectomy is often performed to remove vitreous membranes that reduce vision. Some legally blind patients who could benefit from the procedure are not aware of the possible improvement in vision. The primary disorder that caused the abnormal vitreous humor may also have seriously damaged

TABLE 18-1.
Indications for Vitrectomy

I. Persistent vitreous opacity with legal blindness
   A. Proliferative vitreoretinopathy
   B. Vitreous amyloidosis
   C. Preretinal membranes
   D. Vitreous membranes and strands
II. Complications of cataract extraction
   A. Excision of epiretinal membranes
   B. Pupillary block glaucoma
   C. Loss of vitreous
   D. Incarceration of vitreous in wound with traction
III. Endophthalmitis with vitreous abscess
IV. Trauma
   A. Anterior chamber reconstruction
   B. Intraocular nonmagnetic foreign bodies
V. Complicated retinal detachments
   A. Vitreous adhesion syndromes
      1. Vitreoretinopathy
      2. Massive vitreous retraction
      3. Localized traction
      4. Transvitreal membranes
   B. Giant retinal tears
VI. Persistent hyperplastic primary vitreous
VII. Malignant glaucoma

the retina or caused glaucoma so that substitution of a clear vitreous does not improve vision.

The procedure is of no value if the retina is not functional, but cataract or severe opacification of the vitreous may make evaluation of retinal function difficult. Ideal patients are able to visualize their retinal blood vessels as a penlight moves against the lower eyelid (entoptic visualization). Bright-flash electroretinography should be normal. The visual-evoked potential to bright flash should be normal. The pupillary response and light projection should be normal. The anterior chamber angle and iris should be free of new blood vessels; glaucoma should not be present.

Unfortunately, most patients are not ideal surgical candidates. Light projection may be poor, but light perception must be present. The prognosis is poor if the electroretinogram is nonrecordable. Rubeosis of the iris or anterior chamber angle is often a contraindication. Patients with dense membranes attached to the retina or generalized retinal detachment have a

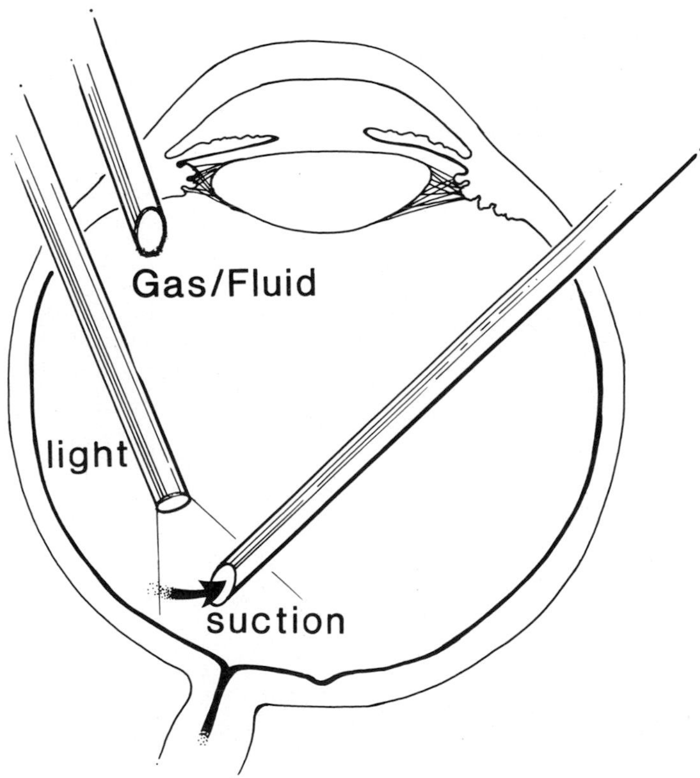

FIG 18-5.
Basic intravitreal surgery unit. The gas/fluid part maintains the intraocular pressure and prevents collapse of the eye. The suction/cutter removes membranes and vitreous. It is guided by the endoscopic light.

poor prognosis. Eyes that have become soft and disorganized (phthisis bulbi) respond poorly. Most of the patients with a good prognosis have improved vision after vitrectomy.

Vitrectomy is performed through a small incision in the pars plana. The eye retains its shape, as vitreous and membranes are removed by suction and cutting, by the simultaneous infusion of saline into the vitreous cavity. The intraocular pressure must be maintained at a near-normal level because the eye collapses if the pressure is too low, and the central retinal artery is closed if the pressure is too high. A pressure of between 25 and 35 mm Hg is considered optimal. The infusion-aspiration is combined with one of several types of scissors or rotating or chopping cutters. (Ultrasound fragmenters, although useful in lens extraction, are usually not helpful in vitrectomy.) In adults, if a clear crystalline lens is present, the operation is usually carried out through a scleral incision in the pars plana about 4 mm posterior to the corneoscleral limbus in the temporal quadrant slightly above or below the horizontal meridian and its long ciliary artery. A cataractous lens is removed with the same or a slightly modified instrument. The small eye in infants necessitates the removal of the crystalline lens even if transparent.

The procedure is performed under direct microscopic observation of the vitreous, the retina, and the instruments within the vitreous cavity. Many types of cutters have been designed to cut membranes with minimal traction on the retina.

The operations may be divided into those in which the anterior vitreous is removed and those in which both the anterior and posterior vitreous is removed. Vitreous membranes may be removed at the same time (Fig 18-5).

Rubeosis iridis and glaucoma are the most common complications. After removal of the lens, an angiogenic factor, possibly that responsible for retinal neovascularization, may have easier access to the iris and may aggravate a preexisting rubeosis iridis or stimulate additional neovascularization.

Glaucoma occurs because of rubeosis iridis or obstruction of the trabecular meshwork by the cell membranes of erythrocytes (ghost cells) that persist after a vitreous hemorrhage. The cells cannot enter the anterior chamber when the lens is present; however, after lens extraction and vitrectomy with rupture of the anterior hyaloid face, these cells are free to circulate through the eye. Glaucoma occurs in as many as one third of the eyes that have had vitrectomy-lens extraction. To provide clear media, every effort must be made to irrigate the vitreous cavity adequately at the time of surgery.

BIBLIOGRAPHY

Book

Morse PH: *Vitreoretinal disease,* St Louis, 1989, Mosby–Year Book.

Article

Lindgren G, Sjödell L, Lindblom B: A prospective study of dense spontaneous vitreous hemorrhage, *Am J Ophthalmol* 119:458-465, 1995.

19

INTRAOCULAR INFLAMMATIONS

Inflammations of the inner eye may be divided as follows: suppurative or nonsuppurative; endogenous or exogenous (mainly trauma); and infectious or noninfectious. The suppurative types include panophthalmitis, in which the entire eye including the sclera and cornea is inflamed, and endophthalmitis, in which the outer layers of the eye are minimally inflamed and the globe does not rupture.

Nonsuppurative inflammations may occur because of exogenous or endogenous causes. The causative exogenous agent is introduced from the outside directly into the eye through an incision or laceration in the cornea or sclera. Endogenous inflammations result from the following: (1) an autoimmune response of intraocular tissue; (2) a systemic disease or abnormality; or (3) an intraocular abnormality, such as a hypermature cataract.

A variety of terms are used to describe intraocular inflammations (Table 19-1).

The iris and anterior portion of the ciliary body share a common blood supply and are often inflamed simultaneously (iridocyclitis). The posterior portion of the ciliary body and the anterior choroid and retina may be inflamed simultaneously (intermediate uveitis). Inflammations of the posterior choroid rarely affect the anterior uvea but often extend to the adjacent retina (chorioretinitis).

Inflammatory cells from an anterior uveitis enter the aqueous humor and may adhere to the cornea (keratic precipitates). Inflammatory adhesions between the iris and the anterior lens capsule (posterior synechiae) may distort the circular shape of the pupil. If the entire pupillary circumference is bound to the lens by adhesions (iris bombé), the flow of aqueous humor from the posterior to the anterior chamber is blocked and the iris balloons forward, causing a secondary pupillary block glaucoma.

Inflammation of the choroid often affects the overlying retina, resulting in a loss of vision. Inflammatory cells and protein from the ciliary body and choroid may cloud the vitreous humor and reduce vision.

SUPPURATIVE INFLAMMATION

A suppurative intraocular inflammation (Table 19-2) is caused mainly by pyogenic (pus-producing) bacteria and rarely by fungi. In exogenous infection the organisms are introduced into the eye after an accidental or surgical penetrating wound, after rupture of a corneal ulcer, or through a thin filtering bleb after glaucoma surgery. A septicemia from any cause may infect the eyes and must be considered in any sudden loss of vision in a patient with other signs of systemic infection, particularly after genitourinary surgery or dental procedures. Endogenous septic emboli may infect the eye in bacterial endocarditis or during the bacteremic stage of meningococcic meningitis.

Panophthalmitis.—Panophthalmitis is an acute suppurative inflammation of the inner eye with necrosis of the sclera, and sometimes the cornea. The causes are mainly bacterial. The incubation period is only a few hours, and the disease follows a fulminating course. The eyelids are red and swollen, and there is severe chemosis of the conjunctiva. Extension to the orbit may cause proptosis. The cornea is often a whitish mass of necrotic tissue. If there has been a laceration or surgical incision, pus exudes from the wound. There may be severe ocular pain, and the globe may rupture. The signs gradually subside, and the eye becomes a shrunken mass of fibrous tissue (phthisis bulbi).

Although often not successful, treatment must be prompt and vigorous. Because the causative organism and its antibiotic sensitivity are not known, broad-spectrum antibiotics to which penicillinase-producing staphylococci and gram-negative bacteria are sensitive are used systemically, topically, subconjunctivally, and intraocularly. The pus from the wound, the aqueous humor, and the vitreous humor are stained and cultured. Initial treatment is based on the findings of the Gram stain, but in about half the patients no organism is found. A vitrectomy removes microbes and leukocytes. Filtration of the intraocular irrigating fluid through a Millipore filter may concentrate the organisms for staining and identification.

Initial antibiotic therapy is modified as necessary on the result of culture and antibiotic sensitivity of the organism. Systemic corticosteroids may reduce the fibroblastic response to inflammation. When bacterial infection is suspected and intravitreal antibiotic therapy is indicated, vancomycin (1 mg; see Chapter 2) is often used initially. Gram-negative organisms cause suppurative intraocular inflammations far less often than gram-positive organisms do. Intravitreal aminoglycosides damage the retina and should be used only for infections by proven gram-negative organisms.

Endophthalmitis.—Endophthalmitis is a suppurative inflammation of the intraocular contents in which not all layers of the globe are affected and in which the eye does not rupture. Endophthalmitis follows penetrating wounds of the eye (either surgical or accidental), metastatic infections, or intraocular foreign bodies. The onset is less violent than that of panophthalmitis, and the inflammation gradually increases in severity. Fungi, necrosis of intraocular tumors, and retained intraocular foreign bodies often cause a purulent endophthalmitis. Leukocytes may accumulate in the anterior chamber (hypopyon), and the vitreous body may be filled with inflammatory cells. Treatment is the same as for panophthalmitis.

TABLE 19-1.
Intraocular Inflammation

I. Suppurative
   A. Entire eye (panophthalmitis)
   B. Interior of eye (endophthalmitis)
II. Nonsuppurative
   A. Panuveitis
      1. Iris, ciliary body, choroid, retina, vitreous
   B. Anterior uveitis
      1. Iris (iritis)
      2. Pars plicata ciliaris (anterior cyclitis)
      3. Iris and pars plicata ciliaris (iridocyclitis)
   C. Intermediate uveitis
      1. Pars plana ciliaris and adjacent choroid and retina (pars planitis)
   D. Posterior uveitis
      1. Choroid (choroiditis [focal, multifocal, or diffuse])
      2. Choroid and retina (chorioretinitis)
      3. Retina and choroid (retinochoroiditis)
      4. Vitreous humor (vitreitis)

TABLE 19-2.
Suppurative Intraocular Inflammations

I. Exogenous
   A. Intraocular infection with pus-producing bacteria after accidental or surgical penetrating wound, rupture of corneal ulcer, or microbial invasion of filtering bleb after glaucoma surgery
II. Endogenous
   A. Septic emboli in bacterial endocarditis, meningococcemia, bacteremia, viremia, and fungemia; septic emboli after dental or urologic surgery
   B. Spread from adjacent structure: orbital abscess, pharyngeal phycomycosis

NONSUPPURATIVE INTRAOCULAR INFLAMMATION

Nonsuppurative inflammations of the inner eye may have an exogenous or endogenous cause (Table 19-3). Exogenous, nonsuppurative inflammations mainly follow injuries to the eye, chemical burns of the eye, and inflammation of the cornea. Endogenous, nonsuppurative inflammations may occur secondary to a local ocular disease or may have no obvious cause, often because of a presumed intraocular autoimmune reaction, which accompanies a systemic disease.

In the past, acute inflammation was classed as a nongranulomatous type of uveitis and chronic inflammation was classed as a granulomatous type of uveitis (Table 19-4). Nongranulomatous inflammations were considered to be the result of previous systemic infection, particularly by streptococci. Granulomatous inflammations were thought to be caused by delayed hypersensitivity (see Chapter 25) such as that which occurs in tubercle infection in a previously infected individual. Granulomas, however, do not occur in most chronic inflammations, even those that have a prominent epithelioid cell reaction.

Symptoms and signs of retinitis and uveitis.—The symptoms of nonsuppurative uveitis vary with the portion of the uveal tract involved. Visual loss is the main symptom of foveal edema, or intermediate and posterior uveitis. Anterior uveitis may initially cause pain, photophobia, and lacrimation. Pain is common in anterior iridocyclitis and is particularly severe when associated with keratitis. It centers in the periorbital and ocular region and is aggravated by exposure to light and by pressure on the eye. Photophobia varies in severity and may be so severe that the eyelids cannot be opened to examine the eye. Lacrimation is usually proportionate to the degree of photophobia. Decreased vision occurs because of exudation of cells, protein-rich inflammatory fluid, and fibrin into either the anterior chamber or vitreous body. Inflammation of the choroid beneath the fovea centralis causes a marked decrease in vision that is disproportionate to the apparent severity of choroidal inflammation. Choroidal inflammation, which is distant from the posterior pole, although damaging to the overlying retina, may cause only minimal changes in the peripheral visual field. Severe inflammation of both the anterior and posterior portions of the inner eye causes swelling of the

TABLE 19-3.
Nonsuppurative Inflammation of the Uvea (Iris, Ciliary Body, and Choroid) and Retina

- I. Exogenous
  - A. Foreign body granuloma; chemical burns; contusions
  - B. Ocular surgery
- II. Endogenous
  - A. Ocular immune reaction
    1. To intraocular contents
       - a. Hypermature cataract; phacoanaphylactica; granulomatous scleritis
    2. Primary ocular autoimmune disorder
       - a. Sympathetic ophthalmia; birdshot retinochoroidopathy; heterochromic iridocyclitis; idiopathic uveitis (iridocyclitis, intermediate uveitis); posterior uveoretinitis; serpiginous choroiditis
    3. Systemic autoimmune disorders with ocular inflammation
       - a. Vogt-Koyanagi-Harada disease; ankylosing spondylitis; rheumatoid arthritis (juvenile, adult); Reiter syndrome; Behçet disease; bowel disease (ulcerative colitis, Whipple); Wegener granulomatosis; lupus erythematosus
    4. Systemic autoimmune disorders with ocular signs
       - a. Insulin-dependent diabetes mellitus
       - b. Hyperthyroidism
       - c. Sjögren syndrome
       - d. Multiple sclerosis
       - e. Myasthenia gravis
       - f. Cicatrizing conjunctivitis
    5. Infectious systemic disease with ocular immune reaction
       - a. Bacteria
         Treponema pallidum: retinitis; *Mycobacterium tuberculosis, M. leprae:* chorioretinitis; *Borrelia burgdorferi* (Lyme disease); *Rickettsia rickettsii; Propionibacterium acnes*
       - b. Viruses
         Human immunodeficiency virus (HIV); herpes simplex; varicella-zoster (acute retinal necrosis); cytomegalovirus (retinitis); rubeola (retinitis [subacute sclerosing panencephalitis])
       - c. Fungi
         Candida sp.: retinochoroiditis; *Cryptococcus neoformans;* choroiditis; *Coccidioides immitis:* choroiditis; *Histoplasma capsulatum* (chorioretinitis)
       - d. Parasites
         Toxoplasma gondii (retinochoroiditis); *Pneumocystis carinii:* choroiditis; *Toxocara canis* (larva): toxocariasis; *Taenia solium* (larva): cysticercosis
    6. Noninfectious inflammations
       - a. Sarcoidosis; juvenile xanthogranuloma; familial chronic granulomatous disease of childhood; lymphoma; granuloma annulare

TABLE 19-4.
Characteristics of Acute and Chronic Uveitis

	Chronic	Acute
	Anterior uvea	
Pain, photophobia	Minimal or absent	Severe
Vision	Gradual reduction	Abrupt reduction
Course	Protracted, remissions, and exacerbations	Self-limited, (1-6 weeks), often recurrent
Keratic deposits	Heavy, coalescent, often "mutton fat," crenated margins, macrophages, phagocytized pigment	Pinpoint
Aqueous humor	Few cells, often large, variable aqueous flare	Many cells, intense aqueous flare, sometimes protein coagulation
Iris nodules and precipitates	Frequent	None
	Posterior uvea	
Retinal and subretinal edema	Usually slight or moderate and localized around exudates	Marked and generalized, with blurring of neuroretinal margins and retinal vascular bed
Choroidal exudates	Heavy massive exudates with edges blurred by surrounding retinal and subretinal edema	No heavy massive exudates, occasionally localized areas of deeper infiltration
Secondary retinal involvement	Almost invariable, with retinal destruction	None or limited to pigment epithelium and rods and cones
Residual organic damage	Heavy glial scars with massive pigment surrounding the lesion	None or fine granular changes in pigment epithelium with damage to neuroepithelium and superficial gliosis
Anterior segment changes	Sometimes mutton-fat keratic deposits	Usually none
Vitreous changes	Usually heavy vitreous blurring; heavy veil-like opacities frequent	Slight to intense general blurring, fine, stringlike, fibrinous opacities

optic disk (papillitis) and central cystoid edema that reduce vision.

Ciliary injection.—Dilation and congestion of the anterior ciliary arteries that nurture the iris and ciliary body are referred to as ciliary injection, which must be distinguished from conjunctival injection seen in conjunctivitis (see Chapter 12). The severity varies with the site of inflammation. Little or no ciliary injection occurs in intermediate or posterior uveitis. In severe anterior iridocyclitis there may be associated episcleral and conjunctival injection and conjunctival edema. In less severe inflammation there is a deep circumcorneal injection with a violet hue. The injection fades in the conjunctival fornix and does not blanch when 1:1,000 epinephrine is instilled in the cul-de-sac.

Exudation into the anterior chamber.—Inflammation of the iris and ciliary body releases prostaglandins, particularly from the anterior ciliary body, and breaks down the blood-aqueous barrier, so that increased protein, fibrin, and inflammatory cells enter the aqueous humor. The protein causes a translucence of the aqueous humor, called aqueous flare, which can be seen with the biomicroscope. The lymphocytes are suspended in the aqueous humor and, because of thermal convection currents, rise when close to the iris and descend near the cooler cornea. Keratic precipitates adhere to the corneal endothelium. Two main types occur: (1) large, greasy-appearing ("mutton-fat") keratic precipitates composed of epithelioid cells, macrophages, and phagocytized pigment cells; and (2) small, white, punctate accumulations composed of lymphocytes. Clumps of macrophages occur at the pupillary margin (Koeppe nodules), on the surface of the iris (floccules of Busacca), on the lens surface, and in the anterior chamber angle. Occasionally in acute iridocyclitis so many granulocytes are present that a hypopyon forms, or, rarely, diapedesis of erythrocytes causes a hyphema.

Iris changes.—In acute iridocyclitis, the pupil may be constricted or in mid-dilation. The iris may be edematous with its pattern blurred ("muddy") and the capillaries engorged. In chronic iridocyclitis, nodules may originate from proliferation of the iris pigment epithelium or infiltration of the iris with round cells and macrophages. Typical granulomatous nodules such as tubercles or sarcoid nodules may be found. Their resolution may be followed by a patchy area of iris atrophy. Diffuse iris atrophy with loss of iris pattern follows prolonged iridocyclitis and may involve both the stroma (mesodermal) and pigment (ectodermal) layers.

Posterior synechiae.—These adhesions bind the iris to the anterior lens capsule. They cause a small, irregular pupil that does not constrict to light in the area of the adhesions. Sometimes small or large clumps of iris pigment remain on the anterior lens capsule or cornea, a sign of past or present iritis or ocular trauma.

Intraocular pressure.—Uveitis decreases the secretion of aqueous humor; the intraocular pressure is usually low. Glaucoma may occur by one of several mechanisms. Topical instillation of corticosteroids in genetically susceptible individuals increases resistance to outflow from the anterior chamber, as happens in open-angle glaucoma. The trabecular meshwork may be inflamed or occluded with inflammatory cells and protein in severe acute iridocyclitis. Repeated or prolonged inflammation damages the trabecular meshwork and leads to a permanent glaucoma that is similar to open-angle glaucoma.

Pupillary block by posterior synechiae causes an angle-closure glaucoma by preventing the passage of the aqueous humor from the posterior to the anterior chamber (iris bombé). Peripheral anterior synechiae may form between the iris and the cornea because of a shallow anterior chamber, exudate between the two structures, or edema of the root of the iris or ciliary body.

The treatment of glaucoma complicating uveitis requires a balance between measures directed against the increased intraocular pressure and those used to treat the inflammation. If increased intraocular pressure is caused by corticosteroids, their use is reduced. The pupil is not constricted. Carbonic anhydrase inhibitors are used systemically and often combined with the local instillation of epinephrine and topical beta blockers. In iris bombé, the ballooning iris may be opened by a laser iridotomy. Ocular surgical procedures that are necessary because of peripheral anterior synechiae or damage to the trabecular meshwork should be postponed until cessation of the inflammation.

Cataract.—Systemic or topical corticosteroid administration for a long period, particularly in patients with rheumatoid arthritis, may cause posterior subcapsular cataracts identical to those caused by uveitis. The typical cataract in uveitis (complicated cataract) occurs in long-standing cyclitis and affects the subcapsular region at the posterior pole. In particularly severe cyclitis, the cataract may involve both the anterior and posterior subcapsular regions.

Keratitis and keratopathy.—Corneal involvement may occur in several ways. The corneal and anterior uvea may be nearly simultaneously inflamed in herpes simplex keratitis (see Chapter 25), herpes zoster ophthalmicus, and syphilitic interstitial keratitis. Iridocyclitis, sometimes with hemorrhage, is a late complication of severe herpes simplex keratitis.

Prolonged iridocyclitis damages the corneal endothelium, causing folds in Descemet membrane, haziness, and stromal and epithelial edema. Continued edema is followed by vascularization of the cornea.

Band keratopathy, in which there is a progressive deposition of calcium in the Bowman zone in a horizontal band across the cornea, often complicates uveitis in young persons. It has been described principally in pauciarticular juvenile rheumatoid arthritis (Still disease), but it also occurs in older individuals after severe ocular uveitis. The calcium may be removed with chelating agents, but if the cause is not eliminated, it recurs.

Vitreous opacities.—A variable degree of clouding of the vitreous humor occurs in posterior uveitis and retinitis. The inflammation of adjacent choroid and retina causes exudation of inflammatory cells suspended in a protein-rich fluid, which sometimes contains erythrocytes. Vitreous opacities consist of cell aggregates, coagulated exudate, fibrin, and strands of degenerated vitreous fibrils.

Ophthalmoscopically, vitreous opacities appear as black dots and strings silhouetted against the background of the red fundus reflex. In severe inflammations they may be so dense as to obscure all details of the fundus, including the red reflex. They are best studied by means of a biomicroscope combined with a concave lens to neutralize the refractive power of the cornea.

Cystoid macular edema.—In this abnormality the capillaries of the central retina become abnormally permeable, with localized accumulation of inflammatory fluid into cystlike swellings (see Chapter 17). Vision is markedly reduced. A uveitis in the region of the ora serrata (intermediate uveitis, pars planitis, or cyclitis) is a common cause of this complication.

Retinal detachment.—Fibrovascular proliferation after exudation into the vitreous may create vitreous traction bands that detach the sensory retina. Severe effusion from the uveal tract may elevate the retina in a uveal effusion.

Chorioretinitis may cause a periphlebitis in the overlying retinal veins. Peripheral sea-fan–shaped neovascularization similar to that seen in sickle cell disease may occur and cause secondary traction or rhegmatogenous retinal detachment.

LOCAL OCULAR DISEASE WITH UVEITIS

Many inflammations of the uvea and retina are secondary to a variety of local disorders: (1) infections in or chemical burns of adjacent tissues; (2) hypermaturity or surgery of the crystalline lens; (3) ocular trauma; and (4) intraocular tissue necrosis or degeneration.

Inflammation of adjacent tissues.—Severe infections of the conjunctiva or cornea may involve the uvea by direct extension or by entry of the exotoxin into the eye (the infection may be bacterial, viral [often herpes simplex], or fungal). Herpes zoster ophthalmicus is associated with both uveitis and keratitis. Alkali burns of the cornea evoke a severe iridocyclitis.

Orbital abscess extending along the vortex veins or meningitis extending along the sheaths of the optic nerve may also cause inflammation of adjacent tissues.

Diseases of the lens.—Hypermature cataract, with release of lens proteins through the lens capsule, causes phacolytic uveitis. The prognosis is good if the lens is removed. In endophthalmitis phacoanaphylactica, an autoimmune process, the eye has become sensitive to its own lens protein. Usually, the sensitization occurs after traumatic rupture of the lens capsule or extracapsular lens extraction. Retained lens protein stimulates B lymphocytes to produce lens antibodies. After extracapsular extraction of the lens in the fellow eye, an antigen-antibody reaction follows. It is not a true anaphylactic reaction since IgE is not involved. Treatment consists of topical corticosteroids and removal of all retained lens material. Retention of the lens nucleus or particles after extracapsular lens extraction may cause inflammation.

Trauma.—Sympathetic ophthalmia is a rare, bilateral, diffuse, nonnecrotizing granulomatous uveitis that usually follows perforating injuries or surgery of one eye and prolapse of the iris or ciliary body (see Chapter 8). It is an autoimmune sensitization with T cell–mediated hypersensitivity (type IV). T lymphocytes are possibly directed at surface membrane antigens shared by photoreceptors, retinal pigment epithelial cells, and choroidal melanocytes.

Other types of trauma that may result in inflammation include a retained intraocular foreign body; contusion damage from blunt trauma; chemical injury (miosis, vascular dilation, and increased permeability are mediated by substance P and not prostaglandins); blood within the eye after trauma or hemorrhagic intraocular disease; and perforation of the lens capsule.

Heterochromic cyclitis.—This is a nongranulomatous iridocyclitis occurring in an eye lighter in color than the fellow eye.

Blind eyes with degenerative changes.—Often these eyes have a chronic uveitis, and a decision must be made as to whether enucleation is preferable to continued inflammation and discomfort.

Necrosis of intraocular tumor.—In most instances the cause of the uveitis is obvious. Ultrasonography and computed tomography are valuable in demonstrating a tumor if the fundus cannot be seen.

UVEITIS AND RETINITIS

Nonsuppurative inflammation of the inner eye is a complicated topic that is not easily divided into either uveitis or retinitis. Inflammation of the iris and the ciliary body (iritis, cyclitis, and iridocyclitis) often does not affect the choroid and retina. Many of these inflammations, however, reflect a cellular autoimmune response similar to those that affect the choroid and retina.

The immature cells of the immune system (T cells of the thymus and B cells of the bone marrow) are exposed to self-antigens during their maturation and develop a tolerance for them. External antigens (nonself) are transported to lymph nodes and the spleen, where they stimulate an immune response. Cells of the immune system are tolerant of self-antigens but react to nonself-antigens. Loss of discrimination between self- and nonself-antigens by the immune system results in reactions against self-antigens, a series of disorders known as autoimmune diseases.

UVEITIS

Uveitis may be divided into three types on the basis of its location: (1) anterior uveitis, which includes iritis, cyclitis, and iridocyclitis; (2) intermediate uveitis, which involves the peripheral anterior portions of the choroid and retina, and the posterior termination of the ciliary body (the pars plana); and (3) posterior uveitis or choroiditis.

Anterior uveitis.—This is a nonsuppurative, self-limited, often recurrent inflammation of the iris and ciliary body. It is characterized by edema, capillary dilation, and an exudation of polymorphonuclear leukocytes, which are quickly replaced by lymphocytes. There are acute and severe inflammatory signs with a sudden onset, severe symptoms, and a tendency to spontaneous remission. The disease may not recur or may continue chronically.

The inflammation may be exogenous or endogenous. Exogenous causes include ocular contusion, which often produces a transient anterior uveitis (traumatic iridocyclitis), alkali burns of the external eye, and an intraocular foreign body. There are numerous endogenous causes, but idiopathic iridocyclitis constitutes the most frequent type of inflammation. Intraocular blood and its degradation products and necrotic intraocular tissue may produce a uveitis. In most instances, there is no obvious ocular or systemic cause. Noninfectious systemic disorders, ranging from arthritis to infectious diseases, may be associated with iridocyclitis of varying degrees of severity. Uveitis is often not diagnosed, although present in rubella, rubeola, or mumps.

Acute anterior uveitis (iridocyclitis) has the signs and symptoms of the red eye. Angle-closure glaucoma, keratitis, or conjunctivitis are usually readily excluded. The diagnosis is confirmed by biomicroscopic observation of keratic precipitates, aqueous flare, and cells.

The endogenous etiologic cause may be immediately evident when associated with systemic disease, but in many instances it is impossible to demonstrate a cause. Often the etiologic factor is diagnosed only by exclusion of other possible causes; in patients, such as those with arthritis or genitourinary tract disease, the practitioner knows only that the uveal tissue is inflamed, as are other tissues. The uveal inflammation may be caused by a different condition than a concurrent systemic disease, even if the disease is often associated with uveal inflammation.

Many patients in whom the cause of uveitis is not found have only a single attack; others are seen with chorioretinal scars or anterior segment lesions from asymptomatic inflammations that have occurred previously. In conditions such as heterochromic cyclitis and glaucomatocyclitic crises, no systemic abnormality ever is found and etiologic studies are not helpful.

Recurrent or chronic anterior uveitis is a progressive inflammation with cellular infiltration chiefly by mononuclear cells, macrophages, and epithelioid cells. There is tissue necrosis and repair by fibrosis. The inflammation has a torpid and persistent course with minimal external signs of inflammation. Mutton-fat keratic precipitates form, and there is a mild aqueous flare with but few cells in the aqueous humor. There is a marked tendency for the formation of posterior synechiae and reduced vision.

The inflammation may be caused by microbes or parasites or may occur with many autoimmune disorders. There are many strictly local causes.

Intermediate uveitis.—Intermediate uveitis (pars planitis; chronic cyclitis; peripheral uveitis) is a frequent, serious, chronic, often bilateral (80%) inflammatory disease that occurs in children and young adults. It originates at the pars plana of the ciliary body and the periphery of the retina and causes a fibrovascular proliferation, particularly at the inferior portion of the choroid and retina. There is cellular exudation into the adjacent vitreous humor with an exudate ("snowbank") over the inferior pars plana ciliaris. There are periodic remissions and exacerbations. Vision is reduced because of the cells in the vitreous, and cystoid macular degeneration often reduces vision further.

Uniocular inflammation is usually treated with subtenon injection of a long-acting corticosteroid (methylprednisolone acetate) administered monthly. Binocular involvement is usually treated with oral corticosteroids. In patients who fail to respond to corticosteroid therapy, transscleral cryotherapy to the inflamed uvea may be helpful. Continued progression may require treatment with cyclosporine or cyclophosphamide. The eyes respond favorably to removal of cataractous lenses and vitrectomy. Some 45% of the patients have a mild inflammation and a favorable prognosis.

Posterior uveitis.—Posterior uveitis (choroiditis, chorioretinitis) at its onset appears ophthalmoscopically as an ill-defined grayish yellow or grayish white choroidal opacity, which is surrounded by the normal colored fundus. The lesions may be single or multiple. The overlying sensory retina becomes edematous and opaque and is so often inflamed that the lesion is described as chorioretinitis. Inflammatory cells and exudate may burst through the pigment epithelium and sensory retina to cloud the vitreous, which further obscures the ophthalmoscopic details of the lesion.

With healing, the margins of the lesion of choroiditis become more sharply defined and the vitreous clouding clears. If the choroid has been the main site of the lesion, it appears as a whitish yellow area stippled with pigment. When the retinal pigment epithelium has been destroyed, a patch of white scar occurs that consists of either a fibrous replacement of retina and choroid or stark, white sclera over which both the retina and choroid have been destroyed. The retinal pigment epithelium proliferates, particularly at the margins of the lesions, and the final ophthalmoscopic appearance is often one of white sclera surrounded by clumps of black pigment. Pigment proliferation does not always occur after severe inflammation, presumably because of destruction of the retinal pigment epithelium. The melanocytes of the choroid do not proliferate.

RETINITIS

The retina is often affected in inflammations of the adjacent choroid and is obviously involved in suppurative infections of the eye, such as panophthalmitis and endophthalmitis. Scleritis and iridocyclitis may affect the retina secondarily, but the severity of the primary inflammation dominates the clinical picture.

A perivasculitis with infiltration of lymphocytes and plasma cells affects retinal venules. An exudative retinopathy occurs in carbon monoxide poisoning. Exogenous retinitis may result from fungal infections and septic emboli.

The pandemic of the acquired immunodeficiency syndrome (AIDS) has resulted in the emergence of cytomegalovirus retinitis as the most frequent cause of retinal inflammation, with retinal toxoplasmosis also being common. A noninfectious retinal vasculopathy develops in some 45% of patients with CD4 counts of less than 50 cells/mm^3 and some 16% of patients with higher CD4 cell counts (see Chapter 25).

Noninfectious retinal vasculopathy.—Patients with AIDS (see Chapter 25) who are also infected with cytomegalovirus (see this chapter), toxoplasmosis (see this chapter) and those having severe uveitis (see Chapter 19) may develop an associated inflammation and ischemia of the retina. The retinal veins are particularly affected. Visual acuity is reduced secondary to macular edema and vitreous opacities. The ophthalmoscopic view of the fundus is obscured by inflammatory cells and protein in the vitreous humor. Cotton-wool spots of ischemic retina and deep, round, superficial, flame-shaped hemorrhages occur. The retinal veins are dilated and on fluorescein angiography stain and leak fluorescein. The margins of the optic disk are obscured, and macular edema reduces vision.

Treatment is difficult, and the disorder is prolonged. In the absence of AIDS, systemic and subconjunctival corticosteroids may control the inflammation. Some patients require immunosuppressive therapy (see Chapter 3). Patients with AIDS and retinal vasculopathy are at increased risk to develop cytomegalovirus retinopathy and should be studied for cytomegalovirus infection so that prophylactic viral chemotherapy can be initiated before severe retinal infection occurs.

Cytomegalovirus retinitis.—The cytomegalovirus is not a pathogenic organism in individuals with a competent immune system. In patients with AIDS, however, cytomegalovirus is a major cause of morbidity and mortality, and the retina is the major site of infection in 15% to 20% of patients with AIDS.

The virus causes a sharply defined retinitis with confluent gray granular patches of necrotic retina. When untreated, the necrosis spreads centrally and peripherally with focal retinal hemorrhages and retinal detachment. One or both eyes may be affected. Skilled ophthalmoscopic examination is required to detect minimal infection. Without treatment the entire retina is inflamed within 6 weeks.

Treatment is with intravenous foscarnet or ganciclovir, which suppress virus replication but do not eliminate the virus. Despite maintenance therapy, eventual relapse appears inevitable. Fulminant lesions are associated with a poorer visual outcome than are indolent lesions. Intraocular ganciclovir may be more effective than intravenous therapy. Surgical treatment of retinal detachment may preserve vision for longer periods. Blindness from cytomegalovirus retinitis has devastating consequences, and practitioners who treat AIDS patients should be familiar with its current therapy complications, and be able to recognize relapsing infection.

Pneumocystis carinii* infection.—Pneumocystis carinii* is a saprophyte of humans and animals with characteristics related more closely to fungi than protozoa. It causes a pneumocystosis in some 80% to 90% of all patients with AIDS and is a common cause of death. Treatment is difficult. Trimethoprim-sulfamethoxazole and parenteral pentamidine isethionate are used; adverse reactions are common. During treatment a cytomegalovirus infection is often reactivated and patients develop a necrotizing hemorrhagic retinitis. Treatment with ganciclovir must begin promptly to prevent necrosis of the fovea and permanent loss of central vision. Treatment is continued indefinitely because the ocular infection recurs when the medication is discontinued.

Necrotizing herpetic retinopathy.—This condition, also known as the acute retinal necrosis syndrome, may affect one or both eyes of otherwise healthy individuals of either sex of any age. It is characterized by an acute peripheral necrotizing retinitis, retinal arteritis, and a severe panuveitis. Most instances are caused by infection with varicella-zoster virus or the herpes simplex virus. The retinal inflammation caused by the cytomegalic virus in AIDS is usually, but not always, clinically different from necrotizing herpetic retinopathy.

The disorder often begins with a severe iridocyclitis that is disproportionately painful for the degree of inflammation evident. Deep multifocal yellow-white patches of retinal necrosis develop in the retinal periphery outside of the temporal vascular arcade and rapidly spread circumferentially. There is a prominent retinal arteritis, with sheathing and occlusion of the blood vessels, and retinal hemorrhages. The vitreous is turbid with inflammatory cells and the optic disk is swollen. Inflammatory cells cloud the anterior chamber. After 4 or 5 weeks the condition begins to regress, with sharply delineated areas of pigment proliferation. Retinal holes occur at the junction of normal and inflamed retina, and a proliferative retinopathy complicates a rhegmatogenous retinal detachment. In about 35% of the patients the fellow eye becomes involved in a similar process within 6 weeks. Repair of the retinal detachment is complicated by the vitreoretinopathy, and visual results may be poor because of optic atrophy, macular edema, and macular abnormalities.

Diagnosis may be based on the detection of varicella-zoster virus DNA or herpes simplex virus DNA in the aqueous humor or the vitreous humor by use of the polymerase chain reaction. In infected patients the level of antibodies to these viruses in the aqueous humor exceeds the blood level. Administration of acyclovir (2 × 15 mg/kg/day to 10 mg/kg every 8 hours) prevents the development of new lesions. Early laser photocoagulation of the retina may minimize retinal detachment.

Toxoplasmosis.—Toxoplasmosis is an infectious disease caused by an obligate intracellular protozoan, *Toxoplasma gondii.* The organism is capable of infecting a wide range of mammals, birds, and reptiles. The cat family is the definitive host. Transmission occurs readily after ingestion of toxoplasmosis cysts in pork or lamb or oocysts from cat feces.

Two types of disease occur: congenital and acquired. Infection of the nonimmune pregnant woman results in transmission of the organism to the fetus. If the fetus is infected during the first trimester of pregnancy, there is often spontaneous abortion. Infection after the first trimester may result in severe fetal ocular and neurologic sequelae. (Nonimmune women should be identified at the beginning of pregnancy, informed as to how to prevent infection, and followed up serologically until delivery.) The congenital infection is characterized by bilateral retinochoroiditis, strabismus, epilepsy, and psychomotor retardation.

Acquired toxoplasmosis may be asymptomatic or cause a nonspecific febrile illness with lymphadenopathy. Subsequent compromise of the immune system by AIDS or immunosuppressive drugs may activate congenital or acquired infections.

Congenital toxoplasmosis causes microphthalmia, a necrotizing retinochoroiditis, iritis, optic atrophy, and vitreous disorganization. Necrosis of the central nervous system causes nystagmus and ocular muscle palsy with strabismus. The retinal lesion often destroys the fovea centralis with loss of central vision.

Infants with less severe toxoplasmosis infections have areas of chorioretinal atrophy with retinal pigment proliferation in both eyes. If the fovea centralis is involved, esotropia may occur or the eyes may be straight although vision is poor. The inactive lesions are sharply demarcated, and contiguous areas of chorioretinal atrophy have pigmented borders (Fig 19-1), which are located mainly at the posterior pole. The vitreous is clear, and there is no active inflammation. The retinal lesions may remain quiescent throughout life or recur 10 to 20 years later in retina adjacent to healed lesions. Presumably delayed inflammation follows rupture of a cell that contains the active parasite.

In immunocompromised patients, ocular toxoplasmosis is usually a new infection and not the reactivation of a congenital lesion. There are no healed or pigmented lesions of the congenital infection, and the organism causes a nonspecific retinochoroiditis. It is important to distinguish the necrotizing retinopathy of toxoplasmosis from that caused by the cytomegalovirus. The toxoplasmosis lesion has smooth, nongranular borders and a thick, densely opaque retinal opacification in contrast to that caused by cytomegalovirus. The polymerase chain reaction gene amplification technique with the use of *Toxoplasma* ribosomal DNA from the aqueous humor or vitreous humor promises more precise and rapid diagnosis than indirect methods used previously.

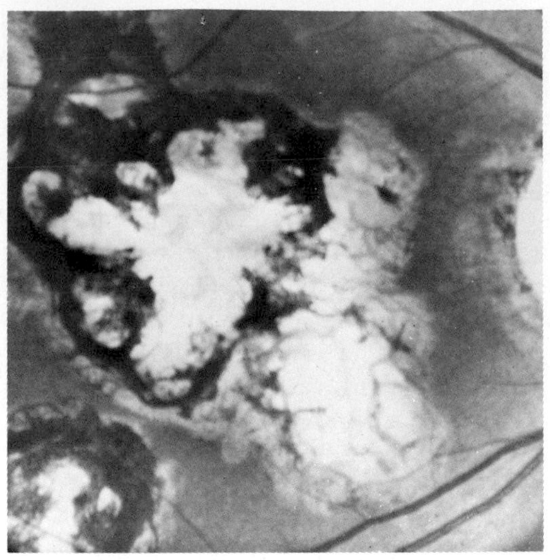

FIG 19-1.
Recurrent toxoplasmosis in a 39-year-old woman. Visual acuity in this eye is counting fingers at 2 feet. There is a series of contiguous lesions, some with marked pigment proliferation and others so severe that the pigment epithelium has been destroyed and the sclera may be seen.

The treatment of choice for systemic or ocular toxoplasmosis is clindamycin and pyrimethamine, which inhibit folic acid metabolism of the protozoa but require leucovorin to prevent bone marrow depression.

Prompt diagnosis after birth and avoidance of prolonged neonatal hypoxia and uncorrected increased intracranial pressure, combined with treatment of the toxoplasmosis infection, may provide normal development of many, although not all, severely infected infants.

Acute posterior multifocal placoid pigment epitheliopathy.—This self-limited disorder is characterized by a rapid loss of central vision, particularly in young women. Ophthalmoscopically, there are many flat or slightly elevated light yellow halos surrounding deeper

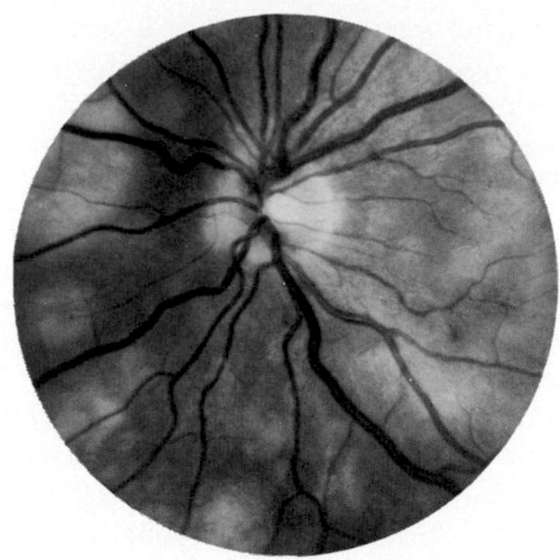

FIG 19-2.
Acute posterior multifocal placoid pigment epitheliopathy with multiple lesions deep to the sensory retina.

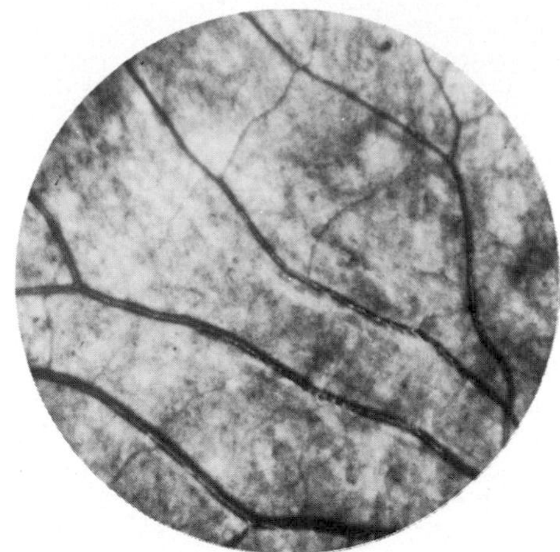

FIG 19-3.
Areas of pigmentation and depigmentation of the peripheral retina in fetal rubella.

yellow centers at the posterior pole (Fig 19-2). Vision improves within 2 to 3 weeks and the yellow lesions disappear, but there is an extensive degeneration of the retinal pigment epithelium. The sensory retina and choroid are normal. Fluorescein and indocyanine green angiography suggest that the arterioles that enter the lobules of the choriocapillaris (see Fig 1-13) are obstructed during the acute stage. The adjacent retinal pigment epithelium degenerates secondary to ischemia.

The disease particularly affects young women who often have an upper respiratory tract illness 1 or 2 weeks earlier. There may be an associated mild uveitis with keratic precipitates and aqueous humor flare and cells in the vitreous. Erythema nodosum and episcleritis may occur. Rarely, headache and cells in the cerebrospinal fluid suggest a mild cerebral vasculitis. Cerebral vasculitis may occur months or even years after an attack. The cause is not known but the history of an earlier upper respiratory tract illness suggests a viral infection.

Toxocariasis.—The larva of the common roundworm of the dog or cat may cause an eosinophilic granuloma of the retina (see Chapter 25). It appears as a whitish elevated area approximately the size of the optic disk. The dark-colored larva, which excites little cellular or pigmentary reaction, may sometimes be seen in the mass. Bands of retinal fibrosis radiate from the mass. Less common is a chronic endophthalmitis, which may lead to enucleation because of a diagnosis of retinoblastoma.

Rubella.—Ocular fetal rubella involves predominantly the retinal pigment epithelium and causes a slight disturbance in the melanin distribution. Ophthalmoscopically, there are discrete areas of pigmentation and depigmentation (Fig 19-3). The electroretinogram is of limited value, since it may be normal, subnormal, or nonrecordable. The retinopathy does not progress, in contrast to primary retinal degenerations (see Chapter 25).

AUTOIMMUNE UVEORETINITIS

Penetrating injuries of the eye have been recognized for many years as causing an inflammation of the uveal tract and retina (sympathetic ophthalmia [see Chapter 8]). This inflammation is differentiated from antibody-mediated inflammation, such as that which occurs after immunization with crystalline lens antigen followed by incision of the lens capsule. More recently, many different systemic disorders are recognized as being associated in some patients with ocular inflammations, optic neuritis, or retinal neovascularization (Table 19-5). The advances in identifying the actions of the different components of the immune system have resulted in recognition of many ocular disorders induced by immune system responses.

In experimental animals, immunization with purified retinal antigens (or the transfer of retinal-antigen-activated CD4+ lymphocytes)

TABLE 19-5.
Eye Diseases Associated with Alteration of the Immune System

Primary ocular disease
Sympathetic ophthalmia
Lens-induced uveitis
Intermediate uveitis (pars planitis)
Vogt-Koyanagi-Harada disease
Idiopathic uveitis
Iridocyclitis
Posterior uveoretinitis
Birdshot chorioretinopathy
Systemic disorders with ocular involvement
Ankylosing spondylitis
Rheumatoid arthritis
Juvenile
Adult
Behçet syndrome
Sarcoidosis
Reiter syndrome
Wegener granulomatosis
Lupus erythematosus
Bowel disease
Whipple disease
Ulcerative colitis
Sjögren syndrome
Cicatrizing conjunctivitis (ocular cicatricial pemphigoid)

produces a uveoretinitis that provides insight into a variety of human ocular disorders.

Experimental autoimmune uveoretinitis.—Experimental autoimmune uveoretinitis describes the inflammatory reactions of the retina and uveal tract induced by injecting one of several different retinal antigens into the footpad of a suitable experimental animal. The animal must have an intact cell-mediated immune system (the inflammation cannot be induced in nude rats), and the spleen must be present. A variety of retinal antigens may be used (see Chapter 2): arrestin (previously S-antigen); interphotoreceptor binding protein; transducin; retinal pigment epithelium; and others.

Immediately after injection there is a short period of inflammation of the uvea and retina that is mediated by CD4+ lymphocytes (T-helper cells) which recognize antigen presented by major histocompatibility class II interaction (see Chapter 25). This inflammation subsides within 1 or 2 days, but approximately 14 days after the injection of the antigen, there is a severe inflammation of the entire uvea and retina with lymphocytes in the aqueous humor and vitreous humor. An inflammatory retinal detachment may occur. Some 2 weeks later there is necrosis of the photoreceptor layer of the retina.

The delayed inflammation is mediated by CD4+ cells, which recognize the antigen presented by major histocompatibility class II antigens. There is activation of CD8+ lymphocytes (cytotoxic cells). Interferon-gamma (IFN-gamma) induces the expression of major histocompatibility class II antigens (HLA-DR and HLD-DQ) by the retinal pigment epithelium and the endothelial cells of the retinal blood vessels. Interleukin 2 (IL-2), a cytokine produced by T cells, activates additional T cells and natural killer cells.

Oral tolerization is an experimental therapy in which minute amounts of the antigen that induce the autoimmune response are given orally. By pretreatment it is possible to prevent or to modify the severity of an autoimmune experimental uveoretinitis that uses the same antigen. Similarly, oral administration of the same antigen after induction of the autoimmune response may induce a remission of the inflammatory signs. In a few instances of Behçet disease, oral administration of minute amounts of arrestin has ameliorated the inflammation. It is evident that the complicated immune responses provide many possible modes of effective therapy other than the corticosteroids and immunosuppressive agents.

OCULAR AUTOIMMUNE DISORDERS

It is convenient to discuss the specific disorders associated with retinal and uveal autoimmune reactions as those that appear limited to the eye and those having both ocular and systemic manifestations (see Table 19-3).

Idiopathic uveitis.—Inflammations of the iris, ciliary body, and choroid not associated with any systemic disorder are discussed earlier in this chapter. In many instances the cause is not evident, and, except in exceptional circumstances, the intraocular fluids or tissues are not removed for special testing. Treatment often is empiric with topical or systemic corticosteroids, and the inflammation gradually subsides.

If the inflammatory cells visible with the biomicroscope are large, it is assumed that they are epithelioid cells and that the inflammation reflects a T lymphocyte response. If the cells are small, it is assumed that they are plasma cells and that the inflammation is a B cell response.

Unfortunately, the inability to learn the cause of many intraocular inflammations may lead the practitioner to neglect testing for disorders for which there is specific therapy. The diagnosis of "idiopathic uveitis" should be made only after other possible causes are excluded.

Sympathetic ophthalmia.—Sympathetic ophthalmia (uveitis) is a bilateral, diffuse, proliferative intraocular inflammation that follows a penetrating injury of the eye or intraocular surgery by 5 days (minimum) to many years (usual, 3 weeks to 3 months). It is considered the initial example of an autoimmune ocular inflammation, but the exact ocular antigen is not known. The inflammation is characterized by epithelioid cells, multinucleated giant cells, lymphocytes, and sometimes eosinophils. The injured eye is the exciting eye and the fellow eye is the sympathizing eye.

Usually an indolent uveitis persists in the exciting eye after a penetrating injury or ocular surgery (often in an eye that has required repeated intraocular surgery). The fellow eye then develops a mild photophobia and redness that steadily become worse. Once the inflammation is established, removal of the exciting eye is not beneficial. Removal is contraindicated since this eye may ultimately provide better vision than the sympathizing eye. Fluorescein angiography discloses many areas of fluorescein leakage that surround areas of nonperfusion. Enucleation of a badly injured and blind eye before the onset of inflammation prevents sympathetic ophthalmia. It is never necessary to remove an injured eye before expert opinion is obtained concerning the need for removal (see Chapter 8).

Birdshot retinochoroidopathy.—This is a specific bilateral inflammation of the retina, choroid, and their blood vessels. It has its onset in adults aged 35 to 69 years (mean, 46 years) with no sexual predilection. Numerous depigmented spots in the fundus, cystoid macular edema, disk edema, inflammatory cells in the vitreous, and retinal vascular leakage occur. Multiple spots in the choroid vary in size, shape, and color. Initially the spots are creamy-yellow but become white, atrophic, sharply circumscribed lesions. More than 80% of the patients have HLA-B29 compared to 7% of the general population.

Diagnosis is based on the characteristic appearance of the bilateral choroidal lesions combined with two or more signs of papilledema, vitreitis, retinal vasculitis, and macular edema. Small doses of cyclosporine (2.5 to 5.0 mg/kg daily) may control the inflammation, and azathioprine (1.5 to 2.0 mg/kg daily) may be added if necessary. The inflammation is presumably an autoimmune reaction to retinal arrestin (see Chapter 2).

Heterochromic iridocyclitis (Fuchs).— This is mainly a chronic, monocular, insidious inflammation of the iris and ciliary body that affects mainly young persons. There are no symptoms, ciliary injection, or adhesions of the iris to the lens (posterior synechiae). Attention is often directed to the eye as the iris becomes lighter in color than its fellow.

The anterior border layer of the iris (see Chapter 1) loses its surface markings. Its pigment is lost in irregular patches ("motheaten") and the iris is thinned. Numerous small keratic precipitates dot the corneal endothelium, but an aqueous flare is faint or absent. Cataract is common, but extraction usually gives excellent visual results. Glaucoma is less common but is often not responsive to medical treatment. Plasma cells and lymphocytes predominate and suggest an abnormality of B lymphocytes.

OCULAR AND SYSTEMIC AUTOIMMUNE DISORDERS

A number of inflammations of the retina and uvea occur in association with systemic diseases or are associated with other signs and symptoms that together constitute a syndrome. Some are associated with particular HLA antigens (see Chapter 25), particularly HLA-B27, -DR5, -B5, -A11, and -A29. A disordered immune mechanism is responsible for some of these syndromes, but the frequent inability to obtain intraocular tissue for diagnosis limits the search for the causative mechanism.

Ankylosing spondylitis.—Ankylosing spondylitis is an inflammatory disease of the joints that affects mainly men (75%) who often have a family history of arthritis. It has its onset in late adolescence or early adulthood, often with ill-defined low back pain that may escape diagnosis. Spondylitis of the cervical spine may make it awkward or impossible for patients to place their heads in position for biomicroscopy. The HLA-B27 allele is present in more than 90% of affected individuals compared to 8% in the unaffected population.

The ocular inflammation has a rapid onset with redness and pain. Usually only one eye is inflamed, but both eyes are affected. Between episodes the inflammation resolves completely. There is a tendency for posterior synechiae and cystoid macular edema but never cataract or secondary glaucoma.

Juvenile rheumatoid arthritis.—Rheumatoid arthritis in individuals less than 16 years of age may have an onset with fever, morbilliform rash, and leukocytosis. The onset, particularly in girls, is before 5 years of age. Monoarticular disease occurs more frequently than in adults. Boys with the pauciarticular pattern, the B27 allele, and recurrent iridocyclitis probably represent a juvenile form of ankylosing spondylitis.

Girls have an increased frequency of antinuclear antibodies. They have a bilateral, chronic iridocyclitis that is refractory to treatment. Band keratopathy, posterior synechiae, cataract, and glaucoma occur.

Reiter disease.—Reiter disease is composed of nongonococcal sterile urethritis, polyarthritis, and conjunctivitis or iridocyclitis. Genitourinary symptoms usually precede ocular or rheumatic features. The cause of the disease is not known, but bacillary dysentery has preceded the inflammation in some patients. Some 20% of individuals who have the HLA-B27 allele will develop Reiter syndrome after a *Shigella* gastroenteritis. HLA-B27 antigen is found in 92% of patients with the full syndrome. The syndrome occurs in patients with AIDS.

The conjunctivitis is usually mucopurulent with preauricular adenopathy, chemosis, eyelid edema, and conjunctival hemorrhage. It resolves in 8 to 10 days. Anterior uveitis is initially monocular but becomes bilateral in recurrences. Scleritis, episcleritis, cystoid macular edema, and optic neuritis have been described.

Vogt-Koyanagi-Harada syndrome.—This is a systemic disease characterized by bilateral uveitis, dysacousia, meningeal irritation, whitening of patches of hair (poliosis), vitiligo, and retinal detachment (Harada). It is associated with HLA-DR4 and HLA-Dq4, which are in strong linkage disequilibrium in the Japanese. Some 8% of all uveitis in Japan may be of Vogt-Koyanagi-Harada type.

The disease is initiated by a severe headache, deep orbital pain, vertigo, and nausea. Days or weeks later a posterior uveitis develops in one eye, followed in several days by a similar inflammation in the fellow eye. An iridocyclitis follows iris nodules, mutton-fat keratic precipitates, and many cells and much protein in the anterior chamber. An exudative retinal detachment may occur in some patients. Magnetic resonance imaging discloses a diffuse thickening of the choroid with intense enhancement after administration of gadopentetate. There is loss of hearing in most patients.

After several months the inflammation gradually decreases with depigmentation of localized areas of the hair of the scalp and sometimes a patchy alopecia.

Behçet disease.—This rare (in the United States) chronic disease is classically associated with painful aphthous ulceration of the mouth (canker sores), similar urethral ulceration, skin lesions, thrombophlebitis, and aneurysms of major arteries. It is associated with HLA-B51. In some 50% of the patients there are circulating antibodies to oral mucous membranes. T lymphocyte abnormalities suggest a continuous formation of an unknown antigen. It may occur in one of two forms: (1) a chronic mucocutaneous type and (2) a neuro-ocular form that may lead to blindness and death.

The mouth and genital region are ulcerated in the mucocutaneous form, and there is an associated conjunctivitis but no uveitis. Erythema nodosum, thrombophlebitis, cutaneous vasculitis, and papulopustular eruption in the extremities are seen.

The neuro-ocular form includes conjunctivitis, iritis, iridocyclitis (sometimes with hypopyon), keratitis, retinal vasculitis, papilledema, and ischemic optic neuropathy. Meningoencephalitis with general or focal neurologic deficits occurs. The lesions of the mucocutaneous type are sometimes present.

Patients with either type of disease may develop thromboses and multiple aneurysms of major arteries. Natural killer cell activity and serum interferon levels are decreased during ocular exacerbations. Interferon therapy, or cyclosporine, sometimes combined with prednisolone, is often effective.

INFLAMMATION WITHOUT INFECTION OR AUTOIMMUNITY

Sarcoidosis.—Sarcoidosis is an acute or chronic multisystem immune reaction to an unknown antigen that apparently originates outside of the body. The disease is characterized most frequently by pulmonary infiltrates, a hilar adenopathy, and lesions of the eye and skin. There are widespread epithelioid cell (macrophage) granulomas that resemble a tubercle, but are without caseation. In the United States most patients are black, and sarcoidosis is most prevalent in the Southeastern United States in both blacks and whites. It is more frequent in women than in men and mainly affects individuals between the ages of 20 and 40 years. Sarcoidosis occurs in an acute active type and in a persistent fibrotic type. The acute type occurs in individuals less than 30 years of age. Initially there is an abrupt, transient polyarthralgia with erythema nodosum. Iridocyclitis may initiate the acute disease. There are many mutton-fat keratic precipitates and early formation of broad, flat posterior synechiae. Sarcoid nodules may occur in the iris stroma or at the pupillary margin.

Chronic sarcoidosis has an insidious, poorly recognized onset with cough, dyspnea, and sometimes hemoptysis. Fever, weight loss, and arthralgia may be the initial signs. Cutaneous plaques, papules, and subcutaneous nodules may occur. Lupus pernio may be present with skin plaques, scars, and keloids. Peripheral areas of sharply defined ("punched-out") chorioretinitis or intermediate chorioretinitis (pars planitis) may occur. Intermediate uveitis results in inflammatory cells in both the anterior chamber and the vitreous humor. Periphlebitis and arteritis occur with focal accumulations of exudates that resemble candle-wax drippings. There may be large "snowball" opacities in the vitreous humor. The intraocular inflammation is resistant to treatment and may be complicated by secondary glaucoma and cataract.

Papillitis, granulomatous optic neuropathy, and retrobulbar neuritis may cause optic atrophy. Papilledema may occur spontaneously or reflect increased intracranial pressure. Optociliary shunt vessels may be prominent on the optic disk. The optic atrophy may result from inflammation or compression of the optic nerve, or glaucoma secondary to intraocular inflammation. A keratoconjunctivitis identical to Sjögren syndrome may occur. The lacrimal and salivary glands may be swollen.

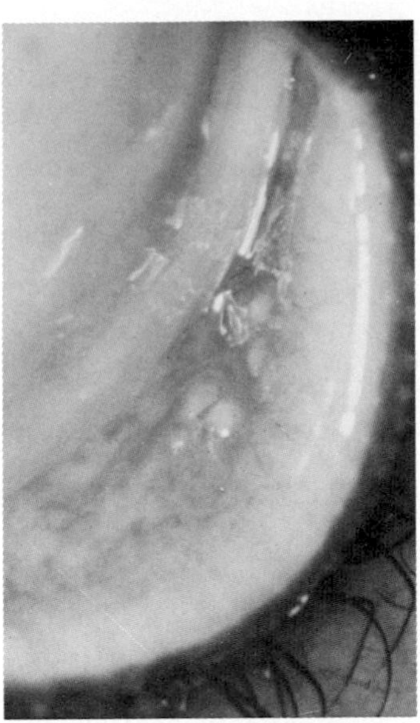

FIG 19-4.
Sarcoid nodules in the inferior cul-de-sac of a 23-year-old woman with advanced sarcoidosis.

Intracranial sarcoidosis is symptomatic in about 5% of the patients. Nearly all patients show intracranial abnormalities with magnetic resonance imaging with gadolinium enhancement. The basal leptomeninges, the region surrounding the hypothalamus, and the cranial nerves, particularly the facial nerve, may be affected. The serum angiotensin-converting enzyme, calcium, and uric acid levels are increased. There is an anergy in the response to skin testing. In both types of sarcoidosis the inferior conjunctival fornices may contain minute, translucent, slightly yellow, elevated lesions that resemble follicles (Fig 19-4). Serial section of such a nodule or of a biopsy specimen of tissue from the inferior cul-de-sac may disclose a typical granuloma without caseation.

Many CD4+ lymphocytes accumulate in the alveoli of the lungs of patients with sarcoidosis and may be recovered by bronchoalveolar lavage. Study of these cells suggests that active sarcoidosis is characterized by a selective activation and accumulation of antigen-specific V (for variable) beta expressing CD4+ T cells. The activated cells initiate a cascade of immune reactions that culminate in the typical pulmonary granuloma of sarcoidosis.

TABLE 19-6.
Special Testing in Uveoretinitis

Blood
- ELISA (enzyme-linked immunosorbent assay): cytomegalovirus; Lyme disease *(Borrelia burgdorferi); Toxocara, Toxoplasma gondii* (IgM antibodies); nematodes
- HLA antigens
- Human immunodeficiency virus (AIDS)
- Syphilis: rapid plasma reagin test
- Varicella-zoster; other viruses

Fluorescein angiography
- Acute multifocal posterior placoid epitheliopathy; birdshot retinochoroidopathy; multiple evanescent white dot syndrome; serpiginous choroidopathy; Vogt-Koyanagi-Harada disease

Vitreous aspiration and uveoretinal biopsy
- ELISA: vitreous humor aspirate: cytomegalovirus, acute retinal necrosis (herpes simplex, varicella-zoster); *Toxocara* larva; nematodes
- Polymerase chain reaction: viruses of acute retinal necrosis
- Cytologic examination: reticulum cell sarcoma
- Anaerobic and aerobic cultures: suppurative inflammation
- Anaerobic culture: *Propionibacterium acnes* after intraocular lens insertion
- Fungal cultures

After Elliott JH: *Introduction to uveitis.* In Albert DM, Jakobiec FA, editors: *Principles and practice of ophthalmology,* vol 1, Philadelphia, 1994, WB Saunders.

DIAGNOSTIC MEASURES

Suppurative inflammations require immediate collection, Gram stain, and culture of the intraocular exudate followed by intraocular antibiotic therapy based upon the Gram stain. Ocular examination should readily disclose inflammations secondary to heterochromic iridocyclitis, penetrating injuries, or abnormalities of the crystalline lens or sclera. The possibility of inflammation being a manifestation of AIDS must always be considered. The causative factor is usually not sought in the first attacks of acute anterior uveitis, which respond promptly to therapy with topical corticosteroids and 1% atropine solution. Recurrent or persistent inflammations are managed as chronic inflammations (below).

In chronic and recurrent inflammations, the medical history and physical examination are directed particularly to cutaneous and mucous membrane lesions, joint inflammation in rheumatoid arthritis and ankylosing spondylitis, and genitourinary tract infection. On the basis of ocular findings, a variety of diagnostic procedures are often suggested (Table 19-6).

Fluorescein angiography may be helpful in retinitis and posterior uveitis. In exceptional instances in which specific treatment would be based on a specific diagnosis, a pars plana vitrectomy or a chorioretinal biopsy may provide diagnostic tissue for DNA hybridization, polymerase chain reaction, monoclonal antibodies, and electron microscopy.

BIBLIOGRAPHY

Books

Nussenblatt RB, Whitcup SM, Palestine AG: *Uveitis: fundamentals and clinical practice,* ed 2, St Louis, 1996, Mosby–Year Book.

Opremcak EM: *Uveitis. A clinical manual for ocular inflammation,* New York, 1994, Springer-Verlag.

Pepose JS, Holland GN, Wilhelmus K: *Ocular infection and immunity,* St Louis, 1996, Mosby–Year Book.

Tabbara K, Nussenblatt R: *Posterior uveitis. Diagnosis and management,* Newton, Mass, 1995, Butterworth-Heinemann.

Articles

DeRemee RA: Sarcoidosis and Wegener's granulomatosis: a comparative analysis, *Sarcoidosis* 11:7-18, 1994.

Jett BD, Jensen HG, Atkuri RV, Gilmore MS: Evaluation of therapeutic measures for treating endophthalmitis caused by toxin-producing and toxin-nonproducing *Enterococcus faecalis* strains, *Invest Ophthalmol Vis Sci* 36:9-15, 1995.

Mann RM, Riva CE, Stone RA, Barnes GE, Cranstoun SD: Nitric oxide and choroidal blood flow regulation, *Invest Ophthalmol Vis Sci* 136:925-930, 1995.

The Studies of Ocular Complications of AIDS Research Group in Collaboration with the AIDS Clinical Trials Group: Combination foscarnet and ganciclovir therapy vs monotherapy for the treatment of relapsed cytomegalovirus retinitis in patients with AIDS: the cytomegalovirus retreatment trial, *Arch Ophthalmol* 114:23-33, 1996.

Vitale AT, Rodriguez A, Foster CS: Low-dose cyclosporin A therapy in treating chronic, noninfectious uveitis, *Ophthalmology* 103:365-374, 1996.

20

THE OPTIC NERVE

Each optic nerve (N II) is composed of the axons of ganglion cells of each retina. Each nerve extends from the optic disk, within the eye, to the optic chiasm. Axons that originate from the nasal one half of each retina decussate in the optic chiasm and join with the uncrossed axons from the temporal one half of the fellow eye to form the optic tract. The axons in the optic tract synapse in the lateral geniculate body (form and movement) and in the pretectal nuclei (pupillary constriction). The axons become myelinated immediately posterior to the lamina cribrosa (see Chapter 1).

The optic nerve may be divided into four parts: (1) intraocular, about 1.0 to 2.0 mm in diameter and 1.0 mm long; (2) intraorbital, about 3.0 to 4.0 mm in diameter as the result of myelination and meningeal coverings, and 20 to 30 mm long; (3) intracanicular, about 5.0 mm long; and (4) intracranial, about 10 mm long.

The surface of the intraocular portion of the optic nerve, the optic disk, is the major ophthalmoscopic landmark of the ocular fundus. Here the axons of retinal ganglion cells make a nearly right-angle turn to enter the posterior scleral canal and exit from the eye together with the central retinal vein. Just nasal to the vein the central retinal artery enters the eye, through a depression in the central portion of the optic disk, the physiologic cup. The edges of the physiologic cup are concentric with the scleral canal and are lined with astrocytes. When these are sparse, the perforations of the lamina cribrosa are visible. The size of the optic disk correlates with the diameter and radius of curvature of the cornea; large optic disks are mainly in eyes with large, flat corneas. The size of the physiologic cup mirrors the size of the posterior scleral canal, and its shape indicates the angle the optic nerve makes with the globe. The surface of the optic disk is nurtured by capillaries from the central retinal artery, but the remainder of the intraocular portion of the optic nerve receives its blood supply from branches of the posterior ciliary arterioles.

The surface of the optic disk is at the same level as the surrounding retina, and the word *papilla* (Latin for pimple or nipple) is a misnomer that persists in many words (papilledema, papillomacular, papillitis, peripapillary) that relate to the optic disk.

The intraorbital position of the optic nerve is S-shaped to permit rotations of the eye. It is surrounded by meninges. The dura mater and arachnoid mater merge with the sclera anteriorly. At the optic canal the dura mater splits to continue as the orbital periosteum, to fuse with the annulus of Zinn, and to continue with the arachnoid and pia (and subarachnoid space) into the intracranial cavity. The optic nerves are myelinated, beginning at the lamina cribrosa, and divided by the collagen septa of the pia mater that carry nutrient blood vessels. The central retinal artery and vein pass through the meningeal covering of the optic nerve about 12 mm posterior to the globe.

Within the optic canal the optic nerve is accompanied by the ophthalmic artery and postganglionic sympathetic nerves. The optic nerve is firmly fixed to bone by its meningeal covering.

The intracranial portion of the optic nerve is a short bridge between the optic canal and the optic chiasm.

SYMPTOMS AND SIGNS OF OPTIC NERVE DISEASE

Loss of vision is the main symptom of optic nerve disease. The central retina provides some 90% of the axons of the optic nerve, and if these are affected visual acuity is decreased, often with disturbed color vision. Disorders that affect the optic nerves anterior to the decussation in the chiasm impair vision in one eye only and cause an afferent pupillary defect (see Chapter 7). Disorders in the chiasm or the optic tract affect vision in both eyes.

Pain occurs only in retrobulbar neuritis, in which there is pain deep in the orbit when the eye rotates or when pressure is applied to the eye. Visual acuity and color vision are decreased, an afferent pupillary defect is present, and the disk appears normal. The causes of papillitis are similar to those of retrobulbar neuritis, but there is no pain and the optic disk is swollen. In anterior ischemic optic neuropathy, vision is reduced and the optic disk is edematous and pale, often with splinter hemorrhages. The fellow eye often has an exceptionally small physiologic cup. Vision is often normal in papilledema, and diagnosis is based on the ophthalmoscopic appearance of the swollen disk and retina. In optic atrophy the diagnosis is based on a correlation of an abnormal visual field with a pale, abnormal optic disk.

Ophthalmoscopy plays a major role in the diagnosis of optic nerve abnormalities since the optic disk may be viewed directly. The central artery is slightly to the nasal side of the disk with the vein to its temporal side. A small whitish depression is located near the center of the disk (optic cup, physiologic cup). Surrounding the optic cup is the neural rim, a tissue composed of axons, columns of astrocytes, and capillaries, which give the rim a pink appearance. The margins of the optic disk are usually regular. In some normal eyes the retinal pigment epithelium and choroid do not extend to the disk, and a crescent of sclera is visible. In other eyes the retinal pigment epithelium terminates short of the disk so that the choroid is visible.

The physiologic cup transmits the central retinal artery and vein but appears white without other blood vessels. It is often conspicuous and symmetrically located within the central optic disk. It may be absent, which suggests a small scleral canal, or extend obliquely toward the nasal side of the eye. The cup/disk ratio is the ratio of the horizontal width of the optic cup to the horizontal width of the optic disk. A high ratio in one or both eyes, or a much higher ratio in one compared to the fellow eye, is an important sign in the diagnosis of glaucoma.

Neovascularization of the surface of the optic disk occurs in diabetes mellitus, branch and central vein occlusion, obstruction or insufficiency of the internal carotid artery, pulseless disease (Takayasu disease), and other diseases associated with ischemia. New vessels are derived from the posterior ciliary arteries and not the retinal blood vessels. In optic atrophy the neuroretinal rim of the disk that surrounds the physiologic cup loses its blood vessel and becomes white.

DEVELOPMENTAL ANOMALIES

Myelinated (medullated) nerve fibers.— Myelination of the anterior visual system begins in the lateral geniculate body at 5 months' gestation. It reaches the chiasm at 6 to 7 months, the intraorbital optic nerve at 8 months, and the lamina cribrosa at birth. Sometimes (0.1%) the process does not stop but continues from the optic disk over the sensory retinal surface (Fig 20-1). Ophthalmoscopy discloses a white, glistening opacity with soft, feathered edges, that contrasts sharply with the adjacent red fundus.

The myelination involves only a small segment of the retina, usually near to the optic disk. The absence of pigment proliferation, the feathery edges, and the normal visual field differentiate myelinated nerve fibers from chorioretinitis. Rarely, a patch of myelinated nerve fibers is visible on the surface of the retina, and the retina surrounding the optic nerve is not myelinated. There are no symptoms, and treatment is not indicated.

Hyaloid artery.—The hyaloid artery is the major vascular system of the embryonic eye. After the fetal fissure closes, the artery is enclosed in the eye at the optic disk. Its anterior

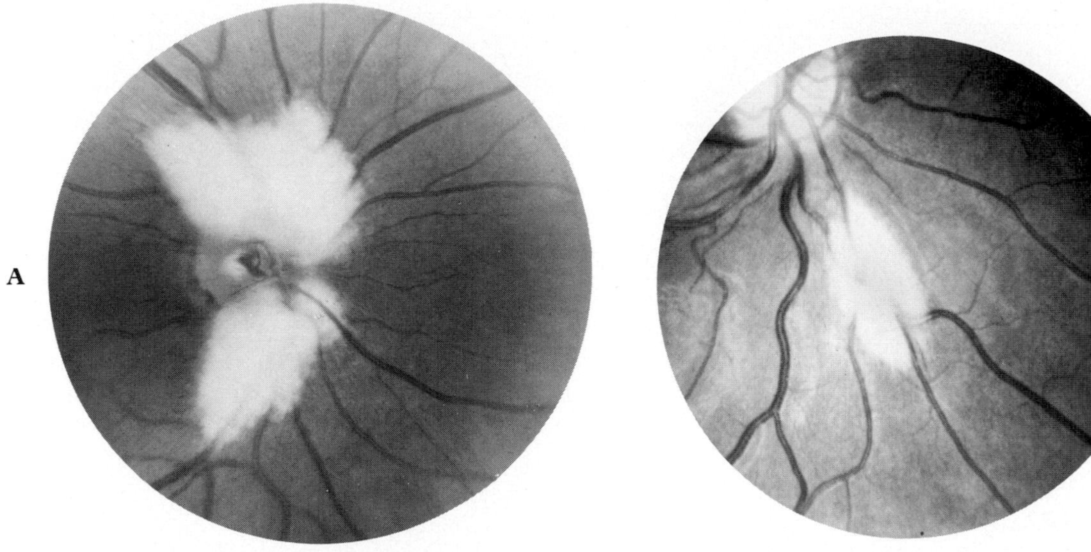

FIG 20-1.
A, Myelination of the optic nerve encroaching over margins of the optic disk. **B,** Small patch of myelination of peripheral retinal nerve fibers.

communication provides the tunica vasculosa of the lens, which begins to atrophy at the 60-mm stage and is complete by 8½ gestational months. The ophthalmoscopic appearance of the remnants of the tunica vasculosa lentis allows an estimate of the gestational age of premature infants. The muscae volitantes of the vitreous humor are minute residual fragments of the hyaloid system.

At the 100-mm stage of fetal development the hyaloid artery forms a fusiform enlargement, the bulb, from which the retinal blood vessels originate. The bulb is surrounded by a small mass of neuroglia, the Bergmeister papilla, which begin to atrophy at the end of the seventh month to form the physiologic cup of the optic disk.

Persistence of the primary vitreous results from failure of the hyaloid vascular system to regress. The crystalline lens develops abnormally, and there are secondary changes in the globe and fetal retina. The condition is the most common abnormality to be confused with retinoblastoma. Occasionally a short stub of the hyaloid artery projects into the vitreous cavity from the center of the disk. It is usually of no clinical significance, although it may rarely be a source of vitreous hemorrhage. Failure of a Bergmeister papilla to atrophy fully may slightly elevate the center of the optic disk.

Drusen.—Two kinds of drusen (German pl. *druse:* stony nodule, geode) occur in the intraocular portion of the optic nerve. Optic nerve drusen are (1) common drusen and (2) giant drusen. Both differ from retinal drusen (see Chapter 17).

Common drusen are laminated, calcareous, acellular accretions. They are the result of axonal degeneration with calcification. When deep in the disk, they may blur the disk margins, which is differentiated from papilledema by the absence of dilated veins. The blood vessels may trifurcate rather than bifurcate on the optic disk surface. Drusen autofluoresce and may be seen more clearly in red-free (green) light. In adults they enlarge and approach the surface of the disk and give it an irregular, nodular appearance (Fig 20-2). Drusen often cause visual field defects but rarely reduce visual acuity. Hemorrhage on the disk, adjacent retina, or vitreous rarely occurs. Computed tomography, magnetic resonance imaging, and ultrasonography demonstrate them well. The optic nerve sheaths are not distended as in papilledema. Drusen must not be confused with more serious lesions of the optic nerve. Angioid streaks (see Chapter 17), pigmentary degeneration of the retina, and optic atrophy are associated with common drusen. They are rarely familial.

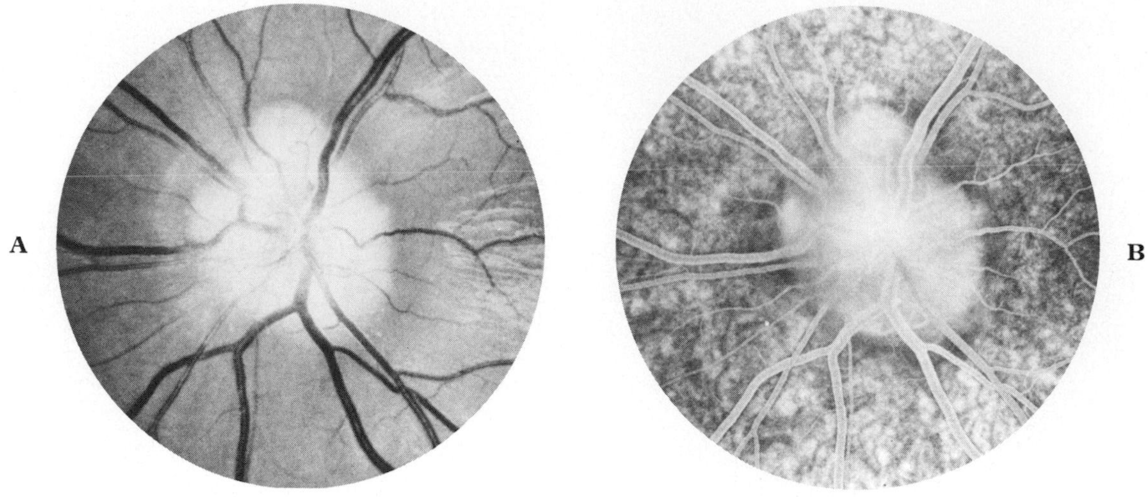

FIG 20-2.
Common drusen of the optic nerve. **A,** Blurred optic disk margins without venous congestion. **B,** Late phase of fluorescein angiography with drusen clearly evident without vascular leakage.

The second type of drusen is giant drusen, which are astrocytic hamartomas that occur with tuberous sclerosis (see Chapter 26).

Pseudopapilledema.—The terms pseudopapilledema, pseudoptic neuritis, and pseudophthalmitis describe a congenital abnormality of the optic disk in which the disk margins are blurred by heaped nerve fibers, accentuated by an excess of glial tissue. The disk has a dirty, grayish appearance with ill-defined margins, frequently most marked on its nasal side. It occurs in severely hyperopic eyes. Vision is not impaired. The retinal nerve fiber layer and the retinal blood vessels are normal. The condition is not progressive and requires no treatment. Drusen of the optic nerve may also blur the disk margin.

Hypoplasia of the optic nerve.—This is a developmental abnormality in which the numbers of ganglion cells and their axons in the retina are reduced. There is no reduction in the supporting tissues of the optic nerve. It may be unilateral (20%) or bilateral (80%), be associated with other developmental defects, or occur as an isolated defect.

Vision is usually reduced, often with a pendular nystagmus, and there is esotropia. The optic disks appear small and surrounded by a pigmented ring and a halo that approaches the size of the normal disk. The retinal blood vessels are of normal size and distribution. There may be severe structural defects of the eye (microphthalmos, colobomas, aniridia), nystagmus, and marked hyperopia.

Midline craniofacial abnormalities occur, often septo-optic dysplasia. There are sagittal midline defects of the central nervous system that include agenesis of the corpus callosum and the septum pellucidum. Abnormalities of the pituitary hormones include reduced growth hormone levels and diabetes insipidus. Most cases are sporadic, although familial cases occur. Some instances are associated with the maternal use of insulin, other medications, illegal drugs, or illness during pregnancy.

Colobomas and pits of the optic disk.—Incomplete closure of the fetal fissure causes optic nerve defects that range from a deep physiologic cup, to a pit in the optic nerve, to a deeply excavated optic nerve (Fig 20-3), which may be associated with colobomas of the choroid and iris. Vision is often reduced. A coloboma appears as a discrete, focal, glistening white, bowl-shaped excavation of the inferior portion of a vertically enlarged optic disk. There is no disturbance of the retinal or choroidal pigmentation. There may be associated ocular defects and failure of the eye to develop normally. The condition is mainly unilateral, but bilateral colobomas of the optic disk occur as an autosomal dominant hereditary defect.

The morning glory anomaly of the optic disk is characterized by a funnel-shaped excavation of the optic disk that is surrounded by chorio-

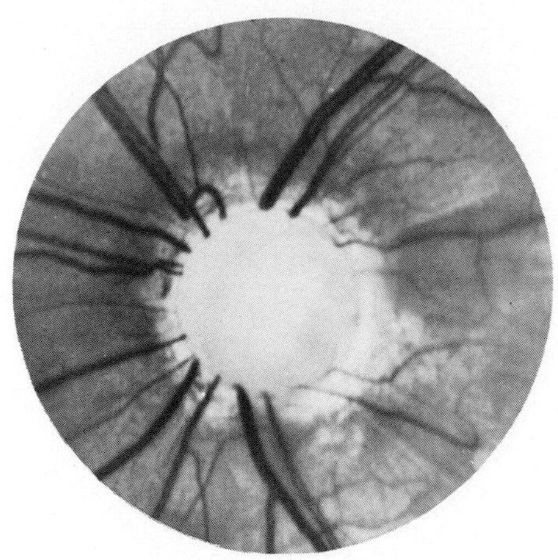

FIG 20-3.
Coloboma of the optic disk in a 19-year-old man with a visual acuity of 20/40. This condition is transmitted as an autosomal dominant defect. Patients are particularly prone to develop a central serous choroidopathy that suggests a communication between the subretinal space and the subarachnoid space.

retinal pigment proliferation and proliferated glial tissue above or in the excavated optic nerve. Anomalous, straight retinal vessels extend peripherally from the margin of the round scleral canal. There may be associated retinal vascular anomalies, severe myopia, and retinal detachment without retinal holes. The posterior sclera may be deficient with optic nerve protruding into it. Females are affected twice as often as males. Midline defects include cleft lip and palate, basal encephalocele, hypertelorism, and agenesis of the corpus callosum. Pituitary dwarfism is a rare complication. Unlike colobomas of the optic disk, the morning glory anomaly is rarely a familial disorder.

Pits in the optic disk are probably incomplete colobomas of the optic nerve. They are usually single and are located in the inferotemporal region of the optic disk. The pit appears darker than the surrounding tissue and is usually round or oval. The pit may be shallow or as deep as 8 mm. It varies from one eighth to one third the size of the disk. A small central scotoma is often present. The pit communicates with the subarachnoid space of the meningeal coverings of the optic nerve. About one third of the affected patients develop a central serous choroidopathy, presumably because of seepage of cerebrospinal fluid into the subretinal space. Treatment is difficult and often not successful. Photocoagulation to the temporal margin of the optic disk combined with intravitreal injection of an expanding gas (C_3F_8) reattaches the retina in about 75% of the occurrences.

Optociliary shunt vessels.—These are markedly dilated veins on the surface of the optic disk that occur as sequelae to gradual obstruction of the central retinal vein behind the lamina cribrosa. They shunt venous blood from the retinal circulation to the choroid, the vortex veins, and the superior and inferior ophthalmic veins. The disk is swollen and vision is reduced. The vessels may occur in meningioma of the optic nerve coverings, glioma, drusen, arachnoid cysts, sarcoid of the optic nerve, and chronic atrophic papilledema. They may follow resolution of a branch retinal vein obstruction.

PAPILLEDEMA

Papilledema is a passive swelling of the optic nerve that occurs secondary to increased pressure in the subarachnoid space of the meningeal coverings of the brain and the optic nerves. The subarachnoid space that surrounds the optic nerve must be patent for papilledema to occur, and thus an atrophic optic nerve is not affected. The central retinal vein passes through the meningeal sheath as it exits from the optic nerve, and thus papilledema impedes venous flow. The increased pressure in the optic nerve sheath slows, but does not stop, slow transport in axons with resultant axonal swelling, particularly in the region of the lamina cribrosa. The swelling produces a secondary but minimal reduction in fast axonal transport.

Papilledema may be divided into four stages: (1) early; (2) fully developed; (3) chronic; and (4) atrophic.

Papilledema begins with hyperemia of the optic disk and (usually) loss of spontaneous pulsation of the central retinal vein. The retina adjacent to the optic disk loses its light reflexes and appears deep red without luster. Small radial hemorrhages may occur on the margin of the disk. The margins of the optic disk may be blurred.

In the fully developed condition (Fig 20-4), the margins of the optic disk are blurred and elevated above the surface of the retina. The retinal veins are engorged, dusky red, and splin-

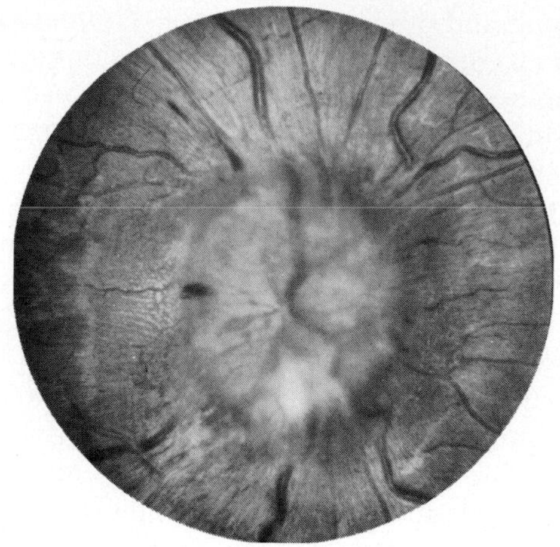

FIG 20-4.
Chronic papilledema in a 33-year-old woman with idiopathic intracranial hypertension. Visual acuity was 20/20 in each eye, and the papilledema disappeared spontaneously.

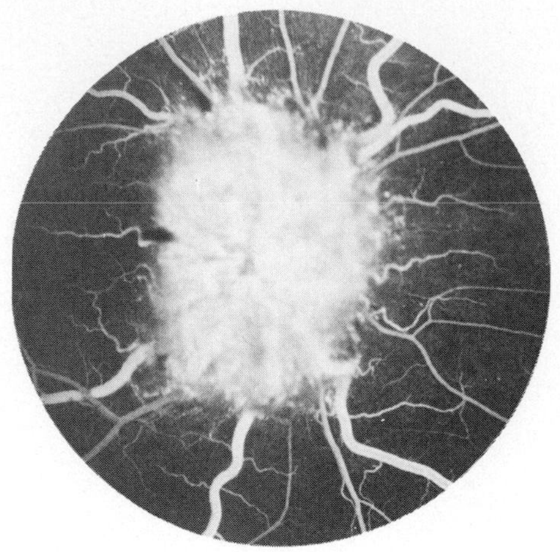

FIG 20-5.
Fluorescein angiography of papilledema. Dye shows the dilated veins and outlines the hemorrhages. There is fluorescein leakage, which never occurs from normal optic disk vessels.

ter hemorrhages occur adjacent to the disk margin. Increased pressure on the eye does not induce pulsation of the retinal veins. There may be cotton-wool patches (ischemic infarcts of the retina), hard exudates (chronic retinal edema residues), and retinal hemorrhages. Capillaries on the surface of the optic disk leak fluorescein (Fig 20-5). The swollen disk displaces the sensory retina, and the blind spot is enlarged on visual field testing. Magnetic resonance imaging discloses distention of the optic nerve sheaths.

If the papilledema persists the hyperemia disappears and the optic disk has a gray, milky appearance from secondary to neuronal degeneration and gliosis. Finally there is an atrophic (secondary) optic atrophy with sheathed, narrow retinal blood vessels and a grayish gliosis of a shrunken and inconspicuous optic disk.

The severity of papilledema is often proportionate to the increase in the intracranial pressure. Papilledema, however, is not an invariable accompaniment of increased intracranial pressure. When papilledema fails to develop although the intracranial pressure is increased, the subarachnoid space surrounding the optic nerve is probably not patent. Similarly, if the flow of cerebrospinal fluid from the brain to the spinal cord is blocked in a patient with increased intracranial pressure, there may be papilledema with a low pressure found on lumbar puncture.

Headache is the earliest symptom of increased intracranial pressure. It has no localizing value except in meningioma, which sometimes causes local pain at the site of the tumor. The headache is sometimes aggravated by coughing and straining. In the late stages there may be unconsciousness with generalized motor rigidity and dilation of both pupils. Visual symptoms may be limited to transient obscurations of vision sometimes aggravated by a change in the position of the head. Rarely there is a paresis of one or both lateral recti muscles (abducent nerve [N VI]) or superior oblique muscles (trochlear nerve [N IV]). In the late stages the optic atrophy results in a complete loss of vision.

Papilledema is caused by a variety of disorders (Table 20-1). Brain tumors located below the tentorium are more likely to cause papilledema than those located above. Papilledema may occur in blood dyscrasias and in hypertensive cardiovascular disease. In hypertensive cardiovascular disease, the retinal cotton-wool spots and the arteriolar constriction serve to distinguish hypertensive papilledema from that caused by intracranial neoplasms. Papilledema is seen in idiopathic intracranial hypertension (pseudotumor cerebri), congenital hydrocephalus, craniosynostosis, and after head injury. Pulmonary insufficiency, particularly that asso-

TABLE 20-1.
Some Causes of Papilledema

I. Space-occupying intracranial lesions
II. Idiopathic intracranial hypertension
III. Development disorders: craniostenosis, aqueduct stenosis (adult type), syringomyelia
IV. Vascular hypertension, heart failure
V. Microbial infections: meningitis, encephalitis, brain abscess, Lyme disease
VI. Cranial trauma: epidural, subdural, intracranial hematoma
VII. Intracranial vascular abnormalities: sagittal sinus thrombosis, dural sinus thrombosis, superior vena cava syndrome, jugular vein obstruction, carotid-cavernous sinus fistula, subarachnoid hemorrhage
VIII. Toxicity: tetracycline, minocycline, nalidixic acid, oral progestational agents, lead, arsenic, corticosteroid administration and withdrawal, vitamin A, cancer chemotherapy
IX. Metabolic disorders: obesity, diabetic ketoacidosis, hypothyroidism, hypoparathyroidism, Addison disease, scurvy, dialysis disequilibrium
X. Sarcoidosis, lupus erythematosus, syphilis, gastrointestinal hemorrhage, status epilepticus, carcinomatosis meningitis, serum sickness, pulmonary emphysema, Guillain-Barré syndrome, cysticercosis
XI. Hematologic disorders: leukemia, thrombocytopenia, pernicious anemia, iron-deficiency anemia, polycythemia, hemophilia, infectious mononucleosis
XII. Occlusive disease of posterior ciliary arteries, anterior ischemic optic neuropathy, giant cell arteritis

ciated with cystic fibrosis of the pancreas, may cause papilledema.

Treatment must be directed to the cause. Persistent papilledema is associated with secondary optic atrophy and loss of vision. Surgical decompression of the optic nerve is indicated to preserve vision.

Idiopathic intracranial hypertension.— Idiopathic intracranial hypertension (pseudotumor cerebri) occurs predominantly in obese women of the reproductive age group. It is characterized by (1) papilledema; (2) increased intracranial pressure; (3) normal cerebrospinal fluid composition; (4) normal-sized or small cerebral ventricles; and (5) normal results of neurologic examination except for the papilledema and rarely an abducent nerve (N VI) paralysis. The symptoms are those of increased intracranial pressure with transient blurring of vision, and headaches aggravated by coughing and sneezing.

Obesity, menstrual irregularity, and recent weight gain are common, but often no abnormality is evident. Treatment includes reducing diet, diuretics (furosemide, ranitidine, and acetazolamide), pulsed intravenous methylprednisolone for 5 days followed by tapering prednisone, and hyperosmotic agents. Lumboperitoneal shunting of the cerebrospinal fluid is required for intractable headaches with normal ocular function. In patients with progressive loss of central or peripheral vision, with or without headache, the treatment of choice is decompression of the optic nerve.

The optic nerve is exposed through a conjunctival incision, detachment of the medial rectus muscle, and lateral rotation of the globe. By means of a knife, scissors, or laser, multiple, linear, longitudinal incisions are made in the distended meningeal covering of the optic nerve. A cytotoxic agent such as mitomycin is sometimes used to prevent closure of the meningeal fistulas. In about 75% of the patients the headache is relieved, but the remainder require lumboperitoneal shunting of the cerebrospinal fluid.

OPTIC NEURITIS

Optic neuritis is an inflammation of the optic nerve that may occur anywhere in its course from the optic disk to the optic chiasm. The chief causes are infection (often viral), demyelinating diseases (mainly multiple sclerosis), and autoimmune disorders. When the intraocular portion of the nerve is affected, the optic disk is swollen and hyperemic, and the condition is called papillitis or anterior optic neuritis. If the optic disk is normal the condition is called retrobulbar neuritis. If both the optic disk and the adjacent temporal retina are inflamed the condition is called neuroretinitis.

The main symptom is a loss of vision in one eye, sometimes occurring within several hours, in an individual aged 20 to 50 years. The severity of the visual loss varies from a minimal reduction to loss of all light perception. Color vision is markedly reduced. In patients with minimal depression of visual acuity, a marked difference in color vision in the two eyes can be demonstrated by using color plates. An afferent pupillary defect is always present. It is detected by alternate light stimulation of the retina in a dimly illuminated room. The pupil of the affected eye constricts normally in the consensual reaction when the normal eye is stimulated. When the light stimulus is directed quickly to the affected eye, the pupil dilates rather than remaining constricted.

A central or paracentral scotoma is present. Altitudinal defects, arcuate scotomas, or cecocentral scotomas are rare and suggest an optic neuropathy rather than an optic neuritis. Retrobulbar inflammation of the optic nerve in the orbit where it is adjacent to the medial and superior recti muscles causes pain on movement of the eye. There may be tenderness on palpation of the globe through the closed eyelids. This pain, combined with loss of vision, the central scotoma, and the normal ophthalmoscopic appearance of the optic disk, suggests a retrobulbar neuritis.

In papillitis, the disk appears smaller than normal because of diminished contrast with the surrounding retina. The disk margins are obscured, and there is dilation of retinal veins. Flame-shaped hemorrhages may occur on the surface of the disk and the adjacent retina. In severe inflammations, hard, yellow retinal deposits occur, which may be grouped about the fovea centralis in an oval (circinate) pattern. With persistence of the swelling there may be glial tissue proliferation from the disk along the retinal vessels, and any subsequent atrophy is classified as "secondary." Ophthalmoscopically, early papilledema and early papillitis appear the same, but vision is decreased in papillitis and not in papilledema. Additionally, papillitis is unilateral, and inflammatory cells may be seen in the vitreous humor adjacent to the optic disk by using a biomicroscope and a condensing lens.

The visual-evoked response is always abnormal. Computed tomography demonstrates a diffuse swelling of the optic nerve. Magnetic resonance imaging demonstrates both the optic nerve abnormality and patchy areas of loss of tissue in the intracranial lesions of multiple sclerosis.

Irrespective of the portion of the nerve inflamed, the causes are the same (Table 20-2). Painless loss of vision with a central scotoma occurs in disorders affecting the fovea centralis, such as cystoid macular edema and central serous choroidopathy. In optic neuritis an afferent pupillary defect is present, and color vision is more severely depressed than in retinal conditions. A penlight beam directed into the eye for 10 seconds does not further impair vision in optic neuritis, whereas vision is reduced one or more Snellen lines in central serous choroidopathy. Children develop papillitis more frequently than adults. Elderly individuals who develop disk swelling with acute monocular loss of vision probably have an anterior ischemic optic neuropathy.

TABLE 20-2.
Some Causes of Optic Neuritis

- Demyelinative disease
  - Multiple sclerosis
  - Acute disseminated encephalomyelitis
  - Neuromyelitis optica (Devic disease)
  - Diffuse periaxial encephalitis (Schilder disease)
  - Diffuse cerebral sclerosis (Krabbe disease, Pelizaeus-Merzbacher syndrome, metachromatic leukodystrophy)
- Systemic disease
  - Autoimmune encephalitis
  - Lupus erythematosus
  - Infection
    - Viral
      - Upper respiratory, mumps, measles, mononucleosis, herpes zoster
    - Bacterial
      - Syphilis, tuberculosis, meningitis
- Ocular inflammation
  - Keratitis, uveitis, endophthalmitis, orbital cellulitis

It is often not possible to determine the cause of optic neuritis. Within 2 years of an attack of optic neuritis the risk of multiple sclerosis is approximately 20%. Within 15 years the risk is between 45% and 80%. About one third of patients with demonstrable multiple sclerosis develop an optic neuritis sometime in the course of their disease. The visual-evoked potential (see Chapter 2) may be impaired in patients with no history of optic neuritis who have multiple sclerosis with intracranial lesions indicated by magnetic resonance imaging.

The Optic Neuritis Treatment Trial found that pulsed intravenous methylprednisolone followed by oral prednisone accelerated recovery of visual acuity and delayed the onset of multiple sclerosis (see Chapter 28). The patients received intravenous methylprednisolone (250 mg every

6 hours) for 3 days followed by oral prednisone (1 mg/kg of body weight) for 11 days.

White patients with a medical history of optic neuritis in the fellow eye and ill-defined neurologic signs, associated with a family history of multiple sclerosis are at high risk to develop multiple sclerosis. Oral prednisone treatment does not improve the visual outcome, is associated with an increased risk of a new attack of optic neuritis, and is contraindicated.

In severe inflammations of the retina or the choroid, there is often an extension of the inflammatory process to the optic nerve. The primary disease dominates the clinical picture.

OPTIC NEUROPATHY

Optic neuropathy describes abnormalities of the optic nerve that occur as the result of ischemia, toxins, vascular and blood pressure abnormalities, and compression within the orbit. Ischemic disorders are termed "arteritic" when they occur secondary to inflammations of blood vessels, chiefly giant cell arteritis (temporal arteritis). They are termed "nonarteritic" when they are secondary to occlusive disease or other noninflammatory disorders of blood vessels. Optic neuropathy is divided into anterior, which causes a pale edema of the optic disk, and posterior, in which the optic disk is not swollen and the abnormality occurs between the globe and the optic chiasm (Table 20-3).

TABLE 20-3.
Classification of Optic Neuropathy

- I. Anterior (optic disk edematous)
  - A. Ischemic
    - 1. Blood vessel inflammation (arteritic)
  - B. Occlusive
    - 1. Noninflammatory and occlusive blood vessel disease (nonarteritic)
  - C. Idiopathic
    - 1. Compressive
      - a. Tumor: glioma, meningioma, hamartoma, choristoma, malignant tumor
    - 2. Ocular hypotony
    - 3. Toxic
    - 4. Primary tumor of optic disk
- II. Posterior (without optic disk edema)
  - A. Idiopathic
    - 1. Compressive
    - 2. Toxic
    - 3. Infiltrative
    - 4. Hereditary
  - B. Ischemic
    - 1. Blood vessel inflammation (arteritic) (anterior more common)
  - C. Occlusive (nonarteritic)

Ischemic anterior optic neuropathy.— Interruption of the blood flow in the short posterior ciliary arteries that supply the optic disk results in a severe loss of vision, altitudinal visual field defects, and a pale, swollen optic disk, with peripapillary hemorrhages (Fig 20-6). The condition is noninflammatory, is clearly ischemic, and affects the nerve fibers immediately posterior to the optic disk in the prelaminar portion of the intraocular optic nerve (see Chapter 1). The optic disk is smaller than normal, the physiologic cup is small or absent, and there are many branches of retinal blood vessels on the surface of the optic disk. In many respects the disk resembles that seen in pseudopapillitis (in this chapter). The neuropathy is bilateral in 40% of the patients, but recurrence in the same eye is exceptional.

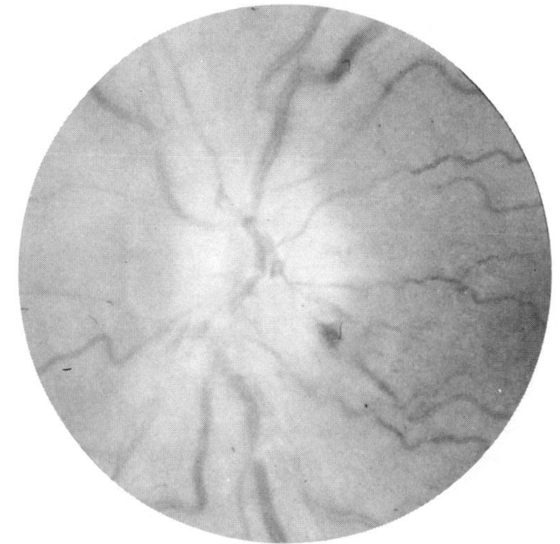

FIG 20-6.
Ischemic optic neuropathy with new small, flame-shaped hemorrhage at the 4 o'clock meridian of the disk.

Ischemic anterior optic neuropathy usually causes a loss of vision that may be sudden or occur over several days. Patients are generally older than those with optic neuritis. There is often loss of the inferior visual field. An afferent pupillary defect is present. The optic disk is swollen and may resemble that seen in papilledema or the swelling may be minimal. Hyperemia of the disk is exceptional, and the disk appears pale. Single or multiple flame-shaped hemorrhages occur near the disk margin. Cotton-wool deposits may be present.

Visual acuity is usually reduced more severely in the inflammatory type. Altitudinal visual field defects are common, with loss of the inferior visual field being more frequent than loss of the superior. An afferent pupillary defect is present. Ophthalmoscopic examination discloses a swollen optic disk that may be so severe as to suggest a papilledema, or there may be mild edema. Hyperemia of the disk is rare, and the disk is usually pale. Single or multiple flame-shaped hemorrhages occur near the disk margin. Cotton-wool patches may be present.

Young patients with abnormally small disks may have recurrent attacks of segmental swelling of the optic disks, with the ischemia ultimately causing blindness. Insulin-dependent diabetes mellitus in some patients with small optic disks is associated with recurrent swelling of the disks. Dilated peripapillary capillaries appear to ameliorate the ischemic process. The hereditary optic neuropathy of Leber, a mitochondrial mutation (see Chapter 26), is also associated with small optic disks.

Posterior ischemic optic neuropathy.—This is an uncommon type of neuropathy, and diagnosis depends largely on exclusion of other causes, chiefly stroke and brain tumor. There are altitudinal visual field defects, sometimes combined with decreased visual acuity. Decreased blood flow in the minute pial vessels supplying the nerve, connective tissue disorders, diabetes mellitus, trauma, and radiotherapy to the orbit have all been described as causes.

Giant cell arteritis.—Giant cell arteritis (temporal arteritis, cranial arteritis) is a chronic, disseminated, inflammatory disease of segments of large and medium-sized arteries that occurs mainly in individuals more than 50 years old. Possibly it is an autoimmune hypersensitivity to the elastic tissue of arteries. It is probably a part of the same disease process as polymyalgia rheumatica, which occurs without arteritis.

Initially, the headache is severe and may be intractable to treatment. The temporal arteries, when affected, become prominent and tender. The cerebral vessels are not affected. There is often erythema of the overlying skin. Pain with chewing or talking is a common complaint. The erythrocyte sedimentation rate is increased; fever may be present.

One to four weeks after the onset of the headache, sudden loss of vision may be caused by inflammation of the central retinal artery or the short posterior ciliary arteries that supply the optic disk. There may be occlusion of branches of retinal arteries, retinal hemorrhage, exudates, and occasionally ocular pain. Often both eyes are affected, the second eye from 1 to 21 days after the first.

Palsies of extraocular muscles, especially of the lateral recti muscles, may occur. Loss of vision may occur in some patients without obvious signs of temporal artery involvement, but biopsy of the temporal artery may indicate the typical histiocytes, epithelioid cells, and multinucleated giant cells in intima and media adjacent to a highly fragmented or absent elastic lamina. Some patients appear curiously unconcerned about the devastating loss of vision.

The diagnosis of giant cell arteritis must be considered in all cases of sudden loss of vision, occlusion of retinal blood vessels, and unexplained ophthalmoplegia in elderly individuals. If ocular symptoms are associated with an increased erythrocyte sedimentation rate, temporal artery biopsy is indicated. Serum alkaline phosphatase and C-reactive protein are increased.

Once vision is lost it seldom improves, but remarkable recovery has been described. Corticosteroids should be administered before visual loss has occurred in the fellow eye. Low dosages of corticosteroids may be required for several years.

Toxic optic neuropathy.—The characteristic finding in toxic lesions of the optic nerve is a scotoma that includes both the blind spot and the fovea (cecocentral scotoma). If the optic disk is swollen these are designated as anterior, and if the disk is not swollen, as posterior. The visual loss is often progressive and an atrophy of the papillomacular retinal nerve fibers results in an optic atrophy involving the temporal portion of the optic nerve.

Deficiencies of a single portion of the vitamin B complex may be responsible: B_{12} (cobalamin), B_6 (pyridoxine), B_1 (thiamine), niacin, or riboflavin. Topical amblyopia may occur in poorly nourished individuals in whom the food staple cassava results in cyanide intoxication. Tobacco-alcohol amblyopia is seen in heavy smokers and alcoholics who are poorly nourished. Lead, methyl alcohol, and many other substances may be causes. A variety of drugs have been implicated: digitalis, Antabuse, quinine, streptomycin, chloramphenicol, ethambutol, and isoniazid.

OPTIC ATROPHY

The nerve fibers of the optic nerve originate in the ganglion cells in the retina and synapse in the lateral geniculate body and the pretectal nuclei. Disease or trauma to the ganglion cells or their axons results in their permanent loss. When severe enough, this loss is visible at the optic disk with the ophthalmoscope. The loss of axons reorients the astrocytes within the optic disk surface, which obscures the capillaries on the surface of the disk, giving it the pale, white color characteristic of optic atrophy. If the lesion causing the optic atrophy is in the retina, an ascending optic atrophy occurs, which terminates in the lateral geniculate body. Descending optic atrophy follows disorders involving optic nerve fibers anterior to their synapse in the lateral geniculate body.

The chief symptom of optic atrophy is reduced central or peripheral vision. Despite marked pallor of the nerve, visual function may seem normal and require refined visual field testing, extensive color vision evaluation, and psychophysical testing to demonstrate an abnormality. Careful study of the nerve fiber layer adjacent to the disk by using a contact lens and the biomicroscope may demonstrate loss of nerve fibers.

The chief symptom of optic atrophy is loss of central or peripheral vision. Inability to demonstrate a defect by means of confrontation fields does not exclude a visual field defect that might require extremely small stimuli to detect.

The atrophy is called primary if there are no ophthalmoscopic signs of preceding edema or inflammation. It is called secondary if there is a preceding papillitis or papilledema. The same conditions may be responsible for either a primary or a secondary optic atrophy; the sole difference is the abnormality of the optic disk that precedes a secondary optic atrophy.

Primary optic atrophy.—In primary optic atrophy the number of nerve fiber bundles in the optic nerve is reduced, and there is a rearrangement of the remaining disk astrocytes into dense parallel layers across the nerve head. The disk margins are distinct and there appears to be a loss of capillaries, although they are demonstrated on fluorescein angiography. The atrophy may be complete or partial. The ophthalmoscopic appearance of pallor does not parallel the severity of the visual field loss.

TABLE 20-4.
Etiologic Classification of Optic Atrophy

I. Glaucoma
II. Retinal ganglion cell or nerve fiber disease
  A. Pigmentary degeneration of the retina
  B. Chorioretinal degenerations, inflammations, atrophy
III. Inflammation
  A. Demyelinating disease
  B. Meningitis, encephalitis, abscess
  C. Tabes dorsalis
  D. Optic neuritis
  E. Metastatic septicemia
IV. Optic neuropathy
V. Papilledema
VI. Toxicity
  A. Chemical: arsenic, lead, methanol, ethanol, quinine, tobacco, chloroquine, ethambutol, chloramphenicol
  B. Vitamin B deficiency: beriberi, pellagra, pernicious anemia
VII. Glioma
  A. Juvenile pilocytic astrocytoma
  B. Adult malignant astrocytoma (glioblastoma)
VIII. Heredity
  A. Leber disease
  B. Dominant juvenile early infantile optic atrophy with diabetes mellitus and sometimes deafness
  C. Behr disease
  D. Glucose-6-phosphate dehydrogenase deficiency—Worcester variant
IX. Trauma

Open-angle glaucoma (see Chapter 23) is the chief cause of primary optic atrophy (Table 20-4). Additionally, the physiologic cup is enlarged so that it extends to the margin of the disk. After central artery occlusion or after quinine poisoning, the optic nerve may appear to be waxy white and the retinal vessels may appear as small white cords. In the late stages of retinal pigmentary degenerations, the disk appears to have a yellowish waxy color with attenuated arteries crossing it. In lesions limited to the central retina, the atrophy involves only the

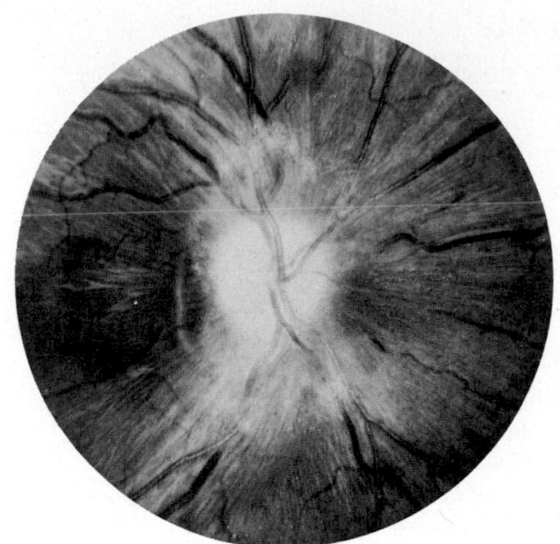

FIG 20-7.
Secondary optic atrophy.

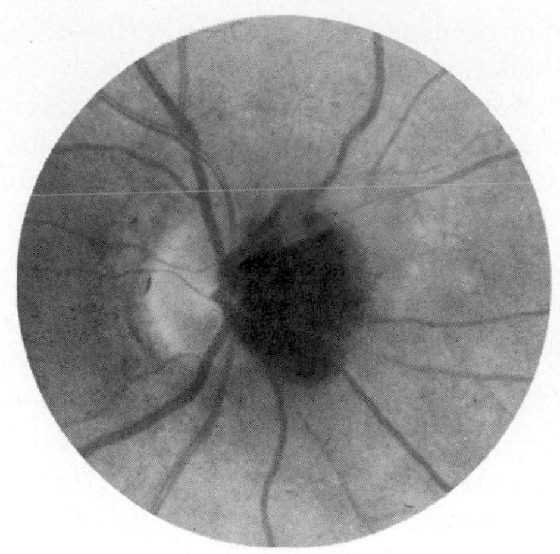

FIG 20-8.
Melanocytoma of the optic disk of the right eye.

papillomacular bundle at the temporal margin of the optic disk.

Secondary optic atrophy.—Secondary optic atrophy is preceded by swelling of the optic disk, caused by papilledema or papillitis. Ophthalmoscopically, the disk margins appear blurred, the lamina cribrosa is obscured, and gliosis of the disk extends over the retina (Fig 20-7). The blood vessels may be obscured and their course distorted by glia.

OPTIC NERVE TUMORS

Retinoblastomas and malignant melanomas of the choroid may extend to involve the optic nerve. Primary optic nerve tumors are uncommon.

Melanocytoma.—A melanocytoma of the optic disk (Fig 20-8) is a heavily pigmented nevus that usually occurs on the inferior temporal portion of the optic disk but may cover the entire disk. It occurs mainly in deeply pigmented individuals. It has but a low malignant potential.

Glioma.—Juvenile gliomas (juvenile pilocytic astrocytomas) have their onset in the first decade of life and are astrocytic hamartomas. The orbital portion of the optic nerve is involved in about half the instances, whereas the tumor is both orbital and chiasmal in the remainder. Orbital tumors cause proptosis. Loss of vision occurs irrespective of the tumor location. About 15% of patients with neurofibromatosis develop an optic nerve glioma.

Adult glioma is a rapidly progressive malignant astrocytoma (glioblastoma) that occurs in middle-aged adults and results in death within 2 years. The tumor is not related to juvenile gliomas.

Optic nerve sheath meningiomas.—Meningiomas affecting the optic nerve originate either from the meningeal coverings of the nerve or extend from the cranial cavity. They cause a slowly progressive loss of vision, optic atrophy, and optociliary shunt vessels. The symptoms and signs are similar to those of sphenoidal ridge meningiomas. Computed tomography demonstrates enlargement of the optic nerve. Women are mainly (5:1) affected; neurofibromatosis is present in about 15%.

BIBLIOGRAPHY

Books

Miller NR: *Walsh and Hoyt's clinical neuro-ophthalmology,* vols 1-4, Baltimore, 1982-1991, Williams & Wilkins.

Spoor TC: *Atlas of optic nerve disorders,* New York, 1992, Raven Press.

Article

Hayreh SS: The optic nerve head circulation in health and disease, *Exp Eye Res* 61:259-272, 1995.

21

THE CRYSTALLINE LENS

The crystalline lens is a transparent, avascular, biconvex structure held in position directly posterior to the iris by zonular fibers. These fibers originate in the crypts between the ciliary processes and insert into the capsule of the lens at its equator. The capsule surrounds the crystalline lens; it is the thickest basement membrane in the body. The anterior capsule is the basement membrane of a single layer of epithelial cells located immediately beneath it. The posterior capsule is the basement membrane of lens fiber cells that have their nuclei near the equator of the lens in the nuclear bow. The majority of lens fibers have lost their cellular nuclei and have migrated inward to form an increasingly compact tissue. A central dense region is formed by the oldest lens fibers (the embryonic lens nucleus) and is surrounded by more recently formed fibers to constitute the lens nucleus. The recently formed lens fibers constitute the lens cortex. The lens metabolism is mainly anaerobic because the lens has no blood vessels. Minimal oxygen is dissolved in the aqueous humor and the vitreous humor surrounding it. The lens is not metabolically inert, has actively multiplying cells at the equator, and synthesizes lens proteins and membranes from amino acids derived from posterior chamber aqueous humor. It maintains a concentration gradient with high potassium, glutathione, ascorbic acid, and inositol levels, and remains relatively dehydrated.

The lens and the cornea are the main refracting surfaces of the eye. The inherent elasticity of the lens causes it to become more spherical as zonular fibers relax when the ciliary muscle contracts, which provides increased refractive power (accommodation). Because of compression of mature fibers in its central portion, the lens gradually loses its inherent elasticity. Usually by the age of 45 years, the loss of elasticity results in diminished accommodation and difficulty in reading and in seeing nearby objects (presbyopia; see Chapter 24).

The crystalline lens proteins are transparent because the lens fibers have a short-range spatial order similar to that of a dense, clear liquid. The only nuclei in the optical axis of the lens are the single layer of cells of the anterior lens epithelium. The main portion of the lens, in the cortex and the lens nucleus, is composed of lens cells (fibrils), which either have their nuclei at the equator of the lens or have lost their nuclei as they matured. Any loss of transparency results in an opacity of the crystalline lens, which is called a cataract. The term lens opacity is less ominous to a patient. Cataracts result from protein denaturation, increased molecular weight of proteins, water clefts, and vesicles between lens fibers.

SYMPTOMS AND SIGNS OF ABNORMALITIES OF THE LENS

The symptoms of abnormalities of the lens relate mainly to vision. In presbyopia, accommodation decreases and the ability to focus on near objects diminishes. Cataracts, in contrast, impair both near and distant vision. In nuclear sclerosis the index of refraction of the lens increases, thus increasing the refractive power of the anterior segment. This added refractive power may induce a myopia and permit the patient to read without glasses (the "second sight" of aging). The myopia reduces uncorrected vision for distance. Rarely, lens opacities in the visual axis cause an optical defect in which two or more blurred images are formed, a monocular diplopia. Opacities caused by the increased water content of the lens decrease vision, but the fluid may migrate or be absorbed, resulting in transient visual improvement. The coincidence of better vision in a patient receiving medication to treat cataract has led to many ineffective nostrums.

A partially dislocated (subluxated) lens may impair vision by substituting irregular refracting surfaces. If the lens is removed from the visual axis through complete dislocation or surgery, the eye loses a major refractive element and becomes severely hyperopic (aphakia). Marked swelling of the lens may obstruct the passage of aqueous humor from the posterior chamber to the anterior chamber and cause a pupillary block glaucoma. An opening in the lens capsule releases lens protein into the aqueous humor and causes uveitis and sometimes a secondary glaucoma.

Ophthalmoscopic examination with a convex lens (+10 D) and the pupil widely dilated discloses cataracts as dark opacities against the red background of the fundus reflex. To visualize the details and location of the opacity requires examination with a biomicroscope. Advanced cataracts (mature) prevent observation of the red fundus reflex.

If the lens is dislocated, the iris loses support and becomes tremulous, the condition of iridodonesis; the anterior chamber is deep. If a lens is dislocated into the vitreous body, it may be seen with the ophthalmoscope in the region to which it has gravitated as a dark sphere that magnifies the retina beneath it or as a black globule if it is cataractous.

DEVELOPMENTAL ANOMALIES

ECTOPIA LENTIS

When the crystalline lens capsule loses the entire support of the zonular fibers, the entire lens dislocates into either the vitreous cavity or the anterior chamber (Fig 21-1). If some, but not all, of the zonular fibers remain attached to the lens capsule, they act as a hinge so that the lens is subluxated from its usual position. Subluxation or dislocation of the lens of one eye is probably secondary to ocular trauma. Bilateral dislocation of the crystalline lens is probably the result of a hereditary or congenital defect.

The lens zonule consists of microfibrils composed solely of fibrillin. The fibrillin gene (FBN-1) is located on chromosome 15 (15q21) in a region flanked by DS15-G103 and CYP 19. Mutations of this gene are seen in a variety of disorders that vary from autosomal dominant lens dislocation to the Marfan syndrome (see below), which has several phenotypes.

Posterior dislocation of the lens is characterized by a deep anterior chamber with a tremulous iris (iridodonesis). The symptoms are mainly optical, since absence of a major refracting element causes the eye to become markedly hyperopic and to lose the accommodation provided by the lens. Migration of a dislocated lens into the anterior chamber causes an acute secondary angle-closure glaucoma. A glaucoma may occur with a lens in the vitreous cavity, but the mechanism is not clear. A subluxated lens often, but not inevitably, dislocates into the vitreous cavity.

The same conditions are responsible for both subluxation and dislocation. Ocular contusion may cause subluxation, particularly in an individual with latent syphilis. Deliberate dislocation or couching of the lens into the vitreous cavity is an ancient (and unwise) surgical procedure still practiced in some parts of the world. Subluxation or dislocation is a regular feature of Marfan syndrome, cystathionine β-synthase deficiency, and spherophakia (Weill-Marchesani). Intraocular tumors, uveitis, severe myopia, and buphthalmos may each be complicated by lens dislocation.

Sometimes a dislocated lens causes only an optical defect that is neutralized with correcting lenses. More often, secondary glaucoma, uveitis, or both necessitate lens removal.

Marfan syndrome.—The Marfan syndrome is a relatively common autosomal disorder of connective tissue. Most instances are caused by a mutation of the fibrillin gene (FBN-1) on chromosome 15q-q21.3. (Fibrillin is a component of elastin and is found in many connective tissues, but the zonule contains only

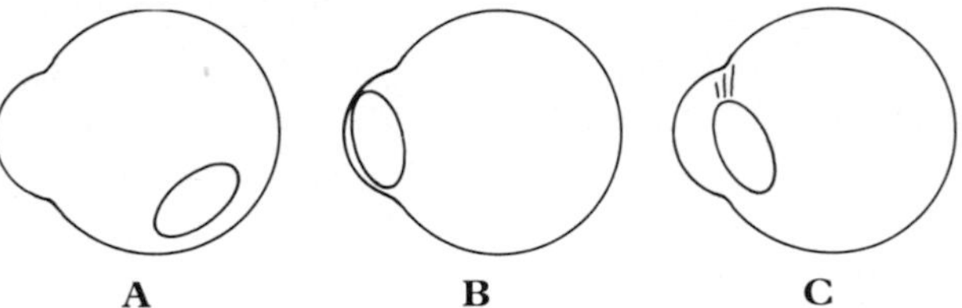

FIG 21-1.
A, Dislocation of the lens into the vitreous cavity. **B,** Dislocation of the lens into the anterior chamber, an abnormality that leads to pupillary-block glaucoma. **C,** Subluxation of the lens, with the remaining zonular fibers acting as a hinge.

fibrillin.) Another fibrillin gene (FBN-2) on chromosome 5 is linked to a Marfan-related disorder, contractural arachnodactyly (spider fingers).

Marfan syndrome has many phenotypes, and 15% to 30% of the patients represent new mutations, often in the offspring of elderly fathers. The frequency of abnormalities of the aorta leading to aortic regurgitation or fatal dissecting aneurysms necessitates a multidisciplinary approach in the care of these patients. The practitioner's attention must not be directed solely to the often conspicuous ocular and skeletal changes.

The major clinical manifestations include the heart and aorta changes, ectopia lentis (subluxation of the crystalline lens), skeletal defects (particularly excessive length of long bones), arachnodactyly, scoliosis, and pectus excavatum (pigeon breast). The pubis-to-sole measurement is characteristically in excess of the pubis-to-vertex measurement, and the arm span is in excess of the height. The more distal bones tend to demonstrate excessive length (arachnodactyly: spider fingers). There is a weakness of the joint capsule, causing flatfoot, hyperextensibility of the joints, recurrent dislocation of the hip, and kyphoscoliosis. Frequently the patient has a long, narrow face, a highly arched palate, and prognathism. The median age of death is in the mid-40s, usually because of aortic dissection and circulatory collapse.

Subluxation of the lens (ectopia lentis) is the major ocular change. Both lenses subluxate early in life, sometimes in utero. The lenses are displaced upward and the inferior zonule is attenuated or fragmented. The zonular fibers superiorly appear shortened and taut. Ectopia lentis may be suspected because of the abnormal mobility of the iris (iridodonesis), which lacks the support of the lens. Downward, but not upward, subluxation of the lens is associated with secondary glaucoma. The lens may be smaller than normal and may be spherical. In some patients, ectopia lentis may be the only sign of the Marfan syndrome.

Patients tend to be myopic and to develop lattice retinal degeneration, which can cause retinal holes and retinal detachment. Heterochromia iridis, translucence of the iris, keratoconus, megalocornea, and blue scleras may be present. In general, surgical removal of the subluxated lens is not indicated. Complications are common, and surgery should be deferred unless necessitated by secondary glaucoma.

The major differential diagnosis includes ectopia lentis, which is also mapped to the fibrillin gene on chromosome 15. Ectopia lentis also occurs in homocystinuria (cystathionine β-synthase deficiency), Stickler syndrome, and Weill-Marchesani syndrome. These conditions are not associated with the skeletal changes of Marfan syndrome.

Homocystinuria (cystathionine β-synthase deficiency).—At least eight different autosomal recessive disorders lead to the urinary excretion of excessive amounts of homocystine. A deficiency of cystathionine β-synthase (chromosome 21q22.3) leads to mental retardation, seizures, vertebral osteoporosis, occlusive vascular disease, and increased risk of thromboembolism. Excessive amounts of homocystine, homocysteine, and methionine are present in the blood. The serum level of cystine is reduced, and cystathionine is absent. The fibrillin of the zonule of the crystalline lens is deficient in both homocystine and homocysteine.

One or both parents are often of Celtic ancestry (Irish, English, Scottish, French). The severity varies in different individuals, but nearly all develop subluxation of the lens between the 3rd and 10th year of age, which is often followed by secondary glaucoma and optic atrophy. Myopia is common and occasionally there is retinal degeneration, retinal detachment, or cataract.

Ectopia lentis is progressive in nearly all patients, and the dislocated lens occasionally causes a pupillary block glaucoma. The lens dislocation is secondary to broken zonular fibers that appear thickened, unlike the thin, elongated fibers in Marfan syndrome. Osteoporosis causes scoliosis, vertebral collapse, genu valgum, pes cavus, and other abnormalities. Mental retardation with delayed psychomotor development occurs in about one half of patients. Thromboembolism may affect large and small arteries and veins, possibly secondary to increased serum homocysteine levels.

Anesthesia for surgery increases the risk of thromboembolism. The skin and hair are fair, and there is a malar flush. Many clinical features suggest Marfan syndrome, but demonstration of the cystathionine β-synthase deficiency in cultured cells distinguishes the two conditions.

There is considerable genetic heterogeneity. Cystathionine β-synthase may be entirely absent, and there may be reduced enzyme activity with normal binding of the cofactor pyridoxal phosphate and reduced enzyme activity with reduced binding of the cofactor. Patients in whom there is no trace of cystathionine β-synthase activity do not respond to administration of pyridoxine, while those with some activity do benefit. Some patients have an abnormally low serum folate concentration that is aggravated by pyridoxine administration. The most common cause of homocystinuria is cystathionine β-synthase deficiency. Homocystinuria also occurs in other genetic disorders, one of which is defective synthesis of cobalamin coenzymes (vitamin B_{12}).

COLOBOMA

A coloboma of the crystalline lens results from loss of the zonular attachments in one segment of the lens equator. The absence of a sector of zonular fibers relaxes the corresponding segment of the lens capsule, which becomes a chord rather than an arc of a circle. There are one or more notches at the equator of the lens and often other intraocular colobomas. The retina may detach.

SPHEROPHAKIA (MICROPHAKIA)

In spherophakia the lens is small with increased anterior and posterior curvatures. The increased curvatures increase its refractive power, causing myopia. The small lens does not adequately support the iris, which is tremulous. When the pupil is dilated, the stretched zonular fibers are easily visible. Subluxation of the lens is common, presumably because the fibers of the zonule weaken and rupture. A pupillary block glaucoma (see Chapter 22) occurs when the small, round lens blocks the flow of aqueous humor through the pupil. Treatment of spherophakia by sector iridectomy is directed mainly to prevention of this pupillary block.

Spherophakia may be part of an autosomal recessive syndrome (of Weill-Marchesani), which is characterized by short stature, short stubby fingers, joint stiffness, and mental retardation. The syndrome constitutes the hyperplastic type of mesodermal dystrophy, in contrast to the Marfan syndrome, a hypoplastic mesodermal defect.

LENTICONUS

Lenticonus is an uncommon defect, rarely inherited as an autosomal recessive characteristic, in which marked thinning of the anterior lens capsule causes a cone-shaped anterior pole of the crystalline lens. An abnormal increase in the posterior curvature of the lens causes lentiglobus. It is usually monocular. Ophthalmoscopically, both conditions cause a dark disk reflex ("oil globule") in the pupillary area.

Anterior lenticonus occurs with familial hemorrhagic nephritis, neural deafness, retinal flecks, spherophakia, and retinal flecks in Alport syndrome.

LENS-INDUCED OCULAR DISEASE

In addition to the glaucoma resulting from deformities or displacement of the lens (phacomorphic glaucoma), secondary glaucoma may result from hypermaturity of the lens (phacolytic glaucoma) or from rapid swelling of the lens (phacogenic glaucoma). Rupture of the lens capsule may be followed by uveitis, or there may be systemic hypersensitivity to lens protein after an extracapsular lens extraction, so that liberation of lens protein in the fellow eye with cataract removed causes a severe intraocular inflammation (endophthalmitis phacoanaphylactica).

Phacogenic glaucoma.—A rapid swelling of the crystalline lens follows hydration of lens fibers in senile intumescent cataract and also follows either surgical or accidental rupture of the lens capsule. A secondary angle-closure glaucoma may ensue, particularly if the anterior chamber is already shallow. The glaucoma must first be controlled medically, and the lens must then be removed.

Phacolytic glaucoma.—Phacolytic glaucoma is secondary to an inflammatory uveitis caused by lens proteins that have leaked from a hypermature cataract. Lens particles and macrophages filled with lipofuscin granules and phagocytes containing lens proteins obstruct the trabecular meshwork. Foamy macrophages are immunoreactive for CD68 protein and HLA-DR and suggest an immune reaction (see Chapter 19). The secondary open-angle glaucoma is intractable to medical therapy. The danger of the glaucoma leads surgeons to remove advanced cataracts before they become hypermature, even though other ocular diseases may preclude restoration of good vision.

Lens-induced uveitis.—Accidental traumatic rupture of the lens capsule liberates lenticular protein within the eye. Although lens proteins are relatively poor antigens, uveitis, sometimes complicated by glaucoma, may develop. Mutton-fat keratic precipitates, posterior synechiae, and, rarely, a pupillary membrane form. Treatment consists of lens extraction and corticosteroid administration. Sometimes after extracapsular cataract extraction, the eyes appear to be sensitized to lens protein. Extracapsular lens extraction with retention of lens material in the second eye then may cause an endophthalmitis (endophthalmitis phacoanaphylactica).

Retention of the lens nucleus or of fragments of the lens in the vitreous cavity after extracapsular lens extraction causes a severe uveitis. The nuclear material must be removed from the eye by means of vitrectomy.

CATARACT

A cataract is any opacity in the crystalline lens. Age-related cataract is a common disorder. In the Framingham, Massachusetts study, 15% of persons 52 to 85 years of age had cataracts that reduced their visual acuity to 20/30 or less. Some 1 million cataract extractions are done annually in the United States, and it is estimated that 5 to 10 million individuals become visually disabled each year because of cataract. Patients who refuse surgery for operable cataracts constitute the second largest group of blind individuals in the United States.

No classification of cataract is satisfactory. They may be classified on the basis of cause, age at onset, severity of opacification, or location of the opacity (Table 21-1). The clinically significant points include (1) severity of visual impairment; (2) the likelihood of visual improvement after cataract extraction; (3) the presence of systemic disease and, if present, whether the disease is related to the cataract development (Table 21-2); and (4) local ocular causes in the absence of systemic disease (Table 21-3).

By definition, cataracts present at birth are congenital and may be hereditary. Cataracts that develop after birth may be associated with ocular disease, trauma, systemic disease, heredity, or aging. Aging is by far the most common cause,

TABLE 21-1.
Methods of Classifying Cataract

I. According to age at onset
   A. Congenital
   B. Infantile
   C. Juvenile
   D. Adult
   E. Age-related
II. According to location of opacity in lens
   A. Nuclear
   B. Cortical
   C. Subcapsular: posterior
III. According to degree of opacity present
   A. Immature: transparent lens fibers are present
   B. Intumescent: swelling of lens with fluid clefts
   C. Mature: opacification of all lens fibers
   D. Hypermature: liquefaction of opaque lens fibers (morgagnian cataract)
   E. After-cataract: opacification of lens capsule or retained lens fibers after extracapsular cataract extraction
IV. According to rate of development
   A. Stationary
   B. Progressive
V. On basis of biomicroscopic appearance
   A. Lamellar
   B. Coralliform
   C. Punctate and many others
VI. On basis of cause (see Tables 21-2 and 21-3)

TABLE 21-2.
Cataract with Systemic Disorders

I. Generalized
  A. Embryopathies (induced in utero)
    1. Maternal infection (rubella first trimester of pregnancy [associated deafness and heart disease], other viruses [cytomegalovirus, mumps, vaccinia, variola, poliomyelitis possible], toxoplasmosis, syphilis)
    2. Maternal drug ingestion, radiation
  B. Marfan syndrome (arachnodactyly, ectopia lentis, mesodermal hypoplasia)
  C. Retinal pigment epithelium degenerations (Laurence-Moon-Biedl: retinitis pigmentosa, obesity, polydactyly, hypogenitalism, deafness, ataxia, oligophrenia)
  D. Systemic infections causing uveitis with complicated cataract
II. Cutaneous
  A. Atopic dermatitis (15 to 25 years of age)
  B. Rothmund syndrome (onset 3 to 6 months of age)
  C. Incontinentia pigmenti (Werner) often with uveitis
  D. Congenital ichthyosis or ectodermal dysplasia
  E. Siemen syndrome
III. Metabolic
  A. Diabetes mellitus (growth-onset diabetes mellitus)
  B. Galactosemia (usually shortly after birth: transferase or kinase deficiency)
  C. Lowe syndrome (oculocerebrorenal syndrome)
  D. Hypocalcemia (with tetany)
  E. Fabry disease
  F. Refsum disease
  G. Glucose-6-phosphate deficiency
  H. Increased plasma tryptophan
IV. Neurologic
  A. Hepatolenticular degeneration (sunflower cataract)
  B. Spinocerebellar ataxia, oligophrenia (Marinesco-Sjögren)
V. Muscular
  A. Myotonic dystrophy (20 to 30 years of age)
VI. Osseous
  A. Mandibulofacial dysostosis
  B. Osteitis fibrosa and skin pigmentation
  C. Stippled epiphysis
  D. Oxycephaly
VII. Chromosomal abnormalities
  A. Down syndrome
  B. 13-15 trisomy
  C. Cockayne syndrome

TABLE 21-3.
Cataract without Systemic Disorders

I. Eye otherwise healthy and no systemic disease
  A. Nearly all aging cataracts
  B. Most cataracts in adults
  C. Many hereditary and congenital cataracts
II. Cataract combined with other ocular disorders but no systemic abnormalities
  A. Congenital and hereditary abnormalities (cyclopia, colobomas, microphthalmia, aniridia, persistent primary vitreous, heterochromia iridis)
  B. Acquired defects and delayed hereditary abnormalities
    1. Miscellaneous ocular diseases (glaucoma, uveitis, retinal separation, pigmentary degeneration of retina, myopia, ocular neoplasms)
    2. Retinopathy of prematurity (cataracts develop after 3 years of age)
    3. Toxicity (corticosteroids systemically or topically, ergot, naphthalene, dinitrophenol, triparanol [MER-29], topical anticholinesterase, phenothiazines)
    4. Ocular trauma
      a. Contusion (Vossius ring [pigment on anterior capsule], posterior subcapsular cataract)
      b. Laceration
      c. Retained intraocular foreign body (iron: siderosis; copper: chalcosis)
      d. Electromagnetic radiation
        (1) Infrared (iris absorption with heat coagulation of underlying lens, also true exfoliation of lens capsule)
        (2) Microwaves (focused high energy, a heating effect)
        (3) Ionizing radiation (cataractogenic dose varies with energy and type, younger lens more vulnerable)
        (4) Ultraviolet radiation
      e. Anterior ocular ischemia after retinal detachment surgery

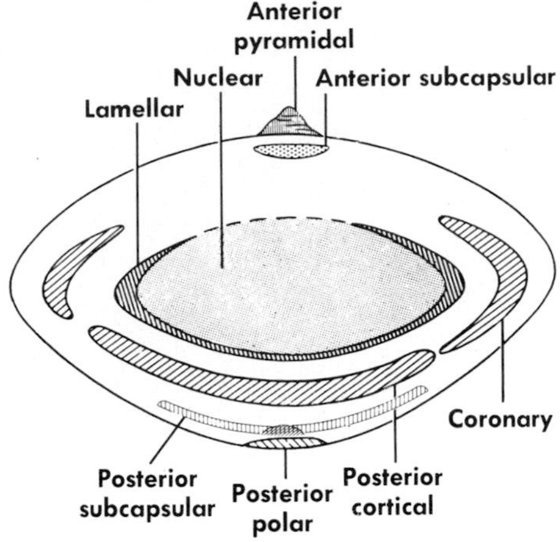

FIG 21-2.
Locations of various cataracts.

and age-related cataracts may occur at a relatively early age.

Cataracts in which all of the lens protein is opaque are termed mature. If some protein is transparent, the cataract is immature. If the protein of the cortex of a mature cataract becomes liquid, the cataract is hypermature. The fluid may escape through an intact capsule and cause the lens to shrink, resulting in a secondary glaucoma (see Chapter 23). Swelling of the lens fibers results in an intumescent cataract.

ACQUIRED CATARACT

Acquired cataracts include those that occur sporadically as a result of toxins, systemic disease, injury, damage from intraocular inflammation, and aging. Many abnormalities cause characteristic morphologic changes that may be distinguished by biomicroscopic examination (Fig 21-2).

Symptoms.—The chief symptom of acquired cataract is a decrease of vision that is not associated with pain or inflammation of the eye. Double vision in one eye (monocular diplopia) may be caused by a lens opacity in the visual axis that splits bundles of light, but this disappears with further decrease in vision. In the early stages, lights may be surrounded by a colored halo.

The dilation of the pupil that occurs in dim illumination improves vision. Glare and constriction of the pupil in bright illumination reduce vision, particularly in patients with posterior subcapsular cataracts that obstruct the visual axis. Patients may complain of spots in the visual field that, unlike those caused by vitreous floaters, remain fixed and do not dart about with movements of the eye. In nuclear cataracts there is often an increase in the refractive power of the lens so that patients may read without glasses.

Examination.—Examination of the lens with the ophthalmoscope may indicate a gross opacity that fills the pupillary aperture or an opacity silhouetted against the red background of the fundus (Fig 21-3). A nuclear opacity is located centrally and usually appears larger than a posterior subcapsular opacity. A peripheral cortical opacity has the appearance of irregular spokes with the optical axis not affected.

Ocular examination is particularly directed toward finding clinical evidence of injury or inflammation to account for the lens opacity. Radiographic examination to demonstrate a metallic foreign body is indicated if there is a history of ocular injury followed by lens opacity. General physical examination and laboratory studies seldom suggest the cause. The main differential diagnosis involves aging, toxins, diabetes mellitus, or other systemic disorders such as hypocalcemia, myotonic dystrophy, or skin disease (see Table 21-1).

Special types.—Many different causes of acquired types of cataract have been described: aging, toxic, traumatic, diabetic, and hypocalcemic. Some have a characteristic appearance in their early stages, but with progression it is not possible to distinguish the various types.

Age-related cataract.—In the Framingham, Massachusetts study, individuals with age-related cataract were likely to have increased serum phospholipid and high nonfasting blood glucose levels, as well as high blood pressure.

With aging, changes in the lens nucleus include the following: (1) increased insoluble protein aggregation; (2) increased nondisulfied covalent cross-links between crystalline polypeptides; (3) oxidation of sulfhydryl groups; (4) increased pigmentation; and (5) blue fluorescence. Age-related cataracts are classified as nuclear sclerosis, cortical, or posterior subcapsular. These changes may occur concurrently but may involve different mechanisms in different parts of the lens.

Nuclear sclerosis, or hard, cataract is an accentuation of a normal condensation process in the lens nucleus. It becomes evident at about

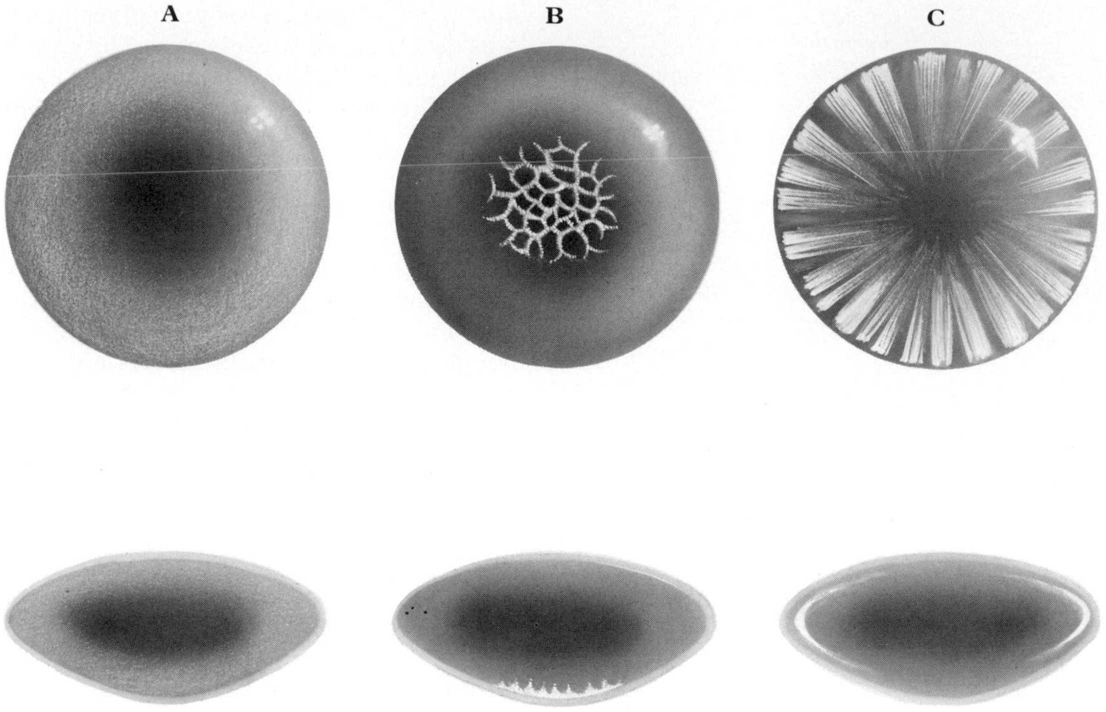

FIG 21-3.
Appearance of various types of aging cataracts. **A,** Nuclear sclerosis. **B,** Nuclear sclerosis and posterior subcapsular cataract. **C,** Nuclear sclerosis and anterior and posterior cortical cataracts.

50 years of age and progresses slowly until the entire nucleus is opaque (see Fig 21-3). Often the earliest change is an increase in the index of refraction of the lens so that there is a decrease in hyperopia or an increase in myopia. The gradual progress of this lens opacity may be associated with improved near vision. This change may lead the patient to believe erroneously that vision is permanently improved—second sight. However, as the opacity progresses, vision for both near and far gradually deteriorates. Since the opacity is located in the visual line, the visual acuity may vary with the pupillary diameter.

A cortical, or soft, cataract involves the lens cortex. Lens fibers are either opaque or hydrated, forming clefts that extend radially to create a spokelike pattern. These opacities tend to involve the equatorial region initially. They may become severe, but if the visual axis is clear, visual acuity is not affected. Gradually, however, the opacities involve the central area of the lens and cause decreased visual acuity.

A posterior subcapsular opacity is the most common type of age-related change. It affects the recently formed lens fibers in the cortical region of the lens adjacent to the posterior capsule, which appear as gold and white granules. Posterior subcapsular cataracts obscure the visual axis early in their formation and disproportionately reduce vision, considering their density and small size.

Traumatic cataract.—Contusion of the eye may cause a posterior subcapsular cataract many months after the original injury, even though the lens capsule has not been grossly injured.

Rupture of the lens capsule invariably causes a cataract. If the opening is microscopic in size, there may be a minute linear opacity corresponding to the opening. More commonly, however, an initial subcapsular opacity extends to involve the entire lens, and grayish lens material extrudes into the anterior chamber. An inflammation of varying severity results. In individuals less than 25 years of age the entire lens may be autolyzed. In patients older than 25 years the nucleus does not absorb and causes a continuing intraocular inflammation.

The effects of a foreign body within the lens depend on its size and rate of oxidation. Glass and plastics are well tolerated. Iron and copper cause characteristic opacities.

Diabetic cataract.—Diabetic cataract is an uncommon type of lens opacity that occurs in poorly controlled growth-onset diabetes mellitus in the second decade of life. The opacity closely resembles "sugar" cataracts in experimental animals. The opacities are bilateral and cortical, predominantly involve the anterior and posterior subcapsular region, and consist of minute dots of varying size, often called "snowflakes." A diabetic cataract may progress to complete opacity (maturity) in less than 72 hours.

Patients with adult-onset diabetes have a slightly earlier onset of age-related cataract than do nondiabetic patients. Surgery is usually uncomplicated, but retinopathy may impair vision.

Hypocalcemic cataract.—Cataracts that are the result of hypocalcemia or hyperphosphatemia develop when the blood calcium falls to a level at which neuromuscular hyperexcitability occurs. The opacities are small, discrete, and iridescent, and are located in the subcapsular region. Correction of the metabolic defect prevents their progression, and transparent lens fibers intrude between the lens fibers, causing the opacities to appear laminated. Not every patient with hypocalcemia develops cataract, and additional metabolic factors may be contributory.

Toxic cataract.—Permanent and transient lens opacities may be produced in experimental animals, particularly weanlings, by various sugars, electrolyte disturbances, and endocrine and dietary deficiencies. For the most part, the correlation with human cataract is remote, although galactose cataract occurs in infants (as well as the susceptible experimental animal). In galactosemia a deficiency of either hexose-1-phosphate uridyltransferase or of galactokinase results in the accumulation of high levels of galactose alcohol (dulcitol) in the crystalline lens (see Chapter 26).

Corticosteroids systemically administered in high doses for long periods, especially in arthritic patients, may cause posterior subcapsular opacities. Prolonged topical administration has the same effect, but there is considerable individual variation. The opacity begins at the posterior pole as highly refractile, multicolored dots that impair vision. Peripheral cortical opacities then develop, but vision is seldom decreased enough to require cataract extraction.

Miotic drugs, particularly anticholinesterases, used topically to treat glaucoma or accommodative esotropia, produce anterior subcapsular opacities. These opacities seldom progress, and they can be distinguished from aging changes only by prospective studies.

Medical treatment.—Lens vacuoles are often the initial change in the development of cataract, but may absorb spontaneously with visual improvement. Lens opacities do not invariably progress, but if they do, their progress is not at a constant rate. Thus, many agents are advocated, particularly in Europe and Asia, to delay, prevent, or reverse cataract formation. Iodine salts, vitamins (particularly vitamins B, C, or E), adenosine triphosphate, various irritating drops reputed to increase ocular blood flow, hormones, organ extracts, reducing agents, aspirin, and many other compounds are used. Aldose reductase inhibitors prevent the accumulation of sugar alcohols in galactosemic or diabetic animals and prevent sugar cataract formation. Photochemical changes in the lens from absorption of ultraviolet radiation, particularly in the range of 310 to 400 nm (see Chapter 7), can be prevented by protective eyeglasses.

During the period of decreasing vision, frequent and accurate refraction will maintain vision at the best possible level. When minute opacities involve the axial area, dilation of the pupil by means of a weak solution of phenylephrine (Neo-Synephrine 2.5%) or 2% homatropine may provide visual improvement. Pupillary dilation must not be used in patients with a shallow anterior chamber in whom there is danger of precipitating angle-closure glaucoma.

Surgical treatment.—Extraction of the lens is indicated in the following instances: (1) when the cataract causes a visual defect that interferes with an individual's vocation or avocation; (2) if the lens threatens to cause a secondary glaucoma or uveitis; (3) to permit visualization of the fundus in order to monitor glaucoma; and (4) to permit adequate visualization of the fundus before photocoagulation, vitrectomy, or retinal surgery.

Many surgeons advocate surgery for monocular cataract in active individuals irrespective of the excellence of vision in the opposite eye. Binocular vision may be restored by insertion of an intraocular lens or by means of a contact lens worn on the operated-on eye.

One of two methods is used to remove an acquired cataract: (1) intracapsular lens extraction, in which the entire lens including its capsule is removed; and (2) extracapsular lens extraction, in which the anterior lens capsule, the nucleus, and the cortex are removed but the posterior capsule and the zonular connections to the lens equator are retained. The intracapsular procedure was the method of choice from 1930 to 1980. Since then, extracapsular extraction has become increasingly popular because of the use of posterior chamber intraocular lenses that require support by the equatorial portion of the lens capsule.

The intracapsular cataract extraction requires an incision of nearly 180° at the superior corneoscleral limbus, which must be closed with a number of interrupted sutures. Voluntary movement of the eyelids and ocular muscles is prevented (akinesia) by local infiltration of the eyelids and orbit with an anesthetic agent.

The extracapsular cataract extraction requires a much smaller incision, sometimes only 3 mm long. Often a valve-type incision (self-sealing) is used, which does not require sutures. The cataract may be removed by suction after ultrasonic disruption (phacoemulsification). Much less local anesthetic is required than for the intracapsular extraction, and many surgeons use only a topical anesthetic. The smaller incision and support provided by the posterior capsule in the extracapsular cataract extraction provide a rapid postoperative recovery and, when an intraocular lens is used, there is early restoration of vision.

Modern extracapsular cataract extraction requires the use of a surgical microscope to visualize the operative field. A large central portion of the anterior lens capsule is removed (capsulorhexis). The dense lens nucleus is fragmented with ultrasound, or it is expressed from the eye through a larger corneoscleral incision. The remaining lens fibers of the cortex are then removed by irrigation and suction. Visual improvement requires that the visual axis is free of opacity and that no excess cortex remains.

A soft (cortical) cataract is removed by one of the variants of mechanical disruption of the lens and aspiration (phacoemulsification). The procedure requires a small (3-mm) incision. The procedure is particularly useful in cataract extraction in eyes in which the lens nucleus is relatively soft. In elderly patients with a hard lens nucleus, phacoemulsification may be time consuming.

Removal of the lens markedly reduces the refractive power of the eye (aphakia) and impairs the efficiency of the eye as an optical instrument. The most evident change is a severe hyperopia that cannot be neutralized by accommodation because the lens is absent. Insertion of an intraocular lens immediately after removal of the cataract often restores normal vision, without the use of spectacles.

Contact lenses in aphakia.—Contact lenses (see Chapter 24) minimize but do not eliminate many of the optical disturbances caused by aphakia. Contact lenses are often better tolerated by cataract patients than by other patients because the sensory nerve supply of the cornea is impaired by the surgical incision. Conversely, many patients are unable to wear contact lenses successfully because of age, parkinsonism, rheumatoid arthritis, or mental deterioration.

Dry eyes, blepharitis, and astigmatism of more than 3 diopters complicate contact lens wear. Patients are fitted after all sutures are removed, when the refraction is stable, usually about 2 or 3 months after surgery. About one fourth of the eyes develop superficial vascularization that extends 1 or 2 mm into the cornea, usually superiorly. In patients with preexisting corneal vascularization, a soft contact lens aggravates the condition or causes vessels not carrying blood (ghost vessels) to carry blood.

Since soft contact lenses correct a maximum of 1.5 diopters of astigmatism, any greater astigmatism must be corrected by means of spectacles or rigid (hard) contact lenses.

Intraocular lens implantation.—Insertion of a clear plastic lens in the visual axis at the time of cataract extraction minimizes the optical problems of aphakia. The main type of lens used is inserted in the posterior chamber and maintained in position by the posterior lens capsule and zonule (Fig 21-4). In the absence of the posterior lens capsule, the intraocular lens may be sutured to the sclera. Anterior chamber lenses may damage the corneal endothelium,

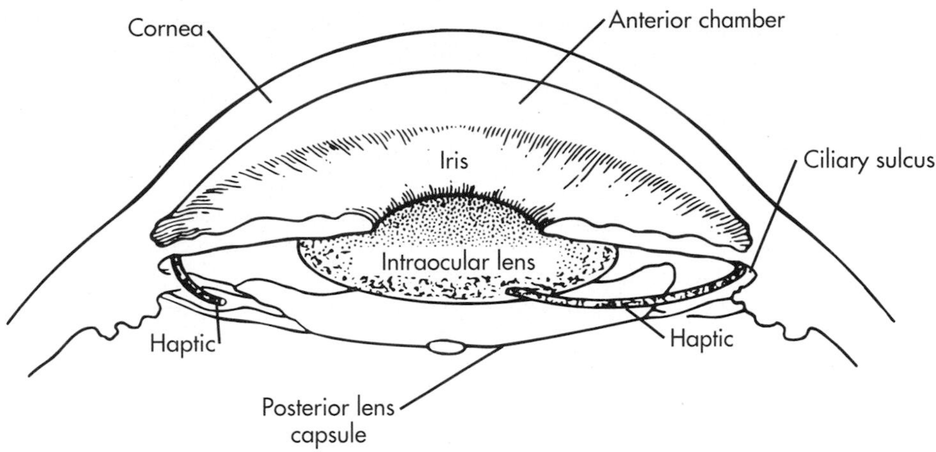

FIG 21-4.
A posterior chamber lens located between the iris and the posterior lens capsule. The haptics, the delicate supporting structures, rest either in the remnants of the capsule of the crystalline lens that is still connected by the lens zonule to the ciliary body or in the recess between the posterior iris and the ciliary body.

even many years after insertion. They are the chief cause of bullous keratopathy and are rarely used.

The refractive power of the intraocular lens used is determined preoperatively by measuring the refractive power of the cornea with a keratometer, and by measuring the length of the eye by means of ultrasound.

The major complication of intraocular lens implantation is damage to the corneal endothelium that results in edema of the corneal stroma (bullous keratopathy). Anterior chamber lenses are seldom used because of this complication. The main complication of posterior chamber lenses is opacification of the visual axis of the retained posterior capsule of the crystalline lens. The opacified visual axis is opened by means of a neodymium-YAG laser.

After-cataract.—The retained posterior lens capsule may become opaque after extracapsular cataract surgery. There are two main causes: (1) lens fibers adjacent to the capsule may not be fully removed at the time of cataract extraction; and (2) the anterior lens capsule that remains after capsulotomy may proliferate over the posterior capsule and obscure the visual axis.

CONGENITAL CATARACT

Every individual has minute nonprogressive lens opacities that do not impair vision. Many hereditary cataracts are recognized by their characteristic structure. These opacities consist of multiple, fine, irregularly shaped opacities in the central or peripheral areas of the lens. The diagnosis is based on their morphologic characteristics as seen with a biomicroscope.

Attention in infancy is directed to cataracts severe enough to impair vision. The questions that arise include the following: (1) Does the opacity involve one or both eyes? (2) Does the visual defect prevent normal schooling? (3) Are there associated ocular defects? (4) Are there associated systemic defects? (5) Are the lens opacities progressive? (6) What is the cause?

General ophthalmoscopic examination shortly after birth should indicate a red fundus reflex. If a red fundus reflex is not seen with the ophthalmoscope, careful examination should be done after the pupils are dilated with 1% phenylephrine and 0.2% cyclopentolate. Ocular examination of infants may be facilitated by nursing a hungry baby or by immobilization. The fundus may be studied with a direct or indirect ophthalmoscope using an infant-size goniolens (Koeppe) that also permits visualization of the lens and anterior chamber angle.

Visual acuity is difficult to assess in infants, but if opticokinetic nystagmus can be elicited, visual acuity likely will be more than 20/60 and surgery will not be required. If retinal blood vessels can be seen with an ophthalmoscope with the pupils dilated, surgery will likely not be necessary and the patient may have normal schooling.

Nystagmus, retinal or choroidal abnormalities, microphthalmia, and strabismus reduce the likelihood of good postoperative vision. Dense cataracts are often removed despite associated ocular defects inasmuch as the 20/200 corrected visual acuity is better than preoperative vision.

Systemic defects should be identified and the progression of the lens opacity observed. The medical and ocular history of other members of the family should be learned. A family study is most rapidly initiated by examining the eyes of parents accompanying an infant. Hearing should be tested. The occurrence of supernumerary fingers and toes, gross abnormality in the development of the bones of the face or skull, or disproportion of the bones of the extremities should be noted. Flaccidity of the muscles should be investigated. Evidence of mental retardation and delayed physical development should be sought, particularly with reference to delayed psychomotor development such as failure to sit, stand, or talk at anticipated age levels.

Laboratory studies may include patient and maternal studies for antibodies against rubella, cytomegalovirus, toxoplasmosis, and syphilis. Galactosemia is excluded by enzyme testing. A reducing substance may be present in the urine. Commercial test tapes are specific for glucose and do not indicate other reducing substances in the urine. Homocystinuria may cause cataract, although it more commonly causes ectopia lentis. It is excluded by means of the cyanide nitroprusside test of urine. A positive test requires chromatography. Reducing substance and albumin may occur in the urine in the oculocerebrorenal (Lowe) syndrome, a moderately common cause of congenital cataract. Aminoaciduria occurs in a variety of congenital disorders associated with cataract. Chromosome analysis is indicated if there are widespread systemic defects in addition to cataracts.

Surgical treatment.—Congenital cataracts should be removed as soon as it is evident that they may impair normal visual maturation. Monocular cataracts are removed shortly after birth, provided the parents can manage the insertion and hygiene of a contact lens.

The anterior lens capsule is opened with a needle knife; the lens cortex is disorganized with a knife, ultrasound, or mechanical cutter with infusion-suction; and the lens cortex is aspirated. The 3-mm incision is large enough to admit the 20-gauge needle that contains the infusion and suction lines and auxiliary devices. If the pupil dilates poorly, it may be enlarged with a cutter. Refraction may be done as soon as the procedure is completed and a contact lens may be prescribed.

Complications.—Early and delayed complications are rare and related to retention of excessive lens cortex that causes an iridocyclitis. The posterior capsule should not be incised, and the structural integrity of the eye is retained.

Retinal detachment, previously a common cause of blindness after congenital cataract surgery, is now rare. It usually occurred 20 or more years after the operation. Intraocular lenses are increasingly popular.

Results.—About 35% of patients with congenital cataracts have an associated serious eye defect that prevents good vision, even after successful lens extraction. Monocular cataract, which in the past was often not removed because of severe amblyopia, may be removed the day of birth or shortly thereafter and vision corrected with a contact lens. Some patients have 20/20 visual acuity in each eye, but binocular vision does not develop.

Special types.—Special types of congenital cataract include lamellar (zonular) and those associated with maternal rubella, oculocerebrorenal (Lowe) syndrome, and galactosemia.

Lamellar (zonular) cataract.—The lens grows throughout life by forming successive layers. Lens fibers may become opaque because of a transient disturbance; with further growth of the lens, these fibers migrate centrally as deep concentric lamellar, or zonular, cataracts. Lamellar cataract is a common type of cataract and may develop up to 1 year after birth (Fig 21-5). It is usually bilateral and is often transmitted as an autosomal dominant defect without any other abnormality. It consists of a series of concentric thin sheets (lamellae) of opacities surrounded by clear lens. There may be riders that extend along the edge from the anterior surface of the opacity to its posterior surface. Depending on the density of the opacity, vision may be good or markedly reduced. Vision may become worse at puberty, necessitating surgery. A unilateral lamellar cataract may follow contu-

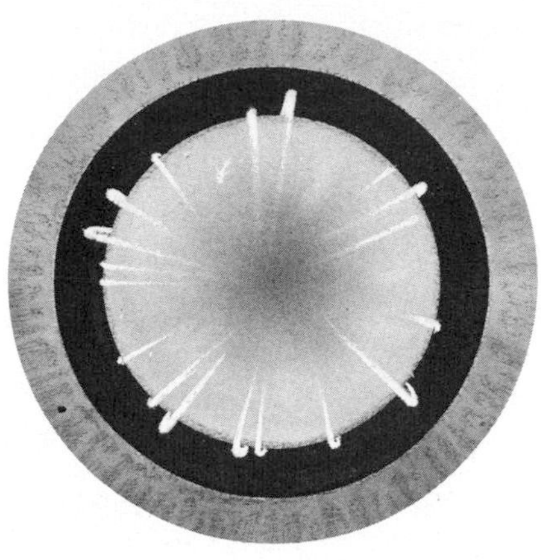

FIG 21-5.
Congenital lamellar cataract with riders.

sion of the eye. Hypocalcemia in infancy causes a bilateral lamellar defect.

Maternal rubella.—Rubella infection during pregnancy may cause widespread fetal ocular and systemic defects (see Chapter 25). The severity of the complications varies with different strains of the virus and is more severe the earlier in the pregnancy the rubella infection occurs. The lens may be entirely opaque, or there may be a central pearly white opacity. Nystagmus, strabismus, corneal opacities, microphthalmia, retinal hyperpigmentation, and glaucoma also occur.

The pupil dilates poorly. The visual results of cataract surgery are often unsatisfactory. The lens may harbor the virus for many years after birth, and all lens cortex should be removed at the initial operation to prevent an endophthalmitis. Nonimmunized health personnel must be protected from infection.

Oculocerebrorenal syndrome of Lowe.—The Lowe syndrome is an X chromosome–linked (Xq25-q26) recessive disorder. Affected infants are born with small opacified crystalline lenses in which the nucleus and cortex are not demarcated. Female carriers of the abnormal chromosome may develop cataracts before 40 years of age.

Microphthalmia and endophthalmos are common, but buphthalmos may follow secondary glaucoma. Visual acuity is rarely better than 20/100, and a pendular nystagmus is present. Corneal keloids may develop (25%) after the age of 4 years and are bilateral in about one half of those affected. Early bilateral cataract extraction combined with vitrectomy is indicated. Keratoplasty for corneal keloids that obstruct the visual axis is seldom successful.

Mental retardation is common but not universal. Head banging, tantrums, aggression, and waving of the hands between the eyes and a light source occur. Neonatal hypotonia may persist into childhood, and deep reflexes are absent after the age of 1 year. Seizures occur in about one half of the patients. A proximal tubular acidosis, aminoaciduria, phosphaturia, and proteinuria develop a few months after birth.

Galactosemia.—Lactose, the main carbohydrate of milk, is hydrolyzed by the enzyme lactase, in the microvilli of the intestine, to its component sugars glucose and galactose. Galactose differs from glucose only in the configuration of the hydroxyl group on carbon 4. Galactose is essential in glycolipids and glycoproteins, and normally nearly all is converted to glucose in a series of three main reactions: (1) Initially the enzyme galactokinase (chromosome 17q21-22 and chromosome 15) catalyzes a reaction in which galactose is phosphorylated by adenosine triphosphate to form galactose-1-phosphate. (2) In a reaction catalyzed by the enzyme galactose-1-phosphate uridyltransferase, the galactose-1-phosphate is converted to uridine diphosphate galactose and glucose-1-phosphate. (3) The enzyme, uridine diphosphate galactose-4-epimerase, reacts with uridine diphosphate galactose to form glucose. Three inherited abnormalities of galactose metabolism result in disorders in which there is a deficiency in one of the three enzymes essential in the conversion of galactose to glucose (see Chapter 26).

Transferase deficiency (reaction 2 above) is the most common abnormality and causes classic galactosemia. There is failure to thrive, jaundice, and punctate cataracts that progress to complete opacification of the crystalline lenses within months if galactose is continued in the diet. Mental retardation is common. Hyperbilirubinemia or *E. coli* sepsis, which often occur simultaneously, signal the need for galactose testing. In women, ovarian failure occurs. Effective treatment requires early recognition of the abnormality combined with removal of milk and milk products from the diet.

Galactokinase deficiency causes a less severe systemic disturbance with hepatomegaly and gastrointestinal disturbances. Zonular cataracts (see above) occur. About 10% of individuals who require cataract extraction before the age of 40 years demonstrate a galactokinase deficiency in their erythrocytes.

Epimerase deficiency is the most uncommon disorder of galactose metabolism. It is detected only by increased levels of galactose-phosphate in erythrocytes. Since galactose is an essential component of systemic glycoproteins and glycolipids and is not available by epimerase conversion from glucose, it is necessary to provide small amounts of galactose in the diet.

BIBLIOGRAPHY

Books

Brown NAP, Bron AJ: *Lens disorders: a clinical manual of cataract diagnosis,* Newton, Mass, 1995, Butterworth-Heinemann.

Jaffe NS, editor: *Atlas of ophthalmic surgery,* ed 2, St Louis, 1996, Mosby–Year Book.

Murrill CA, Stanfield DL, Van Brocklin MD, editors: *Primary care of the cataract patient,* Norwalk, Conn, 1994, Appleton & Lange.

Article

Brady KM, Atkinson CS, Kilty LA, Hiles DA: Cataract surgery and intraocular lens implantation in children, *Am J Ophthalmol* 120:1-9, 1995.

22

THE GLAUCOMAS

The glaucomas are a complicated group of disorders that are mainly, but not always, characterized by an increased intraocular pressure. The adequacy of drainage of the aqueous humor through the trabecular meshwork divides many types into an open-angle or an angle-closure glaucoma. Those that occur early in life are mainly secondary to abnormalities of the anterior segment of the eye and are considered developmental or congenital glaucomas. Those caused by an inflammation, tumor, injury, or a similar disorder are classed as secondary glaucomas (Table 22-1).

The abnormality results in a progressive excavation of the optic disk, optic atrophy, and characteristic defects of the visual field. The intraocular pressure is usually increased, but the degree of increase associated with optic nerve changes is not the same in every eye. Approximately one sixth of the patients never demonstrate increased intraocular pressure.

Clinical attention in glaucoma is directed to two major factors: (1) the intraocular pressure; and (2) the intraocular portion of the optic nerve. The intraocular pressure depends on the ease of drainage of the humor from the eye and, less importantly, the rate of secretion of the aqueous humor by the ciliary body. (Note that the intraocular pressure can be directly measured only by inserting a cannula into the eye, a method never used clinically. The tension of the eye, which is measured clinically, is determined by the ease with which the eye can be indented by an applied force.)

The intraocular portion of the optic nerve measures about 1.5 mm in diameter and about 1.0 mm between its surface, the optic disk, and its exit from the eye. It consists of approximately 1 million axons of retinal ganglion cells. Some 90% of these axons originate with ganglion cells in the macular region, which appear to be affected late in the course of glaucoma. The most vulnerable axons appear to be those that originate in the peripheral retina. Possibly all axons are affected equally, but the large number that originate in the macular region make their loss less clinically evident than the loss of peripheral axons.

The ciliary processes of the ciliary body secrete aqueous humor into the posterior chamber. The aqueous humor then flows through the pupil into the anterior chamber and exits through the trabecular meshwork (80%) and the suprachoroidal space (20%). The trabecular meshwork empties into the canal of Schlemm, which empties into aqueous veins, which empty into an episcleral meshwork. Aqueous humor in the suprachoroidal space is absorbed by local blood vessels. Any abnormality of this system of secretion, flow, and drainage of the aqueous humor may result in an increased intraocular pressure. A prolonged increase in intraocular pressure leads to glaucoma, with a primary optic atrophy and excavation of the physiologic cup of the optic disk (cupping) and typical defects of the visual field. If prolonged, the process culminates in blindness.

A prolonged increase in intraocular pressure leads to a primary optic atrophy in which there is

TABLE 22-1.
Classification of the Glaucomas

I. Primary open-angle glaucomas
  A. Variants
    1. Normal tension
    2. Deteriorated ocular hypertension
    3. Juvenile onset (hereditary?)
II. Secondary open-angle glaucomas (see Table 22-6)
III. Angle-closure glaucomas
  A. Variants
    1. Acute
    2. Intermittent
    3. Chronic
IV. Secondary angle-closure glaucomas (see Table 22-8)
V. Hereditary and congenital glaucomas
  A. Abnormal anterior chamber angle
  B. Other ocular abnormalities

marked excavation of the optic disk with abnormalities of its extracellular matrix and loss of astrocytes. Much attention has been directed to an increase in the intraocular pressure, and it remains the chief method of monitoring both primary and secondary glaucoma. Some eyes, however, tolerate an increased intraocular pressure that would rapidly blind other eyes. Other eyes develop the optic nerve atrophy and excavation of the optic disk with what seem to be completely normal ocular tensions (Normal-Tension Glaucoma, this chapter).

The glaucomas are customarily divided into two types: open-angle and angle-closure. If the cause is evident the glaucoma is designated as secondary, but if the cause is not known the glaucoma is designated as primary. In open-angle glaucoma, the aqueous humor has free access to the trabecular meshwork, the drainage apparatus in the anterior chamber angle. In angle-closure glaucoma the peripheral iris is in contact with the cornea or the trabecular meshwork and impairs the outflow of the aqueous humor from the anterior chamber.

Primary open-angle glaucoma is a disease of unknown cause previously called simple glaucoma, chronic glaucoma, glaucoma simplex, compensated glaucoma, and wide-angle glaucoma. It is characterized by two abnormalities: (1) atrophy of the optic nerve with an increased diameter and depth of the physiologic optic cup combined with a decrease in the surface area and volume of the neuroretinal rim ("cupping"); and (2) typical visual field defects. In most instances the intraocular pressure is too high for continued normal function of the optic nerve. In normal-pressure open-angle glaucoma, typical cupping and characteristic visual field defects occur at a level of intraocular pressure that does not damage eyes of most individuals. The anterior chamber angle appears normal to direct observation, and the aqueous humor has free access to the trabecular meshwork.

Angle-closure glaucoma is an anatomic abnormality in which the peripheral iris blocks the trabecular meshwork and prevents the drainage of aqueous humor from the anterior chamber. In the past it has been called acute glaucoma, congestive (decompensated) glaucoma, closed-angle glaucoma, or narrow-angle glaucoma. Two main mechanisms are involved: (1) pupillary block, in which all aqueous humor does not flow from the posterior chamber through the pupil into the anterior chamber; the accumulation of aqueous humor in the posterior chamber causes the peripheral iris to balloon forward and block drainage from the anterior chamber angle; and (2) direct mechanical block of the drainage angle by the root of the iris (plateau iris). The entire anterior chamber may be shallow, or the central anterior chamber may be of normal depth and the angle recess abnormally narrow.

In combined-mechanism glaucoma, features of both open-angle and angle-closure glaucoma are present.

Secondary glaucoma may occur with open-angle, angle-closure, combined-mechanism, and developmental types of glaucoma.

Secondary open-angle glaucoma occurs because of (1) fibrovascular proliferation on the anterior chamber face of the trabecular meshwork, notably in rubeosis iridis; (2) cells or tissue blocking the pores in the trabecular meshwork; (3) abnormalities within the trabecular meshwork from edema, trauma, or corticosteroid administration; or (4) increased pressure in the episcleral venous network into which aqueous humor drains from the canal of Schlemm.

Secondary closed-angle glaucoma occurs with one or more of the following: (1) contracture of fibrovascular membranes in the anterior chamber; (2) pupillary block with interference with flow of aqueous humor from posterior to anterior chamber; and (3) closure of the anterior chamber angle as the result of a forward shift of the peripheral iris.

In secondary combined-mechanism glaucoma, an additional abnormality is superimposed on an eye that has features of both open-angle and angle-closure glaucoma. In secondary developmental glaucoma an abnormality of the iris, pupil, or trabecular meshwork is superimposed on an eye with an anterior chamber that retains its fetal configuration.

SYMPTOMS AND SIGNS

Open-angle glaucoma is usually asymptomatic. The intraocular pressure slowly increases over several years or more, and although it may reach a high level, corneal edema and ocular pain do not occur. In the early stages of disease the peripheral vision is not affected; abnormalities can be demonstrated by careful measurement of the visual field to show the field defects characteristic of glaucoma. Estimation of the visual field by confrontation testing is of no value.

Ophthalmoscopy discloses an increased diameter and depth of the physiologic cup of the optic disk. There is gradual loss of the neuroretinal rim, pallor of the disk, and nasal displacement of the blood vessels within the physiologic cup. In red-free light, a thinning of the retinal nerve fiber layer may be detected. Flame-shaped hemorrhages may occur at the margin of the optic disk.

The symptoms of angle-closure glaucoma are mainly related to a sudden increase in intraocular pressure and the rapidity with which it occurs. There may be repeated attacks of ocular pain and blurred vision occurring after a prolonged time in darkness, after emotional upset, or with any condition that dilates the pupil.

The rapid increase in intraocular pressure causes an edema of the corneal epithelium that results in blurred vision and halos surrounding lights (iridescent vision). The initial attacks are often spontaneously relieved by pupillary constriction that occurs normally during sleep or in bright illumination. (The supine position [face upward] in sleep may relieve an angle-closure attack by permitting the iris-lens diaphragm to fall away from the anterior chamber angle.) After repeated attacks or without previous symptoms, the iris remains adherent to the cornea and the angle remains closed, resulting in reduced vision and a red, painful eye. Severe prostrating head pain, usually unilateral, may be confused with migraine, impending rupture of a carotid artery aneurysm, and similar causes of hemicrania. There may be nausea, vomiting, and symptoms suggestive of an acute abdominal surgical emergency.

Angle-closure glaucoma is diagnosed on the basis of (1) increased intraocular pressure combined with (2) an anterior chamber angle in which the aqueous humor does not have access to the trabecular meshwork (closed). When the chamber angle is not closed, the pressure is normal unless previous attacks have damaged the trabecular meshwork or caused adhesions between the iris and the peripheral angle (peripheral anterior synechiae).

The developmental glaucomas are often associated with congenital ocular and systemic anomalies and rare syndromes. These are often characterized at their onset by tearing, photophobia, and blepharospasm. The increased intraocular pressure is secondary to a congenital and sometimes hereditary abnormality of the anterior chamber angle. It retains its fetal configuration with the root of the iris attached to the trabecular meshwork or with the trabecular meshwork covered with a thin membrane. When the glaucoma occurs before the age of 3 years, the entire eye enlarges (total staphyloma [Greek: a bunch of grapes]; or buphthalmos [Greek: ox eye, obsolete]).

METHODS OF EXAMINATION

Several tests are of particular importance in the diagnosis of glaucoma: (1) tonometry: the measurement of ocular tension; (2) gonioscopy: the observation of the anterior chamber angle; (3) ophthalmoscopy: the evaluation of the color and configuration of the cup and neuroretinal rim of the optic disk; and (4) perimetry: the measurement of visual function in the central field of vision.

Tonometry.—Intraocular pressure can be measured directly only by means of an intraocular cannula connected to a transducer and amplifier. Such testing, in humans, has been done before removal of an eye for disease. The testing is difficult, for it necessitates that the aqueous humor not leak around the cannula and that the

TABLE 22-2.
Factors That Influence Intraocular Pressure

Factors	Association	Comments
Demographic		
Age	Mean intraocular pressure increases with increasing age	May be mediated partially through cardiovascular factors
Sex	Higher intraocular pressure in women	Effect more marked after age 40 years
Race	Higher intraocular pressure in blacks	—
Heredity	Intraocular pressure inherited	Polygenic effect
Systemic		
Diurnal variation	Most people have a diurnal pattern of intraocular pressure	Quite variable in some individuals
Seasonal variation	Higher intraocular pressure in winter months	—
Blood pressure	Intraocular pressure increases with increasing blood pressure	—
Obesity	Higher intraocular pressure in obese people	—
Posture	Intraocular pressure increases from sitting to inverted position	Greater effect with eyes below horizontal
Exercise	Strenuous exercise lowers intraocular pressure transiently	Long-term training lessens effect
Neural	Cholinergic and adrenergic input alters intraocular pressure	—
Hormones	Corticosteroids increase intraocular pressure; diabetes associated with increased intraocular pressure; eyes soft with diabetic acidosis	—
Drugs	Many drugs alter intraocular pressure	—
Ocular		
Refractive error	Myopic individuals have higher intraocular pressure	Higher intraocular pressure with longer axial length
Eye movements	Intraocular pressure increases if eye moves against resistance	—
Eyelid closure	Intraocular pressure increases with forcible closure	—
Uveitis	Intraocular pressure decreases unless aqueous humor outflow affected more than inflow	—
Intraocular surgery	Intraocular pressure generally decreases unless aqueous humor outflow affected more than inflow	—

From Hoskins HD Jr, Kass MA: *Becker-Shaffer's diagnosis and therapy of the glaucomas,* ed 6, St Louis, 1989, Mosby–Year Book, p 81. Used by permission.

normal pressure equilibrium of the eye not be disturbed.

Clinically the intraocular pressure is measured indirectly by determining the response of the eye to an applied force, the ocular tension. Accurate measurement requires that the patient abstain from alcoholic beverages for 12 hours before the test and from smoking marijuana for at least 24 hours. Ingestion of more than 500 mL of fluid should be avoided for at least 4 hours before testing.

Many different factors affect intraocular pressure (Table 22-2). Despite these variations it remains one of the most sensitive measurements in clinical medicine.

The instruments used are divided into two

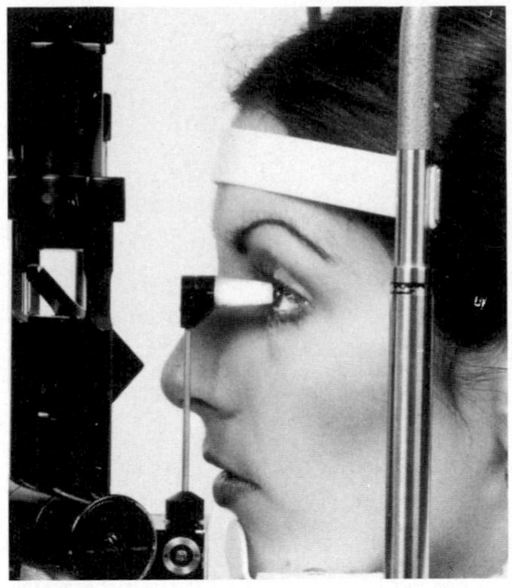

FIG 22-1.
Measurement of the ocular tension with a Goldmann applanation tonometer. This method is more sensitive than Schiøtz tonometry, but it requires an expensive biomicroscope.

major groups. Applanation tonometers measure the force required to flatten a standard area of the cornea. Indentation tonometers measure the deformation of the globe in response to a standard weight applied to the cornea. It is possible to transfer infectious agents with both types of instruments, and the tonometer head must be sterilized between patients.

The Goldmann applanation tonometer is the international standard (Fig 22-1). It measures the force required to flatten an area of the cornea 3.06 mm in diameter. The flattened area is viewed with a biomicroscope through a split prism after instillation of a topical anesthetic and fluorescein. A trained examiner is able to measure the ocular tension accurately. The tension may be overestimated if the cornea is thickened with scar, if the examiner presses on the globe, or if the patient rotates the eye upward more than 15° or widens the palpebral fissure excessively. The tension may be underestimated if an inadequate amount of fluorescein is used, if tonometry is repeated, or if the cornea is thick because of edema.

Modifications of the Goldmann tonometer are battery operated and portable, and may use microprocessors (Perkins, Draeger, Mackay-Marg, Tono-Pen).

Noncontact tonometers measure the deformation of the light reflex of the cornea caused by a puff of air. They do not require topical anesthesia, which may modify the ocular tension, and are easy to use.

The Schiøtz tonometer (Fig 22-2) measures the ease with which the cornea may be indented by the plunger of the instrument. It is an inexpensive, sturdy instrument that is sometimes provided to the patient for home use. A soft eye is easily indented, indicating a low pressure; a hard eye is less easily indented. The amount of indentation and the pressure have been calibrated in enucleated eyes. Generally indentation tonometry is adversely influenced by more factors than applanation tonometry but has the advantages of greater ease and less costly instrumentation. A known weight is placed on the cornea (Fig 22-3), and the intraocular pressure is estimated by measuring its indentation. The weight consists of a plunger, one end of which slides through a hole in a concave plate that rests on but does not press on the cornea. The other end of the plunger is connected to a needle that crosses a scale. The more the plunger indents the cornea, the higher the scale reading, and the lower the ocular tension.

The entire instrument weighs at least 16.5 g, and this can be increased to 19 g and to 21.5 g. Resting this weight on the eye increases the intraocular pressure and distends the ocular coats (scleral rigidity). Eyes with a high ocular rigidity (severe hyperopia or long-standing glaucoma) give falsely high readings. Eyes with a low rigidity (severe myopia, miotic therapy, retinal detachment surgery both with and without compressible intraocular gas) give falsely low readings. It is possible to estimate ocular rigidity by using two different weights for Schiøtz measurements. An electronic Schiøtz tonometer is used for continuous measurement in tonography.

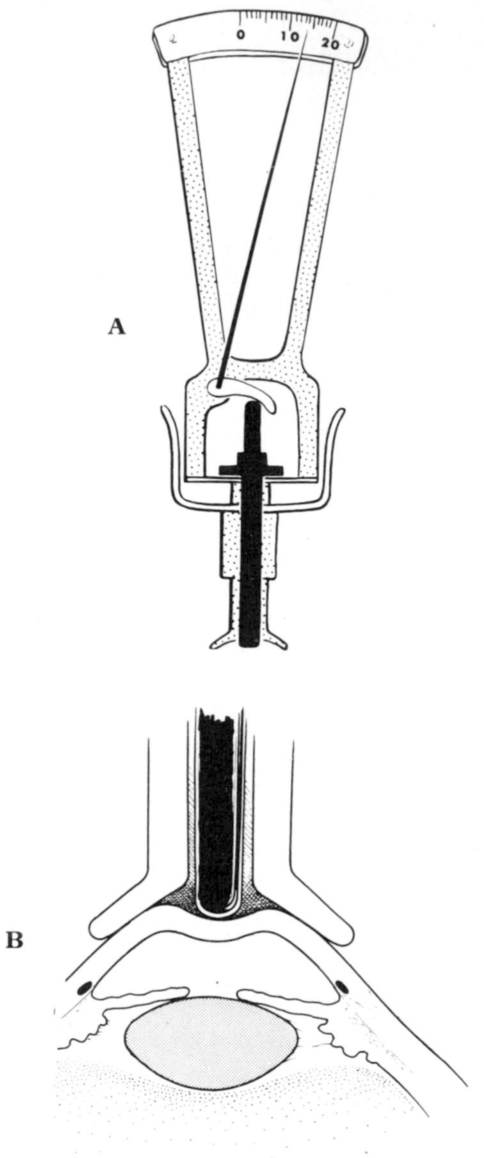

FIG 22-2.
A, Schiøtz tonometer in which the plunger (shown in black) measures the ease of indentation of the cornea. **B,** Indentation of the anesthetized cornea by the plunger of the tonometer to measure ocular tension.

Normal individuals have a mean intraocular pressure of about 15 ± 3 mm Hg. Untreated eyes with open-angle glaucoma and field loss have a mean intraocular pressure of 22 ± 5 mm Hg. Intraocular pressure tends to increase with aging and to be higher in women than in men.

The ocular tension (which reflects the intraocular pressure) varies with the pulse and respiration. Additionally, the tension of the normal eye may vary by as much as 6 mm Hg during a 24-hour period. This 24-hour variation (diurnal) may be much greater in individuals with glaucoma than in healthy individuals.

Adequate evaluation of glaucoma may require measurement of tension at different hours to learn the maximum pressure. Such measurements are particularly important in individuals who seem to have well-controlled glaucoma but who demonstrate progressive abnormalities of the optic nerve.

Gonioscopy.—The opaque corneoscleral limbus prevents direct visualization of the angle of the anterior chamber and its trabecular meshwork. The region may be examined by use of a contact lens combined with either a mirror or a prism (Fig 22-4). Inspection of the anterior chamber angle is essential to the diagnosis of either an open angle or a closed angle. An angle-closure mechanism can be diagnosed only if the angle is observed to be closed, which causes the intraocular pressure to be elevated. Earlier self-limited attacks of angle-closure glaucoma may have produced adhesions between the iris and the angle (peripheral anterior synechiae, goniosynechiae), which suggest the diagnosis. Gonioscopy has also been used in the development of an effective surgical procedure for infantile glaucoma and in the diagnostic evaluation and treatment of many types of glaucoma.

Gonioscopy may be direct or indirect. Direct gonioscopy uses a goniolens to neutralize the corneal refraction. The patient is supine, and a light source and hand-held microscope are used. In indirect gonioscopy a gonioprism is used in combination with a biomicroscope. Direct gonioscopy causes less distortion of angle structures and permits a view of deeper structures within a narrow chamber angle (which is also aided by the supine position). Indirect gonioscopy provides better illumination and magnification. Indentation through the sclera of the region of the ciliary body combined with gonioscopy may be particularly useful.

Ophthalmoscopy.—Ophthalmoscopic examination of the optic disk and the nerve fiber layer of the retina adjacent to the optic disk is of major importance in open-angle glaucoma (see this chapter).

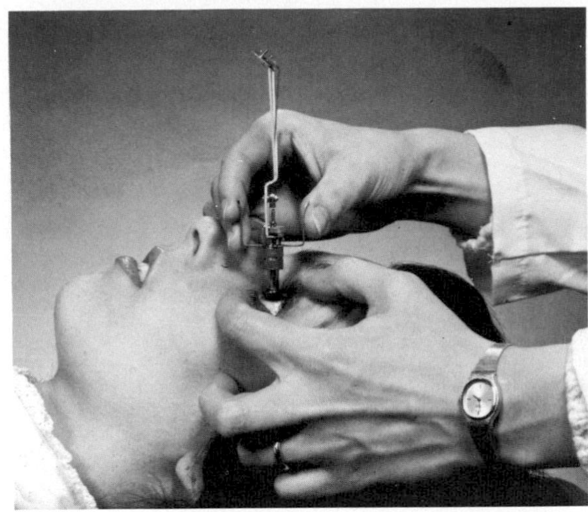

FIG 22-3.
Measurement of ocular tension with a Schiøtz tonometer. The examiner must be careful not to exert pressure on the globe through the eyelids.

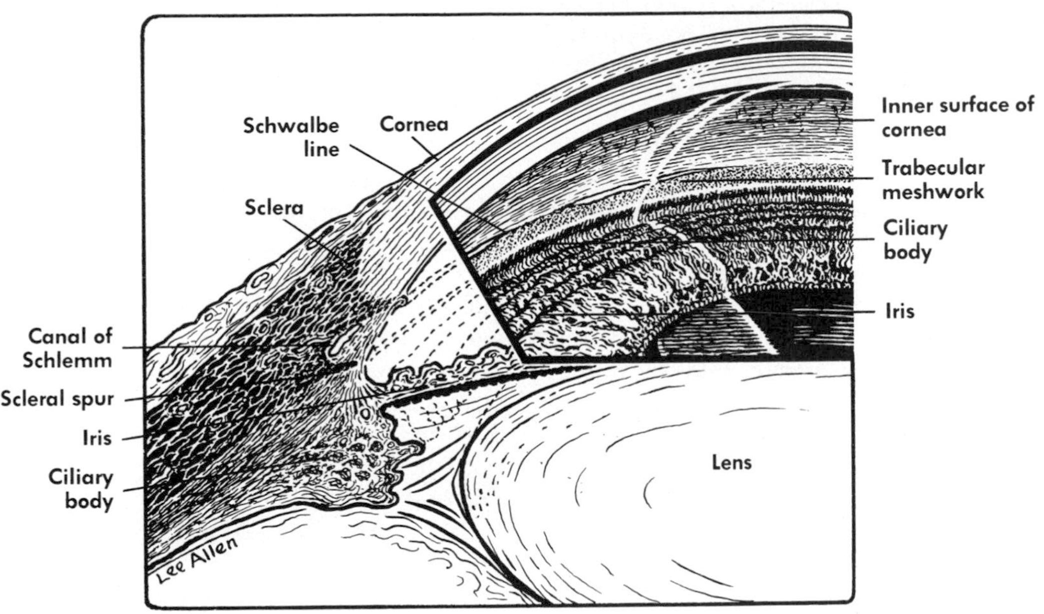

FIG 22-4.
Correlation of the anatomy of the chamber angle with its gonioscopic appearance. The trabecular meshwork, which opens into the canal of Schlemm, is bounded anteriorly by the line of Schwalbe and posteriorly by the scleral spur. *(Courtesy of Lee Allen, University of Iowa.)*

Perimetry.—The appearance of the optic disk must be correlated with measurement of the field of vision. Perimetry is most useful in the diagnosis of early glaucoma and in documenting the control or the progression of the disease. The visual field defect is usually proportionate to the severity of the optic nerve atrophy. In the early stages of glaucoma, visual field defects may be transient and present only when the intraocular pressure is high. As the disease progresses, the defects become permanent.

Visual fields are measured by using kinetic (moving) and static test objects. Kinetic techniques utilize a tangent screen or an arc or bowl

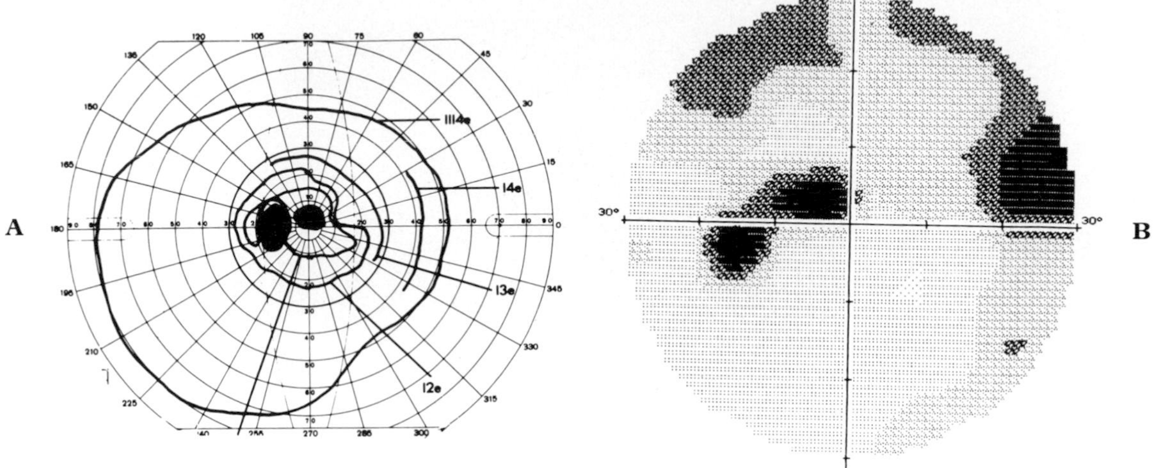

FIG 22-5.

Comparison of Goldmann visual field **(A)** and automated threshold perimeter record **(B)** in the same patient. A paracentral scotoma and a nasal step are demonstrated with each test. The Goldmann testing requires a skilled examiner, while the computer testing may be monitored by a less skilled technician. The Goldmann examination is less accurate and sensitive than the computer testing. The computer examination requires a more reliable and alert patient. (*After Hoskins HD Jr, Kass MA:* Becker-Shaffer's diagnosis and therapy of the glaucomas, *ed 6, St Louis, 1989, Mosby–Year Book.*)

perimeter. The test object moves from a nonseeing area to a seeing area, and the patient signals when it is perceived.

Static perimetry uses nonmoving (fixed) target lights. In suprathreshold perimetry, a target is shown for 0.5 to 1.0 second, and the targets the patient fails to see are recorded. In threshold static perimetry, the luminance of the target light is increased until the patient is just able to see it and the luminance of the light is recorded (Fig 22-5).

Both kinetic and static perimetry require an intelligent and cooperative patient. Kinetic perimetry is best performed by the practitioner or a highly trained and skilled technician. The computerized perimeter used for static perimetry is costly and the examination is time consuming. Patients may require several training sessions before reliable results are obtained. Static perimetry records the number of correct responses to a light stimulus, the number of times a patient stops accurate fixation, the number of responses without a stimulus (false-positive responses), and the number of times a patient fails to respond to a maximal visual stimulus in a seeing area (false-negative responses).

Conditions other than glaucoma must be considered in evaluation of a visual field. Constriction of the pupil may exaggerate defects. Refractive errors must be corrected for an accurate response. The threshold sensitivity is reduced in aging. Ocular abnormalities, such as corneal scarring or cataract, may induce erroneous responses. The patient's alertness, cooperation, and comprehension influence the results, as do the selection of the testing program and the skill of the examiner.

The nasal visual field is most susceptible to glaucomatous change (Fig 22-6). It corresponds to axons that originate from ganglion cells located temporal to the foveola. These axons arch above and below the large mass of nerve fibers that originate in the fovea centralis. The nerve fibers temporal to the fovea centralis do not cross a horizontal line that extends from the fovea centralis to the extreme periphery (temporal raphe). In glaucoma, these axons, which originate from an arc-shaped region of the temporal retina, lose their function, resulting in an island of blindness in the nasal field of vision, called an arcuate scotoma. The axons from ganglion cells in the fovea centralis are more numerous or more resistant to loss of function, and good

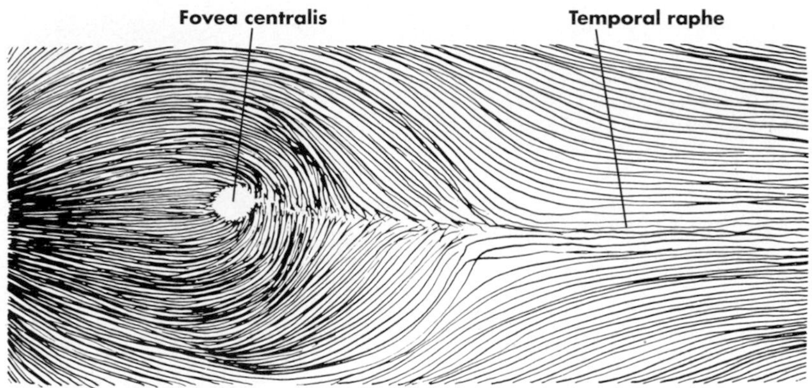

FIG 22-6.
The distribution of the nerve fiber layer at the posterior pole. Nerve fibers from the fovea centralis pass almost directly to the optic nerve, and nerve fibers from the peripheral retina arch above and below them. The nerve fibers do not cross the temporal raphe, which extends laterally from the fovea centralis to the retinal periphery. The raphe divides the peripheral retina into superior and inferior portions. Atrophy of these nerve fibers causes a nerve fiber bundle defect in the nasal visual field. (*From Vrabec F: The temporal raphe of the human retina,* Am J Ophthalmol *62:927, 1966. Used by permission.*)

central vision may be retained despite advanced glaucoma and retention of only 5° to 10° of the visual field.

PRIMARY OPEN-ANGLE GLAUCOMA

Primary open-angle glaucoma (simple glaucoma, glaucoma simplex, compensated glaucoma, chronic glaucoma, or chronic simple glaucoma) is a bilateral condition in which, without treatment, there is progressive excavation of the optic disk (cupping), with optic atrophy and a typical visual field defect. There are periods when the intraocular pressure is abnormally high. There is no grossly visible obstruction between the anterior chamber and the trabecular meshwork. In the United States open-angle glaucoma is one of the chief causes of blindness in adults.

The causes are not known but may be related to (1) an inadequate outflow of aqueous humor from the anterior chamber; (2) an inadequate vascular perfusion of the intraocular portion of the optic nerve; or (3) an imbalance between the level of the intraocular pressure and the level of the vascular perfusion pressure of the intraocular portion of the optic nerve. There are different degrees of severity and, unquestionably, many individuals have undiagnosed and mild types of open-angle glaucoma.

Symptoms and signs.—Open-angle glaucoma tends to become evident after 35 years of age. It has no particular sex predisposition. External examination of the eye does not indicate an abnormality such as that which may be recognized in angle-closure glaucoma.

Open-angle glaucoma is characterized by an almost complete absence of symptoms and a chronic, insidious course. Halos around lights and blurring vision occur only when there has been a sudden increase in intraocular pressure, and many patients never have visual symptoms. Visual acuity remains good until late in the course of the disease; thus, measurement of visual acuity is of no value as a screening test.

Ophthalmoscopy.—Evaluation of the ocular disk and nerve fiber layer of the retina is essential in the diagnosis of open-angle glaucoma. Both the monocular direct ophthalmoscope and the binocular indirect ophthalmoscope usually provide too little magnification for adequate evaluation. The use of either a fundus contact lens to neutralize corneal refraction or a +60 or +90 field lens combined with a biomicroscope (slit-lamp) has the advantage of magnification of a stereoscopic image. Fundus photography gives a permanent record. The confocal scanning laser ophthalmoscope provides a three-dimensional image of the optic disk. The inherent error of subjective evaluation

TABLE 22-3.
Some Ophthalmoscopic Signs in Glaucoma

I. Optic disk
  A. Physiologic cup
    1. Increased diameter; depth
    2. Cup-disk ratio
      a. More than 0.6
      b. Difference of more than 0.2 between two eyes
    3. Increased cup-to-disk margin
    4. Notching of cup
    5. Exposure of lamina cribrosa
    6. Exposed blood vessels within cup (baring)
  B. Neuroretinal rim
    1. Pale with cupping
II. Retinal blood vessels
  A. Peripapillary splinter hemorrhages
  B. Arterial pulsation
  C. Displacement of nasal blood vessels
  D. Dilated veins
III. Nerve fiber layer of retina
  A. Decreased fibers (red-free light)
  B. Peripapillary atrophy

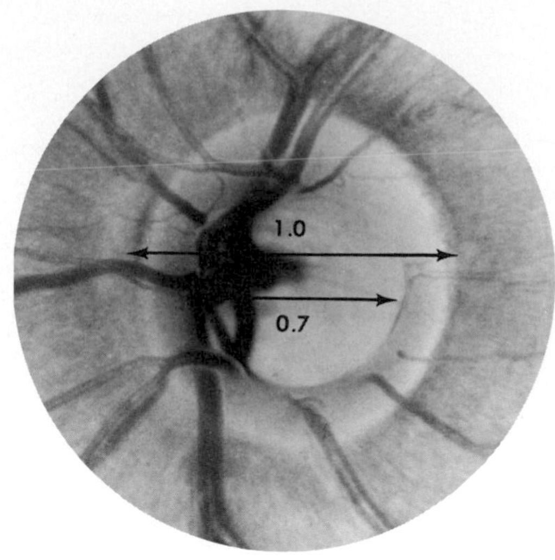

FIG 22-7.
The optic disk with the neuroretinal rim that surrounds the optic cup. The horizontal cup-disk ratio is the ratio of the diameter of the cup to the diameter of the disk. In this illustration, the cup-disk ratio is 0.7.

is minimized but not eliminated by such quantitative measurements.

The normal optic disk is slightly oval vertically. The central area may contain a depression, the physiologic cup, that is of lighter color than the surrounding nerve. In some eyes the cup is stark white and the lamina cribrosa may be seen at its base. The cup is surrounded by the orange-red neuroretinal rim, the nerve tissue between the margin of the cup and the margin of the disk. Optic nerve cupping in glaucoma is the result of loss of nerve fibers, astrocytes, and extracellular elements, which results in an increase in the size of the cup (Table 22-3).

The size and shape of the optic disk are determined by the size and shape of the posterior foramen of the sclera. Except in congenital abnormalities (see Chapter 20), it is oval, with its vertical measurement slightly greater than the horizontal. It measures from 1.0 to 1.7 mm in width, with the larger measurements paralleling those of a cornea of a larger diameter and flatter curvature.

The shape of the physiologic optic cup is determined by the angle the posterior foramen makes with the sclera. Its width reflects the width of the neural rim, and its depth reflects the volume of extracellular matrix and astrocytes. The horizontal ratio of the cup to the disk (Fig 22-7), expressed as a decimal, tends to be the same in both eyes of an individual and to be similar in family members. A difference of more than 0.2 in the cup-disk ratio between the two eyes suggests glaucomatous atrophy.

Examination of the optic disk for glaucoma is directed particularly to (1) the width and depth of the optic cup; (2) the width and the shape of the neural rim with attention to its narrowing or absence (notching) in the inferior or superior temporal quadrants; (3) streak hemorrhage on the disk margin; and (4) exposure of blood vessels within the optic cup. Stereoscopic photographs of the optic cup provide the most accurate records of the optic disk, and drawings of the disk are next best.

The axons of the retinal ganglion cells that have their nuclei located immediately above and below the fovea centralis are the most severely affected. Possibly the large number of ganglion cells in the fovea centralis protects them from damage, or the damage caused cannot be detected with current methods of examination. The loss of the axons that originate above and below the fovea centralis results in a narrowing of the neural margin of the optic cup that increases the diameter of the optic cup. The narrowing begins as a pit, then progresses to a notch of the neural rim most commonly affect-

A 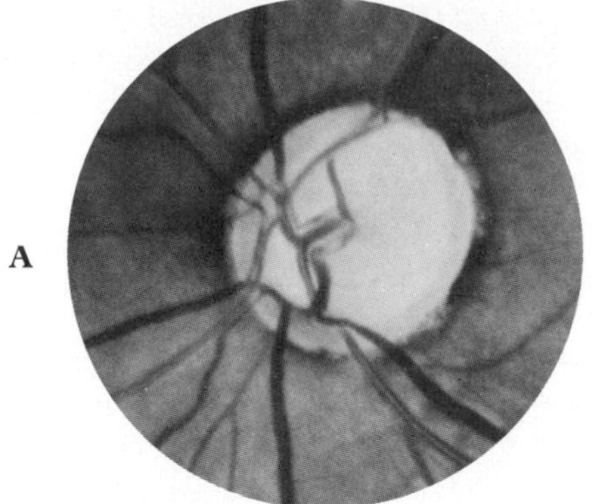

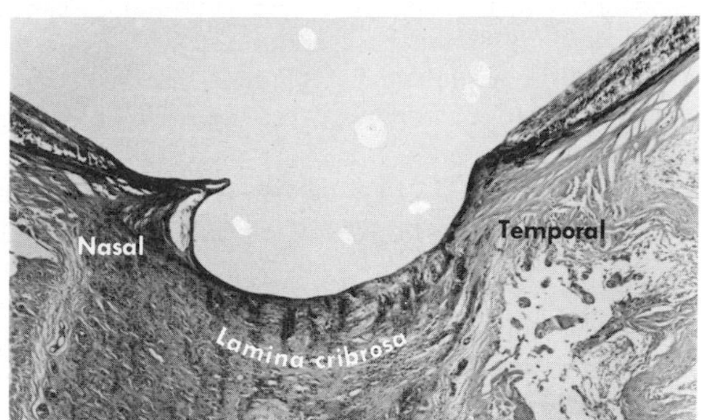 B

FIG 22-8.
A, Optic atrophy with glaucomatous excavation of the optic disk. The temporal neuroretinal rim has disappeared entirely because of glaucomatous atrophy. The blood vessels are displaced nasally and the blood vessels at the base of the optic cup are exposed ("bared"). **B,** Histologic section of advanced optic atrophy and glaucomatous excavation ("bean pot" excavation). The lamina cribrosa is characteristically bowed away from the eye.

ing the inferior temporal margin initially and then the superior temporal margin.

The loss of the neural rim increases the width of the optic cup and increases its depth. The increase in the width of the optic cup increases the cup-disk ratio (see Fig 22-7). A cup-disk ratio of more than 0.7 occurs in less than 2% of normal persons and is considered to be suggestive of open-angle glaucoma. The ratio and any change are more easily determined by measurements on a screen of the projected figure of a slide illustrating the disk. Usually the margin of the optic cup is easily seen but the periphery of the optic disk is more difficult to determine. Many experts regard the determination of the cup-disk ratio as unreliable, because of the inability to determine the exact outer margin of the disk.

An increase in the depth of the optic cup exposes the lamina cribrosa at the floor of the cup as a conspicuous white tissue containing grayish white spots. The temporal wall of the cup slopes gradually from the margin of the optic disk to the lamina cribrosa, which becomes concave with progression of the cupping. The nasal margin is steeper than the temporal.

The incidence of linear (streak) hemorrhages at the margin of the optic disk obviously reflects the frequency of examination, since they are absorbed quickly. When examined quarterly, about 10% of patients with open-angle glaucoma have hemorrhages at the margin of the optic disk, compared to 35% of those with normal-tension glaucoma.

As the optic cup enlarges, blood vessels normally concealed within the substance of the optic nerve become exposed (bared). Blood vessels that were once visible on the surface of the optic disk may disappear from view as they pass on the steep displaced nasal wall of the optic cup. In the untreated eye, the optic disk eventually becomes entirely atrophic and excavated (Fig 22-8).

The nerve fiber layer of the retina may be seen with a direct ophthalmoscope with a bright illumination or with the biomicroscope and a +90-diopter field lens. A red-free filter (green) enhances its appearance. The nerve fiber layer is best seen in dark-skinned, young individuals and becomes increasingly difficult to see with aging and decreased pigmentation. The skilled observer may detect a localized (uncommon) or diffuse (common) loss of nerve fibers in glaucoma.

Fundus photography with a wide-angle lens, blue or green filters, and high-resolution black-and-white film often demonstrates the nerve fiber layer.

NORMAL-TENSION GLAUCOMA

This is an ocular abnormality in which the ocular tension is consistently normal, although at the upper end of the normal range. The optic disks, however, develop the typical excavation of primary open-angle glaucoma combined with the characteristic visual field defects. Patients are often women more than 60 years of age. The anterior chamber angles appear normal, and there are no contributing ocular or systemic diseases. Most instances are detected because of the optic disk abnormality, but streak hemorrhages at the disk margin occur more frequently than in primary open-angle glaucoma.

Possibly the abnormality reflects an imbalance between the arterial perfusion pressure of the optic disk and the intraocular pressure. It may follow a vascular shock or may be the result of a vascular insufficiency of the optic nerve and constitute a chronic ischemic optic neuropathy. Medical treatment of vascular hypertension may lower the arterial perfusion pressure of the optic disk vasculature and result in optic atrophy.

Treatment is directed to the reduction of the ocular tension and any primary medical condition, such as too rigorously treated high blood pressure.

OCULAR HYPERTENSION ("GLAUCOMA SUSPECT")

This is a condition in which the intraocular pressure is consistently 21 mm Hg or more in both eyes in individuals who have open angles, normal optic disks, and normal visual field. Such individuals are more likely to develop glaucoma than the average person. Some practitioners call this early primary open-angle glaucoma; others believe that the patient has potential glaucoma; still others believe the eyes are normal but have pressures at the upper end of the normal distribution of ocular pressures. Some patients gradually develop normal ocular tensions without treatment.

Most patients do not develop optic disk excavation or visual field defects. The likelihood of developing glaucoma, however, is greater with higher tensions, increased age, or higher cup-disk ratios. When all of these factors are unfavorable, about 10% to 15% of the patients develop a visual field defect within 5 years.

Usually patients with pressures consistently less than 24 mm Hg are observed only. Patients with pressure of more than 30 mm Hg are usually treated with a beta-adrenergic antagonist. Patients with pressure in the intermediate range are treated if they have unfavorable factors such as myopia, diabetes mellitus, vascular disease, a family history of glaucoma, or large or asymmetric optic cups.

OPEN-ANGLE GLAUCOMA: MEDICAL TREATMENT

A wide variety of topical and systemic medications are used to treat open-angle glaucoma (see Chapter 3, The Autonomic Nervous System). Many of the compounds used are exceptionally potent and have widespread systemic actions. The practitioner must always be alert that symptoms in any patient being treated for glaucoma may be the result of the eye medications.

The treatment of primary open-angle glaucoma, once mainly medical, is changing. Argon laser trabeculoplasty (see this chapter) is minimally more effective if used immediately after the diagnosis of open-angle glaucoma rather than after medical treatment. About 20% of eyes so treated never require medication for glaucoma in contrast to 15% of the eyes treated with topical timolol before laser trabeculoplasty.

Surgery is required if the intraocular pressure is persistently increased or if there is progression of glaucomatous changes of the optic disk or visual field despite apparent adequate control of the glaucoma. Long-term topical medication is associated with a subclinical conjunctival inflammation and adversely affects subsequent filtration surgery. Glaucoma is unquestionably well advanced when optic atrophy and the concomitant visual field defects are detected. There is thus an increasing tendency to recommend surgery to manage primary open-angle glaucoma. The patients selected for early surgery must have ocular tensions that have been repeatedly demonstrated to be in a range that leads to glaucomatous optic atrophy.

Patients with diabetes mellitus, a family history of glaucoma, a large optic cup, any cardiovascular abnormality, and old age are at increased risk to develop cupping of the optic disk, optic atrophy, and loss of vision.

Medical treatment of open-angle glaucoma presents the same difficulties as the treatment of any asymptomatic chronic disease. Drugs that constrict the pupil may aggravate the visual loss caused by incipient cataract or, in younger

TABLE 22-4.
Suggestions for the Medical Management of Glaucoma

Maintain familiarity with the general physical condition of the patient and any changes that have occurred since the previous visit.
Record all medications used by the patient. Learn at each visit any change in the medications or in the frequency of their use.
Consider the possibility that progression of the glaucoma reflects inadequate vascular perfusion of the optic nerve rather than increased intraocular pressure.
Consider the possibility that the patient faithfully uses the medication prescribed to treat the glaucoma only in preparation for an office visit and measurement of the ocular tension.
So as to recognize random fluctuations in intraocular pressure, initiate or change topical therapy in one eye only.
If treatment is not effective, change the medication rather than adding to the ineffective regimen.
Adjust any treatment program to one that the patient will follow.
Use the lowest concentration of medications, the least frequent times of administration, and the smallest number of medications that will control the glaucoma.
Observe patients to be certain they know how to instill eyedrops.
Provide written instructions recording the names of medications, the appearance of the bottles and their tops, the frequency of administration, and the times of administration.
Communicate with the practitioners managing the patient's general health.
Learn from patient about expense, inconvenience, and possible medication-induced side effects.
If medical treatment is not effective, consider the possibility that the patient is not using medications as directed.
Educate patients about glaucoma and the side effects of the medications they are using.
Stop treatment in one eye periodically to learn if the medications are still effective.
Measure the intraocular pressure at different times during the day and at different times after the administration of medication.
Recommend that patients comparison shop to learn the least expensive and most convenient pharmacies.

After Hoskins HD Jr, Kass MA: *Becker-Shaffer's diagnosis and therapy of the glaucomas,* ed 6, St Louis, 1989, Mosby–Year Book, p 83. Used by permission.

individuals, induce a painful spasm of the ciliary muscle combined with sustained accommodation, causing temporary myopia. Patients may have difficulty remembering to use their medications, a problem often aggravated when several different medications are prescribed for daily use. If the glaucoma is not well controlled, the intraocular pressure is increased, and the visual field defects are progressing, more frequent examination is required. Some patients do not use prescribed medications until a few days before examination, and the examiner may be perplexed by the progression of glaucoma damage in an eye with apparent well-controlled glaucoma. Long-term use of different combinations of eyedrops is a significant risk factor for failure of laser trabeculoplasty or filtration surgery.

Ocular examination is usually indicated at least three times annually for well-controlled open-angle glaucoma. The ocular tension is measured, the ophthalmoscopic appearance of the optic disks is evaluated, and the optic cup and neuroretinal rim are photographed or sketched. Perimetry and gonioscopy should be repeated annually.

The medical treatment of glaucoma is directed toward increasing the outflow of aqueous humor from the anterior chamber or from the uveoscleral pathways, reducing the volume of aqueous humor secreted, or a combination of these. The management of any chronic disease, particularly one without symptoms, is a difficult task for both the patient and the practitioner (Table 22-4).

Primary open-angle glaucoma is treated by one or more different classes of drugs (Table 22-5). The practitioner must be assured that the patient knows how to instill eyedrops in the conjunctival sac. Patients should be instructed to close their eyes for 2 minutes after instilling the eyedrops and to squeeze their inner canthi with their fingers to occlude the lacrimal puncta to minimize systemic absorption and to increase corneal penetration through longer contact.

Medical treatment should begin with the minimum frequency and concentration of the drug that will maintain intraocular pressure in the normal range, prevent visual deterioration, and prevent the development or progression of atrophy of the optic nerve. Treatment is often

TABLE 22-5.
Medications Used in the Therapy of Open-Angle Glaucoma

I. Beta-adrenergic receptor antagonists
  A. Nonselective (beta-1 and beta-2 receptors)
    1. Timolol (Timoptic) (0.25% and 0.5%) (Timoptic-XE) (0.5%: gel-forming solution)
    2. Levobunolol (Betagen) (0.5%)
    3. Metipranolol (Optipranolol) (0.3%)
  B. Beta-1-selective
    1. Betaxolol (Betoptic) (0.5%)
  C. Beta-1-selective with intrinsic sympathomimetic activity
    1. Carteolol (Ocupress) (1%)
II. Cholinergic drugs
  A. Parasympathetic mimetic
    1. Pilocarpine (1% to 4%)
    2. Carbachol (0.75% to 3%)
  B. Anticholinesterase
    1. Physostigmine (Eserine) (0.25% ointment; 0.25% and 0.5%)
    2. Echothiophate iodide (Phospholine Iodide)
    3. Demecarium bromide (Humorsol) (0.12% to 0.25%)
    4. Isoflurophate (Floropryl) (0.025% ointment)
III. Carbonic anhydrase inhibitors
  A. Oral agents
    1. Acetazolamide (250 mg)
    2. Dichlorphenamide (Daranide) (50 mg)
    3. Ethoxzolamide (Cardrase) (125 mg)
    4. Methazolamide (Neptazane) (25 and 50 mg)
  B. Topical agents
    1. Dorzolamide hydrochloride (Trusopt) (2.0%)
IV. Adrenergic agonists
  A. Alpha and beta receptors
    1. Epinephrine (0.5% to 2%)
    2. Dipivefrin hydrochloride (Propine) (0.1%)
  B. Alpha-2 receptors
    1. Apraclonidine hydrochloride (Iopidine) (1%)
V. Prostaglandin analogues
  A. Prostaglandin F2-alpha-analogue (Latanoprost) (0.12%)
VI. Miscellaneous
  A. Ca^{2+}-channel blockers

initiated with a beta-adrenergic receptor antagonist, such as timolol instilled twice daily. If this is not adequate, dipivefrin (Propine), a conjugated epinephrine-adrenergic agonist, may be added. (The additive effects in reducing intraocular pressure by instillation of both an adrenergic receptor antagonist and an agonist suggest that their effects may not be on the adrenergic system.) If not effective, 1% or 2% topical pilocarpine or a carbonic anhydrase inhibitor may be added. Topical 3% or 4% pilocarpine is sometimes substituted if weaker strengths of the drug are not effective.

Beta-adrenergic receptor antagonists.— Therapy for open-angle glaucoma is often initiated with a beta-1 and beta-2 (nonselective) adrenergic receptor antagonist that reduces the secretion of aqueous humor by the ciliary body. Nonselective adrenergic receptor antagonists decrease the high-density lipoprotein cholesterol level, which is inversely correlated with the incidence of coronary heart disease. Blockade of the beta-1 adrenergic receptors reduces the heart rate and may be a factor in falls in the elderly. Blockade of the beta-2 receptors decreases bronchodilation, and the compounds are contraindicated in patients with bronchial asthma.

Timolol maleate (Timoptic).—This was the first commercially available beta-blocker. It is used topically in a concentration of 0.25% or 0.5%. It does not affect pupil size or accommodation and is well tolerated by most patients. It is contraindicated in patients with asthma, other obstructive pulmonary disease, or cardiac conduction defects. Some patients with previously undetected pulmonary or cardiac disease will develop symptoms that are not immediately recognized as drug related. The initial reduction of pressure is not maintained in some patients, and the ocular pressure returns to pretreatment levels in several days. In other patients control of pressure is lost after 3 to 12 months. Central nervous system symptoms of depression, anxiety, or confusion are experienced in some patients. Levobunolol (Betagen) and metipranolol (Optipranolol) have actions similar to those of timolol. Metipranolol is rarely associated with acute anterior granulomatous uveitis, accompanied by increased intraocular pressure in some patients.

Betaxolol (Betoptic).—This is a beta-selective adrenergic receptor antagonist that does not decrease high-density lipoprotein cholesterol levels. It has the same ocular pressure-lowering properties as other beta-blockers and possibly has less effect on the bronchial system.

Adrenergic receptor agonists.—Topical instillation of epinephrine in a 0.5% to 2%

solution decreases secretion of aqueous humor and improves the aqueous outflow. Epinephrine is moderately irritating to the eye and may cause black adenochrome pigmentation of the conjunctiva and maculopathy in aphakic eyes. Epinephrine solutions are used either alone or in combination with cholinergic-stimulating drugs, often pilocarpine.

Dipivefrin (Propine).—This is a conjugated epinephrine. It penetrates the cornea readily and may be used topically in a 0.1% concentration. It is often the drug of choice to supplement timolol treatment.

Apraclonidine.—This is an alpha-2 adrenergic receptor agonist. It lowers the intraocular pressure in both normal and glaucomatous eyes. It is used hourly before and after laser treatment of the anterior ocular segment in the prophylaxis of the transient increase in intraocular pressure. Often, a local allergic contact dermatitis and follicular conjunctivitis limit its usefulness for long-term glaucoma therapy.

Carbonic anhydrase inhibitors.—Carbonic anhydrase inhibitors reduce the secretion of aqueous humor by the ciliary processes. A drug of this class is often prescribed to supplement the effects of topical medications. Acetazolamide is the compound commonly selected for initial use. The drug is effective 2 hours after administration and its maximum action continues for 6 hours. Time-release capsules (Sequels) are effective for 12 hours. Paresthesia, with numbness and tingling of the extremities, and anorexia often necessitate a reduction of the dose or substitution of a different carbonic anhydrase compound.

Carbonic anhydrase inhibitors that penetrate the cornea have been developed for topical instillation in glaucoma therapy. Dorzolamide, a substituted sulfonamide that reduces the intraocular pressure after topical instillation, was made available in 1995. There is cross-sensitivity with other sulfonamides. There may be ocular discomfort after instillation (33%), superficial punctate keratitis (15%), and cutaneous and ocular hypersensitivity reactions (10%).

Cholinergic agonists.—Two main groups of cholinergic agonists that are used in ophthalmology include: (1) acetylcholine and carbachol, a synthetic choline ester; and (2) naturally occurring alkaloids, principally pilocarpine, which mimic the action of acetylcholine on postganglionic parasympathetic nerves.

Acetylcholine chloride.—A 1% solution (Miochol) is instilled in the anterior chamber in intraocular surgery to constrict the pupil rapidly.

Carbachol.—Carbachol is used topically in a solution of 0.75% to 3.0% in the treatment of open-angle glaucoma. A 0.01% solution (Miostat, Intraocular) is instilled in the anterior chamber to constrict the pupil in intraocular surgery. Some patients develop a tolerance to the ocular pressure-lowering effects of pilocarpine, and carbachol is substituted. After several months of carbachol therapy, the patient is again responsive to the ocular effects of pilocarpine.

Pilocarpine.—Pilocarpine is the traditional medication for initial therapy of open-angle glaucoma. It has been mainly replaced by the beta-adrenergic receptor antagonists group ("beta-blockers"). It is used topically in a 1% to 4% solution. Pilocarpine therapy should begin with the lowest concentration that will maintain normal ocular tension and prevent optic nerve atrophy. Because of its effect on constricting the pupil, it is often used in the management of angle-closure glaucoma (see this chapter). The pupillary constriction often decreases vision in patients with minor degrees of cataract. In individuals less than 40 years of age, pilocarpine often causes a transient (1 to 2 weeks) spasm of the ciliary muscle with an aching pain in the eyes and an artificial or increased myopia from increased accommodation.

Anticholinesterase agents.—The action of acetylcholine at cholinergic nerve endings is terminated by the action of the acetylcholinesterases. The anticholinesterase agents either inhibit or abolish the hydrolysis of acetylcholine by the cholinesterases at cholinergic receptor sites, and thus enchance the effects of acetylcholine. In addition to topical use in open-angle glaucoma and accommodative esotropia (see Chapter 24), the drugs are used systemically in the treatment of paralytic ileus, urinary bladder atony, and myasthenia gravis. Many compounds have been synthesized for use as insecticides or nerve gasses.

Eserine (physostigmine salicylate).—This is used topically in a 0.25% or a 0.5% solution or 0.25% ointment, mainly at bedtime, to supplement the action of pilocarpine. Patients become tolerant of its effects after prolonged use. Additionally, it may cause conjunctival irritation and follicular hypertrophy.

Echothiophate iodide (Phospholine Iodide).—Echothiophate iodide (0.03%, 0.06%, 0.125%, and 0.25%) is active against the true cholinesterase of the sphincter pupillae muscle. It causes an intense miosis, with a maximum effect in 4 to 6 hours that persists up to 24 hours. It is used twice daily, usually in 0.03% to 0.06% concentrations. It depletes systemic nonspecific anticholinesterases and may cause prolonged respiratory depression in general anesthesia with the use of succinyl chloride. Toxic reactions may follow the use of procaine, which, like succinyl chloride, is hydrolyzed by the nonspecific anticholinesterases. Its use is contraindicated in angle-closure glaucoma, bronchial asthma, gastrointestinal spasm, vascular hypertension, myasthenia gravis, and Parkinson disease. Long-term topical administration may cause anterior subcapsular cataracts.

Children in whom echothiophate iodide is used in the treatment of accommodative esotropia (see Chapter 23) may develop pupillary cysts. The cysts are prevented by instillation of 2.5% phenylephrine eyedrops. Children may experience episodes of acute abdominal pain that mimics acute appendicitis.

Despite the side effects, echothiophate iodide is useful in the treatment of open-angle glaucoma, some secondary open-angle glaucomas (this chapter), and accommodative esotropia.

Demecarium bromide (Humorsol).—This is used topically in a 0.12% or 0.25% solution every 12 to 48 hours in the management of open-angle glaucoma. It is effective in some patients who do not respond to echothiophate but tolerance occurs readily.

Isoflurophate (DFP; Floropryl).—This is administered topically in a 0.025% ointment or as a 0.01% to 0.10% solution in peanut oil. Hypersensitivity reactions are common and the drug is easily inactivated.

OPEN-ANGLE GLAUCOMA: SURGICAL TREATMENT

In open-angle glaucoma in which the trabecular meshwork is clearly visible, the preferred initial surgical procedure is laser trabeculoplasty. Its major indication is glaucoma in which the optic disk and visual field are normal. The procedure is most effective in eyes in which the trabecular meshwork is pigmented.

The argon laser is usually used. The eye is anesthetized with a topical anesthetic, and the trabecular meshwork is viewed through an antireflective coated four-mirror gonioprism. Usually a 50-μm spot size and 0.1-second duration are used. A power setting is used that will blanch the surface of the trabecular meshwork that faces the anterior chamber but will not form bubbles. Usually an initial power of 400 mW is selected, and this is increased in 200-mW increments until a visible reaction is observed. The power is then reduced by 100 mW and used for treatment if it produces a reaction. Individual surgical preferences vary, but often 45 to 50 burns are spaced evenly over one half of the anterior trabecular meshwork. After 4 weeks, the fellow one half of the trabecular meshwork is treated.

The main immediate complication is a transient increase in intraocular pressure. Apraclonidine, a relatively selective alpha-2-agonist in a 1% concentration administered 1 hour before and immediately after laser therapy, decreases the frequency and degree of increase in intraocular pressure. Acetazolamide and other glaucoma medications are less effective. Despite a normal pressure 1 hour after treatment, a marked increase in intraocular pressure may occur 8 to 12 hours after laser therapy. Patients with severe glaucomatous optic nerve damage should be seen 24 hours after laser therapy. Other complications are relatively minor: transient iritis, peripheral anterior synechiae, hyphema, and transient corneal opacities. Intraocular pressure control is achieved in about 85% of all patients, but most (75%) continue to require antiglaucoma medications. Control may be lost with passing time, and laser trabeculoplasty is often not effective with additional application.

Trabeculectomy.—Trabeculectomy is the filtering operation of choice in many centers. An operating microscope is used, and a superficial flap of sclera is fashioned to expose the scleral side of the trabecular meshwork. A portion of the meshwork is then excised and the scleral flap replaced. A filtering bleb often develops after surgery. The chief advantage of the operation is the immediate formation of the anterior chamber after the procedure that prevents the development of peripheral anterior synechiae. Excessively low pressure (hypotension), cystic conjunctival blebs, cataract, and bullous keratopathy occur less commonly after trabeculectomy than after other filtering operations.

The application of mitomycin C (0.5 mg/mL) on a surgical sponge to the scleral flap for 3 minutes increases the rate of success in decreasing intraocular pressure but is associated with a higher incidence of postoperative hypotony. 5-Fluorouracil must be injected subconjunctivally for 5 to 14 days postoperatively and gives similar results.

Procedures to destroy a portion of the ciliary epithelium to reduce the volume of aqueous humor secreted are usually limited to secondary types of glaucoma, particularly neovascular and inflammatory, and eyes in which previous surgical procedures have been unsuccessful. Often the procedures are performed in eyes with minimal remaining vision. In such desperate instances some surgeons prefer to use a glaucoma valve filtration or to repeat a filtering procedure using mitomycin C.

The ciliary epithelium may be destroyed by a variety of methods. In eyes that have a large iridectomy or in aniridia, in which the ciliary processes may be observed, a transpupillary photocoagulation with laser energy may be used. Laser energy may be delivered to the ciliary processes directly by means of a fiberoptic probe (endolaser) with illumination coupled to the laser or provided by a separate fiberoptic probe.

In cyclocryotherapy a freezing probe is applied to the sclera over the ciliary body. The neodymium:YAG (Nd:YAG) laser is used to apply laser energy through the sclera to the ciliary body. Cyclocryotherapy causes a greater inflammation than the Nd:YAG laser but may reduce the intraocular pressure more effectively.

TABLE 22-6.
Some Types of Secondary Open-Angle Glaucoma

I. Pigment dispersion syndrome
II. Exfoliation syndrome
III. Corticosteroid-induced
IV. Ocular trauma
  A. Angle-recession
  B. Contusion
  C. Chemical
  D. Thermal
  E. Surgical (see below)
V. Lens-induced
  A. Lens fragments (particles)
  B. Phacolytic
  C. Phacoanaphylaxis
VI. Intraocular surgery
  A. Cataract extraction
    1. Retained viscoelastic solution
    2. Intraocular gas
    3. Alpha chymotrypsin
    4. Uveitis
    5. Hyphema
    6. Vitreous prolapse
  B. Laser therapy
    1. Anterior chamber angle
    2. Retina
  C. Vitrectomy
  D. Retinopexy
    1. Intraocular gas
    2. Scleral shrinkage
    3. Scleral implant
VII. Intraocular bleeding
  A. Ghost-cell (erythrocyte membranes)
  B. Hemolysis
  C. Hemosiderin
  D. Hyphema
VIII. Uveitis
  A. Heterochromia of Fuchs
  B. Glaucomatocyclitic crisis
  C. Prolonged or recurrent inflammation
IX. Intraocular tumor
X. Increased episcleral vein pressure
  A. Thyroid disease
  B. Superior vena cava pressure
  C. Carotid-cavernous fistula
  D. Orbital tumor

SECONDARY OPEN-ANGLE GLAUCOMA

Secondary open-angle glaucoma is the condition in which an ocular disorder causes a persistently high intraocular pressure and the aqueous humor has free access to the trabecular meshwork. It may be monocular or affect both eyes. In the early stages the optic disk and visual fields are normal. There are many causes (Table 22-6) that may be obvious, or the increased intraocular pressure may be erroneously attributed to primary open-angle glaucoma.

Pigment dispersion syndrome.—This is a condition in which the iris pigment epithelium releases pigment that is deposited on the corneal endothelium in a vertical line (Krukenberg spindle), on the surface of the trabecular meshwork, and on the posterior lens capsule at the equator. The loss of pigment from the iris causes a transillumination defect in which there are radial, spokelike, midperipheral defects in the iris. Dilation of the pupil with mydriatics or strenuous exercise releases pigment into the anterior chamber, sometimes with an increase in intraocular pressure.

The pigment dispersion syndrome affects mainly men in their early 20s who are myopic. Their eyes are larger than average, the anterior chambers are deeper, and the posterior surface of the iris tends to be in contact with the ciliary processes or the lens zonule. Retinal detachment is slightly more frequent than in unaffected eyes, and miotic eyedrops should never be used. Implantation of a posterior chamber lens after cataract extraction may induce a secondary pigment dispersion syndrome, particularly in patients with diabetes mellitus.

Some 15 to 20 years after the onset of the pigment dispersion syndrome, approximately 35% of those affected develop a frank open-angle glaucoma identical to the primary type. Medical treatment is often not effective, and surgery is required to prevent progression.

Exfoliation syndrome (pseudoexfoliation of the lens capsule; glaucoma capsulare).—This syndrome is characterized by the deposition of flaky, translucent, fibrillar material most conspicuously seen on the anterior lens capsule and pupillary opening, but also on both surfaces of the iris, zonule, trabecular meshwork, ciliary body, corneal endothelium, and the orbital blood vessels. Sometimes the fibrillar material forms a membrane on the anterior iris surface. There is an increased density of the exfoliative material in the matrix of iris vessels combined with adventitial and ensdothelial cell degeneration. The prevalence increases with aging.

The source of the fibrillar material is not known, but it is also found in the skin, myocardium, liver, gallbladder, kidney, and meninges. It is apparently related to an otherwise asymptomatic generalized disorder of basement membrane metabolism.

When glaucoma occurs, it is similar to primary open-angle glaucoma but far more difficult to control with medication. Laser trabeculoplasty is often successful. Filtration surgery is often complicated by severe intraocular inflammation. The pupil dilates poorly, the lens zonule is fragmented and unstable, and the cataract extraction is associated with many complications.

True exfoliation of the lens capsule previously occurred in glassblowers, who faced intense heat from molten glass. The iris absorbed the heat and transmitted it to the lens capsule, causing a splitting of its zonular lamellae.

Corticosteroid-induced glaucoma (cortisone glaucoma; steroid glaucoma).—This is caused by topical and, less frequently, systemic administration of corticosteroid preparations to susceptible individuals. It may be self-limited but may cause severe cupping of the optic disk, optic atrophy, and persistent increase in the intraocular pressure.

Clinically it is indistinguishable from primary open-angle glaucoma. It may be erroneously considered a complication of the disorder for which corticosteroid treatment is indicated. Certain groups of individuals are particularly susceptible to corticosteroid-induced glaucoma: (1) some patients with primary open-angle glaucoma and their first-degree relatives; (2) patients with diabetes mellitus; and (3) patients with severe myopia.

The mechanism is not known. It has been attributed to alterations of cyclic adenosine monophosphate (cAMP) in the anterior segment or to one or more of the following changes in the trabecular meshwork: (1) decreased proteolytic activity; (2) glycosaminoglycan deposition; and (3) decreased phagocytic activity.

Effective treatment requires that the administration of corticosteroids be discontinued. It may be necessary to excise corticosteroid deposits of earlier subconjunctival injections.

Angle-recession glaucoma.—This is a monocular abnormality that occurs 30 or more years after blunt trauma to the eye. Gonioscopic examination discloses the ciliary body band to be irregularly widened secondary to an original tear between the longitudinal and circular muscles of the ciliary body. Often the patients do not recall the original injury until prompted by the typical ocular signs.

Treatment is difficult, as the eyes respond poorly to medical therapy and to laser trabeculoplasty. A trabeculectomy may be required soon after the diagnosis.

Lens-induced glaucoma.—Lens-induced secondary glaucoma of the angle-closure type results when a swollen lens closes the anterior chamber angle (phacomorphic glaucoma) or when a dislocated lens blocks the flow of aqueous humor through the pupil. Lens-induced secondary open-angle glaucoma is caused by (1) leakage of lens proteins from a hypermature cataract (phacolytic glaucoma); (2) sensitization of the uvea to lens proteins after rupture of the lens capsule (phacoanaphylaxis); and (3) blockage of the trabecular meshwork by lens particles.

***Phacolytic glaucoma.*—**This occurs in patients with cataract, in which all lens fibers are opacified (hypermature), which results in the formation of proteins of high molecular weight. These proteins escape through the intact lens capsule and block the trabecular meshwork. Macrophages attracted to the proteins further obstruct the angle. There is an associated iritis with white clumps in the anterior chamber but without keratic precipitates. The hypermature cataract must be removed to correct the glaucoma and inflammation. An extracapsular cataract extraction and a posterior intraocular lens correct the glaucoma and inflammation and restore vision.

Phacoanaphylaxis.—This is a rare autoimmune granulomatous inflammation in which the uvea is sensitized to lens proteins released through accidental laceration of the lens capsule or extracapsular lens extraction.

Lens particle glaucoma.—This follows disruption of the lens capsule by accidental trauma or cataract surgery. There is a severe iritis and a high intraocular pressure with an edematous cornea. The aqueous humor, which may be removed by paracentesis, contains macrophages and lens material. If the glaucoma and iritis do not respond to medical measures, surgical removal of the lens material is necessary.

***Cataract surgery.*—**Removal of the opacified crystalline lens commonly causes an increased intraocular pressure. The breakdown of the blood-aqueous barrier secondary to the opening and manipulation of the eye may cause a transient increase in intraocular pressure with pain within several hours of surgery.

Failure to remove viscoelastic substances from the eye, pigment release by iris manipulation, or air in the anterior chamber may cause glaucoma. Rarely vitreous in the anterior chamber causes a secondary open-angle glaucoma.

Posterior capsulotomy using the laser typically increases intraocular pressure 2 to 4 hours after treatment. Usually apraclonidine or acetazolamide, and a beta-adrenergic antagonist are administered before and after the procedure to minimize the increase. Eyes with preexisting glaucoma are particularly vulnerable and patients with optic nerve damage must be observed closely. Tension should be measured 2 to 4 hours after the procedure and 1 and 7 days later in patients with preexisting glaucoma. Increased pressure is less severe after laser therapy to the retina than after trabeculoplasty but is managed in the same ways as after laser posterior capsulotomy.

Ocular injuries.—Contusion of the eye results in a marked immediate increase in intraocular pressure that persists for 30 to 45 minutes. If hemorrhage follows contusion, a secondary glaucoma may ensue. It results from blockage of the trabecular meshwork by erythrocytes and macrophages containing hemoglobin products. Contusion may result in tears in the ciliary body and recession of the chamber angle. The majority of such eyes do not develop glaucoma. Some develop what clinically appears to be monocular open-angle glaucoma from 1 month to 10 years after the injury.

Chemical burns of the eye cause glaucoma through destruction of episcleral veins, damage to the trabecular meshwork, scleral shrinkage, inflammation, and release of prostaglandins. The usual medical therapy is often not successful. Scarring of the external eye prevents successful external filtration and often procedures to limit ciliary body secretion or drainage through a glaucoma valve are required.

Free blood in the eye causes a secondary open-angle glaucoma through one of several mechanisms. Ghost cells (erythrocyte membranes) migrate from hemorrhage in the vitreous to the anterior chamber and block the trabecular meshwork. Medical therapy is often effective, but when necessary, repeated irrigation of the anterior chamber removes the cells. Hemolytic glaucoma results when macrophages phagocytize erythrocyte debris and occlude the trabecular meshwork. Glaucoma may occur in hemosiderosis after trabecular endothelial cells phagocytize degenerated erythrocytes. Rebleeding in traumatic hyphema is often followed by a secondary open-angle glaucoma. Aspirin must not be used to relieve pain, and antifibrinolytic agents (epsilon-aminocaproic acid [Amicar] or tranexamic acid) are used prophylactically.

Intraocular inflammation.—Iridocyclitis may cause a secondary glaucoma by blocking the trabecular meshwork with inflammatory cells, protein, and fibrin. There may be an inflammation of the trabecular meshwork (trabeculitis) causing irreversible damage to the meshwork and a permanent open-angle glaucoma. The disease course is the same as that of open-angle glaucoma.

Heterochromic iridocyclitis (of Fuchs) is a nongranulomatous, chronic anterior uveitis in which the affected eye is lighter in color than the fellow eye. There is an associated secondary glaucoma and frequently a posterior subcapsular cataract. Both the glaucoma and the cataract with which the uveitis is associated may be aggravated by corticosteroids used locally in the treatment of the uveitis.

Glaucomatocyclitic crisis is a unilateral acute inflammation of the uveal tract in which the signs of a rapid increase in intraocular pressure predominate. There is corneal edema with blurring of vision and marked decrease in the coefficient of outflow facility. The disease is distinguished from angle-closure glaucoma in that the angle is open. The inflammation may be confined to the trabecular meshwork with minimal inflammatory signs. Systemic indomethacin may terminate the attack.

Miscellaneous types.—A carotid-cavernous sinus fistula increases the episcleral venous pressure and impairs aqueous outflow, resulting in increased intraocular pressure.

Rectus muscle fibrosis in thyrotropic exophthalmos increases intraocular pressure when the contralateral muscle contracts. The pressure is normal when the normal muscle is not contracting. Usually the inferior rectus muscle is restricted, and on upward gaze the intraocular pressure increases and erroneously high tensions are recorded. In downward gaze the tension is normal. Any proptosis may increase episcleral venous pressure, decrease aqueous humor outflow, and increase intraocular pressure.

Primary open-angle glaucoma and retinal detachment occur in the same eyes by chance, since they are both common conditions or are secondary to a common underlying cause, such as accidental or surgical trauma, proliferative retinopathy, or retrolental fibroplasia. Open-angle glaucoma may follow scleral buckling or vitrectomy procedures to correct the retinal detachment. Treatment of glaucoma with miotics may cause retinal holes, and the peripheral retina of patients with open-angle glaucoma should be studied by means of indirect ophthalmoscopy before treatment is initiated.

ANGLE-CLOSURE GLAUCOMA

Angle-closure glaucoma is an abnormality in which the intraocular pressure increases because the outflow of aqueous humor from the anterior chamber is mechanically impaired by apposition of the iris to the peripheral cornea, the trabecular meshwork, or both. The condition has been designated in the past as narrow-angle, acute congestive, and uncompensated glaucoma. No term is ideal because the intraocular pressure is normal when the angle is open and pressure is increased only when a major portion of the angle is closed. Adhesions between the iris and trabecular meshwork and peripheral cornea (peripheral anterior synechiae or goniosynechiae) decrease aqueous outflow.

The disease incidence is one quarter as frequent as open-angle glaucoma in the United States and Europe. It is more common than open-angle glaucoma in Asia. In American white individuals it is approximately three times more common in women than men, but in African-Americans the incidence is the same in men and women.

The disease occurs because of a familial anatomic defect that causes a shallow anterior chamber. The peripheral iris often inserts on the extreme anterior edge of the ciliary body, causing the anterior chamber angle to be shallow and placing the iris close to the trabecular meshwork. The corneal diameter may be small and the eye hyperopic. The lens is closer to the cornea than usual, and with the normal increase in size of the lens with aging, it becomes even closer. This iris appears to bow forward so that its surface closely parallels the posterior convexity of the cornea (Fig 22-9). This may be observed by shining a penlight into the anterior chamber from the temporal side of the eye. A shadow, which is not

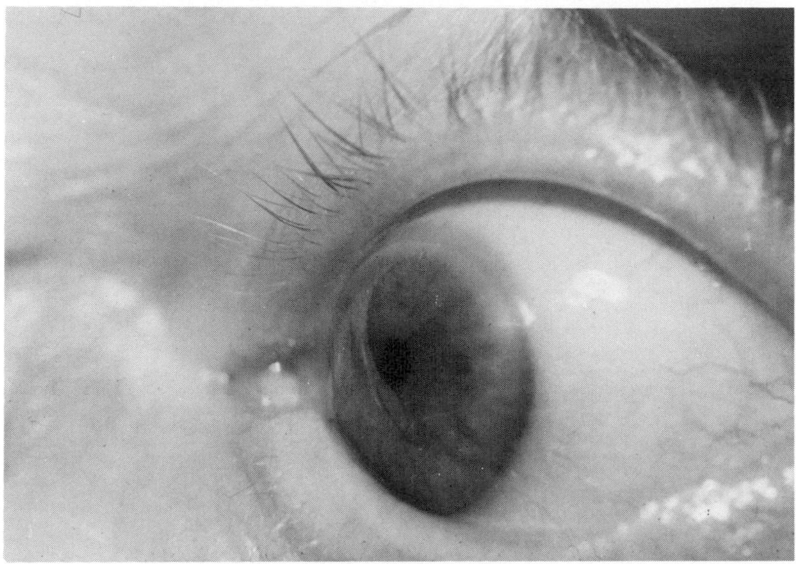

FIG 22-9.
Shallow anterior chamber angle observed from the temporal side. The diagnosis of angle-closure glaucoma requires observation of a closed angle when the tension is increased.

present in the normal eye, is cast by the nasal portion of the convex iris.

Increased intraocular pressure occurs when there is anterior displacement of the peripheral iris. This displacement causes the iris to block the trabecular meshwork and prevents the exit of aqueous humor. Two conditions operating singly or together may cause this displacement: (1) decreased flow of aqueous humor through the pupil causes a relative pupillary block with accumulation of aqueous humor in the posterior chamber, causing the peripheral iris to balloon forward and crowd into the anterior chamber angle; and (2) anterior insertion of the iris to the ciliary body (plateau iris) results in so little space between the trabecular meshwork and iris that dilation of the pupil squeezes the iris against the trabecular meshwork. The central anterior chamber may be deep, although the periphery is shallow.

Patients who have a central anterior chamber depth that measures 2.5 mm or less are likely candidates for the development of angle-closure glaucoma. The shallow anterior chamber may be recognized by the decreased distance between the posterior surface of the cornea and the anterior surface of the iris. Patients with such an anatomic condition may be without symptoms for many years, and it may be impossible to provoke an increase in intraocular pressure. With aging and the gradual increase of the size of the lens, the margin of safety decreases, and such patients may have attacks of increased intraocular pressure. Many patients with a shallow anterior chamber never develop a rapid increase in intraocular pressure. Such eyes, however, must be observed carefully to avoid an acute angle-closure episode. Patients should be warned, particularly concerning blurred and hazy vision that may be combined with rainbows (halos) around lights and pain. Some patients without symptoms have intermittent angle closure that causes progressive peripheral anterior synechiae, which causes a chronic angle-closure glaucoma.

Provocative testing.—Provocative testing seeks to determine under controlled conditions whether an abnormal increase in ocular tension occurs in combination with closure of the anterior chamber angle. The tests may not increase the intraocular pressure even in eyes that have had previous attacks of angle-closure glaucoma or in eyes that are destined to have attacks. The sensitivity and the specificity of the tests have not been determined. Occasionally, eyes with open-angle glaucoma respond with increased pressure to provocative tests for angle-closure glaucoma.

In the dark-room prone test, the patient lies face down or sits with head forward (resting on the arms or hands) in a dark room. The pupil dilates in the dark. Gravity, in the face-down

TABLE 22-7.
Differential Diagnosis of Angle-Closure Glaucoma

	Angle-Closure Glaucoma	Acute Iritis	Acute Conjunctivitis
Pain	Severe, prostrating	Moderate to severe	Burning, itching
Injection	Ciliary type that is more intense near the corneoscleral limbus and fades toward fornices: not constricted with 1 : 1,000 epinephrine; vessels do not move with conjunctiva, are violet in color; individual vessels not distinguishable		Conjunctival type that is most intense in fornices and fades toward corneoscleral limbus: eye whitened with 1 : 1,000 epinephrine; vessels superficial, move with conjunctiva, are bright red; individual vessels evident
Pupil	Semidilated; does not react to light	Miotic; reaction delayed or absent	Normal
Cornea	Steamy; iris details not visible	Usually clear with deposits on posterior surface sometimes visible	Clear and normal
Secretion	Watery	Watery	Stringy pus
Onset	Sudden	Gradual	Gradual
Vision	Markedly reduced	Slightly reduced	Normal
Intraocular pressure	Increased	Normal or soft unless secondary glaucoma	Normal

position, shifts the iris-lens diaphragm toward the cornea, closes the angle, and increases the intraocular pressure in individuals susceptible to angle-closure attacks. The patient must not sleep, which constricts the pupil. A positive test is an increase of the ocular tension of 10 mm Hg or more combined with gonioscopic observation of closure of the anterior chamber angle.

Dilation of the pupils for ophthalmoscopy may precipitate an attack of angle-closure glaucoma in susceptible eyes. The examiner must be assured that the pupils of individuals with shallow anterior chambers have returned to normal size after examination of the fundi. Usually the instillation of a miotic after examination prevents attacks.

ACUTE ANGLE-CLOSURE GLAUCOMA

Acute angle-closure glaucoma is often preceded by attacks of markedly increased intraocular pressure, which spontaneously resolve, often with sleep. Initially there is blurred, iridescent vision; spontaneous relief does not occur, the intraocular pressure continues to increase, and the symptoms become more severe. A ciliary type of injection (Table 22-7) is present, and there may be profuse lacrimation. Epithelial corneal edema is marked, and epithelial bullae form, giving the cornea a steamy appearance. The blood-aqueous barrier breaks down, and there is increased protein in the aqueous humor. The blood vessels of the iris stroma are dilated, and the pupil is in mid-dilation and does not react to light. Severe systemic symptoms include nausea, vomiting, and malaise. The symptoms may be aggravated by systemic absorption of eyedrops used in the treatment of the acute angle-closure attack.

If the attack persists, peripheral anterior synechiae (adhesions) form between the root of the iris and the cornea (Fig 22-10). After several days, these synechiae almost entirely destroy the drainage meshwork. Adhesions (posterior synechiae) form between the iris and the lens, and if the attack is not relieved, necrosis of the sphincter pupillae muscle results in a permanently semidilated pupil. Fluid vesicles form in the anterior subcapsular region of the lens and may persist as white flecks (glaucoma flecks). When present they indicate a previous attack of an

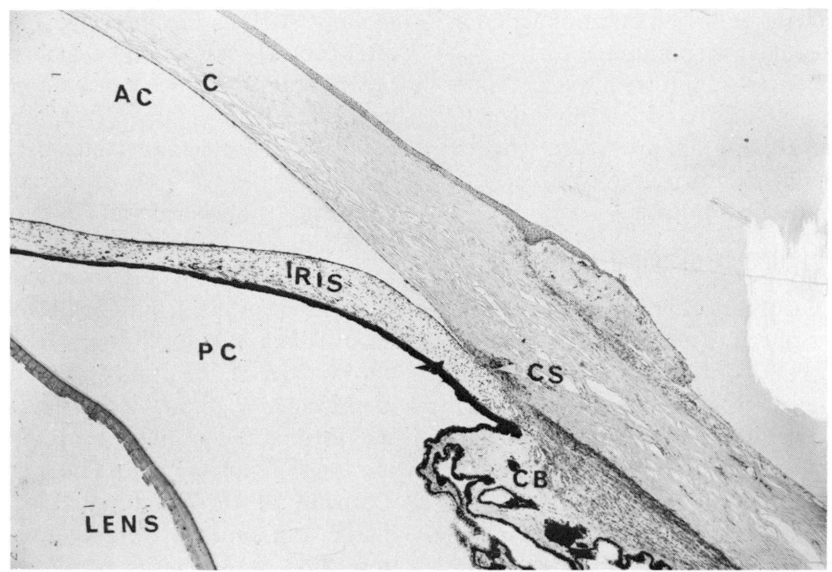

FIG 22-10.
Angle-closure glaucoma with anterior synechiae excluding the anterior chamber angle, *AC,* from the trabecular area and the canal of Schlemm, *CS.* The posterior chamber, *PC,* is larger than normal. *C,* Cornea. *CB,* Ciliary body. (Hematoxylin and eosin; ×38.)

acute increase in intraocular pressure. If the condition is untreated, vision progressively deteriorates and a blind, painful eye develops. Optic atrophy with pallor of the nerve occurs relatively early, but excavation occurs late in angle-closure glaucoma.

CHRONIC PRIMARY ANGLE-CLOSURE GLAUCOMA

This is a type of glaucoma in which the patient never has a severe acute congestive attack but has intermittent periods of partial closure of the anterior chamber angle and increased intraocular pressure. Symptoms may be absent, or there may be periodic subacute episodes of mild congestion and iridescent vision. Beginning superiorly, the iris gradually occludes the trabecular meshwork. Eventually the pressure is at a level of 40 mm Hg or more. The presence of peripheral anterior synechiae distinguishes the condition from open-angle glaucoma. A peripheral iridotomy may cure the condition if more than one quadrant of the angle is free of anterior peripheral synechiae. If the angle remains occluded, a filtering operation is indicated.

Diagnosis.—An angle-closure glaucoma is characterized by abnormally increased intraocular pressure and a closed angle demonstrated by gonioscopy. Acute iritis and acute conjunctivitis are disorders to be differentiated.

ANGLE-CLOSURE GLAUCOMA: MEDICAL TREATMENT

Angle-closure glaucoma is treated surgically by creating an additional opening in the iris so that aqueous humor may flow unimpeded from the posterior and anterior chamber.

An acute attack requires that the intraocular pressure be brought to normal before surgery. The patient should not sleep and should remain in a brightly illuminated room in the supine (face-up) position. Hyperosmotic agents increase the plasma osmolarity and withdraw fluid from the eye through the uveal and retinal blood vessels. Glycerine (1.0 to 1.5 g/kg of body weight) in lemon juice is given orally. It has an onset of action in 20 to 30 minutes and a maximum effect in 45 to 120 minutes. A goniolens or cotton-tipped applicator is used to apply pressure for 30 seconds to the center of the anesthetized cornea. The anterior aqueous humor is displaced toward the peripheral anterior chamber, which may force aqueous humor through the closed angle.

Ocular tension is measured after 30 minutes. If it is still high, mannitol in a 10% or 20% solution (1.0 to 2.0 g/kg of body weight) is administered intravenously. It has an onset of action in 10 to 20 minutes and a maximal effect in 30 to 60 minutes. Intravenous mannitol always reduces the intraocular pressure. At the conclusion of the infusion, gonioscopy is done to learn whether the angle is open. Pilocarpine (2.0%) may be instilled to constrict the pupil.

ANGLE-CLOSURE GLAUCOMA: SURGICAL TREATMENT

The angle-closure mechanism may be eliminated by a peripheral iridotomy in which the accumulation of aqueous humor in the posterior chamber is prevented. The argon or the Nd:YAG laser is customarily used for this. The opening in the iris prevents the pressure in the posterior chamber from exceeding that of the anterior chamber and prevents pupillary block. Laser iridotomy is performed after control of the acute attack when signs of ocular congestion have disappeared.

In patients with shallow angles who have never had an attack of angle-closure glaucoma, an iridotomy probably ensures freedom from attack. Since the anatomic predisposition occurs in both eyes in primary angle-closure glaucoma, a laser iridotomy is made in both eyes even though one eye has been symptom-free. Prophylactic laser iridotomy is suggested for patients who have never developed an acute attack, in those who are distant from medical care, and in eyes with anterior peripheral synechiae indicating prior closure of the angle without symptoms.

A laser iridotomy may be performed with one of several different types of laser. Topical anesthesia is used. A contact lens with a small condensing lens to focus the beam on the iris is used. The iridotomy is made in the mid-iris on the nasal or temporal superior side. Techniques differ, depending on the type and energy of the laser.

SECONDARY ANGLE-CLOSURE GLAUCOMA

The secondary angle-closure glaucomas are those conditions in which contact of the iris with the peripheral cornea or the trabecular meshwork prevents the aqueous humor from draining from the eye (Table 22-8). They occur in an anterior form with contraction of membranes in neovascular glaucoma, trauma, aniridia, and endothelial syndromes. Posterior forms occur with pupillary block secondary to lens abnormalities such as intumescence, in subluxation, after cataract extraction because of iris-vitreous block, or with a block caused by an intraocular lens. They may occur without pupillary block in ciliary block (malignant glaucoma), with cysts of the ciliary body, in contracture of tissue in retrolental fibroplasia, and with persistent hyperplastic primary vitreous.

Neovascular glaucoma.—Neovascular glaucoma results from the development of a fibrovascular membrane over the anterior chamber surface of the trabecular meshwork. The membrane originates from new blood vessels that form at the pupillary margin and surface of the iris (rubeosis iridis). The location suggests diffusion of the vascular endothelial growth factor and other growth factors through the pupil from the posterior ocular segment. Common causes include central retinal vein occlusion (see Chapter 17) and diabetic retinopathy (see Chapter 27). Many other vascular, neoplastic, and inflammatory conditions may be responsible. The eye is often blind and painful.

TABLE 22-8.
Some Types of Secondary Angle-Closure Glaucoma

I. Abnormalities of anterior chamber angle
  A. Contracture of membranes in angle
    1. Rubeosis iridis
    2. Iridocorneal syndrome
    3. Posterior polymorphous corneal dystrophy
    4. Ocular contusion
      a. Uveal edema
      b. Intraocular hemorrhage
  B. Inflammatory membranes
  C. Closure of angle
    1. Ciliary block
    2. Malignant glaucoma
    3. Scleral buckle
    4. Intraocular tumor
    5. Retinal photocoagulation
II. Pupillary block
  A. Crystalline lens abnormalities
    1. Swollen (intumescent)
    2. Anterior dislocation
  B. Iris-vitreous
    1. After cataract extraction
  C. Iris-crystalline lens
    1. Complete posterior synechiae
III. Congenital abnormalities
  A. Aniridia
  B. Persistent hyperplastic primary vitreous
  C. Rieger anomaly
  D. Axenfeld anomaly

The initial sign is a faint aqueous flare caused by abnormal permeability of the iris vasculature. Small tufts of new blood vessels at the pupillary margin are followed by new blood vessels on the surface of the iris and trabecular meshwork. Contraction of a fibrous neovascular membrane causes adhesions (peripheral anterior synechiae) between the iris and trabecular meshwork. In time the entire angle is occluded. Treatment is difficult. The eyes are often blind from the causative disease. Photocoagulation of the retina may cause regression of new iris blood vessels. Topical instillation of 1% atropine and corticosteroids combined with a contact lens to protect the corneal epithelium may relieve pain in a blind eye. Cyclocryotherapy or Nd:YAG laser destruction of the ciliary epithelium may reduce the intraocular pressure and relieve pain. A retrobulbar injection of alcohol relieves pain for several months but often causes an unsightly ocular muscle palsy.

Malignant glaucoma.—Malignant glaucoma (ciliary block glaucoma) may occur after surgery for angle-closure glaucoma, after a filtering procedure for open-angle glaucoma, or cataract extraction in an individual with a narrow anterior chamber angle. Immediately, or within a year, the anterior chamber becomes shallow or obliterated, and the intraocular pressure is increased. Miotics aggravate the condition. Initial treatment consists of maximal dilation of the pupil by means of topical atropine and phenylephrine combined with systemic acetazolamide and intravenous mannitol infusion. Failure of medical therapy requires aspiration of vitreous humor from the anterior chamber and its replacement with air. If the anterior chamber remains flat after surgery, a partial anterior vitrectomy with an infusion-aspiration cutter may be curative. Fluid vitreous may be aspirated from the center of the eye.

Failure of the anterior chamber to reform after cataract or glaucoma procedures and other anterior segment surgery or after a penetrating injury of the eye is a serious complication because the root of the iris comes into contact with trabecular meshwork. If the condition persists, peripheral anterior synechiae form and a secondary glaucoma occurs that is particularly recalcitrant to treatment. The condition is far easier to prevent by careful closure of ocular wounds than it is to treat once it is established.

After injury or anterior segment surgery, particularly lens extraction complicated by faulty wound healing, there may be down-growth of conjunctival or corneal epithelium to cover the trabecular meshwork, iris, and ciliary processes and cause a severe glaucoma, often intractable to treatment.

Secondary angle-closure glaucoma caused by pupillary block occurs when the vitreous or an intraocular lens blocks the pupillary aperture after lens extraction in which the peripheral iridectomy is nonfunctional. Inflammatory adhesions of the iris to the lens or to the vitreous face in aphakia may also cause a pupillary block. Dislocation of the lens into the anterior chamber blocks the pupil and causes a similar secondary glaucoma.

DEVELOPMENTAL GLAUCOMAS

The developmental glaucomas are ocular disorders in which a primary or secondary abnormality in the trabecular meshwork results in increased intraocular pressure (Table 22-9). In primary congenital glaucoma (primary infantile

TABLE 22-9.
Anatomic Classification of Developmental (Congenital) Glaucoma

- Trabecular meshwork abnormalities (trabeculodysgenesis)
  - Flat iris insertion (most primary developmental glaucomas)
    - Anterior insertion
    - Posterior insertion
    - Mixed insertion
  - Concave iris insertion
- Iris abnormalities
  - Anterior stroma
    - Hypoplasia (primary developmental glaucoma, Axenfeld and Rieger anomalies)
    - Hyperplasia (Sturge-Weber syndrome)
  - Anomalous iris blood vessels
    - Superficial (usually with iris hypoplasia)
    - Persistent tunica vasculosa lentis
  - All iris layers
    - Holes, coloboma, aniridia
- Corneal abnormalities
  - Peripheral (mainly Axenfeld syndrome)
  - Midperipheral (usually Rieger syndrome)
  - Central (Peters syndrome, anterior staphyloma, anterior chamber cleavage syndrome)
  - Dimensions (microcornea, macrocornea)

Modified from Hoskins HD Jr, Shaffer RN, Hetherington J: Anatomical classification of the developmental glaucomas, *Arch Ophthalmol* 102:1331-1336, 1984.

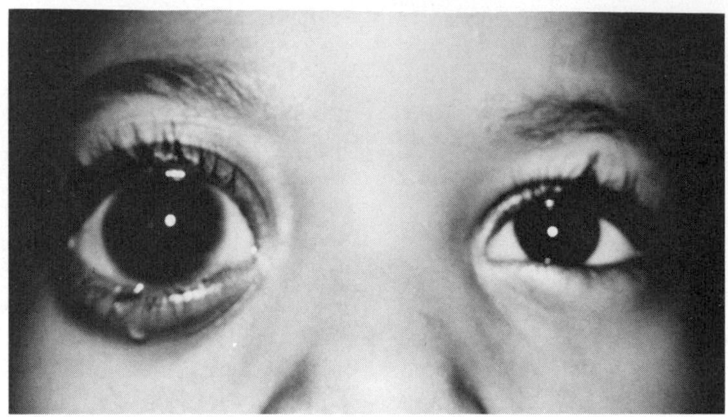

FIG 22-11.
Marked enlargement of the right eye of a 3-year-old girl with infantile glaucoma.

TABLE 22-10.
Glaucoma Associated with Congenital Anomalies

Aniridia
Broad-thumb syndrome
Chromosomal abnormalities
Homocystinuria
Lowe syndrome
Marfan syndrome
Maternal rubella
Microcornea
Neurofibromatosis
Pierre Robin syndrome
Persistent hyperplastic primary vitreous
Spherophakia
Sturge-Weber syndrome
Secondary glaucoma in infants
Retrolental fibroplasia
Tumors
Retinoblastoma
Juvenile xanthogranuloma
Inflammation
Trauma

Modified from Hoskins HD Jr, Shaffer RN, Hetherington J: Anatomical classification of the developmental glaucomas, *Arch Ophthalmol* 102:1331-1336, 1984.

glaucoma) the trabecular meshwork is abnormal and there are no associated ocular or systemic disorders that could cause an increase of the intraocular pressure. A secondary glaucoma in infants may follow uveitis, juvenile xanthogranuloma, retinoblastoma, trauma, persistent hyperplastic vitreous, and retrolental fibroplasia. Other developmental glaucomas are associated congenital structural disorders or abnormalities of the iris and cornea (Table 22-10).

Primary congenital glaucoma is not associated with other ocular or systemic malformations. A fundamental defect in the trabecular meshwork, often combined with insertion of the iris into the meshwork rather than into the scleral spur, leads to increased intraocular pressure. There is photophobia, lacrimation, and blepharospasm as the result of corneal edema. The edema causes a ground-glass opacification that obscures the pattern of the iris. The corneal diameter increases from 10.5 mm to 12 mm or more and the breaks in Descemet membrane appear as glasslike ridges on the posterior cornea. The anterior chamber is deeper than normal. There is an optic atrophy with excavation. Ocular tension may be roughly approximated by using topical anesthesia and a pneumotonometer. Accurate measurement requires general anesthesia with agents other than ketamine, halothane, or succinylcholine, which increase the intraocular pressure. Tension should be measured as soon as the patient is fully anesthetized. The readings may be inaccurate because of the pressure-lowering effect of the anesthetic.

If not treated adequately, the entire eye enlarges in a total staphyloma (Fig 22-11). There is severe optic atrophy with excavation of the optic disk.

Most cases of primary developmental glaucoma are sporadic, but approximately 10% reflect an autosomal recessive inheritance. A polygenic pattern is suggested, however, by the more frequent occurrence in boys (65%) than girls and a markedly variable penetrance in different families.

The preferred surgical treatment of congenital glaucoma is the goniotomy procedure, in which an incision is made into the region of the trabecular meshwork under direct visual control by using a goniolens. Trabeculotomy may be effective if goniotomies fail or cannot be performed because of a hazy cornea.

Patients must be carefully observed postoperatively to be certain the glaucoma is controlled. Intraocular pressure must be determined and the corneal diameters carefully measured with attention directed to breaks in the Descemet membrane. Successful treatment may reverse optic disk cupping. Repeated examinations are required to monitor the ocular tensions, vision, and refractive error.

BIBLIOGRAPHY

Books

Alward WLM: *Color atlas of gonioscopy,* London, 1994, Wolfe.

Drance SM: *Ocular update to glaucoma and drug treatment,* Amsterdam, NY, 1995, Kugler Publications.

Drance SM, editor: *Optic nerve in glaucoma,* Amsterdam, NY, 1995, Kugler Publications.

Higginbotham EJ, Lee DA, editors: *Management of difficult glaucoma,* Cambridge, Mass, 1994, Blackwell Scientific Publications.

Hodapp E, Parrish RK II, Anderson DR: *Clinical decisions in glaucoma,* St Louis, 1993, Mosby–Year Book.

Hoskins HD, Kass MA: *Becker-Shaffer's diagnosis and therapy of the glaucomas,* ed 6, St Louis, 1989, Mosby–Year Book.

Kaufman PL, Mittag TW: *Glaucoma,* St Louis, 1994, Mosby–Year Book.

Quigley HA: *Diagnosing early glaucoma with nerve fiber layer examination,* New York, 1996, Igaku-Shoin.

Ritch R, Shields MB, Krupin T, editors: *The glaucomas,* ed 2, St Louis, 1996, Mosby–Year Book.

Articles

Alm A, Widengard I, Kjellgren D, Soderstrom M, Fristrom B, Heijl A et al: Latanoprost administered once daily caused a maintained reduction of intraocular pressure in glaucoma patients treated concomitantly with timolol, *Br J Ophthalmol* 79:12-16, 1995.

Caprioli J: Clinical evaluation of the optic nerve in glaucoma, *Trans Am Ophthalmol Soc* 92:589-641, 1994.

Dreyer EB, Chaturvedi N, Zurakowski D: Effect of mitomycin C and fluorouracil-supplemented trabeculectomies on the anterior segment, *Arch Ophthalmol* 113:575-580, 1995.

Lee WR: The pathology of the outflow system in primary and secondary glaucoma, *Eye* 9:1-23, 1995.

23

OCULAR MOTILITY

Normal human eyes are spaced 50 to 65 mm apart and are anatomically located so as to be directed straight forward. Because of this horizontal separation the images differ slightly in each eye. The two slightly different images are superimposed (fused) in the brain, and an object is perceived as having height, width, and depth, a stereoscopic image. To be superimposed and perceived in three dimensions, the horizontal separation of the eyes must be neither too little nor too great. Each eye must be directed simultaneously to the same object. The image of each eye must have about the same degree of clarity and size, and have approximately the same refraction. The retinal axons from the nasal one half of each retina decussate at the chiasm, and each side of the brain must be functional.

To fuse these slightly different (disparate) images into one requires sensitive and intact sensory and motor mechanisms. The sensory mechanism provides the visual sensation of form, color, direction, and motion of the stimulus. It consists of the retina and its complicated connections in the brain combined with the muscles of the ciliary body and the iris that control the clarity and amount of light entering the eye. The 12 striated extraocular muscles maintain the direction of the two eyes on the same object. An abnormality in either the sensory or the motor system may lead to faulty vision, abnormal position of the eyes, or both.

TERMINOLOGY

The terms used to describe the relationships between vision and the position of the two eyes are complicated.

Phoria.—A phoria (Greek: movement, range) is the ocular condition in which an eye deviates from parallelism when fusion is interrupted. Orthophoria is the ideal condition in which the eyes are directed simultaneously to the same point of fixation at both near and distance when fusion is suspended.

Heterophoria.—Heterophoria is the condition in which the eyes are directed simultaneously to the same point of fixation at either near or far only when fusion is present. When fusion is interrupted, the eyes are not parallel.

Esophoria refers to the tendency to medial deviation of the eyes, which becomes evident when binocular vision (fusion) is prevented. Binocular vision is prevented when one eye is covered. The deviation is observed by the rotation made by the eye (recovery movement) when it is uncovered. Exophoria refers to lateral deviation when fusion is suspended; and hyperphoria refers to upward deviation. (The higher eye is described, and the term hypophoria is not used.)

Tropia.—A tropia (Greek: a turning) is the condition in which two eyes when open are not directed simultaneously to the same object. Esotropia refers to inward deviation of the nonfixing eye. Exotropia refers to outward deviation of the nonfixing eye. Hypertropia refers to upward deviation. (The higher rather than the lower eye is designated.) Cyclotropia refers to deviation (torsional) in which the upper end of the vertical corneal meridian deviates temporally (excyclotropia) or nasally (incyclotropia).

Esodeviation describes an inward turning of the eyes, which may be either an esotropia or an esophoria. If one eye deviates inward when both eyes are open (and fusion is thus possible) an esotropia is present. If the eyes are straight when both are open but one eye turns inward when covered (and fusion is thus interrupted) an esophoria is present. Exodeviation describes an outward turning of the eyes, which may be an exotropia or an exophoria. If one eye deviates outward when both eyes are open (and fusion is thus possible) an exotropia is present. If the eyes are straight when both are open and one eye turns outward when covered (and fusion is thus interrupted) an exophoria is present.

Strabismus, heterotropia.—Strabismus or heterotropia (squint, crosseyes, walleye) is the condition in which both eyes are not directed to the same object at either near or far, or both, despite both eyes being open and uncovered so that fusion is possible. Strabismus may be divided into (1) paralytic (nonconcomitant), in which one or more muscles are weakened so that their normal action is impaired by mechanical factors or faulty nervous connections; and (2) nonparalytic (concomitant), in which the ocular muscles and their innervation are normal. Secondary overaction or underaction of individual muscles in nonparalytic strabismus may simulate a paralytic strabismus.

Strabismus is termed intermittent or periodic if there are periods when the eyes are parallel. It is termed constant if the eyes are never parallel. Strabismus is monocular if the same eye always deviates and the fellow eye always fixates. It is alternate when either eye deviates while the fellow eye fixates. An accommodative strabismus is one in which the degree of crossing varies with the amount of accommodation. A sensory strabismus is one in which an impaired image causes the deviation.

Concomitance.—Concomitance refers to equal deviation in all directions of gaze. A nonconcomitant deviation is one in which the deviation varies in different directions of gaze. Nonparalytic strabismus is initially a concomitant strabismus, but it may become nonconcomitant because of secondary contracture, overactions, and inhibitions of ocular muscles. At the time of onset, paralytic strabismus is always nonconcomitant but may eventually become concomitant and make it difficult to determine which muscle is weakened.

Duction movements.—Duction movements describe the rotation of one eye: adduction (rotation nasally), abduction (rotation toward the temple), sursumduction (elevation), deorsumduction (depression), excycloduction (rotation of upper pole of cornea toward the temple), and incycloduction (rotation of upper pole of cornea nasally). Rotations in an oblique direction, such as up and in or down and out, are combinations of horizontal and vertical rotations. Duction movements are usually observed by covering one eye and directing attention to the uncovered eye.

Additional terms are defined at the end of this chapter.

DIAGNOSTIC MEASURES

The different tests to measure visual acuity, ocular movements, binocular function, and possible ocular deviation may be confusing. Their apparent complexity may lead to the erroneous conclusion that diagnosis and management of a strabismus are so difficult that treatment should be delayed until a patient is old enough to cooperate with subjective testing. This delay may result in poor vision from strabismic amblyopia or other sensory abnormalities. Examination and treatment are indicated in any infant whose eyes are not aligned at all times during waking hours after 6 months of age. Diagnostic measures emphasize two major areas: (1) the ocular deviation and (2) the visual (sensory) status.

For the first 6 months after birth, the eyes of all infants deviate at times. Most of the time the eyes are straight and remain so after 6 months of age.

If one eye deviates constantly during the first several months of life, the fundi must be examined after pupillary dilation (0.5% cyclopentolate, 1% phenylephrine). The examination is easily accomplished by means of an indirect ophthalmoscope. If there is no ocular obstacle to distinct image formation, such as cataract, hereditary macular degeneration, retinoblastoma, or chorioretinitis, attention is directed to preventing amblyopia (see discussion on amblyopia

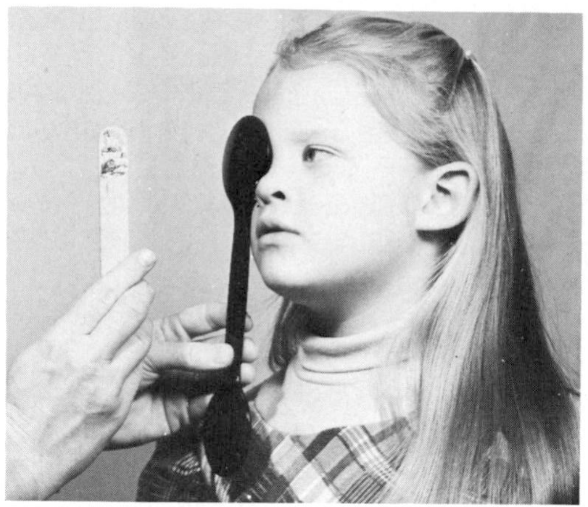

FIG 23-1.
The cover-uncover test with an accommodative target. The individual fixes on details on the target, and the eye is covered for a few seconds and then uncovered. The test should be performed for near and distance fixation and with and without corrective lenses.

later in this chapter). If the infant uses either eye (alternates), there is no primary ocular abnormality or both eyes are affected equally.

A strabismus that develops after the eyes have been parallel suggests either an accommodative strabismus or development of some obstacle to normal vision in the eye. The younger the infant, the more likely there is some obstacle to vision. Ophthalmoscopy and refraction are indicated. By the time an infant is 4 to 6 months old, a meaningful, complete eye examination is possible.

Corneal reflection test.—The deviation may be estimated by observing the reflection of light from the cornea of the deviating eye. The cornea has a radius of approximately 5.5 mm, and each millimeter of displacement of the reflection is equal to about 7° or 15 prism diopters of deviation of the visual axes. Thus, if the reflection from the deviating eye is at the corneoscleral limbus, the deviation is about 38.5° (5.5×7).

The test is more accurately performed by having the patient fixate on a small light with the examiner observing the deviating eye. Prisms are then placed in front of the fixating eye until the light reflection is centered in the deviated eye (Krimsky test).

Cover-uncover test.—The presence or absence of an ocular deviation is determined by the cover-uncover test (Fig 23-1). First, the examiner observes the patient and determines whether or not one eye is preferred for fixation. The patient's attention is then directed to a fixation target. In infants this may be a light or a moving toy. After the age of 3 or 4 years a small picture or letters may be used to stimulate accommodation and convergence. Test objects for both near and far measurements should be used. The eye that appears to be fixing is covered for a few seconds with the palm of one's hand or some other occluder. As the eye is covered, attention is directed to the uncovered eye (Fig 23-2). If there is no movement, binocular fixation was present before covering. If the uncovered eye moves to fix, a latent deviation was present before the fellow eye was covered. Attention is then directed to the covered eye as it is uncovered. If the eye moves to fixate (fusional movement) and the previously uncovered eye does not move, heterophoria is present. If there is no movement of either eye and the eye that was covered is deviated, an alternating strabismus is present. If the eye that was covered assumes fixation and the fellow eye deviates, a nonalternating monocular heterotropia is present, and the eye that was covered is preferred for fixation.

This test is of more than theoretic importance. If either heterophoria or orthophoria is present, the patient has fusion. If heterotropia is present, the individual is either seeing double or suppressing the image from one eye.

Prism and cover test (alternate cover test).—If the cover-uncover test indicates that either a heterophoria or a heterotropia is present, the prism and cover test is used to measure the amount of deviation. While the patient maintains fixation, one eye is covered and then uncovered as the fellow eye is immediately covered. Attention is directed to the movement made by the covered eye as it is uncovered. If the eye has been turned inward while under the cover and moves outward to fix when it is uncovered, either an esophoria or an esotropia is present. If the eye has been turned outward under the cover and moves inward when the cover is removed, an exophoria or an exotropia is present.

Prisms of increasing strength are then placed in front of one eye until the eyes do not move when one is covered and the fellow eye maintains fixation. The movement is neutralized because the prisms move the image of the fixation object onto the foveola. After the age of

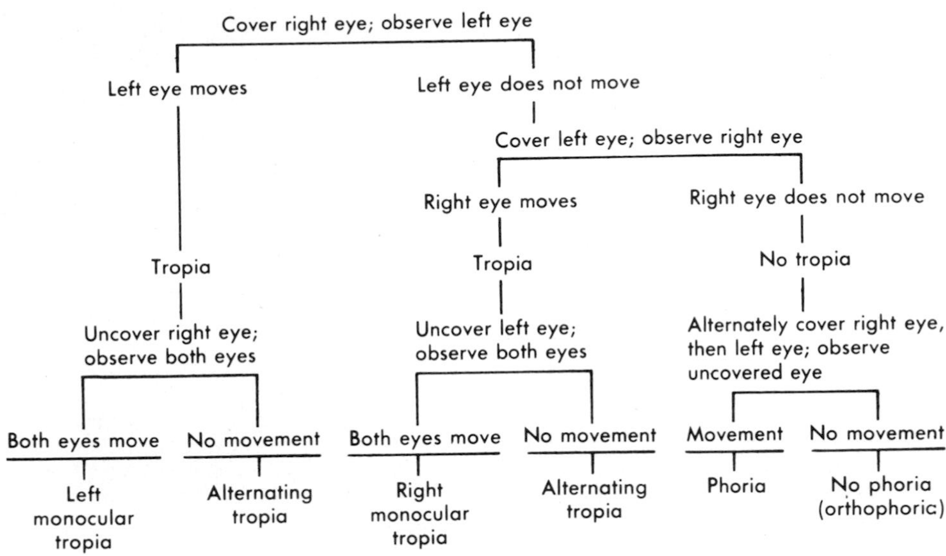

FIG 23-2.
Diagnosis of phorias and tropias by using the cover-uncover test.

3 years, to ensure maximal accommodation, small pictures or letters are used for near fixation and the 20/30 line is used for distance fixation. The test is carried out with the patient wearing corrective lenses and without correction at near and far.

TREATMENT OF STRABISMUS

The treatment of strabismus is directed toward (1) determining the type of deviation; (2) determining the cause of the deviation; (3) the development of normal vision; and (4) the alignment of the visual axes.

Determining the type of deviation.—The initial examination tells whether the extraocular movements are normal or whether there is one or more paretic or underacting ocular muscle. The direction of any deviation is learned by the corneal reflection test, the cover-uncover test, and the prism and cover test.

Determining the cause of the deviation.—Normal newborn infants have parallel eyes most of the time but have occasional episodes of gross misalignment of the eyes. The initial medical examination of a newborn should indicate that the orbits are normal, the eyes are directed straight ahead, and that the cornea, iris, and pupil are normal.

By the age of 6 months the eyes should be parallel at all times. Normal eyes should move fully, the corneal reflection and cover-uncover tests should indicate parallelism, and the pupils should be black and constrict to light. A complete examination including pupillary dilation is indicated if the eyes are not normal. There should be no delay to await a time when the infant can cooperate with vision testing.

Most deviations in infancy are severe inward deviations that are initially alternating but quickly become monocular. Examination must exclude a marked difference in refraction (anisometropia) as the cause. Examination with the indirect ophthalmoscope will exclude cataract, macular abnormalities, and retinoblastoma as a cause. Early surgery to correct the deviation and measures to prevent strabismic amblyopia (which see) are customary.

Accommodative esotropias usually develop after the age of 2 years in a child who has had previously straight eyes. Particular attention must always be directed to exclusion of a paretic muscle caused by intracranial disease. Rarely a paresis of a lateral rectus muscle occurs and then disappears spontaneously. Often correcting lenses are prescribed if an accommodative esotropia cannot be distinguished from a combined accommodative-nonaccommodative type. If eyes have been parallel until the age of 3 years, there is less likelihood of amblyopia and other visual abnormalities.

Development of normal vision.—Normal development of stereoscopic vision requires binocular, simultaneous use of each foveola during a critical time that occurs early in life. In infants

TABLE 23-1.
Causes of Amblyopia

Causes
Strabismus
Esotropia
Exotropia (rare)
Hypertropia (rare)
Anisometropia
Hypermetropia
Myopia
Astigmatism (rare)
Aniseikonia (rare)
Visual deprivation
Unilateral
Cataract (monocular)
Blepharoptosis
Opaque cornea
Hyphema
Vitreous cloudy
Prolonged patching (nonsupervised)
Prolonged atropine eyedrops
Bilateral
Cataract
Nystagmus

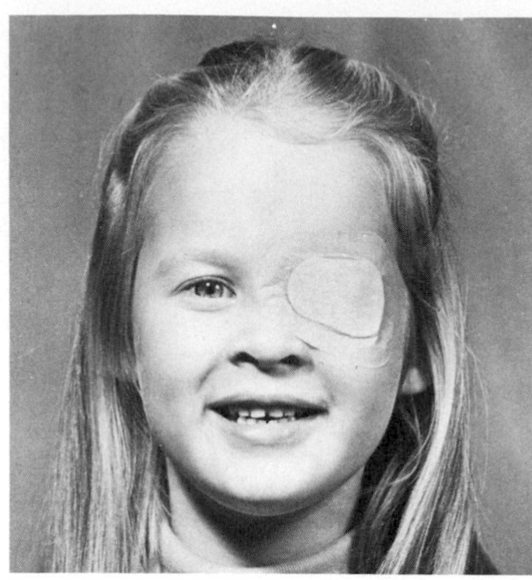

FIG 23-3.
Occlusion of the better eye to force use of the poorer eye in strabismic amblyopia.

with monocular cataracts this time occurs before 3 months of age.

In the experimental animal, unilateral deprivation of vision for 2 weeks during the first 12 weeks of life causes severe structural changes in the visual system that are particularly evident anatomically in the lateral geniculate body. Visual acuity is reduced in the deprived eye. The cell layers of the lateral geniculate bodies innervated by the deprived eye are up to 30% smaller than those in the adjacent layers from the nondeprived eye. Binocularly driven cells are absent in the visual cortex, which derives 90% of its input from the nondeprived eye. The decreased input from the deprived eye is caused by synaptic inhibition in the occipital cortex.

Amblyopia.—Amblyopia is a condition in which a unilateral or bilateral decrease in form vision (visual acuity) occurs that is not fully attributable to organic ocular abnormalities. It is caused (Table 23-1) by deprivation of form vision, abnormal binocular interaction, or both, during visual immaturity (birth to 6 years of age). It may be reversed in some individuals by therapeutic measures. The decreased visual acuity impairs pursuit (following) movement when the amblyopic eye is used for fixation. The visual acuity of the amblyopic eye is better when test letters are viewed singly rather than in a series. In decreased illumination the visual acuity of an amblyopic eye is unchanged, whereas an eye with reduced visual acuity caused by an organic disease may show a marked decrease.

The diagnosis of amblyopia in infants and extremely young children is difficult. Measurement of the preference for fixation of the habitually fixating eye as compared with the habitually deviating eye is helpful. The habitually fixating eye is covered and then uncovered. If it immediately resumes fixation, amblyopia is probably present in the fellow eye. If the normally deviating eye maintains fixation through the next blink of the eyelids, amblyopia is unlikely. An infant may also object when the eye with better vision is covered.

The correction of amblyopia depends on the maturity of the visual system at the onset and the duration of the abnormal visual experience. Treatment is by occlusion of the better eye (Fig 23-3) to force use of the poorer eye. Because of the sensitivity of the visual system in infants to deprivation during the first year of life, patching should follow a pattern of 3 days for the sound eye and 1 day for the amblyopic eye. Between 1 and 3 years of age, the sound eye may be patched 4 days and the amblyopic eye 1 day. Since the previously amblyopic eye may become the better eye and the patching may induce amblyopia in the covered eye, patients must be examined at least once every 2 weeks. After 3 years of age, the patching period may be extended if visual acuity is measured frequently. Patching is carried out until there is no further improvement in visual acuity for 3 months. If visual acuity decreases after patching is terminated, patching should be reinstituted until the visual improvement is sustained. Often this requires intermittent occlusion until the patient is 9 or 10 years of age.

Instillation of atropine solution eyedrops for an extended period or prolonged patching of one eye for a disease or injury should be avoided in children and infants under 5 years of age. If instillation of atropine eyedrops in one eye is essential, the eyedrops should also be instilled in the sound eye to avoid a sensory imbalance. Amblyopia induced by occlusion of the sound eye during visual immaturity is reversible, but prolonged occlusion may induce a permanent iatrogenic amblyopia.

Orthoptic treatment provides binocular vision through correction of suppression, amblyopia, and anomalous retinal correspondence and enhances the development of fusional amplitudes and stereopsis. Orthoptists participate in the diagnosis and nonsurgical correction of sensory and motor anomalies of the eyes under the direction of a practitioner. In the United States they are college-trained individuals who have specialized in orthoptics in a university eye department and have been certified by the American Orthoptic Council.

Eye exercises to correct an esotropia or esotropia are of no value. When convergence is insufficient, fusion exercises with base-out prisms of increasing power will improve the ability to converge and relieve symptoms.

Correction of alignment.—Surgery is indicated to align the visual axes and thus permit the potential for binocular vision, and to improve appearance. In general, overacting muscles are weakened and underacting muscles are strengthened.

When vision is equal in the two eyes, it is desirable to perform symmetric surgery, normally carrying out the same surgical procedure on both eyes rather than limiting the surgical correction to one eye. Usually, the better the fusion, the less surgery is required to achieve a cosmetic and functional result.

In esotropia, in which vision is approximately equal in the two eyes and in which retinal correspondence is normal, bilateral recessions of the medical recti muscles are usually preferred. In congenital esotropia with marked deviation, this is usually done at about 6 months of age.

In older patients with concomitant esotropia in which vision in one eye is poor and cannot be improved, the best results are probably achieved by resecting the lateral rectus muscle and recessing the medial rectus muscle in the amblyopic eye. If this is not adequate to align the eyes, a similar procedure may be carried out in the fellow eye.

In alternating exotropia, each lateral rectus muscle is recessed if the divergence is mainly for distance and the eyes are parallel for near, provided vision and fusion are good. If the exotropia is monocular, the deviation is the same for near and far, and fusion is poor, the initial procedure is recession of the lateral rectus muscle and resection of the medial rectus muscle in one eye.

The surgeon's aim is to perform the minimal procedure that will correct the strabismus. Some patients require several procedures, which commonly occurs because correction of a horizontal or vertical deviation uncovers anomalies that could not be diagnosed earlier. Usually at least 6 months should elapse between procedures to permit the correction to stabilize.

PARALYTIC STRABISMUS

The motor nerves to the eye may be affected in a variety of abnormalities caused by trauma, hemorrhage, cerebral edema, ischemia, inflammation, neoplasm, aneurysms, or demyelination. Impairment of a motor nerve or its nucleus results in a failure of the eye to move in the field of action of the muscle or muscles it innervates. A strabismus is present and, if binocular vision is developed, there is a diplopia.

Inability to move both eyes in the same direction (right or left, up or down) is a gaze palsy. The eyes remain parallel and there is no double vision. Sometimes a gaze palsy and isolated ocular muscle palsy occur simultaneously.

Structural anomalies of an ocular muscle, conjunctiva, or Tenon capsule may cause contracture of a muscle or prevent its antagonist from rotating the eye. The signs are those of paralysis of the normal antagonist. Thus, in thyroid myopathy, fibrosis and contracture of

TABLE 23-2.
Head Position with Paralysis of an Individual Extraocular Muscle

Muscle	Face Turn		Chin		Heat Tilt	
	Normal Side	Side of Paralyzed Muscle	Up	Down	Normal Side	Side of Paralyzed Muscle
Medial rectus		✓				
Lateral rectus		✓				
Superior rectus		✓	✓			✓
Inferior rectus		✓		✓		✓
Superior oblique	✓			✓	✓	
Inferior oblique	✓		✓			✓

muscles that insert on the inferior surface of the eye prevent upward rotation. In blowout fractures of the orbit, the tissues in the inferior portion of the orbit may be trapped in the floor of the orbit and the eye cannot rotate upward.

The forced duction test is necessary to diagnose a physical restriction of ocular rotation. In the forced duction test, the conjunctiva is anesthetized with a topical anesthetic reinforced by 4% cocaine solution on a cotton pledget applied to the conjunctiva near the corneoscleral limbus. This conjunctiva is then grasped with toothless forceps, and the eye is passively rotated to determine its freedom of movement. Children may require general anesthesia.

An abnormally short superior oblique muscle tendon or contracture of the muscle after injury makes the inferior oblique muscle on the same side appear paralyzed because the eye cannot be elevated in adduction. The forced duction test indicates the contracture of the superior oblique muscle.

A paralytic strabismus is a misalignment of the visual axes that results from paresis (weakness), paralysis, or restriction of one or more extraocular muscles. When the eye with normal extraocular muscles is used to fixate, the affected fellow eye is in the position of primary deviation. When the affected eye is used to fixate, the normal fellow eye is in the position of secondary deviation. The secondary deviation (affected eye fixating) is greater than the primary deviation because the affected eye with faulty motor innervation or muscles requires an excessive innervational impulse to maintain fixation. The excessive innervational impulse is distributed to the normal muscles of the fellow eye (Hering's law of equal innervation) and causes an overaction.

In general, paralytic strabismus in an adult with previously single binocular vision causes double vision (diplopia), which is most marked when the eyes are rotated into the field of action of the affected muscle. Diplopia does not occur in individuals who have never developed stereoscopic vision.

To neutralize diplopia, the face may be turned, the chin elevated or depressed, and the head tilted toward the right or left shoulder (ocular torticollis) (Table 23-2). In paralysis of the medial rectus muscle or the lateral rectus muscle, the face is turned toward the field of action of the abnormal muscle. The head is not tilted, nor is the chin elevated or depressed. Thus with either the right medial rectus muscle or the left lateral rectus muscle, the face is turned toward the left side. In this position, fixation is maintained without contraction of either the right medial rectus muscle or the left lateral rectus muscle.

In paralysis of either the inferior oblique muscle or the superior oblique muscle, the face is turned slightly toward the opposite (normal) side. In paralysis of all of the ocular recti muscles, the face is turned to the side of the affected muscle.

The chin is elevated or depressed in the direction of action of the vertical ocular muscles. Thus, the chin is elevated in underactions of the superior rectus muscle and inferior oblique muscle and depressed when the inferior rectus muscle and the superior oblique muscle are affected.

The head is tilted toward the side of the affected muscle in paralysis of all of the vertical muscles except the superior oblique muscle. The head is tilted toward the normal side in paralysis of the superior oblique muscle.

A superior oblique muscle paralysis is detected by tilting the head toward the side of the paralyzed muscle, which causes the eye to rotate upward. The superior rectus muscle and the superior oblique muscle are both intorters of the eye. When the head is tilted toward the normal side, an equal innervational impulse is transmitted to both muscles. The eye rotates upward because of the action of the superior rectus muscle.

The diagnosis of the specific muscle involvement in a paralytic strabismus may be difficult. The history may indicate the cause to be injury, inflammation, tumor, aneurysm, or thyroid oculopathy. The onset of multiple sclerosis may be associated with muscle palsy. Myasthenia gravis may be limited to ocular muscles.

Oculomotor nerve.—Complete paralysis of the oculomotor nerve (N III) causes a blepharoptosis of the upper eyelid (levator palpebrae superioris) and paralysis of the medial rectus, superior rectus, inferior rectus, and inferior oblique muscles (external ophthalmoplegia). The pupil is dilated (mydriasis) and does not constrict to light or convergence, and there is loss of accommodation (cycloplegia). Mydriasis and cycloplegia constitute an internal ophthalmoplegia. When the unimpaired fellow eye fixes, the paralyzed eye rotates outward and downward because of the intact action of the lateral rectus muscle (N VI) and the superior oblique muscle (N IV) (see Chapter 1).

Oculomotor nerve paralysis caused by an aneurysm or neoplasm often involves the pupil as well as ocular muscles (total ophthalmoplegia). When oculomotor paralysis is caused by a medical condition such as diabetic neuropathy, the pupil is often (75%) spared. The pupil and the ciliary muscle are usually not affected in lesions in the oculomotor nerve nucleus. Ophthalmoplegia caused by a lesion in the brain stem is often associated with lesions of other cranial nerves.

Involvement of the fibers of the oculomotor nerve as they pass through the red nucleus causes Benedikt syndrome, in which there is homolateral oculomotor paralysis, contralateral dyskinesia, and an intention tremor of the opposite arm only. There may be an associated contralateral hemianesthesia.

Interruption of oculomotor nerve (N III) axons near the ventral surface of the brain in the cerebral peduncle results in homolateral N III paralysis, contralateral hemiplegia, and paralysis of the tongue and the muscles of the lower face (Weber syndrome). Interruption of the oculomotor nerve in the cavernous sinus is likely to be associated with interruption of the trochlear (N IV) and abducent (N VI) nerves.

The peripheral oculomotor nerve is likely to be involved in aneurysms of the circle of Willis, tumors of the base of the brain, meningeal carcinomatosis, and chronic meningitis caused by herpes zoster, syphilis, or tuberculosis. The nerve is usually spared in purulent meningitis, which is more likely to involve the abducent (N VI) nerve. All motor nerves to the eye are involved in cavernous sinus thrombosis, and the motor involvement is likely to precede pupillary involvement.

The syndrome of the superior orbital fissure involves all motor and sensory nerves of the eye and the sympathetic nerves. It may be produced by suppuration in the sphenoidal sinus, skull fracture, hemorrhage, or tumor. The innervation of both the sphincter and dilator muscles of the pupil is affected and pupillary dilation does not occur.

Aberrant regeneration of nerve fibers after paralysis of the oculomotor nerve may cause a variety of abnormalities. The pseudo–von Graefe abnormality follows interruption of the nerve fibers originally distributed to the inferior rectus muscle regenerating into the levator palpebrae superioris muscle. On attempts to look downward the eye does not rotate downward, but the upper eyelid retracts. Aberrant regeneration of the superior branch of the oculomotor nerve to the superior rectus muscle into the levator palpebrae muscle causes the upper eyelid to retract on attempts to rotate the eye upward. In sleep the upper eyelid is elevated, and the normal Bell phenomenon does not rotate the eye upward. Aberrant regeneration of the branch to the medial rectus muscle into the innervation of the sphincter pupillae muscle causes the pupil to constrict on attempts to adduct the eye.

Trochlear nerve.—Disorders of the trochlear nerve (N IV) affect the superior oblique muscle, which rotates the eye downward when it is adducted. Diplopia is particularly marked in reading. The affected eye is higher than the sound eye; the head is tilted to the sound side, the face is rotated to the sound side, and the chin is depressed. The head in this position is moved to the field of action of the muscle to minimize double vision. When the head is tilted to the affected side, the affected eye moves higher. (The superior rectus muscle and the superior oblique muscle are intorters of the eye and rotate the 12 o'clock meridian of the cornea inward.) When the head is tilted to the affected side, each muscle is stimulated equally to intort the eye. The superior oblique muscle is paralyzed; the unaffected superior rectus muscle then elevates the affected eye.

After superior oblique muscle paralysis, there may be early secondary contracture of the inferior oblique muscle. This results in a hypertropia in upward gaze that is greater than that in downward gaze.

Abducent nerve.—Disorders of the abducent nerve (N VI) or the lateral rectus muscle, which it innervates, prevent rotation of the eye laterally beyond the midline. The unopposed action of the medial rectus muscle results in a paralytic esotropia. On attempts to abduct the eye, the palpebral fissure may widen. The long intracranial course of the abducent nerve and its angulation over the sphenoid bone make it vulnerable in increased intracranial pressure, purulent meningitis, and skull fracture.

The Gradenigo syndrome is caused by an osteitis of the petrous tip of the pyramidal bone and follows mastoid and middle ear infections on the homolateral side. It is associated with sixth cranial nerve paralysis, deafness, and pain on the same side of the face from fifth cranial nerve inflammation. Acoustic neuromas (neurofibromatosis) are associated with deafness, sixth cranial nerve paralysis, facial paralysis caused by seventh cranial nerve involvement, and papilledema.

Internuclear ophthalmoplegia.—When the paramedian pontine reticular system commands the eyes to turn to the right or left, the ipsilateral abducent nucleus is stimulated and the stimulus passes via the medial longitudinal fasciculus to the contralateral medial rectus muscle subnucleus of the oculomotor nucleus (Fig 23-4). Disruption of the medial longitudinal fasciculus disconnects the oculomotor subnucleus that innervates the medial rectus muscle from the abducent nucleus. Then on horizontal gaze to the right or left, the abducting eye (ipsilateral lateral rectus muscle) rotates laterally but may demonstrate a coarse jerk nystagmus. The adducting eye (contralateral medial rectus muscle) remains in the primary position since a signal through the medial longitudinal fasciculus does not reach its nucleus. Convergence, which is not mediated by impulses through the medial longitudinal fasciculus, may or may not be affected. In early internuclear ophthalmoplegia, adduction may be slowed and there is an exodeviation in lateral gaze to the side of the lesions and orthophoria in primary gaze.

Bilateral internuclear ophthalmoplegia in young adults is most commonly caused by multiple sclerosis. In older individuals, occlusive vascular disease is most common. It also occurs with brain stem tumors, syphilis, encephalitis, and trauma and may be stimulated by myasthenia gravis. Unilateral internuclear ophthalmoplegia is the result of an infarct of a small branch of the basilar artery. Internuclear ophthalmoplegia involves conjugate horizontal gaze only.

The retraction syndrome.—The retraction syndrome of Stilling, Türk, and Duane is secondary to the absence of the abducent nucleus and nerve (N VI) that normally innervates the lateral rectus muscle. The muscle is innervated instead by the inferior division of the oculomotor nerve (N III) that also innervates the medial rectus, inferior rectus, and inferior oblique muscles. In the most common type, on attempts to adduct the eyes, both lateral recti muscles contract as do the medial recti muscles.

The eyes retract into the orbits and the palpebral fissures narrow (pseudoptosis). There may be an esotropia with a head turn and an upshoot or downshoot of the eye on adduction. On attempts to abduct the eyes, the palpebral fissure widens but the eye does not rotate outward. Women are more frequently affected (60%) than men. The left eye is affected (75%) more commonly than the right eye, and the condition is bilateral in 20% of the patients. Other ocular abnormalities include cataract, iris and pupil anomalies, persistent hyaloid artery, amblyopia, and choroidal colobomas. Labyrinthine deafness, facial defects, cleft palate, and

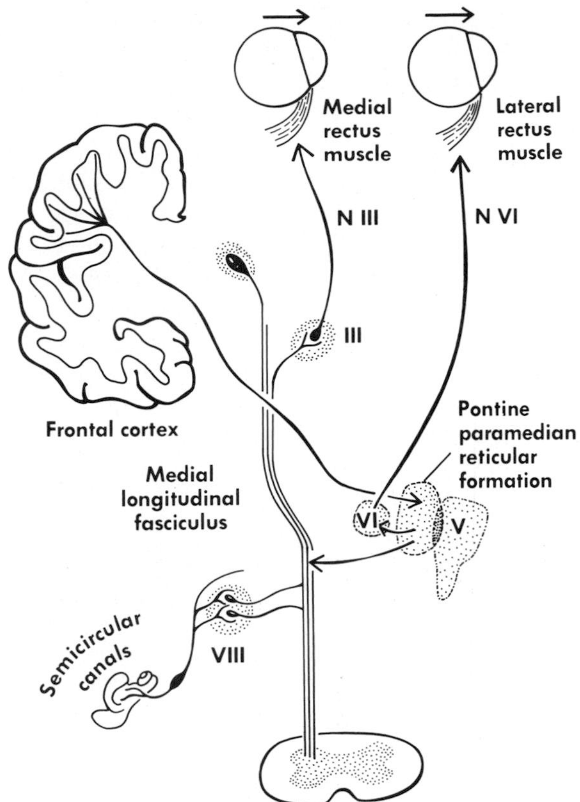

FIG 23-4.

The medial longitudinal fasciculus connects the pontine paramedian reticular formation with the subnucleus of the contralateral oculomotor nerve *(N III)* that serves the medial rectus muscle. On conjugate horizontal gaze to the right, impulses originate in the left frontal optomotor cortex. They decussate in the region of the internal capsule to synapse in the pontine paramedian reticular formation. Impulses pass to the abducent nucleus on the same side and to the medial longitudinal fasciculus on the opposite side. This impulse passes to the portion of the oculomotor nucleus serving the left medial rectus muscle. In internuclear ophthalmoplegia a lesion in the medial longitudinal fasciculus impairs transmission from the pontine paramedian reticular formation to the contralateral medial rectus muscle.

malformations of the external ear, hands, and feet occur.

PARALYSIS OF GAZE

Gaze palsy.—Supranuclear lesions in the frontal lobe result in inability to direct the eyes to the contralateral side. The eyes rotate toward the side of the lesion. In bilateral lesions of the frontal lobe the patient is unable to turn the eyes in any direction but is able to maintain fixation and following movements. (Thus, in testing for abnormalities in conjugate ocular movements [gaze], the examiner should observe the voluntary movements of the eyes and not have the patient follow the movements of a test object.)

Tumors in the midbrain or the pineal body produce Parinaud syndrome, in which there is supranuclear conjugate palsy of vertical gaze (inability to elevate or to depress the eyes on command). Often the pupils are dilated and do not constrict to light; papilledema is usual.

A lesion in the pontine center for lateral gaze that is located near the abducent nucleus causes inability to direct the eyes to the side of the lesion with the eyes rotating to the opposite side.

Oculomotor apraxia is a gaze abnormality in which the eyes rotate in a direction opposite to which the head turns. After the head turn stops, the eyes rotate to the object of fixation. It may occur in ataxia-telangiectasia, in Gaucher disease, or as an isolated defect.

NONPARALYTIC STRABISMUS

In nonparalytic strabismus the eyes move normally because there is no weakness of the extraocular muscles. The angle of deviation is therefore the same in all fields of gaze.

However, with continued deviation, secondary abnormalities may develop, with overaction or underaction of some ocular muscles in some fields of gaze. There may be a superimposed A or V deviation in which the angle of deviation differs markedly in upward and downward gaze.

Esotropia and exotropia are the major types of nonparalytic strabismus.

NONPARALYTIC ESOTROPIA

In esotropia the nonfixing eye deviates inward. It may be divided into nonaccommodative and accommodative types. Additionally, there may be combinations of these two types.

Nonaccommodative esotropia.—Nonaccommodative esotropia (Fig 23-5) may be divided into those types with no abnormality of image formation and those types in which there is an abnormality in image formation (sensory interference) in one or both eyes (Table 23-3). Most patients have obvious abnormality of ocular image formation or perception, and other factors cannot be demonstrated. The deviation appears shortly after birth. There is often a familial history of strabismus. The deviation is often more than 50 diopters and is the same for both near and distance (basic esotropia). There may be a short period after birth in which there is alternate fixation, but the deviation tends to become monocular. The angle of deviation tends to remain relatively constant and is not modified by corrective lenses nor by anticholinesterase agents. Amblyopia and abnormal retinal correspondence commonly develop. The children rarely develop stereopsis or fusion even

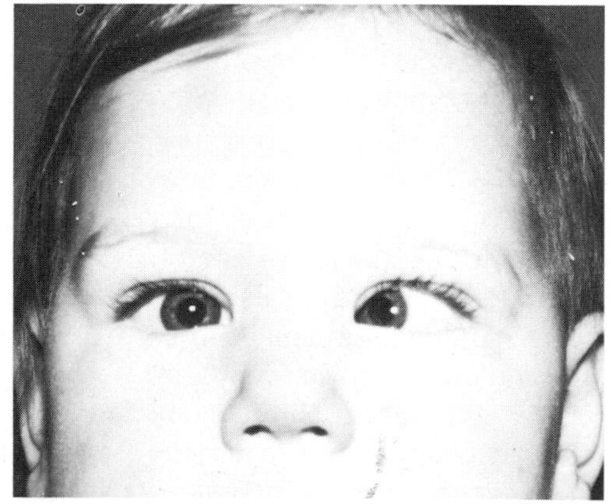

FIG 23-5.
Esotropia with the right eye fixing and the left eye deviating.

TABLE 23-3.
Nonaccommodative Esotropia

I. No sensory abnormality
  A. Onset at birth or shortly thereafter
  B. Familial
  C. No variation with accommodation
  D. Abnormal sensory mechanisms common
    1. Strabismic amblyopia
    2. Abnormal retinal correspondence
    3. Defective binocular vision
  E. Ocular deviation
    1. Nearly equal for near and far
    2. No effect using convex lenses
  F. Treatment
    1. Exclude neurologic and ocular disease
    2. Prevent abnormal sensory mechanism
      a. Mainly patching of eye with better vision
      b. Pleoptics (rare in United States)
    3. Surgery to correct deviation
II. Sensory abnormality
  A. Onset after disease or injury
  B. Possible hereditary eye disease impairing vision
  C. No variation with accommodation
  D. Defective vision in one or both eyes
    1. Marked anisometropia
    2. Corneal opacity
    3. Monocular cataract
    4. Retinal disease
    5. Optic nerve or tract disease
  E. Ocular deviation
    1. Equal for near and far
    2. Monocular fixation using eye with better vision
    3. May develop exotropia
  F. Treatment
    1. Lenses if anisometropic (contact lenses, if necessary, as required in monocular aphakia); cataract extraction in first 24 hours of life followed by immediate contact lens wear
    2. Cosmetic surgery to straighten eyes
    3. Correction of condition causing defective vision, if possible

after early effective surgery to align the visual axes.

Often there is cross-fixation, with the infant using the left eye to look to the right and the right eye to look to the left. This fixation pattern encourages equal use of the eyes and discourages the development of amblyopia and abnormal retinal correspondence. Cross-fixation may lead to the erroneous belief that a bilateral lateral rectus muscle palsy is present, since the child cross-fixates rather than abducts the eyes in lateral gaze. With one eye covered to prevent cross-fixation, ocular movements are full.

Treatment.—In the treatment of nonaccommodative esotropia, it is important (1) to evaluate the neurologic status of the child to exclude cerebral palsy and (2) to exclude opacities of the cornea, lens, and vitreous; unequal refractive errors; and retinal and choroidal disease. Treatment must be started before 6 months of age. Spontaneous improvement does not occur.

When amblyopia has developed, the abnormality is treated by occlusion of the habitually fixing eye to force use of the nonfixing eye, which is essential to develop central vision in each eye. Patching converts monocular strabismus to an alternating type. This conversion, a sign of visual improvement, may concern parents who believe that the crossing involved only one eye. Surgery is recommended during the early months of life to maximize fusion; although stereopsis is seldom attained, the peripheral fusion attained is often adequate to provide straight eyes for life.

Some patients with congenital nystagmus and esotropia may neutralize nystagmus and improve vision by rotating the eyes to the right or to the left. The patient may rotate the fixing eye in a maximally adducted position to see better (the nystagmus compensation or blockage syndrome). This type of esotropia usually has its onset in early infancy and is preceded by nystagmus. There may be pseudoparalysis of the lateral recti muscles, and as the fixing eye moves from adduction to abduction, there is a nystagmus.

Sensory abnormality.—Children born with an abnormality that interferes with clear ocular images often develop esotropia. A severe monocular deviation is present for both near and far. The infant uses the better eye. It is important to diagnose the cause of the sensory disturbance. A life-endangering retinoblastoma may cause sensory interference and amblyopia.

When retinal disease is present, cosmetic alignment of the eyes is the only treatment of value. Alignment may be delayed until just before the child enters school because there is no possibility of providing binocular vision. Since there is no fusion, the eyes tend to deviate outward in later life, and surgery for esotropia to make the eyes parallel in childhood may accelerate the development of exotropia (consecutive exotropia).

Accommodative esotropia.—Accommodation is the process by which the eye increases its refractive power to provide clear vision of nearby objects (see Chapter 2). In hyperopia (see Chapter 24) the individual must accommodate to see both distant and nearby objects. Accommodative esotropia is an excessive inward deviation of the eyes stimulated by accommodation. Recall that the eyes both normally turn inward to maintain fixation on any nearby object. In accommodative esotropia the eyes converge excessively when the individual accommodates to maintain a clear image of an object.

There are two types of accommodative esotropia: (1) refractive and (2) nonrefractive (Table 23-4). Both types have their onset after 1 year of age, usually between 2 and 3 years of age. The onset is abrupt in a child who previously had parallel eyes. The deviation is brought about by an attempt to visualize objects clearly, and the amount of crossing varies with activity and fatigue. There is often a family history of ocular deviation. Initially the esotropia is often intermittent and subsequently it becomes constant.

The cover-uncover test demonstrates the inward deviation of the eyes. A penlight used for fixation does not stimulate accommodation adequately to demonstrate an intermittent accommodative esotropia. A small picture used for fixation requires accommodation for clarity and demonstrates the inward deviation of the eyes.

The angle of deviation may be different for near and far fixation and upward or downward gaze (inconcomitance). Early in the development of the deviation there may be double vision, but this double vision usually disappears quickly as the child learns to suppress the image from the deviating eye.

Refractive accommodative esotropia.—This is caused by uncorrected hyperopia com-

TABLE 23-4.
Accommodative Esotropia

- I. Onset after 1 year (average, 2½ years)
- II. Familial
- III. Sensory mechanisms often normal
- IV. Ocular deviation
  - A. Greater for near than far
  - B. Originally intermittent but tends to become constant
- V. Refractive type
  - A. Normal accommodative-convergence/ accommodation ratio (AC/A)
  - B. Decreased by convex lenses that decrease accommodation
  - C. Treatment: decrease stimulus to accommodation
    1. Full hyperopic correction
    2. Bifocal lenses
    3. Miotics
    4. Orthoptic training
- VI. Nonrefractive type
  - A. High accommodative-convergence/ accommodation ratio (AC/A)
  - B. Deviation same for near and far
  - C. Not decreased by convex lenses
  - D. Treatment
    1. Surgery to provide alignment
- VII. Combined accommodative and nonaccommodative esotropia
  - A. Onset after neglected accommodative esotropia
  - B. Familial
  - C. Abnormal accommodative mechanisms
  - D. Abnormal sensory mechansism common
  - E. Ocular deviation
    1. Monocular fixation
    2. Tends to increase initially; exotropia common in adulthood
  - F. Treatment
    1. Optical correction of accommodative component
    2. Surgery for nonaccommodative deviation

bined with enough fusional ability to ensure binocular vision. The uncorrected hyperopia requires excessive accommodation to maintain a clear retinal image, which evokes excessive convergence. The decreased ability to fuse slightly dissimilar retinal images combined with excessive accommodation causes esotropia. If the fusion is adequate, the inward deviation remains latent (esophoria).

Treatment consists of full correction of the refractive error often combined with bifocal correction for near (Fig 23-6). This treatment may be combined with topical instillation of anticholinesterase drugs into each eye. The anticholinesterase drugs decrease the angle of deviation by facilitating contraction of the ciliary muscle to increase the curvature of the crystalline lens (accommodation) without stimulating the excessive convergence. Since the drug facilitates accommodation, fewer nerve impulses are required for clear vision. Fewer convergence impulses are generated and the amount of accommodative convergence is reduced.

Often 0.06% echothiophate (Phospholine Iodide) combined with 2.5% phenylephrine is used. Phenylephrine (an alpha-adrenergic agonist) prevents the development of cysts on the pupillary border of the iris that may become so large as to interfere with vision. Echothiophate binds pseudocholinesterase. In children it may cause episodes of acute abdominal pain that simulates the pain of acute appendicitis. There may be prolonged apnea after administration of succinylcholine as a muscle relaxant in general anesthesia.

Orthoptic training is valuable for teaching the child to maintain parallel fixation without corrective lenses. This may be a difficult task, because a child may suppress the image of the deviating eye.

Nonrefractive accommodative esotropia.—This is caused by a faulty synkinesis between accommodation and convergence. The effort to accommodate causes an excessive convergence. With the refractive error fully corrected, there remains a marked deviation of the eyes at near.

Miotics do not modify the angle of strabismus. Nonrefractive accommodative esotropia often requires surgery.

Accommodative esotropia may be combined with a nonaccommodative esotropia, in which case surgery must be directed to the nonaccommodative portion of the esotropia.

NONPARALYTIC EXOTROPIA

In nonparalytic exotropia (exodeviation) the nonfixing eye deviates toward the temple (Table 23-5). If the deviation is about the same for far and near, the exotropia is basic. If the deviation is at least 15 prism diopters more for distance than near, the deviation is a divergence excess. If

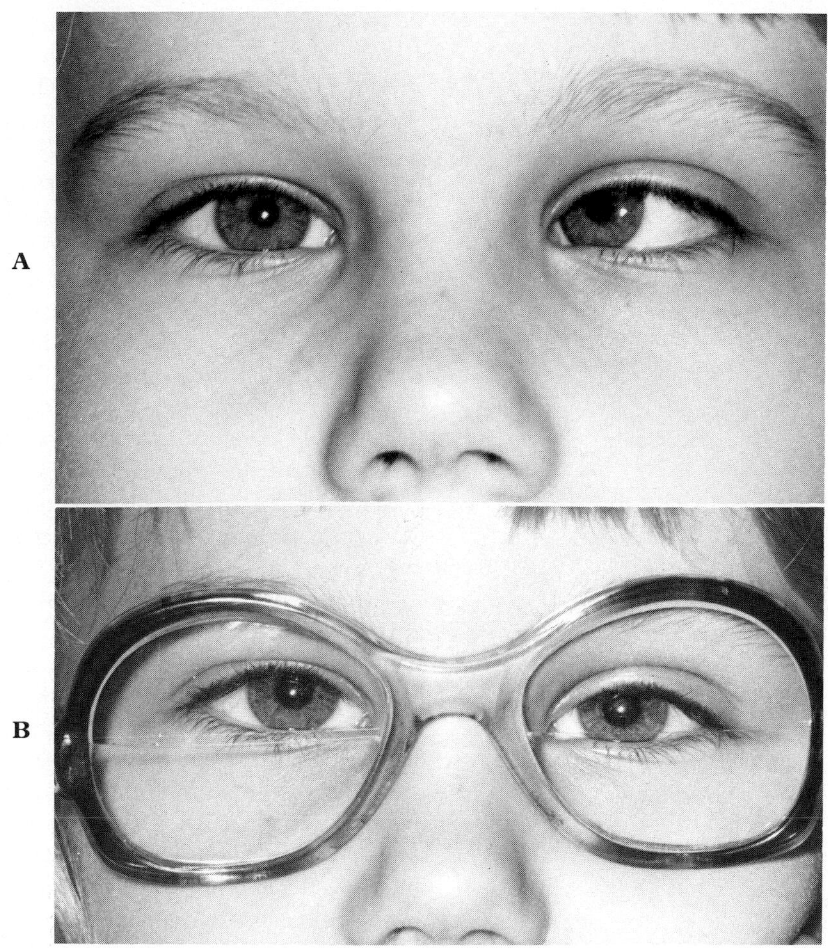

FIG 23-6.
An accommodative esotropia in a 5-year-old girl. **A,** Without optical correction, an esotropia is present. **B,** When hyperopia is corrected, the eyes are parallel.

the deviation is greater at near than distance, the deviation is a convergence insufficiency. (Deviations greater at distance than near involve divergence; deviations greater at near than distance involve convergence).

The usual exotropia begins as an exophoria, becomes an intermittent exotropia, and usually (75%) progresses to a manifest exotropia. Secondary exodeviations occur in adults as the result of reduced visual acuity in one eye and may follow esotropia after surgery (consecutive exotropia) or occur spontaneously. Individuals with uncorrected myopia do not accommodate for clear vision at near, and the inadequate impulse to converge may cause an exotropia that is corrected by lenses that neutralize the myopia. In craniosynostosis (see Chapter 15) the deformity of the skull places the eyes far apart, and there is often inadequate convergence that results in an exotropia.

Exophoria → intermittent exotropia → constant exotropia.—This is the most common type of exotropia. It begins at birth to 5 years of age. Initially the eyes are parallel, but on the cover-uncover test a marked exophoria is evident. This period of straight eyes is important as it permits normal visual development. Thus, amblyopia and abnormal retinal correspondence are not as common as they are in nonaccommodative types of exotropia. With growth of the face, an intermittent exotropia occurs, first at distance and then at near. Initially the exotropia is precipitated by fatigue and visual inattention. Suppression of the deviating retinal image

TABLE 23-5.
Nonparalytic Exotropia

I. Exophoria → intermittent exotropia → constant exotropia
   A. Onset at birth to 5 years of age
   B. Familial
   C. No accommodative element
   D. Sensorial mechanisms proportional to binocularity established before constant exotropia (often normal)
   E. Deviation
      1. Greater for far than near
      2. Exophoria and exotropia measurements the same
      3. Aggravated by fatigue
   F. Treatment
      1. Exotropia: surgery
      2. Exophoria: observe for constant exotropia
II. Acquired exotropia
   A. Variable age at onset
   B. Often nonfamilial
   C. Deteriorated esotropia; after surgical correction of esotropia (consecutive exotropia)
   D. Sensory impairment common
   E. Ocular deviation
      1. Equal for near and far
      2. Convergence poor
      3. Often monocular fixation
   F. Treatment: surgery
III. Accommodative (uncorrected myopic exotropia)
   A. Onset after 5 years of age
   B. Familial
   C. Uncorrected myopia minimizes accommodation required for near work
   D. Sensory mechanisms normal
   E. Ocular deviation
      1. Greater for far than near
      2. Initially intermittent but tends to become constant
   F. Treatment: stimulation of accommodation by correcting myopia with lenses

leads to inhibition of fusion and constant exotropia (Fig 23-7).

When there are long periods (75% of the time) of deviation, treatment is usually surgical. Correction of myopia increases accommodation of near and provides sharp retinal images that encourage fusion. Surgical correction is indicated in infants who develop an early exotropia of more than 20 diopters with little tendency to alignment. In adults with a large-angle exotropia, surgery is indicated as soon as the diagnosis is established.

Acquired exotropia.—Acquired exotropia occurs because of defective vision in one eye or because of an exophoria in which parallel eyes cannot be maintained by fusion (deteriorated exophoria).

Sensory impairment exotropia.—Decreased vision in one eye often leads to exotropia. If the sensory loss occurs in infancy, an esotropia occurs. With passing years the eye diverges. As the eyes pass from esotropia to exotropia, there is a phase in which the visual axes are parallel, which leads to the faulty hope that the esotropia has disappeared. The eyes continue to diverge more, finally developing a constant exotropia that may recur after surgery. In an older person an esotropia never develops. Rather, soon after visual impairment, the eye diverges.

Accommodative exotropia.—This is a relatively uncommon disorder that occurs because of uncorrected myopia, which decreases the need for accommodation for near work. The decrease in accommodative effort minimizes normal convergence, so the eyes tend to turn outward. Since most infants are hyperopic at birth, the condition occurs after visual maturity. Sensory anomalies are uncommon. It may occur in adolescents who are myopic and choose to have poor vision for distance rather than wearing spectacles or contact lenses. There may be a family history of myopia. Symptoms are minimal. Examination shows an intermittent outward deviation of the eyes, which becomes constant if the condition is neglected. The correction of the myopia with concave lenses or contact lenses is the only effective treatment.

A AND V SYNDROMES

A and V syndromes are ocular deviations in which the severity of esotropia or exotropia is more marked on looking either upward or downward. An A-esotropia is greater looking upward than downward. A V-esotropia is greater looking downward than upward. An A-exotropia is greater looking downward than upward. The V-exotropia is greater looking upward than downward.

The cause of the abnormality varies. In A types of both esotropia and exotropia there is often, but not always, overaction of both supe-

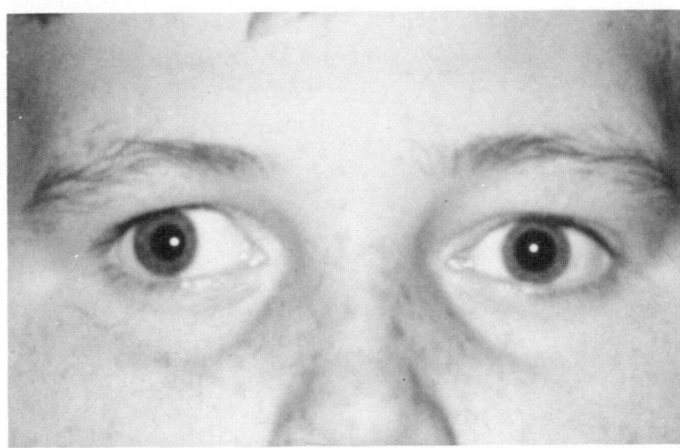

FIG 23-7.
Exotropia that began as a large-angle exophoria, passed through a stage of intermittent exotropia, and then became a constant exotropia, with suppression of the image in the deviating eye.

rior oblique muscles (N IV). In V types of both esotropia and exotropia there is often, but not always, overaction of both inferior oblique muscles. Overaction of the superior oblique muscle causes the adducting eye to deviate downward. Overaction of the inferior oblique muscle causes the adducting eye to deviate upward. The visual axes tend to converge on downward gaze so that in V-esotropia there may be overaction of the medial recti muscles. In V-exotropia there may be overaction of the lateral recti muscles.

A or V patterns occur in 50% of patients with esodeviations or exodeviations. The amount of deviation is measured with the prism cover test at 15° upgaze and 25° downgaze. An A-esotropia is present if there is 15 prism diopters more esotropia on looking upward than looking downward. An A-exotropia is present if there is 15 prism diopters less exotropia on looking upward than downward. A V-esotropia is present if there is 10 prism diopters more of esotropia on looking downward than on looking upward. A V-exotropia is present if there is 10 prism diopters less of exotropia on looking downward than on looking upward.

V-esotropia is the most common, followed by A-esotropia, V-exotropia, and A-exotropia. Recession and resection of the horizontal muscles are done to correct the esodeviation or exodeviation. To enhance the effect of these procedures, the new insertions of the horizontal muscles are displaced upward or downward. The medial recti muscles are always displaced toward the apex of the A or V, thus upward in A patterns and downward in V patterns. The lateral recti muscles are displaced away from the apex, irrespective of whether a recession or resection is done. Recession of the inferior oblique muscles may be done if these muscles are overactive in V pattern anomalies.

PSEUDOSTRABISMUS

Pseudostrabismus is a condition in which the eyes appear crossed to the observer although they are actually parallel. The center of the pupil is normally slightly temporal to the visual axis. When the eye fixates on a penlight beam, the reflection from the cornea usually is on the nasal portion of the pupil and a positive angle kappa (Fig 23-8) is present. If large enough, a positive angle kappa simulates the appearance of an exodeviation or reduces the apparent amount of an esodeviation. If the corneal reflection is temporal, a negative angle kappa (rare) is present that may stimulate the appearance of an esodeviation or a decrease in the apparent amount of an exodeviation.

The appearance of an ocular deviation in pseudostrabismus may be also caused by (1) an extra fold of skin at the inner canthus of each eye (epicanthus [see Fig 9-2]); (2) a broad, flat nose; (3) eyes that are exceptionally close together; or (4) an oval-shaped palpebral fissure. Each of these conditions conceals some of the white sclera at the medial side of the eye and simulates the appearance of an eye deviated inward. The

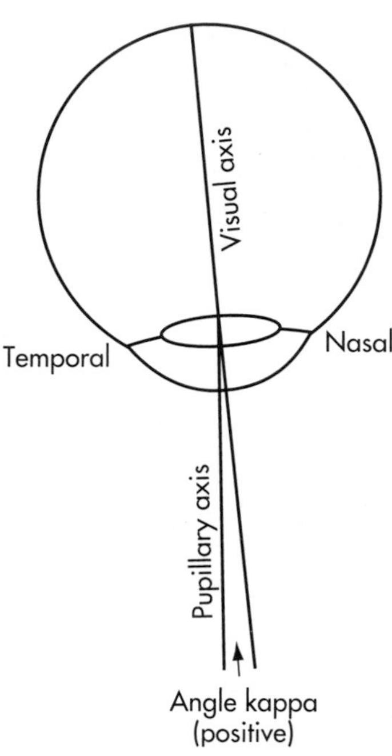

FIG 23-8.
The angle kappa is present when the visual line (axis), the line that extends between an object in space and the fovea centralis, does not pass through the center of the pupil. When the visual axis is nasal to the center of the pupil (the common location) the angle kappa is positive. A positive angle kappa may simulate the appearance of an exodeviation. When the visual axis is temporal to the center of the pupil, a negative angle kappa is present. A negative angle kappa may simulate the appearance of an esodeviation.

cover-uncover test indicates that the visual axes are parallel, and the sole treatment is reassurance. As the child's face grows, the appearance disappears. In pseudoexotropia the appearance is caused by retinal abnormalities that displace the fovea centralis. The retinopathy of prematurity is a common cause, although preretinal membranes and other such abnormalities may be at fault.

MICROTROPIA (MONOFIXATION SYNDROME)

The term microtropia is applied to exceptionally small deviations that cause amblyopia, abnormal retinal correspondence, suppression of central vision, and defective stereopsis.

There is no gross strabismus, but the sensory abnormalities of strabismus are present. The cover-uncover test shows no ocular recovery movement (movement of redress). When the test is repeated with a 4-diopter prism with its base either in or out, there is similarly no recovery movement. Sometimes a severe anisometropia is present. Examination with a special direct ophthalmoscope that projects a pattern into the patient's eye indicates that the patient does not use the fovea to fixate in one eye.

In children up to 6 years of age the amblyopia is corrected by occluding the fixing eye. Microtropia is present in nearly all patients with nonaccommodative esotropia after corrective surgery and accounts for their inability to attain central fusion.

MORE TERMINOLOGY

Following are additional technical terms to supplement those defined earlier in this chapter.

Visual axis.—The visual axis is an imaginary line that connects an object in space with the fovea centralis. In an individual with normal ocular, sensory, and motor systems, the visual axis of each eye intersects at the same object in space (fixation point) and there is binocular perception. If the visual axes are not directed simultaneously to the same object, only one eye is fixing.

The line of direction.—This is a line that connects an object in space with its image on the retina. It corresponds to the visual axis when it connects an object with the fovea centralis.

Retinal correspondence.—Whenever a retinal element is stimulated, the stimulus is perceived as having direction, which localizes the stimulus in space. Retinal elements that project in exactly the same direction are corresponding retinal elements. An object that stimulates corresponding retinal elements in each eye is perceived as a single object. When an object stimulates different retinal elements it is seen as double.

When the corresponding retinal elements are only slightly separated horizontally (disparate) and receive the same stimulus, the stimulus is perceived singly with the sensation of depth (stereopsis). Stereopsis requires the use of both eyes and is restricted to a maximum distance of about 125 to 200 meters. Monocular clues provide additional information concerning depth, including (1) motion parallax (when one looks at a scene with one eye and moves one's head or eye, far objects move more than close objects); (2) linear perspective (parallel lines seem to approach each other in the distance); (3) overlays of contours (interposition of a close object in front of a more distant object); and (4) highlights, shadows, size of close objects, and color of distant objects (bluish haze of distant mountains).

Anomalous retinal correspondence.— Anomalous retinal correspondence is a binocular condition in which corresponding retinal elements do not project in the same direction. Thus the foveolas of the two eyes have different directional values so that the foveola of one eye corresponds to an extrafoveal region of the fellow eye. Abnormal retinal correspondence involves directional values of the two eyes and is sometimes associated with normal visual acuity in each eye.

When the eyes cross, the angle formed by the intersection of the visual axis of each eye is the angle of strabismus. The objective angle of strabismus is that angle measured by the prism cover test (or a similar test). The subjective angle is that angle in which the patient indicates perception of the direction of the visual axis of each eye. When the subjective angle and objective angle are the same, normal retinal correspondence is present. If the subjective angle and the objective angle of strabismus are different, anomalous retinal correspondence is present. If the patient perceives the visual axes to be parallel (subjective angle of zero) when the visual axes are not parallel, the anomalous retinal correspondence is harmonious. If the subjective angle is not zero and does not equal the objective angle of strabismus, the anomalous retinal correspondence is nonharmonious or disharmonious.

Motor correspondence.—In version movements of the eyes, the eyes move simultaneously from eyes front (primary position) to the right, left, up, or down (secondary positions). The nerve impulse for version is always sent simultaneously and equally to the muscles responsible for the movement (Hering's law of equal innervation). Thus, in rotating the eyes to the right, the right lateral rectus muscle and the left medial rectus muscle each receive an equal innervational impulse to contract. Isolated impulses to the muscles of one eye only or to a single ocular muscle do not occur.

In convergence and divergence (vergence movements) the medial recti muscles and the lateral recti muscles receive simultaneous and equal nervous stimuli for contraction and relaxation. The divergence and convergence movements align the eyes in such a way as to maintain binocular fixation and stereopsis.

Fusional vergence.—This term is applied to the movements of convergence or divergence that occur when an object is imaged on slightly disparate horizontal parts of the retina.

Fusion-free position.—This is the position of an eye when it is covered or when vision is otherwise obscured to eliminate binocular vision.

Suppression.—Suppression is that condition in which the image originating on the retina of one eye does not enter consciousness. Rifle users, microscopists, and others who use one eye may, without conscious effort, intermittently ignore the image from the nonfixing eye. If the eyes do not fixate simultaneously on the same object, the stimulation of noncorresponding retinal elements causes a retinal rivalry. To avoid double vision (diplopia) there is cortical suppression of the sensory input from the deviating eye. Visual acuity may be good in each eye when used separately, but the image of the eye that is not being used is suppressed.

Eccentric fixation.—This is a monocular condition (usually) in which the foveola is not used for fixation because of amblyopia or disease of the fovea centralis. A special ophthalmoscope (Visuscope), which projects a fixation target on the fundus, may indicate that an area adjacent to the foveola is used for fixation rather than the foveola. The retinal area used by each patient varies widely. The more distant from the foveola, the poorer the visual acuity. Severe eccentric fixation is evident if an eye remains deviated when the fellow eye is covered. The prognosis for visual improvement is much poorer when amblyopia is associated with eccentric fixation.

Accommodative - convergence / accommodation ratio.—When fixing distance objects, the visual axes are parallel and accommodation is required only to compensate for hyperopia that may be present. Fixation on an object closer than 20 feet requires convergence of the visual axes and accommodation. The amount of accommodative convergence divided by the amount of accommodation indicates the responsiveness of an individual's con-

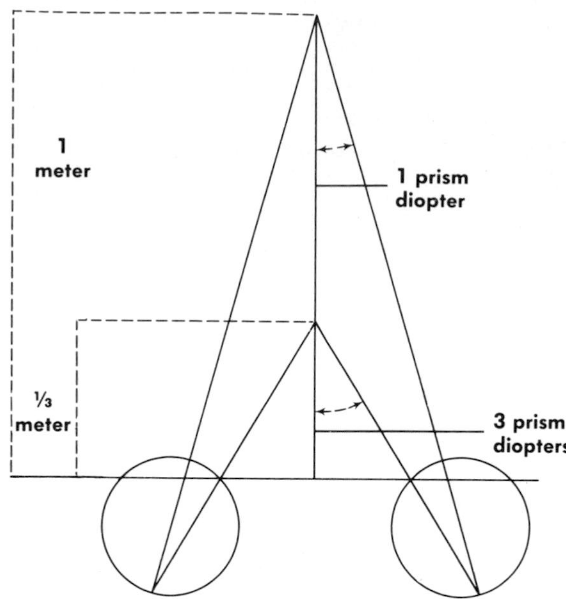

FIG 23-9.
Prism diopters of accommodation. At 1 meter the eyes must accommodate 1 prism diopter. If the eyes are 5.2 cm apart, they must exert 5.2 prism diopters of accommodative convergence.

vergence to a particular amount of accommodation.

Accommodative convergence is measured in prism diopters. It is found by multiplying the interpupillary distance in centimeters by the distance of the object of attention expressed in prism diopters (Fig 23-9) (the prism diopter is the reciprocal of the distance expressed in meters: ½ meter is 2 diopters; ⅓ meter is 3 diopters). Thus, if an individual without an error of refraction has an interpupillary distance of 5.5 cm and the object of attention is ⅓ meter (3 diopters of accommodation) distant, he or she will exert 16.5 (5.5 × 3) diopters of accommodative convergence. The accommodative-convergence to accommodation ratio (AC/A) is 16.5 ÷ 3 prism diopters of accommodation or 5.5. An AC/A ratio equal to the pupillary distance in centimeters is the ideal. Most individuals have a lower value but are able to maintain binocular vision by means of fusional convergence.

The AC/A ratio may be measured by the heterophoria or gradient lens method. Heterophoric testing requires measurement of the interpupillary distance. The deviation is measured for far and near with the patient wearing full correction of any refractive error. The following equation is then used:

$$\frac{AC}{A} = \text{Interpupillary distance (in cm)} + \frac{\text{Deviation for near} - \text{Deviation for far}}{\text{Accommodation at near}}$$

Inward deviations are positive numbers, and outward deviations are negative numbers. Thus, if the interpupillary distance is 5 cm and the deviation for near is 10 prism diopters of esotropia and for far 4 prism diopters of esotropia, the equation would read:

$$\frac{AC}{A} = 5.0 + \frac{10 - 4}{3} = 7.0$$

Alternatively, a gradient method may be used in which the amount of deviation for near is measured first with full correction and then with a concave lens over the correction. The deviation is measured by using a series of convex and concave spherical lenses, the results are plotted on a graph, and the slope of the best fitting lines is the AC/A ratio. The following formula may be used:

$$\frac{AC}{A} = \frac{\text{Deviation with concave lens} - \text{Deviation without concave lens}}{\text{Power concave lens}}$$

The AC/A ratio is not affected by eye muscle surgery or orthoptic treatment of the patient.

Cycloplegics increase the ratio by reducing accommodation. Miotics lower the ratio by decreasing the need for accommodation. Bifocals decrease the need for accommodation when near objects are viewed, and thus excess accommodative convergence does not occur. Spectacle-corrected refractive errors change the patient's near point of accommodation and thus affect the AC/A ratio.

BIBLIOGRAPHY

Books

Cogan DG: *Neurology of ocular muscles,* ed 2, Springfield, Ill, 1978, Charles C Thomas.

Cogan DG: *Neurology of the visual system,* Springfield, Ill, 1980, Charles C Thomas.

Good WV, Hoyt CS: *Strabismus management,* Newton, Mass, 1995, Butterworth-Heinemann.

Pratt-Johnson JA, Tillson G: *Management of strabismus and amblyopia. A practical guide,* New York, 1994, Thieme Medical Publishers.

Veronneau-Troutman S: *Prisms in the medical and surgical management of strabismus,* St Louis, 1994, Mosby–Year Book.

von Noorden GK: *Binocular vision and ocular motility: theory and management of strabismus,* ed 5, St Louis, 1996, Mosby–Year Book.

von Noorden GK, Helveston EM: *Strabismus. A decision making approach,* St Louis, 1994, Mosby–Year Book.

Wright KW, editor: *Pediatric ophthalmology and strabismus,* St Louis, 1995, Mosby–Year Book.

24

OPTICAL DEFECTS OF THE EYE

When a ray of light passes from one transparent medium to another, its velocity decreases in a more dense medium and increases in a less dense medium. If the transparent medium is bounded by surfaces that are not perpendicular to the ray of light, then, in addition to the change in velocity, the emerging ray has a different direction than the entering ray. This change in direction is called "refraction." It is proportionate to the sine of the angle formed by the light ray to the surface of the refracting medium and the velocity of light in this medium. (The index of refraction is the ratio of the velocity of light in a vacuum to the velocity of light in another medium.) The greater the change in the velocity of the light as it passes from one medium to another, the greater will be its refraction.

The diopter is the standard unit to express the refractive power of optical lenses. It is the reciprocal of the distance, expressed in meters, between a lens and its focus (its focal length). Thus, if the focal length of a lens is 0.20 m (20 cm), its power in diopters is 5.0 D (1 ÷ 0.20 = 5.0 D) (Fig 24-1).

A ray of light entering the eye is refracted by the cornea, and then, after passing through the aqueous humor, it is refracted by the crystalline lens. The anterior surface of the cornea is the major refractive surface of the eye. The cornea has a fixed focal length (focus), but the curvature of the lens changes in accommodation so that the human eye provides clear images of objects located both near and far from the eye.

Optically, the crystalline lens consists of layers of transparent proteins having different optical densities (indices of refraction). It acts as though it were composed of a series of lenses within the lens capsule, so that its total refraction is greater than that of any individual layer. With accommodation (see below) in the youthful human eye, the refractive power of the crystalline lens increases from about 19 to 33 diopters because of a change in its thickness and curvature.

A refractive error of the human eye is determined by (1) the variation in the normal radii of curvature of the cornea and (2) the variation of the normal axial length of the eye. These elements are usually correlated so that long eyes have less refractive power and short eyes have more refractive power, which minimizes any refractive error. Thus, it is an oversimplification to regard a myopic eye as one that is too long or a hyperopic eye as one that is too short. Instead, the refractive power of the cornea and lens and the length of the eye are not correlated. Refractive errors of less than 5 diopters are generally considered to be a biologic variation. Refractive errors of more than 5 diopters are generally considered to be abnormal and to result from developmental anomalies, genetic factors, or both.

ACCOMMODATION

Accommodation is the process by which the refractive power of the anterior lens segment increases so that a near object may be distinctly imaged on the retina. The increased refractive power results from an increased curvature of the

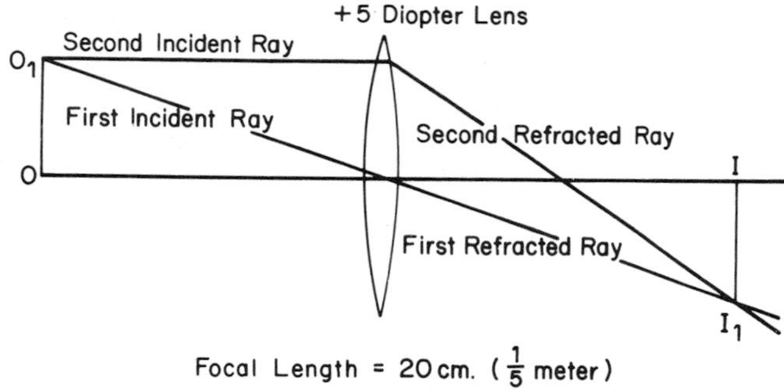

FIG 24-1.
Parallel rays from an object O-O_1 form an image I-I_1 20 cm (0.5 m) from a 5.0-diopter lens. A diopter is derived by dividing 1 by the focal length of a lens expressed in meters ($1 \div 0.20 = 5.0$).

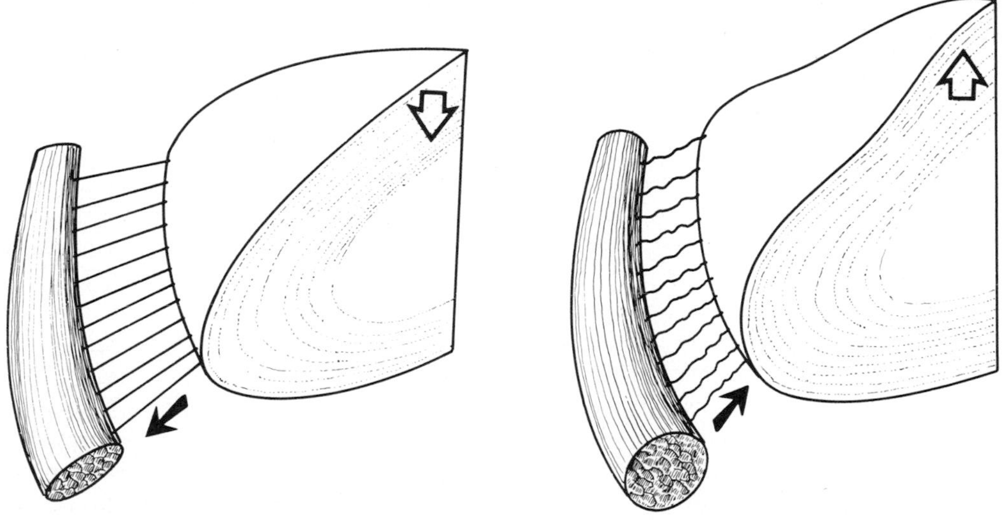

FIG 24-2.
Accommodation. The zonule attaches at the equator of the lens to its anterior and posterior capsule and to the ciliary body between the ciliary processes. When the circular portion of the ciliary muscle is at rest it has a maximum diameter and exerts tension on the zonule to maintain the lens with a minimum curvature, thickness, and refractive power. The diameter of the ciliary muscle is smaller when it contracts, and the tension on the zonule is less. The relaxed zonule results in the inherent elasticity of the lens to become more spherical and thicker, thus increasing its refractive power. The stimulus to accommodation is a blurred retinal image that causes contraction of the ciliary muscle.

central portion of the anterior surface of the lens in response to contraction of the circular portion (mainly) of the ciliary muscle. The ciliary muscle is attached to the lens capsule by zonular fibers. When relaxed the diameter of the circular muscle is maximal, the zonular fibers are taut, and the convexity of the lens surface is minimal. The diameter of the circular muscle decreases with contraction and thereby causes the zonular fibers to relax (Fig 24-2). The relaxation allows the lens (chiefly the central portion of the anterior surface) to become more convex because of inherent elasticity of the anterior capsule.

The stimulus to accommodation is a blurred retinal image. One may imagine a continuous feedback mechanism in which the brain signals the amount of accommodation required and, through stimulation of the short ciliary branches of the oculomotor nerve (N III), constricts or relaxes the circular muscle so that the eye almost

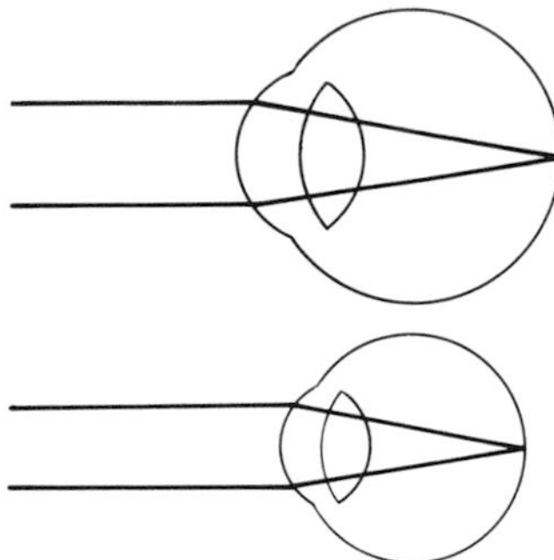

FIG 24-3.
Two emmetropic eyes. The refractive power of the cornea and lens is so correlated with the length of the eye that parallel rays of light are focused on the retina. The eye below has much more refractive power than the eye above, although both are emmetropic. If such a difference were present in the right and left eyes, there would be a difference of image size, called aniseikonia.

instantly adjusts to provide clear vision at whatever distance.

With aging, the lens capsule becomes less elastic and the lens nucleus becomes harder and less compressible, so that the lens becomes less spherical with relaxation of the zonule. This causes a gradual loss of accommodation. The process begins shortly after birth and continues thereafter until about 50 years of age, when only 1 diopter of accommodation remains (presbyopia). The process is mainly the result of changes in the lens, but there may be decreased strength of the ciliary body musculature with aging.

Convergence is associated with accommodation and pupillary constriction (the near reaction). This is not a reflex but an associated reaction of synkinesis that occurs because branches of the inferior division of the oculomotor nerve (N III) innervate the medical recti, ciliary, and sphincter pupillae muscles.

EMMETROPIA

Emmetropia is that optical condition in which an eye does not have an error of refraction, so that without accommodation, rays of light parallel to the optical axis on entering the eye are brought to focus on the fovea centralis (Fig 24-3). (The optical axis is the imaginary line that passes through the centers of curvature of the surfaces of an optical system and are not refracted.) The refractive powers of the lens and cornea are correlated with the length of the eye. Clinically, emmetropia rarely occurs because such an exact correlation is exceptional.

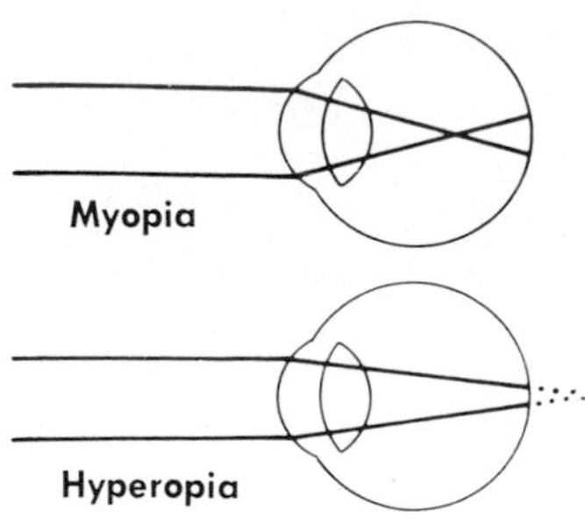

FIG 24-4.
The two major types of refractive error (ametropia).

REFRACTIVE ERRORS (AMETROPIA)

A refractive error is that optical condition in which parallel rays of light from an object an infinite distance from the eye do not come to focus (form an image) exactly at the fovea centralis (Fig 24-4). The refraction of an eye is the result of the refractive powers of the cornea and lens correlated with the length of the eye. It matters little (within limits) whether the refractive power is large or small, provided that a particular power is associated with an eye of such a length that parallel rays of light that reach the eye come to a focus on the fovea centralis.

(Technically, a refractive error is present when the plane of the second principal point of the ocular refractive system [the posterior principal focus] does not coincide with the fovea centralis.)

Hyperopia or myopia may be present. If the refraction is different in different meridians of the eye, astigmatism is present. It may be myopic or hyperopic. If the ametropia is the result of an abnormality in the length of the eye, it is axial ametropia. If the ametropia is the result of a variation in the refractive power of the cornea or lens, it is refractive ametropia.

SYMPTOMS AND SIGNS OF REFRACTIVE ERROR

Decreased visual acuity, which may be fully corrected by means of lenses, is the cardinal sign of a refractive error. If lenses cannot correct vision, an organic cause must be sought. In myopia, vision is decreased for distance and is normal for near. In hyperopia, vision may be normal or slightly decreased for both near and far. Since accommodation may compensate for hyperopia, there is often no relationship between vision without lenses and the amount of the hyperopia.

Many symptoms are attributed to refractive errors. Because vision and the eyes figure prominently in psychologic mechanisms, symptoms may be difficult to interpret. Ocular discomfort is a vague symptom that refers to almost any unpleasant sensation occurring in or about the eyes. Asthenopia, eyestrain, and visual fatigue are terms used to describe complaints related to any symptom originating in the head or eyes, which the patient attributes to use of the eyes. These include burning, itching, increased sensitivity to light, decreased efficiency, various aches, and fatigue.

Headache, irrespective of its cause, is commonly and erroneously attributed to refractive errors. If a refractive error contributes to headache, the discomfort should be related to sustained use of the eyes and relieved when the eyes are not used. It is unlikely that a headache present on awakening in the morning can be ascribed to excessive use of the eyes the evening before. Individuals living in unpleasant situations from which they cannot escape may develop tension headaches that they attribute to the use of the eyes. Migraine is never caused by a refractive error.

HYPEROPIA

Hyperopia is that refraction condition of the eye in which, with accommodation suspended, parallel rays of light are intercepted by the retina before coming to focus (Fig 24-5).

The condition occurs because the refractive power of the cornea and lens is inadequate for the length of the globe (refractive) or the globe is too short (axial) for the amount of refractive power present. Accommodation increases the refractive power of the lens and may compensate for hyperopia.

There are no specific signs of hyperopia. In axial hyperopia the cornea may be smaller than normal, and the globe itself may be small.

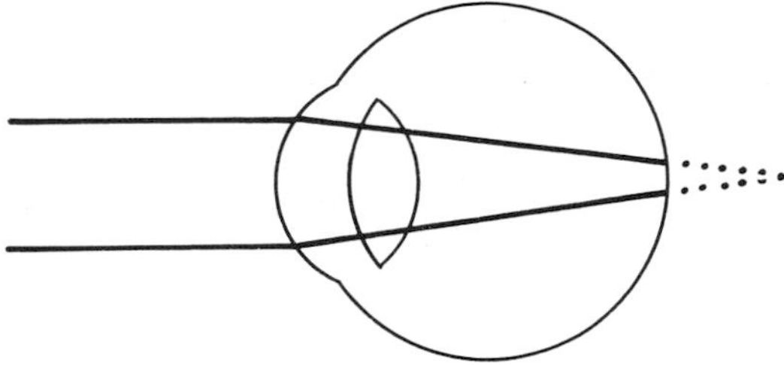

Refractive hyperopia

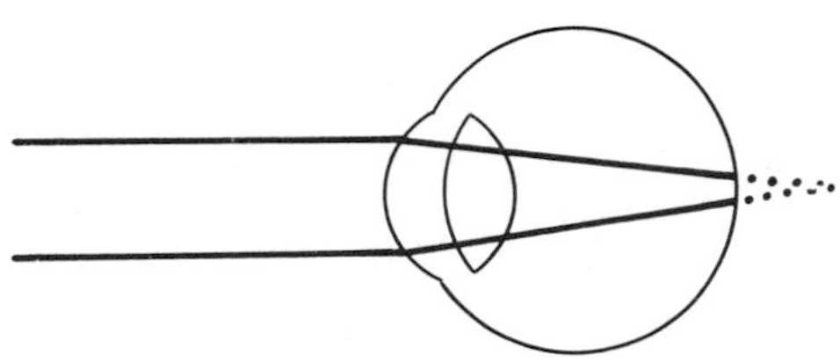

Axial hyperopia

FIG 24-5.
Hyperopia. Both eyes are hyperopic. *Top,* The eye is hyperopic because the refractive power of the cornea and lens is not adequate to focus light on the retina. *Bottom,* The hyperopia occurs because the eye is too small for the amount of refractive power of the anterior segment. Accommodation may increase the refractive power of the anterior segment so that a distinct image is formed on the retina.

Hyperopia that exceeds 5 diopters may be associated with blurring of the optic disk margin, called pseudopapilledema. The disk is not elevated, but the margins are blurred and indistinct and the physiologic cup is absent. This condition is distinguished from early papilledema by the normal caliber of veins, their normal pulsation, and the absence of retinal edema, hemorrhages, and progression. Inflammation of the optic nerve at the level of the disk (papillitis) is usually unilateral and causes decreased vision, a central scotoma, and an afferent pupillary defect.

Hyperopia may be compensated by the accommodation, which increases the refractive power of the lens. If accommodation does not compensate for the hyperopia, vision is blurred. Ocular symptoms may originate with excessive sustained accommodation required for clear vision. There is no direct relationship between the symptoms and the amount of accommodation required to neutralize a hyperopia. Since a portion of accommodation must be used to neutralize the refractive error for distance and additional accommodation is required for near work, the symptoms may be aggravated during or after near work.

Hyperopia is classified as follows:

1. Total hyperopia is the amount of hyperopia present with all accommodation suspended, a condition produced by paralysis of the ciliary muscle by means of a cycloplegic drug, such as atropine (see Chapter 2).
2. Manifest hyperopia is the maximum hyperopia that can be corrected with a convex lens when accommodation is active.
3. The difference between total and manifest hyperopia is the latent hyperopia.

Since accommodation for near is related to convergence of the eyes, the increased accommodation required to neutralize hyperopia may stimulate an excessive degree of convergence. This excessive convergence is manifested as a tendency for the eyes to deviate inward (esophoria [see Chapter 23]).

Convex lenses are prescribed when visual acuity is decreased, when a convergence excess causes esophoria or esotropia, or when hyperopia causes symptoms. If visual acuity is good, muscle balance is normal, and there are no symptoms, correction of the hyperopia is not necessary, irrespective of its severity.

MYOPIA

Myopia is that optical condition in which rays of light entering the eye parallel to the visual axis come to a focus in front of the retina (Fig 24-6). The condition occurs (1) because the refractive power of the cornea and lens is too great for the length of the eye or (2) because the eye is too long for the refractive power present. Patients with uncorrected myopia do not accommodate to improve vision because accommodation shifts the focus even further anterior to the retina and blurs vision further. Myopia may be divided into three types: (1) physiologic myopia; (2) pathologic or degenerative myopia, previously called progressive or malignant myopia; and (3) lenticular myopia. Physiologic myopia may be either refractive or axial. Degenerative myopia is axial; lenticular myopia is refractive.

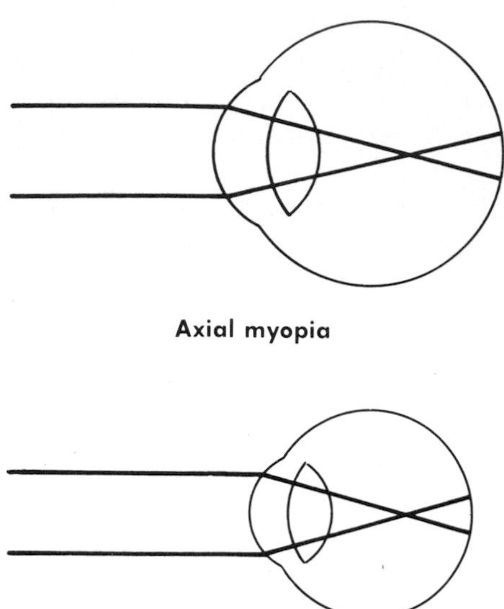

FIG 24-6.
Myopia. Both eyes are myopic. *Top,* The eye is myopic because it is too long for the amount of refractive power present. *Bottom,* The eye is myopic because the refractive power is too great for the length of the eye. Increased accommodation increases the refractive power of the anterior segment and aggravates the myopia.

Physiologic myopia, the most common type, occurs because of inadequate correlation of the refractive power of the cornea and lens with the length of the globe, both of which are within their normal distribution curves. It has its onset usually between 5 and 10 years of age but may begin as late as 25 years of age. It gradually increases until the eye is fully grown, about 18 years of age. It seldom exceeds 6 diopters.

Pathologic (degenerative) myopia is an abnormality in which the axial length of the eye is excessive, primarily because of overgrowth of the posterior two thirds of the globe. Commonly, pathologic myopia begins as a physiologic myopia, but rather than stabilizing when the globe is adult size, the eye continues to enlarge.

The first ophthalmoscopic sign of myopic degeneration is a crescent of the optic disk that begins at the temporal side and progresses to surround the disk (Fig 24-7). Staphyloma of the posterior pole causes degeneration of Bruch membrane, which creates branching, reticular lines (lacquer cracks) that may cause foveal

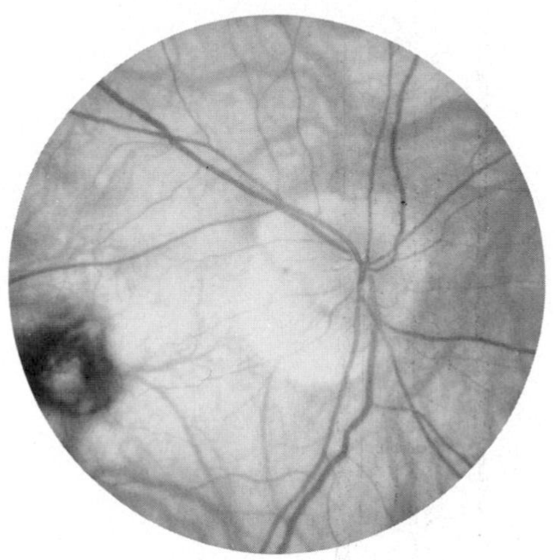

FIG 24-7.
The ocular fundus in pathologic (degenerative) myopia. The sclera is bared in the region surrounding the optic nerve, the choroid is easily visible (depigmentation in situ), and there is pigment proliferation (Fuchs spot) at the fovea centralis.

hemorrhage. Later a subretinal neovascular membrane may develop with vascular leakage and hemorrhage. With resorption of a foveal hemorrhage, hyperpigmentation develops in the fovea centralis (Fuchs spot). Degeneration of the retinal pigment epithelium (depigmentation in situ) and choroid exposes the sclera. The peripheral retina may show lattice degeneration and retinal breaks, increasing the risk of retinal separation. Pigment migration may simulate healed chorioretinitis.

Increase in the refractive power of the crystalline lens (lenticular myopia) increases the refractive power of the anterior segment. Increased refractive power occurs in uncontrolled diabetes mellitus and in nuclear sclerosis, an aging change of the lens. Drugs such as hydralazine and chlorthalidone (antihypertensives) and the phenothiazines may also increase the refractive power of the lens.

Myopia is neutralized by concave lenses. Corrective lenses should be prescribed for patients dissatisfied with poor visual acuity. Wearing corrective lenses has no apparent effect on the progression of myopia. A decrease in myopia requires a decrease in the axial length or refractive power of the eye, and this does not occur spontaneously.

If a patient with myopia wears a corrective lens with more refractive power than is necessary to neutralize the myopia, the individual may compensate by increased accommodation. Vision is clear and often there are no symptoms. When accurate lenses are provided, such individuals may show an apparent decrease in myopia. Optical correction, whether contact lenses or spectacles, with or without bifocal segments, and whether the myopia is overcorrected or undercorrected, does not affect its progression.

Tightly fitted hard contact lenses may temporarily reduce the corneal curvature and thus temporarily decrease the severity of myopia. The refractive error reverts to its previous state after use of the contact lens is discontinued.

Since physiologic myopia is a variation in growth, many remedies may be associated with the termination of the growth process, and credit is often given to the remedy. Studies of treatment to correct or arrest myopia have not been controlled, and double-masked methods and adequate experimental designs have been ignored. Often, there has been no matched control group or an excessive number of patients have been lost to follow-up.

Fusing the upper to the lower eyelid in macaque monkeys to prevent form vision but not light perception causes axial myopia in immature but not adult monkeys. The elongation of the eye is caused by an alteration of the visual input and is mediated by the nervous system. A similar elongation occurs in infants with blepharoptosis, hemangiomas of the eyelids, and opacities of the ocular media.

Ocular hypertension (see Chapter 23) is more common in myopia than in hyperopia. When present, many practitioners initiate prophylactic treatment with a beta-adrenergic antagonist at lower levels of ocular tension than they do in hyperopia. The visual acuity may be maintained at its best possible level in patients with degenerative or progressive myopia by frequent optical correction. To detect peripheral retinal holes and degeneration (see Chapter 17) the peripheral retina must be examined annually. The pupils must be fully dilated and the peripheral fundus studied using an indirect binocular ophthalmoscope combined with scleral depression.

Radial incisions partially through the thickness of the peripheral cornea (radial keratotomy) or excimer laser ablation of the central corneal stroma (photokeratectomy) (see Chapter 11) to decrease the refractive power of the

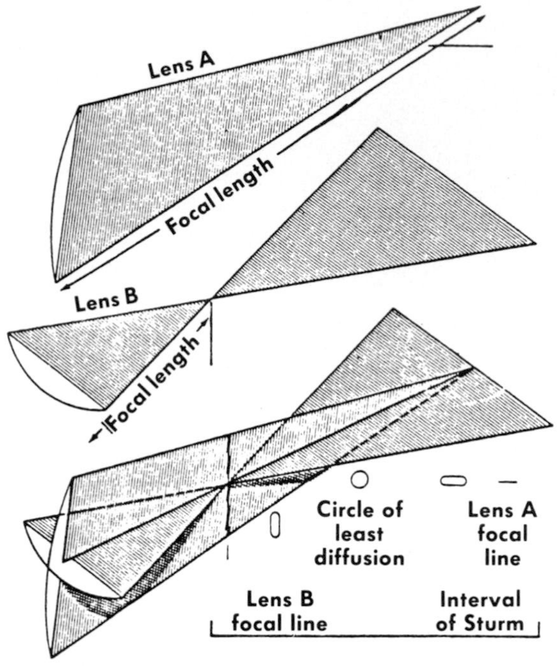

FIG 24-8.
Refraction by two cylindrical lenses, *A* and *B*, of unequal strength. Cylindrical lens *B* has the greatest convexity, and hence a vertical line is focused first. Parallel rays of light are focused as a line rather than as a point. The combination of two cylindrical lenses of unequal power forms two major focal lines corresponding to their refractive power. The distance between the focal lines is the *interval of Sturm.* A circle of least diffusion is located between the focal lines at an area where the diverging and converging tendency of the light rays is the same. It is located between the two focal lines and is closer to the stronger cylinder in proportion to the strength of the component cylinders.

cornea have become exceptionally popular. Initially, such procedures were used only in patients with less than 2 diopters of myopia. Now far more severe degrees of myopia are treated. Most patients are delighted that they are able to discard the lenses used to correct distance vision, even though vision may be poorer than with optical correction. Initially, only patients who were unable to tolerate contact lenses were considered for the operation, but today patients with all degrees of myopia have the procedure.

Excimer ablation of the central corneal stroma destroys the overlying epithelium, which rapidly regenerates, but it also destroys the Bowman zone, which does not regenerate. There is a longer period of discomfort after photoablation of the cornea than there is with radial keratotomy. Much discomfort and corneal inflammation is avoided by surgical removal of a button of corneal epithelium and the attached Bowman zone. The exposed corneal stroma is then treated with photoablation, and the corneal button is reattached.

ASTIGMATISM

Astigmatism is an optical condition in which the refracting power of a lens (or an eye) is not the same in all meridians. Thus, if the refracting power of the eye is 58 diopters in the vertical and 60 diopters in the horizontal meridian, 2 diopters of astigmatism is present. Parallel rays of light do not focus at a point. To aid graphic reconstruction, one considers one focal line corresponding to the 60-diopter meridian and another corresponding to the 58-diopter meridian. The distance separating these focal lines is the interval of Sturm (Fig 24-8). (There is actually a series of images with cylindrical lenses contributing to each.)

Astigmatism is regular when the meridians of minimal and maximal refraction are at right angles to each other and irregular when the meridians are not at right angles to each other. Ocular astigmatism is simple when one meridian is on the retina, simple myopic when the other meridian is anterior to the retina, and simple hyperopic when the other meridian is intercepted by the retina before coming to focus. In compound myopic astigmatism, both meridians are in front of the retina. In compound hyperopic astigmatism, both meridians are intercepted by the retina before coming to a focus. In mixed astigmatism, one focal line is focused in front of the retina and the other focal line is intercepted by the retina.

Regular astigmatism occurs because the cornea has two different radii of curvature at right angles to each other. This may occur as a biologic variant or may result from the weight of the upper eyelid resting on the eyeball, from surgical incisions into the cornea, from trauma and scarring of the cornea, or from tumors of the eyelid such as a chalazion pressing on the globe.

Irregular astigmatism, in which the cornea has three or more different curvatures, occurs in corneal scarring and keratoconus. In keratoconus the cornea becomes cone-shaped with the apex of the cone below and nasal to the corneal center. Variations in the radii of curvature of the crystalline lens induce minor degrees of astigmatism (lenticular astigmatism). The condition is detected in patients who wear hard contact lenses that neutralize corneal astigmatism.

The symptoms caused by astigmatism vary considerably. A distinct retinal image cannot form (Fig 24-9), but the circle of least diffusion may be imaged or first one focal line and then the other is focused on the retina. The changes in accommodation cause symptoms. Severe astigmatism may cause the optic disk to appear oval rather than nearly circular when viewed with the ophthalmoscope while small changes cause no signs.

Astigmatism is neutralized by cylindrical lenses (Fig 24-10). The amount of astigmatism that should be corrected is debated. Some believe that even minor degrees of astigmatism require correction. If, however, visual acuity is good and there are no symptoms, correction is not indicated. Hard contact lenses may be used to correct irregular astigmatism. In keratoconus, if vision is markedly reduced and if the vision cannot be corrected with contact lenses, a corneal transplant should be considered (see Chapter 11). Conversely, a patient with corneal scarring should have a trial with a contact lens before a corneal transplant or photoablation is recommended.

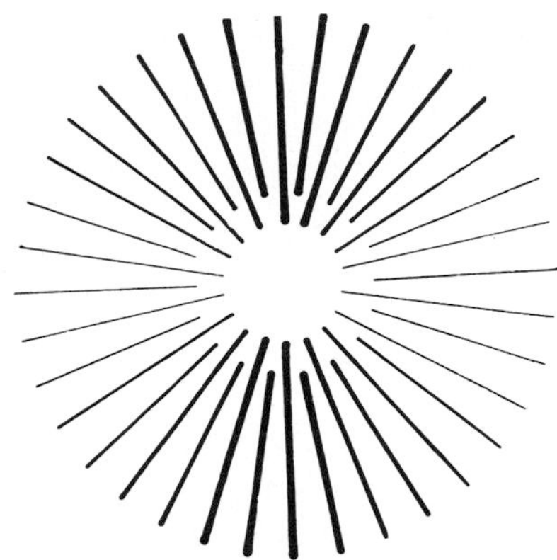

FIG 24-9.
The astigmatic dial as seen by a patient with astigmatism. The thick black lines are focused on the retina, whereas the thin lines lie in front of the retina.

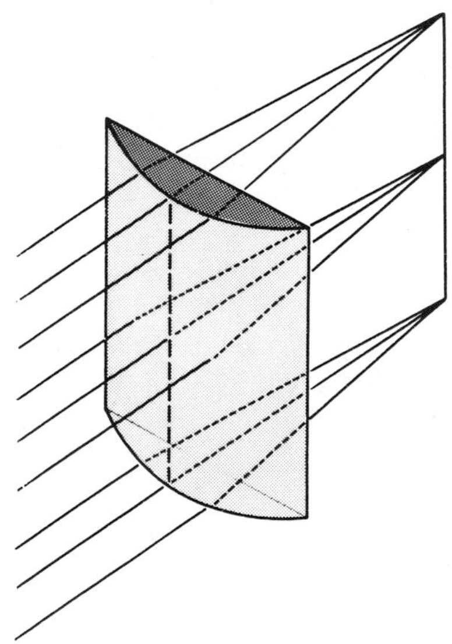

FIG 24-10.
Cylindrical lens. The line of focus parallels the axis of the lens.

PRESBYOPIA

Accommodation increases the refractive power of the anterior segment through an increased curvature and thickness of the lens. The change in the shape of the lens occurs because of its inherent elasticity in response to contraction of the annular ciliary muscle, which reduces its diameter and relaxes the zonule. With each year of life, the lens loses some of this elasticity, decreasing the amount of accommodation. There is about 14 diopters of accommodation at 10 years of age and only 2 diopters of accommodation by 50 years of age. The decrease occurs gradually, but with only 2 diopters of accommodation, small objects viewed closer than 0.5 m from the eye are blurred.

The optical condition of decreased accommodation with aging is known as presbyopia. The loss of accommodation occurs in all individuals, irrespective of their refractive error. However, a myopic individual may compensate for presbyopia by removing the lens that corrects the distance vision. Near vision is poorer in a hyperopic individual if the spectacles that correct the hyperopia are removed.

The chief symptom of presbyopia is inability to see near work distinctly, which is aggravated in dim illumination and with attempts to read small print. The individual is frequently annoyed at having to place reading matter farther away from the eyes than previously. The need to use nearly all accommodation for clear near vision may cause ocular discomfort. There are no external signs of presbyopia except the general appearance that indicates the individual is more than 40 years of age.

Presbyopia is treated by means of convex lenses added to the distance correction. The power of the lens required for clear vision for near work varies with an individual's habits, age, occupation, length of arms, and the distance the patient prefers to see near work clearly. Generally, the weakest possible convex lenses are prescribed to permit the individual to carry on vocational and avocational tasks. Bifocal or trifocal (multifocal) lenses are prescribed not as an additional burden to middle-aged persons, but so that it will not be necessary to wear separate lenses for near and for far vision. If an individual requires lenses for distance, bifocal or trifocal lenses should be worn as early as they are indicated. An individual who does not become accustomed to bifocal lenses relatively early in the development of presbyopia frequently has unnecessary symptoms when multifocal lenses are prescribed in later years. If distance lenses are not required, an individual may get along well with lenses, such as half glasses, that correct the presbyopia solely. Nonetheless, because of the restricted focus of reading lenses, many individuals who do not need a distance correction wear multifocal lenses so that distant objects can be seen without removing the lenses.

APHAKIA

When the crystalline lens is not in the visual axis, rays of light entering the eye are refracted solely by the cornea. Surgical removal of the lens is the usual cause of aphakia, but dislocation of the lens out of the pupillary area may occur in systemic disease, such as Marfan syndrome, or after trauma. Since the lens is one of the two refracting portions of the eye, its removal causes severe hyperopia and a loss of accommodation.

The chief symptom is decreased vision for both far and near. Since accommodation is not possible, there are no symptoms of ocular discomfort.

The condition may be diagnosed by the loss of the reflected image from the surface of the lens and by excessive movement of the iris because of loss of support by the anterior lens capsule (iridodonesis).

Aphakia is corrected today by means of an intraocular lens placed immediately behind the iris after an extracapsular cataract extraction (see Chapter 22), which preserves the posterior lens capsule. Sometimes vision is good for both near and far without glasses, but usually an additional convex lens is required for near work.

When aphakia of one eye is corrected with ordinary spectacle lenses, usually having a power of about 10 diopters, the image in the aphakic eye is 25% to 33% larger than in the fellow eye. If the fellow eye has normal vision, single binocular vision is usually not possible because of the difference in size of the retinal images (aniseikonia). The difference in image size may be reduced to somewhat less than 10% by means of a contact lens.

Intraocular lenses are usually inserted at the time of cataract extraction. An extracapsular lens extraction with implantation of a posterior chamber intraocular lens is usually performed. A secondary implant is made in aphakic eyes, usually eyes that have had an intracapsular lens extraction. Intraocular lenses provide a normal-sized image and obviate the optical problems of aphakia.

ANISOMETROPIA

Anisometropia is that condition in which the refractive error of each eye is different. Minor differences are nearly universal, but when there is a difference of more than 2 diopters, the difference in the size of the image in each eye may cause symptoms. Often such patients are asymptomatic until bifocal lenses are prescribed. When the eyes rotate downward to use the bifocal segment, the difference in power of the two lenses induces a vertical prism, so that one ocular image is above the other. This may cause a vertical diplopia and severe ocular symptoms that may be neutralized by prescribing the appropriate prism in the reading segment or by using separate lenses for near and distance.

Severe anisometropia is a common cause of amblyopia (see Chapter 23) because of the developing infant's failure to use the eye with the greater refractive error. Failure of central vision to develop leads to strabismus. Even when the visual acuity can be corrected to normal with lenses, binocular vision may fail to develop, and the anisometropia produces no symptoms, because the retinal image from one eye is suppressed.

Aniseikonia.—Aniseikonia is that optical condition in which the size or shape of the retinal images of the two eyes are different. A difference of 0.5 diopter in the refractive error gives a retinal image size difference of about 1%. Most individuals can tolerate a difference of up to 5% without ocular discomfort. Symptoms result from aniseikonia only if binocular vision is present. Thus, many individuals who have markedly different refractive errors in the two eyes do not have symptoms because they suppress the image in one eye. Patients may prefer to use only one eye when reading or watching moving objects. All symptoms are entirely eliminated by covering one eye, as is true of all disorders of binocular vision.

MEASUREMENT OF THE REFRACTIVE ERROR

The amount of refractive error may be estimated by many methods. There may be typical ophthalmoscopic signs in myopia, but the severity of ametropia cannot be measured accurately by means of the ophthalmoscope.

Ophthalmoscopy.—The estimation of ametropia by means of the ophthalmoscope is not accurate. In hyperopia the disk may appear smaller than normal, and a pseudopapilledema may occasionally be present. In myopia the disk may appear larger than normal. In degenerative myopia a scleral myopic crescent may be present, there may be attenuation of the retinal pigment epithelium with a prominent choroidal pattern, and there may be areas of pigment proliferation. In astigmatism the optic disk may appear oval rather than round.

Retinoscopy.—Retinoscopy (skiaskopy) is an objective method of measurement of the refractive error. A skilled retinoscopist is able to measure refractive errors rapidly and exactly. The basic principle is to substitute lenses in front of the patient's eye so that merging rays of light reflected from the retina are brought to a focus at the examiner's eye. The light is directed into the patient's eye by the rays of a light source that has an aperture for observation. It is the single most useful method of measuring ametropia. It is most useful in children and in individuals who have poor discrimination or who respond slowly.

Automated refracting instruments combine electronic sensors and microcomputers to measure the refractive error either objectively or subjectively. Generally the results are similar to those obtained by retinoscopy.

Subjective methods.—Subjective methods for estimating refractive errors depend on the patient's responses to changes in lenses. In one method, called fogging, a convex lens, much in excess of that required for distinct vision, is placed in front of the eyes until accommodation relaxes. The power of the convex lens is then gradually reduced until vision is at about the level of 20/40. The patient's attention may then be directed to an astigmatic dial and a concave cylinder placed with its axis at right angles to the axis described as darkest. Subjective testing requires discrimination of moderately small changes in vision by an individual who has moderately rapid reaction times. It is most accurate in patients who are presbyopic.

Keratometry.—The keratometer is an instrument used to measure the radius of curvature (K reading) of the anterior surface of the central optical portion of the cornea. In principle it measures the size of the corneal image of an object of known size that is a fixed distance from the cornea. It is used in contact lens fitting and is combined with ultrasonography before cataract extraction to determine the refractive power of an intraocular lens to be inserted surgically.

Corneal tomography provides a record in colors of the curvature of the entire anterior surface of the cornea. The information is particularly useful in planning surgical correction of astigmatism before keratotomy.

Cycloplegia.—As has been seen, accommodation may increase the refractive power of the eye by as much as 15 diopters. Paralysis of accommodation by means of drugs (cycloplegia) permits measurement of the refractive error uncomplicated by changes in accommodation. Cycloplegia is indicated in children, in patients with strabismus, in patients in whom active accommodation makes accurate measurement of the refractive error difficult, and in patients with cloudy ocular media in whom accurate retinoscopy is not possible through the undilated pupil. Cyclopentolate (Cyclogyl 0.5%) is used in infants and children, and often tropicamide (Mydriacyl 1%) is used in adults.

Since ophthalmoscopic examination of the retinal periphery is not possible through the undilated pupil, many practitioners insist that a complete ocular examination include pupillary dilation and study of the peripheral retina by means of an indirect ophthalmoscope (see Chapter 17). Phenylephrine eyedrops (2.5%) dilate the pupil without reducing accommodation. Pupillary dilation may induce acute angle-closure glaucoma in patients with shallow anterior chambers. The practitioner should be assured that the pupils of patients with shallow anterior chambers are constricted after dilation for ophthalmoscopic examination.

OPTICAL DEVICES

Lenses may provide correction for hyperopia, myopia, astigmatism, presbyopia, and muscle balance. They may be impact resistant, tinted, polarized, antireflective, or various combinations.

Spectacles generally have the following functions: (1) improvement of vision by correction of refractive errors; (2) relief of symptoms by decreasing the amount of accommodation required for clear vision; (3) prismatic alignment of the visual axes in patients with exotropia or nonaccommodative esotropia or correction of an abnormal accommodative-convergence ratio (see Chapter 23); (4) magnification of the retinal image to compensate for subnormal vision; and (5) protection of the eye from mechanical trauma or radiant energy.

Lenses are prescribed to relieve the symptoms that result from astigmatism, to reduce the excessive accommodative effort that may be required in hyperopia, or to improve vision in myopia. Lenses are prescribed to correct anomalies of divergence or convergence that result from disorders of accommodative convergence and cause intermittent crossing of an eye with loss of binocular vision.

Spectacles do not induce or prevent refractive errors. Although there may be no improvement in visual acuity, accommodative esotropia may be corrected by an appropriate lens. Some individuals prefer blurred vision to wearing spectacles, whereas others choose contact lenses. Some individuals complain of ocular discomfort but refuse to wear the lenses that would relieve their symptoms; there is no help for them.

Impact-resistant lenses.—All optical lenses sold in the United States, unless specifically excluded by the prescriber, must be tested to resist the impact of a ⅝-inch-diameter steel ball dropped from a height of 50 inches. Impact-resistant glass lenses are either chemically treated or case-hardened by heating followed by rapid cooling. Plastic lenses do not shatter, but those made of polymethylmethacrylate scratch easily, whereas polycarbonate plastics are exceptionally scratch- and impact-resistant. Industrial safety lenses must be at least 5 mm thick and mounted in an industrial-type frame that minimizes backward displacement of the lens.

Absorptive and reflective lenses.—All spectacle lenses transmit, absorb, and reflect electromagnetic energy. A crown glass spectacle lens absorbs short ultraviolet (ultraviolet B: 290 to 320 nm), transmits about 20% of long ultraviolet (ultraviolet A: 320 to 400 nm), and transmits nearly all visible light (400 to 700 nm) and infrared (700 to 10,000 nm).

Glass and plastic lenses may be coated or impregnated with metallic oxides to reflect or absorb different regions of visible light, ultraviolet rays, and infrared rays selectively. Antireflective lenses are coated with a thin layer of magnesium fluoride that reduces reflections from the surface of lenses. Mirrored surfaces reduce the transmission of light by about 75%. Polaroid lenses, which absorb plane-polarized sun rays reflected from flat surfaces, are used by motorists and fishermen. Photosensitive lenses contain silver salts that darken in ultraviolet and lighten indoors. They strongly absorb ultraviolet.

Generally, strongly tinted green, yellow, neutral gray, and brown lenses effectively filter out ultraviolet rays. Blue-tinted lenses absorb ultraviolet poorly. Neutral gray lenses reduce light transmission, do not impair color values, and are used for color-deficient individuals. Yellow-tinted lenses are good haze filters (haze has a high proportion of blue light) and are used by hunters.

Lenses with light transmissions between 5% and 20% provide much comfort to patients with albinism, cone degeneration, aniridia, mydriasis, and photophobia caused by keratitis, uveitis, or keratoconjunctivitis sicca. Cataract is more common in individuals exposed to high levels of ultraviolet rays for prolonged periods, and such individuals should wear protective lenses. Short-term exposure to ultraviolet radiation, as with a sunlamp, may cause a painful keratitis. Infrared radiation is absorbed by the cornea and by protective lenses, which then act as a secondary source of radiation. Thus, the steel and glass industries use manufacturing methods to protect the worker.

Lenses that reduce light transmission should not be worn at night. Lenses designed for industrial protection should be used only within that industry since they may markedly reduce visual acuity.

Many authorities believe that excessive exposure to sunlight is an etiologic factor in age-related macular degeneration and age-related cataract. Dark-skinned and brown-eyed individuals are mainly spared susceptibility to malignant melanoma of the skin, which is responsible for 42,000 deaths a year in the United States. Possibly, these individuals are also less susceptible to sunlight-induced ocular disorders. In the United States there are millions of fair-skinned, blue-eyed individuals, mainly descendants of Northern Europeans who now live in sun-drenched regions. Many have been exposed to excessive sunlight for decades. When such individuals develop age-related ocular disorders or cutaneous malignancies, the practitioner may attribute their development to previous exposure to sunlight. Similar conditions, however, develop in individuals who have lived in regions of limited sunlight, and the practitioner often has no means of learning their cause. Wearing protective eyewear and broad-brimmed hats to protect the eyes, using topical sunscreens, and avoiding excessive sunlight to protect the skin are sensible precautions but difficult to inculcate in a sun-worshipping populace (see Chapter 8).

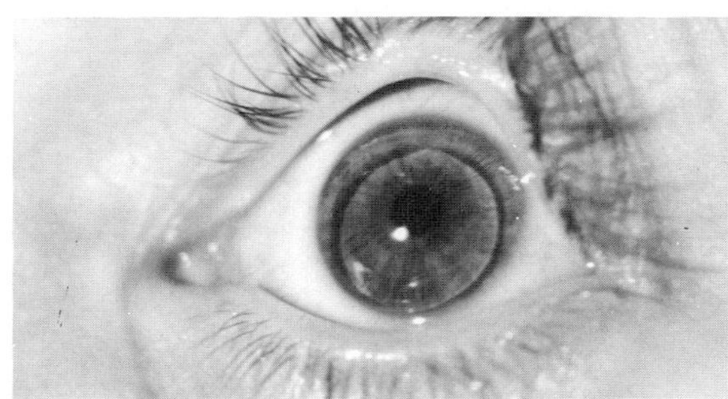

FIG 24-11.
Corneal contact lens. The lens floats on the precorneal tear film. It is outlined by shadows.

Contact lenses.—Contact lenses are worn beneath the eyelids anterior to the cornea (Figs 24-11 and 24-12) and sometimes anterior to both the cornea and sclera. They may be hard (rigid) or soft. They are used to neutralize ametropia, to protect the healing cornea, to conceal unsightly damaged eyes, and to deliver medications to the eye. They vary in diameter from 7.0 mm (corneal) to 15 mm (scleral). Soft lenses are flexible and permeable to the atmosphere so that they do not deprive the cornea of the oxygen required to maintain its transparency. Hard lenses are rigid or semiflexible and the older types are not permeable to atmospheric oxygen, which limits their wearing time.

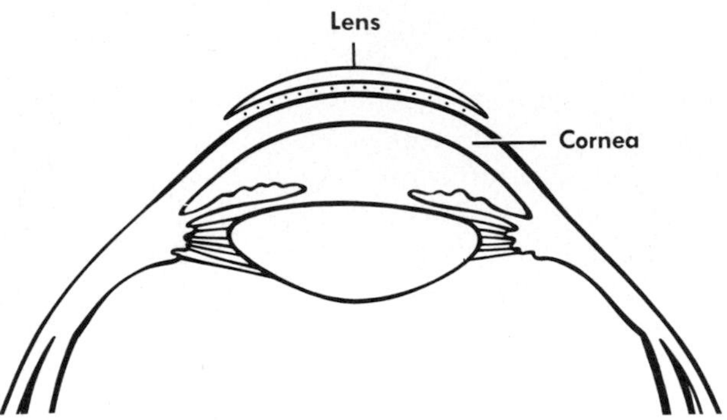

FIG 24-12.
An aspheric contact lens with a back surface that parallels the surface of the eye.

Contact lenses are not appropriate for children unable to manage the lens hygiene, including insertion and removal of the lens. Contact lenses should not be used by individuals who have recurrent conjunctival or corneal infections; anesthetic corneas; inadequate tears; multiple allergies; or are exposed to excessive dirt, dust, or smoke.

Hard contact lenses have good optics; offer clear, crisp vision; are durable; and are relatively easy to clean. They correct major errors of refraction, are available in bifocals, and may neutralize moderate degrees of astigmatism. They are available either as gas permeable or non–gas permeable; the former are more comfortable but more expensive than the latter. Patients must adjust to their use, and they are seldom suitable for intermittent wear. After extended wear, they modify the corneal curvature so that, after their removal, spectacle-corrected vision may be blurred for 7 to 10 days.

Soft contact lenses are more comfortable, require little adjustment to their use, and are easier to insert and remove than hard lenses, but are more fragile. Patients adapt readily to them, and they are suitable for intermittent wear. They do not correct astigmatism and provide poorer corrected vision than do hard lenses. Extended-wear soft contact lenses may be worn for periods of up to 7 days without removal. Because of the risk of infection, however, daily removal and cleansing is recommended.

Soft contact lenses are hydrophilic and absorb lens cleaning solutions, topical medications, and chlorinated water in swimming pools and slowly release them into the eye. They stain with topical epinephrine, fluorescein, and rose bengal solutions.

Successful wear of soft or hard contact lenses requires careful, intelligent personal hygiene and cleaning of the lenses. Eye makeup must be removed daily. If creams or oils are used to remove makeup, they must be thoroughly removed from eyes, eyelids, and hands before removing lenses. The eyelashes, eyelids, and hands must be thoroughly cleaned before lenses are inserted. Lenses should be stored in a clean storage case containing a sterile washing solution. Instructions for cleaning soft contact lenses must be followed meticulously. Careless hygiene of contact lenses or failure to remove them at night may result in severe fungal or bacterial keratitis.

Some individuals who would benefit from contact lenses are not sufficiently motivated to wear them successfully. Individuals should not be given contact lenses if they cannot remove them or do not wish to remove them for cleaning. Some elderly patients cannot handle or see their lenses, and their eyes are frequently dry. Contact lenses should not be worn by patients with conjunctivitis, keratitis, marginal blepharitis, anesthetic corneas, or dacryocystitis. Patients who damage their eyes repeatedly while using contact lenses should not wear them.

Soft scleral contact lenses with a diameter of 15 mm (bandage lenses) are used to protect the cornea in the treatment of recurrent epithelial erosions, ocular cicatricial pemphigoid, and alkali burns. Collagen corneal shields that dissolve in 12, 24, or 72 hours may be treated to release medication into eyes with keratitis. Lenses with an iris and pupil painted on the surface may be used to conceal scarred, unsightly blind eyes. Tinted lenses may be used to change the apparent color of an eye, or a lens may be used to conceal an iris coloboma.

Giant papillary conjunctivitis is a condition in which wearers of (usually) soft contact lenses develop increasing ocular discomfort and itching when wearing their lenses. Eversion of the upper eyelid discloses giant papillae. The cause is unknown but may be a hypersensitivity to lens deposits or irritation to the conjunctiva. The patient must discontinue the use of soft contact lenses and substitute hard, gas-permeable contact lenses. A different system of lens cleaning must be used, thimerosal preservatives must be avoided, and the patient must follow a meticulous lens cleaning method. The condition may persist for months, and it may be necessary to stop wearing contact lenses.

Superficial new blood vessels may extend a millimeter or so onto the peripheral cornea in wearers of soft contact lenses. The condition is of no clinical significance. New blood vessels in the stroma or extending beyond the perilimbal region are best treated by use of a hard, gas-permeable lens that is removed each night at bedtime.

Infectious agents may be introduced into the cornea through epithelial abrasions caused by a contact lens. Contact lenses that are worn night and day for long periods are particularly liable to induce infection. Ocular infections may be erroneously neglected by those who believe their symptoms are caused by wearing contact lenses.

Visual aids for the partially sighted.— Subnormal vision may be aided by various telescopes for distance vision and magnifying devices that increase the size of the retinal image. The two basic devices are (1) a Galilean telescope to bring the object closer to the observer and (2) an optical device to bring the observer closer to the object, usually by means of a magnifier lens. This may be in the form of a spectacle lens, stand magnifier, projection magnifier, or television reader. A reading addition of +5 diopters added to the distance correction brings close work near to the eye and often provides unusually effective magnification.

Diagnosis of the ocular condition that causes reduced vision and an understanding of the occupational needs of the individual must be correlated with the selection of the type of correction. Some patients may benefit from dilation of the pupil or pupillary constriction. Many practitioners lack the patience, special equipment, and optical devices required for testing.

A hand magnifier may be extremely useful. Some patients benefit from the use of a jeweler's loupe. Successful use of reading aids is correlated with the cause of loss of vision and the motivation and personality of the patient. Patients with visual reduction caused by vitreous hemorrhage and retinitis proliferans do poorly compared with those who have isolated central retinal lesions. Optimistic, self-reliant patients accept optical aids much better than those who are hostile, pessimistic, and sedentary.

BIBLIOGRAPHY

Books

Bennett E: *Contact lens problem solving,* St Louis, 1995, Mosby–Year Book.

Bennett ES, Henry VA: *Clinical manual of contact lenses,* Philadelphia, 1994, Lippincott-Raven.

Curtin BJ: *The myopias. Basic science and clinical management,* Philadelphia, 1985, JB Lippincott.

Kastl PR, editor: *Contact lenses. The CLAO guide of basic science and clinical practice,* vols I, II, III, IV, New York, 1995, CLAO.

Ruben M, Guillon M, editors: *Contact lens practice,* London, 1994, Chapman & Hall Medical.

Article

Krueger RR, Talamo JH, McDonald MB, Varnell RJ, Wagoner MD, McDonnell PJ: Clinical analysis of excimer laser photorefractive keratectomy using a multiple zone technique for severe myopia, *Am J Ophthalmol* 119:263-274, 1995.

PART IV

SYSTEMIC DISEASES AND THE EYE

25

INFLAMMATION, IMMUNOLOGY, AND MICROBIOLOGY

The skin of the eyelids forms an effective mechanical barrier to microbial invasion; organisms (except papovavirus [warts]) can penetrate only through a break in the skin or through an arthropod vector. The glands of the margin of the eyelid may become infected if their excretory ducts are blocked and the increased moisture may favor colonization of pathogenic organisms. The conjunctiva provides the same defenses as other mucous membranes. The tight junctions of the intact corneal epithelium prevent the penetration of fluids, and its smooth surface prevents adherence of microorganisms. The orbital fascia effectively prevents suppuration of the external eye from penetrating the orbit proper, but infections may rupture into the orbit through the thin walls of the nasal accessory sinuses or may be introduced through a penetrating injury. The intraocular contents may be affected by suppurative infections (endophthalmitis and panophthalmitis), or granulomatous disease (sarcoidosis), or may participate in a variety of immune reactions (retinitis, choroiditis).

Despite constant exposure and moisture that favor microbial survival, the cornea and conjunctiva are protected by a number of systems that neutralize this innate susceptibility to infection. Evaporation of tears reduces the temperature of the ocular surface and inhibits microbial growth. (Patching an infected eye provides an incubator for microbial growth.) Every few seconds the eyelids close and sweep across the exposed cornea and conjunctiva, keeping them moist and renewing the tear film. Blinking sweeps away microorganisms on the surface of the eye and does not allow them to adhere to epithelial cells and colonize. The desmosomes of the epithelial cells combined with their basement membrane prevent colonization of microorganisms or inhibit extension if colonization begins. The heterogeneous, indigenous microbial flora of the ocular surfaces (mainly *Staphylococcus epidermidis*, *Haemophilus* sp., and *Staphylococcus aureus*) may minimize the opportunity for other microorganisms to adhere and colonize. Microflora may compete for attachment sites and nutrients, produce products toxic to foreign organisms, and stimulate the immune system to express class II histocompatibility (DR) molecules on macrophages.

Tears mechanically dilute the concentration of microorganisms on the ocular surface and wash them into the lacrimal drainage system. Immunoglobulin A (IgA) is synthesized by the lacrimal gland (secretory IgA) as well as plasma cells of the bone marrow. It neutralizes viruses and inhibits bacterial adherence to the conjunctiva. The lactoferrin of tears chelates iron required for bacterial growth. The lysozyme (muramidase) of tears has a limited bacteriolytic action but its action is enhanced by complement, which damages bacterial cell walls.

Microorganisms may invade the conjunctiva and cornea from adjacent tissues or may be deposited by flies, fingers, contact lenses, cosmetics, contaminated eyedrops, or surgical instruments. A minor injury may disrupt the continuity of the epithelial surfaces, and microorganisms may adhere to the disrupted cell layer and colonize.

The environment influences the type of external eye disease in a community. Trachoma is prevalent in dry, hot deserts where flies abound and personal hygiene is poor. Onchocerciasis blinds thousands in the rain forests of Africa and Central America where the black fly is prevalent. Suppurative keratitis from bacterial, fungal, or amebic infection occurs after the commensal organisms or defense mechanisms have been disturbed by exposure, trauma, eyelid dysfunction, topical medications, or immune suppression.

INFLAMMATION

Inflammation is the reaction of living tissue to injury. The injury may be infectious (bacterial, viral, fungal, parasitic, or rickettsial); immune; ischemic; or traumatic (mechanical, electromagnetic, or chemical). Inflammation involves complex alterations of blood vessels and the localization of fluids and blood cells, particularly leukocytes. It is closely related to the process of repair. A variety of cells (Table 25-1) and chemical mediators (Table 25-2) may be involved.

Acute inflammation is the immediate (seconds to minutes), transient (3 to 5 hours) vascular and cellular response to injury. An initial vasoconstriction is followed by increased blood flow (vasodilation). Increased vascular permeability results in swelling of the injured tissues with the accumulation of plasma and leukocytes. For 24 to 48 hours neutrophils predominate, but they are then replaced by monocytes. Acute inflammation may (1) subside; (2) form an abscess; (3) heal with scarring; or (4) become chronic. Chronic inflammations may be either nongranulomatous or granulomatous. A nongranulomatous chronic inflammation is characterized initially by a cellular infiltrate of lymphocytes and macrophages that occurs in some instances of iridocyclitis. With time, macrophages are converted to epithelioid cells or giant cells (fused macrophages), surrounded by lymphocytes, plasma cells, and proliferating fibroblasts. Sometimes macrophages form the small (2-mm maximum dimension) nodule that characterizes a granulomatous inflammation.

The major cellular elements of inflammation include the leukocytes (granulocytes and lymphocytes), the auxiliary cells, and the mononuclear phagocytes. The chief chemical mediators include the major histocompatibility complex, complement, the cytokines involved in immune inflammations, and the immunoglobulins.

TABLE 25-1.
Cells Involved in Inflammation and Immune Reactions

- Leukocytes
  - Phagocytes
    - Granulocytes
      - Polymorphonuclear neutrophils
      - Eosinophils
    - Lymphocytes
      - B cells
      - T cells (CD4+)
        - Class II major histocompatibility complex
          - Restricted
        - Cytotoxic T cells (CD8+)
          - Class I major histocompatibility complex
            - Restricted
      - Large granular (natural killer; null) cells
- Auxiliary cells
  - Basophils
  - Mast cells
- Mononuclear phagocytes
  - Microphages (monocytes) (intravascular)
- Multinuclear phagocytes
  - Macrophages (tissues)
    - Epithelioid cells
    - Giant cells
    - Dendritic cells (lymphoid tissue)
    - Langerhans cells (skin)
    - Histiocytes (connective tissue)

Leukocytes

Phagocytic granulocytes.—The neutrophils and eosinophils are phagocytic granulocytes.

Neutrophils.—Neutrophils are the most numerous leukocyte; the normal adult produces some 80 million new neutrophils each minute. In the circulation their half-life is 6 to 7 hours. The cells mature in the bone marrow, and only enough are produced as are necessary for physiologic functions. The mature cell contains lysosomal factors that kill gram-negative bacteria and polypeptides (defensins) with antimicrobial activity against bacteria, fungi, and some viruses. In infection and immune processes, neutrophils are mobilized from the bone marrow by the complement factor $C3_e$, interleukin-1, tu-

TABLE 25-2.
Some Chemical Mediators in Inflammation

Histamine (mainly from basophils and mast cells)
Serotonin (mainly from platelets)
Platelet activating factor (from basophils, neutrophils, macrophages)
  Released platelet mediator: increased vascular permeability; neutrophil activation; smooth-muscle contraction
Neutrophil chemotaxis
Kinin system
  Hageman factor of blood clotting stimulates bradykinin
  Tissue injury or fibrinolytic (plasmin) system stimulates kallidin, which generates bradykinin and lysylbradykinin
  Dilation of veins; increased vascular permeability; smooth-muscle contraction
Complement
  Classic pathway (antibody activated)
  Alternate pathway (microorganism activated)
  Mast cell degranulation
    Histamine; leukotrienes; prostaglandins; thromboxanes
Arachidonic acid metabolites
  Cyclo-oxygenase pathway
    Prostaglandin E2
  Lipoxygenase pathway
    Leukotriene B4
    Leukotriene D4
Cytokines (active in immune-mediated inflammation)
  Interferon-gamma
    Macrophage activation
    Differentiation of T and B lymphocytes
    Increased class I major histocompatibility complex expression
  Lymphotoxin (tumor necrosis factor-beta)
  Interleukin-10, -5, -12
  Migration inhibition factor

mor necrosis factor-α, the colony-stimulating factor, and cytokines. The neutrophils adhere to the endothelium of capillaries in the region of an inflammatory stimulus and then migrate into the tissues. Immunoglobulin G (IgG) mobilizes neutrophils and complement to generate chemotactic factors that phagocytize pathogenic material. After 1 to 4 days the neutrophils die and are replaced by monocytes.

Eosinophils.—Eosinophils share many functions with neutrophils but have a longer life than neutrophils and have no active role in infections, except those caused by invasive parasites. They are primarily bound in tissues together with mast cells bearing immunoglobulin E (IgE). Unlike neutrophils, eosinophils may recirculate. The eosinophil's granule contains a peroxidase that oxidizes many substances, including microorganisms and a major basic protein with histaminase activity. They modulate the reaction of immediate hypersensitivity, asthma, and cutaneous allergies and are a major factor in immunity to parasitic infection.

Lymphocytes.—Lymphocytes consist of (1) B cells (for bursa of Fabricius derived cells; often designated as bone marrow derived, where they mature together with other constituents of blood); (2) T cells (for thymus maturation cells); and (3) large granular lymphocytes, which lack the surface markers of T cells and B cells.

B cells.—B lymphocytes produce antibodies (immunoglobulins). Their surface antigen receptors are membrane-bound antibodies, which are activated by soluble antigens to produce effector cells that secrete antibodies.

T cells.—T lymphocytes are stimulated by peptide antigens attached to proteins encoded by the major histocompatibility complex to secrete cytokines (lymphokines). Cytokines are protein hormones that promote the proliferation and differentiation of T cells, B cells, and inflammatory cells. They are divided on the basis of their surface markers into helper cells (CD4), cytolytic cells (CD8), and many more. (CD is the abbreviation for cluster of differentiation and describes the group of monoclonal antibodies, which characterize surface molecules of various cells. Some 110 are described.) T4+ lymphocytes that respond to antigens presented by class II major histocompatibility complex surface proteins are helper cells. They secrete the cytokines interferon-gamma, lymphotoxin-2, and interleukin-2. These cytokines generate a strong intracellular immune reaction against intracellular pathogens. T8+ cells that respond to antigens presented by class I major histocompatibility complex surface proteins are classed as cytolytic. They secrete the cytokines interleukin-4, -5, -9, -10, and -13. These cytokines promote the development of a humoral response by B lymphocytes to generate specific responses against extracellular pathogens.

Large granular lymphocytes.—Large granular lymphocytes (natural killer cells or null cells) lyse tumor cells and virus-infected cells by a mechanism that does not involve antigens.

TABLE 25-3.
HLA Antigens Associated with Ocular Disorders

Systemic Disorder	HLA Antigen	Ocular Disorder
HLA class I–associated disease		
Ankylosing spondylitis	B27	Uveitis
Reiter disease	B27	Uveitis or retinitis
Acute-onset uveitis	B27	Acute anterior uveitis
Sympathetic ophthalmia	A11	Bilateral uveitis
Birdshot retinochoroidopathy	A29	Bilateral uveitis
Behçet disease	B51	Ophthalmopathy
HLA class II–associated disease		
Sjögren syndrome	DQB1*0201	Keratoconjunctivitis
Graves ophthalmopathy	DR3	Thyroid ophthalmopathy
Insulin-dependent diabetes	DR3	Ophthalmopathy
Myasthenia gravis	DR3	Ocular muscle weakness
Multiple sclerosis	DRB1*1501; DQB1*0602	Optic neuritis, retinopathy
Optic neuritis	DRB1*1501	Optic neuritis
Rheumatoid arthritis	DR4	Keratoconjunctivitis sicca

They do not mature in the thymus and are activated by cytokines produced by CD4 lymphocytes and other mechanisms.

Basophils and mast cells.—These are auxiliary cells, the basophils being the circulating counterpart of tissue-bound mast cells. Both types of cells bind IgE and secrete their granules, the effector mediators of immediate hypersensitivity. Mast cells are divided into two phenotypes: (1) mucosal-bound in the gastrointestinal tract and (2) connective tissue–bound in the lung and serosal tissues.

Mononuclear phagocytes

The mononuclear phagocytic system consists of monocytes within circulating blood, which enter tissues to differentiate into macrophages ("big eaters"). Macrophages in connective tissue are histiocytes, Langerhans cells in the skin, dendritic cells in lymphoid tissues, and microglia in the nervous system. Within a granuloma, macrophages are modified into epithelioid cells, and Langerhans cells are modified into giant cells. Their proliferation is governed by interferon-gamma produced by CD4+ lymphocytes (T-helper cells).

The major histocompatibility complex (human leukocyte antigen system, HLA).—The surface of nearly every nucleated cell, except the corneal endothelium and some embryonic cells, contains peptide markers that characterize every protein contained within the cell. The peptides are cradled in a groove on the surface of molecules encoded by the major histocompatibility complex or human leukocyte antigen system (HLA), which is located on the short arm of chromosome 6, band p21.3. It encodes two general classes of molecules, class I and class II.

Class I molecules are present on virtually all nucleated cells, while class II molecules are normally expressed only on B lymphocytes and macrophages (see Table 25-1). Antigens associated with class I molecules (HLA-A, HLA-B, and HLA-C) are recognized by CD8+ cytolytic lymphocytes. These lymphocytes are the principal immunologic defense mechanism against viruses and tumors. They ensure that any cell synthesizing viral or mutant proteins is marked for recognition and destruction by CD8+ cells.

Class II–associated antigens (HLA-DP, HLA-DQ, and HLA-DR) are recognized by CD4+ helper T lymphocytes only after accessory cells (macrophages and dendritic cells) have converted the antigens of the proteins to peptides (antigen processing) combined with stimulation of the CD4+ cells. The response of T cell activation by a peptide plus the major histocompatibility complex is as follows: (1) activation of a variety of genes; (2) expression of new surface molecules; (3) cytolysis of viruses or tumor cells or the secretion of effector cytokines; and (4) proliferation of cells specifically directed against the peptide that originated the signal.

There are about 20 different allelic combinations at the HLA-A locus, about 30 at the HLA-B locus, and 6 at the HLA-C locus. There are about 11 HLA-DP, HLA-DQ, and HLA-

DR loci. Specific combinations of HLA loci occur together more frequently than expected by chance (linkage disequilibrium). Thus, in white individuals, HLA-A1, HLA-B8, and HLA-Dw3 combination occurs much more frequently than predicted by the gene frequencies of these alleles in the population. Susceptibility to many rheumatic disorders, particularly sacroiliitis, spondylitis, and Reiter syndrome, is associated with HLA-B27 (Table 25-3). Not all individuals with the haplotype develop the disorder, and not everyone with the disorder has the haplotype.

Complement.—The complement system is composed of a series of functionally linked, heat labile, plasma proteins and membrane receptors that activate inflammation and mediate a humoral immunity response. (Complement lyses bacteria or erythrocytes coated with antibody and hence "complements" the lytic action of antibody.) The proteins of the complement system must first be activated by either the classic pathway or the alternative pathway to generate enzymes called C3 convertases. Only antigen-antibody complexes activate the classic pathway. The alternative pathway does not require antigen-antibody and may be considered an intrinsic amplification system of the complement system.

The principal biologic functions of the activated proteins of the complement system are as follows: (1) lysis of foreign organisms by polymerizing complement protein on the cell surface and disrupting the integrity of the cell membrane; (2) binding of complement protein (opsonins) to the cell surface followed by phagocytosis by leukocytes that express specific receptors for these opsonins; (3) proteolytic fragments of complement protein, which (a) degranulate mast cells causing the release of vasoactive amines of the immediate hypersensitivity reaction; and (b) enhance the antigenic responses of B lymphocytes; and (4) solubilizing immune complexes or clearing them from the circulation.

Cytokines.—Cytokines are protein hormones that mediate and regulate the immune and inflammatory responses of natural and acquired immunity. They are released by mononuclear cells and lymphocytes in response to contact with a specific antigen. Mononuclear phagocytes release cytokines (monokines) in microbial infection in natural immunity. Antigen-activated T lymphocytes produce cytokines (lymphokines) in the responses of specific immunity.

The cytokines released by mononuclear phagocytes in the responses of natural immunity to infectious agents are interferon-alpha and interferon-beta, tumor necrosis factor, interleukin-1, interleukin-6, and the leukocyte chemokinesis and chemotaxis molecules.

The cytokines of the specific immune response are divided into (1) those that regulate lymphocyte activation, growth, and differentiation; (2) those that regulate immune-mediated inflammation; and (3) those that regulate hematopoiesis.

Lymphocyte regulation is mainly provided by interleukin-2, interleukin-4, and transforming growth factor. Immune-mediated inflammation is mainly regulated by interferon-gamma, lymphotoxin, interleukin-10, -5, and -12, and the migration inhibition factor. Hematopoiesis is stimulated by c-kit ligand (stem cell factor), interleukin-3, granulocyte-macrophage colony-stimulating factor, monocyte-macrophage colony-stimulating factor, granulocyte colony-stimulating factor, and interleukin-7.

Antibodies.—Antibodies are protein molecules, called immunoglobulins, that specifically recognize and bind to antigens. They protect the individual against microbial infection and other agents that cause disease (the humoral immune system). There are five different classes of immunoglobulin: IgG, IgA, IgM, IgD, and IgE. On the basis of their concentration in the serum, there are four separate subclasses of IgG: IgG1 (60% to 70%); IgG2 (15% to 20%); IgG3 (5% to 8%); and IgG4 (1% to 5%). There are two subclasses of IgA: IgA1 and IgA2.

Most antibodies (as many as a billion different ones) belong to the IgG class, which are distributed equally between the blood and the tissues. IgG is present in both the tears and the aqueous humor. It has the longest half-life of the immunoglobulins. It is transferred across the placenta and provides immunity to the newborn infant during the first 4 to 6 months of life. The IgG1 and the IgG3 subclasses are the antibodies to protein antigens and the IgG2 to carbohydrate antigens. The first three activate the classic complement component of the immune response, and IgG4 activates the al-

TABLE 25-4.
Immunologic Disorders

Type of Hypersensitivity	Abnormal Immune Mechanism	Mechanism of Tissue Injury	Ocular Disorder
Type I	Immunoglobulin E (immediate)	Mast cell (IgE) mediated	Hay fever, vernal giant-cell conjunctivitis
Type II (antibody mediated)	Immunoglobulins M & G (IgM & IgG) against tissue cells and surface antigens	Complement activation of neutrophils & macrophages; abnormal receptors	Autoimmune diseases
Type III (immune-complex mediated)	Circulating antigen-antibodies (IgM & IgG)	Complement recruitment & activation of leukocytes	Chlamydial infection, *Staphylococcus* immune rings of cornea
Type IV (T lymphocyte mediated)	CD4+ lymphocytes	Activated macrophages & cytokines	Delayed hypersensitivity
	CD8+ lymphocytes	Cytolysis & cytokines	Target cell lysis

ternate pathway. Antibodies of the IgG class promote opsonization of microbes, and the IgG1 and IgG3 antigen-antibody complexes increase chemotaxis, phagocytosis, mediator release, and cytotoxicity.

Exocrine IgA is the major antibody of mucous membranes, including the conjunctiva. It consists of two IgA molecules joined by a secretory piece that is synthesized by the lacrimal gland and other local epithelial cells. The secretory piece (T piece for transport piece) prevents proteolysis of IgA and allows it to act as an antibody in fluids that contain proteolytic enzymes. IgA is not strongly bactericidal or bacteriostatic but may coat epithelial cells and prevent the entry of antigens from the surfaces of mucosal cells.

Immunoglobulin M (IgM) is the largest of the immunoglobulins (macroglobulin) and is confined to the bloodstream. It is the first antibody to be formed after exposure to an antigen. Its short half-life, however, prevents a sustained humoral immune response. Rheumatoid factor, isohemagglutinins (anti-A and anti-B), and the antibodies against gram-negative somatic antigen (O) are of the IgM type.

IgE is widely distributed to plasma cells in the mucosa of the gut, respiratory tract, and conjunctiva. It may function in the local immunity of mucosal surfaces. In allergies and parasitic diseases, IgE is bound to mast cells and basophils. Linkage of antigens to these antibodies degranulates the cells with the release of histamine, heparin, and other vasoactive amines of humoral hypersensitivity and anaphylaxis. The conjunctiva reacts in hay fever conjunctivitis and vernal conjunctivitis.

IgD is expressed on the surface of most B lymphocytes together with IgM. It may function in the clonal activation of B lymphocytes.

Immunologic disorders

An uncontrolled, excessive, or misdirected reaction of the immune system to antibodies, complement, or phagocytes (mainly mast cells) may induce a variety of disorders, often described as hypersensitivity reactions (Table 25-4). Immediate hypersensitivity is caused by immunoglobulin E degranulating mast cells with the release of their vasoactive amines. In type II hypersensitivity reactions (antibody mediated), IgM or IgG antibodies react either with an individual's own antigens (self-antigens) or with foreign antigens either deposited in self-antigens or cross-reactive with them to activate the complement system, neutrophils, and macrophages. In type III hypersensitivity reactions (immune-complex mediated), antibodies form immune complexes with circulating antigens and are deposited in tissues where they activate inflammatory mediators. Type IV hypersensitivity reactions (T-cell mediated) are of two types. In the delayed hypersensitivity type, activated CD4+ lymphocytes release cytokines and stimulate macrophages. In the cytolytic type, CD8+ lymphocytes lyse cells and release cytokines.

Immediate hypersensitivity.—Immediate hypersensitivity (anaphylactic hypersensitivity, type I hypersensitivity) is initiated by IgE stimulation of tissue mast cells and circulating basophils. When a specific antigen reacts with IgE on the surface of mast cells and basophils, they release histamine, eosinophil chemotactic factor, proteolytic enzymes (trypsin), and heparin. Histamine increases vascular permeability and contracts smooth muscle; trypsin activates complement; heparin inhibits blood coagulation; and eosinophils are attracted to the region.

When first exposed to an antigen, B lymphocytes produce IgE, which binds to the surface of mast cells and basophils. When the antigen is reintroduced, it binds to the IgE and the mast cells, and basophils release their mediators. Antigens include pollens, drugs (particularly penicillin), and microbial products, especially those of parasites and worms.

Hay fever conjunctivitis is a typical reaction in which there is massive conjunctival edema. Vernal conjunctivitis and giant-cell papillary conjunctivitis, in which basophils are prominent, and atopic keratoconjunctivitis are ocular examples of the immediate type of hypersensitivity. Asthma, anaphylaxis, urticaria, allergic rhinitis, and sinusitis are examples of systemic immediate hypersensitivity.

Antibody-mediated hypersensitivity.— Antibody-mediated hypersensitivity (type II) occurs mainly when IgM and IgG antibodies develop against an individual's own tissues or cell surfaces. The normal action of antibodies in neutralizing an antigen, activating the complement system, and recruiting inflammatory cells is then directed against an individual's own tissues. The reactions may be limited to a single tissue, as in autoimmune intraocular inflammations (see Chapter 19); ocular cicatricial pemphigoid (see Chapter 10); Sjögren syndrome (see Chapter 13); Graves disease (see Chapter 27); insulin-dependent diabetes mellitus (see Chapter 27); and myasthenia gravis (see Chapter 9). A number of other systemic disorders are secondary to related autoimmune mechanisms.

Immune complex disease (type III hypersensitivity).—Immune complexes normally form in response to a variety of microbial and foreign antigens and are rapidly phagocytized. Sometimes the antigen-antibody or antibody-antibody (rheumatoid factor, cryoglobulin) are deposited in a tissue and activate the complement system, causing an inflammation. Staphylococcal catarrhal keratitis, immune rings in the cornea, and chlamydial infections may reflect ocular immune complex deposition. Rheumatoid arthritis, vasculitis, and systemic lupus erythematosus are each caused by deposition of immune complexes in the tissues.

Delayed hypersensitivity (CD4+ lymphocyte mediated; CD8+ lymphocyte mediated); type IV.—Delayed hypersensitivity is mediated by T lymphocytes. CD4+ helper cells are responsible for delayed hypersensitivity reactions, and CD8+ cytotoxic cells are responsible for cell-mediated cytolysis. These lymphocytes activate mononuclear phagocytes (macrophages) as effector cells. The positive tuberculin skin test in an individual with healed primary tuberculosis is the classic example of delayed hypersensitivity. Delayed hypersensitivity reactions occur in transplant rejection, tuberculosis, and trachoma.

Cell-mediated cytolysis prevents proliferation of tumor cells. It may be demonstrated by the absence of delayed hypersensitivity (anergy) in patients with acquired immunodeficiency syndrome (AIDS) who have developed Kaposi sarcoma or in patients with malignant tumors.

BACTERIAL INFECTIONS

The bacterial kingdom, Procaryotae, is characterized by living organisms that do not have a membrane-bound nucleus or other intracellular organelles. A relatively rigid plasma membrane encloses cytoplasm that contains nucleoplasm with deoxyribonucleic acid (DNA) and ribosomes of the 70s type. The rigid cell wall gives a shape to the organism (spherical [cocci], cylindrical [bacilli], and helical [spirochetes]) and also stains typically with the Gram stain.

GRAM-POSITIVE BACTERIA

Gram-positive bacteria (Table 25-5) may be cocci or bacilli (rods), which may be sporulating or nonsporulating. The cocci include two important families: (1) the Micrococcaceae, which contains the widespread genus *Staphylococcus,* and (2) the Streptococcaceae, with the genus *Streptococcus,* which has many species. Gram-positive bacilli (rods) rarely cause ocular disease but are sometimes wrongly dismissed as contaminants, although pathogenic.

The most common gram-positive bacilli found on culture are members of the *Corynebacterium* group ("diphtheroid"). *Corynebacte-*

TABLE 25-5.
Gram-Positive Bacteria of Ophthalmic Interest

Family Micrococcaceae
- Genus *Micrococcus*
  - Species *M. luteus:* conjunctivitis
- Genus *Staphylococcus*
  - Species *S. aureus:* blepharitis; keratitis; panophthalmitis
  - Species *S. epidermidis:* blepharitis; sties; chalazion; endophthalmitis
- Genus *Streptococcus*
  - Species *S. pyogenes:* conjunctivitis
  - Species *S. pneumoniae;* hypopyon keratitis; dacryocystitis

Family Bacillaceae
- Genus *Bacillus*
  - Species *B. anthracis:* malignant pustule eyelid
  - Species *B. cereus:* panophthalmitis
- Genus *Clostridium*
  - Species *C. botulinuum:* food poisoning; N III and N VI paralysis
  - Species *C. tetani:* tetanus; panophthalmitis
  - Species *C. perfringens:* keratitis; endophthalmitis

Family Lactobacillaceae
- Genus *Listeria*
  - Species *L. monocytogenes:* keratitis; endophthalmitis; septicemia

Family Propionibacteriaceae
- Genus *Propionibacterium*
  - Species *P. acnes;* keratitis; endophthalmitis

Family Actinomycetaceae
- Genus *Actinomyces*
  - Species *A. israelii:* dacryocanaliculitis

Family Mycobacteriaceae (acid-fast)
- Genus *Mycobacterium*
  - Species *M. tuberculosis:* uveitis; phylctenules; periphlebitis
  - Species *M. leprae:* keratitis; anterior uveitis

Family Nocardiaceae
- Genus *Nocardia*
  - Species *N. asteroides (Leptothrix):* cat-scratch fever; keratitis

Coryneform bacteria
- Genus *Corynebacterium*
  - Species *C. diphtheriae:* postdiphtheritic paralysis
  - Species *C. xerosis:* foamy conjunctival secretion
  - Miscellaneous: "diphtheroids"

rium xerosis is found in the foamy secretion that collects at the canthi of the elderly. *Corynebacterium diphtheriae,* now a rarity because of immunization, was a cause of membranous conjunctivitis and postdiphtheritic oculomotor and abducent nerve paralysis. *Listeria monocytogenes* causes puerperal septicemia, and septicemia and meningitis in both newborn and the immune compromised patient. It is an important cause of a delayed postoperative endophthalmitis and keratitis. *Bacillus cereus,* a spore-forming gram-positive rod that is considered to be nonpathogenic, is a cause of a fulminating panophthalmitis in drug addicts and after penetrating injury of the eye. *Bacillus anthracis* causes anthrax and a malignant pustule of the eyelid.

Clostridium botulinum, a cause of food poisoning, releases a potent neurotoxin that paralyzes skeletal muscle including the muscles of the eyelids and eyes. Diplopia may be the first sign of systemic infection. The toxin is used in the treatment of ocular muscle palsies. *Clostridium tetani,* a spore-forming bacillus, is a cause of a devastating wound infection, largely prevented by prophylactic immunization and wound debridement. *Clostridium perfringens* is a cause of panophthalmitis and keratitis. *Propionibacterium acnes,* part of the normal microbial flora of the skin, may cause keratitis or endophthalmitis.

Staphylococci.—The staphylococci are gram-positive, catalase-positive spherical cocci that often appear in grapelike clusters in stained smears. Ocular smears, however, often show pairs and single cocci combined with many neutrophils. Three species are common: *S. aureus, S. epidermidis* (formerly *albus*), and *S. saprophyticus.* Most strains of *S. aureus* produce toxins (leukocidin, necrotoxin, and hyaluronidase), as do occasional strains of *S. epidermidis.* These two strains are differentiated by the usual golden color produced by *S. aureus* on solid culture media and its production of coagulase and other extracellular enzymes. Coagulase-negative staphylococci, mainly *S. pyogenes,* are relatively avirulent, but they contaminate implanted heart valves and hip prostheses.

Staphylococcal infection is common in chronic blepharitis, suppurative infection of the glands of Zeis (hordeolum or sty), and chalazia (meibomian gland). Catarrhal marginal ulcers of the cornea occur in staphylococcal conjunctivitis secondary to a type III hypersensitivity reaction to immune complexes of staphylococcal exotoxin.

Acute *Staphylococcus* conjunctivitis is less common than that caused by the *Streptococcus* and *Haemophilus* species. Most staphylococci found in hospitals produce beta-lactamases that inactivate all beta-lactam antibiotics, including the cephalosporins. Staphylococcal infections of the skin of the eyelids (see Chapter 9) do not require antibiotic treatment but respond to local skin hygiene.

Streptococci.—The streptococci are gram-positive, nonmotile, non–spore-forming, catalase-negative, spherical, ovoid, or lancet-shaped cocci that often occur in pairs (diplococci) or chains. Chain formation is uncommon in ocular infections, and bacteriologic diagnosis is based on the results of culture on blood agar to demonstrate hemolysis. Gram-stained streptococci may be confused with staphylococci. Pathologic strains of streptococci produce either partial (alpha) or complete (beta) hemolysis when cultured on blood agar. In contrast to staphylococcal infections that produce a purulent exudate, streptococcal infections usually produce a thin, watery exudate.

Streptococcus pyogenes (group A; beta-hemolytic) causes pharyngitis, impetigo, septicemia, conjunctivitis, keratitis, erysipelas, glomerulonephritis, scarlet fever, bronchopneumonia, puerperal sepsis, and postinfectious rheumatic fever. A streptococcal conjunctivitis may form a pseudomembrane and extend into the cornea with a stromal abscess and hypopyon. A post-streptococcal glomerulonephritis may cause vascular hypertension that affects the retinal blood vessels. After the onset of the rash in scarlet fever, severely ill patients may develop ecchymoses and petechiae. Erysipelas mainly affects the skin of the face and head of elderly persons. The affected areas are glistening red, swollen, and sometimes versicolored. The skin of the eyelids may be infected.

Streptococcus pneumoniae (the "pneumococcus") is alpha-hemolytic and serologically divided into 84 different serotypes, some of which are gathered into serogroups. Type 1 and types 3 to 8 are mainly implicated in lobar pneumonia in adults. Less pathogenic types are a part of the normal microbial flora of the respiratory tract. They are gram-positive, oval or spherical organisms that generally have tapered ends (lance-shaped) and grow in pairs.

The organism may cause an acute, mild conjunctivitis in children. An infected lacrimal sac in chronic dacryocystitis may serve as a reservoir for organisms that cause a pneumococcal keratitis.

TABLE 25-6.
Gram-Negative Bacteria of Ophthalmic Interest

- Family Neisseriaceae
  - Genus *Neisseria*
    - Species *N. gonorrhoeae:* ophthalmia neonatorum; purulent conjunctivitis
    - Species *N. meningitidis:* conjunctivitis; endophthalmitis
    - Species *N. sicca:* conjunctivitis
  - Genus *Moraxella*
    - Species *M. lacunata:* indolent ulcer; conjunctivitis
    - Species *M. nonliquefaciens:* indolent ulcer; conjunctivitis
    - Species *M. acinetobacter* (Tribe: Mimeae, sp. *polymorpha*): endophthalmitis; conjunctivitis
  - Subgenus *Branhamella*
    - Species *B. catarrhalis:* conjunctivitis
- Family Pseudomonadaceae
  - Genus *Pseudomonas*
    - Species *P. aeruginosa:* necrotic keratitis
- Family Bacteroidaceae
  - Genus *Haemophilus*
    - Species *H. influenzae:* conjunctivitis; orbital abscess (children)
    - Species *H. aegyptius* (Koch-Weeks bacilli): conjunctivitis
  - Genus *Bacteroides*
    - Species *B. fragilis:* endophthalmitis; keratitis
- Family Enterobacteriaceae
  - Genus *Escherichia:* keratitis; panophthalmitis
  - Genus *Salmonella:* iritis; keratitis; panophthalmitis
  - Genus *Klebsiella:* keratitis; panophthalmitis
  - Genus *Proteus:* keratitis; panophthalmitis
  - Genus *Yersinia*
    - Species *Y. pestis:* plague; hemorrhagic chemosis
- Unassigned family
  - Genus *Brucella:* uveitis?; optic neuritis?; nummular keratitis
    - Species *B. melitensis*
    - Species *B. abortus*
    - Species *B. suis*
  - Genus *Bordetella*
    - Species *B. pertussis:* conjunctival and retinal hemorrhages
  - Genus *Francisella*
    - Species *F. tularensis:* necrotic conjunctiva Parinaud ulcer)

GRAM-NEGATIVE BACTERIA

The cell walls of gram-negative bacteria (Table 25-6) are far more sensitive to cell wall disruption and generally less sensitive to antibiotics than those of gram-positive organisms. Neisseriaceae is the major family of gram-negative cocci and cocci-bacilli. It includes the genera *Neisseria, Moraxella* (with its subgenera *Moraxella* and *Branhamella*), *Acinetobacter,* and *Kingella. Pseudomonas aeruginosa,* the most frequently isolated human pathogen of the genus *Pseudomonas,* is an important cause of keratitis and hospital nosocomial infections. A large group of gram-negative facultatively anaerobic rods are normal inhabitants of the human large intestine. Included in this group are the genera *Escherichia* and *Klebsiella,* which are common causes of opportunistic infections. Additional genera are *Salmonella, Proteus,* and *Yersinia.* The genus *Haemophilus* (family Bacteroidaceae) includes *H. influenzae* and *H. aegyptius* (Koch-Weeks bacillus), which cause conjunctivitis.

Neisseria.—This genus includes two important disease-producing species, *N. gonorrhoeae* and *N. meningitidis,* each of which may cause conjunctivitis. Each produces a protease for IgA, the major immunoglobulin of the tears. *Branhamella catarrhalis* and *B. sicca* (genus *Moraxella*) are generally nonpathogenic but may cause conjunctivitis.

Neisseria gonorrhoeae.—These are gram-negative cocci, usually arranged in pairs with flattened adjacent surfaces and oval ends. There are more than 30 different serotypes useful in classifying the organisms in epidemiologic and virulence studies. Humans are the only reservoir, and the organism may infect the mucous membranes of the urethra, vagina, anal canal, pharynx, and conjunctiva. The organisms have developed resistance to many antibiotics, and effective therapy must be based on current information.

Gonorrheal conjunctivitis (see Chapter 12) is a purulent inflammation of the conjunctiva that has an incubation period of 2 to 5 days. It is a major cause of blindness, particularly in the Middle East, where it complicates trachoma. After an incubation period of 3 to 5 days, patients develop a serous discharge that quickly becomes purulent. Extreme conjunctival chemosis and periorbital edema prevent the drainage of pus. The central cornea may perforate, resulting in panophthalmitis or corneal scarring.

Ophthalmia neonatorum (see Chapter 12) is the term applied to any conjunctival inflammation occurring during the first 10 days of life. The most common causes in the United States are *Chlamydia trachomatis* (inclusion conjunctivitis), *Streptococcus pneumoniae, Neisseria gonorrhoeae,* and species of the *Haemophilus* genus.

Gonorrheal conjunctivitis must be treated promptly. Gram or immunofluorescent staining permits identification of the gram-negative intracellular diplococcus 48 hours before the results of conventional cultures are available.

Gonococcemia is the most common complication of genitourinary infection. It occurs soon after infection or later during menstruation. There is fever, polyarthralgia affecting the knees, wrists, and ankles, and skin lesions varying from petechiae to necrosis. There may be a catarrhal conjunctivitis or a severe acute iridocyclitis. Reiter syndrome (urethritis, arthritis, and ocular inflammation) is a more likely cause of this triad than gonorrhea, particularly in patients with histocompatibility antigen HLA-B27. Gonococcemia is diagnosed by culture or specific immunofluorescent antibody staining of blood, cerebrospinal fluid, synovial fluid, or skin lesions.

Neisseria meningitidis.—These gram-negative aerobic and facultative anaerobic organisms appear as biscuit-shaped diplococci. They are antigenically divided into the A, B, C, D, W135, X, Y, Z, and 29e groups. Their natural habitat is the human nasopharynx, and they cause meningitis and bacteremia in susceptible individuals.

Ocular involvement during meningococcemia consists of conjunctival petechiae and ecchymosis. A purulent conjunctivitis may occur. Intraocular embolization may cause a panophthalmitis that requires prompt treatment to prevent necrosis of the tissues of the inner eye followed by shrinkage of the globe (phthisis bulbi). Meningitis may be associated with ocular muscle paralysis and optic nerve inflammation. The organism may cause a purulent conjunctivitis in the absence of systemic infection that is distinguished from the gonococcus by cultural characteristics.

Moraxella.—Members of the genus *Moraxella* of the family Neisseriaceae are the cause of infections in children. *Moraxella lacunata* causes conjunctivitis and keratitis (indolent ulcer). The species *Branhamella* is a common cause of otitis media and may cause conjunctivitis.

Haemophilus influenzae.—This is a gram-negative, aerobic and facultative anaerobic, pleomorphic coccobacillus to rod-shaped organism. It requires blood factors X (hemin) and V (nicotinic adenine dinucleotide) for culture. It does not cause influenza, a viral infection, but may cause meningitis, pneumonia, and an acute orbital infection in infants, usually by extension from an infected paranasal sinus. *Haemophilus aegyptius* (Koch-Weeks bacillus), possibly a subspecies, causes acute or subacute conjunctivitis, particularly in tropical regions.

Pseudomonas.—The genus *Pseudomonas* is a complex of free-living, ubiquitous, opportunistic, gram-negative, aerobic bacilli of soil and water. *Pseudomonas aeruginosa* is the most common pathogen, and only *Staphylococcus aureus* and *Escherichia coli* cause more nosocomial hospital infections. *Pseudomonas aeruginosa* infects tissues after skin or mucous membrane injury or immunocompromised patients with malignancy, cystic fibrosis, or AIDS.

Pseudomonas aeruginosa keratitis may follow minor injuries to the corneal epithelium, particularly in wearers of soft contact lenses who neglect to remove the lenses daily or who use contaminated contact lens solutions. Radiation of the eye, tracheostomy, or an intensive care environment may predispose to *Pseudomonas* keratitis (see Chapter 12).

ACID-FAST BACTERIA

Mycobacterium

The genus *Mycobacterium* consists of many different nonmotile, encapsulated rods that stain with difficulty but, once stained, resist decolorization with strong mineral acids (acid-fast). The genus contains many species, most of which are nonpathogenic to humans. *Mycobacterium tuberculosis* and *M. leprae,* which cause clinical tuberculosis and leprosy, have infected humans for eons. Nontuberculosis mycobacteria, particularly *M. avium-intracellulare,* may cause systemic infection in immunocompromised hosts, particularly patients with AIDS. Human and bovine varieties are pathogenic for humans, whereas murine and piscine varieties cause tuberculosis in rodents and fish but not in humans. The avian (bird) variety rarely causes human disease.

The clinical and pathologic changes of tuberculosis depend on the tissue involved and the degree of hypersensitivity of the host. Generally, the initial or primary lesion is an asymptomatic process, healing or progressing in a short time, and characterized by an inconspicuous parenchymal lesion and tissue necrosis (caseation) of the draining lymph nodes. During this period there is lymphohematogenous dissemination of the entire body. The development of cellular immunity (hypersensitivity type IV) stops the primary process. In most individuals the infection remains quiescent. In others, after a period of latency of variable duration, there is a hematogenous spread of the organism and the clinical condition of tuberculosis.

In individuals who have developed cellular immunity to the organism (tuberculin sensitive), the process is more persistent than the primary infection. There is severe parenchymal inflammation and only a minor effect on the regional lymph nodes. Clinical tuberculosis, an infection that waned a decade ago, is now more widespread in the United States, particularly among the aged, immigrants, and patients with AIDS.

The skin of the eyelids may be infected in lupus vulgaris or, more rarely, in other cutaneous manifestations of tuberculosis, each of which may spread to the conjunctiva and the cornea.

Phlyctenular disease involves the conjunctiva and the cornea. In many instances it appears to be a cell-mediated reaction to tuberculoprotein (tuberculin) or other antigens and is responsive to local instillation of corticosteroids.

Previously, chronic uveitis was often thought to be caused by tuberculosis when it occurred in an individual who was hypersensitive to tuberculin. Chronic iridocyclitis causes mutton-fat keratic precipitates, minute nodules at the pupillary margin (Koeppe nodules), and posterior synechiae. Choroiditis destroys the adjacent retina, and inflammatory cells are released into the vitreous body. A posterior subcapsular cataract frequently develops.

Retinal periphlebitis may be complicated by neovascularization and recurrent vitreous hem-

TABLE 25-7.
Spirochaetales

Family Spirochaetaceae
Treponema
T. pallidum: syphilis
T. pertenue: yaws
Borrelia burgdorferi
Lyme disease
Endemic and relapsing fever
Family Leptospiraceae
Leptospira (Leptospirosis)

orrhage. Photocoagulation of the area surrounding periphlebitis is used to destroy new blood vessels. Unabsorbed blood is removed by vitrectomy.

Hansen disease (leprosy).—This disease is caused by an acid-fast rod, *Mycobacterium leprae,* similar to the agent that causes tuberculosis. About one third of the patients with Hansen disease have ocular complications. The infection predominantly involves the skin, superficial nerves, nose, and throat. It occurs as two principal types: (1) the lepromatous (LL, cutaneous), with depressed cellular immunity and frequent ocular involvement; and (2) the tuberculoid (TT, neural), with systemic immunity and ocular complications caused by neuroparalytic keratopathy.

The eyes are affected late in the course of the lepromatous type of disease. There may be an initial superficial infection and conjunctivitis, episcleritis, or keratitis. An insidious chronic iritis and granuloma formation cause loss of vision. Eventually, complicated cataract and ocular atrophy occur. Involvement of the skin of the brows causes alopecia of the eyebrows. Facial nerve paralysis causes ectropion of the lower eyelids and weakness in elevation of the eyebrows.

Spirochetes

The order Spirochaetales contains two families: Spirochaetaceae, which contains two human disease-producing genera, and Leptospiraceae, which contains one genus (Table 25-7). The spirochetes are mobile, slender helices that contain one or more coils. *Treponema pallidum* is the cause of syphilis and *Borrelia burgdorferi* is the cause of Lyme disease and relapsing fever. Leptosporosis is a zoonotic disease, predominantly of dogs in the United States. Conjunctivitis and iritis in humans are attributed to cell-mediated hypersensitivity to leptospiral antigen.

Treponema pallidum.—This spirochete causes acquired syphilis, usually by direct body contact. Congenital syphilis is transferred through the placenta of a pregnant syphilitic mother. Ocular involvement is seen in untreated or inadequately treated patients. Undetected syphilis is the more frequent cause of ocular inflammation. It must be considered in every instance of chronic ocular infection of unknown cause.

Acquired syphilis.—Untreated acquired syphilis is divided into primary, secondary, and tertiary stages. The primary and secondary stages are infectious. The chancre, the primary lesion of syphilis, occurs after 21 days (extremes of 10 to 90 days) at the site of entry of treponemes. A painless papule breaks down to form an ulcer with indurated margins and regional adenopathy. The eyelids may be the site of the chancre.

The iris and the ciliary body are inflamed early in the secondary stage and late in the tertiary stage. A severe iridocyclitis is associated with a skin rash and occurs in the fourth to the sixth month after the chancre. Broad, flat posterior synechiae occur between the stromal layer of the iris and the lens.

The tertiary stage of syphilis occurs 10 or more years after the chancre, or it may never occur. It is characterized by a small number of organisms, extensive parenchymal destruction, gumma formation, and connective tissue proliferation.

Tabes dorsalis is a degenerative disease of the central nervous system characterized by signs of involvement of the posterior columns of the spinal cord and the cranial nerves. Ataxia is common, as is posterior root pain, with paroxysmal attacks at night involving the legs, abdomen, arms, and face. Slight inequality in size of the pupils and a sluggish reaction may be the only signs. Fully developed Argyll Robertson pupils are diagnostic of tabes dorsalis (see Chapter 7).

Congenital syphilis.—Congenital syphilis is an infection caused by *Treponema pallidum.* The infection is acquired in utero and is characterized by diffuse systemic involvement without a primary lesion. Symptoms are usually present 2 to 6 weeks after birth, but fatal lesions resembling pemphigus may be present at birth. A severe, persistent rhinitis usually develops, followed in a week by a maculopapular skin eruption. The infant's general nutrition suffers, and the infant is thin, snuffling, and irritable.

The clinical signs of congenital syphilis appear at puberty. The Hutchinson triad includes (1) pegged secondary dentition, particularly notching of the upper central incisors; (2) nerve-type deafness; and (3) interstitial keratitis. Other signs are collapse of the bridge of the nose as a result of necrosis of the nasal septum from syphilitic rhinitis, splenomegaly, lymphadenopathy involving the epitrochlear nodes, saber tibia, and exostosis of the tibia and the cranial bones.

Syphilitic interstitial keratitis is an inflammation of the corneal stroma that occurs with an associated anterior uveitis. The disease, which affects boys predominantly (60%), occurs between 5 and 20 years of age. It begins with anterior uveitis and corneal endothelial edema. After about 2 or 3 weeks there is acute pain, photophobia, and lacrimation. All corneal layers are affected, with corneal edema and cellular infiltration of the stroma. This stage of the inflammation lasts but a short period and is followed by vascular invasion of the cornea from the periphery. The invading vessels, which appear to be pushing the haze in front of them, ultimately meet to form a "salmon patch." As soon as the vessels meet, symptoms and inflammation subside. When healing is complete, faint gray lines of empty blood vessels (ghost vessels) persist in the cornea. There may be late degenerative changes, with band keratopathy, keratoconus, or secondary glaucoma. In many instances a penetrating corneal transplant will restore useful vision in healed syphilitic interstitial keratitis.

Lyme borreliosis.—This is an immune-system–mediated multisystem infection caused by the spirochete *Borrelia burgdorferi,* which is transmitted by the bite of *Ixodidae* ticks (the mouse is the preferred host of the larval tick, and the deer is that of the mature tick). The major focus of the tick is from Maryland to Massachusetts in the Eastern United States, Minnesota and Wisconsin in the Midwest, and the midsection of the West Coast. All states have reported cases, and the disorder is sporadic in Europe.

After an incubation period of 3 to 30 days, the initial stage begins with nonspecific flulike symptoms that usually (75%) accompany a characteristic skin lesion at the site of the tick bite, erythema chronicum migrans. The skin lesion begins as a macule or a papule with an expanding bright red margin, sometimes with rings, and a center that becomes blue before it disappears. Conjunctivitis, choroiditis, retinal edema, and papillitis may occur. The signs and symptoms may disappear over several weeks.

A second stage occurs with excruciating headaches, cranial nerve paralysis, and motor or sensory radiculoneuropathy. A fluctuating atrioventricular heart block or a complete heart block may develop. Without treatment, patients develop arthritis of large joints, particularly the knees. An encephalopathy may develop with impaired memory, mood, and sleep. Ocular inflammation may occur in all stages.

The enzyme-linked immunosorbent assay (ELISA) may be negative in the first stage, and its sensitivity is reduced by antibiotic therapy. Erythema migrans combined with involvement of two or more organ systems with or without a positive antibody test suggests the diagnosis. Physicians should be alert to unusual types of conjunctivitis, keratitis, iridocyclitis, retinal vasculitis, or disk edema in individuals who have been within endemic areas. Treatment consists of oral doxycycline in adults and in children more than 8 years old, and amoxicillin in younger children.

VIRAL INFECTIONS

Viruses (Table 25-8) are intracellular parasites that may infect and cause disease in all living organisms. Human viruses, which range in size from 17 nm (picornavirus) to 300 nm (poxvirus) demonstrate marked species and organ specificity. They consist of a genome, composed of either ribonucleic acid (RNA) or deoxyribonucleic acid (DNA) that is surrounded by a protective protein shell, the capsid. Sometimes the shell is surrounded by an envelope composed of both protein and lipid derived from the host cell. The complete virus particle is virion.

To initiate an infection, a virion attachment protein on the virus surface interacts with a

TABLE 25-8.
Virus Infections and the Eye

Family Name and Nucleic Acid	Systemic Disease	Ocular Disease
Family Herpesviridae, DNA		
Subfamily Alphahepresvirinae		
Genus simplex virus		
Human herpesvirus 1 (herpes simplex virus, type 1 [HHV-1])	Encephalitis Facial vesicles	Keratitis Retinitis
Human herpesvirus 2 (herpes simplex virus, type 2 [HHV-2])	Genital warts	Keratitis
Genus varicellavirus	Chickenpox (children)	Eyelid vesicles
Human herpesvirus 3 (varicella-zoster virus)	Zoster (adults)	Zoster keratitis Episcleritis
Subfamily Betaherpesvirinae	Hepatosplenomegaly	Retinitis
Genus cytomegalovirus	Brain damage	
Human herpesvirus 5 (HHV-5) (human cytomegalovirus [CMV])	Death (AIDS)	
Subfamily Gammaherpesvirinae	Mononucleosis	Optic neuritis
Genus lymphocryptovirus		Dacryoadenitis
Human herpesvirus 4 (Epstein-Barr virus)	Burkitt lymphoma	Orbital metastasis
Unassigned		
Human herpesvirus 6 (human beta-lymphotropic virus)		
Family Adenoviridae, DNA		
Genus mastadenovirus		
Human adenovirus, 42 serotypes		
Subgenus A		
Serotypes 12, 18, 31	No pathogenicity	
Subgenus B		
Serotypes 3, 7, 11, 16, 21, 34, 35	Acute respiratory disease 3, 7, 14, 21; pharyngitis 3, 7, 14; urinary tract 11; infection (AIDS) 34, 35	Epidemic keratoconjunctivitis
Subgenus C		
Serotypes 1, 2, 5, 6	Acute pharyngitis; pneumonia 1, 2; hepatitis after liver transplant (children) 1, 2, 5	
Subgenus D		
Serotypes 8, 9, 10, 13, 15, 17, 19, 22, 23, 24, 26, 27, 29, 30		Epidemic keratoconjunctivitis 8, 11, 19, 27
Family Papovaviridae, DNA	Warts	Eyelid warts
Subfamily papillomavirinae		
Genus papillomavirus		
Human papillomaviruses (HPV) 1-58		

specific receptor on the surface of the target cell. The virus then penetrates the cell through endocytosis or direct translocation across the plasma membrane. The virus may remain latent in the cell without any sign, or it may be stimulated to replication by a physiologic, biochemical, environmental change or trauma.

Virus diseases associated with petechial hemorrhages may cause subconjunctival hemorrhage or ecchymosis of the eyelids. Iridocyclitis

TABLE 25-8 (cont.).

Family Name and Nucleic Acid	Systemic Disease	Ocular Disease
Family Picornaviridae, RNA		
Genus enterovirus		
Poliovirus	Poliomyelitis	
Coxsackievirus A		Hemorrhagic conjunctivitis, 24
23 serotypes		
ECHO (enteric cytopathogenic human orphan)		Hemorrhagic conjunctivitis, 70
32 serotypes		
Family Paramyxoviridae		
Genus paramyxovirus	Mumps	Corneal edema Optic neuritis
Genus morbillivirus	Measles	Keratitis, uveitis
Family Retroviridae, RNA		
Tumor viruses		
Genus not named		
Human T cell leukemia		
HTLV-I	Adult T cell leukemia	
HTLV-II		
Lentivirinae		
Human immunodeficiency virus (HIV: HIV-1; HIV-2)	Acquired immunodefidiency syndrome (AIDS)	
Family Togaviridae, RNA		
Genus rubivirus	Rubella Fetal defects	Microphthalmia, cataract, retinopathy

may occur with any viremia but may not be diagnosed because of the mildness of the iridocyclitis and the severity of the systemic disease.

Viruses that affect the skin, such as the virus of warts, may involve the eyelid margin and cause a secondary chronic conjunctivitis or keratitis. Respiratory tract viruses may migrate through the nasolacrimal passages to cause conjunctivitis or keratoconjunctivitis. Viruses that affect the mucous membranes, such as herpes simplex, infect the conjunctiva and corneal epithelium. Viruses that affect the central nervous system may impair the nerves to the eye and cause extraocular muscle palsies, optic neuritis, or papillitis.

HERPESVIRIDAE

This is a group of large-enveloped DNA viruses that become latent after primary infection. The infection becomes recurrent with reactivation of the virus, which occurs despite an immune response that produces antibodies.

The family Herpesviridae includes three subfamilies: (1) alphaherpesvirinae; (2) betaherpesvirinae; and (3) gammaherpesvirinae. The subfamily alphaherpesvirinae includes four members: the viruses of herpes simplex, herpesvirus hominis 1 and herpesvirus hominis 2; the varicella-zoster virus (herpesvirus 3), the causative agent of varicella (chickenpox) and herpes zoster (shingles); and herpes B virus, which infects monkeys and rarely humans. The subfamily betaherpesvirinae includes a single member, the cytomegalovirus (herpesvirus 5). The subfamily gammaherpesvirinae includes the Epstein-Barr virus (herpesvirus 4), the causative agent of infectious mononucleosis, and the agent of the Burkitt lymphoma. Herpesvirus 6 causes roseola (exanthem subitum) and possibly other disorders. Antibodies to herpesvirus 7 are widely distributed in humans but have not been identified with any disease.

Herpes simplex viruses.—The herpes simplex viruses include two subtypes, herpesvirus 1 and herpesvirus 2, that share many common antigens and cannot be distinguished by the usual serologic tests. Herpesvirus 1 produces lesions of the mouth, cornea, central nervous system, and the skin above the waist. Herpesvirus 2 is transmitted mainly as a venereal infection and involves the genitalia and the skin below the waist. In about one third of patients between 15 and 24 years of age, herpesvirus 1 invades the genital region. Occasionally, herpesvirus 2 involvement of the mouth or cornea may occur.

Infection usually occurs after 6 months of age, when maternal antibodies have disappeared. Usually, there is gingivostomatitis accompanied by adenopathy, fever, and malaise. In many cases, the primary infection either does not cause clinical signs or is so minor as not to be recalled. After the primary disease, the virus remains latent in ganglia, particularly the gasserian (N V). If atopic eczema is present, a severe, widespread disease may occur (eczema herpeticum, Kaposi varicelliform eruption). Systemic infection in individuals without antibodies may cause meningoencephalitis. Visceral herpes simplex usually occurs in newborns infected by their mothers who have recurrent herpetic vulvovaginitis.

After the primary infection, subsequent disease is entirely local and without systemic signs. Reactivation and migration of the virus cause vesicles on an erythematous base that recur at the same site in each individual. The most frequent manifestation is a fever blister (herpes labialis, herpes facialis, "cold sore"), which often infects a mucocutaneous junction. Reactivation causes an initial sensation of burning and irritation at the involved site followed by reddish papules that vesiculate within 24 hours. The vesicles then becomoe purulent (frequently with localized adenopathy), scale, and heal without a scar.

The eye may be the site of a primary infection in a child. More commonly it is the site of recurrent (reactivation) disease. Primary infection of the eye occurs in children and begins as a unilateral follicular conjunctivitis with a preauricular adenopathy and malaise. The disease may be confined to the conjunctiva, or the cornea may be involved with superficial punctate erosions or a single vesicle. Both types develop into a typical dendritic (branching) keratitis (see Chapter 12).

Herpesvirus 1 keratitis is reactivated by stress, fever, ultraviolet light, and immunosuppression, both iatrogenic and disease related. There is an initial foreign body sensation in the eye, and the experienced patient usually knows the disease has recurred. Vesicles occur initially but are usually ruptured by the time the patient is seen. A dendritic pattern can be demonstrated on the cornea using a fluorescein strip or sterile solution. Treatment is by mechanical removal of corneal epithelium and frequent topical administration of antiviral agents.

Varicella-zoster virus.—The varicella-zoster virus (herpesvirus 3) causes chickenpox in susceptible individuals, mainly children. In adults, mainly those past 50 years, reactivation of the latent virus causes herpes zoster (shingles) and acute retinal necrosis.

Chickenpox (varicella).—Chickenpox is an acute contagious disease characterized by a vesicular exanthem involving predominantly the hands and trunk. It develops in crops over a period of 1 to 5 days and is associated with malaise and fever. In adults a varicella pneumonia may develop. Vesicles may occur on the eyelids and rarely on the conjunctiva and the cornea. A mild iridocyclitis may occur. Chickenpox in patients with AIDS may be fatal and must be treated promptly with intravenous acyclovir.

Zoster.—Zoster is an infectious process of the dorsal root or extramedullary cranial nerve ganglia characterized by a circumscribed vesicular eruption and neurologic pain in the areas supplied by the sensory nerves that extend to the affected ganglia. Chickenpox is the primary infection in the nonimmune host. After the disease, the virus remains latent in the sensory ganglia for the life of the patient. If immunity is impaired the infection recurs locally; the virus replicates and migrates along sensory nerves to the skin or eye, causing the lesions of herpes zoster (shingles). Zoster is most common after 50 years of age but also occurs in younger individuals. It may appear in the course of severe and debilitating systemic illness. Patients with lymphosarcoma and reticulum cell sarcoma are particularly susceptible.

Herpes zoster ophthalmicus is an infection and inflammation of that portion of the skin and eye innervated by the gasserian ganglion that transmits ophthalmic division fibers of the trigeminal nerve (N V_1). The initial symptom is often a severe, unilateral, disabling neuralgia in the region of distribution of the nerve. Several days later there is a vesicular eruption with much swelling and tenderness. The vesicles rupture, causing hemorrhagic areas that heal in several weeks and leave deep-pitted scars. Pain usually disappears in about 2 weeks. In a small percentage of patients a postherpetic neuralgia that is resistant to treatment persists for many years. Zoster usually increases immunity so markedly that thereafter the virus remains permanently latent.

Zoster lesions of the cornea occur in two forms: (1) acute epithelial keratitis and (2) corneal mucous plaque keratitis. Acute epithelial keratitis is characterized by small, fine, multiple dendritic or stellate lesions in the peripheral portion of the cornea. They are always associated with conjunctivitis and resolve within 4 to 6 days. Corneal mucous plaque keratitis appears as a whitish gray, sharply defined plaque on the surface of the cornea that can be lifted with ease.

Superficial and deep corneal opacities occur. Anterior uveitis causes folds in Descemet membrane and keratic precipitates. Episcleritis may occur. The disease may persist for months and slowly regress, leaving a residue of round corneal infiltrates in the anterior corneal stroma. Secondary glaucoma occurs in about 20% of the patients and paresis of extraocular muscles in about 10%.

Treatment is often not satisfactory. Adults, particularly those more than 60 years of age, should avoid exposure to children with chickenpox. Topical corticosteroids and atropine may be helpful. Acyclovir (4 g/day for 10 days) limits inflammation but does not prevent postherpetic neuralgia.

Progressive outer zone retinal necrosis is caused by the varicella-zoster virus in patients with AIDS. There are multiple, peripheral, deep retinal lesions that become confluent and cause a retinal detachment. Blindness occurs in two thirds of the patients.

Epstein-Barr virus.—The Epstein-Barr virus (herpesvirus 4) causes heterophil-positive infectious mononucleosis. This is a contagious disease with a benign though commonly protracted course that predominantly affects young adults. Fever and pharyngitis occur initially, and there is associated lymphadenopathy and hepatitis with or without icterus. Atypical lymphocytosis is associated with some infections. There is a high serum concentration of heterophilic antibodies against sheep erythrocytes as well as development of antibodies against the Epstein-Barr virus.

Follicular or membranous conjunctivitis, subconjunctival hemorrhages, nodular episcleritis, uveitis, nummular keratitis (stacked coins), periorbital edema, optic neuritis, retinal edema, and hemorrhages have been described. In some epidemics, lacrimal gland inflammation (dacryoadenitis) is prominent. It causes a painful swelling, with redness of the outer one third of the upper eyelid and typically S-shaped curve of the upper eyelid margin. Involvement of the central nervous system may cause extraocular muscle paralysis, nystagmus, hemianopsia, and disturbances of conjugate movement.

Treatment is symptomatic, and the disease is usually self-limited.

Cytomegalovirus.—The cytomegalovirus (herpesvirus 5) infects most of the population but is usually asymptomatic. After infection the virus remains latent in tissues and becomes activated when the immune system is compromised in AIDS, organ transplantation, and cancer chemotherapy. Congenital infection in the newborn is often fatal, and survivors may be mentally retarded and deaf (10%). Symptomatic cytomegalic inclusion disease occurs in 25% of fatal instances of AIDS.

The ocular lesions of cytomegalic inclusion disease vary from an isolated area of chorioretinitis to one that disorganizes the globe. The diagnosis is based on the demonstration of larger than normal cells, with typical inclusions found in the urine, saliva, tears, or any tissue specimen. In the mother of an affected infant, a complement-fixing antibody titer equal to or greater than 1:64 is diagnostic. The affected infant demonstrates a rising titer after 4 months of age.

An acute cytomegalic necrotizing hemorrhagic retinitis may cause irreversible retinal damage and loss of vision in adults. Men are affected more frequently than women. It occurs frequently in clinically advanced AIDS (elsewhere in this chapter). Other causes include transfusion, direct spread from other patients, and reactivation of a latent infection. Treatment with ganciclovir (5 mg/kg/day intravenously) resolves the retinitis, but the inflammation recurs when treatment is stopped.

In renal transplant patients, the inflammation is often superimposed on a retina already damaged by vascular hypertension. There are hard yellow deposits, retinal edema, hemorrhages, and vascular occlusion. An optic atrophy may follow. The infection is self-limited. Effective therapy is not available.

Cytomegalic virus mononucleosis is an acute febrile illness with splenomegaly, hepatic involvement, and atypical lymphocytes. The heterophil test is negative, and Epstein-Barr antibodies do not develop.

ADENOVIRUS

The group of adenoviruses is composed of at least 42 serologically distinct human types of large DNA viruses, which mainly cause acute infection of the respiratory tract and the conjunctiva. There are many animal and avian strains that do not cause human diseases.

Adenovirus types 8, 11, 19, and 37 cause epidemic keratoconjunctivitis in adults. Other strains may cause sporadic keratoconjunctivitis. In children, type 8 causes systemic disease with fever, respiratory or gastrointestinal signs, and a conjunctivitis without corneal opacities. Adenovirus types 3 and 7 cause an acute respiratory disease, pharyngoconjunctival fever, and simple follicular conjunctivitis.

Epidemic keratoconjunctivitis.—Adenovirus types 8, 19, 11, and 37 cause epidemic keratoconjunctivitis in the United States. This is an acute infection of the cornea and conjunctiva that may occur in families and industrial settings. Occasionally, endemics in eye clinics and offices are spread by ocular secretions, contaminated eyedrops, and instruments, particularly tonometers. Contaminated ocular anesthetics and fluorescein solutions are common sources. Personnel who treat patients with inflamed eyes must avoid infecting themselves and others by adequate and frequent handwashing, careful cleansing of instruments, and avoidance of contamination of eyedrops by using single instillation disposable containers.

At the onset only one eye is affected. The conjunctiva is markedly injected and chemotic with tender preauricular lymph nodes. The fellow eye may become inflamed within 5 days or may escape infection. About 8 days later, a painful punctate keratitis occurs that is quickly followed by coalescence of the lesions and subepithelial inflammation. Within 3 or 4 days, these develop into white, faint corneal opacities (maculae) that persist for many months with reduction in vision. Eventually the opacities clear and vision is restored. Treatment is symptomatic.

Pharyngoconjunctival fever.—Pharyngoconjunctival fever is an acute sporadic or endemic disease that may affect all age groups, but particularly children. Adenovirus type 3 is the most common cause, but other adenovirus types have been implicated. The serum of infected patients contains group-specific antibodies. It occurs in all seasons of the year but is more common in summer and is often associated with infection transmitted in contaminated ponds and swimming pools. The incubation period is 5 to 7 days, and fever and other symptoms last 3 to 5 days. Clinical manifestations vary markedly in different individuals and in epidemics. A usually mild nasopharyngitis is associated with a cervical or maxillary lymphadenopathy. A fever that may reach 39° C persists 3 to 14 days. Headache referable to the sinuses, catarrhal otitis, lassitude, malaise, and sometimes gastrointestinal disturbances occur.

The conjunctivitis is acute, sometimes nonpurulent, and monocular. Follicle hyperplasia is marked in the lower cul-de-sac. Chemosis and injection are most apparent over the palpebral conjunctiva. Preauricular lymphadenopathy may be present.

MOLLUSCUM CONTAGIOSUM

Molluscum contagiosum is an infectious tumor caused by a genus of the Poxviridae family. It causes multiple, discrete nodules in the epidermal layer of the skin. The nodules are painless and often pearly white with an umbilicated center that contains a small white cone. Humans are the only host of the virus, and children are affected most commonly. It may be an opportunistic tumor in AIDS.

The tumors may occur on the skin and margins of the eyelids and may cause blepharitis. Release of an incomplete virion into the conjunctival sac may cause keratitis or a follicular conjunctivitis.

PAPOVAVIRIDAE FAMILY (VIRUS WARTS)

Virus warts (verrucae vulgaris) are contagious viral tumors caused by members of the A genus of the Papovaviridae family. They cause common warts and juvenile warts in school-age children and plantar warts in adolescents and young adults. They are characterized by the development of one or more circumscribed, elevated growths, with a hyperkeratotic, papillomatous surface. When located on the eyelid the lesions scrape the cornea, or epithelial debris contaminates the tears and causes a chronic conjunctivitis.

More than 40 different types of human papillomavirus (HPV) are associated with cutaneous, genital, and cutaneous papillomas. Carcinomas of the skin in renal transplant recipients have contained nucleotide sequences HPV-5, and carcinomas of the eyelids have been associated with HPV-16 or -18 infection. The nodule of the eyelid must be excised to heal any keratitis.

PARAMYXOVIRIDAE FAMILY

The Paramyxoviridae family includes the measles virus, the mumps virus, several parainfluenza viruses, the respiratory syncytial virus, and a pathogen of chickens, the Newcastle disease virus, which may accidentally infect humans.

Measles (rubeola).—Measles is a contagious viral disease characterized by prodromal symptoms of fever, cough, coryza, conjunctivitis, and Koplik spots (bluish gray dots on a red base). In 3 to 5 days a maculopapular rash appears. The conjunctivitis is nonpurulent and may be associated with Koplik spots, particularly on the semilunar fold. There are multiple punctate erosions of the cornea, which cause a severe photophobia. The patient who has photophobia is made more comfortable by either darkness or colored glasses. Permanent corneal scarring does not occur unless there is secondary microbial infection.

Sometimes measles or another acute contagious disease of childhood is the precipitating event in the appearance of strabismus. The primary cause of the squint is already present, and the disease seems only to accelerate its appearance or to transform an intermittent or latent type into a continuous type of strabismus.

Immunization has almost eliminated measles in the United States. During the incubation period, the administration of gamma globulin may prevent or modify the disease in the nonimmune individual. Subacute sclerosing panencephalitis is a slow viral infection caused by either the rubeola virus or a closely related virus.

Mumps.—Mumps is an acute contagious viral systemic disease characterized mainly by a painful enlargement of the salivary glands, most commonly the parotid glands, and, after puberty, by orchitis. Lymphocytic meningitis, pancreatitis, and involvement of other viscera rarely occur. Mumps may eventually trigger type I diabetes mellitus in young children (see Chapter 27).

Transient corneal edema decreases visual acuity. There are no associated ocular inflammatory signs. A uveitis or dacryoadenitis may occur. The only sign of meningeal involvement may be optic neuritis, or there may be widespread extraocular muscle palsy.

TOGAVIRIDAE FAMILY

Viruses of this family cause several types of equine encephalitis and rubella (German measles).

Rubella (German measles).—Rubella is a mild contagious disease characterized mainly by an evanescent, maculopapular skin eruption beginning on the face and neck, spreading to the trunk and extremities, and fading in 3 days. There may be mild pharyngitis and postauricular adenopathy, sometimes accompanied by slight fever, malaise, lassitude, and myalgia. Conjunctivitis is common and consists of bilateral bulbar chemosis and injection. Keratitis is exceptional. Fetal or childhood rubella may predispose to type I diabetes mellitus.

Rubella causes severe congenital defects in infants of mothers who contract the disease early in pregnancy. Infection between the second and sixth weeks of pregnancy causes cardiac malformation, microphthalmic cataract, and retinal pigment epithelium degeneration. Infection any time during the first trimester of pregnancy up to the fifth month may cause deafness and mental retardation with extensive brain necrosis. A chronic viral infection may persist as long as 3 years after birth, causing further systemic deterioration as well as serving as a nidus of infection for pregnant mothers.

Retinitis and congenital cataract are the most common ocular disorders. Microphthalmia results from infection early in pregnancy. Fetal uveitis causes iris atrophy, which may prevent pupillary dilation.

The cataract is usually nuclear, cortical (complete), and bilateral. Aspiration of the cataract may be followed by chronic endophthalmitis centered around lens remnants, with the severity proportional to the amount of lens cortex remaining in the eye. Inability to dilate the pupil complicates lens extraction. A sector iridectomy, which is almost always indicated, often results in significant visual improvement. The pupil may be enlarged with vitrectomy cutting instruments.

The retina has a mottled appearance (salt-and-pepper), which is caused by hyperpigmentation and hypopigmentation of the retinal pigment epithelium. The optic disks and blood vessels are normal. Fluorescein angiography shows a diffuse hyperfluorescence throughout the posterior eyegrounds, reflecting a widespread loss of pigment of the retinal pigment epithelium. Vision and electroretinograms are normal.

Prevention of rubella infection in pregnant women has eliminated rubella embryopathy. Children should be immunized with rubella vaccine to minimize transmission and so that girls will be immune when they reach childbearing age. The vaccine can infect the fetus and may be used in sexually active women only when pregnancy can be excluded (as during menstruation or immediately after childbirth) and continued nonpregnancy can be ensured for 3 months. After immunization, the hemagglutination-inhibition test indicates the presence or absence of immunity to rubella.

PICORNAVIRIDAE FAMILY

This family consists of two genera, the genus Enterovirus and the genus Rhinovirus, an important agent of the common cold. The genus Enterovirus is subdivided into polioviruses, coxsackieviruses, and echoviruses. Newly discovered members are no longer classified as coxsackieviruses or echoviruses but are numbered serially beginning with enterovirus number 68.

The polioviruses cause acute anterior poliomyelitis. Bulbar poliomyelitis may cause external ophthalmoplegia with opsoclonus. The coxsackieviruses and echoviruses may cause an aseptic meningitis (viral meningitis) in which there may be paralysis of muscles innervated by the oculomotor and abducent nerves together with papilledema.

TABLE 25-9.
Frequent Infective Organisms in Patients with AIDS

Retina and choroid
- Viruses: cytomegalovirus; herpes simplex; varicella-zoster
- Protozoa: *Toxoplasma gondii; Pneumocystis carinii*
- Fungi: *Fusarium* sp.; *Histoplasma capsulatum; Cryptococcus neoformans; Candida albicans; Sporotrichum schenckii*
- Bacteria: endogenous; *Nocardia* sp.; *Mycobacterium tuberculosis; Mycobacterium avium* complex
- Spirochete: *Treponema pallidum*

External eye
- Viruses: herpes simplex; molluscum contagiosum; varicella-zoster
- Parasite: Microsporidia
- Fungi: *Candida albicans*
- Chlamydia: *Trachomatis;* serotype L2 (lymphogranuloma venereum)
- Bacteria: *Staphylococcus* sp.; *Pseudomonas* sp.; *Capnocytophaga* sp.

Hemorrhagic conjunctivitis.—This is a specific violent inflammatory conjunctivitis first reported in Africa in 1969. The infection has spread eastward and was endemic in Florida. It is caused by a member of the picornavirus group, enterovirus 70.

ACQUIRED IMMUNODEFICIENCY SYNDROME

The acquired immunodeficiency syndrome is an acquired infection of the cells of the immune system by a retrovirus, the human immunodeficiency virus (HIV-1). Initially, infection of CD4+ lymphocytes causes an impaired immunity. Eventual depression of other components of the immune system then reduces the host resistance to many infectious organisms (Table 25-9) and a variety of malignancies.

The symptoms of human immunodeficiency viral infection begin 3 to 6 weeks after the virus has invaded the host, with a mononucleosis-like syndrome that includes fever, myalgia, lymphadenopathy, and fatigue. These symptoms resolve without treatment, and the individual may enter a period of latent infection that continues for many years. During this period there is a gradual diminution of CD4+ T cells to 500/μL, and the individual may develop early symptomatic disease with a generalized lymphadenopathy, thrush, zoster, thrombocytopenia, and molluscum contagiosum. As the CD4+ cell count decreases, the patient becomes increasingly sus-

TABLE 25-10.
Ocular Disorders and AIDS

Conjunctiva
- Abnormal blood vessels: dilated capillaries; microaneurysms; isolated vascular fragments
- Altered blood flow: "sludging"
- Kaposi sarcoma
- Squamous cell carcinoma
- Infections

Eyelids
- Kaposi sarcoma
- Infections

Cornea
- Infections
- Peripheral melting
- Keratitis
- Keratoconjunctivitis, culture negative
- Keratitis sicca

Uvea
- Infections
- Iridocyclitis
  - Reiter syndrome
- Treatment of *M. avium* complex
- Lymphoma
- Choroidal effusion

Retina
- Vasculopathy: cotton-wool spots; hemorrhages; microaneurysms; ischemia
- Infections (see Table 25-9)
- Vasculitis
- Absent or diminished electroretinogram

Vitreous humor
- Vitreitis

Optic nerve
- Ischemic neuropathy
- Papilledema
- Optic atrophy

Orbit
- Kaposi sarcoma
- Pseudotumor
- Burkitt lymphoma
- Eosinophilic granuloma
- Cellulitis

Neuro-ophthalmic
- Oculomotor nerves
- Skew deviation
- Opsoclonus
- Pupillary abnormalities

ceptible to a variety of serious opportunistic infections, neurologic changes, and neoplasms.

Ocular complications of AIDS may be noninfectious or infectious (Table 25-10). More than 65% of all patients develop retinal cotton-wool patches sometime in the course of the disease. These cause no symptoms and are seen on routine ophthalmoscopic examination. Isolated, flame-shaped blot, or blot hemorrhages with a pale center may occur. The cotton-wool patches and hemorrhages appear and disappear entirely independent of the general course of the disease. Punctate hemorrhages in association with an opaque retina suggest an infection with the cytomegalovirus, toxoplasmosis, or other opportunistic infection.

Cytomegalovirus retinitis is the most common intraocular infection in patients with AIDS. It is a progressive destructive retinitis that, if not treated, destroys the entire retina, affects the fellow eye, and causes blindness. Approximately 20% of patients with AIDS are affected, often without initial symptoms of a retinal disorder. Many patients develop a retinal detachment even after the active infection appears quiescent.

The lesions are either indolent or fulminant. The indolent lesion appears in the fundus periphery as a circular or oval opacification of the retina with a trace of retinal hemorrhage at its borders. The center may be atrophic. The fulminant lesion is more common at the posterior pole. It is densely opaque, with marked hemorrhages, and often inflammatory vascular sheathing. Treatment with intraocular foscarnet, ganciclovir, or both, suppresses the virus, which promptly reactivates if the treatment is stopped. Treatment seemingly only delays a relapse, which seems inevitable if the patient survives. (Intravenous, rather than intraocular injections, and intraocular inserts are being tested.)

Retinal toxoplasmosis in patients with AIDS must be differentiated from cytomegalovirus retinitis because toxoplasmosis is treated with pyrimethamine and does not respond to foscarnet or ganciclovir. The necrotizing retinitis of toxoplasmosis is a densely opaque, thick, yellowish white lesion, with smooth nongranular margins. Retinal hemorrhage is uncommon, but there are many inflammatory cells in the vitreous and anterior chamber. Unlike in patients with intact immune systems and ocular toxoplasmosis, the retinal lesions in patients with AIDS are not adjacent to retinochoroidal scars.

Kaposi sarcoma may affect the conjunctiva or orbit; the tumor occurs most commonly in homosexual men with AIDS. The vascular tumor varies in size and appears as a deep red, smoothly elevated mass in the inferior cul-de-sac that suggests a hemangioma. Treatment is indicated only for the cosmetic blemish. Within the

TABLE 25-11.
Chlamydiae and Rickettsiae

Chlamydiales
Chlamydia psittaci: psittacosis (parrot fever)
C. trachomatis
Serotypes A, B, Ba, C: trachoma
Serotypes D, E, F, G: in women: cervicitis
Pulmonary infiltration, cough: infants born to mothers with cervicitis
Serotypes D-K: in men: urethritis
Serotypes D, E, F, G: inclusion conjunctivitis
Serotypes L-1; L-2; L-3: lymphogranuloma venereum
Rickettsiales
Rickettsia
Typhus (3 species: epidemic typhus, etc.)
Spotted fever (8 species: Rocky Mountain spotted fever, etc.)
Scrub typhus (1 species and 3 serovars: trench fever, Q fever)

orbit, Kaposi sarcoma causes proptosis, blepharoptosis, ocular muscle palsies from motor nerve involvement, and conjunctival edema and infection.

CHLAMYDIAE AND RICKETTSIAE

These obligate intracellular parasites contain a large order, the Rickettsiales, and a small order, the Chlamydiales (Table 25-11). The Rickettsiales have three families and many members. The Chlamydiales have one family and two members. All are gram-negative organisms that can multiply only within living cells. Except for epidemic typhus, in which the natural cycle is humans and lice, all other Rickettsiales have an insect vector and animal host. Chlamydiales are parasites of humans and birds that are transmitted by contact.

Rickettsiales.—These organisms are transmitted by various arthropods to humans and cause an acute febrile illness and usually a skin rash. Vaccines have been prepared against some of the microorganisms, and the tetracyclines (doxycycline or minocycline) and chloramphenicol are effective therapeutically.

The ocular changes caused by infections with this family have been best described in epidemic louse-borne typhus fever (*Rickettsia prowazekii* transmitted by the human louse, *Pediculus humanus*) and Rocky Mountain spotted fever (*Rickettsia rickettsii,* transmitted by animal ticks). At the onset of the disease, conjunctival hyperemia may occur, sometimes with subconjunctival hemorrhages. Marked retinal venous engorgement with edema of the optic disk and retina may occur during the second and third weeks of the fever. Venous engorgement may be severe enough to cause a retinal hemorrhage, which may rupture into the vitreous body. Cotton-wool spots and arterial occlusion may be observed.

The diagnosis of rickettsial disease depends on clinical signs in regions where the diseases are endemic.

Chlamydiales.—This order has only one genus, *Chlamydia,* divided into two species, *C. trachomatis* and *C. psittaci. Chlamydia trachomatis* infects the epithelial cells of the cornea, conjunctiva, pulmonary tract, urethra, and cervix of humans. *Chlamydia psittaci* infects birds and causes pneumonia in humans.

All species of *Chlamydia* have an antigen detectable by complement-fixation tests. Serotyping indicates that genital isolates are generally serotypes D to G in women (silent cervicitis) and serotypes D to K in men (nongonococcal urethritis). Ocular isolates in trachoma areas are generally antigenic groups A, B, Ba, and C. Lymphogranuloma venereum is caused by serotypes L-1, L-2, and L-3.

The infective particle, the elementary body, enters an epithelial cell by phagocytosis. These fragile reticulate bodies are responsible for intracellular replication that develops into a crescent-shaped mass of resilient elementary bodies (inclusion bodies) that stain with specific immunofluorescence. Further multiplication ruptures the cell, and the elementary bodies are transmitted from one host cell to another.

Trachoma.—Trachoma is a chronic follicular conjunctivitis caused by *C. trachomatis,* which affects the upper eyelid and causes conjunctival and corneal scarring and blindness. The disease, which has been recognized since antiquity, affects 400 million people; 20 to 40 million are blinded. In the United States, it is prevalent mainly in Indians in the Southwest. Rural children are infected, and the combination of poverty, flies, lack of water, heat, crowding, and dust causes severe infection.

Communicable ophthalmia is a mixed infection in which the chronic conjunctival inflammation caused by trachoma is combined with a chronic purulent conjunctivitis. Flies transfer the infection from one child to another, and the disease becomes recurrent.

Inclusion conjunctivitis.—This conjunctivitis is caused by *Chlamydia trachomatis,* which causes a urethritis in men and an asymptomatic cervicitis in women. It is a common sexually transmitted infection of the adult genital tract. Adult inclusion conjunctivitis is transmitted to the eye by fingers and fomites and occasionally by the water in swimming pools ("swimming pool conjunctivitis"). The neonate is infected during passage through the birth canal. The conjunctivitis is purulent in the newborn and mucopurulent and follicular in the adult.

Typical inclusion conjunctivitis in the neonate develops as a purulent conjunctivitis 5 to 14 days after birth. There is eyelid and conjunctival swelling, purulent discharge, and conjunctival hyperemia. The untreated disease persists 3 to 12 months and usually heals without sequelae, although there may be mild tarsal conjunctival scarring and superficial corneal neovascularization. The neonatal infection may be prevented by instillation of erythromycin ointment in the conjunctival cul-de-sac at birth. It is not prevented by silver nitrate (Credé) prophylaxis. Treatment in the neonate consists of administration of tetracycline topically and erythromycin systemically for 6 weeks. The mother should be treated for cervicitis and the father for urethritis even if asymptomatic.

Adult inclusion conjunctivitis is an acute follicular inflammation with preauricular adenopathy. The follicles, unlike those of trachoma, are more marked in the lower eyelid and do not contain follicular material. Untreated, the disease may continue for months and cause corneal neovascularization and marginal infiltrates. The genitourinary tract serves as a reservoir for the infection. Ocular treatment is by means of topically applied tetracycline ointment or drops and systemic tetracycline. Systemic erythromycin should be substituted for tetracycline in children whose permanent teeth have not erupted, in pregnant women, and in nursing mothers.

Lymphogranuloma venereum.—Lymphogranuloma venereum is a contagious venereal disease transmitted by *C. trachomatis* serotypes L-1, L-2, and L-3. It is manifested initially by a vesicle that bursts, leaving a grayish ulcer, followed by regional lymphadenitis that is frequently suppurative. Mild to severe constitutional signs may be present during the stage of adenitis. The disease is common in Central America, South America, and Southeast Asia. It is sexually transmitted, and men are affected 20 times more often than women.

Primary infection of the eyelid, occurring venereally or through accidental contamination in a laboratory worker, causes an ulcerative lesion of the eyelid or conjunctiva and preauricular adenopathy (Parinaud oculoglandular syndrome). Hematogenous spread of the disease may cause uveitis, keratouveitis, or sclerokeratitis. Tetracyclines, sulfonamides, and chloramphenicol are recommended for therapy.

FUNGAL INFECTIONS

Fungi grow as either unicellular organisms (yeasts) or multicellular, filamentous colonies (molds). Some pathogenic fungi grow as yeasts at 37° C and as molds at 25° to 30° C (thermal dimorphism). Oculomycosis is caused by fungi that are opportunistic pathogens. The most severe fungal infections occur in patients without deficiencies of the immune system. Trauma is an etiologic factor in more than one half of cases.

Fungi infect the eye and its adnexae in four main ways: (1) superficially to produce conjunctivitis, keratitis, and lacrimal obstruction; (2) by extension from infection in neighboring skin, paranasal sinuses, or the nasopharynx; (3) by direct intraocular introduction during surgery or by accidental penetrating trauma, particularly with plant material; or (4) by hematogenous or lymphatogenous routes in patients with pulmonary, cutaneous, or generalized mycosis.

Presumed ocular histoplasmosis is considered a common cause of subretinal neovascularization. *Candida* endophthalmitis may develop in patients with indwelling catheters who receive antibiotics for a long time. Fungal, viral, bacterial, and protozoal infections may develop in immune-suppressed patients.

Superficial infection.—Fungi may be introduced into the cornea by an epithelial abrasion or a foreign body, frequently consisting of vegetable matter. Instillation of corticosteroids reduces tissue resistance to infection. A fluffy white spot of inflammatory cells first appears in the anterior stroma and, with necrosis, melts into a shallow ulcer with a sterile hypopyon.

There may be satellite stromal lesions. There is severe ciliary and conjunctival injection, but corneal neovascularization is absent or occurs late. The necrosis gradually involves the entire cornea, which may perforate.

The main causative organisms are *Fusarium, Aspergillus,* and *Candida.* Other causative fungi include *Acremonium (Cephalosporium), Penicillium,* and *Coccidioides immitis.* Treatment is by local and systemic antifungal agents. Medical therapy is frequently not effective, and the cornea does not heal until covered with a conjunctival flap.

A fungus conjunctival inflammation usually occurs secondary to keratitis. In tropical areas, *Rhinosporidium* may produce polyps of the conjunctiva.

Unilateral, persistent tearing with patent lacrimal passages characterizes infections of the canaliculus. The lower canaliculus is usually involved. The punctum is dilated, and its margins are elevated and inflamed. There is tearing and itching with a slight conjunctivitis medially. Diagnosis is often delayed until a lacrimal probe grates against concretions of hardened colonies of fungi in the infected canaliculus.

The skin of the eyelids may be infected by any of the fungi that cause a dermatomycosis. Extension of fungus infection into the orbit may cause a cellulitis and retrobulbar neuritis. Some inflammatory granulomas of the orbit may also be caused by fungi.

Intraocular infection.—Fungal endophthalmitis after intraocular surgery originates from fungal contamination of the air in an operating room, from the surgical instruments and solutions, or from the conjunctival sac and eyelids of the patient. Mucormycosis extends directly from the nasal pharynx in debilitated patients who have ketoacidosis.

A variety of fungal infections of the uvea and retina are seen in patients with immune suppression after organ transplant. Fungal endophthalmitis has an incubation period of several weeks to several months and follows an indolent course. The anterior vitreous and uvea are predominantly involved. The aqueous humor is clouded with inflammatory cells, and a hypopyon may be present. Small gray-green areas or white infiltrates resembling small balls of cotton are present in the anterior vitreous. The pupils gradually fill with an inflammatory mass, and the vitreous humor is converted to a granuloma. The therapeutic effect of antifungal agents is variable and unpredictable. Removal of the vitreous humor by vitrectomy may save the eye by reducing the number of organisms and inflammatory cells present and permitting increased penetration of drugs.

The slow, indolent progression distinguishes mycotic endophthalmitis from bacterial endophthalmitis.

Rhino-orbitocerebral phycomycosis.—This is a rapidly lethal infection caused by fungi such as *Mucor, Basidiobolus, Mortierella,* and *Rhizopus.* The nose or nasopharynx is the usual route of entry. The infection occurs in debilitated individuals with ketoacidosis, who develop facial swelling, proptosis, eyelid edema, and total ophthalmoplegia and blindness. Coma develops, and death occurs within 1 week. Mucormycosis occurs in adults with diabetes mellitus, whereas the other species may be the cause in debilitated infants and children. The infection occurs in individuals with severe underlying disease, commonly diabetes with ketoacidosis, or leukemia, carcinomatosis, or bacterial infection. The inhaled spores initially cause a nasopharyngitis with infarction of vessels to the skin that causes a black, ulcerated eschar on the skin, palate, or nasal mucous membrane. Visual loss, proptosis, and ophthalmoplegia occur. Facial or orbital pain in a susceptible individual and coma in a diabetic patient that does not respond to metabolic correction are important signs. Treatment consists of systemic antifungals and antibacterials, extensive surgical debridement, and correction of acidosis.

Immunosuppression.—Many fungi may cause a choroiditis or retinitis in patients with AIDS, or those receiving corticosteroids and immunosuppressive agents to suppress graft rejection. *Aspergillus* and *Candida* are the most commonly involved causal organisms. More uncommon are *Nocardia, Coccidioides,* and others. Men are more commonly affected than women. An unrelated renal donor, increasing age, and leukopenia all predispose the individual to infection. Ocular inflammation is not severe, and attention may be directed to the eyes because of decreased vision. The mild chorioretinitis causes minimal cellular reaction, and there is little tendency for extension.

Hematogenous *Candida* endophthalmitis may follow antibiotic therapy, immunosuppressive therapy, cardiac and abdominal surgery, use of intravenous catheters, and drug abuse. The organisms may be in the bloodstream without causing parenchymal involvement, and treatment is not required. Sometimes systemic *Candida* may be diagnosed because of a chorioretinitis, which reflects an underlying systemic candidiasis. The chorioretinitis consists of many white, fluffy, circumscribed exudates with a filamentous border located in the choroid and retina and extending into the vitreous. Additional ocular lesions include retinal hemorrhage, hypopyon, iritis, papillitis, and ciliary body abscess. Patients may be asymptomatic or have loss of vision, pain, and redness. The histologic lesion is a combination of suppurative and granulomatous inflammation that begins in the choroid and extends into the retinal pigment epithelium and overlying retina. Antifungal agents are used to treat patients with ocular or systemic *Candida* infections, but patients with candidemia only are not treated.

Presumed ocular histoplasmosis.—Histoplasmosis is a mild to lethal systemic disease caused by *Histoplasma capsulatum*. It manifests itself mainly as an asymptomatic acute primary respiratory tract infection or rarely as a chronic pulmonary disease with cavitation that resembles tuberculosis. Uncommonly the infection is disseminated, with widespread systemic involvement. Infection is common in rural dwellers of the Mississippi Valley and the great river valleys of South America, Africa, and Asia, but it is rare in Europe. The fungus is common in soil contaminated with bird droppings.

The presumed ocular histoplasmosis syndrome consists of (1) a lesion of the central retina; (2) a (usually) quiescent chorioretinitis adjacent to the optic disk; and (3) peripheral areas of chorioretinal atrophy. Patients are usually first seen when a neovascular membrane disturbs the fovea centralis, at which time the lesions adjacent to the optic disk and peripheral lesions are entirely healed and asymptomatic.

The central lesion is usually a subretinal neovascular membrane adjacent to or beneath the fovea centralis. There may be fresh blood at the periphery of the lesion (Fig 25-1). If untreated the neovascular membrane progresses, destroys the overlying fovea centralis, and involutes during a period of 2 years. Surgical excision of the membrane before extensive foveal damage yields better results than similar surgery in age-related macular degeneration, presumably because the vascular membrane is confined to the choroid and has not invaded the retinal pigment epithelium.

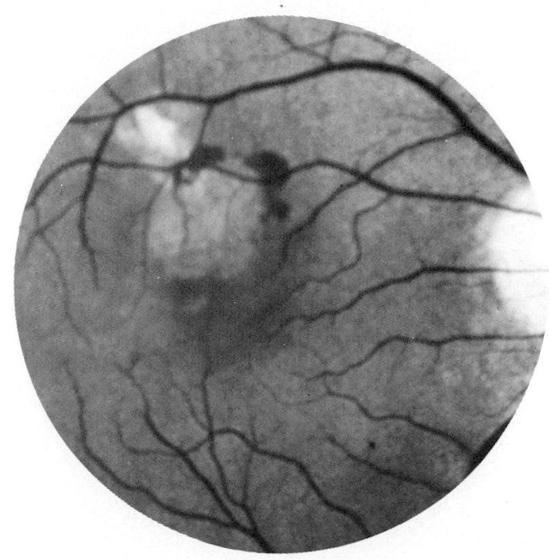

FIG 25-1.
The central fundus lesions of presumed ocular histoplasmosis in a 61-year-old woman. The lesions had been quiescent for many years before a recent decrease of vision. The edge of the optic disk is at the right margin. The white area in the 11 o'clock meridian marks an area of chorioretinitis that has destroyed the retinal pigment epithelium to expose the sclera. The gray region below appears green on ophthalmoscopy and indicates subretinal neovascularization. The darkest region is intraretinal blood.

The lesion adjacent to the optic disk is usually observed only after healing. It may affect a segment of the optic disk (juxtapapillary) or surround the entire disk (peripapillary; Fig 25-2). There is marked atrophy of the choroid and retinal pigment epithelium with mild pigment proliferation.

The areas of peripheral chorioretinal atrophy ("histo spots") vary in size from a minute dot to an area as large as the optic disk. They indicate a healed chorioretinitis with destruction of the choroid and retinal pigment epithelium. Like the lesion adjacent to the optic disk, they are not symptomatic.

Presumed ocular histoplasmosis does not occur in patients with symptomatic systemic

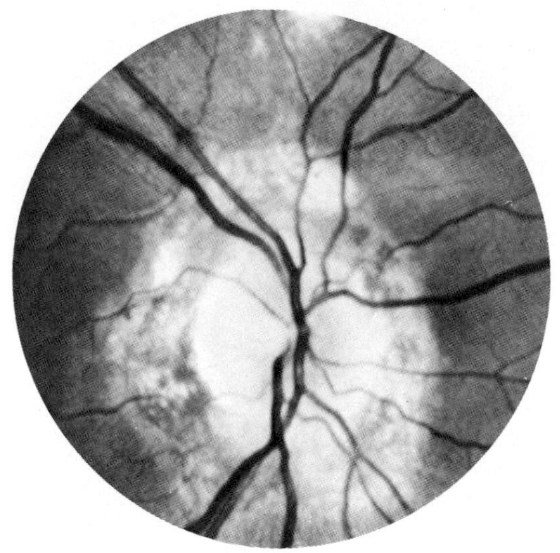

FIG 25-2.
Peripapillary chorioretinitis and the punched-out atrophic lesion (above) of presumed histoplasmosis syndrome in a 33-year-old woman.

histoplasmosis, but there is cutaneous hypersensitivity to histoplasmin. The organism is not found within the affected eyes or the excised subretinal membranes. Presumably the syndrome is associated with a hypersensitivity to antigens associated with the histoplasmosis organism.

METAZOAN AND PROTOZOAN DISEASES

The kingdom Animalia is divided into two subkingdoms, the Metazoa and the Protozoa. The subkingdom Metazoa includes all multicellular animals in which the cells are differentiated to form tissues. The subkingdom Protozoa includes a diverse group of unicellular animals or aggregates of undifferentiated cells that replicate by asexual division.

Metazoan infection of humans is by worms (helminths). Additionally, the larvae (but not the fly) of two-winged flies and gnats are parasitic and may multiply within human tissue in myiasis. Infection of humans by protozoa is widespread, and one such infection, malaria, affects millions each year. Other protozoan infections include toxoplasmosis, *Acanthamoeba* sp. keratitis in soft contact lens wearers, *Pneumocystis carinii* pneumocystosis in AIDS (often with an associated cytomegalovirus hemorrhagic retinitis), leishmaniasis trypanosomiasis, *Entamoeba histolytica* amebiasis, and others.

METAZOAN INFECTION

The main metazoan infections of humans are caused by nematodes (roundworms) and two groups of flat worms, the trematodes (flukes) and the cestodes (tapeworms). The majority cannot multiply within the human host, with two exceptions. The larva of *Strongyloides* may become infectious within the human gut, resulting in an overwhelming autoinfection, and the larva of the dog tapeworm may multiply within a hydatid cyst.

Nematodes (roundworms)

There are an estimated 500,000 species of nematodes that may become parasitic in virtually all arthropods, mollusks, plants, and vertebrates. Typically, nematodes are elongated, cylindric, nonsegmented worms that taper more or less at the head and tail and have a complete digestive tract. They vary from minute filiform worms to 1.5 m in length. Most human infections are acquired by ingestion of the eggs, but hookworm and *Strongyloides* larvae actively invade the skin.

Ocular infection occurs because of invasion of the eye by the larvae of nematodes that are parasitic in lower animals, most commonly the roundworms of the dog and cat.

Visceral larva migrans.—This term is applied to the invasion of nematode larvae into tissues other than the skin. The common roundworm of the dog and, less frequently, of the cat *(Toxocara canis* and *Toxocara cati)* are common causes of ocular disease. Visceral larva migrans also describes the disease produced by the wandering worms of *Ascaris lumbricoides* and other nematodes.

Toxocariasis is acquired by the ingestion of *Toxocara* eggs that contain the infective second-stage larvae. The eggs are excreted by puppies and lactating bitches and require 2 or 3 weeks' development in the soil before becoming infective. The eggs hatch in the patient's small intestine, and the larvae migrate to the liver through the portal circulation. Some may enter the lungs and then the systemic circulation. When larvae exceed the diameter of a blood vessel, they actively bore through the vessel wall. Many larvae become encapsulated in muscle and may

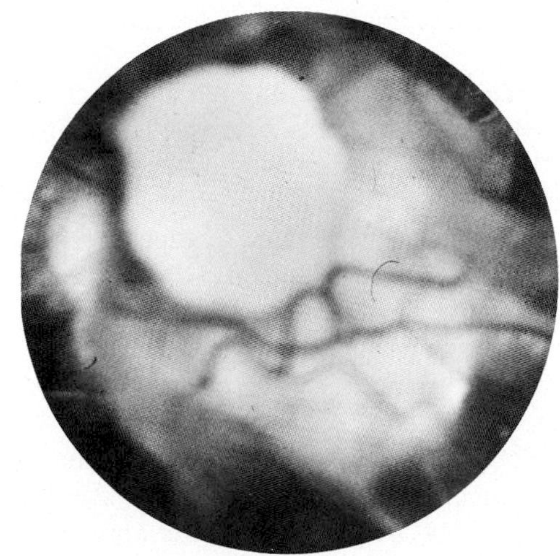

FIG 25-3.
Granuloma of the retina in toxocariasis. The white mass extends into the vitreous cavity and obscures the optic disk.

produce infection years later when the capsule ruptures.

The clinical picture of toxocariasis varies with the number of eggs ingested, the frequency of reinfection, and the distribution of larvae. Typically, human visceral larva migrans is seen in boys, aged 6 months to 4 years, who have contact with puppies and who eat dirt (geophagia). There is a fever, pallor, coughing or wheezing, lassitude, anorexia, and weight loss. There may be hepatomegaly, pruritic eruption over the trunk and legs, and transient subcutaneous nodules. Most patients have a leukocytosis, with 50% to 90% eosinophils and high levels of IgG and IgM.

Ocular lesions are unusual in patients with concurrent or previous visceral larva migrans. The average age of patients with ocular involvement is 8.6 years rather than the 6 months to 4 years in patients with visceral larva migrans. Usually only one eye is infected, with loss of vision, pain, and strabismus. The lesion varies from a granuloma that resembles a retinoblastoma to an endophthalmitis. The granuloma appears as a white, round lesion, about the size of the optic disk, in the retina or pars plana (Fig 25-3). Traction lines in the retina radiate from the lesion. Fibrous bands may extend from the central retina to the pars plana. Rarely, the larvae can be seen. The lesion may be flat, or it may protrude into the vitreous cavity. Multiple retinal granulomas, posterior uveitis, vitreous hemorrhage, and optic atrophy may occur. A granulomatous retinitis may be confused with a retinoblastoma. Peripheral retinitis may cause an inflammatory falciform fold of the retina. Rarely the optic disk is invaded by the larva. Visceral larva migrans should be suspected in any child with pica, fever, eosinophilia, hepatosplenomegaly, and signs of a multiple system disease.

An increased titer of the ELISA test, prepared with larval antigens and with serum that has been absorbed on *Ascaris* antigen, is highly diagnostic. The indirect hemagglutination and bentonite flocculation tests are less diagnostic. Serum tests may be negative in patients with infection limited to the eye because only a few larvae entered the body and lodged in the eye. Titers of the vitreous and aqueous humors are elevated. There is no specific therapy. Children with pica should not be exposed to contaminated environments and infected dogs and cats.

***Ascaris lumbricoides*.—**This giant (30 cm long) intestinal roundworm affects children predominantly. There is no intermediate host, and infection occurs because of ingestion of eggs. The eggs hatch in the bowel, and the migrating larvae may cause pneumonia, encephalitis, or meningitis. Infection of the eye causes an intraocular inflammation that varies in severity from iridocyclitis to endophthalmitis. Ingested eggs hatch in the small intestine and the larva are carried to the liver. From here they migrate to the heart and then to the lungs and trachea and are eventually swallowed. The adult worm matures in the small intestine. Ingestion of hundreds of eggs may be followed by an enlarged liver, pneumonitis, and a generalized toxicity.

In the bowel the worm may be asymptomatic or cause intestinal disorders varying in severity from mild colic to obstruction and perforation. Sensitization to the worms or their products may cause allergic manifestations, mainly asthma or urticaria.

The ocular inflammation of the larval migration is nonspecific but may be suspected because of the violent ocular tissue reaction often combined with an eosinophilia, depending on the number of worms in the circulation. In enucleated eyes the lesions resemble those of either Coats disease or endophthalmitis. The larvae may be found in histologic sections.

***Necator americanus*.**—*Necator americanus* (New World hookworm) is a nematode common in the southeastern United States. *Ancylostoma duodenale* (Old World hookworm) is common in Africa, Asia, and South America, where there may be overlapping of species. There is no intermediate host. In moist soil, eggs develop into larvae that readily penetrate the skin. The cutaneous invasion produces a severely pruritic cutaneous eruption, "ground itch." The larvae ultimately reach the lungs, enter the pharynx, and are swallowed. They develop into mature worms in the intestinal tract. An iron-deficiency anemia develops, along with malaise, fever, and anorexia. The disease is diagnosed by discovery of ova in the stools. Treatment is with tetrachloroethylene.

The ocular signs are those described in visceral larva migrans. In the past, *Toxocara canis* infections were thought to be caused by the hookworm. The anemia may be associated with retinal hemorrhage.

Trichinellosis.—Trichinellosis is an infestation of striated muscles by the larvae of the nematode *Trichinella spiralis,* which infects a large group of animals of which swine are the chief human reservoir.

The encysted larvae are ingested in undercooked pork and develop in the intestine into sexually mature adults. Eggs develop and hatch in the female nematode, which releases about 1,500 larvae during a 6-week period. The larvae enter the general circulation about 7 days after an individual has eaten infected meat and are widely distributed to all tissues. There is an initial gastroenteritis, diarrhea, abdominal pain, and vomiting followed by muscle weakness and pain. Edema is frequently localized to the orbit, particularly the upper eyelid. Ocular muscle infestation causes pain on ocular rotations. There may be subconjunctival hemorrhages and petechial hemorrhages in other regions.

Muscle tenderness, eosinophilia, and orbital edema suggest the diagnosis. The larvae may be found in biopsy specimens 10 days after infection. The intradermal skin test becomes positive about the third week after infection.

Filariasis.—The filariae are slender, threadlike nematodes that have a tendency to colonize in a specific part of the human body. The female worms produce embryos, microfilariae, which live in the blood or skin. Bloodsucking arthropods, their intermediate hosts, spread the infection.

***Onchocerca volvulus*.**—Ocular onchocerciasis (river blindness) is a chronic filarial infection that occurs endemically in Mexico, Guatemala, Venezuela, and equatorial, sub-Saharan Africa. It has been estimated to affect more than 40 million people, and in some communities as many as 40% of the adult population are blind with ocular onchocerciasis. The infection is transmitted from person to person by bites of infected black flies of the genus *Simulium* (buffalo gnats). Infected larvae are injected into the skin or subcutaneous tissue, which causes nodules (cercoma) of pathognomonic appearance.

The microfilariae of *Onchocerca* may be seen beneath the bulbar conjunctiva or as squirming yellowish threads in the aqueous humor. Microfilariae in the cornea cause a superficial punctate keratitis. A sclerosing keratitis, continuing over a 20- to 30-year period is the chief cause of blindness. Inflammation of the iris is common, and generalized atrophy of its pigmented layers gives it a spongy appearance. The ocular posterior segment lesion is variable. It occurs rarely in areas where there is adequate dietary vitamin A. There is circumscribed atrophy of the choroid, clumping of retinal pigment, perivascular sheathing, and optic neuritis, which is followed by a secondary optic atrophy. Death of the microfilariae causes a severe inflammatory reaction.

A single dose of the parasiticide, ivermectin, may be administered once or twice each year. The drug is well tolerated and entire populations are treated. Ivermectin does not kill the adult worms encysted in a nodule and may elicit severe systemic reactions in patients infected with a concurrent *Loa loa.* Tourists planning to visit infested regions should be warned of the dangers of bathing in local lakes and streams, some of which have been developed as recreational areas.

Loiasis.—*Loa loa* (African eye worm) is a threadlike nematode measuring 30 to 70 × 0.3 mm. It lives in the subcutaneous tissue of humans, travels from place to place beneath the skin, and causes a creeping itch sensation. The disease is limited to West and Central Africa. The vectors are day-biting flies. The worm is responsive to warmth, and in persons sitting before a fire, the worms move to the face and the eyes. Native populations are often asymptomatic and the allergic responses are seen in visitors and expatriates.

In the eye the adult worm resembles a piece of surgical catgut beneath the conjunctiva or swimming in the anterior chamber. There is local irritation, chemosis, and lacrimation, all of which disappear quickly when the worm moves to deeper tissues. The subconjunctival worm may be removed after it is captured with a ligature.

Calabar swellings are painless, edematous, erythematous, subcutaneous nodules that occur as an allergic reaction to metabolic products of the worm or from injured or dead worms. There is a marked eosinophilia and localized angioedema. Systemic antihistamines or corticosteroids give relief. Diethylcarbamazine eliminates microfilariae from the blood but not the adult worm. Ivermectin is also effective and possibly less toxic than diethylcarbamazine.

Cestodes (tapeworms)

Tapeworms have flat segmented bodies and consist of a head (scolex) and a series of segments (proglottids). They cause human illness at one of two stages in their life cycle: (1) the adult stage in which the mature worm is attached to the intestinal wall and (2) the larval stage in which there are enlarging larval cysts in various tissues. The intestinal type may cause no symptoms or only symptoms of gastrointestinal disturbances. The visceral type follows ingestion of tapeworm eggs, which hatch in the intestine and release larvae that penetrate the bowel wall and spread the infection through the bloodstream. The two main types of visceral involvement with tapeworms are (1) echinococcus, or hydatid, cysts and (2) cysticercosis.

Echinococcosis (hydatid disease).— Echinococcus cysts form part of the inflammatory response to the larvae of *Echinococcus granulosus,* a minute tapeworm parasitic in dogs, coyotes, and jackals. Eating contaminated feces by swine, cattle, or humans leads to hydatid cysts of the liver, lungs, kidney, brain, orbit, eye, and other organs. The cyst develops into hundreds of adult worms. Cyst development is slow and induces the symptoms of a slowly developing tumor. Diagnosis may be based upon magnetic resonance imaging of the tumor, which discloses hypodensities and hyperdensities, scattered calcification, daughter cysts, and internal septae. The cyst fluid is highly irritating and infectious and should not be evacuated. Orbital cysts, which are more common than intraocular cysts, cause a proptosis with related signs. The intraocular cyst appears as a white pea-sized mass within the vitreous body, or there may be progressive, solid retinal detachment. Surgical excision is the only effective therapy. Care must be taken not to rupture the cyst and release toxic and infectious fluid.

Cysticercosis.—Cysticercosis in humans is caused by infection with eggs of *Taenia solium* (pork tapeworm) or *Taenia saginata* (beef tapeworm). *Taenia solium* infection is common in regions where pigs are raised and human feces is used as fertilizer. The infection is endemic in Central America, particularly Guatemala; South America, particularly Ecuador; Eastern Europe; and Southern California. In Los Angeles, cysticerci of the brain is the leading cause of epilepsy. Mexican immigrants are mainly infected.

The cyst is usually 0.5 to 1 cm in diameter and can develop in almost any tissue body. Most commonly, lesions within the cerebrum, the subarachnoid space at the base of the brain, or the ventricles cause the signs and symptoms of an expanding tumor. There may be headache, papilledema, decreased vision, hemiparesis, and seizures. The cyst in the eye appears as a translucent oval body 6 to 18 mm in length, without a capsule, in which the head of the larva may be seen as a white spot. It may occur in the choroid, causing a retinal detachment, float free in the vitreous humor or anterior chamber, or be found beneath the conjunctiva or in the orbit. Removal is the only therapy, but rupture of the cyst is followed by a violent inflammation.

PROTOZOAN INFECTIONS

The chief protozoan infections of ophthalmic concern are toxoplasmosis, *Acanthamoeba* keratitis, and *Pneumocystis carinii* pneumocystosis, which may be associated with a reactivation of a latent cytomegalovirus infection and cause a necrotizing hemorrhagic retinitis.

Toxoplasmosis.—Toxoplasmosis is an infectious disease caused by an obligate intracellular protozoan, *Toxoplasma gondii.* The organism is capable of infecting a wide range of mammals, birds, and reptiles. The cat family is the definitive host. Transmission occurs readily

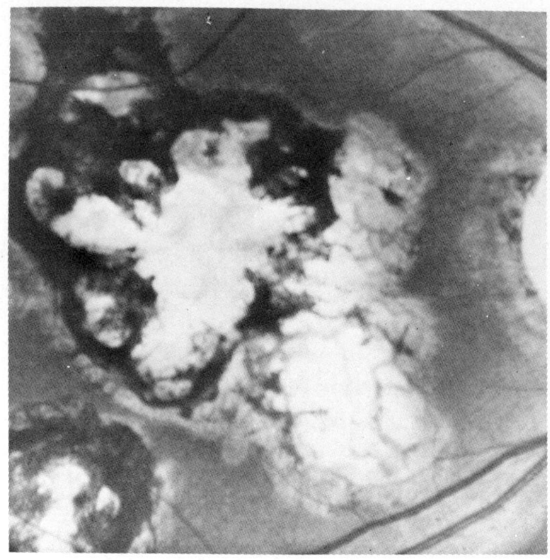

FIG 25-4.
Recurrent toxoplasmosis in a 39-year-old woman. Visual acuity in this eye is counting fingers at 2 feet. There is a series of contiguous lesions, some with marked pigment proliferation and others so severe that the pigment epithelium has been destroyed and the sclera may be seen.

after ingestion of toxoplasmosis cysts in pork or lamb or oocysts from cat feces.

Two types of disease occur: congenital and acquired. The congenital disease is characterized by a bilateral necrotizing neuroretinopathy, deafness, and brain necrosis. Acquired infections may be asymptomatic or cause a lymphadenopathy, fever, and malaise. In patients with AIDS or neoplasms of the lymphatic system or who are being treated with immunosuppressive drugs, acquired toxoplasmosis causes severe damage to the brain, muscles, heart, liver, or lungs. Most ocular toxoplasmosis is either congenital or an activation of a congenital lesion. Ocular toxoplasmosis lesions, mainly retinochoroiditis, may be an acquired infection in AIDS.

Congenital toxoplasmosis occurs in utero during the first 7 months of pregnancy. The mother transmits the infection to the fetus, which may result in an abortion or stillbirth, or an infant with clinical signs of toxoplasmosis. Severe congenital toxoplasmosis causes microphthalmia, necrotizing retinitis and choroiditis, optic atrophy, iritis, visual loss, and vitreous disorganization. Central nervous system necrosis causes nystagmus and extraocular muscle palsy.

Infants with less severe toxoplasmosis infections have areas of chorioretinal atrophy with retinal pigment proliferation in both eyes. If the fovea centralis is involved, esotropia may occur or the eyes may be straight although vision is poor. The inactive lesions are sharply demarcated, and contiguous areas of chorioretinal atrophy have pigmented borders (Fig 25-4), which are located mainly at the posterior pole. The vitreous is clear, and there is no active inflammation. The retinal lesions in some children remain quiet throughout life. In others, inflammation recurs 10 to 20 years later in an area adjacent to a healed lesion.

The active ocular lesions vary considerably in an adult who was infected in utero but has no systemic signs. The retinal inflammation occurs because of rupture of a pseudocyst and infection of adjacent cells. There is a generalized nonspecific retinochoroiditis with many vitreous exudates and veils. The retinal and choroidal atrophy with surrounding pigment proliferation of infantile inflammation is rarely seen. The disease tends to be bilateral, recurrent, and chronic. Treatment is often difficult because organisms are encysted, and tissue edema, inflammation, granuloma formation, and relative avascularity prevent access of the drugs to the organisms. *Toxoplasma* antibody titers are low.

In patients with an immune system deficiency, ocular toxoplasmosis is usually a new infection and not the reactivation of a congenital lesion. There are no healed and pigmented congenital retinal scars, and the organism causes a nonspecific retinochorioretinitis.

The treatment of choice for systemic or ocular toxoplasmosis is pyrimethamine or clindamycin. Pyrimethamine inhibits folic acid metabolism of the protozoa and requires leucovorin to prevent bone marrow depression. Minocycline may be substituted for clindamycin. In the absence of an acute systemic disease, the ocular inflammation is treated with low doses of corticosteroids.

***Acanthamoeba* keratitis.**—*Acanthamoeba* are free-living amebae with no known insect vectors or human carrier states. They rarely cause a fatal meningoencephalitis in patients with skin or pulmonary lesions and an impaired immune system. They are an important cause of severe corneal ulcers in patients who wear soft contact lenses. Often there is a history of poor contact lens hygiene and cleansing of the lenses with tap water or homemade saline solutions.

The ulcer resembles that caused by fungi and is associated with severe conjunctival injection and a flare and cells in the anterior chamber. The organisms may be demonstrated with ink–potassium hydroxide staining of corneal specimens. Corneal debridement combined with oral administration of a broad-spectrum antifungal agent, itraconazole, and topical application of 0.1% miconazole hourly has been effective treatment.

Pneumocystis carinii.—*Pneumocystis carinii* is a saprophyte of humans and animals with characteristics of both fungi and protozoa. It causes a pneumocystosis in some 80% to 90% of all patients with AIDS and is a common cause of death. Others susceptible to *P. carinii* pneumocystosis include patients immunocompromised after organ transplantation, those with lymphoma and leukemia in remission, and malnourished children.

Treatment is difficult and usually requires specific treatment of the infection and inhibition of the pulmonary immune response, usually using corticosteroids as adjunctive therapy. Trimethoprim-sulfamethoxazole is usually administered parenterally. In patients allergic to this medication, pentamidine is used although it may cause hypotension, hypoglycemia, blood dyscrasias, vomiting, and renal damage. During treatment a cytomegalovirus infection is often reactivated and patients develop a necrotizing hemorrhagic retinitis. Treatment with ganciclovir must begin promptly to prevent necrosis of the fovea and permanent loss of central vision. Treatment is continued indefinitely because the ocular infection recurs when it is stopped.

BIBLIOGRAPHY

Books

Abbas AK, Lichtman AH, Pober JS: *Cellular and molecular immunology,* ed 2, Philadelphia, 1994, WB Saunders.

Caspi RR, Nussenblatt RB: *Natural and therapeutic control of ocular autoimmunity: rodent and man.* In Coutinho A, Kazatchkine MD, editors: *Autoimmunity: physiology and disease,* New York, 1994, Wiley-Liss.

Ehrlich GD, Greenberg SJ: *PCR-based diagnostics in infectious disease,* Cambridge, Mass, 1994, Blackwell Scientific Publications.

Epstein MA, Achong BG, editors: *The Epstein-Barr virus,* New York, 1994, Springer-Verlag.

Joklik WK, Willett HP, Amos DB, Wilfert CM, editors: *Zinsser microbiology,* ed 20, Norwalk, Conn, 1992, Appleton & Lange.

Mims CA et al: *Pathogenesis of infectious disease,* London, San Diego, 1995, Academic Press.

Pepose JS, Holland GN, Wilhelmus KR: *Ocular infection and immunity,* St Louis, 1995, Mosby–Year Book.

Reeves G, Todd I: *Lecture notes on immunology,* Cambridge, Mass, 1996, Blackwell Scientific Publications.

Roitt IM, Brostoff J, Male DK: *Immunology,* ed 3, St Louis, 1993, Mosby–Year Book.

Salyers AA, Whitt DD: *Bacterial pathogenesis: a molecular approach,* Washington, 1994, ASM Press.

Sell S, Berkower I, Max EE: *Immunology, immunopathology, and immunity,* Norwalk, Conn, 1996, Appleton & Lange.

White DO, Fenner FJ: *Medical virology,* ed 4, San Diego, 1994, Academic Press.

Articles

Holland GN, Tufail A: New therapies for cytomegalovirus retinitis, *N Engl J Med* 333:658-659, 1995.

Karma A, Seppälä I, Mikkilä H, Kaakkola S, Viljanen M, Tarkkanen A: Diagnosis and clinical characteristics of ocular Lyme borreliosis, *Am J Ophthalmol* 119:127-135, 1995.

Kirsch LS, Arevalo JF, DeClercq E, Chavez de la Paz E, Mungia D, Garcia R, Freeman WR: Phase I/II study of intravitreal cidofovir for the treatment of cytomegalovirus retinitis in patients with the acquired immunodeficiency syndrome, *Am J Ophthalmol* 119:466-476, 1995.

Luttrull JK, Wan WL, Kubak BM, Smith MD, Oster HA: Treatment of ocular fungal infections with oral fluconazole, *Am J Ophthalmol* 119:477-481, 1995.

26

HEREDITARY DISORDERS

The human genome (the complete set of chromosomes derived from one parent) is estimated to contain 3 billion base pairs of deoxyribonucleic acid (DNA). An individual inherits one copy of this genome from each parent. The DNA is contained in 23 pairs of chromosomes, each of which contains between 30,000 and 150,000 different gene sequences, which specify the structure of a protein. Each gene is situated at a specific site, or locus, on each chromosome. At least 4,300 single-gene mendelian disorders have been recognized in humans. Some 20% of these affect the eye only, or the eye is the major target of apparently unrelated, multiple clinical effects of a single mutant gene.

Genes that occupy the same position (locus) on an identical pair of chromosomes (autosome) are alleles. When both members of a pair of alleles are identical, the individual is homozygous for that gene pair; when they are different, the individual is heterozygous for that gene pair. The genotype describes the genetic constitution of an individual. The phenotype describes the physical, physiologic, and biochemical characteristics of an individual, which are determined by that individual's genotype.

Each human cell (except gametes formed in meiosis) has 22 pairs of homologous (autosomal) chromosomes and one pair of sex chromosomes, which are homologous in the female (XX) and dissimilar in the male (XY). Each parent contributes 22 autosomal chromosomes and one sex chromosome to each normal offspring. A male offspring receives a Y chromosome from his father and an X chromosome from his mother. A female offspring receives an X chromosome from each parent.

Genetic disorders generally fit into one of four categories: (1) chromosomal disorders; (2) abnormalities of a single gene (monogenic); (3) abnormalities of two or more genes often combined with external factors (multifactorial); and (4) abnormalities in a gene or genes transmitted by the mitochondria.

Chromosomal disorders involve an absence, excess, or abnormal arrangement of one or more chromosomes that produce a deficiency, or an excess of genetic material that affects multiple genes. Monogenic or mendelian abnormalities are determined primarily by a mutation of a single gene and cause a permanent heritable change in genetic material. Multifactorial disorders are caused by abnormalities of two or more different genes that combine with various exogenous or environmental factors. The mitochondrion is transmitted exclusively by the ovum of the mother and codes for 37 genes that play a major role in body metabolism. There is one set of chromosomes in the nucleus of each cell but thousands of copies of mitochondria in some cells.

CHROMOSOMAL ABNORMALITIES

Chromosomal abnormalities result from (1) an excess or a loss of one or more chromosomes (aneuploidy); (2) breakage and loss of a piece of a chromosome (deletion); (3) breakage of two chromosomes with transfer and fusion of parts of the broken fragments into each other (translocation); (4) abnormal splitting of the centromere during mitosis so that one arm is lost and the other duplicated (isochromosome formation); and (5) chromosomal mosaicism so that one individual possesses two different chromosomal cell lines.

The number and the structure of the chromosomes of an individual (the karyotype) can be ascertained by growing skin fibroblasts or peripheral blood lymphocytes in tissue culture and then preparing single metaphase cells for microscopy. Special staining permits identification of each individual chromosome by its characteristic banding pattern.

Chromosome parts are classified as follows: the first number is the number of the chromosome; X is the chromosome derived from either parent in a female offspring or from the mother in a male offspring; Y is the chromosome derived from the father in a male offspring. Thus, XX designates the sex chromosome of a female and XY designates the sex chromosome of a male. Cen is the centromere; p is the short arm; q is the long arm; ter indicates a terminal end; pter indicates the terminal end of a short arm; qter indicates the terminal end of the long arm; if there is an extra chromosome its number is preceded by a "+." If a chromosome is missing its number is preceded by a "–." The band is designated first by a p or a q and then the band number.

A locus is the location of a gene on a chromosome, a sequence of DNA on a chromosome of unknown function (an anonymous DNA segment), a fragile site, a break point, a marker, or other distinguishable sequence by which a site can be specified. The letter D designates an anonymous DNA segment. The number or the letters X or Y following indicate either the chromosome number or the sex chromosome on which the segment is located. The type of sequence is indicated by a letter: S for a single copy sequence followed by a number unique for the location of the sequence on the chromosome; F for a family of homologous sequences on one or more chromosomes. Thus, D15S12 indicates the 12th single copy anonymous sequence assigned to chromosome 15.

With any abnormality of an autosomal chromosome, there may be low birth weight for gestational age, failure to thrive, and mental retardation. The following ocular abnormalities may occur: hypertelorism, small palpebral fissures that slant downward and inward, blepharoptosis, strabismus, epicanthus, corneal opacities, colobomas of the iris and choroid, microphthalmia, and anophthalmia.

Down syndrome (trisomy 21).—Down syndrome is the most common chromosomal disorder and the most common cause of mental retardation that can be recognized at birth. Some 93% to 96% of affected individuals have an extra copy of chromosome 21. There is a triplication of a region of chromosome 21 around D21S55 in 21q22 (Down chromosome region). It is present commonly as a free chromosome. Rarely, there is a fusion of the long arm of chromosome 21 (Robertsonian fusion) or a partial reciprocal translocation. In 2% to 4% of the cases there are two populations of cells (mosaicism), one of which has an extra chromosome 21.

There is a gradual linear increase in incidence with increasing maternal age and a rapid logarithmic type of increase after about 33 years of age. In mothers between ages 20 and 30 years the risk increases from about 1 in 2,000 live births to 1 in 900. At 35 years of age, the incidence rises to 1 in 350 and by 40 years to 1 in 110. After 46 years of age, the risk increases to 1 in 25. Males with Down syndrome are sterile, but women occasionally reproduce.

Mental retardation and generalized muscle hypotonia may occur in all. A neuronal degeneration, histologically identical with that seen in Alzheimer disease, occurs in adulthood. There are many physical findings. Adults are short and fat. The mouth is open with a thick, protruding, furrowed tongue, and broad, dry, fissured lips. The teeth are irregular. The head is small and there is hypoplasia of the nasal bones with a flat nasal bridge. The ear lobes are small or absent and the ear is folded or dysplastic. There is loose skin on the nape of a short neck. The hands are short and broad and the fifth finger is short and incurved. Congenital heart disease is common and there is a high rate of leukemia.

The palpebral fissure is almond-shaped; the outer canthus is higher than the medial canthus (mongoloid slant), and epicanthal folds are present. The iris is hypoplastic, and in early life, white areas are present (Brushfield spots). Cataract occurs in about 60% of the patients. Esotropia, nystagmus, myopia, and blepharitis are common. Teenagers may develop keratoconus, often complicated by an acute corneal hydrops (edema) that heals with severe scarring.

Irrespective of the refractive error or the degree of skin or iris pigmentation, the ophthalmoscopic appearance of the fundus is similar to that in myopic or blond individuals. The pigmentation of the retinal pigment epithelium and choroid is scanty, and the choroidal vasculature is easily visible. The large number of retinal vessels crossing the disk margin gives it a pinker color than usual.

Trisomy 18 syndrome.—Trisomy 18 syndrome (Edwards syndrome) occurs about one third as often as the Down syndrome. Duplication of most of chromosome 18q (18w12.1-qter) results in severe signs, while duplications that affect only the distal one half of 18q cause a mild anomaly. It is most common in females (3 : 1) born to mothers more than 40 years of age. The birth weight is low, and there is failure to thrive, hypertonicity, and mental deficiency. The mandible and mouth are abnormally small, ventricular septal defects are present, and umbilical and inguinal hernias are common. The life span is usually less than 3 months. Ocular hypertelorism, prominent epicanthal folds, and blepharophimosis are common. There may be microphthalmia, uveal colobomas, corneal opacities, congenital glaucoma, and abnormal optic disks.

Trisomy 13 syndrome.—Trisomy 13 syndrome (Patau syndrome) includes severe psychomotor retardation, arhinencephaly, sloping forehead, cleft lip and palate, renal defects, and capillary hemangiomas. There are many ocular abnormalities: microphthalmia; coloboma of the iris, choroid, and optic nerve; retinal dysplasia; optic nerve hypoplasia; persistent hypoplastic primary vitreous; cataract; cyclopia; corneal opacity; ocular hypertelorism; absent eyebrows; and intraocular cartilage. Embryonic or fetal hemoglobin is common. Few affected infants live more than a year.

Cat-eye syndrome.—This is an abnormality with a chromosomal duplication within chromosome 22 (22pter-q11.2). There is a coloboma of the iris, motor retardation, hypertelorism, antimongoloid slant of the palpebral fissures, microphthalmia, and sometimes optic atrophy. Preauricular skin tags and fistulas, abnormal ears, congenital heart disease, renal abnormalities, and anal atresia may occur.

DELETION SYNDROMES

Partial deletion of the short arm of chromosome 4 (Wolf-Hirschorn) is associated with profound mental and growth retardation, hypertelorism (simulating exophthalmos), blepharoptosis, exotropia, epicanthal folds, and coloboma of the iris. Hemangioma of the brow is common, as are cryptorchidism and hypospadias.

Deletion of the short arm of chromosome 5 is characterized by a high-pitched, weak, shrill catlike cry (cri du chat) of the infant during the first few weeks of life, the result of laryngomalacia. There is severe mental and growth retardation with microcephaly. The infant's face is round, the inner canthus is higher than the outer, and epicanthus, hypertelorism, and alternating esotropia are present.

Deletion of the short arm of chromosome 18 is associated with mental retardation, hypertelorism, epicanthal folds, strabismus, blepharoptosis, and rarely cataract. Deletion of the long arm of chromosome 18 is associated with midface hypoplasia and frequent eye defects, such as glaucoma, strabismus, nystagmus, tapetoretinal degeneration, and optic atrophy.

Hereditary deletion of band 13q14.3 combined with inactivation of its allele on the corresponding chromosome leads to retinoblastoma (see Chapter 17). Similarly, a small group of patients with Wilms tumor have a deletion on chromosome 11, band p13. Generally the Wilms tumor in such patients occurs in association with bilateral aniridia. A specific locus for aniridia exists at chromosome 11p13, but not every patient with aniridia and this deletion develops Wilms tumor (see Chapter 16).

Turner syndrome.—Patients with Turner syndrome (gonadal dysgenesis) receive an X chromosome from the mother but lack the X chromosome from the father. Individuals are unambiguously female but have infantile genitalia, primary amenorrhea, infertility, and a short stature. Patients with Turner syndrome who are heterozygotes for X chromosome–linked color blindness will express the defect because of the absence of the normal fellow X chromosome to inactivate the X chromosome. Additionally, strabismus, blepharoptosis, blue sclera, cataract, and corneal arcus occur in more than one third of these patients.

MONOGENIC (MENDELIAN) DISORDERS

Monogenic disorders are caused by a gene in which a permanent heritable change in genetic material has occurred (Table 26-1). The gene defect is dominant if the gene can be fully expressed in the phenotype by a gene present on only one chromosome of a homologous pair of chromosomes. If the gene defect requires a mutant gene at the same locus of each of a pair of homologous chromosomes to be expressed, the defect is recessive. If the defect is carried on sex chromosomes, it is sex-linked or X chromosome–linked. Autosomal defects are transmitted on the 22 pairs of nonsex chromosomes. Both males and females are affected, and both can transmit the abnormality to both sons and daughters.

Autosomal dominant disorders are those conditions that can be expressed in the heterozygous states. In families with 100% penetrance (regular dominance), the trait appears in every generation, the trait is transmitted to 50% of the offspring, there is an equal sex incidence, and unaffected persons do not transmit the trait to their children. Some inherited autosomal dominant genes do not affect an individual because of lack of penetrance. Other autosomal dominant genes are not fully expressed in the phenotype, a variable expressivity that may cause a partial or arrested (forme fruste) type of the disorder.

Autosomal dominant disorders are manifested from one generation to the next. Except in the instance of fresh mutations, each affected individual has a parent who is affected and may have affected siblings. An affected individual and a normal mate will transmit the gene to half of their offspring; both sexes will be equally affected. Autosomal dominant conditions involve mainly structural or nonenzymatic proteins. Generally, the disorders are less severe than those that occur with autosomal recessive traits. Autosomal dominant ocular disorders (Table 26-2) include most corneal dystrophies, aniridia, some congenital cataracts, some retinitis pigmentosa pedigrees, and vitelliform macular degeneration (Best disease).

Autosomal recessive traits are transmitted by clinically normal phenotypes, each of whom contributes an abnormal gene. The carrier of a single defective gene (heterozygous), although clinically normal, may show minimal evidence of the defect such as a deficiency of the enzyme, which occurs in carriers of Tay-Sachs disease or galactosemia. When both parents are heterozygous for a recessive trait, one fourth of the offspring will be homozygous for the abnormal allele, one fourth will be normal, and one half will be heterozygous for the recessive trait. Most inborn errors of metabolism are autosomal recessive disorders, as are oculocutaneous albinism, and some instances of retinitis pigmentosa (Table 26-3). In general, those affected with autosomal recessive conditions have clinically more severe abnormalities than those that involve dominant inheritance. Since related individuals are more likely to be heterozygous for the same abnormal gene, consanguinity is more likely to produce offspring affected by a recessive disorder.

Defects that are carried on the sex chromosomes may be heterozygous or homozygous in the female and hemizygous in the male. The female, with two X chromosomes, may be either a heterozygous or a homozygous carrier for an X chromosome defect and demonstrate either recessive or dominant transmission. An abnormal X chromosome is always expressed in the male, whether dominant or recessive, because there is no corresponding X chromosome to suppress expressivity of the abnormal X chromosome. The homozygous female transmits an abnormal X chromosome to all her children. Her sons will express the trait, and her daughters will be carriers and transmit the trait. The heterozygous female transmits an abnormal X chromosome to one half of her sons and daughters. The hemizygous male transmits an abnormal X chromosome only to his daughters.

The male has one X chromosome and thus carries only half the complement of X chromosome–linked genes found in the female. There can be no father-to-son transmission, because the male transmits a Y chromosome to his sons and an X chromosome to his daughters. All daughters of an affected male will inherit the defective gene (see Table 26-1). Half the children of the daughter will inherit the defective gene. The abnormality will be expressed in the sons, while the carrier daughters (first-generation carriers) will transmit the gene to one

TABLE 26-1.
Chromosome Location for Some Ocular Tissues and Some Ocular Disorders

Location	Ocular Tissue or Disorder
X Chromosome	
Xpter.p22.2	Craniofrontonasal dysplasia
Xp22.3	Ocular albinism
Xp22.3-p22.1	Retinoschisis
Xp22.2	Microphthalmia with linear skin defects
Xp22.2-p22.1	Corneal dermoids
Xp22	Aicardi syndrome
Xp21.3-p21.2	Retinitis pigmentosa
Xp21.1	Retinitis pigmentosa
Xp21.-p11.3	Cone dystrophy
Xp21	Oregon eye disease
Xp11.4	Norrie disease
Xp11.4-p11.23	Äland island eye disease
Xp11.3	Congenital stationary night blindness
Xp11.3	Retinitis pigmentosa
Xp11-21	Incontinentia pigmenti
Xp11.3	Retinitis pigmentosa
Xp	Cataract, congenital
Xcen-q21	Arrestin
Xq28	Incontinentia pigmenti (type 2)
Xq12.q13	Menkes disease
Xq21.2	Choroideremia
Xq21.3-q22	Megalocornea
Xq22	Fabry disease
Xq26.1	Oculocerebrorenal (Lowe) syndrome
Xq26.3-q27.1	Albinism with deafness
Xq27-q28	Anophthalmos with mental retardation
Xq28	Blue cone monchromacy
Xq28	Green cone pigment
Xq28	Mucopolysaccharidosis II (Hunter)
Xq28	Incontinentia pigmenti
Xq28	Myopia
Xq28	Red cone pigment
Chromosome Number 1	
1p36.3	Homocystinuria 3
1p36-p36.2	Ehlers-Danlos syndrome VI
1p36.2-p36.1	Neuroblastoma suppressor
1p36-p35	UPD galactose-1-epimerase deficiency
1p32	Neuronal-1 ceroid lipofuscinosis, invantile
1p31	Retinal pigment epitheolium specific protein
1p22-p21	Zellweger syndrome
1p21-p13	Stargardt macular degeneration
1p13	Transducin
1p	Pheochromocytoma
1q2	Cataract (zonular pulverulent)
1q21	Gaucher disease
1q21-q22	Glaucoma, open-angle
1q32	Retinitis pigmentosa and deafness (Usher)
1q42	Fanconi syndrome
1q42	Xeroderma pigmentosum
1q42-qter	Choroideremia
Chromosome Number 2	
2pter-p25.1	Iris coloboma
2q24-q37	Arrestin
2q31	Ehlers-Danlos syndrome
2q33-q35	Cataract, Coppock-like
2q33.qter	Cerebrotendinous xanthomatosis
2q34	Ehlers-Danlos syndrome
2q35	Waardenburg syndrome

TABLE 26-1 (cont.).

Location	Ocular Tissue or Disorder
Chromosome Number 3	
3p26.p25	von Hippel-Lindau syndrome
3q24	Retinoic acid receptor
3q21.33	G_{M1}-gangliosidosis
3q21.33	Mucopolysaccharidosis IV
3q21.33	Epidermolysis bullosa
3p21	Transducin
3q2	Alkaptonuria
3q21-q24	Rhodopsin
3q21-q22	Retinol-binding protein
3q22-q23	Blepharophimosis, epicanthus, and blepharoptosis
Chromosome Number 4	
4p16.3	Mucopolysaccharidosis I (Hurler)
4p16.3	Phosphodiesterase
4p16.3	Night blindness
4p14-q13	Cyclic nucleotide-gated channel (rod)
4q21-q23	Mucolipidoses II, III
4q25-q27	Rieger syndrome
4q28.q31	Anterior segment mesenchymal dysgenesis
Chr 4	Phosphodiesterase
Chromosome Number 5	
5q11-q13	Maroteaux-Lamy syndrome
5q13	Sandhoff disease
5q22-q33.3	Groenouw corneal dystrophy (type I); lattice type combined granular-lattice type
5q31.3-q33.1	G_{m2}-gangliosidosis
5q32-q31.1	Manidbulofacial dysostosis (Collins)
5q34-q35	Craniosynostosis
Chromosome Number 6	
6p21.3	Ankylosing spondylitis
6p21.3	Insulin-dependent diabetes mellitus 1
6p21.3	Paget disease, bone
6p21.1-cen	Retinal degeneration (peripherin)
6p21.1cen	Retinitis punctata albescens
6p21.1cen	Macular dystrophy
6q13-q15	Ocular albinism
6q14.q16.2	Macular degeneration (North Carolina type)
6q25.q26	Cone dystrophy
Chromosome Number 7	
7p21.3-p21.2	Craniosynostosis
7p21-p15	Macular dystrophy, dominant cystoid
7p15.1-p13	Retinitis pigmentosa
7p13	Greig cephalopolysyndactyly
7p	Godenhar syndrome
7q	Retinitis pigmentosa (autosomal dominant)
7q11.24	Zellweger syndrome
7q21.11	Mucopolysaccharidosis VII
7q22.1	Osteogenesis imperfecta
7q22.1	Ehlers-Danlos syndrome
7q31.3-q32	Blue cone pigment
Chromosome Number 8	
8p11-q21	Retinitis pigmentosa
8q21.1	Zellweger syndrome
8q24	Epidermolysis bullosa, Onga tpe
8q24	Macular dystrophy, atypical vitelliform

Continued.

TABLE 26-1 (cont.).

Location	Ocular Tissue or Disorder
Chromosome Number 9	
9p23	Albinism, brown (tyrosinase-related protein I)
9p13	Galactowe-1-phosphate uridyltransferase (galactosemia)
9q31-q33	Dysautonomia (Riley-Day)
9q33-q34	Tuberous sclerosis
9q34.1	Xeroderma pigmentosum, type A
Chromosome Number 10	
10q.112	Multiple endocrine neoplasia IIA, IIB
10q21-q22	Metachromic leukodystrophy
10q21-q22	Gaucher disease
10q23-q24	Retinol-binding protein
10q25-q26	Crouzon craniofacial dysostosis
10q26	Gyrate atrophy, choroid and retina
Chromosome Number 11	
11p15.5	Hemoglobin beta (sickle cell anemia)
11p15.5	Thalassemias
11p15.5	Insulin
11p15.5	Wilms tumor 2
11p15.4-p15.1	Niemann-Pick disease A, B
11p13	Aniridia
11p13	Peters anomaly
11p13	Rod outer segment membrane protein, retinitis pigmentosa
11p13	Wilms tumor
11p	Retinitis pigmentosa and deafness (Usher)
11q	Insulin-dependent diabetes mellitus
11q13	Vitelliform retinal dystrophy (Best)
11q13	Neovascular vitreoretinopathy
11q13.5	Retinitis pigmentosa and deafness (Usher)
11q14-q21	Tyrosinase (albinism)
11q22.3q23.1	Ataxia telangiectasia
Chr 11	Congenital glaucoma
Chromosome Number 12	
12q11-q13	Epidermolysis bullosa
12q12-q13	Peripherin
12q12-q13	Hermansky-Pudlak syndrome
12q13.11-q13.2	Stickler syndrome
12q14	Sanfilippo syndrome
Chromosome Number 13	
13q12.2-q13	Möbius syndrome
13q14-q31	Letterer-Siwe disease
13q14.1-q14.2	Retinoblastoma suppressor gene
13q14.3-q21.1	Hepaticolenticular degeneration (Wilson)
13q33	Xeroderma pigmentosum
Chromosome Number 14	
14q24q31	Cataract, anterior polar
14q31	Graves disease
14q32	Usher syndrome
Chr 14	Sanfilippo disease, type III C
Chr 14	Rod monochromacy
Chromosome Number 15	
15q11.12-q12	Albinism, oculocutaneous
15q15	Sorbitol dehydrogenase (congenital cataract)
15q21.1	Fibrillin I (Marfan syndrome)
15q23-q24	Tay-Sachs disease
15q23-q24	G_{m2}-gangliosidosis
Chr 15	Xeroderma pigmentosum

TABLE 26-1 (cont.).

Location	Ocular Tissue or Disorder
Chromosome Number 16	
16p13.3	Cataract, congenital, with microphthalmia
16p13.3	Tuberous sclerosis
16p12	Neuronal ceroid lipofuscinosis, juvenile
16q21	Bardet-Biedl syndrome
16q21.1	Cataract
16q22.1	Fish-eye disease
16q24.3	Mucopolysaccharidosis IVA
Chromosome Number 17	
17q11.2	Neurofibromatosis 1 (von Recklinghausen)
17q21-q22	Galactokinase 1 (galactosemia)
17q21.31-q22.05	Osteogenesis imperfecta
17q21.31-q22.05	Ehlers-Danlos syndrome
17q23	Glycogen storage disease II (Fanconi)
Chromosome Number 18	
18p	Sphingomyelinase (Niemann-Pick disease, type C)
18q21-q22.2	Cone-rod dystrophy
18q22-pter	Multiple sclersois
Chromosome Number 19	
19cen-q13.1	Mannosidosis
19q13.1-q13.11	Green/blue iris color
19q13.1	Malignant hyperthermia
19q13.3	Myotonic dystrophy
Chromosome Number 20	
20p13	Diabetes insipidus
Chromosome Number 21	
21q21	Alzheimer disease
21q22.3	Homocystinuria
21q22.3	Down syndrome
Chromosome Number 22	
22q11	Cat-eye syndrome
22q11	Hurler-Scheie mucopolysaccharidosis
22q12.2	Neurofibromatosis type 2
22q13.1-qter	Sorsby fundus dystrophy
Mitochrondria	
Location (nt)	
3307-4262	Leber optic atrophy
4470-5511	Leber optic atrophy
5729-5657	Progressive opthalmoplegia
5826-5761	Progressive ophthalmoplegia
9207-9990	Leber optic atrophy
9991-10058	Leber optic atrophy
10405-10469	Leber optic atrophy
10760-12137	Leber optic atrophy
14673-14149	Leber optic atrophy
Multiple deletions	Kearns-Sayre syndrome
Multiple deletions	Pearson syndrome
Multiple deletions	Neuropathy, ataxia, retinitis pigmentosa
Multiple deletions	Cerebrotendinous xanthomatosis

Modified from McKusick VA, Amberger JS: *Genetic map of the human genome: the autosomes and X, Y, and mitochondrial chromosomes.* In Scriver CR, Beaudet AL, Sly WS, Valle D, editors: *The metabolic and molecular basis of inherited disease,* ed 7, New York, 1995, McGraw-Hill.

TABLE 26-2.
Some Autosomal Dominant Disorders with Ocular Signs

Albinism (rarely)
Aniridia
Cataract (some)
Corneal dystrophies (most)
Marfan syndrome
Neurofibromatosis 1 and 2
Osteogenesis imperfecta
Tuberous sclerosis
Vitelliform retinal degeneration
von Hippel-Lindau disease (usually)

TABLE 26-3.
Some Autosomal Recessive Abnormalities with Ocular Signs

Abetalipoproteinemia
Albinism, oculocutaneous
Alkaptonuria
Ankylosing spondylitis
Ataxia-angioectasia
Cataract
Cone dystrophy
Ehlers-Danlos syndrome
Galactosemia
Glaucoma
Gyrate atrophy of retina and choroid
Hemoglobinopathies
Macular degeneration
Metachromic leukodystrophy
Multiple sclerosis
Neurofibromatosis
Organelle mutation
Lysosomal storage
Peroxisome
Mitochondria
Retinitis pigmentosa
Retinoblastoma
Tay-Sachs disease
Usher syndrome
Waardenburg syndrome

fourth of their sons. An X chromosome–linked disease is evident in the female when the condition is recessive and there are allelic genes on the X chromosome. A recessive gene may be expressed if only one X chromosome is present, as in the Turner syndrome.

The Y chromosome in the male seems devoid of genetic information beyond testicular differentiation and regression of the anlage of the uterus. The X chromosome contains genetic information and, since the female derives one X chromosome from each parent, there is an excess of genetic material. This excess is compensated in each cell by a random inactivation of one of the X chromosomes. Thus, every female cell has one active and one inactive X chromosome (Barr body) that is derived from one or the other parent. The active paternal cells may manifest themselves in some X chromosome–linked disorders. For example, in X chromosome–linked ocular albinism, the carrier mother's iris may transilluminate. In choroideremia the mother's peripheral fundus is pigmented.

Multifactorial inheritance governs many characteristics, such as height, refraction, and intelligence, that vary over a wide range. Many genes on many chromosomes are responsible. There is no sharp distinction between normal and abnormal phenotypes. Proof of this type of inheritance is difficult to establish, but strabismus, some refractive errors, glaucoma, and many other conditions are examples.

DISORDERS OF CARBOHYDRATE METABOLISM

Clinically, diabetes mellitus is the most important abnormality of carbohydrate metabolism (see Chapter 27). Insulin-dependent diabetes (type I) appears to require susceptibility gene(s) that may be located on the short arm of chromosome 6. The disease is precipitated by a humoral and cell-mediated autoimmune attack on the beta cells of the islets of Langerhans of the pancreas.

Non–insulin-dependent diabetes mellitus (type II) is not an autoimmune phenomenon, but there is impaired release of insulin by the beta cells of the islets of Langerhans combined with a cellular insulin resistance. Some patients may have a slowly evolving insulin-dependent diabetes. Many patients are obese, as are their mothers. There is a strong familial tendency to the disorder, but the genetic mechanisms are not clear.

A variety of other hereditary disorders affect carbohydrate metabolism (Table 26-4). Galactosemia is an enzymatic abnormality in which the conversion of the hexose sugar, galactose, to glucose is faulty. The glycogen storage diseases do not have conspicuous ocular defects. In Gierke (type I) glycogen storage disease (glucose-6-phosphatase deficiency), peripheral corneal clouding and patchy paramacular yellowish deposits have been described. In Pompe disease (type II) glycogen storage disease (acid-

TABLE 26-4.
Some Disorders of Carbohydrate Metabolism

Diabetes mellitus
  Type I (insulin-dependent; juvenile)
  Type II (growth-onset)
Galactosemia
  Classic (hexose-1-PO_4 uridyl transferase)
    Cataracts, mental retardation, hepatosplenomegaly, vomiting, dehydration
    Galactose in urine; albuminuria; aminoaciduria; erythrocyte deficiency of hexose-1-PO_4 uridyl transferase
  Galactokinase type
    Cataracts
      Reducing substances in urine; erythrocyte deficiency of galactokinase
Epimerase type
  Asymptomatic (erythrocytes only)
    Symptomatic (liver, erythrocytes, fibroblasts)
      Signs and symptoms of classic type
Hepatoretinal glycogenesis (Gierke)
  Peripheral glycogen corneal deposits; retinal deposits; retarded growth; adiposity; hepatomegaly; eruptive xanthoma
  Hypoglycemia; hyperglyceridemia; acidosis; hypercholesteremia; hyperuricemia
Generalized glycogenesis (Pompe)
  Ocular glycogen deposition; lethal; anorexia; heart and nervous involvement; enlarged tongue
  Deficiency of alpha glucosidase and acid maltase?
Glucose-6-PO_4 deficiency
  Red-green color perception deficiency; optic nerve atrophy; hemolytic anemia
  X chromosome–linked

alpha-glucosidase deficiency), glycogen occurs in the corneal endothelium, the extraocular muscles, the ciliary muscle, the retinal ganglion cells, and the pericytes of the retinal capillaries.

Galactosemia.—Galactosemia is an autosomal recessive abnormality in which the enzymatic conversion of galactose to glucose is impaired. Galactose, a hexose sugar, differs from glucose only in the configuration of the hydroxyl (OH) group of the fourth carbon atom. Although galactose is a component of many complex and essential polysaccharides, nearly all dietary galactose is converted to glucose in a sequence of three enzymatic reactions.

Dietary galactose is first phosphorylated by the enzyme galactokinase to yield galactose-1-phosphate. Galactose-1-phosphate is converted to the nucleotide sugar uridine-diphosphate-galactose by the enzyme galactose-1-phosphate uridyl-transferase. Uridine-diphosphate-galactose is converted to glucose-1-phosphate by the enzyme uridyl-diphosphate galactose-1-epimerase.

There are three types of galactosemia, depending on which one of the three enzymes is deficient: (1) galactokinase deficiency, a rare type (chromosome 17q21-22); (2) transferase deficiency, the classic usual type (chromosome 9p13), which also includes a Duarte variant; and (3) epimerase deficiency, the rarest type (chromosome 1).

Galactokinase deficiency is an autosomal recessive disorder characterized by cataracts, galactosemia, galactosuria, and usually an absence of any additional systemic signs. Sometimes there is increased urinary galactitol that suggests that the enzyme aldose reductase reduces excess galactose to its alcohol. Heterozygous galactokinase deficiency may be associated with early adulthood cataracts in individuals whose diets include much milk. Cataracts may be delayed in all types of galactosemia in those exceptional individuals who have never had milk in their diet.

Transferase deficiency is an autosomal recessive disorder. The afflicted children are usually normal at birth, but cataracts have been found in the fetus at the fifth month of gestation. Usually shortly after birth, as the infant begins to receive milk feeding, problems develop. There are severe systemic signs with vomiting, diarrhea, jaundice, hepatomegaly, feeding problems, and failure to thrive. There may be abdominal distention and sometimes ascites. Cirrhosis may develop. Mental retardation occurs early.

Progressive cataracts occur early. There is an initial increase in the refractive power of the lens nucleus, not unlike that which occurs in the nuclear sclerosis of aging. On ophthalmoscopic examination, the crystalline lens appears to contain a droplet of oil in its center. As the cataract progresses the lens cortex is affected. If galactose is removed from the diet, cataracts either will not develop or, if already present, will not progress.

The cataracts are secondary to the accumulation of galactose alcohol (galactitol) within the lens. The galactose-1-phosphate is converted from the sugar by the action of galactokinase and diffuses freely into the crystalline lens. Here it is converted to its alcohol by the enzyme aldose reductase. The galactose alcohol formed diffuses poorly out of the lens, the lens imbibes water, and cataract follows. In experimental animals fed an excess of galactose, the administration of an aldose reductase inhibitor (sorbinil) prevents the development of cataracts. The cataracts in humans with galactose transferase deficiency reflect the accumulation of the sugar alcohol in the lens, while the systemic abnormalities are the result of the accumulation of galactose-1-phosphate.

Epimerase deficiency occurs in two forms: (1) asymptomatic, in which the enzyme is absent in the erythrocytes only; and (2) symptomatic, in which the enzyme is absent in the liver, erythrocytes, and skin fibroblasts, causing the symptoms of classic galactosemia.

Reducing substances, without glucose present, may be demonstrated in the urine of all types. Diagnosis is based on specific galactose enzyme activities in the infant and both parents. Treatment involves the exclusion of all milk and milk-containing foods. A milk substitute for infants contains casein hydrolysate and soybean preparations. Organ meats must be avoided. If treatment is instituted early, mental retardation, cataract formation, and liver dysfunction may be avoided.

DISORDERS OF LIPID METABOLISM

Defects of lipoprotein metabolism manifest themselves mainly in cardiovascular disorders. Several, however, show ocular abnormalities that vary from corneal arcus, corneal opacities, pigmentary degeneration of the retina, to premature central retinal artery atherosclerosis.

Corneal arcus.—Corneal arcus (gerontoxon, embryotoxon, arcus senilis, arcus juvenilis) is a deposition of phospholipids and noncrystalline cholesterol in the peripheral cornea and adjacent sclera. Generally it appears as a deep, often partial, yellowish white ring in the corneal periphery, concentric to the corneoscleral limbus (Fig 26-1). Its peripheral margin is sharp, whereas its inner margin is poorly defined. Corneal arcus begins in the upper and lower portions of the cornea and may extend to form a complete ring. It involves all layers of the cornea except the epithelium and is usually most marked in Descemet membrane and least marked in midstroma.

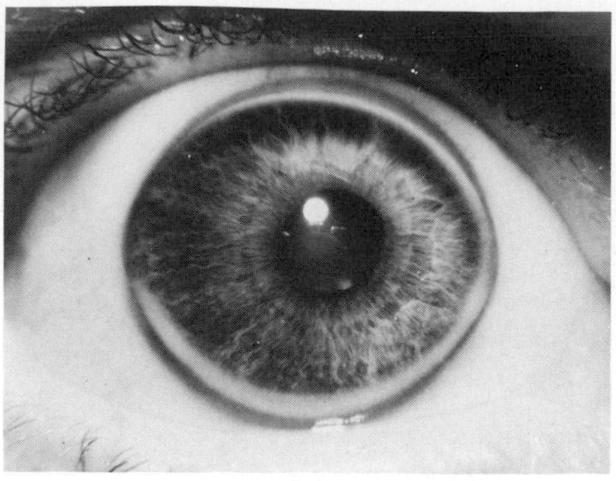

FIG 26-1.
Corneal arcus begins at the corneal periphery above and below and progresses to involve the entire corneal circumference.

Corneal arcus accompanies aging, but the occurrence of corneal arcus or xanthelasma in any person less than 50 years of age, should prompt a study of the lipid metabolism.

Xanthelasma (xanthoma palpebrum).—Xanthelasma consists of multiple, soft-yellowish deposits in the skin of the inner aspects of the upper and lower eyelids. They occur mainly in middle-aged to elderly individuals, often women, who do not have an abnormal lipid metabolism. Xanthelasma, however, occurs together with arcus cornealis in advanced lipid abnormalities. The deposits tend to cluster around blood vessels and sometimes infiltrate the vessel wall. They are easily excised or ablated with a laser but may recur.

Chylomicronemia.—Chylomicrons are synthesized and assembled from several apoproteins, dietary triglycerides, and cholesterol in the intestinal wall. They are delivered into the blood from the thoracic duct. They bind to lipoprotein lipase on the surface of the capillary endothelium and lose their lipids. In several rare inherited disorders, chylomicrons are not catabolized and accumulate in the blood. The blood has a milky appearance, and if refrigerated overnight a creamy supernatant is evident. There may be repeated attacks of abdominal pain with pancreatitis, hepatosplenomegaly, and eruptive cutaneous xanthomatosis.

Secondary types of chylomicronemia may occur in several familial disorders, including lipoprotein lipase deficiency, apolipoprotein

C-II deficiency, and deficiency of lipoprotein lipase inhibitor. Precipitating factors in susceptible individuals include diabetes mellitus, alcohol abuse, and medication with thiazides or estrogens. Often the diagnosis is suspected when blood is withdrawn in the course of an investigation for abdominal pain and found to be lipemic. Abdominal pain, sometimes with pancreatitis and a triglyceride level that may exceed 2,000 mg/dL, are common.

Lipemia retinalis.—This is a rare transient condition in which the retinal blood vessels are abnormal in an individual with chylomicronemia. The blood vessels of the ocular fundus appear orange-red and the arterial light reflex is lost. The arteries and veins have a similar appearance although the difference in diameter persists. Vision is not affected.

Abetalipoproteinemia.— Abetalipoproteinemia (Bassen-Kornzweig syndrome) is an autosomal recessive disorder characterized by an absence of circulating lipoproteins (chylomicrons, very-low-density lipoproteins, and low-density lipoproteins). Each contains a B apoprotein, a protein of high molecular weight. There is a failure of transport vitamin E to peripheral tissues. Abetalipoproteinemia is not a defect of lipid biosynthesis or of the gene for B apolipoprotein, but rather it is caused by a mutation of the gene that codes the 97-kCd subunit of the microsomal triglyceride transfer protein.

Males are mainly affected. Lipoprotein lipase and lecithin-cholesterol acyltransferase activities are severely reduced. A severe anemia responsive to replacement therapy with iron or folic acid may be present.

From 50% to 100% of all circulating erythrocytes have an abnormal shape (acanthocytosis). Malabsorption of fat from the gastrointestinal tract leads to vomiting, diarrhea, and failure to gain weight normally in the neonatal period. Spinocerebellar degeneration may occur in childhood in the absence of vitamin E (tocopherol) therapy. Deep tendon reflexes are lost, gait is ataxic, and a positive Romberg sign is common.

Impaired dark adaptation occurs initially followed by pigmentary degeneration of the retina, which resembles classic retinitis pigmentosa, and occurs in childhood or early adulthood. There is pigment clumping in the central retinal region and bright dots in the periphery. Macrophages ingest lipofuscin in the degenerating retina. Angioid streaks may occur. The severity of the retinal degeneration parallels the severity of the neurologic impairment. Dissociate nystagmus on lateral gaze, blepharoptosis, ophthalmoplegia, and anisocoria may occur. In contrast to retinitis pigmentosa, cataract occurs rarely.

Tocopherol administration in doses of 1,000 to 2,000 mg/day to infants may prevent neurologic and ocular changes. Administration of water-soluble vitamin A may be useful. Treatment of older children and adults may prevent progression of, but not reverse, neurologic damage. Restriction of triglycerides in the diet minimizes gastrointestinal tract symptoms.

Tangier disease (familial high-density lipoprotein deficiency).—Premature corneal arcus or diffuse clouding of the cornea may direct attention to rare autosomal recessive conditions in which there is either a deficiency or an absence of high-density lipoprotein in the plasma combined with an absence of A-1 lipoprotein. There is a marked variation of the genotype and the phenotype.

In homozygous Tangier disease, A-1 azoprotein is absent, plasma cholesterol level is low, and the level of triglycerides is normal. Cholesteryl esters accumulate in many tissues, and the tonsils are streaked with orange-red deposits. There are hepatosplenomegaly, lymphadenopathy, and peripheral neuropathy. Corneal arcus occurs early in adult life or, alternatively, the cornea is clouded with many fine dots of varying size located deep in the stroma. In heterozygous Tangier disease, the premature corneal arcus may be the sole sign.

Familial fish-eye disease.—In this condition a severe diffuse clouding of the cornea gives the appearance of the eyes of a boiled fish. There is a deficiency of lecithin-cholesterol-acyltransferase. Anemia, proteinuria, hyperlipidemia, and increased risk of arteriosclerosis are present.

DISORDERS OF COLLAGEN

Collagen is the most abundant protein in the body. More than 28 different genes dispersed to at least nine chromosomes encode more than 16 different types of collagen. Collagen is composed of three chains of proteins that are wound in a triple helix to form a long molecule.

Collagen I is the most abundant and is the major or only component of skin, tendon, ligament, cornea, sclera, blood vessels, and hollow viscera. The major collagen abnormalities with ocular manifestations are Marfan syndrome (dislocated lenses) (see Chapter 21), Ehlers-Danlos disease (hyperextensible joints), osteogenesis imperfecta (blue scleras), and several abnormalities involving a defective structure of the vitreous humor (collagen II). Most are autosomal dominant disorders.

The Marfan syndrome.—This is an autosomal dominant abnormality of the fibrillin gene on chromosome 15q15-q21.3. Fibrillin is a component of the elastin of many tissues. The major change is in excessive length of long bones, and there is subluxation of the crystalline lenses. The most important change is in the aorta, which leads to aortic regurgitation or fatal dissecting aneurysms. The Marfan syndrome is discussed in Chapter 21.

Osteogenesis imperfecta.—This is a heterogeneous group of defects of the structure of procollagen. Some 90% of the patients have a missense mutation in one of the two genes that code for type I procollagen. There is extensive variation in the phenotype. Osteogenesis imperfecta is associated with severe bone fragility, abnormal teeth, deafness, and blue (or sometimes dark gray) scleras. Type I, the most common, is an autosomal dominant defect, in an individual with blue scleras and normal teeth who may experience a few to more than 50 bone fractures (mainly long bones) before puberty. There is early onset of deafness, joints are hypermobile, tendons may rupture, and aortic valves are thin and sometimes incompetent.

In a rare autosomal dominant type (IV), the scleras are of normal appearance, but the bone disease is considerably more severe. Infants with a grossly abnormal skeleton die at or near birth (type II), while the rare survivor joins children with a progressively severe deformity (type III).

The blue scleras are evident at birth and may be dark blue; with aging, they become gray-blue. The color—described as robin's egg blue, slate blue, or Wedgewood blue—is caused by thinning of the sclera, which permits the underlying uvea to become partially visible. The collagen fibers of the cornea and sclera are immature and have fewer cross-striations than mature collagen. The eyes are often hyperopic, with keratoconus, megalocornea, and faint corneal opacities with corneal arcus. The extreme thinning of the ocular coats (fragilitas oculi) predisposes the eye to rupture with minor trauma.

Ehlers-Danlos syndrome.—This is a heterogeneous group of at least 10 different syndromes of defective connective tissue synthesis that are usually, but not always, transmitted as an autosomal dominant condition. There is hypermobility of the joints, fragility of the skin, hyperextensibility of the skin, bruising, and poor wound healing. Minor trauma often causes gaping skin wounds that must be repaired with adhesive bridges or long sutures because of the friable skin.

Genetic defects vary from mutations of the type III collagen gene (Ehlers-Danlos type IV), mutations of the lysyl hydroxylase gene (Ehlers-Danlos type VI), to mutations of the type I collagen gene (Ehlers-Danlos type VII A and type VII B).

The skin of the eyelids may be involved with epicanthal folds and easy eversion of the eyelids. Esotropia, myopia, microcornea, and blue scleras are common. There may be keratoconus, ectopia lentis, proliferative retinopathy, retinal hemorrhages, and tractional retinal detachment.

NEUROCUTANEOUS SYNDROMES (PHACOMATOSES)

A wide variety of hereditary disorders predominantly involve the nervous system and skin with widely distributed ocular, intracranial, and cutaneous tumors. Pheochromocytoma may occur with all. Most are transmitted as autosomal dominant disorders.

A variety of disorders are included: (1) neurofibromatosis type 1 (von Recklinghausen) and neurofibromatosis type 2 (bilateral acoustic neurofibromatosis); (2) tuberous sclerosis (Bourneville-Pringle); (3) encephalotrigeminal angiomatosis (Sturge-Weber); (4) retinal and cerebellar hemangioblastoma (von Hippel-Lindau); (5) ataxia telangiectasia (Louis-Bar); and (6) encephalo-ocular arteriovenous shunts (Wyburn-Mason).

Neurofibromatoses.—The neurofibromatoses consist of at least two clinically and genetically distinct autosomal dominant disorders of neural crest cells. Both are caused by a disruption or mutation of tumor suppressor genes that normally encode proteins that regulate cell differentiation.

Neurofibromatosis type 1 (von Recklinghausen).—Neurofibromatosis type 1 is an autosomal dominant abnormality that becomes symptomatic in childhood. It is characterized by multiple tumors that originate from the Schwann cells of peripheral nerves and more rarely from astrocytes of the central nervous system. The gene for neurofibromatosis 1 is assigned to chromosome 17q11.2, which encodes the protein neurofibromin. Its action in suppressing tumors appears to be derived through modulation of the phosphorylation of a cellular proto-oncogene p21-*ras*. Its expression is altered in a variety of human malignancies that are not related to neurofibromatosis.

Schwann cell tumors of peripheral nerve sheaths of the skin cause large masses but are seldom otherwise symptomatic. There are characteristic light brown skin lesions (café au lait spots) and freckles of the axillary region, of other intertriginous regions, and surrounding the nipples. Small grayish neuromas (hamartomas) of the hypoplastic iris (Lisch nodules) are diagnostic.

Other ocular changes include corneal nodules and corneal nerve enlargement, fibroma molluscum, or plexiform neuromas that cause thickness of the eyelids and orbital tumors. There may be blepharoptosis, trichosis, strabismus, proptosis (sometimes pulsating), visual failure, buphthalmos, and glaucoma. Astrocytic hamartomas of the retina and the optic disk appear as small hemispheres resting on a white, refractile, slightly uneven base. Optic nerve glioma is the most common tumor of the anterior visual system associated with neurofibromatosis type 1, but not every central nervous system glioma in childhood is secondary to neurofibromatosis. Magnetic resonance imaging is superior to computed tomography in demonstrating the intracranial lesions of neurofibromatosis.

Neurofibromatosis type 2.—This is an autosomal dominant disorder (chromosome 22q12.2) that becomes symptomatic when the patient is in the teens or the twenties with tinnitus or a hearing loss as the result of vestibular schwannomas. Sometimes there are gliomas, meningiomas, and Schwann cell tumors of the spinal cord. Posterior subcapsular cataracts in one or both eyes are a significant association. (One of the genes coding beta lens crystalline is also assigned to the 22q12 region.) Café au lait spots and skin tumors may rarely occur with neurofibromatosis 2. Other ocular changes have not been described. The cataract, occurring in the teens, may be an early sign of the disorder.

Tuberous sclerosis (Bourneville).—Tuberous ("potato-like") sclerosis is an irregular autosomal dominant and sporadic disorder with characteristic skin lesions (adenoma sebaceum-angiofibroma); mental retardation; seizures; and hamartomas in the brain, heart (rhabdomyosarcoma), kidneys (angiomyolipoma), and other organs. There is loss of heterozygosity on chromosome 16p13.3 that may contain a gene that functions as a tumor suppressor gene.

Symptoms begin during the first 3 years of life, and most patients die before the age of 21 years. Congenital patches of hypopigmented skin occur on the trunk and limbs. Pedunculated tumors may occur on the eyelids and palpebral conjunctiva. Astrocytic hamartomas of the retina appear initially on smooth, grayish white masses that develop into elevated, nodular tumors with a granular (mulberry-like) surface. Glial hamartomas of the optic disk ("giant drusen") tend to calcify. Astrocytic hamartomas of the brain, which account for the seizures and mental deficiency, tend to calcify ("brainstones") in more than half of the cases. Before calcification they are most easily demonstrated with T_2-weighted magnetic resonance imaging, whereas computed tomography demonstrates the calcified lesions.

Encephalotrigeminal angiomatosis (Sturge-Weber).—This is a congenital, rarely hereditary, disorder. There is a capillary or cavernous hemangioma (nevus flammeus, port-wine stain), usually but not always along the distribution of the ophthalmic branch of the trigeminal nerve; a cavernous hemangioma of the choroid that causes glaucoma; and a hemangioma of the meninges often associated with intracranial calcification. If the skin lesion is confined to the ophthalmic branch of the trigeminal nerve, the intracranial hemangioma often affects the meninges of the occipital lobe. If the skin lesion affects the maxillary or mandibular branches of the trigeminal nerve, the intracranial lesion often affects the parietal and frontal lobes. Mental retardation and focal seizures on the side opposite the skin lesion are common.

Retinal cerebellar hemangioblastomatosis (von Hipple-Lindau).—This is an autosomal dominant disorder (chromosome 3p26.p25). Retinal capillary angiomas, usually multiple, affect one or both eyes. Ophthalmoscopic examination discloses a reddish, slightly elevated tumor about the size of the optic disk, or smaller. It is nourished by a large artery and vein. Coagulation of the tumor by means of photocoagulation or transscleral diathermy prevents hemorrhages, deposits, and secondary glaucoma. Similar angiomas may occur in the cerebellum and spinal cord. Cysts of the pancreas, kidneys, epididymus, liver, lung, adrenals, bone, omentum, and mesocolon may occur as well as renal carcinomas, pheochromocytomas, and meningiomas. Manifestations vary widely among kindreds.

Ataxia telangiectasia (Louis-Bar).—This is an autosomal recessive disorder characterized by cerebellar ataxia, ocular and facial telangiectases, widespread immunologic disorders, and endocrinopathy. A muted gene, ATM, is mapped to chromosome 11q22.23. There is a chromosomal instability and susceptibility to acute leukemia and lymphoma. Individuals who are heterozygous for ataxia telangiectasia are mildly predisposed to cancer and to radiation hypersensitivity. Cancer predisposition is three- to fourfold that of the general population. The relative risk for breast cancer in carrier women is fivefold that of unaffected women.

A progressive truncal ataxia begins in infancy with an unsteady gait and a pendular nystagmus. There is difficulty in learning to walk. Dilated blood vessels (telangiectases) of the conjunctiva may be mistaken for conjunctivitis. Subsequently, the cheeks, ear lobes, and upper neck develop telangiectases. The stature is short and there is premature aging. Ovarian dysgenesis and gonadal tumors are common. The thymus is absent or degenerated with a severe deficiency of the humoral and cellular immune responses, which causes recurrent sinusitis and upper respiratory infections. A cutaneous anergy is present. The IgA and IgE are absent or reduced. There is persistence of alpha fetoprotein and carcinoembryonic protein. The increased sensitivity to radiation injury must be considered in the management of the frequent malignancies. Patients usually die during their teens.

Encephalo-ocular arteriovenous shunts (Wyburn-Mason).—This is a familial abnormality in which there are no capillaries between the arteries and veins of the retina, mid-brain, and face. The resulting aneurysms and angiomas cause ocular muscle paralysis, pulsating exophthalmos, and intracranial calcification.

DISORDERS OF AMINO ACID CATABOLISM

Ocular signs occur in several (of more than 60) disorders of amino acid catabolism in which intermediate products accumulate within tissues. Tyrosine accumulates in tyrosinemia, and homogentisic acid produced in the catabolism of tyrosine accumulates in alkaptonuria. The absence or deficiency of the enzyme tyrosinase leads to albinism (see the following section). Homocystinuria results from faulty metabolic conversion of methionine to cysteine.

Oculocutaneous tyrosinemia (tyrosinemia type II).—This is an autosomal recessive disorder of tyrosine aminotransferase, the first enzyme of tyrosine catabolism. The gene is located on chromosome 16q22-22.3 and its expression is confined to the cytoplasm of the hepatocytes. Tyrosine crystallizes in the epithelium of the cornea during the first months of life (Fig 26-2), and there is lacrimation, photophobia, pain, and ciliary injection. There are corneal erosions and ulcers, sometimes with corneal and conjunctival plaques. The associated decreased vision may lead to poor vision and exotropia. Painful hyperkeratotic plaques occur on the palms and soles. Mental retardation may occur. Systemic corticosteroids aggravate the disorder.

A low-tyrosine and low-phenylalanine diet, commercially available, ameliorates the signs and symptoms.

Gyrate atrophy of the choroid and retina (hyperornithinemia).—Ornithine, a nonprotein amino acid, originates from dietary arginine. It is the ligand of a mitochondrial transport protein and is normally catabolized to glutamic acid by the enzyme ornithine-delta-aminotransferase (chromosome 10q26). A deficiency of this enzyme causes gyrate atrophy of the choroid and retina.

Sharply defined circular areas of complete chorioretinal atrophy, with scalloped edges, begin at the age of 7 to 9 years. These extend

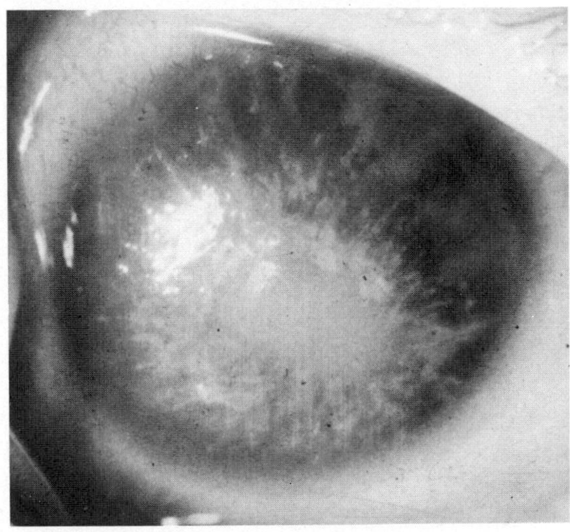

FIG 26-2.
Bilateral corneal ulceration secondary to tyrosinemia II in a 4-week-old male infant. *(Courtesy of Robert P. Burns, MD.)*

centrally and peripherally to involve the entire fundus. There is myopia, night blindness, loss of peripheral vision, and eventual blindness at 25 to 35 years. Posterior subcapsular cataracts develop in the late teens.

The ornithine level is increased 10 to 20 times in the plasma, cerebrospinal fluid, and urine. Plasma levels of glutamate, glutamine, lysine, creatinine, and creatine are reduced. An arginine-restricted diet and the administration of creatine may be helpful. Administration of vitamin B_6 reduces plasma ornithine levels.

Alkaptonuria and ochronosis.—Alkaptonuria is an autosomal recessive disorder (chromosome 3q2) in which homogentisic acid, an intermediary product in the catabolism of phenylalanine and tyrosine, accumulates because of the absence of the enzyme homogentisic acid oxidase, which is normally present in the liver and kidney.

In affected individuals, homogentisic acid is actively excreted by the kidney and appears in the urine (alkaptonuria) in large amounts. It causes the urine to have a dark color or to become dark after standing, provided the urine is alkaline and large amounts of ascorbic acid are not simultaneously excreted. Homogentisic acid reduces Benedict reagent and may give false-positive results for reducing substance in the urine.

Clinically alkaptonuria is characterized by homogentisic acid in the urine and generalized pigmentation of cartilage and other connective tissue (ochronosis), which in turn causes arthritis. The pigmentation is most prominent in the eyes, ears, and nose, and it becomes evident between 20 and 30 years of age. The ocular pigmentation is the result of deposits of homogentisic acid metabolites in the collagen bundles of the cornea, sclera, and elastic tissue of the conjunctiva. The deposits appear on both globes in the palpebral fissure just anterior to the insertions of the horizontal recti muscles; they are oval and have a slate-gray pigmentation. Biomicroscopy of the cornea discloses tiny round, golden brown deposits at the level of the Bowman zone within the palpebral fissure. The concha and the antihelix of the ears are a drab blue-gray. Arthritis develops with aging and is more severe in men than in women.

There is a tendency toward calcification of the heart valves with mitral and aortic valvular heart disease. Advanced atherosclerosis and myocardial infarction are a common cause of death.

ABNORMALITIES OF COPPER TRANSPORT

Copper is an essential element in many enzymes. It is absorbed from the intestine, stored in the liver, and excreted in the bile. In hepaticolenticular degeneration (Wilson disease) and Menkes steely-hair disease there is impaired incorporation of copper into two closely related enzymes, probably secondary to mutations of intracellular copper transport proteins. Despite an accumulation of copper in many tissues, a functional copper deficiency is present.

HEPATICOLENTICULAR DEGENERATION

Hepaticolenticular degeneration is an autosomal recessive disorder (chromosome 13q14.3) of faulty copper transport that results in accumulation of copper in the liver with eventual deposition in the brain (particularly the basal ganglia [lenticular degeneration]), cornea (Kayser-Fleischer ring), renal tubules, heart and skeletal muscle, bones, and joints. The rust-colored ring at the periphery of the cornea occurs in most adults with central nervous system symptoms.

Initially Wilson disease produces signs of liver disease with episodes of jaundice, vomiting, and malaise. Acute hemolytic anemia is more likely caused by Wilson disease than any other condition. As copper is released from the overloaded liver cells it may cause renal stones, renal tubular acidosis, cardiomyopathy, pancreatic disease, osteoporosis, and osteomalacia. Typically liver signs develop between 8 and 16 years of age, and other complications follow. In some patients the accumulation of copper in the liver leads to liver failure and death at age 8 to 10 years without clinical involvement of other organs. Wilson disease must be excluded in all children and young adults with chronic liver disease.

The Kayser-Fleischer ring consists of a green to yellow or brown ring at the corneoscleral limbus at the level of Descemet membrane. The peripheral margin of the ring always sharply ends at the termination of Descemet membrane (Schwalbe line). The ring begins in the upper portion of the cornea and extends circumferentially. It consists of dense accumulations of unequal-sized copper granules in Descemet membrane. The ring is visible only in Descemet membrane, although the entire corneal stroma contains a markedly increased amount of copper. Gonioscopic examination may be necessary to see the ring in early corneal involvement. Its early recognition is important because specific therapy can prevent hepatic and neurologic involvement.

Less common (20%) is a sunflower cataract involving the anterior and posterior lens capsules. With biomicroscopy it appears as a powdery deposit of brilliantly colored material—browns, reds, blues, greens, and yellows—that is located in the visual axis with deposits radiating peripherally, resembling the petals of a sunflower.

Neurologic signs involve the following: (1) degeneration of the nucleus lentiformis (the part of the corpus striatum comprising the putamen and globus pallidus that lies just lateral to the internal capsule), with spasticity, rigidity, dystonic deformities, disturbances of gait, dysarthria, dysphagia, or drooling; or (2) Westphal disease with tremor a major symptom. The sole manifestation may be a psychotic illness, usually of abrupt onset. The patient may have a bizarre personality, with grossly inappropriate social behavior, deterioration of schoolwork, a severe neurosis, or a disorder indistinguishable from schizophrenia or manic-depressive psychosis. Personality disorders may occur in the absence of motor involvement, and jacksonian epilepsy or hemiplegia may occur, as may a coma that persists for several weeks.

Nystagmus, cranial nerve palsies, and other ocular movement disorders do not occur despite extensive cerebral degeneration. Night blindness and degenerative changes in the peripheral retina seem to be unrelated to the primary disorder; however, retinal function has not been systematically studied.

The diagnosis must be considered in all patients with chronic liver disease, particularly children and young adults. Measurement of the copper content of liver biopsy cells reliably establishes the diagnosis. In patients with neurologic disease the plasma ceruloplasmin level is reduced, nonceruloplasmin copper concentration is increased, and urinary excretion of copper is increased. Intravenous radioactive copper (^{67}Cu) is minimally bound to plasma ceruloplasmin. The Kayser-Fleischer corneal ring is highly diagnostic but has also been found in patients with primary biliary cirrhosis.

Treatment consists of copper chelation with penicillamine, which may have to be administered for 6 months before there is clinical improvement. Successful treatment results in disappearance of the Kayser-Fleischer corneal ring and amelioration of the hepatic and neurologic symptoms. Liver transplantation is required in irreversible liver disease.

There is linkage to esterase D and the retinoblastoma locus on chromosome 13 in the region of 13q14 (D13S10). Siblings of patients with

Wilson disease must be examined for liver disease, neurologic disease, and corneal rings because there is a one in four risk of having the disease. Heterozygotes do not develop clinical abnormalities.

MENKES STEELY-HAIR DISEASE

Menkes steely-hair disease is an X chromosome–linked (Xq12-q13) recessive disorder of a copper-transporting adenosine triphosphatase gene. It is characterized by cerebral degeneration, seizures, spasticity, hypothermia, "kinky" and depigmented hair, depigmented skin, osteoporosis, and fragmentation of the internal elastic lamina of blood vessels that rupture and occlude. Individual hairs are twisted, white, and coarse and break easily. The face is typical, with pudgy cheeks, sagging jowls, blond skin, and eyebrows and eyelashes with scanty, stubby, broken hairs. The children do not thrive and usually die in infancy. There is no effective treatment.

The eyes develop normally but the children are blind by the age of 6 months. Ganglion cells in the retina are markedly reduced and there is an optic atrophy. There are microcysts of the pigment epithelium of the iris. The mitochondria of the retinal pigment epithelium, surviving ganglion cells, and inner segments of photoreceptors are swollen with an electron-dense substance within the matrix of the mitochondria. The elastic tissue of Bruch membrane is reduced.

ALBINISM

Albinism (Latin *albus:* white) is a hereditary disorder characterized by an absence or deficiency of the enzyme tyrosinase, which is essential for the synthesis of melanin pigmentation. A variety of tissues may be affected: (1) the skin and eyes (oculocutaneous albinism); (2) the eyes only (ocular albinism); and (3) the skin only (cutaneous albinism) (Table 26-5).

The melanocytes, which synthesize the pigment melanin in cytoplasmic vacuoles in the skin, mucous membranes, hair, choroid, ciliary body, retinal pigment epithelium, iris, pia mater, arachnoid, and inner ear, are normal. The melanocytes of the retinal pigment epithelium and its anterior extension the iris originate in the ectoderm of the outer layer of the optic cup. All other melanocytes originate from melanoblasts of the neural crest that migrate to peripheral sites during embryonic development. The melanocytes are normal both in structure and number in albinism, but tyrosinase is absent or deficient. Tyrosinase normally oxidizes tyrosine to 3.4 dihydroxyphenylalanine (dopa) and then to a quinone. Melanin is formed nonenzymatically in a reaction that requires zinc. The absence or deficiency of the enzyme tyrosinase causes a failure of melanin synthesis that results in depigmented skin, hair, eyes, lateral geniculate body, and other structures. (Gene mutations that cause defects in the proliferation or structure of melanocytes cause hypopigmentation in conditions such as piebaldism, vitiligo, and other disorders often associated with reduced pigmentation of the skin and hair. Tyrosinase is not deficient and the conditions are not albinism.)

TABLE 26-5.
Classification of Albinism

Oculocutaneous albinism
Tyrosinase-negative (type I A; classic; tyrosinase absent)
Tyrosinase-positive (type II B; tyrosinase deficient)
Hermansky-Pudlak syndrome
Yellow-mutant type (Amish)
Prader-Willi syndrome (mutation of P-protein [transporter of tyrosine]; deletion of chromosome 15q; ceroid-lipofuscin-like pigment in lysosomes)
South African type
Ocular albinism
X chromosome type (Nettleship-Falls)
X chromosome type with sensorineural deafness (Xpp22.2-22.3: DSX452 locus; allelic variants or contiguous gene defects)
Autosomal recessive
Minimal pigment type
Cutaneous albinism

Oculocutaneous albinism.—Oculocutaneous albinism is an autosomal recessive abnormality, linked to chromosome 15q11.q13. It is divided into some 26 genotypes and many phenotypes. The major types are (1) tyrosinase-negative in which there is no tyrosinase activity in any tissue and which affects races about equally; and (2) tyrosinase-positive in which tyrosinase is present but in reduced amounts, and which is more common among black individuals.

In tyrosinase-negative albinism there is no visible pigment in the eyes, skin, or hair. There is no tyrosinase activity in any tissue. The iris is gray-blue and translucent to light directed through the sclera (transillumination). There is a prominent red reflex from the fundus, and the eye appears pink. The fovea is hypoplastic, and there is no central light reflex from the foveola. Visual acuity is at the level of 20/200 or less with no tendency to improvement with aging. There is a severe pendular nystagmus and marked photophobia. Strabismus is present in about 90% of tyrosinase-negative albinos. Esotropia is common (80%); the eyes diverge in the remaining individuals. The strabismus and nystagmus are aggravated by prolonged exposure to bright sun. The hair is snow-white and the skin is pink-white. The irides may be translucent in white individuals heterozygous for tyrosinase-negative albinism (60%); in black individuals the irides are usually normal (75%).

Tyrosinase-positive albinism is the most frequent type. Some melanin pigment is evident in the eyes, hair, and skin, and pigmentation of a yellow-red pheomelanin increases in late childhood.

Infants resemble tyrosinase-negative albinos, but with aging the phenotype extends from the appearance of tyrosinase-negative albino to lightly pigmented individuals. The hair is usually white in infancy and darkens to yellow or light tan with age. The eyes tend to darken with age. The iris in white individuals transilluminates in infancy, often with spokes. In black individuals the iris appears normal. Nystagmus is present in all but is less severe than in tyrosinase-negative albinism. Visual acuity is reduced but tends to improve with age.

Ocular albinism.—This occurs as a deficiency of melanin that is limited to the iris and the retinal pigment epithelium. The two types are transmitted mainly as an X chromosome–linked disorder (Xp22.2-22.3; locus DX5422) or rarely as an autosomal recessive disorder. An autosomal dominant type with deafness is associated with cutaneous brown macules that resemble freckles. The ocular fundi of women heterozygous for the X chromosome–linked albinism may show a mosaic pattern of abnormal pigmentation as the result of random X chromosome inactivation. Some patients with X chromosome–linked ocular albinism have a deficiency in red-green color vision, but their mothers do not have a mosaic fundus.

The severity of depigmentation varies, and the fundus may resemble a blond fundus with the choroidal vasculature visible. The foveal reflex is absent. The iris transmits light to a variable degree. Some but not all female carriers have a partial iris transillumination and may have coarse pigment in the midperiphery of the fundus. The pigmentation of the fundus of the female carrier may be caused by lyonization of the X chromosome. The associated pendular nystagmus may be diagnosed as a congenital nystagmus rather than being recognized as the result of the ocular albinism. The outstanding symptom is photophobia with extreme intolerance to light. Ophthalmoscopic examination indicates a bright orange-red reflex with prominent choroidal vessels that are normally obscured by the retinal pigment epithelium. The retinal blood vessels are normal.

Autosomal recessive ocular albinism is characterized by decreased vision, photophobia, nystagmus, diaphanous irides, and light-yellow fundi. The parents sometimes have diaphanous irides.

Individuals with tyrosinase-negative oculocutaneous albinism and ocular albinism have misrouted axons of retinal ganglion cells, so that some temporal retinal axons decussate in the optic chiasm. Magnetic resonance imaging indicates no abnormality of the intracranial portion of the optic nerves, the chiasm, or the corpus callosum. The lateral geniculate body has three rather than six layers. The geniculocortical pathway (lateral geniculate body to occipital lobe) is also misrouted.

The treatment of albinism is directed toward the accurate correction of the refractive error and any strabismus present. The vision for near is frequently better than distance vision and normal schooling is possible. The use of strong convex lenses for near work may be helpful. Tinted lenses with deeply tinted temples reduce the amount of light that enters the eye. Pigmented contact lenses with a clear pupillary area simulate the appearance of the normal iris but do not improve vision. They are helpful in reducing photophobia.

Albinoidism is a hereditary deficiency of pigmentation in which vision is normal, the iris pigmented, and nystagmus absent. It may be associated with deafness. There is sparse pigmentation in a number of different hereditary abnormalities: Menkes steely-hair syndrome, Apert syndrome, phenylketonuria, and the Waardenburg-Klein syndrome.

Hermansky-Pudlak syndrome.—This consists of tyrosinase-positive oculocutaneous albinism, hemorrhagic diathesis caused by defective platelets, and accumulation of ceroidlike material in the reticuloendothelial system, oral mucosa, and urine. The hair is white to dark red-brown, the iris is blue-gray and not translucent, and the eyes reflect the albino red appearance. Nystagmus, photophobia, reduced vision, and foveal hypoplasia occur. Hemorrhagic episodes are common, and administration of aspirin and related drugs is contraindicated. The disorder is secondary to deletions of chromosome 15q11.2-12, sometimes called the human P gene, which corresponds to the pink-eye deletion of the mouse. Possibly a P-protein transports tyrosine.

HEMOGLOBINOPATHIES

Hemoglobin consists of a protein molecule, globin, bound to four molecules of heme, an iron and protoporphyrin compound. The globin is composed of four amino acid chains that differ in the sequence and composition of their constituent amino acids. Six different globin chains (alpha, beta, gamma, delta, epsilon, and zeta) occur in normal human hemoglobin at some stage of development. The genes concerned with alpha and beta globin are on chromosome 16 (alpha) and 11 (beta).

Normal adult hemoglobin consists mainly (97%) of hemoglobin A (Hb A), which has a pair of alpha chains and a pair of beta chains. Normal adults also have a minor amount (2%) of hemoglobin composed of a pair of alpha chains and a pair of delta chains (Hb A_2). Fetal hemoglobin (Hb F), which is normally found in trace amounts (1%) after birth, contains a pair of alpha chains and a pair of gamma chains.

An alteration in the sequence of amino acids in the amino acid chains may cause changes in the shape, oxygen affinity, electrophoretic mobility, pliability, solubility, and life span of the hemoglobin molecule. Most variations of clinical importance (Table 26-6) involve the beta chain. The variants are tabulated according to the position in the amino acid chain in which the amino acid substitution has occurred. Thus, sickle hemoglobin (Hb S) is designated $\alpha_2\beta_2{}^{6\ glu \rightarrow val}$ indicating that valine has been substituted for glutamic acid in the sixth position of the beta chain of globin. Hb C has a structure of $\alpha_2\beta_2{}^{6\ glu \rightarrow lysine}$

TABLE 26-6.
Hemoglobinopathies of Major Ophthalmic Interest

Sickle cell anemia: SS disease ($\alpha_2\beta_2{}^{6\ glu\rightarrow val}$ and $\alpha_2\beta_2{}^{6\ glu\rightarrow val}$)
  Each parent provides Hb S
Sickle cell trait: SA disease ($\alpha_2\beta_2{}^{6\ glu\rightarrow val}$ and $\alpha_2\beta_2$)
  One parent provides Hb S and one parent provides normal Hb A
Sickle cell disease: SC disease ($\alpha_2\beta_2{}^{6\ glu\rightarrow val}$ and $\alpha_2\beta_2{}^{6\ glu\rightarrow lysine}$)
  One parent provides Hb S and one parent provides Hb C
Hemoglobin C trait: AC disease ($\alpha_2\beta_2$ and $\alpha_2\beta_2{}^{6\ glu\rightarrow lysine}$)
  One parent provides normal Hb A and one parent provides Hb C
Sickle cell β-thalassemia: S-β-thalassemia ($\alpha_2\beta_2{}^{6\ glu\rightarrow val}$ and $\alpha_2\delta_2$)
  One parent provides Hb S and one parent provides β-thalassemia

SICKLE CELL SYNDROMES

Sickle cell anemia, or homozygous Hb S disease, occurs when each parent provides a gene for hemoglobin S. From 70% to 98% of the individual's hemoglobin is hemoglobin S and the remainder is hemoglobin F. Deoxygenated hemoglobin polymerizes to form a gel and subsequently a crystal, which results in an elongated, distorted erythrocyte, the sickle cell. The cell passes through capillaries with difficulty, which is responsible for sluggish blood flow, tissue hypoxia, and infarction. Patients with sickle cell anemia experience symptoms caused by hemolytic anemia and microvascular thrombi. Vascular thrombi result in strokes, retinal infarcts, atrophy of the spleen (with resultant susceptibility to bacterial infection), aseptic necrosis of bones, inability to concentrate urine, priapism, and placental insufficiency with spontaneous abortion. Bone and organ infarction cause episodic painful crises.

In sickle cell trait, Hb SA disease, one parent provides the gene for sickle cell hemoglobin (Hb

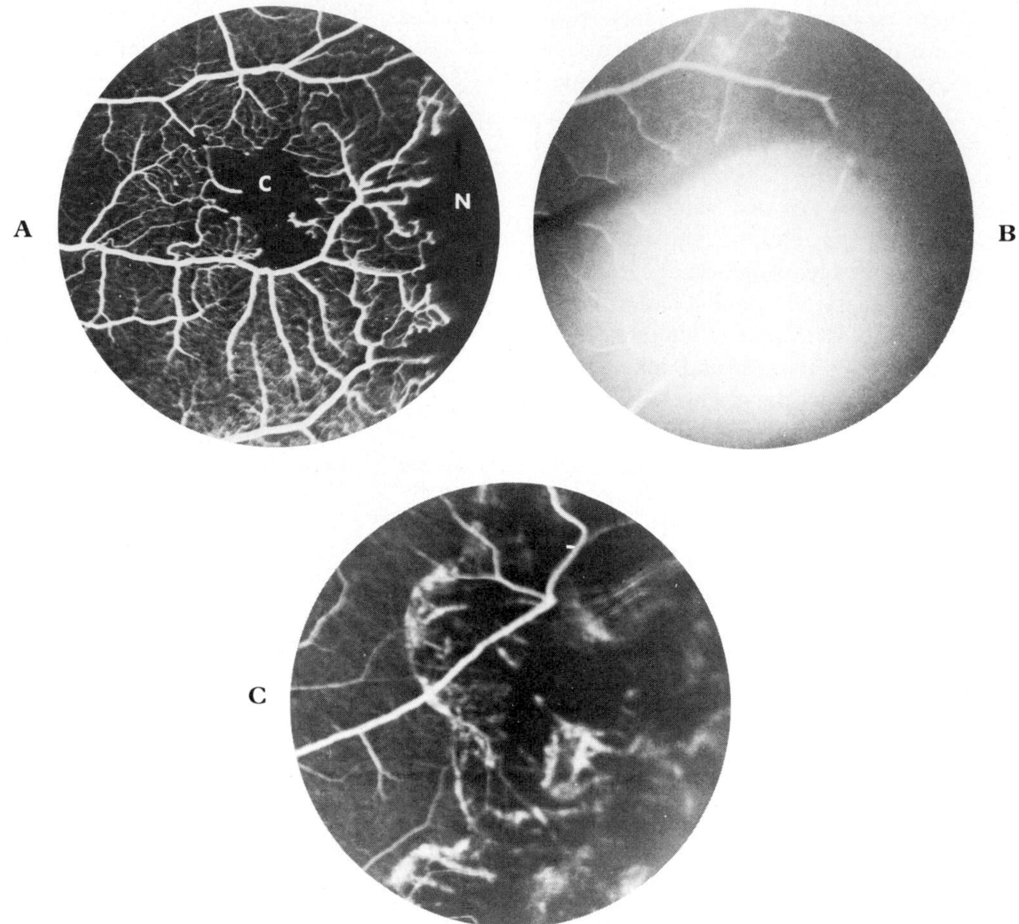

FIG 26-3.

A, Late venous angiogram in a 23-year-old woman with Hb SC disease. Because of arteriolar occlusion there is a central area *(C)* of failure of capillary filling with fluorescein. There is distal occlusion in the periphery and early neovascularization adjacent to this area *(N)*. **B,** In the extreme periphery, new blood vessels leak fluorescein. **C,** The new blood vessels have been destroyed by xenon photocoagulation of the retina.

S) and the other provides a gene for normal hemoglobin (Hb A). In sickle cell disease, Hb SC disease, one parent provides the gene for sickle cell hemoglobin and the other for hemoglobin C. The resultant Hb SC results in the most severe retinopathy caused by sickle cell syndrome.

The ocular lesions are caused by thrombi in the conjunctival or retinal arterioles. The conjunctival changes have no symptoms. They consist of multiple, short, comma-shaped, or distorted isolated capillary segments that do not seem to be connected to the vascular network. Conjunctival changes are most marked in Hb SS anemia, mild in Hb SC disease and rare in Hb SA trait.

The retinal changes are the result of occlusion of the arterioles of the peripheral retina. Initially there is capillary occlusion, and the retina peripheral to the occlusion appears white because of edema. The edema is followed by narrowing of the peripheral arterioles and tortuosity of the veins. An occluded arteriole ends abruptly, and the retina beyond appears avascular (Fig 26-3). Salmon-patch hemorrhages in the peripheral retina are followed by retinoschisis as blood absorbs. The retinoschisis is lined with iridescent hemosiderin-filled macrophages (iridescent deposits). The retinal pigment epithelium proliferates at the margins of chorioretinal atrophy to create black sunburst lesions at the ocular equator.

The zone between the ischemic and normal retina is the site of arteriolar-venular anastomosis that is followed by neovascularization on the surface of the retina. The new blood vessels initially lie flat on the retina and have a sea-fan configuration. These new blood vessels continue to grow and, with collapse of the vitreous, are drawn into the vitreous cavity, and subsequently rupture with vitreous hemorrhage.

Patients with Hb SC disease are the most vulnerable to retinal complications. Generally, retinal infarction is uncommon in Hb SS anemia and Hb SA trait.

Persons of Mediterranean or African ancestry who develop hemolytic anemia, angioid streaks, peripheral retinal neovascularization, or recurrent vitreous hemorrhages should have hemoglobin electrophoresis. Correction of rhegmatogenous retinal separation in patients with hemoglobinopathies is difficult, because encircling bands may cause anterior segment ischemia. Subsequent sickling with anterior ciliary artery occlusion may cause anterior segment necrosis. The risk may be minimized by preoperative exchange transfusion. Tractional retinal detachment and persistent vitreous hemorrhage are managed by vitrectomy.

Photocoagulation of newly formed blood vessels by means of a xenon arc or argon laser photocoagulator may minimize vitreous hemorrhage.

THALASSEMIA SYNDROMES

The thalassemia ("the sea") syndromes are hereditary abnormalities in which the rate of normal hemoglobin synthesis is impaired and in which there may be too few alpha or beta chains. The major group occurs because of a deficiency in the rate of synthesis of beta chains (beta-thalassemia) and their substitution by delta chains. A deficiency of alpha chains (alpha-thalassemia) is more difficult to recognize and less clinically severe.

Hemolytic anemia and deposition of iron in spleen, liver, and kidneys dominate the systemic aspects of the condition. The onset is in infancy, and the children have flat hypoplastic facies with prominent epicanthal folds. There may be neovascularization of the peripheral retina as in sickle cell disease. The thalassemia syndromes may be combined with sickle cell hemoglobinopathies.

GENETIC DISORDERS OF CELLULAR ORGANELLES

The eukaryotic cell is surrounded by a plasma membrane and contains a membrane-bound nucleus, in which DNA is stored and replicated. The cell contains an integrated endoplasmic membrane system consisting of (1) endoplasmic reticulum, which synthesizes proteins; (2) the Golgi apparatus, which modifies many proteins received from the endoplasmic reticulum and transfers them within the cell; (3) secretory vesicles and granules, which receive proteins from the Golgi apparatus and release them from the cell surface; (4) endosomes, which receive materials from outside the cell; and (5) lysosomes, which degrade exogenous material from endosomes and endogenous intracellular elements. Lysosomes contain more than 50 different enzymes that degrade glycolytic bonds in a mildly acid medium. Hereditary absence or deficiency of a particular enzyme leads to an accumulation of undigested material within a cell, a lysosomal storage disease (Table 26-7).

Two intracellular organelles do not directly communicate with the endoplasmic membrane system: (1) mitochondria, which participate in intermediary metabolism and generate most of the adenosine triphosphate required for cellular activity; and (2) peroxisomes (microbodies), which initiate the synthesis of a variety of enzymes, provide enzymes that generate hydrogen peroxide and degrade very long-chain fatty acids, and participate in the synthesis of plasmalogens and bile acids. Gene mutations of mitochondrial enzyme systems produce widespread disorders of oxidative phosphorylation or fatty acid oxidation. Peroxisome disorders result in multiple enzyme deficiencies with anomalies of many organ systems.

LYSOSOMAL STORAGE DISEASES

Lysosomes contain 50 or more hydrolases (acid phosphatase, lipase, esterase, phospholipases, sulfatases, peptidases, galactose and glu-

TABLE 26-7.
Disorders of Cellular Organelles with Ocular Changes

- I. Lysosomal storage disease
  - A. Gangliosidosis
    1. Tay-Sachs disease
    2. Sandhoff disease
    3. G_{M2} gangliosidosis
  - B. Mucopolysaccharidosis
    1. Hurler syndrome (MPS I)
    2. Scheie syndrome (MPS S)
    3. Hurler-Scheie syndrome (MPS I H/S)
    4. Hunter syndrome (MPS II)
    5. Sanfilippo syndrome (MPS III)
    6. Morquio A syndrome (MPS IV)
    7. Maroteaux-Lamy syndrome (MPS IV)
    8. Sly syndrome (MPS VII)
  - C. Beta-galactosidase deficiency
    1. G_{M1} disease
    2. Morquio B syndrome
  - D. I-cell disease
    1. Mucolipidosis II
    2. Hurler polydystrophy (MLD III)
  - E. Sphingomyelinase deficiency
    1. Niemann-Pick disease A, B, C
  - F. Cystine storage disease (Fanconi)
  - G. Glycoprotein degradation
    1. Mannosidosis
    2. Sialidosis
    3. Gaucher disease
    4. Fabry disease
    5. Krabbe disease
- II. Mitochondrial disorders
  - A. Kearns-Sayre syndrome
  - B. Pearson syndrome
  - C. Chronic hereditary optic atrophy
  - D. Leber optic atrophy
  - E. Cerebrotendinous xanthomatosis
  - F. Neuropathy, ataxia, retinal pigment degeneration
- III. Peroxisome disease
  - A. Zellweger syndrome
  - B. Refsum disease

cose aminidases, fucosidase and glucosidase, ribonuclease and deoxyribonuclease, glucuronidase, and hyaluronidase) that degrade many biologic substrates in a mild acid medium. More than 40 rare, autosomal recessive disorders are caused by a deficiency or absence of a lysosomal enzyme so that a partially degraded metabolite accumulates within the cell.

Lysosomal storage disorders may affect skeletal growth, mental development, and central nervous system maturation. The severity varies markedly, often depending on the degree of development attained when the accumulation of abnormal metabolic products impairs function. In some patients there are cloudy corneas, a cherry-red spot at the fovea secondary to degeneration of retinal ganglion cells, and optic atrophy. Other individuals develop a pigmentary degeneration of the retina.

In many patients electron microscopy of conjunctival tissue will demonstrate abnormal lysosomes. The enzyme deficiency can be detected in cultured fibroblasts of the affected individual and sometimes by prenatal testing. Analysis of tissue-culture medium will indicate the enzymatic abnormality, and electron microscopy will indicate abnormal lysosomes. Tears, urine, hair follicles, leukocytes, and fibroblasts have been used for enzyme assay. Heterozygote screening is available at many centers for hexosaminidase A and B, the deficient enzymes in Tay-Sachs disease, and Sandhoff disease.

Gangliosidosis

There are at least 12 different glycolipids, which are localized primarily in the gray matter of the brain, in synaptic membranes, and on cell surfaces where they are responsible for cell-cell recognition and blood group composition. Gangliosides are degraded by lysosomal hydrolases, and a hereditary failure of catabolism results in storage of catabolic substrates in lysosomes. Some 55 phenotypes have been characterized.

The main disorders of ganglioside catabolism of ocular concern involve the degradation of G_{M2} gangliosides by hexosaminidase A (HEXA), hexosaminidase B (HEXB), and the G_{M2} activator protein. Hexosaminidase A is composed of alpha and beta subunits, which are encoded on chromosome 15q21-q25.1. Hexosaminidase B is an isoenzyme of hexosaminidase A and is encoded on chromosome 5q13, as is the G_{M2} activator protein. A mutation of hexosaminidase A causes Tay-Sachs disease. A mutation of both hexosaminidase A and B causes Sandhoff disease. In a rare abnormality, the gene for the G_{M2} activator protein is mutated resulting in G_{M2} gangliosidosis, although both hexosaminidase A and B are normal.

Tay-Sachs disease.—Infantile acute G_{M2} gangliosidosis is the most common type of gangliosidosis. It is an autosomal recessive disorder caused by a mutation in the gene coding hexosaminidase A. Infants appear normal at birth but develop a generalized motor weakness 3 to 5 months after birth. The most common initial symptom is a startled reaction to sound (hyperacusis). The infants are beautiful, with long eyelashes, fine hair, and a delicate pink coloring. Vision is affected early. There is inattentiveness, failure to move the eyes, or strabismus. Ophthalmoscopic examination may be normal initially, but soon the macular region shows a whitish area ophthalmoscopically that is approximately 2 disk diameters in size, with a small reddish foveola area (cherry-red spot). Retinal and optic atrophy is followed by blindness. As neurologic involvement progresses, convulsions or a state of decerebrate rigidity may occur. Death from bulbar involvement usually occurs at about 30 months of age.

Storage of gangliosides in the retinal ganglion cells causes the normally transparent retina to appear white at the posterior pole where the ganglion cells are several layers thick. The cherry-red spot results from the normal appearance of the choroidal circulation at the fovea centralis, where the inner retinal layers are absent. Changes in the brain include enormously swollen and distorted ganglion cells.

With light microscopy the neurons of the central, autonomic, and somatic nervous systems appear enormously swollen and distended. Electron microscopically, the neuronal deposits consist of concentric membranes called membranous cytoplasmic bodies. Nerve fibers are demyelinated, which contributes to the optic atrophy.

Sandhoff disease.—This condition is similar to Tay-Sachs disease, but tubular epithelial cells contain lipids. It is distinguished from Tay-Sachs disease by the severe deficiency of hexosaminidase B.

Juvenile G_{M2} gangliosidosis.—The onset is between 2 and 6 years of age, with ataxia, dysarthria, seizures, and eventual decerebrate rigidity. Cherry-red spots and blindness occur late, and patients die between 5 and 15 years of age. Diagnosis is based on demonstration of normal hexosaminidase A and B and a deficiency of the G_{M2} activator protein.

Wide-scale testing is available to detect carriers for the gene for Tay-Sachs disease. Among Ashkenazi Jewish Americans, a carrier rate of 1:31 is estimated. Among American Sephardic Jewish and non-Jewish people, the carrier frequency is 1:300. For Sandhoff disease the carrier rate among Ashkenazi Jewish individuals is 1:500 compared to 1:278 for non-Jewish individuals.

The mucopolysaccharidoses

Glycosaminoglycans (previously called mucopolysaccharides) are major components of cell membranes, cartilage, bone, intracellular cement substance, and other connective tissues. They are degraded by a series of 10 lysosomal enzymes. A hereditary deficiency of one or more of these enzymes results in the lysosomal accumulation of intact or partially degraded glycosaminoglycans, which causes widespread abnormalities (Table 26-8).

Hurler syndrome (MPS I H; Hurler).—The Hurler syndrome is the most severe mucopolysaccharidosis. It affects many systems and is usually evident within 6 to 18 months after birth. It is clinically characterized by extensive skeletal deformities (dysostosis multiplex), limitation of joint movements, umbilical or inguinal hernia, cardiomyopathy, deafness, mental retardation, and severe corneal clouding.

Typically the skull is large, the calvarium thickened, and the orbits shallow. The bridge of the nose is flattened, the nostrils are broad, and the posterior pharynx is occluded. The children are mouth breathers, and they have markedly carious teeth and fetid breath. The facies are apathetic, the tongue is enlarged, and the facial features are coarse (Fig 26-4). The neck is short, and the head appears to rest directly upon the thorax. The abdomen is protuberant. Kyphosis is common, as are deformities of the vertebrae. The broad hands have stubby fingers, and on roentgenologic study, the terminal phalangeal bones are hypoplastic. Limitation of extension of the joints is striking. Roentgenographic examination discloses a long and shallow sella turcica.

Clouding of the cornea is characteristic. The subepithelial area has the appearance of slightly glazed glass. The central cornea is more cloudy than the periphery, although histologically the deep epithelial layers of the periphery are more involved. The normal tension, absence of tearing, failure of the globe to enlarge, and associated physical changes exclude glaucoma as a cause of the corneal clouding. Rarely, primary glaucoma develops. Increased intracranial pressure may rarely occur, but the papilledema cannot be seen through the cloudy cornea. There is retinal infiltration with mucopolysaccharides and an extinguished electroretinogram.

Dermatan sulfate and keratan sulfate are found in the urine and tissues. Fibroblasts synthesize dermatan sulfate, an abnormality that permits diagnosis by means of culture of amniotic fluid. There is increased ganglioside in the brain and decreased β-galactosidase in tissues. Allogeneic bone transplantation slows but does not prevent progression.

Mucopolysaccharidosis I S (MPS I S; Scheie).—The Scheie syndrome is a relatively mild disorder, although the face is typically coarse. Onset is between the ages of 5 and 20 years. Claw hand, pes cavus, and the carpal tunnel syndrome are present. The corneas are

TABLE 26-8.
Mucopolysaccharide Storage Diseases

Type	Eponym	Skeletal Dysplasia	Mental Retardation	Somatic Changes	Corneal Clouding
MPS I H	Hurler	Severe	Severe	Severe	Severe
MPS I S (formerly MPS V S)	Scheie	Slight	Slight to normal	Aortic regurgitation	Severe
MPS I H-S*	Hurler-Scheie	Moderate	Moderate	Moderate	Moderate
MPS II	Hunter†				
	A. Severe	Severe	Severe	Severe	None
	B. Mild	Moderate	Slight to normal	Moderate	With aging
MPS III A	Sanfilippo	Slight	Severe		None
MPS III B	Sanfilippo	Slight	Severe		None
MPS IV	Morquio	Severe	Slight to normal	Aortic regurgitation	Moderate
MPS VI	Maroteaux-Lamy	Severe	Normal	Aortic regurgitation; hydrocephalus	Severe
MPS VII	β-Glucuronidase deficiency (Sly)	Moderate	Moderate	Aortic regurgitation	Severe

*Heterozygous with mutant Hurler gene on one allele and mutant Scheie gene on other.
†Hunter syndrome is inherited as an X chromosome–linked recessive trait; all others are autosomal recessive. Optic atrophy has been reported in all. Pigmentary degeneration of the retina has been described in all but IV and VI.

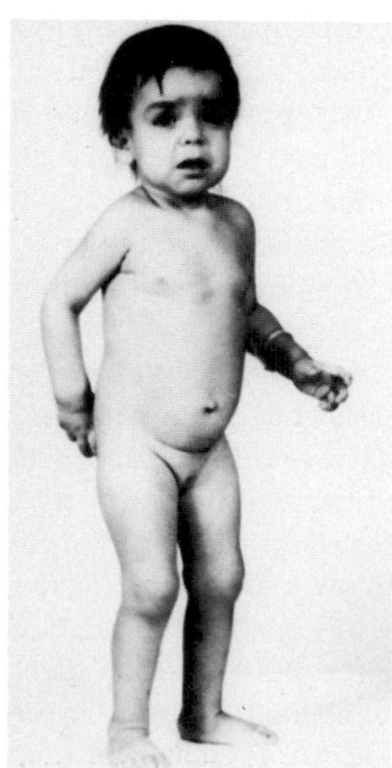

A

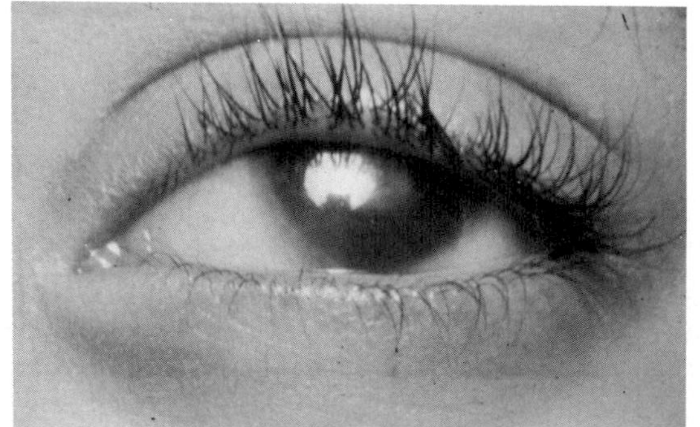

B

FIG 26-4.
A, Typical appearance of a patient with mucopolysaccharidosis (Hurler syndrome). **B,** The cloudy corneas of the mucopolysaccharidosis.

severely clouded, and retinal degeneration and glaucoma may develop. Intelligence and stature are normal. Aortic stenosis and regurgitation may develop.

Mucopolysaccharidosis I H-S (MPS I H-S; Hurler-Scheie).—This is a clinical phenotype that is midway between the mild involvement of the Scheie type and the severity of the Hurler type. One parent contributes an allele for the Hurler type and one parent contributes an allele for the Scheie type. The facial features resemble those of the Hurler type, but intellectual development is usually normal. There is corneal clouding, joint stiffness, deafness, and aortic valve disease. Pulmonary obstruction and cardiac disease cause death.

Mucopolysaccharidosis II (MPS II; Hunter).—The Hunter syndrome is inherited as an X chromosome recessive condition (Xq27-q28). It occurs in mild and severe forms, although the deficiency of iduronidate sulfatase is equally severe in both types. The patients with the severe type have coarse features, short stature, skeletal deformities, and mental retardation. The corneas are grossly clear, but severe retinal degeneration occurs. Otitis media and deafness occur. Severe neurologic degeneration is often complicated by internal hydrocephalus and increased intracranial pressure. Death often occurs between 10 and 15 years of age.

The mild type resembles MPS I S, but intelligence is normal and there is no central nervous system involvement. In adulthood the physical features resemble those of the severe type but progress slowly. Deafness occurs in all patients, and some develop a papilledema without increased intracranial pressure. The corneas may become slightly cloudy in adulthood. Death usually occurs before 50 years of age.

Mucopolysaccharidosis III (MPS III; Sanfilippo).—The Sanfilippo syndrome includes similar abnormalities caused by the mutation of one of four different enzymes required for the degradation of heparin sulfate. The onset is between 2 and 6 years of age, with severe progressive central nervous system deterioration and subtle somatic changes. Speech development is delayed, and patients never speak normally. Deafness develops in many but not all. Initially there are coarse hair, hirsutism, insomnia, delayed development, hyperactivity, and aggressive behavior. Mental deterioration and behavior problems follow. Magnetic resonance imaging demonstrates cortical atrophy. Results of urine tests for mucopolysaccharides are often false-negative, and diagnosis requires blood studies to demonstrate the defective enzyme.

Mucopolysaccharidosis IV (MPS IV; Morquio).—There are two Morquio syndromes. The Morquio A syndrome is a mucopolysaccharidosis, whereas the Morquio B syndrome is a beta-galactosidase deficiency. Both cause short-trunk dwarfism, corneal deposits, and spondyloepiphyseal dysplasia. Intelligence is normal in both.

The teeth are small with a thin enamel that results in caries. A hypoplastic odontoid process can cause atlantoaxial subluxation that requires spinal fusion of the upper cervical spine to prevent a cervical myelopathy.

The Morquio B syndrome is a generalized bone disease, with corneal clouding. There is no central nervous system involvement although spinal cord compression may occur as in the Morquio A syndrome. Intelligence is normal.

The deficiency of beta-galactosidase is identical to that in G_{M1} gangliosidosis, which develops shortly after birth with developmental delay, progressive neurologic deterioration, retinal cherry-red spots, and skeletal changes that resemble those seen in the Morquio A and B syndromes.

Mucopolysaccharidosis VI (MPS VI; Maroteaux-Lamy).—The Maroteaux syndrome is nearly identical to MPS I (Hurler), but the intelligence is normal, and it is caused by a different enzyme deficiency. Calcified aortic and mitral valves have been successfully replaced.

Mucopolysaccharidosis VII (MPS VII; Sly).—The Sly syndrome resembles the Hurler or Scheie syndrome with a wide range of variability. It is characterized by marked coarse metachromatic inclusions in granulocytes.

I-cell disease

Patients with I-cell disease (mucolipidosis II) and pseudo-Hurler polydystrophy (mucolipidosis III) strongly resemble patients with Hurler syndrome or one of its less severe variants. The patients, however, do not excrete mucopolysaccharides in their urine, and their fibroblasts contain dense inclusion bodies.

The serum and other body fluids contain lysosomal enzymes, which lack a mannose-6-

phosphate marker necessary for incorporation into the lysosome. Patients with mucolipidosis II strongly resemble patients with severe Hurler syndrome, but the disease is more rapidly progressive and death occurs at 5 to 8 years of age. Gingival hyperplasia in mucolipidosis II does not occur in mucopolysaccharidosis.

Mucolipidosis III has its onset at 2 to 4 years of age and follows a mild course that permits survival to adulthood. In many respects it resembles one of the less severe mucopolysaccharidoses but without urinary excretion of mucopolysaccharides.

Sphingomyelinase

Sphingomyelin and cholesterol metabolism are closely linked. Sphingomyelin is degraded by the lysosomal enzyme acid sphingomyelinase, a deficiency of which results in Niemann-Pick disease. There are many genotypes and phenotypes, and the exact biochemical nature of many of the disorders is not known.

The Niemann-Pick disease A and B (sphingomyelin-cholesterol lipidoses).— This is a group of disorders in which there is widespread accumulation of sphingomyelin and cholesterol in the reticuloendothelial and nervous systems and in the parenchymal cells of many organs. There is a wide variation in the clinical phenotype and in the extent and nature of the stored substance. In type A, the sphingomyelinase activity is reduced to 10% or less of normal. The condition occurs as an acute infantile form, a subacute form in childhood, and a chronic form in adults. In type B, sphingomyelinase activity is normal or reduced to as much as 20% of normal, but there is visceral and neuronal storage of the same lipid material as in type A Niemann-Pick disease. The acute form occurs between birth and age 2 years, the subacute form in infancy to 18 years, and the chronic form in adulthood.

In the acute infantile form, which may occur prenatally, poor feeding may be the earliest sign followed by retarded mental and physical development. Nearly every organ may be infiltrated with sphingomyelin, and there is enlargement of the liver and spleen, abdominal distention, infiltration of lymph nodes and bone marrow, fever, and yellow-brown skin discoloration. There is a cherry-red spot in one or both retinas, cloudy corneas, and brown discoloration of the lens. The conjunctival stroma contains inclusions.

Type C Niemann-Pick disease is characterized by the lysosomal accumulation of unesterified cholesterol. At about 5 years of age there may be frequent blinking and the onset of a vertical supranuclear paralysis of gaze, which occurs eventually in all patients. Vertical gaze eventually is entirely paralyzed. In many patients there is enlargement of the spleen and liver. There is increasing physical and mental deterioration with severe dysphagia and sometimes psychosis. Death occurs in the late teens.

Cystinosis (Fanconi syndrome)

Childhood cystinosis is an autosomal recessive lysosomal storage disease that results from the failure of cystine transport across the lysosomal membrane. Cystine crystals accumulate within the lysosome until the cell dies. There is widespread deposition of cystine crystals in the renal tubule (Fanconi syndrome), spleen, bone marrow, lymph nodes, cornea, conjunctiva, uvea, and retinal pigment epithelium.

The disease becomes evident between the fourth and sixth months of life. Failure to grow, emesis, recurrent fever, a severe form of rickets resistant to vitamin D in the usual doses, and chronic acidosis result. An amino-aciduria involves many amino acids. There is progressive renal tubule damage, and chronic glomerulonephritis develops. There may be a terminal vascular hypertension and ophthalmoscopic signs of severe vascular hypertension, including papilledema. Death usually results from uremia or intercurrent infections.

Crystalline deposits occurring in the conjunctiva and the cornea are pathognomonic of the disease. Cystine is also deposited in the sclera and iris, where it may cause adhesions between the iris and anterior lens capsule (posterior synechiae). Good illumination and magnification are required for demonstration of the deposits because of their small size. They appear as tinsel-like, fine refractile crystals or fine white dots uniformly scattered over the entire cornea, predominantly in the anterior stroma (although the corneal crystals have the same clinical appearance as the conjunctival crystals, they do not have the same x-ray diffraction pattern and may not be cystine.) Conjunctival crystals are superficial and tend to aggregate in the walls of blood vessels. Photophobia is severe, but visual acuity is initially normal. Ophthalmoscopically there is peripheral retinal patchy depigmentation and pigment clumps that often form small rings. The retinal pigmentary changes precede corneal and conjunctival involvement. Vision is severely impaired in young adults.

Treatment is directed toward correction of the acidosis and dietary supplementation of vitamin D, phosphate, and potassium. Supplementary calcium may be necessary until the skeleton is normal, but hypercalcemia must be avoided. A cystine-free diet may be helpful. In advanced stages, renal transplant is indicated.

The renal changes of the disorder also occur in galactosemia, Wilson disease, fructose intolerance, tyrosinemia, and the glycogen storage disease oculocerebrorenal (Lowe) syndrome.

Benign cystinosis.—Benign cystinosis is an autosomal recessive disorder in which cystine crystals are found in the eye and bone marrow. There are no kidney signs or retinal abnormalities. The cystine level is much lower than in the nephropathic type. Attention is often directed to the disorder only when the crystals are seen in the cornea and conjunctiva.

Disorders of glycoprotein degradation

Lysosomal storage disorders of glycoproteins resemble a mild mucopolysaccharidosis. Most body tissues demonstrate vacuolation of cells, and electron microscopy reveals membrane-bound vacuoles with a conspicuous granular pattern. Those of ocular interest include mannosidosis and sialidosis.

Mannosidosis.—This is a lysosomal storage disease that results from a deficiency of alpha-mannosidase (chromosome 19cen-q13.1). It occurs as an infantile phenotype (type I) and as a juvenile-adult phenotype (type II). In both there is psychomotor retardation. There is cardiac dysfunction, hepatosplenomegaly, and seizures. Connective tissue defects include hernias, diastasis recti, and testicular hydrocele. There is a marked tendency to infections and reduced serum immunoglobulin levels. Initial rapid growth is followed by slow growth.

A posterior cortical lens opacity that resembles the spokes of a wheel when viewed with the ophthalmoscope develops in infancy in many patients. In the juvenile-adult phenotype the lens opacity is punctate. Diagnosis is based on direct measurement of alpha-mannosidase in leukocytes, fibroblasts, or cultured amniotic fluid cells.

Sialidosis.—This name is applied to different disorders: an isolated deficiency of neuraminidase (10pter-q23) and a deficiency of both neuraminidase and beta-galactosidase (3p). The infantile forms of the neuraminidase and beta-galactosidase deficiency (familial neurovisceral lipidosis, infantile G_{M1} gangliosidosis, galactosialidosis) have cherry-red spots of the macula identical with those of Tay-Sachs disease.

Isolated neuraminidase deficiency characterizes the cherry-red spot–myoclonus syndrome. The onset is in the second decade with progressively severe decreased vision, myoclonus, or gait abnormalities. The cherry-red spot occurs in all patients but may not be typical in everyone. Nystagmus, ataxia, and grand mal seizures may occur. The diagnosis is based on the deficiency of neuraminidase in fresh unfrozen fibroblasts, leukocytes, or cultured amniotic fluid cells.

Glucosylceramide lipidosis.—Gaucher disease (chromosome 1) is a lysosomal storage disorder in which glucosylceramide is not hydrolyzed because of a deficiency of beta-glucosidase. The common type, particularly among Ashkenazi Jews, has no ocular signs. Types 2 and 3 may be ushered in by a bilateral fixed strabismus that results in jerky head movements as the infant attempts to fix on a moving object. Severe neurologic involvement causes death by the age of 2 years. Type 3 has a later onset and milder neurologic involvement than type 2 but the same ocular signs. Bone marrow transplantation may cure the disease. Some 75% of the patients develop a brownish yellow, triangular deposit in the bulbar conjunctiva that resembles a pinguecula.

Fabry disease (diffuse angiokeratoma).—Fabry disease is a recessive X chromosome (Xq21.33-q22) lysosomal error of glycosphingolipid catabolism that results from mutations of the alpha-galactosidase A gene. Some 49 different mutations have been described, most of which result in similar phenotypes, but classic and mild abnormalities are described.

The defect leads to the progressive accumulation of the neutral glycosphingolipid globotriaosylceramide in the endothelial cells of blood vessels and smooth muscle cells. There are episodes of excruciating pain in the extremities and fever. Angiokeratomatous skin lesions, particularly affecting the thighs and genitalia, occur in early childhood. Venous aneurysmal dilations and tortuosity on the inferior bulbar conjunctiva occur in both hemizygous males (78%) and heterozygous females (46%). The retinal veins are more tortuous than normal and sometimes segmentally dilated. Central retinal artery or vein occlusion may occur. There are cream-colored whorl-like opacities in the cornea at the level of the Bowman zone in all hemizygotes and most heterozygotes (88%). The corneal opacities are indistinguishable from those seen in patients receiving chloroquine or amiodarone therapy. A granular anterior subcapsular cataract occurs in some hemizygotes, and a white posterior subcapsular branching opacity resembling a herpetic dendrite occurs in both hemizygotes (37%) and heterozygotes (14%). Myopia occurs frequently, especially among heterozygotes.

Galactosylceramide lipidosis (Krabbe disease).—Krabbe is an autosomal recessive abnormality of a glycosphingolipid that is found only in myelin sheaths. After normal initial development, Krabbe disease has its onset between 3 and 6 months of life, and death results from emaciation between 1 and 2 years. The disease begins with hypersensitivity to visual, aural, or tactile stimuli and frequent crying without apparent cause. There is initial spasticity followed by flaccid paralysis. Blindness caused by optic atrophy is common. Deafness may occur. There are numerous multinucleated globoid cells in the white matter of the brain, loss of myelin, and astrocytic gliosis. The protein level of the cerebrospinal fluid is increased, particularly in patients with an early onset. The diagnosis is based on the demonstration of a deficiency or absence of the enzyme galactosyl ceramidase in leukocytes, serum, or cultured fibroblasts.

MITOCHONDRIAL DISORDERS

The mitochondrion is an extranuclear organelle that contains DNA (mtDNA). All mitochondrial DNA is derived from the ovum during the formation of the zygote. All mitochondrial DNA is transmitted exclusively by maternal inheritance. Thus, the mother transmits her mitochondrial genes to all of her children but only her daughters transmit her mitochondria.

The drug zidovudine (AZT) used in the treatment of acquired immunodeficiency syndrome (AIDS) is incorporated into mitochondrial DNA and inhibits its replication. The depletion is reversible when the drug is stopped.

Mitochondrial DNA contains 16,659 base pairs and 37 genes. Thirteen of these genes code for structural proteins of the respiratory chain. Two genes code for ribosomal RNA and 22 code for transfer RNA. Each mitochondrion contains 2 to 10 copies of the mitochondrial genome. Some cells have thousands of mitochondria and contain up to 10,000 copies of the mitochondrial genome. Abnormalities of the mitochondria may result in defects of fatty acid oxidation, defects of pyruvate metabolism, or defects of enzymes of the respiratory chain. Additional biochemical defects occur secondary to the failure of metabolic proteins to enter the mitochondria for processing.

Mitochondrial mutations reflect either a large-scale rearrangement of the mitochondrial DNA or a strategic point mutation that affects transfer RNA genes. Many mitochondrial mutations are associated with an accumulation of mitochondria in skeletal muscles that result in a distinctive appearance ("ragged red fibers") when stained with the modified Gomori trichrome stain. Ragged red fibers are usually not seen with point mutations that affect the 13 genes that code for the structural proteins of the respiratory chain.

The main mitochondrial abnormalities associated with prominent ocular symptoms include the Kearns-Sayre syndrome; Leber hereditary optic atrophy; and the syndrome of neuropathy, ataxia, and retinitis pigmentosa. Short stature and hearing loss are common in all mitochondrial disorders. Ophthalmoplegia, pigmentary degeneration of the retina, and cataract occur sporadically in several other disorders associated with defects in the mitochondrial DNA genome. Exact diagnosis requires appropriate molecular genetic analysis.

Kearns-Sayre syndrome.—This is the prototype of mitochondrial diseases associated with large-scale rearrangements of the mitochondrial genome. The age at onset is after 3 years, and death occurs in the second or third decade. There are blepharoptosis, restricted eye movements, and pigmentary retinopathy. The retinal pigmentation is patchy without bone spicules, and the electroretinogram is not recordable. Many mitochondria may be demonstrated in the outer nuclear layer of the retina. Neurologic signs include uncoordination, mental retardation, and episodes of coma without seizures. Heart block may cause death unless a pacemaker is implanted. Ragged red fibers are present in many patients. Magnetic resonance and computed tomographic imaging of the brain show spongy degeneration and sometimes calcification of the basal ganglia. Lactate and pyruvate levels are increased in the blood and cerebrospinal fluid. Incomplete forms of the Kearns-Sayre syndrome invariably show an ophthalmoplegia often combined with other signs. An ophthalmoplegia, however, may be inherited as a chromosomal gene mutation or as a mitochondrial gene mutation, or may be nonhereditary.

The Pearson syndrome.—The Pearson syndrome has the identical genetic lesion as the Kearns-Sayre syndrome. The onset, however, is in infancy with pancytopenia and altered pancreatic exocrine function. If the infant survives, there may be phenotypic transition from the Pearson syndrome to the Kearns-Sayre syndrome. Alternatively, there may be full recovery of the bone marrow and pancreatic function. The syndrome reflects a mixture of normal and abnormal mitochondria at birth. Full recovery is the result of the proliferation of normal mitochondria in rapidly dividing tissue, such as bone marrow.

Chronic progressive ophthalmoplegia.—Ophthalmoplegia is divided into external, which involves the levator palpebrae oculi muscles and the external oculi muscles; internal, which involves the pupillary muscles; and complete, which involves both. Complete and internal ophthalmoplegia are usually secondary to neurologic lesions. External ophthalmoplegia may be neurologic (myasthenia gravis, myotonic dystrophy, supranuclear palsies, or encephalopathies) or secondary to a mitochondrial abnormality as seen in the Kearns-Sayre syndrome. Other instances are seen with normal mitochondrial DNA but other genetic defects (Bassen-Kornzweig, Refsum, Shy). The condition is dominated by the drooping eyelids that often prevent the two eyes from being used simultaneously and thus minimize the double vision from the ocular muscle paralysis.

Leber hereditary optic atrophy.—The Leber hereditary optic atrophy is the result of a variety of mitochondrial point mutations (see Table 26-1). It is characterized by the sudden onset of bilateral optic neuropathy in young men. The onset is between 20 and 24 years of age, but children as young as 5 years may be affected. Males are affected preferentially with approximately 85% of the patients being young men, a finding that suggests an X chromosome factor. Patients do not have ragged red fibers of skeletal muscle, and the blood and cerebrospinal fluid lactate levels are normal.

Three or more years before the onset of symptoms, the optic disk is edematous and the surrounding arterioles are dilated and develop telangiectasis. When optic neuropathy occurs there is deficient perfusion in attenuated temporal arterioles, atrophy of the temporal portion of the optic nerve, and a glistening white layer overlying the optic disk. Most individuals recover visual acuity to the 10/100 level, but many patients with mild cases may not be examined. Family members may be affected with hyperreflexia, uncoordination, peripheral neuropathy, cardiac conduction defects, and Babinski signs.

Neuropathy, ataxia, and retinitis pigmentosa.—This is an abnormality of infants that is associated with a mitochondrial point mutation that involves the gene for subunit 6 of mitochondrial H^+-ATPase. Development is delayed, and there are pigmentary degeneration of the retina, hyperreflexia, generalized ataxia, and bilateral Babinski signs. The clinical signs are proportionate to the severity of abnormal mitochondrial DNA. The condition is similar to the Leigh syndrome.

Cerebrotendinous xanthomatosis.—This is a rare mitochondrial abnormality of bile acid synthesis in which the mitochondrial gene for 27-hydroxylase is mutated. There are anterior cortical cataracts that may be present by the age of 6 years, xanthelasma, xanthomas of the Achilles tendons, mental retardation of variable severity, spinal cord paresis, cerebellar ataxia, and early atherosclerosis. Cerebrotendinous xanthomatosis has been seen most frequently in Japan. The ataxia occurs after puberty and may be followed by pseudobulbar paralysis, which often results in death. There is a generalized tissue accumulation of cholestanol (cholesterol lacking the 5,6 double bond) and cholesterol, but the blood cholesterol level is nearly normal. Treatment with chemodoxycholic acid reduces the formation of cholestanol.

PEROXISOMES (MICROBODIES)

Peroxisomes are small membrane-bound organelles, sometimes continuous with the tubules of the smooth endoplasmic reticulum, which are present in every eukaryotic cell. They catalyze the beta-oxidation of very-long-chain fatty acids, polyunsaturated fatty acids, and prostaglandins. They initiate the synthesis of plasmalogens, which are abundant in myelin. Peroxisomes contain enzymes that oxidize a variety of substrates to generate hydrogen peroxide. The peroxisome enzyme catalase decomposes the hydrogen peroxide to H_2O and O_2. Other peroxisomal enzymes oxidize fatty acids and synthesize bile acids. Abnormalities of peroxisomes with prominent ocular changes include the cerebrohepatorenal (Zellweger) syndrome and phytanic acid storage (Refsum) disease.

Cerebrohepatorenal syndrome (Zellweger).—The Zellweger syndrome is an autosomal recessive multisystem disorder of peroxisomes that includes primary dysgenesis of the central nervous system, hepatic interstitial fibrosis, and multiple cysts of the renal cortex. Abnormalities of neuronal migration and demyelination cause hypotonia, muscular seizures, and psychomotor retardation. Liver involvement causes jaundice, hepatomegaly, hypoprothrombinemia, and gastrointestinal hemorrhage. A profound hypotonia sometimes suggests the Down syndrome to be the cause.

The forehead is high and bulging, the orbits are widely separated, the palpebral fissures slant upward, and epicanthal folds are present. There may be corneal opacification; glaucoma; cataract; Brushfield spots; nystagmus; rudimentary, irregular, or atrophic optic disks; narrow retinal blood vessels; and irregular retinal pigmentation. Bilateral corneal edema is associated with paracentral iridocorneal adhesions and focal attenuation of Descemet membrane. Selective degeneration of the outer nuclear layers and photoreceptors occurs mainly in the central retinal region. The electroretinogram is nonrecordable.

Liver enzyme and serum iron levels are high. There is a deficiency of peroxisomes in all cells. The basic abnormality may be a failure to process the components essential to the assembly of the protein matrix of the peroxisomes. Death occurs within 1 year of age, often within 3 months of birth.

Phytanic acid storage disease (Refsum disease, heredopathia atactica polyneuritiformis).—Refsum disease is an autosomal recessive abnormality secondary to the systemic accumulation of phytanic acid because of the absence of the enzyme phytanic acid alpha-oxidase. Phytanic acid is derived mainly from the diet (dairy products, beef, lamb, deer and antelope meat, and fat). Chlorophyll is poorly absorbed from the intestine and is not a significant source of phytanic acid. Thus, cooked green vegetables may be used in diets that exclude the major sources of phytanic acid.

The major clinical findings are pigmentary degeneration of the retina, cerebellar ataxia, peripheral polyneuropathy, and high cerebrospinal fluid protein. Retinal pigmentary degeneration, night blindness, and constricted visual fields always occur. In 90% of the patients, there is a peripheral neuropathy, motor weakness, muscular atrophy, loss of deep tendon reflexes, and loss of superficial sensation to pain, touch, or temperature. Onset is in childhood, but diagnosis may be delayed until midlife. The retinal changes are followed by blepharoptosis, foot drop, and loss of deep tendon reflexes. Ataxia, intention tremor, and nystagmus indicate cerebellar involvement. There may be cataract, miotic pupils, anosmia, deafness, and nonspecific changes in the electrocardiogram.

Long remissions occur and exacerbations are triggered by fever, surgery, and pregnancy. Improvement may follow long-term exclusion of dietary dairy fat and cattle fat, but the slow course and tendency to spontaneous remission make evaluation difficult.

A thin layer of lipid occurs in standing urine and serum when the phytanic acid level is markedly increased. Cultured fibroblasts of homozygotes indicate the absence of phytanic acid alpha-oxidase.

Plasmapheresis and exclusion of phytanic acid from the diet stabilize but do not restore lost function.

MISCELLANEOUS GENETIC DISORDERS

INCONTINENTIA PIGMENTI

Incontinentia pigmenti is an X chromosome–linked (Xp11.21) dominant systemic disorder that is lethal in most male embryos and is thus seen clinically mainly (97%) in the female. Within a few days of birth, erythema and bulla of the extremities occur, followed by verrucous lesions that after several months are succeeded by whorled, marbled pigmentation most conspicuous on the trunk. Dentition is delayed and teeth are missing or cone shaped. Microcephaly, seizures, mental retardation, and spastic paralysis may occur.

About one sixth of the affected individuals have a retinal dysplasia with rosettes and fibrous tissue that cause a total nonrhegmatogenous retinal detachment. Esotropia, optic atrophy, cataract, blue sclera, nystagmus, and hyperpigmentation of the conjunctiva and retina may occur. The retinal blood supply may terminate at the equator with a zone of arteriovenous anastomoses, fibrovascular proliferation, and peripheral retinal avascularity. Foveal hypoplasia occurs. One eye is often more severely affected than its fellow and may be microphthalmic. If abnormalities have not occurred by the first year of life, the prognosis for normal vision is good.

HEREDITARY OCULOACOUSTIC CEREBRAL DYSPLASIA

Norrie disease is an X chromosome (Xp11.4-p11.3) recessive abnormality in which newborn males either are born with or develop shortly after birth a gray-yellow or opaque vascularized retrolental vascular mass in each eye. The pupils are dilated, the iris is hypoplastic, and posterior synechiae and ectropion of the pupillary fringe are present. Falciform folds of the retina, retinal detachment, and vitreous hemorrhage may occur. Corneal degeneration begins at about 1 year of age, followed by cataracts at 2 years of age. In early childhood the eyes begin to shrink (phthisis bulbi). Deafness occurs in about 33% and mental retardation in about 66% of those affected.

X-linked familial exudative vitreoretinopathy seemingly results from mutations of the same gene.

METACHROMATIC LEUKODYSTROPHY

This is a group of autosomal recessive disorders in which an arylsulfatase A deficiency causes sulfatides to accumulate in myelin sheaths and cerebral white matter. There is massive urinary excretion of sulfatides. Late infantile, juvenile, adult, and variant forms with multiple sulfatase deficiencies have been described.

Weakness, ataxia, dysarthria, ocular muscle palsies, nystagmus, and severe mental retardation occur. Optic atrophy and grayish infiltration of the central retina with macular cherry-red spots lead to blindness. Membranous lysosomal residual bodies are confined to the ganglion cells of the retina and central nervous system. Material that stains red with toluidine blue (metachromasia) is found in urinary sediment and in ganglion cells, including those of the retina.

NEURONAL CEROID LIPOFUSCINOSIS (BATTEN)

Batten disease is a group of autosomal recessive neurodegenerative disorders characterized by the accumulation of autofluorescent lipopigment in neurons and other cells. Infantile (chromosome 1p32), late infantile, juvenile (chromosome 16p12.1), and adult forms are described. The biochemical defect is unknown. Electron microscopy of skin and conjunctival specimens shows cytoplasmic curvilinear and fingerprint inclusions. Magnetic resonance imaging discloses generalized cerebral atrophy.

There is severe pigmentary degeneration of the retina, attenuation of the blood vessels, and optic atrophy that closely resembles retinitis pigmentosa. The macular region often has a granular appearance. Visual loss may be the initial symptom, followed by motor and mental deterioration. Alternatively, the disease may be initiated by progressive, severe, mixed, myoclonic seizures.

Dietary supplementation with polyunsaturated fatty acids may arrest but not reverse the usual course of the disease.

OCULOCEREBRORENAL SYNDROME (LOWE)

This is an X chromosome–linked (Xq25) recessive abnormality in which the affected male demonstrates hypotonia, mental retardation, osteoporosis, and failure to thrive. There is a renal tubular acidosis and aminoaciduria. Cataracts are present at birth and may involve the entire lens or be confined to the fetal nucleus. The female carrier has punctate lens opacities. Congenital glaucoma occurs in slightly more than 50% of the males. The poor vision causes nystagmus and strabismus. The pupil may be miotic and may not dilate with mydriatics. The maternal (100%) and amniotic fluid (25%) alpha-fetoprotein levels are elevated and without acetylcholinesterase activity.

BIBLIOGRAPHY

Books

Scriver CR, Beaudet AL, Sly WS, Valle D, editors: *The metabolic and molecular basis of inherited disease,* vols I to III, New York, 1995, McGraw-Hill.

Wiggs JL, editor: *Molecular genetics of ocular disease,* New York, 1994, Wiley-Liss.

Articles

Baty BJ, Blackburn BL, Carey JC: Natural history of trisomy 18 and trisomy 13. I. Growth, physical assessment, medical histories, survival, and recurrence risk, *Am J Med Genet* 49:175-188, 1994.

Goldberg MF: The blinding mechanisms of incontinentia pigmenti, *Trans Am Ophthalmol Soc* 92:167-179, 1994.

Guttman DH: New insights into the neurofibromatoses, *Curr Opin Neurol* 7:166-171, 1994.

Johns DR: Mitochondrial DNA and disease, *N Engl J Med* 333:638-644, 1995.

Lee SK, Nicholls RD, Bundey S, Laxova R, Musarella M, Spritz RA: Mutations of the P gene in oculocutaneous albinism, ocular albinism, and Prader-Willi syndrome plus albinism, *N Engl J Med* 330:529-534, 1994.

Spritz RA: Molecular genetics of oculocutaneous albinism, *Hum Mol Genet* 3:1469-1475, 1994.

Tilstra DJ, Byers PH: Molecular basis of hereditary disorders of connective tissue, *Annu Rev Med* 45:149-163, 1994.

27

ENDOCRINE DISEASE AND THE EYE

The endocrine, nervous, and immune systems are the major pathways for the transfer of information between organs and cells in different parts of the body. The endocrine system secretes chemical mediators (peptides or peptide derivatives, steroids, or amines), which govern the reproduction, growth, physiologic homeostasis, and other functions of the individual. These mediators regulate the rate at which enzymes are synthesized, govern the enzymes of metabolism, and alter the permeability of membranes.

Diabetes mellitus is by far the major endocrine disease with ocular changes and is the chief cause of blindness in adults in the United States. Thyroid disease may cause an increase in the volume of the orbital contents, which causes protrusion of the eyes. This effect is compounded by an increased sensitivity to adrenergic hormones, which results in retraction of the eyelids and other ocular signs. Multiple endocrine neoplasia type IIb (medullary thyroid carcinoma, pheochromocytoma, and marked dysmorphic changes) also causes thickened corneal nerves, which permits early diagnosis. Decreased secretion of the parathyroid hormone causes a lowered serum calcium level, neuromuscular hyperexcitability, and bilateral, subcapsular cataracts.

Other endocrine disorders are rarely associated with ocular changes.

DIABETES MELLITUS

Diabetes mellitus is categorized into idiopathic and secondary types. Idiopathic diabetes is divided into two main types: (1) insulin-dependent diabetes mellitus (IDDM, type 1), in which the beta cells of the pancreas, which produce insulin, are destroyed in childhood by an antigen-antibody reaction; and (2) non–insulin-dependent diabetes mellitus (NIDDM, type 2), in which the cells of the body gradually lose their ability to utilize circulating insulin. Type 2 diabetes is further divided into late-onset diabetes, either with (common) or without obesity, or maturity-onset diabetes of the young.

Secondary diabetes complicates diseases of the pancreas or other endocrine organs, a number of specific genetic diseases, pregnancy, and drugs such as glucocorticosteroids, diuretics, and others.

Diabetes mellitus is associated with a number of ocular complications that range from background diabetic retinopathy (see Table 27-1) to proliferative diabetic retinopathy (see Table 27-2), cataract, ophthalmoplegia, iris neovascularization, and others (see Table 27-3).

Diabetes is the major systemic disease that causes blindness in the United States and is the leading cause of blindness in individuals 30 to 70 years of age. The rate of blindness among diabetic persons is 20 times that of the general population. There is a much higher risk of blindness from diabetes in nonwhite women than in either white women or white men. Nonwhite men have the lowest risk of blindness from diabetes. Other risk factors include the age at which the diabetes is diagnosed, the length of time it has been present, renal disease, uncontrolled high blood pressure, pregnancy, poor control of glucose levels, and increased glycosylated hemoglobin levels.

Disease of the capillaries and small blood vessels (microangiopathy) causes retinopathy, nephropathy, and neuropathy. Accelerated atherosclerosis, possibly resulting from microangiopathy of the vasa vasorum, causes coronary insufficiency and myocardial infarction as well as ischemia of the extremities with gangrene of the feet.

Many of the ocular complications of diabetes can be effectively treated if diagnosed at an early stage. Each patient with diabetes should be aware of the possibility of ocular complications and the need for routine eye examinations. Each diabetic patient should have the ocular fundi skillfully examined, with the pupils dilated, at least once each year. The ocular fundi of patients with background diabetic retinopathy should be examined every 6 months, more frequently in patients with more severe complications. Ophthalmoscopic signs of a progressive retinopathy should initiate prompt referral.

About 20% of all patients with diabetes escape the ocular complications of the disease. The factors responsible for this protection are not known. Patients who develop the ocular complications appear to have the same disease and control as those who avoid the ocular changes. In light of the tragic visual toll of diabetes, a search for these protective factors is worthy of study.

INSULIN-DEPENDENT DIABETES MELLITUS

Clinically, insulin-dependent diabetes mellitus has an abrupt onset with thirst, excessive urination, and weight loss despite an increased appetite. It occurs most frequently in persons of Northern European descent, and the incidence peaks between the ages of 10 and 15 years. Before the onset of symptoms, most of the beta cells of the pancreas have been destroyed by a chronic immune-mediated reaction that has been present for years. Cells that secrete glucagon (alpha cells), somatostatin (delta cells), and pancreatic polypeptide are preserved.

Susceptibility to insulin-dependent diabetes is conferred by inheritance of genes of the class I major histocompatibility complex on chromosome 6 (see Chapter 25). The HLA molecules (HLA-DR3 and -DR4) expressed by these genes present antigenic peptides to CD8 (cytotoxic or suppressor) T lymphocytes. Some 45% of white individuals in the United States have these HLA genotypes, but 95% of the patients with insulin-dependent diabetes have at least one. Diet and environmental influences may play a role in that 90% of those afflicted do not have an affected first-degree relative. The frequency is higher among children who were not breast-fed, and the incidence increases in the fall and early winter months. Another gene for susceptibility to insulin-dependent diabetes occurs on chromosome 11 near the genes for insulin growth factor and also on genes that code for the transporter antigen protein (TAP).

Destruction of the pancreatic beta cells creates measurable islet-cell cytoplasmic and insulin autoantibodies and permits prediction of the disease, particularly in those with HLA susceptibility genotypes. In children who have such autoantibodies and the likelihood of developing insulin-dependent diabetes, the risk may be minimized by insulin therapy, which may relieve the pancreatic beta cells of the task of producing insulin and minimize them as a target for immune disease. Other investigative therapies include BCG vaccine to suppress the immune system, nicotinamide to neutralize free radicals, avoidance of cow's milk, and others.

NON–INSULIN-DEPENDENT DIABETES MELLITUS

Clinically, non–insulin-dependent diabetes mellitus becomes evident mainly in obese individuals beyond the age of 40 years, although the metabolic abnormality may have existed long before any clinical signs. It is associated with obesity, high blood pressure, atherosclerosis, aging, and polycystic ovarian disease. There is no association with the major histocompatibility complex as with type 1 diabetes mellitus but the disorder is more strongly familial. Thus, monogenetic twins demonstrate a concordance rate that exceeds 90%.

In the early stages of the disease, there is a resistance to insulin at the peripheral tissue level that induces an increased blood glucose level and stimulates glycogen, lipid, and protein synthesis. The excess blood glucose does not stimulate increased insulin synthesis and release because the beta cells of the pancreas are desensitized to glucose. In the early stages of the disease the excess glucose leads to obesity.

Patients with non–insulin-dependent diabetes mellitus are subject to the same complications as insulin-dependent patients but mainly do not develop ketosis. Weight reduction often reduces blood glucose to normal levels, but in many patients a deficiency of insulin develops, which may require insulin therapy.

RETINOPATHY

Retinopathy is the most important ocular complication of diabetes. The introduction of insulin in 1921, followed by the sulfonamides in 1937 and the antibiotics thereafter, prevented premature death of diabetic persons from coma or infection. Since then the ocular, renal, and cardiovascular effects have emerged as the chief complications of the disease. Diabetic retinopathy is not a result of concurrent atherosclerosis or vascular hypertension but is severely aggravated by systemic factors.

The prevalence of diabetic retinopathy is related to the duration of the disease, the onset of which can be accurately known only in the insulin-dependent type and estimated only in the non–insulin-dependent type. The prevalence of diabetic retinopathy is 17% in patients who have had diabetes for less than 5 years. After 15 years the prevalence is 97% in patients with insulin-dependent diabetes and about 60% in older patients, presumably affected with non–insulin-dependent diabetes. The younger group is more likely to develop proliferative retinopathy, in contrast to the older group of individuals who seem more subject to decreased vision from cystoid macular edema. Retinopathy is rare in children less than 10 years old but occurs after puberty. Careful ophthalmic examination is an important aspect of care, and routine examination of the fundi through the dilated pupils should begin no later than the fifth year after diagnosis of the diabetes. The frequency of subsequent examinations should be determined by the presence or absence of retinopathy, but examinations must be done at least once annually.

The severity of the retinopathy generally parallels the duration of the disease, increasing age, increased glycosylated hemoglobin level (reflecting the blood glucose level in the previous 7 to 8 weeks), vascular hypertension, proteinuria, and lean body mass. Smoking, obesity, and severity of the diabetes appear to be unrelated to the development of retinopathy. Once retinopathy begins, the degree of diabetic control seems to have little effect on its progression. The severity and rapidity of involvement of the two eyes may be unequal, and even in the same eye the retinopathy may progress in one region and regress in another. Severe proliferative retinopathy develops more frequently in younger men, and blindness is more common in men than women before the age of 45 years.

Visual acuity is a deceptive index of the severity of the retinopathy. A single lesion impairing the foveola will reduce form vision, possibly to the level of legal blindness. Conversely, extensive peripheral proliferative retinopathy may severely restrict the peripheral field of vision, but good central vision may be retained. Vitreous hemorrhage from relatively minor neovascularization may severely reduce vision, but vitreous hemorrhage that spares the visual axis may allow good central vision.

Histologically the earliest change of diabetic retinopathy is loss of capillary pericytes (mural cells). Generalized thickening of capillary basement membranes occurs throughout the body, but the loss of pericytes is confined to retinal capillaries. Retinal pericytes are strikingly responsive to insulin in comparison to the endothelial cells of the aorta and retinal capillaries. Pericytes likely regulate regional blood flow, and their loss may impair the integrity of the capillary wall, disrupt the blood-retinal barrier, deplete the endothelial cells, and occlude the capillaries. Blood proteins diffuse into the retinal tissues and the intraocular fluids. Fluorescein angiography indicates failure of capillaries to perfuse regional areas of the retina, with dilation of capillaries in adjacent regions. Capillary microaneurysms occur, followed by the retinal hemorrhages and deposits of diabetic retinopathy.

Retinopathy is clinically divided into (1) background retinopathy and (2) proliferative (neovascular) retinopathy. Except for new blood vessel formation of proliferative retinopathy and its sequelae, the retinal lesions are similar. Older non–insulin-dependent diabetic patients tend to develop more severe retinal microangiopathy of the central retina and macular edema than do younger, insulin-dependent diabetic patients, who tend to develop more neovascular proliferation of the peripheral fundus. Increased vascular permeability and occlusive vascular disease are

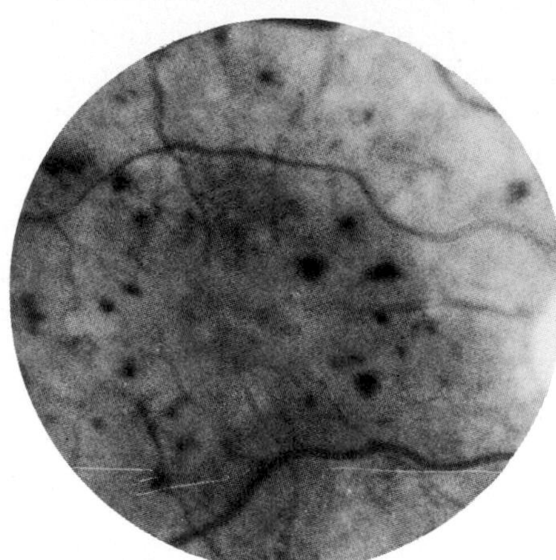

FIG 27-1.
Background retinopathy with preponderance of blot and punctate (dot) hemorrhages.

TABLE 27-1.
Background Diabetic Retinopathy

A. Capillary microaneurysms
B. Retinal hemorrhage(s)
   1. Blot, punctate, splinter (flame-shaped) hemorrhages
   2. Preretinal hemorrhage(s)
   3. Vitreous hemorrhage
C. Intraretinal microvascular abnormalities
D. Hard exudates
E. Soft exudates
F. Macular edema
   1. Retinal thickening
   2. Exudates

more common in the non–insulin-dependent type. In both background and proliferative retinopathy, there are microaneurysms, dot and blot hemorrhages (intraretinal and preretinal) (Fig 27-1), hard exudates, soft exudates (cotton-wool patches of acute retinal ischemia), retinal microangiopathy, increased vascular permeability, retinal edema, capillary dilation, tortuosity, telangiectasis, and irregularities of caliber and configuration.

Background retinopathy.—Background diabetic retinopathy describes the fundus abnormalities evident on ophthalmoscopy and fluorescein angiography in eyes that have not developed new retinal blood vessels on the surface of the retina or extending into the vitreous cavity (Table 27-1). The major ophthalmoscopic changes include (1) capillary microaneurysms; (2) retinal hemorrhages; (3) retinal exudates (hard, waxy); (4) intraretinal microvascular abnormalities; and (5) macular edema.

***Capillary microaneurysms.*—**Capillary microaneurysms of the retina occur most frequently in diabetes mellitus. They also complicate retinal vein closure, Coats disease, arterial hypertension, pernicious anemia, dysproteinemia, and other systemic diseases. Only in diabetes do such large numbers occur. Those associated with diabetes occur on the venous side of the capillary circulation and at the posterior pole of the eye. Microaneurysms associated with diseases other than diabetes occur on the arterial side of the capillary circulation and in the peripheral retina. The microaneurysms of diabetes are also rarely seen (in histologic preparations) in nonocular tissues.

Microscopically, microaneurysms consist of minute spherical red spots with sharp margins that range in size from 20 to 125 μm. They are located on the venous side of the capillary network at the level of the inner nuclear layer. The resolving power of the direct ophthalmoscope is approximately 70 to 80 μm. Thus, the majority of retinal microaneurysms are not seen with the ophthalmoscope. This is evident when the retina is viewed after intravenous injection of fluorescein (Fig 27-2) or is seen histologically in flat retinal sections after trypsin digestion. Microaneurysms may become hyalinized and appear ophthalmoscopically as white dots.

Ophthalmoscopically, microaneurysms are minute, round, sharply circumscribed, red spots that appear similar to hemorrhages. They may be distinguished from deep punctate hemorrhages by their unchanging appearance; their usual location far from blood vessels; their sharp, smooth borders; and a central light reflex.

Microaneurysms are permeable to large molecules and cause retinal edema in the area surrounding them. Near the regions of retinal edema may be hard deposits (exudates) that consist of lipid-laden macrophages and cholesterol. If the microaneurysms are obliterated with laser photocoagulation, the exudate disappears. The development of such edema deposits in the fovea is a serious complication because elimination of the edema does not fully restore visual function.

***Retinal hemorrhages.*—**The retinal hemorrhages of diabetes do not differ from retinal

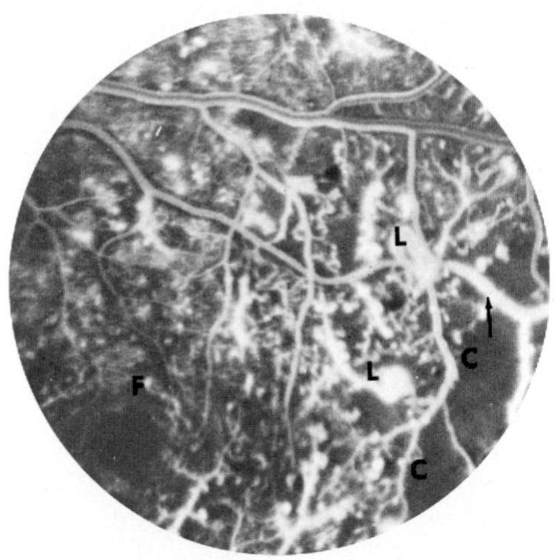

FIG 27-2.
Fluorescein angiography (early venous phase) of the left fundus of a 27-year-old woman with insulin-dependent diabetes mellitus. There are numerous microaneurysms and dilated, kinked, tortuous retinal blood vessels with areas of capillary nonperfusion *(C)* and capillary leakage *(L)* causing retinal edema. The wall of a branch of the superior temporal artery leaks fluorescein *(arrow)*, indicating endothelial damage. The foveola *(F)* is not affected, and visual acuity is 20/20.

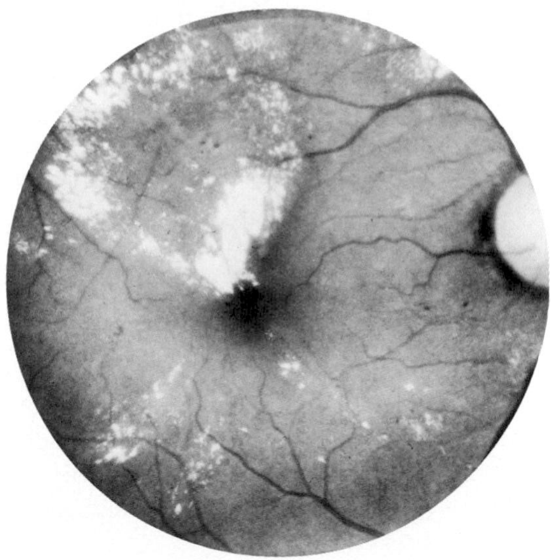

FIG 27-3.
A hard circinate exudate, which surrounds an area of intraretinal microvascular abnormalities. The deposit is immediately above the center of the fovea centralis and required immediate laser therapy to preserve central vision.

bleeding that complicates other conditions. They are described as punctate (dot), blot, globular, and splinter (flame-shaped). Punctate hemorrhages are small areas of bleeding into the inner nuclear layer of the retina, the cells of which are arranged so compactly that the blood cannot spread. Most are larger than microaneurysms and tend to disappear spontaneously. If the bleeding is a little more severe, the blood may spread to the inner plexiform layer and the hemorrhage is larger (blot). More extensive bleeding causes the blood to spread through the central layers of the retina (globular hemorrhage).

Splinter (flame-shaped) hemorrhages are located in the nerve fiber layers of the retina; their shape reflects the distribution of the nerve fibers. Similar hemorrhages are seen in hypertension, blood dyscrasias, papilledema, and central vein obstruction.

Preretinal hemorrhages spread between the internal limiting membrane and the nerve fiber layer of the retina or between the internal limiting membrane and the vitreous (subhyaloid). Some may show a fluid level with bed rest. Acute ocular trauma and subarachnoid and subdural hemorrhage may produce a similar hemorrhage. Preretinal hemorrhages may burst into the vitreous body, causing immediate obscuration of vision.

Intraretinal microvascular abnormalities.—This term originated with fluorescein angiography to describe retinal edema secondary to microaneurysms and capillary closure and leakage with a failure of capillary perfusion (Fig 27-3). The retinal capillaries are dilated, tortuous, irregular, and fragmented and sometimes develop fusiform aneurysms. When located near the fovea, a macular edema develops with impairment of central visual acuity, although the retinopathy may not be otherwise far advanced. Laser photocoagulation of the areas of microangiopathy, but not the fovea, is indicated as soon as the macular edema occurs.

Capillaries may appear normal, irregularly dilated, segmented, or occluded. Possible causes of capillary occlusion include loss of capillary tone, microthrombi, blood sludging, platelet aggregation, edema of the surrounding retina, reduced capillary perfusion pressure, and endothelial proliferation. Blood may be channeled into unaffected capillaries that dilate and become collateral vessels ("shunt vessels") that carry blood past areas of capillary closure. Alternatively, there may be new blood vessels in regions of intraretinal neovascularization. There is leakage of fluid from the capillaries and a retinal edema that eventually thickens the sensory retina.

Dilation of retinal veins occurs sometime before or during the course of nearly every instance of retinopathy. All of the veins or only a branch becomes engorged and dilated, and there may be a granular blood flow. There may be dilated segments of veins ("beading"). Although the picture resembles an impending central vein closure, the veins pulsate normally with pressure on the globe, and there are no adjacent retinal hemorrhages.

Retinal exudates.—Retinal exudates or deposits in diabetes are divided into "hard" or "waxy" deposits (chronic edema residues) and soft exudates (cotton-wool patches).

Hard exudates are yellowish to whitish intraretinal collections of serum and necrotic retina, which are located mainly in the outer plexiform layer. They reflect the exudation of blood lipids through the retinal capillaries or microaneurysms in which the blood-retinal barrier is defective. The exudates often surround an area of retinal edema adjacent to microaneurysms. They appear ophthalmoscopically as sharply defined, yellowish white, shiny, waxy areas. Some coalesce and become confluent while others remain as small irregular dots. They sometimes form a ring that surrounds the fovea centralis ("macular star"). They are composed of cholesterol crystals and lipid-laden macrophages.

Soft deposits (cotton-wool patches; cytoid bodies) are often an early sign of impending proliferative retinopathy. They are superficial, whitish opacities with indistinct, irregular margins that reflect the distribution of the retinal nerve fibers. They are ovoid in shape and variable in size and number. They are located in the posterior fundus and reflect infarction of the retinal capillaries.

Macular edema.—Macular edema is an important cause of loss of vision in both insulin-dependent and non–insulin-dependent diabetes (Fig 27-4). It is initiated by a breakdown of the blood-retinal barrier in the capillaries surrounding the fovea centralis. The macular area is whitened and thickened, and, on fluorescein angiography, spokes may radiate from the fovea centralis.

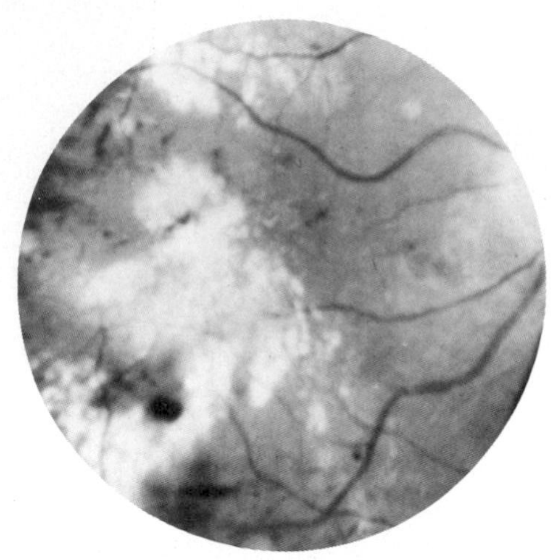

FIG 27-4.
Background retinopathy with hard exudates in the fovea centralis, which have reduced central visual acuity to less than 20/200. The deposits have destroyed the underlying fovea centralis, and effective treatment is not possible.

Macular edema is the main cause of loss of vision in patients with background retinopathy. It is associated with higher levels of glycosylated hemoglobin and more severe retinopathy. In older groups it is more common in women and those with increased diastolic blood pressure. Laser photocoagulation of the retina surrounding the fovea centralis often arrests further decrease of central visual acuity, but vision is seldom completely restored.

Thickening of the retina.—Thickening of the retina reflects retinal edema that may be focal or diffuse. Focal edema usually reflects vascular leakage from a localized group of microaneurysms and more rarely from an area of microvascular abnormalities. Diffuse leakage occurs from a generalized leakage of capillaries throughout the posterior pole. It tends to affect both eyes simultaneously in a similar fashion.

Retinal edema is considered clinically significant and requires laser therapy if the retina is thickened at the fovea centralis or within 500 μm of its center; if there are retinal exudates within 500 μm of the fovea centralis associated with adjacent thickening of the retina; or if

TABLE 27-2.
Proliferative Diabetic Retinopathy

A. Background retinopathy + new blood vessels
B. Preproliferation
   1. Soft exudates
   2. Venous beading
C. New blood vessels onto or above surface of retina
   1. Peripheral to 1,500-μm region surrounding optic disk
      a. Focal
      b. Generalized
   2. Optic disk
   3. Both peripheral and optic disk
D. Fibrous proliferation
   1. Peripheral to 1,500-μm region surrounding optic disk
   2. Optic disk
   3. Both peripheral and optic disk
E. Preretinal hemorrhage(s)
F. Vitreous hemorrhage
G. Retinal detachment (tractional)

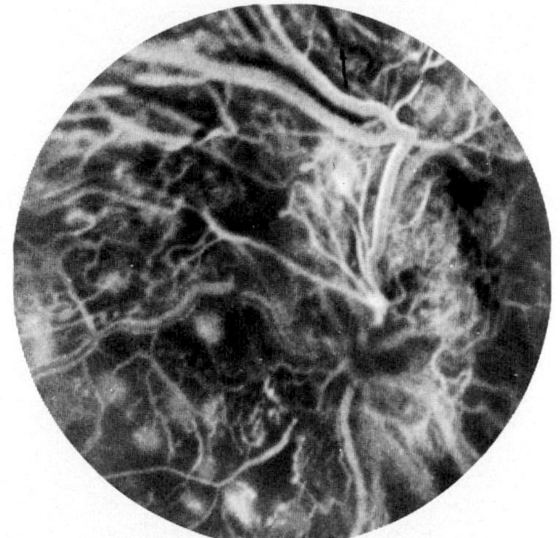

FIG 27-5.
Fluorescein angiography of severe neovascularization at the optic disk. A major retinal vein is occluded additionally *(arrow)*.

there is thickening of the retina that measures 1 disk diameter or more (1,500 μm) within 1 disk diameter of the fovea centralis.

Proliferative retinopathy.—The development of new blood vessels within the substance of and anterior to the retina (Table 27-2) heralds a serious deterioration in the visual prognosis of diabetic retinopathy. New blood vessels also complicate retinal vein occlusion and the retinopathy of prematurity. The new blood vessels usually originate from a retinal vein near an arteriovenous crossing at the posterior pole. The superior temporal vein is the most common retinal location; the inferior temporal, superior nasal, and inferior nasal veins are involved in that order of frequency. Additional blood vessels may proliferate on the surface of the optic disk (Fig 27-5).

Initially, a fine network of vessels develops within the layers of the inner retina. These vessels have a minimal fibrous component, are extremely permeable, and increase in length, caliber, number, and branches. Proliferation of the associated connective tissue causes increasing intervascular opacification. The vessels involute and decrease in size and number as the fibrous tissue becomes more opaque and dense.

As long as the vitreous remains in contact with the inner limiting membrane of the retina, the new vessels spread as a flat sheet on the inner retinal surface (Fig 27-6). If the vitreous contracts, fibrovascular tissue adherent to its retinal surface is torn loose and may rupture blood vessels, resulting in a vitreous hemorrhage. Traction on the fibrovascular tissue by vitreous may cause a tractional, nonrhegmatogenous retinal detachment. If the vitreous is already detached when neovascularization occurs, the blood vessels extend into the vitreous cavity and may cause hemorrhage.

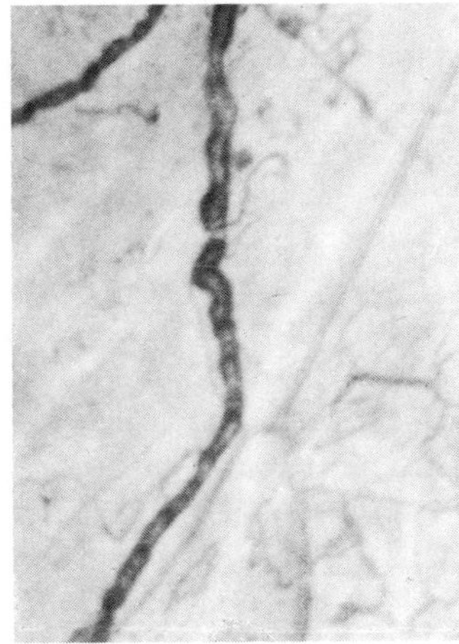

FIG 27-6.
Beading of a retinal vein with extensive neovascularization on the inner surface of the retina.

The process of fibrovascular proliferation followed by vascular involution and fibrous proliferation and contraction continues for many

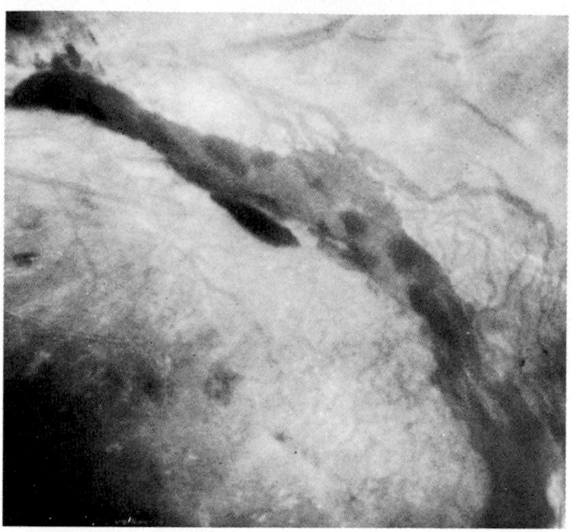

FIG 27-7.
Preretinal hemorrhage with slight hemorrhage escape into the vitreous originating from an area of retinal neovascularization.

years. Eventually, the new vessels are not apparent, and large white fibrous traction bands extend from the surface of the disk to the vascular arcades. Much, if not all, of the retina may be detached. If, however, the foveola remains attached, some patients may maintain excellent visual acuity despite extensive fibrous and tractional retinal detachment.

Vitreous hemorrhage (Fig 27-7) may cause sudden loss of vision or, when less dense, a red mist that obscures vision. In young individuals it may be quickly absorbed, but often after repeated episodes, or in elderly persons the blood persists indefinitely. The hemorrhage may produce a black ophthalmoscopic reflex or cause all fundus details to be blurred. As the blood is absorbed, large vitreous floaters are visible.

The vascular endothelial growth factor stimulates proliferative retinopathy. It is found in an increased amount in the vitreous humor and aqueous humor during active retinal proliferation and diminishes with laser obliteration of new blood vessels. It originates from the retinal pigment epithelium, the retinal pericytes, and new blood vessels of the iris that are induced by ischemia. It is actively angiogenic, and this activity is enhanced by fibroblastic growth factor liberated by death or disruption of retinal cells.

Treatment.—Diabetic proliferative retinopathy and macular edema are the chief causes of blindness in individuals aged 30 to 70 years. Every patient with diabetes must be aware of these complications. Every patient with diabetes should have a competent ophthalmoscopic examination with the pupils dilated at regular intervals. The fundi of patients without retinopathy should be examined annually, while those with background retinopathy should be examined every 6 months. Evaluation of the fundi is recommended at more frequent intervals for patients with proliferative retinopathy, in adolescence, and in pregnancy. Retinal photocoagulation, intensive diabetic therapy, and other measures can delay or prevent the progress of retinopathy and macular edema and prevent blindness from the disease.

Strict control of the blood glucose levels at a consistent physiologic level is the basic, but also the most difficult to achieve, purpose of treatment. Insulin may be administered in divided doses or by means of an insulin pump in an attempt to parallel the secretion of insulin by the pancreas. (Curiously, there is a small early adverse ocular effect of intensive treatment followed by a beneficial effect.) Hypoglycemia may be difficult to avoid. Insulin analogues that enter the bloodstream more quickly than regular insulin may be helpful. Amylin, a pancreatic beta-cell secretion that slows the emptying of the stomach, may prevent hyperglycemia after eating. Alpha-glucosidase inhibitors slow digestion and the absorption of carbohydrates and may minimize hyperglycemia after eating. Pancreas transplantation requires immunosuppression, which limits its usefulness. Implantation of encapsulated islet cells avoids the need for immunosuppression. Aldose reductase blockers and angiogenesis inhibitors are used.

Photocoagulation of the retina is indicated for treatment of new blood vessels of the retina, optic disk, or both. Background retinopathy is treated if it involves or threatens to involve the foveola, irrespective of severity. Local microaneurysms (focal retinopathy) have a better prognosis than diffuse retinopathy. The visual results depend on the integrity of the foveola and the location, extent, and duration of retinal edema and exudates.

The laser is usually used in combination with a biomicroscope and contact lens, which neutralizes the corneal refraction and permits visualization of the fundus. A three-mirror contact lens permits visualization of the peripheral fundus. The foveola is not photocoagulated, and usually burns are not placed any closer than 0.25 disk diameter (375 μm) to the center of the capillary-free zone. The area between the fovea centralis and the disk is photocoagulated cautiously to avoid damage to the nerve fibers of the papillomacular bundle.

New blood vessels more than 1 disk diameter from the optic disk are treated with focal photocoagulation. Often the new blood vessels are near the first bifurcation of the superior temporal vein. The origin of the new blood vessels is surrounded for a distance of about 0.2 disk diameter with photocoagulation of sufficient intensity to produce a slight opacification (coagulation) of the sensory retina. Major blood vessels are not photocoagulated. Treatment is continued until new blood vessels no longer carry blood and may have to be repeated.

In patients with new blood vessels either on the optic disk or next to it, scatter coagulation is usually followed by involution of the vessels, with the fibrous component becoming more prominent. Involution occurs with photocoagulation of a single quadrant, but scatter photocoagulation may be required. Extensive destruction of the peripheral retina impairs dark adaptation and peripheral vision.

Intraretinal microvascular abnormalities in the region adjacent to the foveola cause a rim of hard yellow exudates or retinal edema to reduce vision. Photocoagulation of the vascular component resolves the edema and exudates and, if done promptly, improves vision.

OTHER OCULAR MANIFESTATIONS

Diabetes mellitus induces a variety of changes in the eye and its function. Nearly every ocular structure may be affected (Table 27-3).

TABLE 27-3.
Ocular Complications of Diabetes Mellitus Other Than Retinopathy

- I. Fundus
  - A. Optic nerve atrophy, edema
  - B. Lipemia retinalis
- II. Oculomotor nerves
  - A. Neuropathy with muscle paralysis (pupil frequently spared in N III involvement)
- III. Visual acuity
  - A. Transient variations in refraction
  - B. Photopsia and diplopia in cerebral hypoglycemia
  - C. Decreased accommodation
  - D. Depressed in cataract, vitreous hemorrhage, capillary nonperfusion adjacent to foveola, deposits in foveola, and foveola microangiopathy
  - E. Blindness from tractional retinal detachment, massive vitreous retraction
  - F. Diplopia in ophthalmoplegia caused by neuropathy
- IV. Intraocular pressure
  - A. Decreased in acidosis
  - B. Increased in neovascular glaucoma
- V. Conjunctiva
  - A. Sludging of blood; tortuous, constricted blood vessels
- VI. Cornea
  - A. Wrinkling of Descemet membrane
  - B. Decreased corneal sensation (trigeminal nerve neuropathy)
  - C. Impaired healing
  - D. Abnormal epithelial basement membrane, delayed wound healing
  - E. Punctate keratopathy
- VII. Iris
  - A. Hydrops of pigment epithelium (transient glycogen storage, disappears with normal blood glucose)
  - B. Rubeosis iridis
  - C. Transmission defects in pigment epithelium
- VIII. Lens
  - A. Variation in refractive power (hyperglycemia)
  - B. Snowflake ("sugar") cataract (insulin-dependent diabetes)
  - C. Premature onset of senile cataract

Rubeosis of the iris.—Rubeosis of the iris (Fig 27-8) is a vascular proliferation of the iris vessels that first becomes evident at the pupillary margin and in the anterior chamber angle. It also occurs spontaneously and after central vein closure. If glaucoma occurs, it is often resistant to both medical and surgical treatment. The origin of neovascularization of the iris adjacent to the pupil suggests that the vascular endothelial growth factor from the retina has diffused with the posterior aqueous humor through the pupillary opening.

Hydrops of the iris.—Glycogen may accumulate in the pigment epithelium of the iris. Alcohol-fixed sections of eyes that have been enucleated during a period of high blood glucose

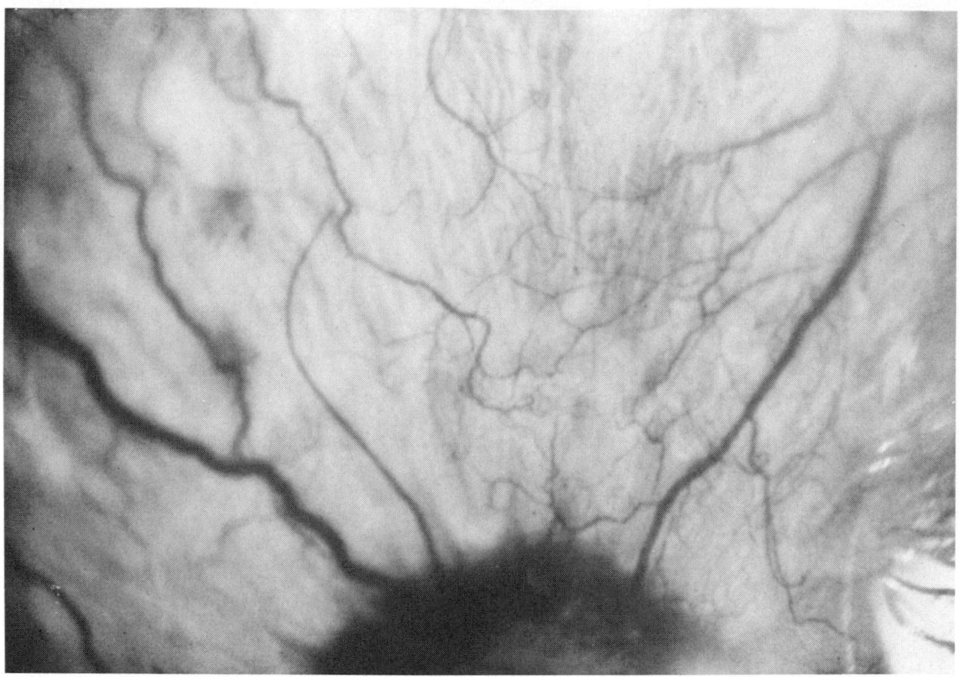

FIG 27-8.
Rubeosis of the iris in a man with insulin-dependent diabetes. Secondary glaucoma as the result of neovascularization of the anterior chamber angle did not develop.

concentration indicate the glycogen in dilated, vacuolated cells (Fig 27-9). Clinically, the condition may be suspected by observing the release of pigment into the anterior chamber after dilation of the pupil or after iridectomy in diabetic persons.

Diabetic cataract.—The lens may be affected in diabetes by transient changes in refractive power, early and more frequent age-related cataract, and juvenile diabetic cataract ("sugar" cataract).

Cataracts secondary to diabetes occur rarely and 10 to 20 years after the onset of insulin-dependent diabetes. Diabetic cataract develops rapidly and decreases vision after it starts. Both eyes are involved, often simultaneously. Typically, the opacity consists of small flaky opacities (snowflakes) and water clefts located in the anterior or posterior cortex immediately beneath the lens capsule. Control of the diabetes with restoration of normal blood glucose levels stops progression of the opacity. In persistent hyperglycemia the entire lens may opacify within 48 hours, but progress is usually more gradual. Diabetic retinopathy may prevent good vision after cataract extraction.

Neuropathy.—Paralysis of ocular muscles innervated by the oculomotor (N III) or abducent (N VI) nerve (Fig 27-10) occurs relatively rarely in diabetes. Characteristically, a middle-aged to elderly individual with mild overt diabetes or chemical diabetes has a sudden onset of diplopia and muscle paralysis associated with a homolateral headache severe enough to lead one to suspect an intracranial aneurysm. There may be a history of previous Bell palsy or similar neurologic disease. Neuropathy involving other areas may or may not be present. Signs of meningeal irritation do not occur. If the oculomotor (N III) nerve is involved, the pupil will most likely be spared (75%), in contrast to pupillary paralysis, which occurs in cerebral tumors and aneurysms. The paralysis disappears spontaneously within several weeks if the diabetes is of short duration, or it persists up to 6 months if the diabetes has been present for a long time, particularly if it has been poorly controlled.

Severe unilateral frontal headache and oculomotor paralysis are characteristic of aneurysms of the intracranial portion of the carotid artery. The sparing of the pupil, the laboratory

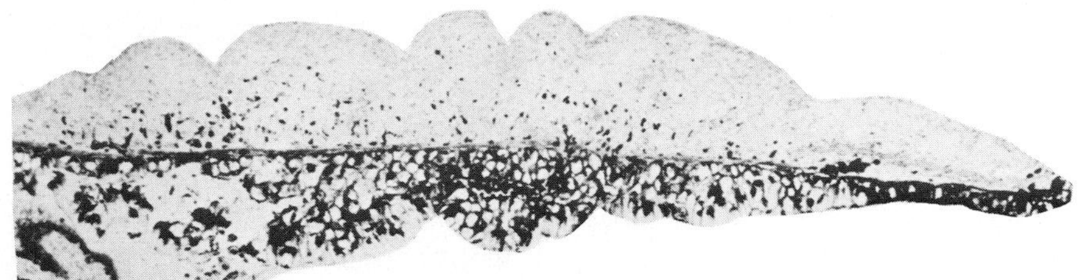

FIG 27-9.
Hydrops of the iris with the accumulation of glycogen in cystlike spaces in the pigment epithelium of the iris.

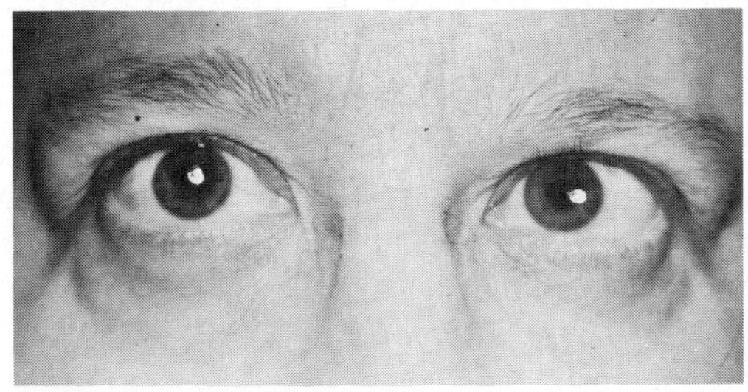

FIG 27-10.
Paralysis of the left lateral rectus muscle in a 62-year-old woman with non–insulin-dependent diabetes mellitus.

signs of diabetes, normal spinal fluid, and absence of meningeal irritation suggest that the disease is caused by diabetes.

Other causes of ophthalmoplegia besides intracranial aneurysms include tumors (magnetic resonance imaging or computed tomography), leukemia (blood cell count), ophthalmoplegic migraine (history), head trauma, demyelinating disease (painless onset), myasthenia gravis (painless onset), and cerebrovascular disease. The cornea may become less sensitive, reflecting a trigeminal neuropathy, particularly in diabetes of long duration.

Variations in refractive error.—Hyperglycemia may be associated with or followed by increased refractive power of the lens, resulting in a change in the refractive error in the direction of myopia. The exact mechanism of the change is not known, but it is assumed that during hyperglycemia there is an increased glucose content of the lens cortex with imbibition of water, causing the lens to become thicker and thus increasing its refractive power. Restoration of the blood glucose level to normal reverses the process. The refractive power of the lens decreases and the refractive error changes in the direction of hyperopia.

The visual acuity parallels the change in refraction. Refraction during hyperglycemia varies, often markedly, from that during an interval of normal blood glucose concentration. Paralysis of accommodation by means of a cycloplegic drug does not affect the induced refractive error. Corrective lenses, often quite different from those usually worn, improve vision to normal. Diagnosis is not difficult in a known diabetic, but the variation in refraction and visual acuity may be the first indication of diabetes mellitus, particularly in the insulin-dependent individual.

A similar change in refractive power may be produced in nondiabetic individuals by drugs, particularly sulfonamide derivatives. An actual change in the total refractive power of the eye, as occurs in diabetes, should be differentiated from that occurring with sustained accommodation (spasm of accommodation), which is neutralized with topical instillation of an eyedrop that paralyzes accommodation (cycloplegic).

Subjective visual symptoms.—During periods of hypoglycemia, patients with diabetes mellitus without organic changes in the eyes may complain of photopsia or of double vision. These symptoms are presumably of cerebral origin and are abolished by increasing the blood glucose level.

Intraocular pressure.—Ciliary body secretion is sensitive to the plasma bicarbonate level. A low intraocular pressure is associated with diabetic acidosis, and the ocular hypotension may be augmented by the concurrent dehydration.

Glaucoma in diabetes is a complication of rubeosis of the iris. Open-angle glaucoma occurs more commonly in patients with diabetes mellitus, but proliferative retinopathy occurs less commonly in diabetic patients with glaucoma.

THYROID GLAND

The thyroid gland is composed of two lobes adjacent to the trachea, which are connected by an isthmus located just below the cricoid cartilage of the trachea. It is the largest endocrine gland of the body and is composed of numerous small follicles that synthesize two metabolically active modified amino acids, thyroxine (T_4) and triiodothyronine (T_3).

Secretion of the thyroid hormones is initiated by the hypothalamus, which secretes the thyrotropic-releasing hormone (TRH). This stimulates the pituitary gland to release the thyroid-stimulating hormone (TSH, or thyrotropin), which binds to receptor sites on the surface of the thyroid gland follicles to form the thyroid-stimulating hormone receptor protein (TSHR). This protein activates a complex regulatory system that mediates most of the biologic actions of the thyroid gland, which include (1) iodide trapping and concentration by the basement membranes of the follicles of the thyroid gland; (2) oxidation of iodide to iodine; (3) iodination of the modified amino acid tyrosyl; (4) coupling of iodated tyrosyl with thyroglobulin (Tg); and (5) formation of the thyroid hormones, thyroxine (the major hormone of the thyroid gland) and triiodothyronine.

Thyroxine, which is not metabolically active, is released from the thyroid gland bound to the serum thyroxine-binding protein (TBG), to a prealbumin (transthyretin, TTR), and to albumin. It is monodeiodinated mainly in the liver, kidney, and brain to triiodothyronine, which is metabolically active only in the free form. Free triiodothyronine binds to specific receptors on nuclear and mitochondrial membranes to induce the transcription of specific target genes to synthesize particular proteins and enzymes.

Thyroid-stimulating immunoglobulins are antibodies to the normal receptor sites of the thyroid-stimulating hormone located on the surface of thyroid follicle cells. These antibodies may mimic the biologic action of the thyroid-stimulating hormone on thyroid function. Specific thyroid-stimulating hormone T lymphocytes occur in the circulation of patients with autoimmune thyroid disease. Similar reactive cells also occur in patients with nonautoimmune thyroid disease and in some entirely healthy patients.

GRAVES OPHTHALMOPATHY

Graves ophthalmopathy occurs in individuals with (1) thyrotoxicosis, (2) Hashimoto thyroiditis, (3) euthyroidism, or (4) hypothyroidism.

Thyrotoxicosis.—Thyrotoxicosis is a generalized systemic disorder secondary to excessive secretion of the thyroid hormones triiodothyronine and thyroxine. Women are predominantly affected (4:1), with the incidence peaking at about 44 years of age. There are sympathetic and calorigenic effects. The sympathomimetic effects include retraction of the upper eyelid, nervousness, tremor, and diarrhea. The calorigenic effects include an increased basal metabolic rate with increased appetite, weight loss, and increased heat production that stimulates heat loss mechanisms, such as tachycardia and increased skin circulation.

The onset of the disease is usually marked by fatigue, tachycardia, and, despite increased appetite, weight loss. There may be a fine tremor of the fingers and tongue, heat intolerance, and excessive sweating. The systolic blood pressure increases, atrial arrhythmias occur, and the pulse pressure widens. In individuals over 40 years of age there may be cardiac failure. Muscle weakness may be severe, but true myasthenia gravis rarely occurs. Serum free thyroxine and triiodothyronine levels are increased, and thyroid-stimulating hormone is absent when measured with the earlier tests and present at a low level when measured with sensitive or supersensitive tests.

Thyroid-stimulating immunoglobulins are antibodies to the normal receptor sites of the thyroid-stimulating hormone located on the surface of the thyroid follicle cells. These antibodies may mimic the biologic action of the thyroid-stimulating hormone on the thyroid function.

The occurrence of the thyroid-stimulating antibodies in patients who have hyperthyroidism suggests that the disease is initiated by an autoimmune abnormality. Current theories relating to the pathogenesis of autoimmune hyperthyroidism relate to (1) an abnormality of the HLA-DW3 genotype (in white patients) that impairs T cell–suppressor functions and allows B lymphocytes to synthesize immune globulins directed against receptor sites for thyroid-stimulating hormone; and (2) depression of T lymphocyte–suppressor function through stress or aging that permits synthesis of antibodies to thyroid-stimulating hormone receptors by B lymphocytes.

Lymphocytic (Hashimoto) thyroiditis.— Lymphocytic (autoimmune) thyroiditis may be responsible for some 10% of the instances of Graves ophthalmopathy in patients seen in the United States. Levels of thyroxine, triiodothyronine, and thyroid-stimulating hormone are in the normal range in the early stages of the disorder. Patients have antibodies to thyroglobulin and thyroid cytoplasmic proteins, which, however, may occur in individuals who do not have thyroid disease or ocular abnormalities. Like other patients with autoimmune disorders, affected patients often have other autoimmune disorders or affected family members. The lobes and isthmus of the thyroid gland are enlarged and firm, and there may be a regional lymphadenopathy. As the disease progresses, the levels of the thyroid hormones decrease, as does that of the thyroid-stimulating hormone. Eventually the patients may become hypothyroid.

Euthyroidism.—Rarely a patient without other physical abnormalities develops Graves ophthalmopathy. Results of all thyroid tests are normal, although some patients may have autoimmune antibodies, as do many patients without signs of thyroid disease.

Hypothyroidism.—About 1% of patients with Graves ophthalmopathy are hypothyroid. Possible causes include thyroidectomy, radioactive ablation of the gland, autoimmune thyroiditis, inadequate iodide intake, and hormonal deficiencies of the hypophysis, pituitary, or thyroid glands. The incidence peaks between the ages of 50 and 65 years. There is fatigue, mental slowness, and lethargy. The skin is dry and thickened, the face pale and puffy, and the lips thickened, and halitosis is common. The thyroxine and triiodothyronine levels are depressed but the thyroid-stimulating hormone level is increased.

ENDOCRINE OPHTHALMOPATHY

The diagnosis of endocrine ophthalmopathy is based on retraction of the eyelid combined with a goiter or laboratory evidence of an abnormality of the thyroid gland (Table 27-4). If retraction of the eyelid is present without evidence of abnormality of the thyroid gland, then the occurrence of exophthalmos, optic nerve dysfunction, or restriction of extraocular movements or physical demonstration of an enlarged muscle will support the diagnosis.

TABLE 27-4.
Diagnostic Criteria for Endocrine Ophthalmopathy

I. Retraction of eyelid (upper eyelid either at or above superior corneoscleral limbus)

PLUS

A. Thyroid gland abnormality
   1. Goiter
   2. Laboratory evidence (see text)

OR

B. Exophthalmos
   1. Exophthalmometer reading 20 mm or greater

OR

C. Optic nerve dysfunction
   1. Reduced visual acuity, color vision, or visual field
   2. Abnormal pupillary reactions

OR

D. Extraocular muscle restriction
   1. Impaired ocular movements
   2. Enlarged muscle
      a. Magnetic resonance imaging
      b. Computed tomography
      c. Ultrasonography

II. Thyroid gland dysfunction (without retraction of eyelid)

PLUS

A. Exophthalmos (see B. above)

OR

B. Restrictive extraocular myopathy (see C. above)

OR

C. Optic nerve impairment (see D. above)

After Bartley GB: The epidemiologic characteristics and clinical course of ophthalmopathy associated with autoimmune thyroid disease in Olmsted County, Minnesota, *Trans Am Ophthalmol Soc* 92:477-588, 1994.

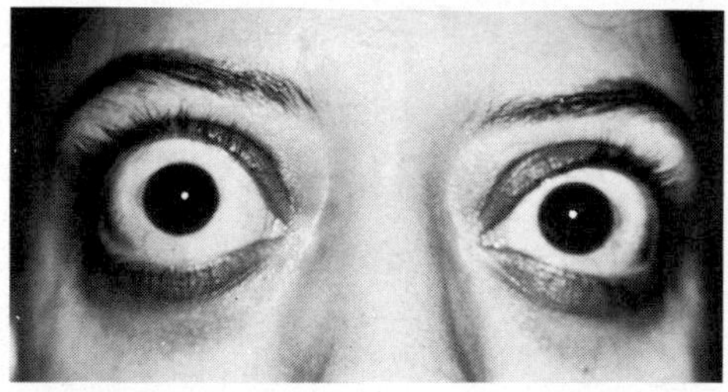

FIG 27-11.
Extreme exophthalmos and eyelid retraction in a 29-year-old woman who developed the condition gradually without signs of orbital congestion or ocular muscle weakness.

If the upper eyelid is not retracted but the laboratory signs of thyroid gland dysfunction are present, then the occurrence of exophthalmos, restriction of ocular movements or demonstration of an enlarged extraocular muscle, or an optic nerve impairment will support the diagnosis of endocrine ophthalmopathy.

In somewhat more than half of the patients with thyrotoxicosis, ocular signs (Table 27-5) appear sometime in the course of the disease. These may be unilateral or bilateral, symmetric or asymmetric, mild or severe. They may precede overt disease or occur long after the thyroid abnormality has been clinically ameliorated. The severity of the ophthalmopathy does not parallel any clinical or laboratory manifestation of the disorder or any abnormality of the thyroid, pituitary, or other endocrine gland.

Retraction of the upper eyelid.—Retraction of the upper eyelid is an important sign of thyroid gland dysfunction (Fig 27-11). The eyelid is symmetrically retracted to the superior corneoscleral limbus or the sclera is exposed in the 12 o'clock meridian. There is widening of the palpebral fissure and infrequent blinking, which cause a wide-eyed staring appearance. There is often failure of the upper eyelid to follow the globe in downward gaze (eyelid lag). Both eyelids are retracted in most patients (55%). In an additional 20% of the patients, the retraction is monocular.

Sympathetic overactivity and contraction of the smooth muscle in the upper eyelid cause retraction of the eyelid. The retraction is aggravated by the instillation of epinephrine eyedrops in the conjunctival cul-de-sac, and it is abolished on one side by blocking the superior cervical

TABLE 27-5.
Ocular Signs of Thyroid Dysfunction

I. Eyelids
   A. Retraction of upper eyelid to level of superior corneoscleral imbus or above (Dalrymple)
   B. Minor eyelid signs (not diagnostic)
      1. Increased retraction in attentive gaze (Kocher)
      2. Increased retraction after adrenergic stimulation
      3. Decreased retraction after adrenergic blockade
      4. Upper eyelid delay in following globe in downward gaze (von Graefe)
      5. Jerky downward movement of eyelid (Boston)
      6. Globe lags behind upper eyelid in upward gaze (Means)
      7. Lower eyelid lags behind globe in upward gaze (Griffith)
      8. Infrequent blinking (Stellwag)
      9. Staring appearance (Dalrymple)
      10. Increased pigmentation of skin (Jellinek)

II. Orbit
   A. Exophthalmos (unilateral or bilateral)
      1. Early signs
         a. Fullness of eyelids (Enroth)
         b. Inability to evert upper eyelid (Gifford)
      2. Established exophthalmos
         a. Compressible
         b. Not compressible (solid)

III. Extraocular muscles (restrictive myopathy)
   A. Limitation of ocular rotation
      1. Restricted upward gaze (common)
         a. Contracture of inferior rectus muscle
      2. Ophthalmoplegia (Ballet)
      3. Convergence weakness (Möbius)
   B. Muscle enlargement
      1. Ultrasonography
      2. Magnetic resonance imaging
      3. Computed tomography
      4. Autoantibodies to extraocular muscle plasma membranes

IV. Optic nerve
   A. Neuritis (papillitis or retrobulbar neuritis)
      1. Reduced vision
      2. Visual field defect
   B. Papilledema
   C. Acquired color vision defect

V. Cornea (complications of exophthalmos)
   A. Rapid drying of precorneal tear film
   B. Keratitis e lagophthalmos (failure of eyelid to cover cornea adequately)

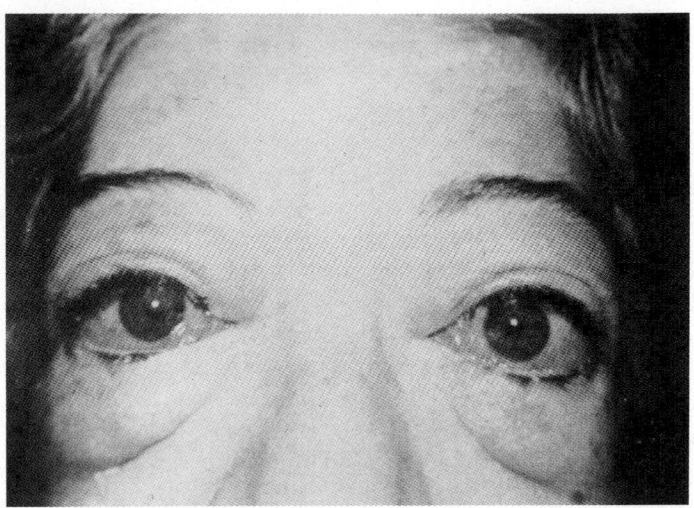

FIG 27-12.
Orbital congestion with eyelid edema, chemosis, and rapidly developing exophthalmos in a 57-year-old woman.

ganglion. The eyelid retraction, however, does not parallel the increase in free triiodothyronine that potentiates the action of epinephrine. The eyelid retraction, however, persists in sleep, general anesthesia, and after correction of excess triiodothyronine, which suggests that sympathetic stimulation of the orbital Müller muscle is not the sole cause. Possibly there is fibrosis of the muscle after prolonged retraction or an associated exophthalmos contributes to the eyelid retraction.

Exophthalmos.—Both orbits are usually involved in thyroid disease, although one orbit may be more severely affected than the other. The exophthalmos develops gradually or suddenly after eyelid retraction, with increased prominence of the eyes, sensitivity to light, and conjunctival hyperemia. Slow development of the exophthalmos allows extreme prominence of the eyes without orbital congestion. Rapid development of the exophthalmos is associated with orbital congestion, often with relatively minor degrees of exophthalmos.

When severe exophthalmos develops rapidly, the globe is not protected by the eyelids and an exposure keratitis occurs (keratitis e lagophthalmos), which can lead to corneal necrosis.

Signs of marked orbital congestion may develop quickly (Fig 27-12). The eyelids become puffy and full. The conjunctiva becomes chemotic and injected. The conjunctival vessels may be so congested as to suggest conjunctivitis. Chemosis (edema) of the palpebral conjunctiva may be marked, and the closed eyelids may not entirely cover the globe. Edema of the conjunctiva may cause ectropion, and tearing becomes a prominent symptom. Orbital congestion may occur without exophthalmos, but more often there is a rapid increase in exophthalmos during this period. If the cornea is not protected by the eyelids, keratitis e lagophthalmos develops, causing rapid loss of vision and loss of the eye from corneal necrosis if it is not effectively treated.

Many histopathologic changes increase the volume of orbital contents. Few orbits have been studied histologically, and the evidence is not adequate to conclude that the process is the same in every patient. The ocular muscles are inflamed, may increase three to six times in mass, and have a pale, swollen, pink appearance. Lymphocytes and plasma cells infiltrate the tissues, and there is deposition of glycosaminoglycans. These increase the water content of the orbital tissues and may be responsible for the exophthalmos. Eventually, fibrous tissue replacement occurs. The cause is not known, but there are specific autoantibodies directed against plasma membranes of extraocular muscles in 60% of patients with exophthalmos.

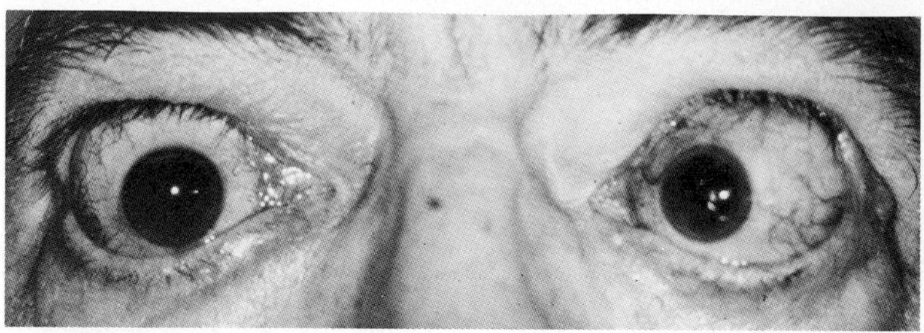

FIG 27-13.
Fibrosis of multiple extraocular muscles in a 68-year-old man. There is contraction of both medial recti muscles and both inferior recti muscles, along with severe exophthalmos and eyelid retraction.

These immune globulins are distinct from thyroid-stimulating antibodies and other antibodies directed against thyroid gland components.

Exophthalmos has not been produced in experimental animals by the administration of thyroid or pituitary hormones (corticotropin [ACTH], gonadotropin, growth hormone, or prolactin). Patients with exophthalmos have antibodies to the plasma membrane of ocular muscles. They do not have antibodies to the plasma membranes of skeletal muscle elsewhere in the body.

Optic nerve dysfunction.—Papilledema, papillitis, and optic neuropathy may develop in some individuals. Papilledema causes an enlargement of the blind spot on visual field testing, but there is no reduction of vision unless neglected for a long period. Papillitis and optic neuropathy (see Chapter 20) cause reduced visual acuity, a central scotoma, and sometimes restriction of the peripheral visual field. Like other ocular complications of Graves disease, the disorders may develop long after the hyperthyroidism has been corrected. Systemic prednisone, which may have to be continued for a long period in large amounts, is the main therapy. Cyclosporine may be used to supplement prednisone or substitute for it in patients in whom corticosteroids are contraindicated. Some patients who do not respond to prednisone benefit from cyclosporine. Orbital decompression with removal of the medial wall of the apex of the orbit or radiation therapy to the retro-orbital tissues is used if medical measures fail.

Extraocular muscle enlargement.—Limitation of ocular movement may develop at any time in the course of thyroid ophthalmopathy. Additionally, severe congestion of the orbit may limit ocular rotations. If there is any interference with the Bell phenomenon, in which the globe is rotated upward and outward with eyelid closure, the cornea may be exposed. A weakness of convergence follows mechanical inefficiency of the medial recti muscles in rotating the exophthalmic globes medially.

Graves disease may be complicated at any time by extraocular muscle fibrosis that frequently follows a moderately severe exophthalmos. Any extraocular muscle may be fibrosed. Frequently, the inferior rectus muscle contracts, which prevents upward rotation of one or both eyes and causes a vertical diplopia. Fibrosis of multiple extraocular muscles (Fig 27-13) may limit ocular rotation so that the head must be turned or tilted to move one eye to the primary position.

Muscular fibrosis and contraction is differentiated from a muscle weakness by the forced duction test. In a contracture of the inferior rectus muscle, the superior rectus muscle appears weakened since the eye cannot be elevated. The forced duction test indicates that contracture of the inferior rectus muscle prevents elevation of the globe.

Ultrasonography, computed tomography, or magnetic resonance imaging demonstrates one or more enlarged extraocular muscles in nearly every case of thyroid exophthalmos (Fig 27-14). Cushing syndrome and acromegaly that cause endocrine exophthalmos do not show muscle enlargement. Often the inferior recti muscles are markedly enlarged, but all muscles may be affected. Demonstration of such muscle enlargement constitutes an important diagnostic

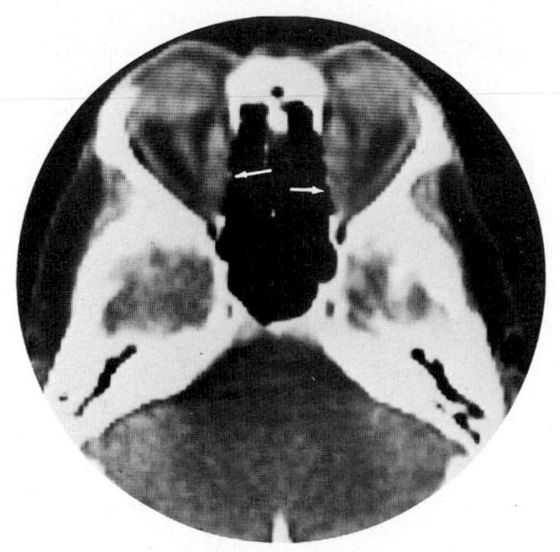

FIG 27-14.
Computed tomography of the orbits demonstrating increased size of medial recti muscles in hyperthyroidism.

method in Graves disease. Ultrasonography may demonstrate ocular muscle thickening and diffuse swelling of orbital fat.

The intraocular pressure varies by more than 3 mm Hg in different directions of gaze. Usually it is higher on upward gaze. Any contracture of an ocular muscle, such as that caused by myositis or muscle entrapment in an orbital bone fracture, may cause increased ocular pressure with a change in the direction of gaze.

Medical treatment.—The treatment of the ocular changes of thyroid disease is difficult. Relief of thyrotoxicosis usually minimizes eyelid retraction, and the exophthalmos appears to regress, although it may well increase 1 or 2 mm. Despite the increase, the eyes appear less prominent without the eyelid retraction. If ocular signs are marked, antithyroid drugs or radioactive iodine should be used in small, fractionated doses to avoid rapid changes in the thyroid status. If the ocular signs of Graves disease are present without clinical signs of hyperthyroidism, antithyroid treatment is not indicated.

Many patients complain of ocular discomfort ("grittiness") and benefit from topical instillation of artificial tears and wearing dark glasses with side arms. Instillation of an ophthalmic ointment at night and, if necessary, taping the eyelids closed prevents dessication of the exposed conjunctiva during sleep.

Elevating the head of the bed on 5-inch blocks may decrease orbital edema. Systemic prednisone often relieves orbital and eyelid edema while having little effect on the exophthalmos. Orbital decompression is the treatment of choice for severe orbital congestion with exposure of the cornea (keratitis e lagophthalmos, Fig 27-15). The floor of the orbit and the medial wall may be removed (Ogura) through a maxillary sinus approach (Caldwell-Luc) or the lateral, medial, and inferior walls through skin and conjunctival incisions.

Keratitis usually requires orbital decompression or tarsorrhaphy, whereas the optic neuritis often responds to systemic corticosteroids. In severe orbital congestion with exposure of the cornea, orbital decompression is the treatment of choice.

Permanent cosmetic improvement of exophthalmos after correction of the hyperthyroidism is not fully satisfactory. If the exophthalmos developed gradually and congestion is not present, a lateral blepharoplasty narrows the palpebral fissure and improves the cosmetic appearance. Retraction of the upper eyelid persisting after correction of the hyperthyroidism has been adequately treated by recessing the Müller smooth muscle of the eyelid.

Correction of the fibrous replacement of an extraocular muscle is often disappointing. The procedure must be delayed until spontaneous improvement is unlikely, usually a year or more after the onset of the muscle weakness. The fibrosed muscle may then be recessed.

MULTIPLE ENDOCRINE NEOPLASIA

Multiple endocrine neoplasia includes three distinct disorders of neural crest differentiation. Multiple endocrine neoplasia type 2B consists of medullary thyroid carcinoma and pheochromocytoma with marked dysmorphic changes. Prominent, enlarged, nonmyelinated corneal nerves occur in every patient with type 2B. Additionally, conjunctival neuromas, thickened eyelids, thickened conjunctival nerves, prominent eyebrows, and impaired pupillary reaction may occur. The body habitus resembles Marfan syndrome. In medullary carcinoma, the thyroid gland secretes calcitonin, which should be measured in all first-degree relatives of patients with this malignancy.

Observation of the thickened corneal nerves may allow diagnosis of multiple endocrine neo-

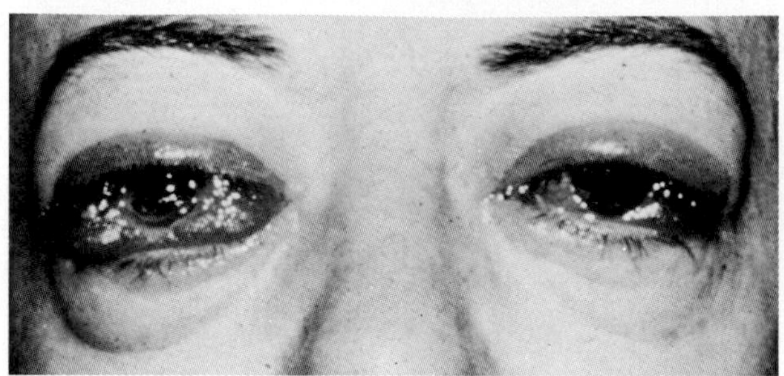

FIG 27-15.
Keratitis e lagophthalmos that developed after amelioration of hyperthyroidism in a 25-year-old woman. Loss of the eye was prevented by lateral (Berke) decompression of the orbit combined with a temporary tarsorrhaphy.

plasia type 2B before the development of neoplasms and unusual physical features.

PARATHYROID GLANDS

The parathyroid glands maintain the concentration of ionic calcium (and secondarily the concentration of inorganic phosphate) of the extracellular fluids. The secretion of the parathyroid glands is closely regulated by the concentration of inorganic serum calcium. Its direct effects, which are probably secondary in health, are on calcium bone resorption and absorption, renal excretion of calcium, and intestinal absorption. A secondary, and more likely important, action is the synthesis of 1,25-hydroxyvitamin D.

Ocular abnormalities secondary to the parathyroid gland malfunction occur mainly in those conditions in which there is an excess or decreased level of calcium in the extracellular fluids.

Hypercalcemia and hypophosphatemia.—In hypercalcemia and hypophosphatemia, calcium crystals are deposited in the cornea and conjunctiva. In the cornea, the deposits are in the Bowman zone and within epithelial cell nuclei. They are usually most marked near the corneoscleral limbus in the palpebral fissure (band keratopathy). The conjunctiva is injected, particularly in the palpebral fissure, and glistening crystals may be seen with the biomicroscope. The crystals disappear when the blood calcium level becomes normal. Computed tomography may demonstrate calcification of the sclera.

Calcification in otherwise normal eyes is seen in juvenile rheumatoid arthritis (Still disease), hyperparathyroidism, milk-alkali syndrome, sarcoidosis, hypervitaminosis D, Graves disease, posturemic phosphate depletion, widespread malignant disease, and myeloma. Calcium deposition occurs locally in conditions of the eye such as uveitis, corneal scarring, and phthisis bulbi.

Hypocalcemia and hyperphosphatemia.—Decreased secretion of the parathyroid hormone results in a lowered serum calcium level, an increased serum phosphorus level, and decreased urinary excretion of both calcium and phosphorus. A decreased serum calcium level causes tetany and neuromuscular hyperexcitability. In milder cases numbness and tingling occur in the extremities or in the area around the lips. Hoarseness may occur. In more severe cases carpopedal spasm and laryngeal stridor are seen. Generalized convulsions are common. Latent tetany is elicited by the Chvostek sign, in which tapping the finger over the facial nerve causes twitching of the muscles of the mouth and, in severe cases, of the nose and eyelids. Carpal spasm follows nerve ischemia when the blood supply to the arm is reduced for 3 minutes by a sphygmomanometer cuff (Trousseau sign).

Cataracts develop when the blood calcium level falls to a level at which neuromuscular hyperexcitability is observed. Lens changes are bilateral and involve lens fibers predominantly in the subcapsular region. As lens damage progresses, small, discrete, punctate opacities and crystals of different shapes and colors develop in the cortical lens near the equator. Similar opacities may be found in myotonic dystrophy, cretinism, and the Down syndrome.

Cataracts do not always develop with hypocalcemia, and the mechanism is unknown.

Calcification of basal ganglia, increased intracranial pressure, and papilledema may occur in hypoparathyroidism. Hypoparathyroidism with convulsive seizures and papilledema must be distinguished from an intracranial space-occupying lesion.

Children with idiopathic hypoparathyroidism (girls, 2:1) develop chronic recurrent keratoconjunctivitis with corneal neovascularization. Superficial moniliasis involving the face and nails occurs simultaneously; later an adrenal insufficiency develops that may be fatal (78%).

THE PITUITARY GLAND

Abnormalities of the pituitary gland may manifest themselves by endocrine hypersecretion or hyposecretion or by local pressure effects. The endocrine abnormalities do not cause major ocular changes, and the local pressure effects (chiasmal syndrome, atrophy of the optic nerve(s) [N II]), visual field defects, and oculomotor nerve paralysis (N III) are discussed in Chapter 28.

BIBLIOGRAPHY

Books

Kahn CR, Weir GC, editors: *Joslin's diabetes mellitus,* ed 13, Philadelphia, 1994, Lea & Febiger.

Olk RJ, Lee CM: *Diabetic retinopathy: practical management,* Philadelphia, 1993, JB Lippincott.

Rayner D, Champion BR, editors: *Thyroid autoimmunity,* Austin, 1995, RG Landes.

Articles

Aiello LP, Avery RL, Arrigg PG, Keyt BA, Jampel HD, Shah ST et al: Vascular endothelial growth factor in ocular fluid of patients with diabetic retinopathy and other retinal disorders, *N Engl J Med* 331:1480-1487, 1994.

Bartley GB: The epidemiologic characteristics and clinical course of ophthalmopathy associated with autoimmune thyroid disease in Olmsted County, Minnesota, *Trans Am Ophthalmol Soc* 92:477-588, 1994.

Diabetes Control and Complication Trial Research Group: Progression of retinopathy with intensive versus conventional treatment in the Diabetes Control and Complications Trial, *Ophthalmology* 102: 647-661, 1995.

Feman SS: The natural history of the first clinically visible features of diabetic retinopathy, *Trans Am Ophthalmol Soc* 92:745-773, 1994.

Maddux BA, Sbraccia P, Kumakura S, Sasson S, Youngren J, Fisher A et al: Membrane glycoprotein PC-1 and insulin resistance in non–insulin-dependent diabetes mellitus, *Nature* 373:448-451, 1995.

Soliman M, Kaplan E, Fisfalen ME, Okamoto Y, DeGroot LJ: T-cell reactivity to recombinant human thyrotropin receptor extracellular domain and thyroglobulin in patients with autoimmune and nonautoimmune thyroid diseases, *J Clin Endocrinol Metab* 80:206-213, 1995.

Yanagawa T, Hidaka Y, Guimaraes V, Soliman M, DeGroot LJ: CTLA-4 gene polymorphism associated with Graves' disease in a Caucasian population, *J Clin Endocrinol Metab* 80:41-45, 1995.

28

THE CENTRAL NERVOUS SYSTEM AND THE EYE

Many disorders of the central nervous system affect the eye or its adnexa. Some are immediately apparent, but others require extensive diagnostic study. Magnetic resonance imaging and computed tomography expedite the diagnosis of many complicated conditions, but their high cost limits their use. The careful examiner, however, can often determine quickly whether there is any abnormality of the cranial nerves serving the eyes.

Even the most cursory physical examination should indicate that (1) the pupils are round and equal and react directly and consensually to light; (2) the eyes are parallel and move to the right and to the left and up and down (by request and not by following the examiner's finger or a light); (3) blinking is normal and the eyelids can be squeezed closed; (4) the ocular media are transparent; (5) the optic disks are flat and of normal color; and (6) the major retinal blood vessels near the optic disks are normal.

PUPILS

The pupils are normally round and approximately equal in size. Both pupils constrict equally when the retina of one eye is stimulated with light (see Chapter 7).

Lesions that affect the afferent pathway between the retina and the optic chiasm more severely on one side than the other result in a relative afferent pupillary defect (Robert Marcus Gunn). When light is directed into the better eye, both pupils constrict promptly. If the light is quickly directed to the fellow eye, both pupils dilate despite the continued retinal stimulation. (Normally the pupils remain constricted and dilate, but slowly, as the retina adapts to the additional light.) The afferent pupillary defect is an important sign of an optic nerve conduction defect or an extensive retinal lesion. The pupillary reaction is normal in strabismic amblyopia, in conversion reactions with simulated loss of vision, cystoid macular edema, and most retinal lesions. It is conspicuous in optic neuritis, and in optic atrophy that is more severe on one side.

Horner syndrome is caused by interruption of the sympathetic nerve fibers to the dilatator pupillae muscle. The pupil is miotic and does not dilate when cocaine is instilled into the eye; there is an associated blepharoptosis and failure of sweating of the face on the involved side. Adie syndrome involves parasympathetic postganglionic nerves of the ciliary ganglion in which the pupil is larger than its fellow and pupillary constriction is absent or delayed. Patients, often women, may notice the anisocoria and seek medical attention. Argyll Robertson pupils (miotic and irregular pupils that do not constrict to light but constrict to convergence) occur in tabes dorsalis.

Unilateral mydriasis and coma after head injury suggest a skull fracture on the side of the dilated pupil. Tumor, intracranial aneurysm, and head injury are more likely to compress pupillary fibers and to cause pupillary dilation (mydriasis) than are diabetic neuropathy or meningitis. With midbrain hypoxia, the pupils dilate, but otherwise the pupils are constricted in sleep and coma. Pupils dilated by systemic or topical instillation of drugs such as atropine, ocular injury, or closed-angle glaucoma do not constrict after instillation of 1% pilocarpine. Pupils dilated because of oculomotor nerve disease or injury constrict readily after instillation of pilocarpine.

OCULAR ROTATIONS

The normal eyes are directed simultaneously to the same point in space and move synchronously to the right and left and up and down (see Chapter 23). Patients should be requested to move their eyes in these directions. To detect a paralysis of gaze, ocular rotations should not be tested by having the patient follow the examiner's finger or an examination light. Full ocular movements indicate intact oculomotor (N III), trochlear (N IV), and abducent (N VI) nerves (see Chapter 23). The ability to squeeze the eyelids tightly closed indicates a functioning facial nerve (N VII).

OPHTHALMOSCOPY

Ophthalmoscopy (see Chapter 6) is an essential portion of the complete physical examination. Usually a direct ophthalmoscope is used and a +10-diopter lens is rotated into its viewing aperture. The examiner directs the light of the ophthalmoscope into the eye at a distance of about 20 cm. Any opacity of the media is seen as a black silhouette against the red fundus reflex. Opacities may occur in the cornea, anterior chamber, lens, or vitreous humor.

While directing attention on the red reflex, the examiner gradually moves closer to the eye, reducing the power of the convex lens in the viewing aperture of the ophthalmoscope. The optic nerve and then the major blood vessels of the retina gradually come into sharp focus.

OPTIC NERVE

Atrophy of the optic nerve (see Chapter 20) may be complete or partial and may be caused by diseases within the eye that affect ganglion cells or their axons in the retinal nerve fiber layer, or by disorders of the optic nerve or optic tract that affect axons in their course to the lateral geniculate body. These lesions are localized as retinal, prechiasmatic, chiasmatic, and those of the optic tract. Prechiasmatic lesions affect one eye only unless two separate lesions affect the two optic nerves.

Optic atrophy, hemianopsia, and reduced visual acuity suggest a lesion of the axons of ganglion cells between the eye and the lateral geniculate body. Optic nerve atrophy preceded by papilledema or inflammation is called secondary. Optic nerve atrophy that is not preceded by inflammation or edema is called primary.

Inflammation of the optic nerve (termed retrobulbar neuritis when it involves the optic nerve posterior to the eye and papillitis when it involves the intraocular portion of the optic nerve) is nearly always monocular and reduces visual acuity. In the retrobulbar variety there are no ophthalmoscopic signs of the disorder, but the pupil constricts poorly or not at all to light stimulation.

Papilledema (see below) is usually bilateral, does not impair vision early in its course, is not present if the lamina cribrosa is clearly visible, and is associated with absence of spontaneous or induced retinal vein pulsation.

Papilledema.—The symptoms of increased intracranial pressure are severe bioccipital and bifrontal headaches that awaken the patient from sleep or are present at awakening. The headache is deep, steady, and dull and is aggravated by coughing, sneezing, or defecating, all of which increase intracranial pressure. Typically, the headache is relieved by vomiting, which occurs without nausea and may or may not be projectile. Signs include incontinence, mental torpor, and unsteady gait. Late vagus nerve effects are slowed pulse, lowered pulse pressure, and increased respiratory rate. There is a clouding of consciousness that varies from a delirium to a psychosis, or somnolence to deep coma.

The main ocular sign of increased intracranial pressure is bilateral papilledema. In the absence of ocular or orbital disease, the most likely cause is an intracranial space-occupying lesion. Many brain tumors do not cause increased intracranial pressure or are diagnosed before it develops. Other ocular signs of increased intracranial pressure occur relatively late. Extraocular muscle paresis, particularly unilateral lateral rectus muscle paralysis, occurs late and is of no localizing value. Initially pupillary constriction to light is normal, but it is lost after prolonged papilledema.

The oculomotor nerve may be compressed at the tentorial notch in herniation of the temporal lobe, which causes unilateral mydriasis and loss of the direct and consensual light pupillary reflex. Subsequently, paresis of the levator palpebrae superioris muscle causes blepharoptosis followed by paresis of other muscles innervated by the oculomotor nerve.

VISUAL PATHWAYS

The visual field (see Chapter 5) is the loci of objects or points in space that can be perceived when the head is fixed and the eyes directed straight ahead. Prechiasmal lesions affect vision in one eye only. A lesion immediately anterior to the chiasm may cause a severe visual field defect in the ipsilateral eye and a minor temporal field defect in the fellow eye because the neurons that originate in the inferior nasal portion of the fellow retina bend into the opposite optic nerve just anterior to the optic chiasm.

A lesion of the chiasm involves decussating nasal fibers and causes loss of vision in the temporal portion of each visual field, a bitemporal visual field defect or, if complete, a bitemporal hemianopsia. A chiasmal lesion that is predominantly lateral may rarely cause a hemianoptic defect in the temporal field of only one eye rather than the usual bitemporal defect.

Lesions posterior to the chiasm involve nerve fibers that originate from the temporal retina on the ipsilateral side (causing a nasal field defect) and from the nasal retina on the contralateral side (causing a temporal field defect). The visual defect is bilateral, a homonymous defect. If complete, it is hemianopsia (half blindness: visual fields are always described in terms of the blind portion of the field). Disturbances of the nasal retina cause temporal visual field defects; disturbances of the temporal retina cause nasal visual field defects. Partial defects that do not involve the entire half of the visual field may be congruous or incongruous. Congruous defects are the same in size, shape, and intensity in the visual field of each eye. They occur in lesions in the geniculocalcarine tract that extends from the lateral geniculate body to the visual cortex. Generally, lesions of the parietal or occipital lobes cause congruous defects. Incongruous visual field defects are bilateral but different in each eye. They occur in lesions in the optic tract, lateral geniculate body, and temporal lobe.

HEADACHES

Disabling headaches are rarely caused by ocular disorders except in the uncommon ocular conditions of acute angle-closure glaucoma or a blind painful eye. Many patients, however, and sometimes their physicians, attribute any discomfort that occurs about the head to an ocular abnormality (see Chapter 4).

Organic headaches may be divided into those that originate from extracranial and intracranial sources (Table 28-1). Iridocyclitis, high in-

TABLE 28-1.
Some Causes of Headache

I. Extracranial causes
  A. Vascular headache
    1. Migraine
      a. Without aura (common)
      b. With aura (Classical)
        (1) Cerebral
        (2) Ophthalmoplegic
        (3) Retinal
    2. Hypertension
  B. Cluster
  C. Tension
  D. Dental
  E. Nasal accessory sinuses
  F. Giant cell arteritis
  G. Blind eye
  H. Angle-closure glaucoma
  I. Temporomandibular joint
  J. Occipitofrontal muscle contracture
II. Intracranial causes
  A. Brain tumor
  B. Subarachnoid hemorrhage
  C. Intracranial dilation and distention
    1. Increased intracranial pressure
    2. Decreased intracranial pressure
      a. Post-lumbar puncture
  D. Inflammation
    1. Zoster
    2. Meningitis
    3. Arteritis
    4. Phlebitis
  E. High altitude
  F. Traction and displacement
    1. Venous sinuses and tributaries
    2. Middle meningeal arteries
    3. Carotid and basilar arteries
    4. Cranial nerve with sensory component
  G. Cranial nerve neuralgia
    1. Trigeminal (N V); tic douloureux
    2. Glossopharyngeal (N IX)

traocular pressure, impending and past herpes-zoster ophthalmicus, and temporal arteritis cause orbital pain. Retrobulbar neuritis is associated with pain behind the eye aggravated by ocular movements. The ocular muscle palsy of diabetic neuropathy begins with severe retrobulbar pain. Refractive errors are commonly thought to cause discomfort and pain in the head, but usually the cause of such pain is vascular, neurologic, or psychogenic.

Intracranial disease, such as brain tumor, subarachnoid hemorrhage, intracranial aneurysms, and incensed intracranial pressure, are uncommon causes of organic headache. The practitioner is usually required to distinguish between conditions such as migraine and its variants, cluster, and tension headaches.

Migraine.—This is a symptom complex of transient (usually), paroxysmal, severe, often unilateral, throbbing headache. There are two main types: (1) migraine without aura (common migraine), and (2) migraine with aura (classic migraine) (aura: in medicine, a neurologic dysfunction of the visual, sensory, speech, or motor systems). Except for the occurrence of the aura the two types are similar.

Migraine without aura is characterized by a severe, throbbing headache, which is aggravated by physical activity. The head pain is initially unilateral but eventually involves the whole head. There is sensitivity to light and sound, nausea, and vomiting. Migraine with aura is initiated by neurologic symptoms, which are often similar with each attack. The visual aura begins as a C-shaped scotoma in the central portion of the visual field (Fig 28-1) which gradually expands and disappears into the periphery. Its edges are colored, serrated, and pulsating. Some patients may experience dysarthria, vertigo, or diplopia. The typical headache without treatment persists some 72 hours, and there may be recurrent attacks over a period of several weeks. Some individuals, mainly middle-aged and older, have only the aura without the headache.

Some migraines with aura are associated with severe and lasting motor, visual, and sensory complications. Some patients develop permanent hemianopsia, hemiplegia, and speech difficulties. Ophthalmoplegic migraine is associated with transient ocular muscle paralysis, blepharoptosis, and pupillary signs, each of which may persist permanently. In migraine of the anterior visual pathway there may be serous chorioretinopathy, vitreous hemorrhage, ischemic papillitis, and optic atrophy.

Mild attacks may be treated effectively with early administration of aspirin or acetaminophen. Nonsteroidal anti-inflammatory drugs such as naproxen sodium or ibuprofen may be effective. Other related nonsteroidal anti-inflammatory drugs may be substituted. Intramuscular ketorolac is an effective, rapidly active analgesic.

Ergotamine preparations are often used but have many side effects. A maximum of 6 mg of ergotamine tartrate may be used in a 24-hour period, with a maximum of 10 mg in 1 week. Intranasal dihydroergotamine may be helpful. Methysergide and propanolol are used as prophylactic therapy.

Serotonin (5-hydroxytryptamine) is probably released from platelets at the beginning of an attack. Sumatriptan binds to some serotonin

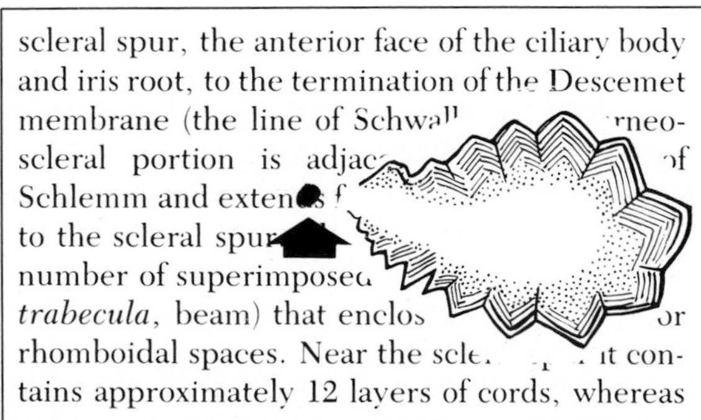

FIG 28-1.
The scintillating scotôma of migraine as projected on the printed page. The arrow points to the fixation point. The scotoma expands and contracts and always involves both eyes.

receptors and inhibits pain arising from cerebral arteries. It must be administered subcutaneously or used intranasally.

Cluster headache.—Cluster headache (recurrent nocturnal headache, paratrigeminal syndrome of Raeder, histamine headache, sphenopalatine neuralgia [Sluder], petrosal, vidian, or ciliary [Charlin] neuralgia) is a sudden, recurrent, excruciating, debilitating pain in one orbit or temple. It occurs chiefly in men between 30 and 50 years of age but may affect all ages and both sexes. Attacks often begin within a few minutes to several hours after falling asleep. There may be lacrimation, conjunctival injection, Horner syndrome, and sweating of the forehead. The nostril on the side of the pain is blocked, followed by rhinorrhea.

The attack lasts 15 to 180 minutes (average, 45 minutes). The attacks occur frequently for days or weeks (hence, cluster) and then disappear, sometimes for years. During a period when attacks are occurring, they may be triggered by alcohol, monosodium glutamate, aged cheeses and meats, chocolate, high altitude, or excessive exercise.

The inhalation of 100% oxygen (9 L/min) through a mask for 10 to 15 minutes aborts most attacks. Attacks may be aborted with many of the same medications used in the treatment of migraine.

Tension-type headache.—Stress and tension in an individual's life do not cause headaches but may exacerbate them. The discomfort is described as dull, pressing, tightening, pounding, and bandlike, affecting both sides of the head. Some patients experience a day-long headache that begins on awakening in the morning. There may be an associated sensitivity to bright lights (not relieved with the tinted spectacles patients often wear), dizziness, and nausea. The patients often overuse analgesics. Treatment is difficult. Many patients have many pairs of glasses that have not relieved the headaches. The use of analgesics should be avoided if possible and narcotics should never be used. Nonsteroidal anti-inflammatory drugs may be useful.

Pseudotumor cerebri.—In this chronic condition, obese young women with a history of menstrual irregularity, often with amenorrhea, develop bilateral papilledema, headache, and high cerebrospinal fluid pressure. The headache is often worse on awakening and is aggravated by coughing and straining. The papilledema (see Chapter 20) may be associated with dimming or blurring of vision. Visual symptoms may be minimal despite severe papilledema. The disorder may persist for years without serious sequelae. Brain tumor must be excluded by magnetic resonance imaging and chronic meningitis by cerebrospinal fluid study.

Papilledema also develops with vascular hypertension; chronic emphysema; meningitis caused by sarcoid, tuberculosis, or carcinomatosis; Addison disease; corticosteroid withdrawal; vitamin A toxicity; and hypothyroidism.

INTRACRANIAL MASS LESIONS

Primary and metastatic neoplasms of the brain, hamartomas, intracranial aneurysms, hematomas, granulomatous inflammations, and parasitic cysts may cause increased intracranial pressure and may induce localizing neurologic defects. Primary neoplasms of the brain may be divided into gliomas, meningiomas, vascular tumors such as angiomas and hemangioblastomas, pituitary tumors, congenital tumors such as craniopharyngioma, hamartomas, teratomas, and adnexal tumors that originate in the pineal body or choroid plexus. Metastatic tumors constitute 10% to 25% of all brain tumors and may originate from almost any primary tumor, most commonly the lung in men and the breast or lung in women.

Gliomas are composed of ectodermal supporting tissue (neuroglia) and are the most common primary brain tumor. They include the histologically benign gliomas of childhood and astrocytomas, ependymomas, oligodendrogliomas, and medulloblastomas. Gliomas in childhood involve the optic nerves and chiasm, may be associated with neurofibromatosis type 1 (von Recklinghausen), and likely constitute a hamartoma that causes proliferation of adjacent neuroglia. The other glioma of childhood is the highly malignant medulloblastoma, whose origin is restricted to the cerebellum mainly in boys (67%) aged 5 to 9 years and again at age 20 to 24 years. The most common type of astrocytoma (50% to 60%) is the highly malignant and uniformly fatal glioblastoma, of which there are several types.

A meningioma is a slow-growing connective tissue tumor of the dura mater. Sphenoidal ridge meningiomas may include structures at the apex of the orbit, and they may invade the orbit. Meningioma of the intraorbital portion of the optic nerve sheath causes proptosis and shunt vessels on the optic disk.

Angiomas are slow-growing congenital vascular malformations. Hemangioblastomas are slow-growing vascular neoplasms most commonly found in the cerebellum. They may be associated with angiomatosis of the retina and cysts of the kidney and pancreas (von Hipple-Lindau syndrome).

Intracranial granulomatous inflammations include tuberculosis; toruloma; sarcoidosis, usually of the meninges; and syphilitic gumma. Cysticercosis caused by the larva of *Taenia solium* or *Taenia saginata* may cause single or multiple cerebral masses.

Focal symptoms.—The brain differentiates from the hollow dorsal neural tube that forms three vesicles (Table 28-2). The structures derived from the forebrain (prosencephalon) are located above the tentorium (supratentorial), while those derived from the hindbrain (rhombencephalon) are located below the tentorium (infratentorial). Structures derived from the midbrain (mesencephalon) may be in supratentorial or infratentorial location.

Supratentorial tumors.—Structures derived from the forebrain include the cerebral hemispheres (frontal, temporal, parietal, and occipital lobes), the chiasm, the pituitary gland, the anterior and middle fossa, and the diencephalon. Visual field defects are common, as are optic atrophy and papilledema. Disturbance of ocular movements is less common than with infratentorial lesions.

Chiasmal syndrome.—The chiasmal syndrome consists of optic atrophy combined with bitemporal visual field defects. It is caused by impairment of nerve conduction at the optic chiasm of axons that originate in the ganglion cells located in the nasal half of each retina. Magnetic resonance imaging (preferred) or computed tomography combined with radioimmunoassay of pituitary hormones makes the diagnosis of lesions that cause the chiasmal syndrome more accurate than previously.

The common causes of the chiasmal syndrome are pituitary adenomas, craniopharyngiomas, and meningioma of the tuberculum sellae. Rarely sarcoidosis, metastatic carcinoma, or Hand-Schüller-Christian disease is the cause. Tumors of the hypothalamus (hamartomas, choristomas, gliomas, and ganglioneuromas) and other midbrain disorders may release pituitary stimulating hormones that cause endocrine effects identical to those caused by pituitary tumors.

TABLE 28-2.
Embryonic Origin of Some Parts of the Brain

- I. Anterior primary vesicle
  - A. Cerebrum
    - 1. Prosencephalon (forebrain)
      - a. Telencephalon (endbrain)
        - (1) Hypophysis
        - (2) Optic nerves and retinae
        - (3) Anterior third ventricle
        - (4) Cerebral hemispheres
          - (a) Corpus striatum
          - (b) Olfactory bulb and tract
          - (c) Cerebral cortex
          - (d) Lateral ventricle
      - b. Diencephalon (interbrain)
        - (1) Thalamus
        - (2) Geniculate bodies
        - (3) Pineal body
        - (4) Posterior third ventricle
    - 2. Mesencephalon (midbrain)
- II. Middle primary vesicle
  - A. Cerebrum
    - 1. Mesencephalon (midbrain)
      - a. Quadrigeminate bodies (colliculi)
      - b. Cerebral peduncles
      - c. Cerebral aqueduct (Sylvii)
      - d. Oculomotor nerve (N III)
- III. Posterior primary vesicle
  - A. Rhombencephalon
    - 1. Isthmus rhombencephalon
      - a. Superior cerebellar peduncles
      - b. Cerebral peduncles
    - 2. Metacephalon (hindbrain)
      - a. Cerebellum
      - b. Pons
        - (1) Medial longitudinal fasciculus
        - (2) Abducens nerve (N VI)
        - (3) Facial nerve (N VII)
    - 3. Medulla oblongata (afterbrain)
      - a. Cranial nerves
        - (1) N IX; N X; N XI; N XII

Pituitary adenomas.—Pituitary tumors produce clinical effects in three ways: (1) endocrine hypersecretion by tumor cells; (2) endocrine hyposecretion secondary to damage to the normal pituitary; and (3) local pressure effects caused by tumor growth into adjacent structures. Superior extension compresses the optic chiasm and causes a bitemporal visual field defect that begins in the superior quadrants. Optic atrophy is delayed. Inferior extension into the sphenoid sinus may cause a cerebrospinal

TABLE 28-3.
Pituitary Gland Adenomas

Differentiated cell (77%)
Prolactin cell (amenorrhea, impotence, galactorrhea)
Growth hormone cell (acromegaly; gigantism)
Corticotropin cell (ACTH excess: Cushing or Nelson syndrome)
Mixed prolactin cell–growth hormone
Thyroid-stimulating hormone (TSH) hyperthyroidism or hypothyroidism
Gonadotropic cell (gonadal failure)
Undifferentiated cell (23%)
Oncocytoma (increased tumor mitochondria content)
Null cell

fluid rhinorrhea that has a higher sugar content than nasal secretions. Lateral extension into the cavernous sinus (often after radiation or incomplete surgical excision of a pituitary tumor) causes oculomotor nerve palsies.

Pituitary adenomas (Table 28-3) may result from differentiated cells (endocrine secreting, 77%) or from undifferentiated cells (without endocrine activity; mainly null cell tumors). Prolactin cell tumors, the most common, occur more frequently in women than men. In women they cause amenorrhea and galactorrhea; in men they cause impotence, gynecomastia, galactorrhea, and hypopituitarism. Growth hormone cell adenomas cause gigantism when they occur before fusion of the epiphyses and acromegaly when they occur after epiphyseal fusion. There are increased serum levels of growth hormone and insulin-like growth factor I. Corticotropic cell adenomas may follow adrenalectomy (Nelson syndrome) or cause Cushing syndrome (moon face, truncal obesity, decreased carbohydrate metabolism, and other signs of excessive secretion of adrenocorticotropic hormone [ACTH]). Some adenomas result in an excess secretion of both prolactin and growth cell hormone. Rare tumors result from untreated primary thyroid failure (thyroid-stimulating hormone [TSH] cell adenoma) and untreated primary gonadal cell failure in Turner or Klinefelter syndrome (gonadotropic cell adenoma).

Visual field defects occur, chiefly in men, late in the course of pituitary adenomas. The field defect initially affects the superior temporal field and then extends to the inferior temporal quadrant (Fig 28-2). The defect may be asymmetric, with one eye being blind and temporal field loss in the fellow eye. Optic atrophy lags behind the visual field defect.

Treatment is highly individualized. Transsphenoidal surgical resection of an adenoma usually reduces abnormal hormone secretion and preserves normal pituitary function. Radiation therapy arrests tumor growth, but complications include optic nerve atrophy, oculomotor nerve palsy, and tropic hormone failure. Bromocriptine reduces the secretion of growth hormone and is used in acromegaly and prolactinomas. Octreotide suppresses growth hormone secretion and insulin secretion but requires daily subcutaneous administration. Minute enlargement of the pituitary gland is detected fairly often by magnetic resonance imaging of the skull. The enlargement is usually stationary and rarely increases in size.

Craniopharyngiomas.—Craniopharyngiomas originate from secretory vestiges of the Rathke pouch, are usually located above the sella turcica, and may extend into the third ventricle. They are the most common cause of hypopituitarism before puberty and the most common type of tumor involving the pituitary gland in children. They occur most frequently in younger children but occasionally are not symptomatic until adulthood.

In children, progressive visual loss may not be noted until internal hydrocephalus with papilledema and behavioral changes occur. Obesity, delayed sexual maturation, somnolence, and diabetes insipidus occur. In adolescents, decreased anterior pituitary secretion may cause dystrophia adiposogenitalis (Fröhlich syndrome), cachexia (Simmonds disease), or dwarfism (Lorain disease). In adults, a fluctuating bitemporal hemianopsia that involves the two eyes unequally occurs. An associated hypopituitarism causes impotence or amenorrhea with loss of libido; obesity; fine, silky skin with loss of body hair; and decreased beard growth in males.

Visual field impairment is typically asymmetric with a tendency for initial involvement of the temporal field. Defects tend to be far advanced in one eye before the fellow eye becomes involved. Because of the cystic nature of the tumor, the visual fields may fluctuate even without treatment. Magnetic resonance imaging provides the most helpful information.

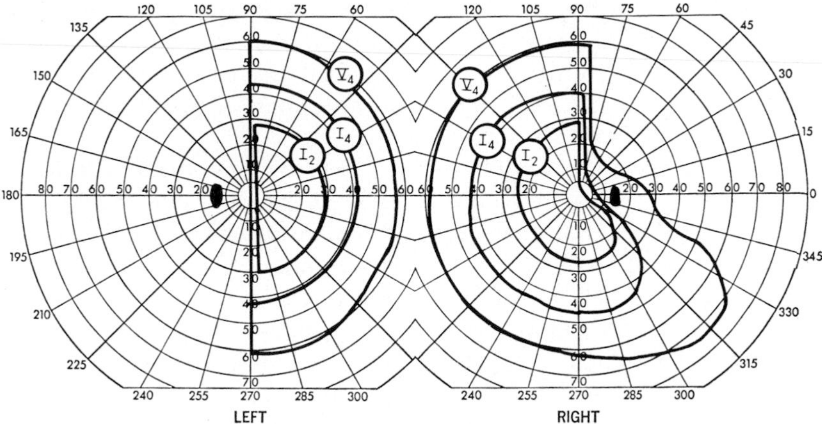

FIG 28-2.
Bitemporal hemianopsia produced by compressive disease of the optic chiasm. The visual field defect is seldom symmetric in the two eyes and here has affected the decussating axons originating in the nasal retina of the left eye far more severely than the nasal axons originating from the right eye. (*From Burde RM, Savino PJ, Trobe JD:* Clinical decisions in neuro-ophthalmology, *ed 2, St Louis, 1992, Mosby–Year Book. Used by permission.*)

Frontal lobe tumors.—The frontal lobe of the brain is concerned mainly with control of body movements. The cardinal sign of frontal lobe lesions is hemiplegia. Voluntary movements of the eye are initiated in the frontal lobe. Lesions affect ocular movements of gaze (conjugate movements). Changes in mentation caused by lesions include apathy, euphoria, amnesia, and confabulation. Unilateral inability to release voluntarily an object placed in the hand (forced grasping) is of localizing importance. Papilledema is the most common ocular sign.

The Foster Kennedy (Robert Foster) syndrome consists of optic atrophy as the result of compression of a tumor combined with papilledema on the opposite side and anosmia. It occurs rarely with frontal lobe tumors but occurs commonly in tumors of the olfactory groove. It has been described in association with sphenoidal ridge meningiomas, intracranial aneurysms, and inflammations.

Temporal lobe tumors.—Lesions of the temporal lobe induce vertigo, confusion, loss of memory, and often trance-like states. Lesions of the dominant lobe impair motor and sensory functions concerned with speech. Lesions in the area between the frontal, parietal, and temporal lobes (Broca) cause inability to express appropriate words (motor aphasia); posterior lesions cause inability to understand the spoken word. Irritative lesions cause unpleasant odors and taste (uncinate fits). Visual field defects are usually incongruous and begin in the superior quadrants of the visual field on the side opposite the lesion. Temporal lobe tumors often cause oculomotor nerve palsy.

Parietal lobe tumors.—Lesions of the parietal lobe cause astereognosia (faulty recognition of shape and form of objects placed in the hand) and loss of position sense and two-point discrimination on the side of the body opposite the lesion. Lesions in the angular gyrus on the dominant side cause loss of visual recognition of words (alexia) and inability to write (agraphia). Visual field defects are homonymous and the same in extent and intensity (congruous) in each eye. Field defects begin in the inferior quadrants of the visual field on the side opposite the lesion.

In parietal lesions, the opticokinetic nystagmus to moving objects is abolished with movements toward the side of the defective field of vision. In movements away from the side of the defective visual field, the opticokinetic nystagmus is normal. In forcible closure of the eyes, patients with parietal lobe lesions may show a deviation of the eyes to the side opposite the lesion.

Lesions of the nondominant parietotemporal lobes cause topographic agnosia in which patients lose the ability to recognize that which was familiar, such as landmarks in their community or the location of buttons on their clothes. There is impairment of ability to construct a diagram, such as the face of a clock (constructional apraxia). There is difficulty in dressing and sometimes failure to recognize faces (prosopagnosia). There may be neglect of the nondominant side, so that a right-handed individual leaves the left side of drawings unfinished or neglects food on the left side of the plate.

Occipital lobe tumors.—Lesions of the occipital lobe induce a congruous homonymous hemianopsia. If the posterior tip of the occipital lobe is involved, the point of fixation is affected. Visual hallucinations with the flashing of many lights may occur. Bilateral lesions of the occipital lobe cause blindness that may be accompanied by denial of blindness (Anton syndrome). Impairment of the association area may cause inability to recognize people and objects (visual agnosia) or to recognize the relationship of objects in space (topographic agnosia).

Infratentorial tumors.—Structures derived from the hindbrain include the cerebellum, pons, and medulla oblongata. Ocular lesions, if present, involve motor nerves to the eye with supranuclear and infranuclear paralysis and various ocular oscillations.

Cerebellar tumors.—Cerebellar tumors cause ataxia, asynergy, dysmetria, and weakness. Ataxia and asynergy are demonstrated by the heel-to-knee test and in testing for diadochokinesis. Dysmetria is demonstrated in the finger-to-finger test. Weakness occurs on the same side. There is a distinct tendency to fall toward the side of the lesion. Acute cerebellar lesions disturb posture, and the patient may be unable to stand or sit up. There is a loss of skeletal muscle tone and coordination.

The earliest ocular sign is jerk nystagmus, which is usually horizontal and accentuated on lateral gaze. Lesions in the vermis cause vertical nystagmus that is accentuated on upward gaze. Papilledema occurs early and may be the initial sign of disease. Other ocular signs are secondary to increased intracranial pressure.

Cerebellopontine angle tumors.—Cerebellopontine angle tumors are mainly acoustic neuromas causing cerebellar signs, with lesions of the trigeminal (N V), abducent (N VI), facial (N VII), and auditory (N VIII) nerves. Impairment of hearing occurs initially, followed by cerebellar signs with nystagmus and then cranial nerve involvement. Facial nerve impairment causes a facial tic followed by blepharospasm. Corneal anesthesia indicates trigeminal nerve involvement. Increased intracranial pressure occurs late.

Tumors of the pons and medulla.—Tumors of the pons and the medulla are likely to cause disturbance of the abducent nucleus or disturbance of horizontal conjugate gaze. Horizontal jerk nystagmus occurs occasionally, combined with vertical nystagmus. It is usually absent when the eyes are in the primary position and becomes more marked as the eyes are turned toward the side of the lesion. Palsies of the oculomotor (N III) nerve are uncommon. Corneal anesthesia from trigeminal nerve involvement is common. Increased intracranial pressure does not occur.

Herniation of the hippocampus through the tentorium causes brain-stem compression. The most common signs are decreasing levels of consciousness, dysarthria, and respiratory distress. Mydriasis is the most important ocular sign and is usually (but not always) on the side of the lesion. Other ocular signs are oculomotor palsy, internuclear ophthalmoplegia, and nystagmus. Blindness occurs if the posterior cerebral arteries are compressed.

Lesions of the midbrain.—Depending upon their location, lesions in this area may cause predominantly supratentorial or infratentorial symptoms and signs. Compression of the aqueduct of Sylvius may occur initially and cause an internal hydrocephalus and papilledema. Impairment of the supranuclear center for gaze, as in Parinaud syndrome, causes paralysis of conjugate upward movement and mydriasis. Lateral extension to the lateral geniculate body causes an incongruous homonymous hemianopsia. The nuclei of the oculomotor, trochlear, and portions of the trigeminal nerve and medial longitudinal fasciculus are located deep in the midbrain.

CEREBROVASCULAR DISEASE

Sudden loss of intracranial neurons may result from ischemia or hemorrhage. Ischemia is caused by local or general abnormalities that decrease the supply of blood to the brain. Emboli originating from the heart valves are the major local causes. The major cause is athero-

TABLE 28-4.
Cerebrovascular Disease

- I. Occlusive vascular disorders
  - A. Thrombotic
    - 1. Intracranial
    - 2. Carotid (transient ischemic attacks)
- II. Cerebral aneurysms
  - A. Infraclinoid
    - 1. Carotid artery within cavernous sinus
      - a. Carotid-cavernous sinus fistula
  - B. Supraclinoid
    - 1. Carotid artery
    - 2. Middle cerebral artery
    - 3. Anterior cerebral artery
    - 4. Basilar artery
- III. Subarachnoid hemorrhage
  - A. Vascular hypertension
  - B. Ruptured supraclinoid aneurysm
  - C. Angiomas and arteriovenous malformations
- IV. Arteritis
  - A. Infectious disease (e.g., syphilis, tuberculosis)
  - B. Idiopathic
    - 1. Giant cell arteritis
    - 2. Wegener arteritis

matous occlusion of the internal carotid artery or its branches (Table 28-4). Intracranial hemorrhage, apoplexy, and stroke are caused by either hypertensive or cardiovascular disease or rupture of berry aneurysms, acquired fusiform aneurysms, or arteriovenous malformations. The hemorrhage may be limited to the cerebrospinal fluid-filled space between the arachnoid and pia membranes (subarachnoid hemorrhage) or may occur within the brain (intracerebral hemorrhage). Subarachnoid hemorrhage may extend into the substance of the brain, and intracerebral hemorrhage may extend into the subarachnoid space, or into the ventricles, or both. Only heart disease and cancer cause more deaths in the United States. Stroke is the most common disorder that affects the central nervous system.

The brain is supplied by two internal carotid arteries and two vertebral arteries (Fig 28-3). The internal carotid artery enters the skull through the foramen lacerum; passes through the cavernous sinus; sends branches to the ophthalmic, anterior choroidal, and posterior communicating arteries; and then bifurcates into the anterior and middle cerebral arteries.

The vertebral arteries enter the skull through the foramen magnum. Medial branches immediately join to form the anterior spinal artery; just distal to this, the posterior cerebellar artery branches off. The vertebral arteries supply the medulla oblongata and pons, and then unite to form the basilar artery.

Carotid artery.—The internal carotid arterial system or its branches supply the frontal and parietal lobes, part of the temporal lobe, the corpus striatum, and the internal capsule. Occlusive disease is associated with contralateral impairment of motor or sensory function of the hand, arm, leg, or lower portion of the face. Ischemia of structures nurtured by the left middle cerebral artery may cause aphasia in right-handed persons. Unconsciousness simulating syncope occurs when an anterior cerebral artery is compromised.

The effects of occlusion of the internal carotid artery proximal to the circle of Willis depend on the adequacy of the collateral circulation. In about 25% of cases of symptomatic stroke, intermittent transient diminution of vision occurs in one eye (amaurosis fugax) as a warning symptom. Amaurosis fugax, a type of transient ischemic attack, consists of sudden constriction of the visual field of one eye that varies from hemianopsia to loss of light perception. The retinal arteries are markedly attenuated during an attack. Vision gradually returns within a few minutes. Permanent visual loss does not occur. Amaurosis fugax may also occur in migraine, impending central artery closure, and giant cell arteritis.

Repeated attacks of amaurosis fugax may cause an ophthalmoscopic picture of cotton-wool patches in one eye, caused by small infarcts secondary to vascular insufficiency. In patients with vascular hypertension, an occluded carotid artery may protect the retinal vasculature from the signs of arteriolar sclerosis, hemorrhages, or papilledema.

Rarely a venous stasis retinopathy develops on the same side as carotid artery insufficiency. Ophthalmoscopically, there are attenuated arteries and veins or, alternatively, dilated and tortuous retinal veins. There may be microaneurysms and flame and blot hemorrhages. New blood vessels may develop on the surface of the optic disk. The intraocular pressure may be high. If the diseased eye is examined without reference to the nearly normal fellow eye, the abnormality might be mistaken for the retinopa-

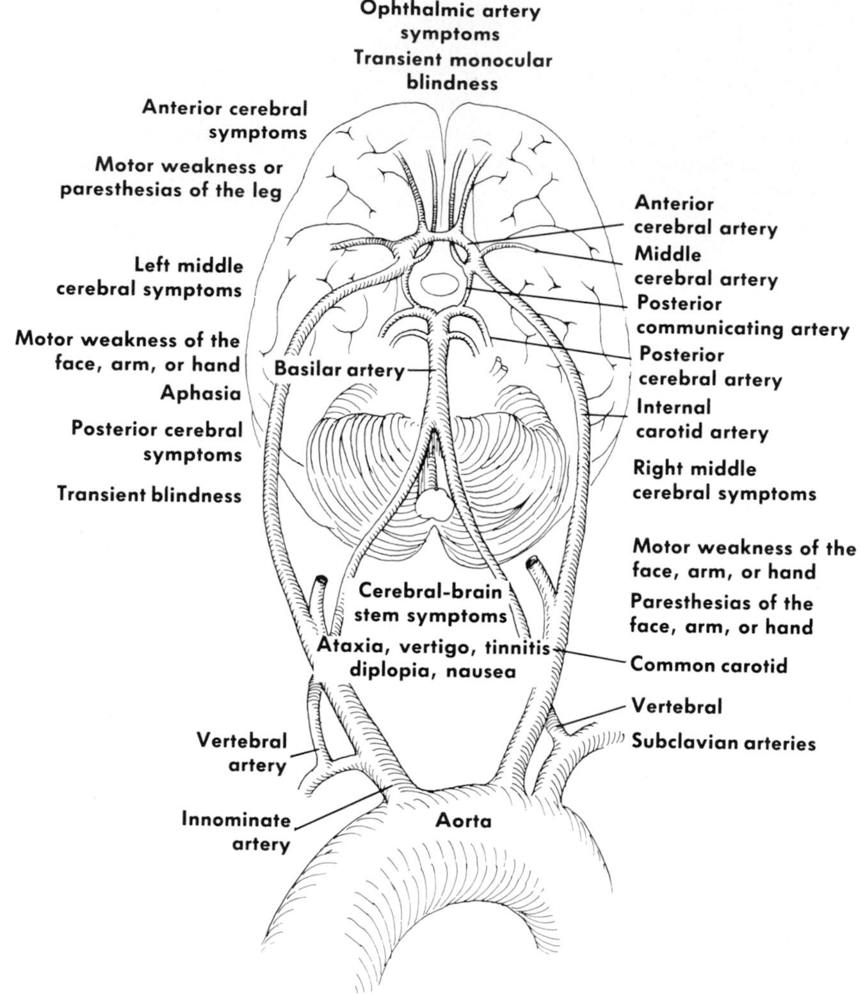

FIG 28-3.
The primary cerebral arteries and the symptoms of transient ischemic attacks in different regions of the brain. Probably less than 20% of individuals have the anatomic configuration illustrated, although it is the most common.

thy of diabetes, impending central vein occlusion, or pulseless disease.

In carotid artery system atherosclerosis, there may be retinal artery emboli that originate from an ulcerating atherosclerotic plaque. Cholesterol emboli appear as bright, yellow-orange plaques near the bifurcation of a retinal arteriole (Fig 28-4). With massage on the globe they tumble to the periphery and disappear. Platelet emboli appear as small white bodies. As they course through the arteries, they may cause the sensation of flashing or shimmering vision.

Pulsation in the affected internal carotid artery may be diminished or absent. Even with complete occlusion of the internal carotid artery, the common and the external carotid artery may be normal to palpation.

A thrill and murmur may occur over the bifurcation of the carotid artery in the neck. A murmur heard with the stethoscope over the fellow eye indicates augmented blood flow through the patent artery. The bruit of occlusive disease of the vertebral arteries is best heard over the supraclavicular area and is sometimes accentuated by turning the patient's head to the opposite side.

Measurement of the pressure in the ophthalmic arteries with the ophthalmodynamometer has its greatest application in carotid artery insufficiency. The measurement is made by

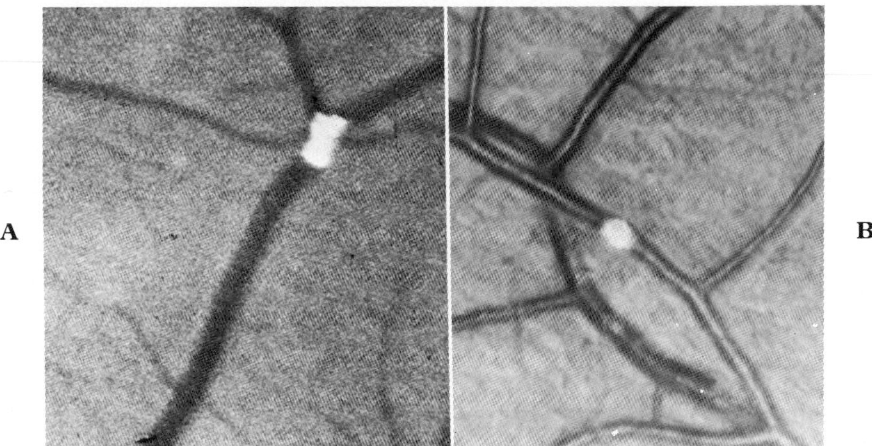

FIG 28-4.
A, Cholesterol embolus (Hollenhorst plaque) at bifurcation of a branch of a retinal artery in a 57-year-old woman with an atheroma of the common carotid artery. **B,** Fibrin embolus in the inferior temporal artery of the left eye of a 23-year-old man with mitral regurgitation after rheumatic heart disease. Four months later, the embolus was no longer present. There were no symptoms.

increasing the intraocular pressure until the central retinal artery is seen to pulsate on the optic disk. Most patients with carotid artery occlusive disease, which reduces the lumen 90% or more, have a 15% to 25% reduction in the systolic pressure of the ophthalmic artery on the side of the occlusive disease. In about one fourth of the patients with proven disease, the pressure is the same or higher on the affected side.

Several noninvasive tests are useful: (1) ultrasound scanning of the carotid arteries using B-mode ultrasound imaging, combined with pulse Doppler analysis of blood flow at each part in the image; and (2) oculoplethysmography to estimate more accurately the pressure within the internal carotid artery than is possible with ophthalmodynamometry.

Compression of the carotid artery may produce syncope suggestive of an insufficiency of the vascular supply of the contralateral anterior cerebral artery. Compression is not recommended and can produce permanent, complete occlusion. In vertebral-basilar artery insufficiency, there may be syncope or convulsive movements.

Cerebral angiography shows the site and extent of the occlusion but carries the risk of permanent complications. It is reserved preferably for distinguishing between carotid occlusive disease, cerebral infarction, and tumor in patients who have symptoms of recent onset and do not have brain infarcts. These patients are good candidates for surgery if necessary.

Vertebral-basilar system.—The vertebral-basilar arterial system supplies the brain stem, cerebellum, occipital lobe, and a portion of the temporal lobe. The vertebral system originates from the two vertebral arteries, which are the first branches of the subclavian arteries. The vertebral arteries traverse the neck in the vertebral canals of the cervical vertebrae and unite within the cranium to form the basilar artery. The basilar artery supplies branches to the brain stem and the cerebellum, and the posterior cerebral artery supplies branches to the occipital lobe. The posterior communicating arteries connect the vertebral-basilar system with the carotid circulation.

Involvement of the cochlear-vestibular system causes vertigo, nausea, and a staggering gait. Auditory system symptoms include partial deafness and unilateral tinnitus. There may be paresthesia, hemiplegia, or hemiparesis. Headache, dysarthria, dysphagia, and hiccupping occur.

Many patients note ocular symptoms for many months before complete occlusion. There may be blurred vision, diplopia, transient homonymous hemianopsia, and scintillating scotomas. Visual blurring is usually bilateral, and occasionally, the individual is momentarily completely blind.

Complete thrombosis causes a congruous homonymous hemianopsia and motor involvement of the eyes. There may be paresis of conjugate gaze, with a conjugate deviation to the opposite side. Intranuclear ophthalmoplegia may be identical with that seen in multiple sclerosis. Horizontal or rotatory nystagmus is frequent. Horner syndrome is sometimes present.

Recognition of the transient symptoms of cerebral ischemia, a transient ischemic attack, is important in preventing the development of a cerebrovascular accident. Differential diagnosis includes migraine, epilepsy, carotid sinus syncope, and Ménière syndrome. Diagnostic steps should include auscultation of the neck for bruit, ophthalmoscopy for emboli, comparison of the radial pulses and brachial blood pressure in the two arms, magnetic resonance imaging, and other noninvasive tests.

Possible causes, such as giant cell arteritis, vascular hypertension, neurosyphilis, systemic lupus erythematosus, polyarteritis nodosa, pulseless disease, and thrombocytopenia from leukemia, must be excluded. A sudden decrease in blood pressure or alteration in the heart rhythm or rate may be the cause.

Surgery to correct ischemic attacks is limited to the extracranial portion of the carotid artery system. It may be indicated for patients who have symptoms of recent onset but who do not have brain infarction or widespread atherosclerotic disease. In other patients, anticoagulation may be used. Aspirin, which decreases platelet adhesiveness, is currently popular. Control of vascular hypertension and investigation of its cause are desirable.

Aortic arch syndrome.—The aortic arch syndrome is a chronic disorder resulting from obstruction of the subclavian and the carotid arteries. It includes pulseless disease, reversed coarctation of the aorta, and the subclavian steal syndrome. Symptoms are caused by insufficiency of the cerebral blood supply and are similar to those described in carotid and vertebral-basilar insufficiency.

Pulseless disease is a giant cell arteritis of the aorta of unknown origin that occurs mainly in young Japanese women. It causes retinal neovascularization, venous engorgement, microaneurysms, and arterial and venous occlusions. The radial pulse is absent. There may be widespread ischemia of the head and the upper extremities.

Reversed coarctation of the aorta occurs in aortic arch occlusion and is a disorder of collateral circulation in which blood reaches the head, neck, and upper extremities through the intercostal, scapular, axillary, posterior and inferior thyroid, inferior epigastric, and internal mammary arteries.

The subclavian steal syndrome results from stenosis or occlusion of the first portion of the subclavian artery. Blood flows up the contralateral vertebral artery and down the opposite vertebral artery to supply the subclavian artery distal to the occlusion. Cerebral ischemia in the area of distribution of the vertebral-basilar system causes symptoms. A bruit in the subclavicular area and reduction of pulse and blood pressure in the ipsilateral arm suggest the diagnosis.

Brachial-basilar insufficiency occurs in patients with occlusive disease of the proximal segment of the subclavian artery who develop transient ischemic vertebral-basilar symptoms when the arm is exercised. The symptoms result, as in the subclavian steal syndrome, from retrograde blood flow through the ipsilateral vertebral artery.

Arterial aneurysms.—Berry aneurysms form most commonly at the anterior portion of the circle of Willis because of a congenital weakness in the wall of the artery. Although the weakness is congenital, the aneurysms do not occur until arterial hypertension aggravates the defect. They are most common at the junction of the internal carotid artery with the posterior communicating artery or middle cerebral artery or with the anterior communicating artery or anterior cerebral artery.

Fusiform aneurysms are caused by atherosclerosis that weakens and results in dilation of the basilar artery or the internal carotid artery in the cavernous sinus (infraclinoid). Symptoms occur suddenly, with severe unilateral headache and pain about the face and eye. Pain in the medial canthal region is common. The pain is caused by meningeal irritation and not by direct involvement of the trigeminal nerve as occurs in infraclinoid aneurysms. Simultaneously with the headache, or within 72 hours, an oculomotor paralysis develops, with blepharoptosis, exotropia, pupillary dilation, and failure of accommodation.

The prognosis for life is poorer with supraclinoid aneurysms than with infraclinoid aneurysms. Death occurs from subarachnoid hemorrhage or from bleeding into the brain. Untreated patients may experience no further episodes, presumably because of intravascular clotting, or they may have recurrent attacks. Recovery with regeneration of the oculomotor nerve is seldom complete. Retraction of the upper eyelid with attempts to look down (pseudo-von Graefe phenomenon) is often present. The pupil may be widely dilated with no constriction to stimulation with light.

Aneurysms of the middle and anterior cerebral arteries.—Aneurysms of the middle and anterior cerebral arteries are particularly likely to cause defects in the visual fields of both eyes and optic atrophy. An anterior cerebral artery aneurysm may cause a bitemporal hemianopsia that begins in the inferior temporal quadrant rather than in the superior temporal quadrant, as in early pituitary gland adenoma. With aneurysm of the middle cerebral artery, there may be loss of vision in one eye and a hemianopsia in the fellow eye. Subarachnoid hemorrhage is common.

Basilar artery aneurysms.—Congenital berry aneurysms may rarely occur at the anterior end of the basilar artery where it divides into the posterior cerebral arteries or at the posterior end where the vertebral arteries join to form the basilar arteries. The basilar artery is also the most common artery in the body to be affected with atherosclerosis.

The symptoms of basilar-vertebral aneurysms are variable and not characteristic. Dizziness, diplopia, and blurring of vision are the most common symptoms. There may be involvement of motor nerves on the brain stem, occipital headache, deafness, memory impairment, and coma. Diagnosis is often not made until autopsy.

Infraclinoid aneurysms.—Dilation of the internal carotid artery within the cavernous sinus occurs most commonly in women during or after the fifth decade of life. The artery gives off no major branches in this location, and atheromatous plaque formation is common. The cavernous sinus contains the motor nerves to the eye and the ophthalmic and maxillary divisions of the trigeminal nerve. An expanding aneurysm thus causes an ophthalmoplegia of all motor nerves and pain and paresthesia in the face. In infraclinoid aneurysms, unlike supraclinoid aneurysms, corneal and facial sensitivity is reduced.

The most conspicuous sign is an insidious, slowly progressive ophthalmoplegia that involves all muscles of one eye. The pupil does not constrict to light but may not be dilated because of interruption of sympathetic nerve fibers on the surface of the artery. Pain is a relatively minor symptom. There is pain or paresthesia of the face, of the side of the head, about the eye, or along the nose on the same side. Corneal anesthesia usually occurs and is usually associated with anesthesia of the face.

The gradual onset is suggestive of tumor, and arteriography is often necessary for exact diagnosis. Large infraclinoid aneurysms are probably reinforced by the walls of the cavernous sinus and do not rupture. Although it is likely that most spontaneous arteriovenous fistulas represent rupture of an aneurysm, usually they are so small before rupture that they do not cause signs of an aneurysm.

If untreated, infraclinoid aneurysms follow one of two patterns. Complete thrombosis of the aneurysm may occur, with resultant spontaneous improvement, but a residual loss of ocular motility. The artery may expand anteriorly within the cavernous sinus, causing erosion of the optic foramen and the superior orbital fissure, with compression and atrophy of the optic nerve and a proptosis. The development of proptosis is frequently concealed by blepharoptosis. Venous drainage of the orbit is not involved, and there is no chemosis or congestion of bulbar vessels. Posterior expansion may involve the petrous portion of the temporal bone and the acoustic nerve, causing ipsilateral deafness.

The treatment of choice is gradual occlusion of the internal carotid artery, provided arteriography indicates adequate filling of the middle and anterior cerebral arteries on the side of the aneurysm from the contralateral carotid artery and provided there is no untoward effect from digital compression of the common carotid artery for 15 minutes. Patients should be less than

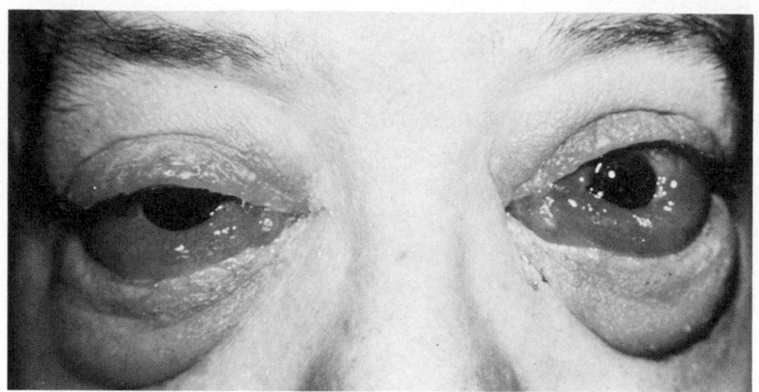

FIG 28-5.
Severe orbital congestion and bilateral proptosis in a spontaneous carotid artery–cavernous sinus fistula in a 57-year-old woman.

60 years of age, and the operative procedure should be done to relieve severe pain, failing vision, or exophthalmos.

Carotid artery–cavernous sinus fistula.—The rupture of an infraclinoid aneurysm shunts blood from the carotid artery into the cavernous sinus, creating an arteriovenous fistula. The arterial blood passes into channels connecting with the cavernous sinus, and congestion of the superior ophthalmic vein draining the orbit causes visual loss, diplopia, headache, and pain.

Carotid-cavernous fistulas are traumatic (75%) or spontaneous. The traumatic fistula follows skull fracture, particularly basilotemporal fracture. A latent period may occur before the onset of symptoms. Spontaneous fistulas occur most commonly in middle-aged women, presumably because of rupture of fusiform aneurysms so small that they did not cause symptoms before rupture. Some follow small fistulas of branches of the internal carotid artery within the cavernous sinus. Symptoms are less severe than those that occur with fistulas of the internal carotid artery, and spontaneous occlusion of the fistula may occur.

The outstanding sign is unilateral or bilateral proptosis (Fig 28-5), which may pulsate. A bruit synchronous with the pulse is heard by the patient as a rushing, roaring sound. The increased venous pressure with stasis causes chemosis (Fig 28-6), eyelid swelling, congested conjunctival and retinal veins, and hemorrhages. The abducent nerve may be involved or, less commonly, the third, fourth, or seventh cranial nerves. Visual failure is common from impairment of arterial and venous retinal circulations. Secondary open-angle glaucoma, although not obvious, may cause visual loss.

Subarachnoid hemorrhage.—The chief causes of spontaneous bleeding into the space between the arachnoid and the pia mater are (1) vascular hypertension, (2) ruptured supraclinoid aneurysms, and (3) angiomas or arteriovenous malformations. Less common causes include blood dyscrasias and necrosis of metastatic or primary brain tumors.

Subarachnoid hemorrhage is characterized by a sudden, violent head pain of shocking severity followed by photophobia and stiffness of the legs. Unconsciousness persisting for a few hours to days may follow. Later there may be rigidity of the neck and spine. Lumbar puncture, in which only a few drops of fluid should be removed, indicates fresh blood.

The ocular signs are mainly those described for unruptured supraclinoid aneurysms. In addition, there may be sudden loss of vision, papilledema, and exophthalmos. An uncommon but pathognomonic ocular sign is bilateral hemorrhage on the surface of the retina (subhyaloid), at the posterior pole adjacent to the optic disk.

Treatment must be individualized, but modern microsurgical techniques have decreased mortality, although the morbidity is still high. Surgical treatment should be carried out immediately in patients who are conscious or semiconscious, provided the collateral circulation is adequate. Gradual occlusion of the common carotid artery in the neck is moderately effective in subarachnoid hemorrhage caused by ruptured aneurysms of the internal carotid or pos-

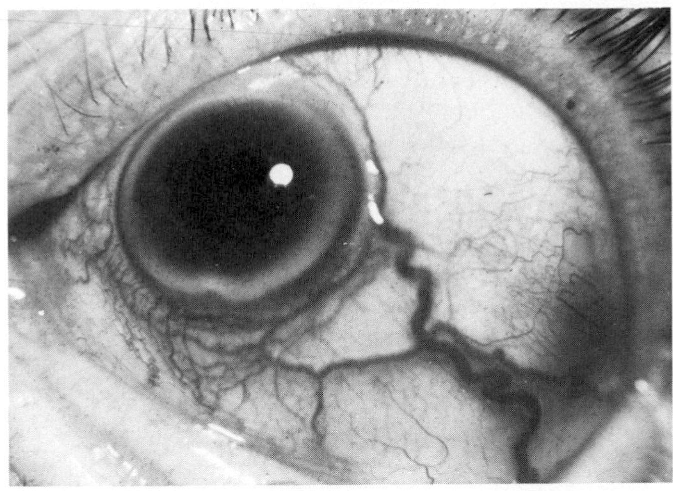

FIG 28-6.
Congested conjunctival vessels in a long-standing carotid artery–cavernous sinus fistula. The dilated blood vessels that surround the corneoscleral limbus are sometimes called "caput medusa."

terior communicating artery. The treatment of choice is exposing the aneurysm and either clipping it, coating it with plastic, or inducing intravascular thrombosis with an electric current, animal hair, or wire in the arterial wall.

Sudden severe headache with confusion followed by deep coma with bloody spinal fluid suggests cerebral hemorrhage. Sudden suboccipital headache, stiff neck, nausea, and vomiting are usually caused by subarachnoid hemorrhage from a ruptured saccular aneurysm. Five or more spontaneous subarachnoid hemorrhages suggest a hemangioma rather than a saccular aneurysm. Increasing headache, drowsiness, confusion, and hemiparesis over a period of a few weeks suggest a chronic subdural hematoma. Progressive symptoms over a long period suggest tumor. Hypertensive encephalopathy, tumors, trauma, and syphilis may cause seizures and stupor.

DIABETES MELLITUS NEUROPATHY

Diabetes mellitus (see Chapter 27) may be complicated by neuropathy involving the cranial motor nerves. There is a severe unilateral headache usually followed by lateral rectus muscle weakness. More rarely there is weakness of muscles innervated by the oculomotor nerve. The pupil is not impaired in 75% of the instances. Diabetes mellitus neuropathy is usually distinguished from supraclinoid aneurysms by isolated paralysis of the lateral rectus muscle, which rarely is solely affected with an aneurysm. The sparing of the sphincter pupillae muscle suggests the likelihood (75%) that a medical condition rather than a neoplasm or aneurysm is the cause.

NYSTAGMUS AND OCULAR OSCILLATION

Oscillation of the eyes may be divided into nystagmus, a biphasic involuntary ocular oscillation that always involves slow eye movements, and nonnystagmus oscillations that are always saccadic or saccadically initiated (fast eye movements: ocular dysmetria, flutter, opsoclonus, myoclonus, and bobbing).

Saccadic eye movements.—These fast eye movements involve the interaction of three groups of neurons within the brain stem: burst cells, tonic cells, and pause cells. Burst neurons located within the pontine and mesencephalic-reticular formation initiate a velocity command (saccadic pulse) that generates tonic neurons that move the eyes from one position to another (saccadic step). Pause cells within the pons then inhibit the burst neurons so that the eyes stop in the new position.

Abnormalities of ocular movement may involve the burst cells, tonic cells, or pause cells. During head rotation, the vestibulocerebellar complex stabilizes the retinal image so that there is no perception of movement. In ocular dysmetria, the saccade either overshoots or undershoots the target so that a corrective movement is required to bring the eyes on target. The mismatch is caused by an imbalance in the burst cell velocity command innervation and pause cells that inhibit burst cells. It is seen in abnormalities of the vestibulocerebellum, such as the Arnold-Chiari deformity with malformed posterior fossa structures, the result of caudad traction and displacement of the rhombencephalon because of tethering of the spinal cord.

Ocular flutter consists of spontaneous, conjugate, to-and-fro saccades that interrupt fixation. Patients often demonstrate flutter when recovering from opsoclonus. Opsoclonus (dancing eyes or lightning eye movements) consists of rapid, involuntary, chaotic, repetitive, unpredictable, conjugate eye movements in all directions. The movements prevent fixation and continue during sleep and in darkness. Opsoclonus occurs with cerebellar and brain-stem disorders. There is an unexplained association between opsoclonus and occult neoplasms, particularly neuroblastoma. Opsoclonus and ocular flutter are attributed to pause cell dysfunction so that burst neurons are not inhibited after a saccade.

Ocular myoclonus consists of rapid bursts of conjugate saccades often associated with myoclonic jerks of other parts of the body. Myoclonus of the eyes and palate occurs in pseudohypertrophy of the inferior olivary nucleus in the medulla.

Superior oblique muscle myokymia causes a monocular, rapid, fine ocular tremor that may be vertical, torsional, or oblique. There may be an associated monocular oscillopsia. The attacks are recurrent, often precipitated by rotating the eyes into the reading position. The condition may be spontaneous or follow trochlear nerve disorders. Therapy with carbamazepine, a membrane-stabilizing drug, may be helpful.

Nystagmus.—This is an involuntary, rhythmic, bilateral oscillation of the eyes. It is usually detected by simple observation of the eyes, but when minimal, it may be observed during ophthalmoscopy, the magnification of the fundus emphasizing the movement. In testing for nystagmus, the ocular movement should be observed in eyes front, right and left, and up and down.

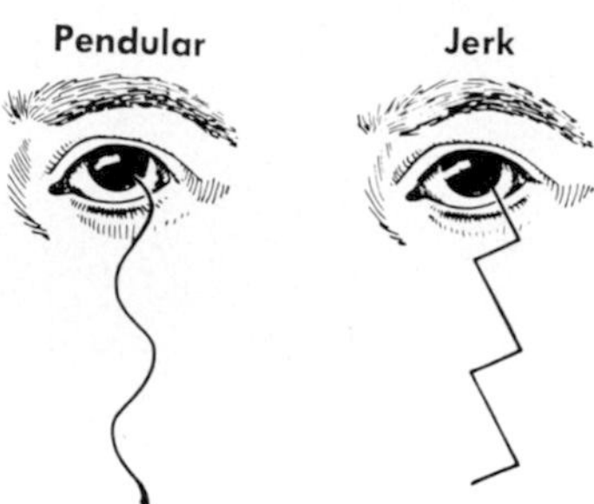

FIG 28-7.
The two general types of nystagmus. The pendular nystagmus has undulating movements of the eyes. The jerk nystagmus shown has a quick phase nasalward and a slow phase templeward. (*From Huber A:* Eye signs and symptoms in brain tumors, *ed 3, St Louis, 1976, Mosby–Year Book. Used by permission.*)

Nystagmus is divided on the basis of its rhythm into pendular and jerk types (Fig 28-7). The rhythm of pendular nystagmus is regular. In jerk nystagmus, there is a slow movement in one direction, followed by a quick recovery movement in the opposite direction.

***Pendular nystagmus.*—**Pendular nystagmus is a to-and-fro oscillation of both eyes that is equal in amplitude and velocity in each direction. Acquired pendular nystagmus in adults reflects vascular or demyelinating disease affecting the brain stem or cerebellum. A head tremor is usual, and there may be a complaint of objects moving (oscillopsia).

Congenital nystagmus is a pendular nystagmus evident at birth or shortly thereafter and is often associated with poor vision. Congenital nystagmus decreases with convergence, and in many cases a direction of gaze angle can be found where nystagmus is minimal (null angle). Patients often turn or tilt the head to place the eyes in the null position. Treatment with prisms or ocular muscle surgery to place the eyes so that they are in the null position may improve vision. Congenital nystagmus may occur without other ocular defects, but often there are gross opacities of the media, or retinal or optic nerve abnormalities. Albinism (see Chapter 26) is often associated with nystagmus. Nystagmus does not occur in eyes in which the congenital defects cause complete absence of light perception.

Physiologic nystagmus is a high-frequency (50 to 100 kHz), low-amplitude (5 to 30 sec/arc), pendular oscillation that occurs during fixation so that different regions of the macula will be stimulated.

Seesaw nystagmus is a conjugate pendular oscillation in which one eye rises and intorts while the fellow eye falls and extorts. It reflects diencephalic dysfunction and occurs in bitemporal hemianopsia from parasellar lesions, brain-stem lesions, and after trauma.

Ocular bobbing is generated by fast downward jerks of each eye (sometimes nonconjugate) followed by a slow drift to midposition. It occurs in comatose patients who have extensive pontine destruction, obstructive hydrocephalus, or metabolic encephalopathy.

Spasmus nutans is a rapid nystagmus of small amplitude that occurs in children between 4 months and 2 years of age. There is an associated head nodding and sometimes abnormal head position. It may be bilateral or unilateral and is the most common cause of unilateral nystagmus in children. It has been attributed to poor illumination, but the cause is unknown. It invariably disappears.

Voluntary nystagmus is a pendular nystagmus in individuals who induce rapid ocular oscillations by extreme convergence. It is of no clinical significance.

Jerk nystagmus.—Jerk nystagmus is a horizontal oscillation that has a slow component in one direction and a rapid corrective movement (saccadic) in the opposite direction. Reference is made to the direction of the rapid component, although the slow movement reflects the basic disability. Jerk nystagmus in the primary position may indicate vestibular dysfunction, whereas that present in other directions of gaze suggests brain-stem or cerebellar disease or drug toxicity.

Opticokinetic nystagmus is a jerk nystagmus induced by a visual pattern, such as black and white stripes, which moves at a constant velocity. There is a slow eye movement in the direction of the moving pattern followed by a fast phase in the opposite direction. Since the subject cannot voluntarily inhibit the eye movements, induction of opticokinetic nystagmus is used to measure vision in infants and children. In homonymous hemianopsia caused by parietal lobe lesions, moving the targets from the seeing side to the blind side does not induce an opticokinetic nystagmus.

Clinically, opticokinetic nystagmus is studied by having the subject look at a rotating drum or television screen in which there are moving figures or alternate white and black lines. More simply, a 20-inch strip of alternate 2-inch red and white squares may be used.

Latent nystagmus is a bilateral horizontal jerk nystagmus elicited by covering one eye or making the brightness or clarity of retinal images unequal in the two eyes. The slow component is in the direction of the covered eye, and the rapid component is in the direction of the open eye. With both eyes open, such patients may have normal vision, but when either eye is covered, visual acuity in the open eye is 20/200 or less. There is no treatment. Strabismus is common in this disorder.

Gaze-evoked nystagmus (end-position nystagmus) is seen when the eyes are turned into an extreme position of gaze. It is horizontal or vertical. The slow component is toward the central primary position, and the fast component is toward the extreme position of gaze. It may occur in normal persons who are debilitated or fatigued. It is common after administration of barbiturates or other tranquilizers and may follow use of phenothiazine and anticoagulant drugs. Multiple sclerosis may cause nystagmus in extreme lateral gaze, and nystagmus may be present in brain-stem cerebellar dysfunction.

Vestibular nystagmus.—This is a jerk nystagmus that follows asymmetric stimulation of the semicircular canals or their central pathways. There are three semicircular canals in each labyrinth: horizontal, superior, and vertical. The innervation of the inner ear controls body musculature and maintains a conjugate deviation of the eyes with changes in position of the head, so that the eyes tend to maintain a primary position in reference to the environment. The major action of the semicircular canals is evident in torsion of the eyes. The semicircular canals function in acceleration or deceleration of the body, in which the eyes tend to oppose a change of position when the body rotates.

Vestibular nystagmus can be conveniently studied by rotation of the body or by caloric irrigation of the external auditory canal, which sets up convection currents in the semicircular canals. Cold water applied to the tympanic membrane induces a jerk nystagmus in which the fast-phase is to the side opposite the ear to which the cold water was applied.

Nystagmus occurs in diseases of the vestibular apparatus, its nuclei, or its central nervous system connections. Peripheral disease may be associated with vertigo, tinnitus, and deafness. The onset is abrupt. The nystagmus is horizontal and tends to decrease in the course of the disease. The common diseases causing peripheral involvement are labyrinthitis and Ménière disease.

Spontaneous vertical nystagmus is virtually always of central origin; spontaneous rotatory nystagmus suggests involvement of vestibular nuclei. Nystagmus may occur in multiple sclerosis, encephalitis, vascular disease (particularly occlusion of the posteroinferior cerebellar artery), and cerebellar and cerebellopontine lesions, which are likely to produce nystagmus that varies with the position of the head. The fast component is toward the side of the lesion.

MULTIPLE SCLEROSIS

Multiple sclerosis is a chronic, inflammatory, neurologic disease characterized by destruction of the myelin of the central nervous system. In most patients acute episodes are followed by remissions with recurrences occurring over many years. Rarely the disease is slowly progressive without remissions from the beginning. In a small number of patients the disease rapidly progresses to death within a year.

The onset occurs mainly between the ages of 15 and 50 years (average, 33 years), but there are extremes in childhood and old age. Typically an attack worsens for 3 to 21 days and then remits over a period of weeks. Recovery in early attacks is usually complete, but subsequently there are residual neurologic defects with progressive deterioration. The prevalence and death rate are relatively high in the northern regions of the United States and Europe. The prevalence is relatively low in the southern United States and Europe, and also in Africa and Asia.

Experimental autoimmune encephalomyelitis is a T lymphocyte autoimmune disease of the central nervous system induced by immunization of experimental animals with myelin basic protein or proteolipid. Some believe it to be a model of multiple sclerosis in humans and some patients have T lymphocytes that react with myelin basic protein. Such lymphocytes, however, occur in healthy individuals. Environmental data suggest the possibility of a viral cause, and such an infection may be combined with an immunologic reaction.

The sites of the foci of demyelination govern the clinical involvement. Classically there is poor vision, with optic neuritis, nystagmus, dysarthria, decreased vibration and position sense, ataxia, weakness or paralysis of one or more extremities, spasticity, and sphincter impairment. Six criteria are generally accepted for diagnosis: (1) the results of neurologic examination are abnormal; (2) at least two separate parts of the nervous system are involved; (3) fiber tract damage (white matter) predominates; (4) there are at least two separate episodes of worsening, separated by at least 1 month, or alternatively slow stepwise progression over at least 6 months; (5) age at onset is between 15 and 50 years; and (6) no other condition can explain the disease process.

Magnetic resonance imaging may supplement clinical criteria. Plaques in the white matter of the brain are easily detected on T_2-weighted sequences. Early in the disease there is a breakdown of the blood-brain barrier, which may be demonstrated by T_1-weighted sequences after the intravenous administration of gadolinium.

Optic neuritis is the initial episode of the disease in 15% of the patients. Of patients hospitalized because of multiple sclerosis, 70% have or have had optic neuritis. Displopia secondary to damage to the third, fourth, or sixth cranial nerve or to internuclear ophthalmoplegia is the initial symptom in another 25% of the patients. Facial hypesthesia, tic douloureux, Bell's palsy, vertigo, and nystagmus may also occur. Sheathing of peripheral retinal veins occurs in about 5% of the patients.

Currently, the National Institutes of Health is sponsoring a number of controlled, double-masked, clinical trials to evaluate the outcome of therapy on slowing the progression, enhancing the recovery, or controlling the symptoms of multiple sclerosis. Current studies include effects of plasma exchange, the administration of pooled immunoglobulins, interferon beta-1b, potassium channel blockers, or sulfasalazine. The results are based on measurement of clinical disability, control of symptoms, and the signal abnormalities on magnetic resonance imaging. Intravenous methyl prednisolone therapy of optic neuritis is followed by a remission of the neuritis and other signs of multiple sclerosis for at least 2 years.

Neuromyelitis optica (Devic).—This is a bilateral, acute optic neuritis and a transverse spinal cord myelitis. The disease may occur at any age. There are prodromal signs of headache, sore throat, fever, and malaise. The visual loss occurs rapidly, and blindness or near-blindness develops within a few days. Paralysis and sensory disturbances caudal to the transverse myelitis occur within a few weeks before or after blindness. Patients may die within a month, or there may be complete remission with recurrences. Most patients develop chronic, relapsing multiple sclerosis, but other types of demyelinative disease may mimic the clinical syndrome.

Subcortical encephalopathy.—Subcortical encephalopathy (Schilder disease) affects children and adolescents and is characterized by progressive involvement of the brain with loss of vision, spastic paralysis, deafness, mental deterioration, and death in a few months to a year. Papilledema occurs in most of the patients.

Postinfectious encephalitis.—Encephalitis may develop after viral infections such as measles, rubella, chickenpox, and mumps. It most commonly follows measles, and the mortality of patients with measles encephalitis is 10%. There may be papilledema, papillitis, or retrobulbar neuritis. Recovery of vision is common.

BIBLIOGRAPHY

Books

Glaser JS, editors: *Neuro-ophthalmology,* ed 2, Philadelphia, 1990, JB Lippincott.

Kupersmith MJ, Berenstein A: *Neurovascular neuro-ophthalmology,* New York, 1993, Springer-Verlag.

Lisak RP, editor: *Handbook of myasthenia gravis and myasthenic syndromes,* New York, 1994, Marcel Dekker.

Meyer FB, editor: *Sundt's occlusive cerebrovascular disease,* ed 2, Philadelphia, 1994, WB Saunders.

Miller NR: *Walsh and Hoyt's clinical neuro-ophthalmology,* ed 4, vols 1-5, Baltimore, 1982-1995, Williams & Wilkins.

Robbins LD: *Management of headache and headache medications,* New York, 1994, Springer-Verlag.

Tomsak RL: *Pediatric neuro-ophthalmology,* Newton, Mass, 1995, Butterworth-Heinemann.

Articles

Kumar KL, Cooney TG: Headaches, *Med Clin North Am* 75:261-282, 1995.

Olesen J: Understanding the biologic basis of migraine, *N Engl J Med* 331:1713-1714, 1994.

Radhakrishnan K, Ahlskog JE, Garrity JA, Kurland LT: Idiopathic intracranial hypertension, *Mayo Clin Proc* 69:169-180, 1994.

Silberstein SD, Lipton RB: Overview of diagnosis and treatment of migraine, *Neurology* 44:S6-S16, 1994.

Wray SH: The management of acute visual failure, *J Neurol, Neurosurg, Psychiatry* 56:234-240, 1993.

Wyllie JP, Wright MJ, Burn J, Hunter S: Natural history of trisomy 13, *Arch Dis Child* 71:343-345, 1994.

APPENDIXES

A

GLOSSARY

aberration (optics) Failure of paraxial and peripheral light rays to focus at same point on axis of optical system because of difference in refraction of different wavelengths of white light (chromatic) or difference in refractive power of different portions of optical system (spherical).

ablepharia Absence of the eyelids.

accommodation Process by which the refractive power of the crystalline lens is increased through contraction of the ciliary muscle (N III), causing an increased thickness and curvature of the lens.

- **amplitude** The difference in diopters of refraction of the eye at rest and when fully accommodated.

accommodative esotropia Inward deviation of the eyes characteristically more marked for near than far and increased by ciliary muscle contraction in accommodation.

achromatopsia Color vision deficiency.

- **atypical** Incomplete achromatopsia with normal visual acuity and no nystagmus.
- **typical** Severe congenital deficiency in color vision with reduced vision and nystagmus.

acorea Absence of pupil.

adaptation Biochemical and neurologic retinal processes by which the eye becomes more sensitive to reduced illumination (dark adaptation or scotopic adaptation) or to increased illumination (light adaptation or photopic adaptation).

after-cataract Opacity of posterior capsule of the crystalline lens after extracapsular cataract extraction. Secondary cataract.

after-image Persistence of visual response after stimulus stops.

agnosia (visual) Inability to recognize objects by sight while retaining the ability to recognize by touch; a sign of lesions of the angular gyrus of the parieto-occipital fissure of the brain.

agraphia (optic) Loss of ability to write.

albinism Inherited deficiency or absence of melanin in skin and hair only (cutaneous); the eyes only (ocular); or the skin, hair, and eyes (universal) caused by an abnormality in tyrosinase required for melanin synthesis.

- **tyrosinase negative** Albinism with an absence of tyrosinase.
- **tyrosinase positive** Albinism with normal tyrosinase, which fails to enter pigment cells.

amaurosis Blindness.

- **fugax** Transient blindness, often monocular.
- **of Leber** Autosomal recessive rod-cone abiotrophy with severely reduced vision and nonrecordable electroretinogram.

amblyopia Decreased visual acuity without detectable organic disease of eye.

- **ex anopsia** Functional, refractive, sensory, or strabismic. Stimulus deprivation amblyopic now preferred.
- **functional** Cortical inhibition as in refractive or strabismic amblyopia.
- **refractive** Secondary to a refractive error, particularly a marked difference in refraction of the two eyes (anisometropia).
- **sensory** Caused by organic disease such as optic atrophy, central retinal degeneration, or cataract.
- **strabismic** Associated with deviation of the eyes that occurs before the establishment of normal visual acuity in each eye; there appears to be active inhibition of perception of the retinal image transmitted by deviating eye.

amblyoscope A reflecting stereoscope used to evaluate binocular vision.

ametropia Optical condition in which, with eyes at rest, the retina is not in conjugate focus with light rays from distant objects (see hyperopia, myopia, astigmatism, presbyopia).

angiography, ocular Photographic documentation of fluorescence of the passage of a dye through the intraocular blood vessels after intravenous injection. A solution of fluorescein is generally used. Indocyanine green absorbs light at 766 nm and fluoresces at 826 nm (near infrared range) and is useful in documenting choroidal vascular abnormalities.

angioid streaks Degeneration of the elastic layer of lamina basalis (Bruch membrane) causing pigmented striations of the ocular fundus; associated with a variety of systemic diseases such as pseudoxanthoma elasticum, sickle cell disease, and osteitis deformans (Paget disease) and several generalized diseases that affect the elastic lamina of blood vessels.

angioscopy Ophthalmoscopic visualization of passage of fluorescein through the intraocular vessels after intravenous injection.

angle Meeting point of two lines or planes or the space bounded by two converging lines or planes that meet.

- **abnormality** That angle between the directional values of the two retinas in space.
- **alpha** The angle between the visual line and the optical axis.
- **deviation** The angle of strabismus in degrees or prism diopters.
- **disparity** The angle between images on two retinas that permits fusion.
- **kappa** The angle between visual axis and center of pupil; it is positive when the pupillary center is nasal to the visual axis, and negative when the pupillary center is temporal to the visual axis.
- **meter** The unit of convergence; the amount of convergence required to view an object binocularly; an object of 50 cm requires 2 diopters of accommodation and 2 meter angles of convergence.
- **visual** The angle subtended by an object at point of observation.

angle-closure glaucoma Ocular abnormality in which the intraocular pressure increases because the aqueous humor is mechanically prevented from draining through the trabecular meshwork of the anterior chamber.

angstrom (Å) Unit of wavelength equal to 10^{-10} m (nanometer now preferred [10^{-9} m]).

aniridia Absence of iris.

aniseikonia Optical condition in which the retinal images in the two eyes are of different sizes.

anisocoria Condition in which the pupils of the two eyes are of unequal size.

anisometropia Condition in which the refractive errors in the two eyes are different.

ankyloblepharon Condition in which the margins of the eyelids are fused together.

anomaloscope Instrument used in refined evaluation of color perception in which one half of a field of color is matched by mixing two other colors.

anomalous retinal correspondence *See* angle.

anomalous trichromatism Defect of color vision in which there appears to be a deficiency of one of the cone pigments.

anophthalmia Absence of the eye.

anterior chamber The space between the peripheral cornea and iris through which the aqueous humor leaves the eye.

aphakia Absence of the crystalline lens of the eye.

aqueous flare Tyndall beam observed with a biomicroscope when excessive protein is present in the aqueous humor of the anterior chamber.

arcuate scotoma Area of blindness in the field of vision of characteristic arc shape; caused by interruption of a nerve fiber bundle in the retina; most often seen in glaucoma.

arcus cornealis Deposition of lipid in the peripheral cornea mainly in the aged (arcus senilis; gerontoxon) and rarely in youth (arcus juvenilis; embryotoxon).

area 17 The primary visual cortex.

area centralis The rod-free area of the retina that contains the fovea centralis.

argyria Discoloration of the skin or mucous membranes produced by prolonged administration of silver salts with deposition of metallic silver in tissue.

asteroid hyalosis Fixed opacities composed of a calcium lipid complex that occur in an otherwise normal vitreous humor; there are no symptoms.

asthenopia Ill-defined ocular discomfort attributed to use of the eyes.

astigmatism Optical condition in which the refractive power is not uniform in all meridians; when regular, there are two main meridians of refractive power; when irregular, there are a number of meridians of different power.

avulsion of caruncle Term usually applied to a laceration involving inner one sixth (lacrimal portion) of lower eyelid with rupture of the inferior canaliculus.

band keratopathy Deposition of calcium in the cornea most marked in the horizontal meridian; occurs in degenerating eyes, hypercalcemia, hypophosphatemia, and juvenile arthritis (of Still).

bedewing of cornea Subepithelial corneal edema, often associated with sudden prolonged increase in intraocular pressure or wearing of contact lenses for an excessively long period (Sattler veil).

Bell palsy Peripheral paralysis of the facial nerve (N VII).

Bell phenomenon Upward and outward rotation of the eyes that occurs in sleep or with forcible closure of the eyelids.

Bergmeister papilla Small mass of glial cells that surrounds the fetal hyaloid artery in the center of the optic disk; occasionally it persists and obliterates the physiologic cup of the optic disk.

biomicroscope Microscope for examining the eye; consists essentially of a dissecting microscope combined with a light source that projects a rectangular light beam that can be changed in size and focus (a slit lamp).

Bitot spot Highly refractile mass with silver-gray hue and foamy surface that appears on the bulbar conjunctiva in vitamin A deficiency.

blenorrhea Discharge from mucous surfaces.

adult Gonorrheal conjunctivitis.

inclusion Chlamydial conjunctivitis.

neonatorum Ophthalmia neonatorum.

blepharadenitis Inflammation of marginal glands of eyelid: meibomian, Moll, and Zeis.

blepharitis Inflammation of the margin of the eyelids; occurs in squamous (seborrheic) and ulcerative forms.

blepharochalasis Relaxation of the skin of the eyelid caused by atrophy of the elastic tissue; the upper eyelid is commonly involved, and a fold of tissue hangs over the eyelid margin.

blepharoclonus Exaggerated reflex blinking.

blepharophimosis Decreased size of the palpebral fissure, often associated with excessive distance between the inner canthi (telecanthus) and drooping of the upper eyelid (blepharoptosis).

blepharoptosis Drooping of the upper eyelid caused by paralysis of the oculomotor nerve (N III) or the sympathetic nerves or by excessive weight of the upper eyelids.

blepharospasm Tonic spasm of the orbicularis oculi muscle, which results in forcible closure of the eyelids.

blepharostat Instrument for holding eyelids apart in eye surgery.

blind spot (of Mariotte) The temporal area of blindness in the visual field marking the site of the optic disk in that portion of the eye in which there are no photoreceptors.

blindness Absence of sense of sight; defined by the United States Internal Revenue Service as reduction of best corrected visual acuity to 20/200 or less in better eye or restriction of the visual field to 20° or less; defined by Social Security Agency as reduction of visual acuity in best corrected eye to 5/200 or less; in industry, reduction of the best corrected visual acuity to less than 20/200.

color *See* achromatopsia, protanopia, tritanopia, deuteranomaly, protanomaly.

cortical Caused by a lesion in the cortex of the visual occipital lobe.

night Inadequate adaptation in reduced illumination so that vision is markedly decreased.

snow Inability to open the eyes to see; secondary to ultraviolet keratitis.

blood-aqueous and -retinal barrier Limitation of diffusion of lipid-insoluble substances by tight junctions of iris vasculature, pigment epithelium of ciliary body, retinal pigment epithelium, and retinal vasculature.

blowout fracture of orbit Fracture of the roof of the maxillary sinus with prolapse of the intraorbital contents into the antrum; there is enophthalmos, blepharoptosis, inability to turn the eye upward, and usually infraorbital anesthesia.

blue sclera Abnormality in which the sclera is thin and has a blue appearance caused by the underlying pigmented choroid.

bobbing Intermittent rapid downward rotation of eyes with slow return to primary position in persons with lower pontine lesions.

Bowman zone Anterior condensation of the corneal stroma.

break up time, tears Time in seconds for dry spot to form on corneal epithelium in absence of blinking.

Bruch membrane Tissue between the choriocapillaris and the retinal pigment epithelium.

Brushfield spots Transient whitish areas in the iris at birth that occur in Down syndrome and in many normal children.

buphthalmos Enlargement of the eye usually occurring as a result of congenital glaucoma.

Busacca floccule Accumulation of macrophages on surface of iris, lens, and anterior chamber angle in anterior uveitis.

campimeter Alternative term for perimeter.

canaliculitis Inflammation of a lacrimal canaliculus, often caused by fungal infection.

candela Unit of luminous intensity; one candela is defined as the luminous intensity of 1/60 of a square centimeter of projected area of a blackbody radiator operating at the temperature of solidification of platinum.

canthotomy Cantholysis, surgical division of the canthus.

capillary-free zone Region of foveola; area adjacent to retinal arterioles.

caput medusae Dilated ciliary blood vessels girdling the corneoscleral limbus in rubeosis iridis.

cardinal points Three pairs of points on axis of an optical system (principal, nodal, and focal) that determine its refractive characteristics.

cardinal positions of gaze Eyes right, eyes right and up, eyes right and down, eyes left, eyes left and up, eyes left and down.

crossed Double vision in which the image from the right eye is observed to the left of the image from the left eye; associated with conditions in which the eyes turn outward.

monocular Diplopia in one eye as a result of opacities in the visual axis.

uncrossed Condition in which the image of the right eye is to the right of the image from the left eye; observed in conditions in which the visual axes of the eye are directed toward each other, as in esotropia.

disciform keratitis Inflammation of corneal stroma, often a secondary stromal involvement in a herpes simplex keratitis.

disease A disorder of body function, systems, or organs composed of an identifiable group of signs and symptoms, a consistent causative etiologic agent, or a consistent anatomic alteration. *See also* syndrome.

Alport Autosomal dominant renal disease with cataract, maculopathy, and deafness.

Alzheimer Progressive atrophy of the cerebral cortex with distinctive histopathologic brain changes (senile plaques) affecting predominantly aging women.

Basedow Thyroid ophthalmopathy.

Behçet Recurrent aphthous ulcers (canker sores) of mouth and genitalia combined with uveitis, iritis, and hypopyon.

Berlin Perimacular retinal edema following trauma (commotio retinae).

Best Familial, congenital macular degeneration.

Bielschowsky-Lutz-Cogan Internuclear ophthalmoplegia with medial rectus muscle paralysis for versions, intact convergence, and nystagmus of abducted eye.

Bloch-Sulzberger Incontinentia pigmenti.

Boeck Sarcoidosis.

Bowen Intraepithelial epithelioma; when the eye is affected, it commonly involves the conjunctiva at the corneoscleral limbus in chronically inflamed eyes.

Bourneville Mental deficiency, tuberous sclerosis, and adenoma sebaceum; glaucoma and conjunctival and retinal tumors may occur.

cat-scratch Infectious lymphadenitis with a localized papule or pustule.

Chédiak-Higashi Recessive albinism with leukocytic inclusions.

Coats Chronic progressive retinal abnormality characterized by retinal deposits and malformation of retinal blood vessels.

Creutzfeldt-Jakob Infectious spongiform encephalopathy with progressive pyramidal and extrapyramidal degeneration and dementia. Can be transmitted by a transplanted cornea.

Crouzon Craniofacial dysostosis.

Devic Subacute encephalomyopathy with severe demyelination of optic nerves.

Eales Retinal phlebitis characterized by inflammation, occlusion, neovascularization, and recurrent retinal hemorrhages, occurring particularly in young men.

Fabry Diffuse angiokeratoma; X chromosome–linked lysosomal storage of sphingolipid.

Farber Galactosyl ceramide lipidosis; lysosomal storage of sphingolipid.

Gaucher Lysosomal storage disease with globusyl ceramide accumulation.

Graves Thyroid ophthalmopathy.

Hand-Schüller-Christian Insidious and progressive abnormality in children characterized by exophthalmos, diabetes insipidus, and softened areas in the bones, particularly in femurs and in bones of the skull, shoulder, and pelvic girdle.

Heerfordt Uveitis, fever, and parotid gland swelling; a manifestation of sarcoidosis.

Hermansky-Pudlak Partial oculocutaneous albinism with bleeding tendency.

Hunter Mucopolysaccharidosis.

Hurler Mucopolysaccharidosis.

inclusion cell Mucolipidosis II.

Jansky-Bielschowsky Late infantile neuronal ceroid lipofuscinosis.

Krabbe Galactosyl ceramide lipidosis; a lysosomal sphingolipidosis.

Kufs Adult neuronal ceroid lipofuscinosis; a lysosomal sphingolipidosis.

Leber Autosomal recessive congenital retinal degeneration.

Leber Mitochondrial mutation with optic neuropathy and optic atrophy occurring at about age 20 years.

Letterer-Siwe Nonfamilial reticuloendotheliosis of early childhood.

Lignac-Fanconi Cystinosis with renal rickets (Abderhalden-de Toni-Debré).

Lindau Angioma of the central nervous system, particularly in the cerebellum, and associated von Hippel-Lindau disease with angioma of the cerebellum, retina, pancreas, and kidney.

Louis-Bar Phacomatosis with ataxia and telangiectasis and widespread T lymphocyte abnormalities.

Maroteaux-Lamy Mucopolysaccharidosis.

Menkes steely hair Defective intestinal copper transport with cerebral degeneration, seizures, spasticity, hypothermia, and depigmented hair and skin.

metachromic leukodystrophy Sulfatide lipidosis and lysosomal storage of glycoprotein.

Möbius (1) Migraine headache with recurrent oculomotor paralysis (ophthalmoplegic migraine).

(2) Congenital facial diplegia with facial and abducent nerve paralysis.

Morquio Mucopolysaccharidosis.

Niemann-Pick Sphingomyelinase deficiency; a lysosomal storage disease with tissue accumulation of sphingomyelin and cholesterol with many phenotypes.

Norman Wood Congenital neuronal ceroid lipofuscinosis.

Oguchi Autosomal recessive night blindness found almost exclusively in Japanese.

Paget Bone thickening and thinning, sometimes with angioid streaks.

Pompe Glycogen storage disease, type II.

Purtscher Traumatic angiopathy of the retina.

Recklinghausen Autosomal dominant neurofibromatosis type I.

Refsum Phytanic acid storage disease.

Sandhoff Gangliosidosis, a lysosomal storage disease, a sphingolipidosis.

Sanfilippo Mucopolysaccharidosis.

Scheie Mucopolysaccharidosis.

sickle cell Abnormality resulting from an alteration in amino acid chains of hemoglobin.

Stargardt Fundus flavimaculatus with atrophic central retinal degeneration.

Sturge-Weber-Dimitri Phacomatosis with encephalotrigeminal angiomatosis.

Tangier Familial high-density lipoprotein deficiency.

Tay-Sachs Gangliosidosis, a lysosomal storage disease, a sphingolipidosis.

Vogt-Spielmeyer-Sjögren Juvenile ceroid lipofuscinosis.

Wilson Hepaticolenticular degeneration.

Wyburn-Mason Phacomatosis with encephalo-ocular arteriovenous shunts.

disparity, retinal The slight difference in retinal images that occurs because of the lateral separation of the two eyes that stimulates stereoscopic vision.

distichiasis Supernumerary row of eyelashes.

districhiasis Two hairs that share a single hair follicle.

divergence Outward rotation of the eyes.

drusen Local pockets of the cytoplasm of the retinal pigment epithelium, which may impinge on Bruch membrane and degenerate, or acellular laminated bodies of the optic nerve.

ductions Ocular rotations of one eye only.

dyscoria Abnormality in the shape of the pupil.

dyslexia Psychologic abnormality in which, despite adequate intelligence, motivation, and instruction, and in the absence of a physical handicap, emotional disturbance, or cultural deprivation, an individual fails to master printed and written language.

dysmetria Ocular overshoot or undershoot of eyes on attempted fixation.

dystrophy Noninflammatory developmental, nutritional, or metabolic abnormality.

ecchymosis Extravasation of blood beneath the skin.

ectasia of sclera Localized bulging of the sclera lined with uveal tissue; staphyloma.

ectopia Displacement or malposition, especially congenital.

ectropion Turning outward of the margin of the eyelid, occurring in spastic, cicatricial, and paralytic forms.

electro-oculogram (EOG) Recording of the standing potential between the retina and choroid.

electroretinogram (ERG) Recording of the action potential that follows stimulation of the retina.

ELISA Acronym for *e*nzyme-*l*inked *i*mmuno*s*orbent *a*ssay. Specific antigens available for variety of organisms.

Eischnig pearls Proliferated anterior lens capsule epithelium after extracapsular cataract extraction.

embryotoxon

anterior Arcus cornealis.

posterior Proliferation of peripheral corneal endothelium at Schwalbe ring.

emmetropia Refractive condition in which no refractive error is present with accommodation at rest.

endophthalmitis Purulent inflammation of the intraocular contents.

enophthalmos Recession of the eye within the orbit.

entropion Inward turning of the eyelid, observed in cicatricial, spastic, and paralytic forms.

enucleation In ophthalmology, the removal of the eye.

epiblepharon Supernumerary fold of skin along lower eyelid margin that turns eyelashes against the globe.

epicanthus Crescentic fold of skin of lower eyelid extending upward at inner canthus.

epidemic keratoconjunctivitis Inflammation of the cornea and conjunctiva caused by adenovirus.

epiphora Tearing as the result of faulty drainage of tears.

episcleritis Localized inflammation of the superficial tissues of the sclera.

epithelial downgrowth Epithelization of the interior of the eye that may follow faulty wound healing of the anterior segment.

esodeviation Inward deviation of the eye.

esophoria Latent inward deviation of the eyes in which, with binocular vision suspended, an eye deviates inward.

esotropia Inward deviation that occurs with both eyes open.

evisceration In ophthalmology, the removal of the intraocular contents with retention of the cornea (sometimes) and the sclera.

excyclodeviation Deviation of upper pole of vertical axis of eye toward the temple (plus cyclodeviation).

exodeviation Outward deviation of the eyes.

exophoria Latent outward deviation of the eyes in which, with binocular vision suspended, an eye deviates outward.

exophthalmos Abnormal protrusion of both eyes.

endocrine Associated with abnormalities of the thyroid gland.

ophthalmoplegic Inability to move the eye because of exophthalmos.

pulsating Associated with a carotid-cavernous fistula.

exotropia Outward deviation of the eyes.

extorsion Temporal rotation of 12 o'clock corneal meridian.

eye

dominant Preferred eye for monocular fixation.

exciting Initially injured eye in sympathetic ophthalmia; the fellow eye is the sympathizing eye.

fixating In strabismus, the eye directed to the object of regard.

reduced, schematic Simplified eye used in optics.

Farnsworth-Munsell color test 84 colored chips arranged in order of increasing hue.

far-point Remotest point where object is clearly seen without accommodation.

field of vision Area simultaneously visible to a motionless eye.

filter In optics, a lens that transmits, reflects, or absorbs selective wavelengths of the electromagnetic spectrum.

filtering operation Procedure designed to establish a fistula between the anterior chamber and subconjunctival space.

fixation Coordinated accommodation and ocular movements that maintain the image of objects on the fovea centralis.

floater Object seen in the field of vision that originates in the vitreous humor; physiologic floaters are muscae volitantes, minute residues of hyaloid vasculature seen in bright, uniform illumination; pathologic floaters may be erythrocytes, inflammatory cells, or fragments of the sensory retina.

fluorescein angiography Serial photography of ocular fundus after intravenous administration of fluorescein solution.

fluorescence Reradiation of light energy by an absorbing substance with increase of wavelength.

focus (1) Point of convergence of light rays; (2) starting point of disease.

fogging Method to determine refractive error in which accommodation is relaxed by means of convex spheres that make the patient artificially myopic.

fovea centralis Rod-free area of the retina that contains the foveola.

foveola Capillary-free area of the sensory retina.

Fuchs black spot Area of proliferation of the retinal pigment layer in the foveal area in degenerative myopia.

Fuchs dystrophy Corneal abnormality in which an initial degeneration of the endothelium is followed sometimes by epithelial and stromal edema and scarring.

funduscope Many organs have a fundus; a more precise term for the instrument used to visualize the interior of the eye is *ophthalmoscope*.

fusion reflex The stimulus to unify similar images that fall on retinal areas that have the same directional value in space.

fusion with amplitude Blending of the similar images from the two foveas into a single perception.

simultaneous central retinal perception (normal correspondence) Ability of the brain to receive and comprehend images from the fovea centralis of each eye simultaneously.

stereopsis Blending of slightly dissimilar images from each eye with the perception of depth.

fusion-free Position of the eyes when binocular vision is suspended.

gaze palsy Paralysis of ocular movements to right and left or up and down.

gerontoxon Arcus cornealis.

glare Sensation produced by brightness within the visual field that is sufficiently greater than the luminance to which the eyes are adapted to cause annoyance, discomfort, or decreased visual performance.

glaucoma An ocular disease in which there is usually increased intraocular pressure with atrophy and excavation of the optic nerve, producing characteristic visual field defects.

goniolens Optical instrument for studying the angle of the anterior chamber of the eye.

goniosynechiae Adhesions between the iris and cornea at the anterior chamber angle.

goniotomy Operation to correct congenital glaucoma in which the trabecular meshwork is incised.

hallucinations Perception without external stimulus that may occur in every field of sensation; formed visual hallucinations are composed of scenes, and unformed (scintillating) hallucinations are composed of sparks, lights, and the like; formed hallucinations characterize temporal lobe disturbances, and unformed hallucinations characterize occipital lobe disorders.

hamartoma Localized tumor composed of an abnormal increase of a single tissue element of tissues normally present in a particular region.

haploscope Instrument that presents separate views to each eye so that they may be fused into a stereoscopic image.

Hassall-Henle bodies Hyaline deposits of Descemet membrane that occur with aging.

hemianopsia Loss of vision in one half of the visual field in one or both eyes.

congruous Hemianopsia in which the hemianopsia of each eye is completely symmetric in extent and intensity.

homonymous Blindness in corresponding parts (right or left) of the visual field of each eye.

hemeralopia Defective vision in bright light.

Henle layer Outer plexiform layer of the retina in the region surrounding the foveola.

Hering's law of equal innervation Nervous impulse to each muscle involved in turning the eyes in the same direction is equal in duration and intensity.

heterochromia of iris Condition in which the irises of the two eyes are different colors.

heterophoria Condition in which there is a latent tendency of the eyes to deviate that is prevented by fusion.

heterotropia Condition in which there is deviation; strabismus.

hippus Spasmodic rhythmic dilation and contraction of the pupil, independent of stimulation with light.

Hollenhorst plaque Cholesterol embolus in retinal artery originating from atheromatous plaque in carotid artery.

homonymous In ophthalmology, having the same side of the field of vision; thus, a right homonymous hemianopsia is right half-blindness and results from a defect involving the nasal fibers of the right eye that decussate and the uncrossed temporal fibers of the left eye; the lesion is on the left side of the brain, posterior to the optic chiasm.

hordeolum Acute inflammation caused by infection of one of the sebaceous glands of Zeis; a sty; the term "internal hordeolum" is sometimes applied to a chalazion.

horopter Plane in space that localizes the visual direction of corresponding retinal points.

Hudson-Stähli line Pigmented iron line of the cornea.

humor, aqueous The watery fluid that fills the anterior and posterior chambers of the eye.

humor, vitreous The gel that fills the vitreous cavity of the eye.

hyalitis Inflammation of vitreous humor. Vitreitis.

hyalosis Degeneration of vitreous humor.

- **asteroid** Numerous small spherical bodies ("snowball" opacities) in the vitreous cavity visible ophthalmoscopically as bright, shiny objects; an age change, usually unilateral and not affecting vision.

hydrops of cornea Severe corneal edema.

hydrops of iris Vacuolization of the iris pigment layer.

hyperopia Refractive state of the eye in which rays of light cannot be brought to focus on the retina except by interposition of a convex lens or by accommodation (farsightedness).

- **absolute** Cannot be neutralized completely by accommodation so that there is indistinct vision both for near and for distance.
- **axial** Caused by abnormal shortness of the anteroposterior diameter of the eye.
- **latent** Portion of total hypermetropia that cannot be overcome, or the difference between the manifest and total hypermetropia.
- **manifest** Amount of hypermetropia indicated by the strongest convex lens a patient will accept while retaining normal visual acuity.
- **total** Entire hypermetropia, both latent and manifest.

hyperphoria Tendency for the eyes to deviate vertically that is prevented by binocular vision.

hypertelorism Excessive width between two organs; in ocular hypertelorism there is increased distance between the eyes (telecanthus).

hypertropia Deviation of the eyes in which one eye is higher than the other.

hyphema Blood in the anterior chamber.

hypopyon Pus in the anterior chamber.

illusion, visual Faulty interpretation of the color, form, size, or movement of visual stimuli.

image Visual impression of an object formed by a lens or mirror.

- **false** In diplopia, the image in the deviating eye.
- **Purkinje-Sanson** The images reflected from anterior and posterior surfaces of the cornea and the lens.
- **real** In optics, the inverted image formed by rays of light after refraction by a convex lens.
- **true** In diplopia, the image received by the nondeviating eye.
- **virtual** In optics, the erect image formed by backward projection of divergent rays from concave lens.

image jump Abrupt shift in field of view as direction of gaze moves across segment line of bifocal lens.

inclusion body Irregularly shaped particles in cytoplasm and nuclei of cells containing virus particles.

incongruous field defects Visual field defects that are different in each eye; occur in lesions involving that portion of the visual pathways anterior to the lateral geniculate body.

incyclodeviation Deviation of the upper pole of the vertical meridian of the cornea toward the nose (negative cyclodeviation).

infrared radiation Portion of the electromagnetic spectrum that has a wavelength between 700 and 10,000 nm.

inner plexiform layer That portion of the retina between the inner nuclear layer and the ganglion cell layer where dendrites of ganglion cells interact with amacrine and bipolar cells.

interstitial keratitis Inflammation of the corneal stroma with neovascularization, often complicating congenital syphilis.

intorsion Nasal rotation of 12 o'clock corneal meridian.

iridectomy Excision of a part of the iris.

- **peripheral** Excision of a portion of the iris near its root.
- **sector** Removal of an entire segment of the iris, usually extending from the pupillary margin to the root.

iridescent vision Perception of halos around lights, particularly in corneal edema.

iridocyclitis Inflammation of the iris and ciliary body.

iridodialysis Separation of the base of the iris from the ciliary body.

iridodonesis Tremulousness of the iris; occurs after loss of support after lens removal.

iridoplegia Paralysis of the sphincter pupillae muscle.

iridoschisis Separation of the mesodermal layer of the iris from the ectodermal layer.

iridotomy Surgical opening through all layers of the iris.

iris bombé Condition in which adhesions between the iris and lens prevent passage of aqueous humor from posterior to anterior chamber causing the iris to balloon forward, often resulting in angle-closure glaucoma.

iris coloboma Absence of a portion of the iris that occurs either as a congenital abnormality or after surgery.

iritis Inflammation of the iris.

irradiance Density of radiant flux incident on a surface.

Ishihara color plates Charts for screening for color discrimination using figures composed of different colored dots.

isopter Curve of equal sensitivity in the visual field.

jaw-winking (Robert Marcus Gunn) Abnormality in which movements of the face cause retraction of upper eyelid, often associated with blepharoptosis

joule Ten million ergs; unit of energy.

K reading Corneal curvature as measured with keratometer.

Kayser-Fleischer ring Golden deposit of copper in the periphery of Descemet membrane observed in hepatolenticular degeneration (Wilson disease).

keratectomy Excision of a portion of the cornea.

keratic precipitates Clumps of leukocytes adhering to the corneal endothelium in uveal tract inflammation; customarily divided into mutton-fat (macrophages and epithelioid cells) and punctate (lymphocytes and plasma cells).

keratitis Inflammation of the cornea.

keratocele Anterior herniation of Descemet membrane through the cornea; descemetocele.

keratocentesis Aqueous humor paracentesis.

keratoconjunctivitis Simultaneous inflammation of the cornea and conjunctiva.

keratoconus Cone-shaped abnormality of the cornea.

keratoglobus Enlargement of the cornea.

keratomalacia Softening of the cornea, often occurring in severe vitamin A deficiency.

keratome Knife with a triangular blade used for corneal incision.

keratometer Instrument for measuring the radius of curvature of the cornea.

keratomileusis Surgical procedure to reshape the cornea to modify refractive error.

keratomycosis Keratitis caused by fungus infection.

keratopathy Noninflammatory disorder of the cornea.

keratoplasty Transplantation of a portion of the cornea.

- **lamellar** Replacement of superficial layers.
- **partial** Replacement of a portion of the cornea.
- **penetrating** Replacement of entire thickness of the cornea; may be partial or total.
- **tectonic** Reconstruction of the cornea.
- **total** Replacement of entire cornea.

keratotomy Incision of the cornea.

- **radial (refractive)** Nonpenetrating radial incisions through peripheral cornea to reduce curvature of optical portion of the cornea and reduce myopia.

Koeppe nodule Accumulation of epithelioid cells at the pupillary margin in chronic uveitis.

Krukenberg spindle A vertical accumulation of pigment on the corneal endothelium.

lacrimation Excessive secretion of tears.

lagophthalmos Abnormality in which the globe is not entirely covered with the eyelids closed.

lambert Unit of luminance.

laser Acronym for *l*ight *a*mplification by *s*timulated *e*mission of *r*adiation; the laser produces a nearly monochromatic and coherent beam of radiation

lens Glass or other transparent material used optically to modify the path of light.

- **achromatic** A compound lens made of two or more lenses having different indices of refraction, so correlated as to minimize chromatic aberration.
- **bandage** Contact lens used to treat corneal disorders.
- **bifocal** Spectacles with two foci, usually arranged with focus for distant vision above and a focus for near vision below.
- **contact** Worn between the cornea and the eyelids.
- **crystalline** Transparent biconvex tissue located behind the pupil and in front of the vitreous.
- **cylindrical** Lens that is a section of a cylinder and used to correct astigmatism.
- **decentered** Lens in which the ocular visual axis does not pass through its optical center.
- **meniscus** Lens that has one concave and one convex surface.
- **prism** Transparent solid with two converging sides; separates white light into its spectral components; bends emerging rays of light toward its base; used to measure or to correct ocular muscle imbalance.
- **safety** Lens resistant to shattering made either of plastic or by means of case-hardening, coating, or lamination.
- **spherical** Concave or convex.
- **toric** Meniscus lens with a cylinder on one surface.

lensectomy Removal of lens by small incision through pars plana (orbicularis ciliaris) of ciliary body.

lenticonus Abnormality of the lens characterized by a conical prominence on the anterior or posterior lens surface.

leukocoria Whitish pupillary reflex caused by intraocular mass.

leukoma Opacity of the cornea; a less severe opacity is a macula, the least severe opacity is a nebula.

adherent Corneal opacity to which the iris is adherent.

levoversion Rotation of eyes to the left.

light That portion of the electromagnetic spectrum (400 to 700 nm) that stimulates the retina and causes a visual sensation.

lightning streaks (Moore) Flashes of light, usually within the temporal field, with movements of eyes that occur after detachment of vitreous humor and caused by impingement of separated vitreous on the retina or by vitreous traction.

Lisch nodules Bilateral hamartomatous nodules of the iris, possibly pathognomonic of neurofibromatosis.

Listing plane Transverse vertical plane perpendicular to the anteroposterior axis of the eye that contains the center of rotation of the eye.

lumen Unit of luminous flux emitted in a solid angle of 1 steradian from a uniform point having a luminous intensity of 1 candela.

lysozyme (muramidase) Antibacterial enzyme found in tears, leukocytes, egg albumin, and plants; mainly destructive of nonpathogenic gram-positive bacteria.

macula corneae Minute corneal opacity.

macula lutea Yellow spot; the retinal region that surrounds the fovea centralis.

mandibulofacial dysostosis Hereditary hypoplasia of zygoma and mandible.

medulloepithelioma, embryonal Tumor of nonpigmented layer of ciliary epithelium.

megalocornea Cornea with a diameter of 12 mm or more.

melanocytoma Nevus with giant melanosomes on the surface of the optic disk.

mesopic Intermediate illumination between daylight (photopic) and twilight (scotopic).

metamorphopsia Condition in which objects appear distorted, usually caused by foveal disturbance.

microaneurysms Capillary outpouchings; occur in the retina in diabetes mellitus, pulseless disease, and hypertension.

microcornea Adult cornea having a diameter of less than 9 mm.

microphakia Anomaly in which the crystalline lens is abnormally small.

microphthalmia Condition in which the eyeball is abnormally small.

micropsia Disturbance of visual perception in which objects appear smaller than normal.

microtropia Strabismus of less than 4°.

millimicron Unit of wavelength equal to 10^{-9} m; nanometer now preferred.

miosis Condition in which the pupil is constricted.

Mittendorf dot Opacity of the posterior lens capsule marking the site of attachment of the atrophied embryonic vasculature.

monochromatism Achromatopsia.

Mooren ulcer Chronic, peripheral, necrotic keratitis in the aged.

morgagnian cataract Hypermature cataract in which the cortex is liquefied, permitting the lens nucleus to move within the lens capsule.

movement

cardinal ocular Eye rotations to the right and left, upward to the right and left, downward to the right and left; the diagnostic positions of gaze. Rotation from primary to secondary position.

cog-wheel ocular Loose, jerky ocular rotations replacing smooth following movements.

conjugate movement of the eye Rotation of the two eyes in the same direction. *See also* version.

disjugate movement of the eyes Rotation of the two eyes in opposite directions, as in convergence or divergence.

fixational ocular Rotation of the eyes during voluntary fixation on an object; tremors, flicks, and drifts may occur.

fusional A reflex movement that tends to move the visual axes to the object of fixation so that stereoscopic vision is possible.

paradoxic movement of eyelids Spontaneous, involuntary elevation or lowering of the eyelids, associated with movement of eyes or jaws.

perverted ocular A condition in which attempts to move eyes affected by partial ophthalmoplegia initiate a movement in another direction.

rapid eye movements (REM) Symmetric, quick, scanning rotations occurring in clusters for 5 to 60 minutes during sleep; associated with dreaming.

saccadic (1) Rapid rotation of the eyes from one fixation point to another as in reading. (2) The rapid correction movement of a jerky nystagmus.

mural cells Pericytes in retinal capillary walls.

muscae volitantes Remnants of the fetal hyaloid system that appear as opacities in the vitreous humor (floaters).

mydriasis Dilation of the pupil.

myectomy Excision of a portion of a muscle.

myocionus, ocular Lightning eye movements; rapid bursts of small ocular saccadic movements that usually follow gaze toward the paretic or ataxic side of the body.

myokymia Persistent quivering of a muscle.

myopia Ocular condition in which parallel rays of light come to focus in front of the retina.

axial Caused by abnormal length of anteroposterior diameter of the eye.

degenerative Associated with conus of optic disk, choroidal stretching, and retinal abnormalities.

refractive Caused by increased index of refraction of the crystalline lens, as in nuclear sclerosis.

myopic crescent Term applied to a conus of the optic disk in myopia.

nanometer (nm) Unit of wavelength equal to 10^{-9} (one one-billionth) m; formerly called millimicron.

nanophthalmos Microphthalmos.

near point Closest point an eye can distinctly perceive an object.

convergence Closest point eyes can converge on an object without double vision.

near reflex Convergence, accommodation, and miosis on viewing a nearby object. Associated actions, not a reflex.

nebula of cornea Translucent corneal opacity.

neuroglia Supporting structure of neural tube composed of astroglia (macroglia), oligodendroglia, and microglia.

neuroretinitis Inflammation of the optic nerve and retina.

neurotrophic keratitis Keratitis occurring because of anesthesia of the cornea.

nodal points Locations in an optical system toward and from which are directed corresponding incident and transmitted rays that make equal angles with the optic axis.

nyctalopia Night blindness.

nystagmus Rhythmic oscillation of the eyeballs, either pendular or jerky.

after-nystagmus That which follows the abrupt cessation of rotation in the opposite direction in the testing of rotatory nystagmus.

ataxic A unilateral nystagmus with impairment of horizontal conjugate movement, most commonly caused by multiple sclerosis.

caloric Jerky nystagmus induced by labyrinthine stimulation with hot or cold water in the ear.

central Reflex from stimulation originating in the central nervous system.

cervical Originating from a lesion of the proprioceptive mechanism of the neck.

congenital (1) Present at birth, caused by lesions sustained in utero or at the time of birth. (2) Inherited, usually X chromosome–linked, without associated neurologic lesions and nonprogressive.

conjugate A nystagmus in which the two eyes move simultaneously in the same direction.

deviational End-position nystagmus.

dissociated Dysjunctive, incongruent nystagmus, or irregular nystagmus; a nystagmus in which the movements of the two eyes are dissimilar in direction, amplitude, and periodicity.

downbeat A vertical nystagmus with a rapid component downward, occurring in lesions of the lower part of the brain stem or cerebellum.

dysjunctive Dissociated nystagmus.

end-position A jerky, physiologic nystagmus occurring normally on attempts to fixate a point at the limits of the field of ocular rotation.

fixation A nystagmus aggravated or induced by ocular fixation, occurring as opticokinetic nystagmus, or resulting from midbrain lesions.

galvanic Involving galvanic stimulation of the labyrinth.

gaze A nystagmus occurring in partial gaze paralysis when an attempt is made to look in the direction of the palsy.

irregular Dissociated nystagmus.

jerk Nystagmus in which there is a slow drift of the eyes in one direction, followed by a rapid recovery movement; it usually results from labyrinthine or neurologic lesions or stimuli.

latent Jerk nystagmus evoked by covering one eye.

ocular Pendular nystagmus with severely reduced vision.

opticokinetic; optokinetic Railroad nystagmus physiologic nystagmus induced by looking at moving visual stimuli.

pendular A nystagmus that, in most positions of gaze, has oscillations equal in speed and amplitude.

positional Occurring only when the head is in a particular position.

rotational Jerk nystagmus originating from stimulation of the labyrinth by rotation of the head around any axis and induced by change of motion.

rotatory A movement of the eyes around the visual axis.

seesaw A nystagmus in which one eye rotates upward as the other rotates downward, often combined with a torsional rotation.

upbeat A vertical jerk nystagmus with a rapid component upward, occurring with brain-stem lesions.

vertical An up-and-down oscillation of the eyes.

vestibular Labyrinthine nystagmus; nystagmus resulting from physiologic stimuli to the labyrinth that may be rotatory, caloric, compressive, or galvanic, or caused by labyrinthal lesions.

ocular deviation

primary Ocular deviation in paralysis of an ocular muscle when the nonparalyzed eye fixes.

secondary Ocular deviation in paralysis of an ocular muscle when the paralyzed eye fixes.

supranuclear Binocular paralysis of the volitional ocular movements.

ocular flutter Involuntary, intermittent, to-and-fro movements of eye occurring in cerebellar disease.

ocular hypotony Decreased intraocular pressure.

ocularist One skilled in the design, fabrication, and fitting of artificial eyes and the making of prostheses associated with the appearance or function of the eyes.

oculist Ophthalmologist.

open-angle glaucoma Condition of increased intraocular pressure in which the aqueous humor has access to the trabecular meshwork.

operculum, ocular The attached flap of a retinal tear.

ophthalmia Inflammation of the eye.

ophthalmodynamometer Instrument for measuring blood pressure in the ophthalmic artery through observation of collapse of the central retinal artery.

ophthalmologist Physician and surgeon who specializes in diagnosis and treatment of disease of the eyes and the correction of refractive errors.

ophthalmoplegia Paralysis of one or more of the ocular muscles.

- **externa** Paralysis of the external ocular muscles.
- **interna** Paralysis of the muscles of the iris and the ciliary body.
- **total** Combination of both internal and external paralysis.

ophthalmoscope Instrument for examining the interior of the eye.

- **direct** Provides an upright image of about 15 diameters magnification.
- **indirect** Convex lens is held in front of the eye and an inverted image is observed; provides a magnification of about four times, but allows examination of a more peripheral portion of the fundus than direct ophthalmoscopy.

opsin The protein of the light-sensitive pigment of retinal rods and cones.

opsoclonus Irregular jerks of the eyes in all directions in cerebellar disease.

optic radiation The intracranial neural pathway composed of axons between the lateral geniculate body and the visual cortex.

optician A professional concerned with design, manufacture, and fitting of spectacles.

optometrist A professional concerned with the provision of primary eye and vision care for the diagnosis, treatment, and prevention of eye disorders and vision problems, and the prescription and adaptation of lenses and other optical aids, the use of visual training, and ocular medications.

optotypes Test symbols of graduated size for measuring visual acuity.

orbital emphysema Air in the orbit; generally follows traumatic rupture of a nasal sinus, particularly the lamina papyracea of the ethmoid bone.

orbital exenteration Removal of all of the orbital tissues, including the eye and its nervous, vascular, and muscular connections.

orbitonometer Instrument for measuring resistance to compression of orbital contents.

orthokeratology A method of molding the cornea with contact lenses to improve unaided vision.

orthophoria Tendency for eyes to be parallel when fusion is suspended.

orthoptics Technique of providing correct and efficient visual responses, usually by the form of visual training; these measures include the treatment of functional amblyopia, management of convergence insufficiency, and muscle imbalance and strabismus.

oscillopsia Oscillatory vision in which objects seem to move back and forth; symptom of multiple sclerosis.

outer plexiform layer That portion of the retina between the inner and outer nuclear layers where dendrites of bipolar cells interact with axons of photoreceptors as modified by horizontal cells.

palsy Paralysis.

pannus A fibrovascular tissue that affects mainly the superior portion of the cornea, a frequent complication of trachoma. Three forms of pannus occur: *crassus* (thick), in which there are many blood vessels and the opacity is very dense; *siccus* (dry), pannus with dry, glossy surface; and *tenuis* (thin), in which there are few blood vessels and the opacity is minimal.

panophthalmitis Purulent inflammation of all parts of the eye.

Panum area Spatial area surrounding the horopter in which objects are viewed with stereopsis; outside this area, diplopia occurs.

papilla Small nipplelike eminence.

- **Bergmeister** Small mass of glial tissue on the surface of the disk.
- **lacrimal** Small conical eminence on the upper and lower eyelid at the inner canthus pierced by the lacrimal punctum; particularly evident in the elderly.
- **optic** Misnomer in that the normal optic disk does not project into the eye.

papilledema Passive edema of the optic disk above the surrounding retina.

papillitis Inflammation of the optic nerve at the level of the optic disk.

paracentesis Puncture of cavity for removal of fluid; anterior chamber keratocentesis.

parallax Apparent displacement of an object resulting from a change in observer's position.

paresis Partial paralysis.

pars planitis Inflammation of ciliary body or peripheral choroid often associated with foveal edema; intermediate uveitis.

perception Conscious mental registry of a sensory stimulus.

perimeter Device to measure peripheral visual field.

perimetry Measurement of the limits of the field of vision.

- **computed** Mapping of the visual field by means of a programmed routine of stimulus and response.
- **kinetic** Perimetry in which the test object moves as its intensity and size remain constant.

static Perimetry in which the size of the test object and its location remain constant as its luminance increases.

persistent hyperplastic vitreous Congenital abnormality of the vitreous humor caused by failure of the hyaloid system to regress.

phacoanaphylaxis Uveitis induced by hypersensitivity to lens protein.

phacoemulsification Fragmentation of the lens with ultrasound combined with aspiration.

phakomatoses Group of hereditary diseases characterized by the presence of spots, tumors, and cysts in various parts of the body; types recognized as associated with ocular findings are tuberous sclerosis, von Hippel-Lindau disease, Recklinghausen disease, Bourneville disease, and Louis-Bar syndrome. *See also* syndrome.

phlyctenule Localized lymphocytic infiltration of the conjunctiva.

phoria Tendency for deviation of an eye when fusion is suspended.

phosphene Sensation of light produced by electrical or mechanical stimulation of the visual system.

photoablation Removal of tissue using the excimer laser.

photon A quantum of light (troland).

photopsia Subjective sensation of lights induced by mechanical or electrical stimulation of retina.

phthisis bulbi Degenerative shrinkage and disorganization of the eye.

pinguecula Small yellowish usually white subconjunctival elevation composed of elastic tissue usually located between the corneoscleral limbus and the canthus.

pits Incomplete coloboma of the optic disk, sometimes associated with central serous choroidopathy.

Placido disk Optical device composed of concentric black and white lines that are reflected onto the anterior surface of the cornea to detect irregular astigmatism.

poliosis Premature graying of hair.

polycoria Occurrence of multiple pupils; true polycoria if openings are surrounded with sphincter muscles.

presbyopia Refractive condition in which there is a diminished power of accommodation because of decreased elasticity of the crystalline lens, as occurs with aging.

prism Lens with two converging sides that splits light into constituent colors and deflects light rays toward its base.

proptosis Forward displacement of any organ, specifically, protrusion of the eyeball(s).

prosthesis Artificial substitute for body part.

protanomaly Form of anomalous trichromatism in which luminosity for long wavelengths is reduced.

protanopia Form of dichromatism in which red and bluish green are confused and relative luminosity is much lower than for a normal observer.

pseudoglioma Any intraocular opacity liable to be mistaken for retinoblastoma.

pseudoisochromatic plate Ishihara color plates.

pseudopapilledema Blurring of optic disk margins in severe hyperopia.

pseudostrabismus Appearance of crossed eyes caused by epicanthal folds or a visual axis not centered in the pupil.

pterygium Abnormality originating in the cornea in which a triangular patch of conjunctiva extends into the cornea; apex of the patch points toward the pupil.

pupil Aperture in the iris of the eye for the passage of light.

Adie Tonic pupil with denervation hypersensitivity and reduced tendon reflexes.

Argyll Robertson Pupil that does not constrict to light but constricts to convergence; pupils are small, unequal in size, and irregular; seen mainly in tabes dorsalis.

cat's eye Pupil with a white reflex when light is directed into it; most commonly associated with retinoblastoma.

Gunn Relative afferent pupillary defect to stimulation by light.

Horner Miotic pupil as a result of impaired sympathetic innervation of dilatator pupillae muscle.

keyhole Pupil with superior coloboma.

pupillary membrane Anomaly of the iris in which the fetal pupillary membrane fails to atrophy; often a persistent strand extends between the iris collarette and the anterior lens capsule; a fibrovascular occlusion after surgery.

Purkinje image Reflected image from surface of cornea and anterior and posterior surfaces of crystalline lens.

Purkinje phenomenon If intensity of illumination is reduced in fields of equal brightness, green becomes brighter than other colors.

Purkinje shift Luminosity curve of dark-adapted individual peaks at 500 nm, whereas the luminosity curve of light-adapted individual peaks at 550 nm; indicates two types of retinal photoreceptors.

quadrantanopsia Loss of one quadrant of the visual field; homonymous inferior considered pathognomonic for parietal lobe involvement; homonymous superior vascular lesion of temporal loop of the visual radiation.

reflex Involuntary, invariable, adaptive response to a stimulus.

accommodative Constriction of the pupils when the eyes converge for near vision; an associated reaction and not a reflex.

acousticopalpebral (cochleopalpebral; auropalpebral; cochleaorbicular) Brief closure of the eyelids in response to a sudden sound.

auditory oculogyric Rotation of the eyes toward the source of a sudden sound.

auricular-palpebral (Kisch) Closure of the eyelids elicited by stimulation of the skin in the deep external auditory canal.

cephalopalpebral Contraction of the orbicularis oculi muscle elicited by tapping on the vertex of the skull.

cerebropupillary (corticopupillary; Haab) Contraction of the pupils when a dark-adapted subject looks at a bright object.

conjunctival (eyelid) Closure of the eyelids induced by touching the conjunctiva (also called corneal reflex).

consensual light (crossed) Constriction of the pupil when the opposite retina is stimulated with light.

direct light Contraction of the sphincter pupillae muscle induced by stimulation of the retina with light (also called pupillary reflex).

eye compression (oculocardiac) Decrease of cardiac rate caused by pressure on the eye.

fixation Direction of the eye so that an image remains on the fovea centralis of each eye.

foveolar Bright dot of light originating from the foveola when an ophthalmoscope light is directed on the region of the fovea centralis.

lacrimal Secretion of tears induced by irritation of the cornea and conjunctiva.

orbicularis oculi (nose-bridge-lid; nose-eye) Contraction of the orbicularis oculi muscle on tapping the margin of the orbit, or the bridge or the tip of the nose.

orbicularis pupillary Constriction of the pupil on forcible closure of the eyelids or attempts to close the eye while the eyelids are held apart.

pupillary Constriction of the pupil in response to light stimulation of the retina.

pupillary-skin (ciliospinal; cutaneous-pupillary; skin-pupillary) Pupillary dilation elicited by scratching the skin of the neck.

red Red glow of light seen to emerge from the pupil when the interior of the eye is illuminated.

supraorbital (McCarthy; trigeminal-facial) Contraction of the orbicularis oculi muscle elicited by tapping the supraorbital nerve.

vestibulo-ocular (doll's eye sign; proprioceptive-oculocephalic reflex) Conjugate rotation of the eyes in the opposite direction to rotation of the head.

refraction Deviation of rays of light when passing from one transparent medium into another of a different density.

retinal detachment Separation of the sensory retina from the retinal pigment epithelium.

combined Including choroid and retina.

rhegmatogenous With hole formation in the sensory retina.

secondary Resulting from tumor or inflammation.

retinal hole Opening in the sensory retina so that there is a communication between the vitreous cavity and the potential space between the sensory retina and the retinal pigment epithelium.

retinitis Inflammation of the retina.

retinoblastoma Malignant retinal tumor of infancy.

retinopathy Noninflammatory degeneration of the retina.

diabetic Retinal hemorrhages and deposits (background retinopathy), or neovascularization of the retina and the optic disk (proliferative retinopathy).

hypertensive Arteriolar constriction with cotton-wool patches and hemorrhages in accelerated hypertension and eclampsia.

retinopathy of prematurity Replacement of sensory retina with fibrovascular tissue, occurring mainly in premature infants having a birth weight of less than 1,500 g.

rubella Pigmentary degeneration in congenital rubella.

venous-stasis Monocular venous dilation and hemorrhages in partial occlusion of carotid or ophthalmic artery.

retinopexy Surgical procedure to correct retinal detachment by means of diathermy.

retinoschisis Retinal abnormality in which the sensory retina splits at the level of the inner plexiform layer.

retinoscopy Objective method of determining the refraction of the eye by observing the movements of the reflection of light from the eye (skiascopy).

retrobulbar neuritis Inflammation of the optic nerve occurring without involvement of the optic disk.

retrolental fibroplasia End-stage of retinopathy of prematurity.

rhegmatogenous With hole formation.

rhodopsin Light-sensitive photopigment of rods.

rubeosis iridis Neovascularization of the iris.

salmon patch Central area of intense vascularization that occurs in interstitial keratitis as the result of the confluence of all blood vessels at the center of the cornea; also retinal hemorrhage in sickle cell disease.

Sattler veil Subepithelial corneal edema that occurs after prolonged wearing of a contact lens.

scintillating scotoma Unformed visual hallucination with flashing, bursting lights occurring in occipital lobe disorders, particularly migraine.

scleromalacia perforans Degenerative condition of the sclera in which localized rheumatoid nodules cause necrosis and perforation of the globe.

sclerosing keratitis Inflammation in which the cornea becomes white and opaque, resembling the sclera.

scotoma Area of blindness in the field of vision.

scotopic adaptation Adaptation of retinal rods to low levels of luminance.

Seidel test Dilution of fluorescein on the surface of the eye caused by aqueous humor leaking through a fistula.

siderosis Chronic inflammation of the eye caused by a retained ferrous foreign body within the eye.

skiascopy Retinoscopy.

slit lamp Biomicroscope.

Snell law of refraction (1) The incident ray, the normal to the surface at the point of incidence, and the refracted ray lie in one plane. (2) For two given media, the sine of the angle of incidence bears a constant relation to the sine of the angle of refraction.

Snellen letter Letter so constructed that at a given distance from the eye it subtends an angle of 5 minutes, with each portion of the letter subtending an angle of 1 minute.

spherical aberration Unequal refraction of light rays that pass through periphery of a lens.

squamous blepharitis Seborrheic inflammation of the eyelid margins.

squint Cross-eyes (strabismus).

staphyloma Ectasia of the sclera lined with the uveal tissue.

stereoscope An instrument that provides two horizontally separated images of the same object to give a single image with an appearance of depth.

Stiles-Crawford effect Light that passes through the center of the pupil of the eye evokes a greater sensation of brightness than an equal amount of light passing through an equal area near the edge of the pupil.

strabismus Abnormality in which the eyes are not simultaneously directed to the same object.

concomitant Deviation of the eyes in which the angle of deviation is the same in all directions of gaze.

nonconcomitant Deviation of the eyes in which the deviation differs in different directions of gaze.

sty Purulent inflammation of a gland of Zeis; hordeolum.

subhyaloid hemorrhage Hemorrhage between the sensory retina and the vitreous body.

subluxation of lens Condition in which a portion of the supporting zonule is absent and the lens lacks support in one or more quadrants.

suppression Physiologic cerebral process whereby the retinal image transmitted by one eye is ignored.

sursumversion Upward rotation of the eyes.

symblepharon Adhesion between the palpebral and bulbar conjunctivas.

sympathetic ophthalmia Nonsuppurative uveitis originating with perforating wound of the uvea followed by a similar uveitis of the fellow eye; the eye secondarily affected is called the sympathizing eye, and the injured eye is called the exciting or activating eye.

synchysis Liquefaction of the vitreous body.

syndrome Group of symptoms and signs that occur together; disease or definite morbid process having a characteristic sequence of symptoms; may affect the whole body or any of its parts. *See also* disease.

A and V Esotropia in which the eyes are closer together in looking up than down (A) or closer looking down than up (V).

Adie *See* pupil.

Alström Pigmentary degeneration of retina without bone spicules, obesity, diabetes, deafness, and normal mentation.

Anton Form of anosognosia in which a patient denies blindness; usually accompanied by confabulation, with the patient claiming to see objects in the blind field.

Axenfeld anomaly Posterior corneal arcus, glaucoma, and hypertelorism.

Balint Inability to fixate objects in the peripheral visual field (oculomotor apraxia).

Bassen-Kornzweig Progressive ataxic neuropathy associated with retinal pigmentary degeneration and a crenated appearance of erythrocytes (abetalipoproteinemia).

Benedikt Hemianesthesia and involuntary movements of a choreiform nature in the extremities on the side opposite the lesion in the medial lemniscus and region of the red nucleus.

Biedl-Bardet Autosomal recessive disorder of the pituitary gland characterized by girdle-type obesity, hypogenitalism, mental retardation, polydactyly, and pigmentary retinal degeneration.

Brown tendon sheath Contracture of superior oblique muscle with apparent paralysis of ipsilateral inferior oblique muscle.

cavernous sinus Thrombosis of the cavernous sinus with oculomotor (N III), trochlear (N IV), and abducent (N VI) nerve palsy; proptosis; and edema of the face and eyelids.

cerebellopontine angle tumor Ataxia, tinnitus, deafness, ipsilateral paralysis of the sixth and seventh cranial nerves, involvement of the fifth cranial nerve, vertigo, and nystagmus.

Chandler Iris atrophy, dystrophy of corneal endothelium, and secondary glaucoma.

chiasmal Optic atrophy and bitemporal hemianopsia.

Cockayne Autosomal recessive pigmentary degeneration of the retina, optic atrophy, photosensitivity, deafness, progeria, and mental retardation.

Cogan (1) Nonsyphilitic interstitial keratitis with associated nerve deafness. (2) Oculomotor (N III) nerve apraxia with absence of voluntary ocular movements with full random movements; fixation by jerky head movements with overshooting.

Cogan-Reese Iris nevi, iris atrophy, and corneal endothelial dystrophy.

Collins (Franceschetti) Mandibulofacial dysostosis.

crocodile tears Spontaneous lacrimation that occurs with the normal salivation of eating; follows facial (N VII) nerve paralysis and is caused by aberrant regenerating nerve so that neurons destined for the salivary glands go to the lacrimal gland.

Crouzon Craniofacial dysostosis with eyes widely separated.

Cushing Pituitary adenoma causing chiasmal syndrome with adrenocorticotropic hormone (ACTH) secretion resulting in endocrine effects of adrenocortical hyperplasia.

Down Mental retardation with retarded growth, flat hypoplastic face, muscle hypotonia, and other abnormalities.

Doyne Autosomal dominant drusen of retinal pigment epithelium.

Duane retraction Simultaneous contraction of the medial and lateral recti muscles on attempts to adduct eye with retraction of the globe and narrowing of the palpebral fissure.

Edward Trisomy 18.

Ehlers-Danlos Overextensibility of joints, hyperelasticity of the skin, fragility of the skin, and pseudotumors after trauma; there may be epicanthal folds, esotropia, blue sclera, glaucoma, ectopic lenses, proliferating retinopathy, and acanthocytosis.

fetal alcohol Specific pattern of growth deficiency, limb defects, hyperplasia of mandible, hypoplasia of maxilla, microphthalmia, epicanthal folds, and later mental retardation in offspring of alcoholic pregnancy.

Fisher Ophthalmoplegia, ataxia, absent reflexes (polyneuroradiculitis).

floppy eyelids Spontaneous eversion of upper eyelids, especially during sleep, causing papillary conjunctivitis, often in obese men.

Foix Ophthalmoplegia, ocular sympathetic nerve paralysis, neuroparalytic keratitis secondary to compression within cavernous sinus.

Foster Kennedy *See* syndrome, Kennedy.

Foville Supranuclear paralysis of ocular rotation to side of facial paralysis and contralateral hemiplegia.

Franceschett (Collins) Mandibulofacial dysostosis.

François Dyscephaly, microphthalmia, and cataract.

Fuchs Unilateral heterochromia, inflammation of the iris and ciliary body, and secondary cataract.

Goldenhar Mandibulofacial dysostosis with epibulbar dermoids and vertebral anomalies.

Gradenigo Palsy of the lateral rectus muscle (N VI) and severe unilateral headache in suppurative disease of the middle ear.

Grönblad-Strandberg Angioid streaks of the fundus and pseudoxanthoma elasticum of the skin.

Gunn (Robert Marcus Gunn) (1) Unilateral blepharoptosis with retraction of eyelids during chewing. (2) Relative afferent pupillary defect.

Hallerman-Streiff Mandibulofacial dysostosis with microphthalmia and congenital cataract (François).

Harada Vogt-Koyanagi syndrome combined with retinal detachment.

hepatolenticular degeneration (Wilson) Abnormality of copper metabolism associated with progressive degeneration of the liver and the lentate nucleus of the brain, mental retardation, and a brownish ring (Kayser-Fleischer) composed of copper at the periphery of the cornea.

Horner Sympathetic nerve paralysis with miosis, blepharoptosis, and anhidrosis of the face.

Hunter X chromosome–linked form of mucopolysaccharidosis (type MPS II) in which the corneas remain clear until the third decade of life.

Hurler (gargoylism) Autosomal recessive mucopolysaccharidosis (type MPS I H) characterized by dwarfism with short, kyphotic spinal column; short fingers; depression of bridge of the nose; heavy, ugly facies; stiffness of joint; cloudiness of the cornea; retinal degeneration; hepatosplenomegaly; and mental retardation.

Hutchinson (1) Interstitial keratitis, deafness, and notched, narrow-edged permanent incisors in congenital syphilis. (2) Neuroblastoma with orbital metastasis.

Irvine-Gass Cystoid macular edema with corneal-vitreous adhesions after cataract extraction.

Jensen disease Chorioretinitis adjacent to the optic disk (juxtapapillary).

Kearns-Sayre Mitochondrial mutation with ophthalmoplegia, pigmentary degeneration of retina, and cardiac conduction defect.

Kennedy (Foster Kennedy) Ipsilateral optic atrophy and contralateral papilledema in frontal lobe tumors, aneurysms, or abscesses.

Lowe Oculocerebrorenal X chromosome–linked glaucoma, cataract, growth and mental retardation, and aminoaciduria.

Marcus Gunn *See* syndrome, Gunn.

Marfan Spider fingers and toes (arachnodactyly), ectopia lentis, cardiovascular defects, and widespread defects of elastic tissue.

Marinesco-Sjögren Autosomal recessive stationary cerebellar ataxia, mental retardation, cataract, and oligophrenia.

Mikulicz Chronic lymphocytic infiltration and enlargement of the lacrimal and the salivary glands.

Millard-Gubler Paralysis of sixth and seventh cranial nerves and contralateral hemiplegia of extremities.

morning glory Unilateral enlarged optic disk with funnel-shaped excavation and elevated annulus of chorioretinal tissue.

Morquio-Brailsford Mucopolysaccharidosis type MPS IV.

orbital apex Oculomotor (N III) nerve paresis and neuralgia resulting from involvement of structures at the apex of the orbit by a tumor, often a neoplasm of the nasopharynx.

osteogenesis imperfecta (van der Hoeve) Bone fragility, blue sclera, and deafness.

Ota nevus Pigmented nevus of the eyelids, nose, and zygomatic and frontal regions.

paratrigeminal (Raeder) Trigeminal (N V) nerve neuralgia; often followed by sensory loss on the affected side of the face, weakness and atrophy of the muscles of mastication, miosis, and blepharoptosis.

Parinaud (1) Necrotic lesion of conjunctiva associated with palpable preauricular lymph nodes. (2) Paralysis of conjugate upward gaze, usually associated with lesions at the level of the superior colliculi.

Peters anomaly Adherent corneal leukoma with absence of Descemet membrane and endothelium.

Pierre Robin *See* syndrome, Robin.

Posner-Schlossman Glaucoma cyclitic crisis; recurrent cyclitis with glaucoma.

Reiter Urethritis, iridocyclitis, arthritis, sometimes with diarrhea in males. Arthritis may persist with recurrence of one or more other disorders.

Rieger Autosomal dominant mesodermal dysgenesis of the cornea and iris; corneal opacities, hypoplastic iris, iridotrabecular adhesions, and posterior corneal arcus occur.

Riley-Day (familial autonomic dysfunction) Reduced or absent tears, postural hypotension, excessive sweating, corneal anesthesia, exotropia, and absence of taste buds.

Robin micrognathia Small tongue, cleft palate, myopia, congenital glaucoma, and retinal detachment.

Rollet Orbital apex syndrome with involvement of the second, third, fourth, fifth, sixth, and sympathetic nerves.

Roth spot Retinal hemorrhage with white center in subacute bacterial endocarditis.

Rothmund (-Thomson; Bloch-Stauffer) Autosomal recessive congenital cataract with skin telangiectasis and pigmentation.

Sanfilippo Mucopolysaccharidosis type MPS III.

Scheie Mucopolysaccharidosis type MPS I S.

Sjögren Keratoconjunctivitis sicca, xerostomia, enlargement of the parotid gland, and polyarthritis.

Stevens-Johnson Erythema multiforme and scarring of the conjunctiva and oral mucosa.

Stilling-Duane-Türk *See* syndrome, Duane retraction.

Usher Autosomal recessive pigmentary degeneration of the retina with nerve deafness.

vitreoretinal, familial exudative Autosomal dominant peripheral pigmentary retinopathy, vascular abnormalities, choroidal atrophy, and vitreous opacities.

Vogt-Koyanagi-Harada Bilateral uveitis, poliosis, vitiligo, alopecia, and dysacousia.

Waardenburg-Klein Autosomal dominant hypertrophy of the root of the nose, heterochromia iridis, white forelock, and deafness.

Weill-Marchesani Short fingers and toes, compact body, glaucoma, and spherophakia.

synechiae Adhesions between the iris and adjacent structures.

anterior Adhesions between the iris and the cornea.

peripheral anterior Adhesions between the root of the iris and peripheral cornea that occlude the anterior chamber angle.

posterior Adhesions between the iris and the lens as occur commonly in uveitis.

syneresis Liquefaction and shrinkage of vitreous humor.

tangent screen Instrument used for the study of the field of vision within 30° of the fixation point; testing is carried out 1 or 2 m from the eye; tangent because it would be tangent to the arc of a perimeter.

tapetoretinopathy Hereditary degeneration of the retinal pigment epithelium and sensory retina.

tarsorrhaphy Operative procedure in which the eyelids are sutured together.

telecanthus Increased distance between medial canthi.

temporal arteritis Giant cell arteritis.

tension, ocular Resistance of coats of eye to deformation by external pressure.

Terrien marginal degeneration Bilateral stromal degeneration of the cornea with gutter formation followed by ectasia.

Thygesson superficial punctate keratitis Bilateral, coarse, multiple, transient epithelial opacities of cornea.

tonography Test to determine the volume of fluid forced from the eye by a constant pressure during a fixed period.

tonometer Instrument to measure ocular tension.

torsion Rotation of eye about its anteroposterior axis.

trabeculectomy A filtering operation for glaucoma by creation of a fistula between the anterior chamber of the eye and the subconjunctival space, through a subscleral excision of a portion of the trabecular meshwork.

trachoma Cicatrizing conjunctivitis caused by *Chlamydia trachomatis.*

TRIC agents Acronym for *tr*achoma and *i*nclusion *c*onjunctivitis, members of the psittacosis-lympho-granuloma venereum-trachoma *(Chlamydia)* group of microorganisms.

trichiasis Condition in which there are ingrown eyelashes.

tritanopia Form of dichromatism in which there are only two cone pigments present and there is a complete insensitivity to blue.

tropia Strabismus.

Uthoff sign Weakness with warming of the body in multiple sclerosis.

uveitis Inflammation of the uveal tract.

vergence Binocular disjunctive rotations of the eyes as in convergence and divergence.

version Binocular conjugate movements of the eyes.

vision

- **binocular** Faculty of using both eyes synchronously, with diplopia.
- **color** Ability to distinguish a large variety of wavelengths of light in the visible spectrum.
- **iridescent** Perception of colored halos around light; occurs because of corneal edema particularly in glaucoma.
- **mesopic** Vision in illumination between photopic and scotopic ranges.
- **photopic** Vision in bright illumination.
- **scotopic** Vision in dim illumination or vision after the biochemical or neurologic changes occurring in dark adaptation.
- **stereoscopic** Vision in which objects are perceived in three dimensions.

visual axis Straight line connecting an object seen with the foveola.

visual field Loci of objects or points in space that can be simultaneously perceived when the eyes are fixed in the primary position; the field may be monocular or binocular.

visuscope Ophthalmoscope that projects a pattern the patient fixates for diagnosis of eccentric fixation.

vitrectomy Surgical removal of the vitreous.

- **closed** Through pars plana incision.
- **open** Through corneoscleral limbal incision.

Vossius lenticular ring Pigment on anterior lens capsule after contusion of eye.

xerophthalmia Dryness of conjunctiva and cornea in vitamin A deficiency.

xerosis Abnormal dryness.

X, Y cells Classes of retinal ganglion cells.

yellow spot Term applied to macula lutea.

yoke muscles Muscles of the eyes that function in rotations in the same direction.

zonulolysis Dissolution of the zonule by α-chymotrypsin in intracapsular cataract extraction.

BIBLIOGRAPHY: APPENDIX A

Dorland's illustrated medical dictionary, ed 28, Philadelphia, 1994, WB Saunders.

Magalini SI: *Dictionary of medical syndromes,* ed 3, Philadelphia, 1990, JB Lippincott.

Roy FH: *Ocular syndromes and systemic diseases,* ed 2, Philadelphia, 1989, WB Saunders.

Stedman's medical dictionary, ed 26, Baltimore, 1995, Williams & Wilkins.

B

A NOTE ON REFERENCES

The Medline system of the National Library of Medicine is unexcelled as a key to searching medical and scientific periodicals. Grateful Med software simplifies the search of the National Library of Medicine's more than 30 biomedical databases. Information concerning Grateful Med is available from the National Library of Medicine:

Medlars Services (800) 638-8480
Public Information (800) 272-4787

Information concerning Internet databases is available from the National Science Foundation:

Telephone: (800) 444-4345
(619) 455-4600
Fax: (619) 455-4640
Internet e-mail: info@is.internic.net

The *American Journal of Ophthalmology,* the *Archives of Ophthalmology,* the *British Journal of Ophthalmology,* and *Ophthalmology* provide current discussion of many clinical conditions. The *Transactions of the American Ophthalmological Society* and *Eye,* formerly *Transactions of the Ophthalmological Societies of the United Kingdom,* are clinically oriented. *Investigative Ophthalmology and Visual Science, Experimental Eye Research,* and *Current Eye Research* provide many basic studies. The *Survey of Ophthalmology,* The *Ophthalmology Clinics of North America,* and the *International Ophthalmology Clinics* offer excellent reviews of clinical topics.

The biochemistry, physiology, and disorders of the normal and diseased eye are extensively described in many monographs, textbooks, and multivolume works. The most recent is the magnificent six volume *Principles and Practice of Ophthalmology* edited by Daniel M. Albert and Frederick A. Jakobiec. It joins several other series: *Duane's Clinical Ophthalmology* (five volumes, looseleaf); Duke-Elder: *System of Ophthalmology* (15 volumes); Miller: *Walsh and Hoyt's Clinical Neuro-ophthalmology* (five volumes); Duane and Jaeger: *Biomedical Foundations of Ophthalmology* (three volumes, looseleaf); Spencer: *Pathology of the Eye* (three volumes); Ryan: *Retina* (three volumes); Scriver, Beaudet, Sly, and Valle: *Metabolic and Molecular Bases of Inherited Disease* (three volumes); and Garner and Klintworth: *Pathobiology of Ocular Disease* (two volumes). Several are available on CD-ROM. There are a host of single volume works that deal with nearly every facet of ophthalmology.

Abstracts of ophthalmic articles are available in the *American Journal of Ophthalmology, Excerpta Medica,* and *Ophthalmic Literature.* Indexes of the *American Journal of Ophthalmology* appeared in 1953, 1963, 1973, 1978, 1983, 1988, and 1993. The *Medical Letter on Drugs and Therapeutics* provides current authoritative commentary.

BIBLIOGRAPHY

Books

Albert DM, Jakobiec FA: *Principles and practice of ophthalmology,* vols 1-6, Philadelphia, 1994, WB Saunders.

Fraunfelder FT, Roy FH: *Current ocular therapy 4,* Philadelphia, 1994, WB Saunders.

Garner A, Klintworth GK, editors: *Pathobiology of ocular disease, a dynamic approach,* New York, 1994, Marcel Dekker.

Grant WM, Schuman JS: *Toxicology of the eye,* ed 4, Springfield, Ill, 1993, Charles C Thomas.

Isenberg SJ, editor: *The eye in infancy,* ed 2, St Louis, 1994, Mosby–Year Book.

Isselbacher KJ, Braunwald E, Wilson JD, Martin JB, editors: *Harrison's principles of internal medicine,* ed 13, New York, 1994, McGraw-Hill.

McLean IW, Burnier MN, Zimmerman LE, Jakobiec FA: *Tumors of the eye and ocular adnexa,* Washington, DC, 1994, Armed Forces Institute of Pathology.

Miller NR: *Walsh and Hoyt's clinical neuro-ophthalmology,* ed 4, vols 1-5, Baltimore, 1982-1995, Williams & Wilkins.

Ryan SJ, editor: *Retina,* ed 2, St Louis, 1994, Mosby–Year Book.

Scriver CR, Beaudet AL, Sly WS, Valle D, editors: *The metabolic and molecular bases of inherited disease,* vol I-III, New York, 1995, McGraw-Hill.

Spalton DJ, Hitchings RA, Hunter PA, editors: *Atlas of clinical ophthalmology,* ed 2, London, 1994, Wolfe.

Tasman W, Jaeger EA, editors: *Duane's ophthalmology,* vols 1-9, Philadelphia, Lippincott-Raven.

C

CENTRAL VISUAL ACUITY: DISTANCE, SNELLEN

Feet	Meters	Reduced	Percent Loss of Central Vision
20/16	6/5	1.2	0
20/20	6/6	1.0	0
20/25	6/7.5	0.8	5
20/30	6/9	0.66	9
20/40	6/12	0.5	15
20/50	6/15	0.4	25
20/60	6/18	0.33	35
20/80	6/24	0.25	40
20/100	6/30	0.2	50
20/200	6/60	0.1	80
20/300	6/90	0.066	85
20/400	6/120	0.05	90
20/800	6/240	0.025	95

Conversion Factors to Obtain SI Units		Conversion Factor to Give cd m^{-2}
Unit	Geometry	Multiply Column Units by
Candela per meter squared (nit or meter-candle)	1 cd m^{-2}	1
Lambert	$(1/\pi)$ cd cm^{-2}	3183
Millilambert	10^{-3} $(1/\pi)$ cd cm^{-2}	3.183
Stilb	1 cd cm^{-2}	10,000
Apostilb	$(1/\pi)$ cd m^{-2}	0.3183
Footlambert	$(1/\pi)$ cd ft^{-2}	3.4258

D

COMMON OPHTHALMIC ABBREVIATIONS

+	Convex lens
–	Concave lens
Δ	Prism diopters
A	Ocular tension by applanation tonometer; initial negative deflection of electroretinogram; accommodation
AC	Anterior chamber
AC/A	Accommodative-convergence/ accommodation ratio
Acc	Accommodation
ARC	Abnormal retinal correspondence; anomalous retinal correspondence
Ax	Axis of cylindrical lens
B	Large positive deflection of electro-retinogram; base of prism
C	Coefficient of facility of outflow in tonography; cylindrical lens
cc	Cum correction (with lenses)
CF	Counting fingers
cyl	Cylindrical lens
D	Diopter; dextro: right
DA	Dark adaptation
dd	Disk diameters (1.5 mm)
E	Esophoria for distance
E′	Esophoria for near
ECCE	Extracapsular cataract extraction
EOG	Electro-oculography
EOM	Extraocular muscles; extraocular movements
ERG	Electroretinography
ET	Esotropia for distance
ET′	Esotropia for near
FC	Finger counting
HM	Hand movements
HT	Hypertropia
I	Luminous intensity
ICCE	Intracapsular cataract extraction
IOL	Intraocular lens
IOP	Intraocular pressure
J-1	Jaeger test type number 1
K	Coefficient of scleral rigidity; refractive power of cornea
KP	Keratic precipitates
LE	Left eye
LP/DT	Light-peak/dark-trough ratio
LPerc	Light perception
LProj	Light projection
NPA	Near point accommodation
NPC	Near point convergence
OD	Oculus dexter: right eye
OS	Oculus sinister: left eye
OU	Oculi uterque: both eyes
PC	Posterior chamber
PD	Interpupillary distance; prism diopters
P_o	Intraocular pressure
RE	Right eye
S	Spherical lens; sinister: left
sc	Sine correctio (without lenses)
TT	Tactile tension of eye
VA	Visual acuity (without correction)
VA_{cc}	Visual acuity with correction
VA_{ph}	Visual acuity with pinhole
VA_{sc}	Visual acuity without correction
VEP	Visual-evoked potential
X	Exophoria
X′	Exophoria near
XT	Exotropia distance
XT′	Exotropia near
YAG	Acronym for yttrium-aluminum-garnet

INDEX

D

Q

R

S